Raymond Smith
1934

THE DISEASES OF INFANTS AND CHILDREN

By

J. P. CROZER GRIFFITH, M.D., PH.D.

Emeritus Professor of Pediatrics in the University of Pennsylvania; Consulting Physician to the Children's Hospital, Philadelphia; Consulting Physician to St. Christopher's Hospital for Children; Consulting Pediatrist to the Woman's, the Jewish, and the Misericordia Hospitals, etc.; Corresponding Member of the Société de Pédiatrie de Paris

and

A. GRAEME MITCHELL, M.D.

B. K. Rachford Professor of Pediatrics, College of Medicine, University of Cincinnati; Medical Director and Chief of Staff of the Children's Hospital of Cincinnati; Director of the Children's Hospital Research Foundation; Director of Pediatric and Contagious Services in the Cincinnati General Hospital

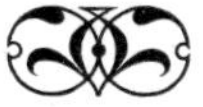

PHILADELPHIA AND LONDON

W. B. SAUNDERS COMPANY

1934

Reprinted April, 1934

MADE IN U. S. A.

PRESS OF
W. B. SAUNDERS COMPANY
PHILADELPHIA

PREFACE

A THIRD edition of our "Diseases of Infants and Children" has become necessary, inasmuch as but few copies of the second edition are still available. This has brought the authors face to face with a serious problem. On the one hand the very favorable reception of the first two editions made it seem advisable to make no change in the construction of the book, but merely to bring it up to date. On the other hand there was an urgent call from many quarters for a one-volume work, which would in its character and in its lesser cost meet the needs of medical students. Our problem has therefore been how to maintain the text-book as a work of reference for pediatric practitioners and writers, and how, at the same time, to fit it for the needs of undergraduate students. We have tried to accomplish this by abbreviating many of the older references which possessed little but historical interest, but retaining those which seemed of most importance. At the same time the diminution in the size of the text-book has made necessary a decided condensation of sentences, and an elimination of all material that could be spared without loss. Every part of the book has been subjected to a critical study, and a very large amount of new pediatric literature has been perused in search for that most useful for our aim. The labor has been arduous, but the authors trust that they have accomplished their purpose, and believe that the text-book should be suitable for undergraduates, and at the same time should serve as a reference text-book for physicians especially interested in pediatric subjects and literature. For the sake of economy of space the references have been placed at the end of the chapters instead of being foot-notes.

CONTENTS

DIVISION I

GENERAL SUBJECTS

CHAPTER I

CHAPTER II

CHAPTER III

CHAPTER IV

CHAPTER V

CHAPTER II

CHAPTER III

CHAPTER IV

CHAPTER V

CHAPTER VI

CHAPTER VII

CHAPTER VIII

CHAPTER IX

CHAPTER X

CHAPTER XI

CHAPTER XII

CHAPTER XIII

CHAPTER XIV

CHAPTER XV

CHAPTER XVI

SECTION II

INFECTIOUS DISEASES

CHAPTER I

CHAPTER II

CHAPTER XXIV

SECTION III

GENERAL NUTRITIONAL AND MISCELLANEOUS DISEASES

SECTION IV

DISEASES OF THE DIGESTIVE SYSTEM

CHAPTER II

CHAPTER III

CHAPTER IV

CHAPTER V

CHAPTER VI

SECTION VI

DISEASES OF THE CIRCULATORY SYSTEM

CHAPTER I

CHAPTER II

CHAPTER III

CHAPTER IV

SECTION VII

DISEASES OF THE GENITO-URINARY SYSTEM

CHAPTER I

CHAPTER V

CHAPTER VI

CHAPTER VII

SECTION IX

DISEASES OF THE MUSCLES, BONES AND JOINTS

CHAPTER I

CHAPTER II

SECTION X

DISEASES OF THE BLOOD, SPLEEN AND LYMPH-NODES

CHAPTER I

CHAPTER II

THE DISEASES OF INFANTS AND CHILDREN

DIVISION I

GENERAL SUBJECTS

CHAPTER I

ANATOMY AND PHYSIOLOGY

THE DIVISIONS OF LIFE

For the purpose of study human life is usually sub-divided somewhat arbitrarily into several stages. A convenient arrangement separates life into *Intra-uterine*, or fetal; *Infancy*, including the *New-born* as a sub-division; *Childhood*, early and later; *Youth* or adolescence, with *Puberty* as the initial period of this stage; *Adult* life, and its sub-division, *Old Age*.

Intra-uterine Life.—Although apparently closely resembling a new-born child, the fetus is in reality so different that it is not capable of independent existence. Many of its organs, though perfect, are not yet active. Circulation is not fully developed and respiration and digestion are entirely in abeyance, oxygen and nutriment being obtained through the maternal blood.

Being so closely dependent upon the mother for its life, it would seem that the condition of her health during pregnancy and her method of living would have an influence on the health of the fetus. There is little statistical evidence to support this view, and entirely healthy infants are often born of sickly mothers. The fetus may, however, directly inherit a feeble constitution from a delicate father or mother, irrespective of the production of debility by other prenatal causes. Actual disease may be transmitted from mother to fetus. This is occasionally true of such infectious disorders as measles, whooping-cough, typhoid fever, malaria, tuberculosis, and very frequently of syphilis. The tendency to rheumatism apparently is directly transmitted, as are certain nervous maladies.

There are, besides, a variety of accidents which may happen to the fetus *in utero*, and various diseases may occur or anomalies of development arise, producing monsters or lesser degrees of malformation, the reason for the occurrence of which is little understood. Other characteristics and disorders of this period are fully discussed in works upon obstetrics and diseases of the embryo and fetus.

The New-born.—The first stage of infancy is that in which the child is designated as *New-born*. By this term is meant the brief period following birth, regarding the exact duration of which there is some variance of opinion. It seems best to apply it to the first two or, at longest, three weeks, since in this period no very distinct alterations show themselves during the process of development. The change from intra-uterine to extra-uterine life is so great that the new-born are very subject to disturbances of health, especially to those accidents and disorders caused by birth or appearing shortly after it. There are also a number of pathologic conditions seen at birth which developed during fetal life (p. 209).

Infancy.—This taken as a whole is a division of life to which various arbitrary and rather confusing limitations have been set. In English-speaking countries infancy is generally considered as lasting until the age of two years, since during this period the important epoch of the first dentition is nearly closed, and features are exhibited, especially in earlier infancy, which differ in many respects from those seen in the later years of child-life. Children in the first year may be called *nurslings.*

Development, both of the body and of the mind, during infancy is very rapid, except that for the first few months there is little discoverable gain in intellectual power. Infants, especially those of an early age, are extremely susceptible to external depressing influences, such as cold and fatigue, often easily affected by drugs, and rapidly exhausted by disease. On the other hand they exhibit remarkable recuperative power when recovery begins.

Childhood.—The term "*Childhood*" covers the period from the close of infancy to puberty. It may be divided into *Early Childhood* from the age of two to that of six years, the latter marking the beginning of the second dentition, and *Later Childhood* from the age of six years to puberty. During childhood growth continues with a rapidity which, though great, is less than in infancy. The mental and physical differences between the sexes become constantly more apparent. The incidence of diseases at different periods of infancy and childhood will be discussed later (p. 170).

Youth.—The term "*Youth*" or "*Adolescence*" is applied to the period extending from puberty to the commencement of adult life; *i. e.*, twenty-one to twenty-five years. The exact time for the development of puberty varies not only with individuals but with race and climate. In general for temperate climates it may be placed at from fourteen to sixteen years for boys and from twelve to fifteen years for girls. Common law puts it at fourteen years for males and twelve years for females. With the oncome of puberty the sexual functions are established, the genital organs increase in size, and the growth of hair begins upon the pubis and later in the axillae. In the female the breasts enlarge and become rounded by a deposit of fat. In the male the voice changes and hair begins to grow upon the face. The psychic characteristics belonging to each sex now become accentuated.

THE NEW-BORN

The infant at birth is more or less covered by a white, waxy substance, the *vernix caseosa,* which protected it during fetal life. This is especially abundant on the flexor surfaces, the back, and in the folds of the body, although some infants have almost none of it upon them. It is composed of the thickened secretions of the sebaceous glands and of scales of epidermis. When it has been removed by washing the skin is found to be thin, smooth, delicate and of a deep-reddish color. The fine hair, or lanugo, characteristic of fetal life has generally largely disappeared in fully developed new-born infants, although many still show a fine soft down.

The flesh should be plump and firm from a good development of subcutaneous fat. The head is proportionately very large and often rather thickly covered with long hair. The eyes are an indeterminate blue, except in dark-skinned races, and are usually kept shut or but half open. The face is expressionless. The chest is small and narrow and the abdomen large and prominent. The arms are short and are held most of the time flexed and pressed against the body in the position maintained in the uterus. The hands are generally closed, but will grasp firmly any object placed in them. The nails are well-developed and project beyond the tips of the fingers and toes. The legs are comparatively small and short, and curved with an outward bow (Fig. 1). This curvature, however, is only apparent, as can be shown by the dissecting away of the muscles (Zschocke[1]). They are much of the time held flexed at the knees and drawn up to the abdomen as in the fetal position. Intellectual activity and the powers of the special senses are practically absent.

DEVELOPMENT

A more detailed study is necessary of the characteristics of the new-born infant and of its development as growth advances. These subjects will be considered in course.

Increase in Weight.—The weight of the normal healthy infant at birth may be taken as from 7 to 7½ lb. (3175 to 3402). (See p. 1090 for abnormally great birth-weights.) The children of primiparae are slightly lighter than those of multiparae, the difference averaging about 5 oz. (142). There is a great range in the weight of the new-born even within physiologic limits. This is shown by the variation in the statistics, as seen in the following table:

Table 1.—Average Weight at Birth

	No. of cases.	Average.	
		Gm.	Lb.
Kézmársky[2]	73	3330	7.34
Ingerslev[3]	3450	3334	7.35
Holt[4]	1158	3330	7.34
Schäffer[5]	94	3151	6.95
Camerer[6]	119	3433	7.57
Peterson[7]	1675	3527	7.78
Griffith and Gittings[8]	226	3456	7.62
Fuhrmann[9]	1000	3337	7.36
Benestad[10]	1979	3466	7.64
Bachman[11]	511	3190	7.03

Male children are somewhat heavier than female, the difference being about 100 to 200 Gm. (3.5 to 7 oz.). Some of the statistics illustrating the differences between the sexes are seen in the following table:

Table 2.—Birth-weight of Male and of Female Infants Respectively

	Males.		Females.	
	Gm.	Lb.	Gm.	Lb.
Ingerslev[3]	3381	7.45	3280	7.23
Gregory[12]	3386	7.46	3331	7.34
Quetelet[13]	3200	7.05	2910	6.41
Altherr[14]	3214	7.08	3077	6.78
Kézmársky[2]	3383	7.46	3284	7.24
Holt[4]	3400	7.49	3260	7.19
Peterson[7]	3595	7.92	3455	7.62
Griffith and Gittings[8]	3494	7.70	3418	7.54
Ramsey and Alley[15]	3391	7.48	3276	7.22
Taylor[16]	3484	7.53	3377	7.44

It has been stated that the birth-weight varies with the season of the year, but evidence is lacking to support this. There is also no statistical proof that the diet of the mother during pregnancy greatly affects the weight of the new-born infant.

Immediately after birth, loss of weight begins in nearly all cases. This depends upon the excretion of meconium and urine, the removal of the vernix caseosa, the excretions of the skin and lungs, the vomiting of allantoic fluid, and the metabolic changes progressing in the tissues. The loss of weight due to metabolic changes may be spoken of as physiologic, and that from other causes as mechanical. The chief loss of a metabolic nature is water from the skin and tissues (Birk and Edelstein;[17] Rot;[18] Benestad;[19] Bailey and Murlin;[20] Bakwin;[21] Coda[22]). In addition there is a loss of body-tissue due to the oxidation of fat and of a small amount of protein and carbohydrate (Benedict and Talbot,[23] Bakwin[21]). The combined weight of meconium, urine and vernix ranges from 3 to 5 oz. (85 to 142) according to the observations of Townsend.[24] A review by Fleischmann[25] of the results obtained by a number of observers showed that the total loss of body weight averaged 222 Gm. (7.83 oz.); *i. e.*, about $\frac{1}{15}$ (6.66 per cent) of the whole weight if we assume this as 3300 Gm. (7.28 lb.). Certain other observations, however, give a loss somewhat greater than this as normal. In an examination of 226 infants made by Gittings and one[8] of us the total average loss equalled about 11 oz. (312), the relative loss being approximately $\frac{1}{11}$ (9 per cent) of the initial weight. It is usually accepted that the heavier the full-term baby, the greater will be the absolute loss of weight and the slower the regain. Adair and Stewart[26] found that the first-born lost a larger percentage of their total body-weight (8 per cent) than did later infants (6.4 per cent). This was due, in part at least, to the fact that the infants of multiparae received larger feedings than those of primiparae. According to Bakwin and Bakwin[27] the initial weight-loss is greater in infants born in winter than those born in summer. The loss of weight is chiefly physiologic, and therefore cannot usually be entirely prevented. Observations carried out by Gittings and one[8] of us on 61 infants confirmed the results of others, that by wet-nursing from the beginning until the mother's secretion is established the initial loss could be reduced very considerably, yet that this offered no distinct advantage. It has also been recommended by a number of writers that artificial feeding be commenced in the first days of life, using solutions of lactose or glucose, milk-mixtures, or other foods, in the effort to prevent the loss of weight; but, as with early wet-nursing, this does not seem to be necessary in healthy infants. Keilmann[28] found that when artificial feeding was commenced immediately after birth, the infants, although losing somewhat less, regained the initial weight more slowly than did those who had been nourished solely at the mother's breast. It should be said, however, that Bachmann's[11] observations in 511 infants do not confirm this view.

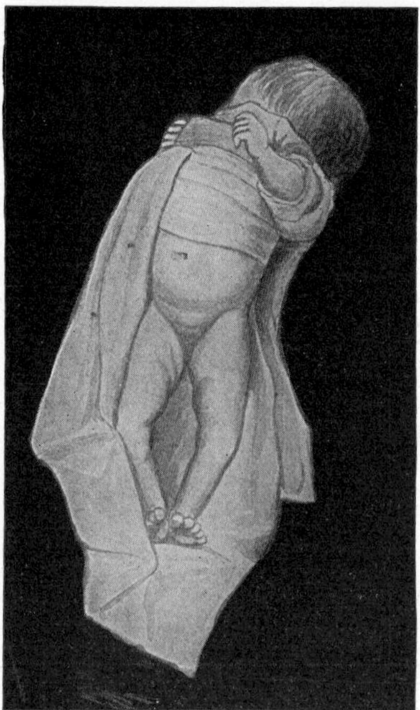

Fig. 1.—Baby a few weeks old, showing the natural curve of the legs with the bending in of the soles. (*From a photograph.*)

The diminution of weight continues until the third or fourth day and sometimes even longer, but this cannot be called physiologic. From 3.5

to 4 per cent of the birth-weight is lost on the first day, and from 2 to 2.6 per cent on the second. The third day usually shows but little loss or the beginning of gain. The original weight is not regained before the eighth or ninth day, and often not until the fourteenth day. In a study upon 600 infants by Schulz,[29] 228, or 48 per cent, had regained their original weight in ten days, illness of a number of the children preventing an earlier average time of regain. On the other hand, in 611 cases recorded by Bergmann[30] only 21.17 per cent regained their birth-weight by the end of the second week, and in the 300 cases of Ramsey and Alley[15] only 25 per cent by the tenth day.

Published statistics regarding the influence of sex are contradictory, some showing a greater loss in males, others in females. In personal[8] studies upon 105 infants, the average loss in boys was somewhat greater and the regain of the initial weight slower in being accomplished. After gain in weight begins increase is rapid, yet the rate of growth progressively decreases making graphic plotting a *curved* line.

It must be remembered that all tables of weight represent only the *average* rate of growth. A considerable variation in the individual child within physiologic limits is possible. The following figures give approximate weights of well-developed breast-fed children during the first year of life. They follow to a considerable extent the investigations of Camerer[6] starting with a birth-weight somewhat higher, viz., 3400 Gm. (7½ lb.), than that given by many investigators.

TABLE 3.—SHOWING INCREASE IN WEIGHT DURING THE FIRST YEAR

Age.	Lb.	Gm.
Birth	7½	3402
1 week	7½	3402
2 weeks	7¾	3473
3 weeks	8	3685
1 month	8¾	3969
2 months	10¾	4876
3 months	12¼	5557
4 months	13¾	6237
5 months	15	6804
6 months	16¼	7371
7 months	17¼	7824
8 months	18¼	8278
9 months	18¾	8505
10 months	19¾	8958
11 months	20½	9299
1 year	21½	9752

Based on these figures it will be noticed that in the last three weeks of the first month and during the second month the gain in weight is about 1 oz. (28) a day, 7 oz. (198) a week; in the third and fourth months slightly over ¾ of an oz. (21) a day, 5½ oz. (156) a week; in the fifth and sixth months ⅔ of an oz. (19) a day, 4⅔ oz. (132) a week, and in the remainder of the first year about ½ oz. (14) a day, 3¾ oz. (106) a week, or 1 lb. (454) a month; except that about the ninth month there is liable to be a temporary diminution in the rapidity of increase. The initial average weight is doubled at the age of five months and nearly trebled by one year.

The average weight of males during the first year is somewhat greater than that of females, amounting at the age of a year to a difference of ½ up to even 1¼ lb. (227 to 567). Infants fed artificially generally gain less rapidly than those at the breast, but this is by no means an invariable rule. This difference depending on the food may sometimes persist during the first three or four years, but very often a healthy infant artificially fed and thriving on its diet will equal the breast-fed child in weight by the end of the first year. Allen and Bagg[31] made an analysis of 500 cases showing that infants who are at birth over the average weight continue to gain faster than do others. The babies of multiparae gain better than do those of primiparae.

There are fewer extended observations made upon the weight of children from the first to the sixth year. Those of Camerer[6] appear reliable. The weights obtained by him are as follows:

TABLE 4.—INCREASE IN WEIGHT FROM THE SECOND TO THE FIFTH YEAR OF LIFE INCLUSIVE
(Camerer)

Age.	Gm.	Lb.
12 months	10,030	22.11
13 months	10,220	22.53
14 months	10,600	23.36
15 months	10,870	23.96
16 months	10,900	24.03
17 months	11,450	25.24
18 months	11,480	25.30
19 months	11,850	26.12
20 months	12,050	26.56
21 months	11,950	26.34
22 months	12,220	26.80
23 months	12,480	27.51
2 years	12,740	28.08
3 years	14,930	32.91
4 years	16,410	36.16
5 years	18,710	41.25

In some studies the figures given are less than this and in others, especially those in private practice, greater. In general the average healthy infant gains in its second year from 5 to 6 lb. (2268 to 2722); *i. e.*, ½ lb. (227) a month or ¼ oz. (7) a day, the increase being greater in the first half. (See chart, p. 9.) In the third and fourth years the child gains about 5 lb. (2268) and in the fifth year about 4 lb. (1814). In tabular arrangement the figures read as follows:

TABLE 5.—GAIN IN WEIGHT FROM ONE TO FIVE YEARS

Age.	Weight.		Gained.	
	Lb.	Gm.	Lb.	Gm.
End of first year	21½	9,752		
End of second year	27	12,247	5½	2495
End of third year	32	14,515	5	2268
End of fourth year	37	16,783	5	2268
End of fifth year	41	18,597	4	1814

Girls continue to be from 1 to 1½ lb. (454 to 680) lighter than boys to the end of this period.

A large number of measurements made upon 167,024 white, healthy and apparently normal children without clothing, from early infancy to the age of six years and in different parts of the United States, were collected and analyzed by the Children's Bureau.[32] A condensation of the published table reads as follows:

TABLE 6.—WEIGHT AND HEIGHT FROM ONE TO SIX YEARS

Age.	Boys.				Girls.			
	Height.		Weight.		Height.		Weight.	
	In.	Cm.	Lb.	Gm.	In.	Cm.	Lb.	Gm.
12 mos. (under 13 mos.)	29½	74.93	21⅜	9,695.53	28⅞	73.34	20	9,071.84
24 mos. (under 25 mos.)	33⅝	85.40	26⅝	12,076.89	33⅛	84.14	25⅛	11,396.49
36 mos. (under 37 mos.)	36⅝	93.02	30¾	13,947.95	36¼	92.07	29½	13,380.96
48 mos. (under 49 mos.)	39¼	99.69	34½	15,648.92	38⅞	98.74	33⅛	15,025.23
60 mos. (under 61 mos.)	41⅝	105.72	38⅛	17,293.19	41⅜	105.09	36⅞	16,726.20
71 mos. (under 72 mos.)	43⅞	111.44	41⅝	18,880.77	43⅝	110.80	40½	18,370.48

Estimating roughly from different sources the combined average weight of the sexes we find children gaining about 4 lb. (1814) in the sixth and seventh years, 4½ lb. (2041) in the eighth, 5 lb. (2268) in the ninth, 5½ to 6 lb. (2495 to 2722) in the tenth and eleventh years, 7 to 8 lb. (3175 to 3629) in the twelfth year, and then from 9 to 10 lb. (4082 to 4536) per year to the age of sixteen years. In tabular form the approximate weight for the different years according to this rate of increase reads as follows:

TABLE 7.—WEIGHT FROM SIX TO SIXTEEN YEARS

Years.	Lb.	Gm.
6	45	20,412
7	49	22,226
8	53½	24,267
9	58½	26,535
10	64	29,030
11	70	31,751
12	78	35,380
13	87	39,463
14	96	43,549
15	106	48,080
16	116	52,617

It will be seen that the child nearly doubles its normal weight at one year by the age of five years, and trebles it by ten years.

The difference, however, which the sexes show in the rate of increase in weight is so decided in later childhood and in youth, that a separate consideration is necessary. The rate of growth continues about the same in each sex until about the age of eight or nine years, at which time the increase in girls is somewhat retarded, and boys advance decidedly beyond them. By eleven years, however, girls begin to gain in weight rapidly, and by twelve years decidedly surpass boys. This continues until the age of fifteen or sixteen years when boys again take and maintain the lead. The relative weights and rates of increase in boys and girls respectively during this period, according to the statistics of Bowditch,[33] Porter[34] and Peckham,[35] can be learned from the accompanying table. The figures of Bowditch are based upon 24,595 observations upon public school-children of Boston; those of Porter upon 30,817 children of St. Louis; and those of Peckham upon 5403 children of Milwaukee. It should be stated,

TABLE 8.—WEIGHT OF BOYS AND GIRLS FROM FIVE TO EIGHTEEN YEARS

Years.	Bowditch.				Porter.				Peckham.			
	Boys.		Girls.		Boys.		Girls.		Boys.		Girls.	
	Pounds.	Kilograms.	Pounds.	Kilograms.	Pounds.	Kilograms.	Pounds.	Kilograms.	Pounds.	Kilograms.	Pounds.	Kilograms.
5	41.09	18.64	39.66	17.99	......	.....	......	.....	41.09	18.64	40.03	18.16
6	45.17	20.49	43.28	19.63	43.54	19.75	41.74	18.93	44.81	20.33	43.12	19.56
7	49.07	22.26	47.46	21.10	47.77	21.67	45.90	20.82	49.10	22.27	46.97	21.21
8	53.92	24.46	52.04	23.44	52.42	23.78	50.44	22.88	53.81	24.41	50.87	23.07
9	59.23	26.87	57.07	25.91	57.45	26.06	55.29	25.08	59.46	26.97	56.44	25.60
10	65.30	29.62	62.35	28.29	62.43	28.32	60.60	27.49	65.35	29.64	62.45	28.33
11	70.18	31.84	68.84	31.23	68.34	31.00	66.47	30.15	70.92	32.17	68.84	31.22
12	76.92	34.89	78.31	35.53	73.73	33.51	74.21	33.66	76.08	34.51	77.82	35.30
13	84.84	38.49	88.65	40.21	80.71	36.61	84.85	38.49	84.89	38.50	87.96	39.90
14	94.91	42.95	98.43	44.65	89.15	40.44	93.23	42.29	95.76	43.43	97.64	44.29
15	107.10	48.59	106.08	48.12	101.90	46.22	102.93	46.69	109.05	49.46	105.87	48.02
16	121.01	54.90	112.03	50.81	113.76	51.60	110.78	50.25	122.06	55.36	110.58	50.16
17	127.49	57.84	115.53	52.41	122.73	55.67	115.98	52.61	130.35	59.12	113.32	51.40
18	132.55	60.13	115.16	52.24	......	.....	......	.....	137.76	62.49	112.48	51.02

however, that there appears to be a variation in different countries for the age at which boys finally surpass girls in weight, European statistics differing somewhat from American.

The figures given (Table 8) for children over five years include clothing. Those for younger periods are without clothing. According to a series of personal[36] estimations made on over 200 children, the average weight of the clothes in the first year is approximately $1\frac{3}{4}$ lb. (794); from one to four years, 2 lb. (907); and from four to six years, $2\frac{1}{4}$ to $2\frac{1}{2}$ lb. (102 to 113). The ratio of the weight of the clothing to the gross weight of the normal child dressed is approximately 16 per cent in the first three months, but after this during the first two years approximately 8 per cent to 10 per cent; and from two to five years 6 per cent. The weight of the clothing in the first two years, according to the studies of Sauer[37] is decidedly less than the figures given. The changes of fashion in the clothing of children which occur from time to time make, of course, decided differences in the weights.

Especially in infancy the influence of any illness upon the weight is very decided. Increase ceases and even rapid loss of weight may occur, depending upon the nature of the disease. There appears to be a positive influence of *season* upon the growth of children. The investigations of Malling-Hansen[38] upon children of from nine to seventeen years showed the most rapid increase occurring from August to December. Others, such as Porter,[39] have largely corroborated this and shown, too, that it applies to young children as well as to infants. Malling-Hansen[38] also called attention to the daily fluctuations, with an increase in weight and a decrease in height during the day and a reversal of these during the night. Some German pediatricians, following Finkelstein,[40] classify infants into *hydrostabile* and *hydrolabile* types, the latter having a tendency to lose weight quickly under a dietary restriction of salt or carbohydrate or following the development of infection or gastro-intestinal disturbance. In addition to these factors race, climate, environment, social status, exercise and, of course, food affect growth. (See also Constitution p. 480.) Hence weight-curves must be considered as average ones only, especially in a country such as the United States. Many of the published weight-curves are too low for ideal standards.

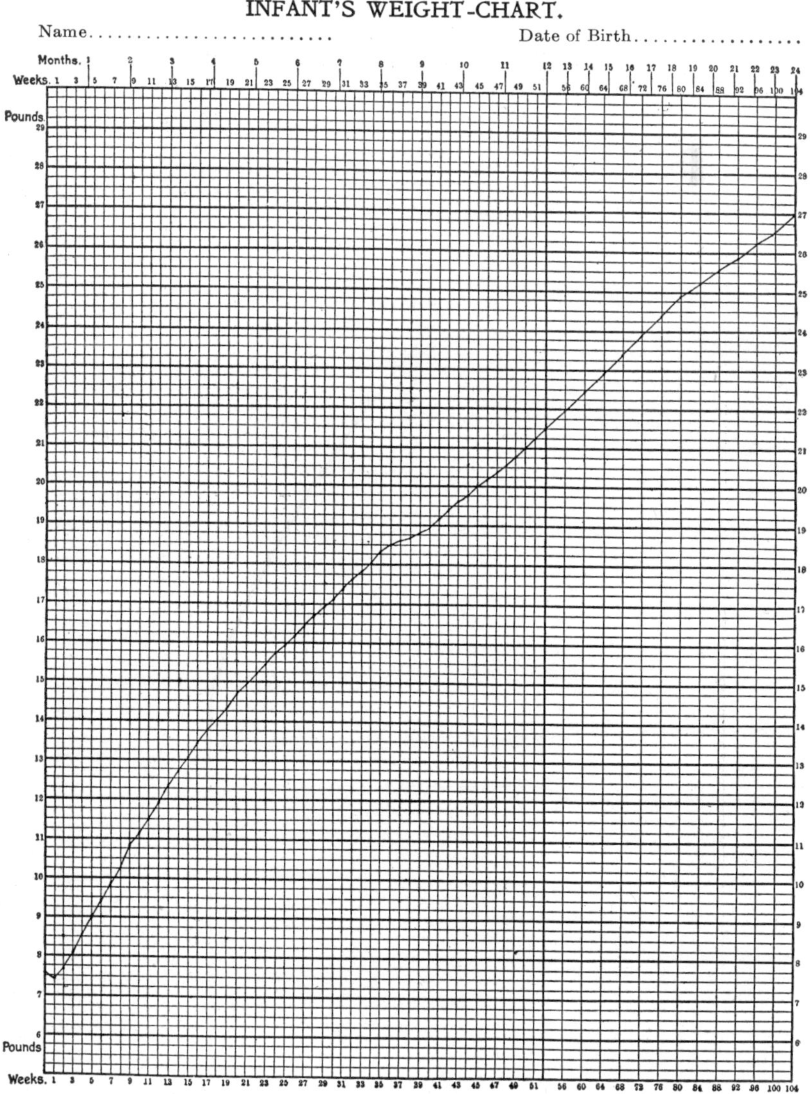

Fig. 2.—Author's weight-chart for the first two years of life. Reduced size. (*Griffith, New York M. J.*, 1899, *March* 4.)

The importance of weighing children regularly during the first two years of life, and especially during the first year, cannot be over-estimated, since cessation of gain is often the earliest sign of illness or of lack of sufficient nourishment. The child should be weighed at least weekly, divested of clothing, or dressed and the weight of the clothes subsequently deducted.

Scales should be used which indicate ounces or grams. Standing spring scales with a scoop or basket attached are very convenient, but some form of balance scale is more accurate. For recording the results a *weight-chart* is a great convenience. The illustration (Fig. 2) is a reduced reproduction of one which we have employed for a number of years. The curve already plotted upon it represents the normal average gain in weight for a healthy breast-fed infant. To economize space the portion for the second

INFANT'S WEIGHT-CHART

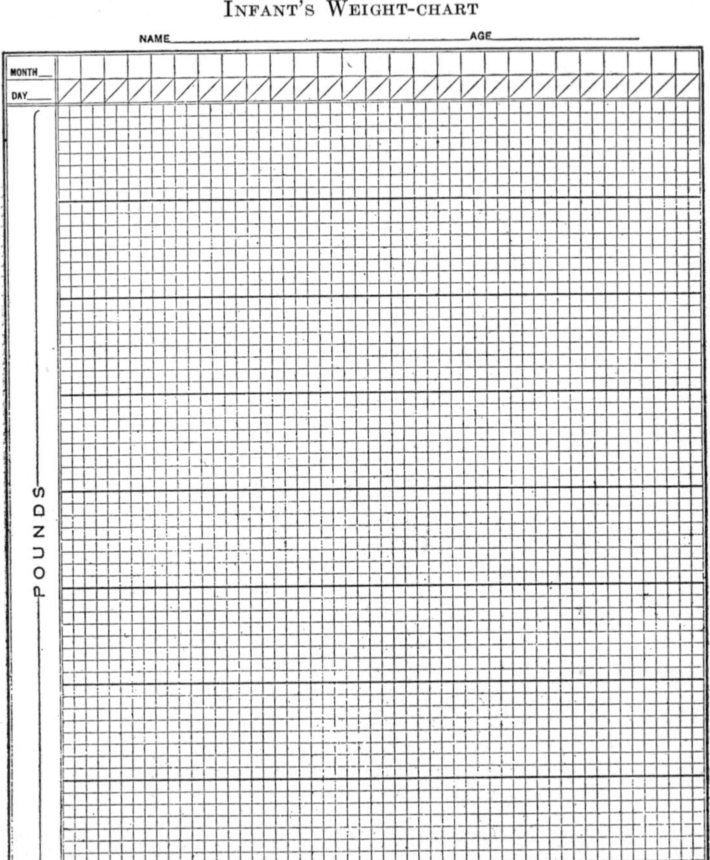

Fig. 3.—Daily weight-chart. To be used for daily weighings at any period of infancy. As employed in the Children's Hospital and in the Children's Medical Ward of the University Hospital, Philadelphia. Reduced size.

year is narrowed one-half, which necessarily distorts the line. A very convenient form for recording daily weighings is that of which a reduced reproduction is shown (Fig. 3).

Length.—Estimations upon growth in length in the first year are much less numerous than those upon weight, and accurate determinations are difficult, causing those of different observers to show decided variations. The average length at birth may be assumed as 49.5 to 50 cm. (19.5 to 20 in.), with males about 0.5 to 1 cm. (0.2 to 0.4 in.) longer than females.

Gain in length goes on rapidly but with decreasing speed. Thus in the first three months, according to Camerer,[6] the gain is 9 cm. (3.5 in.), in the next three months 8 cm. (3.2 in.), and in the third and fourth three-month periods 3 to 5 cm. (1.2 to 2 in.), making a total gain of 24 cm. (9.4 in.) for the year. These figures are somewhat in excess of certain other statistics. Heubner[41] gives the following table for average figures taken from different investigators:

TABLE 9.—GAIN IN LENGTH IN BOYS AND GIRLS
(Heubner)

Age.	Boys.		Girls.	
	Cm.	In.	Cm.	In.
Birth	51.0	20.1	49.0	19.3
1 month	52.5	20.7	51.3	20.2
2 months	55.3	21.8	54.8	21.6
3 months	57.8	22.7	56.7	22.3
4 months	60.1	23.7	58.7	23.1
5 months	61.3	24.1	60.2	23.7
6 months	62.6	24.6	61.5	24.2
7 months	64.6	25.4	63.2	24.9
8 months	65.6	25.8	64.3	25.3
9 months	67.8	26.7	65.4	25.8
10 months	67.0	26.4	67.2	26.5
11 months	69.0	27.2	68.1	26.8
12 months	70.3	27.7	69.2	27.2

As the table shows, the length of male children continues slightly in excess of that of females, the differences at the end of the year equaling about 1 cm. (0.4 in.).

From the ages of one to five years the gain in the second year of life is about 10 cm. (3.9 in.); in the third, 9 cm. (3.5 in.) and in the fourth and fifth years 7 cm. (2.8 in.). The following figures show this in tabular form, assuming the length at one year to be 28 in. (71 cm.):

TABLE 10.—GAIN IN LENGTH IN THE FIRST FIVE YEARS

Years.	In.	Cm.
1	28.0	71
2	32.0	81
3	35.5	90
4	38.25	97
5	41.0	104

Well-cared for children have an optimum length greater than the standards given (Freeman[42]). During this period the difference in length between the sexes continues, but does not increase. (See also Table 6, p. 7.)

From the age of five years onward the combined rate of increase of the two sexes is about 2 in. (5 cm.) a year until the age of eleven years, after which girls slightly exceed boys in height until the age of fifteen years when boys again take the lead. Increase in length is very slight in girls after they reach sixteen years. The normal birth-length is doubled between the ages of four and five years and trebled at about thirteen or fourteen years.

The following table from Bowditch[33] demonstrates the gain in height in boys and in girls respectively. It agrees largely with other extensive observations by Porter,[34] Variot and Chaumet,[43] Peckham,[35] and Tuxford and Glegg.[44]

TABLE 11.—LENGTH IN BOYS AND GIRLS FROM SIX TO EIGHTEEN YEARS OF AGE

Years.	Bowditch.			
	Boys.		Girls.	
	In.	Cm.	In.	Cm.
5	41.57	105.6	41.29	104.9
6	43.75	111.1	43.35	110.1
7	45.74	116.2	45.52	115.6
8	47.76	121.3	47.58	120.9
9	49.69	126.2	49.37	125.4
10	51.68	131.3	51.34	130.4
11	53.33	135.4	53.42	135.7
12	55.11	140.0	55.88	141.9
13	57.21	145.3	58.16	147.7
14	59.88	152.1	59.04	152.3
15	62.30	158.2	61.10	155.2
16	65.00	165.1	61.59	156.4
17	66.16	168.0	61.92	157.2
18	66.66	169.3	61.95	157.3

Growth in length exhibits certain definite *seasonal* relationships, analogous to, though differing from, those affecting weight. (P. 8.) The greatest increase in length, according to the studies of Schmidt-Monnard[45] on children of from two to thirteen years, takes place in July and August, and the least from September to February. Holt[46] found the greatest growth in boys of from six to eighteen years of age taking place from May to November. Increase in length is less influenced by illness than that in weight, except in the case of rachitic children who are often unduly short.

According to Gray[47] American boys have increased in height during the past fifty years.

Relation of Weight to Length.—In recent years much attention has been given by different investigators to the relationship of weight and height, in the effort to determine what should be considered abnormal, especially in the former. The following valuable table has been prepared by the Children's Bureau,[32] based upon the measurements of 167,024 white children without clothes. It shows the normal relationship of weight to height up to the age of six years.

For periods after early infancy one of the most extensive collections of statistics from many different sources is that made by Wood,[48] based upon 250,000 observations on each sex. In the table published by him the age is taken as the nearest birthday, the weight and length are with clothing, but without shoes and with the coats of the boys removed. For measurements taken in this way Wood[49] allows 4 lb. for the clothes (1814.36) of boys and 3 lb. (1360.77) for those of girls. If shoes are worn 1 in. (2.54 cm.) should be deducted.

The standard or normal weight for the height is found where the horizontal line drawn from the height crosses the vertical column under the age. Thus the standard weight for a boy of 57 in. and thirteen years would be 84 lb. The *average* weight will fall nearly in a line drawn obliquely in the table for boys from 36 to 176 lb., and that for girls from 35 to 148 lb. Any figure in the vertical column for a certain age may be considered within the normal range, the figure to be selected as the standard depending upon the height as read in the column on the extreme left. Height, although subject to variation, is so to a much less degree than is weight, and can

TABLE 12.—NORMAL RELATIONSHIP OF HEIGHT TO WEIGHT (*Children's Bureau*)

Height.		Weight.			
		Boys.		Girls.	
In.	Cm.	Lb.	Gm.	Lb.	Gm.
20	50.80	8¼	3,742.13	8⅛	3,685.43
21	53.34	9½	4,309.12	9¼	4,195.63
22	55.88	10½	4,762.72	10½	4,762.72
23	58.42	12	5,443.10	11⅞	5,386.40
24	60.96	13½	6,123.49	13⅜	6,066.79
25	63.50	15	6,803.88	14⅞	6,747.18
26	66.04	16⅝	7,540.97	16⅜	7,427.57
27	68.58	18	8,164.66	17⅝	7,994.56
28	71.02	19⅜	8,788.34	19	8,618.25
29	73.66	20⅝	9,355.33	20¼	9,185.24
30	76.20	22	9,979.02	21¼	9,638.83
31	78.74	23¼	10,546.01	22⅝	10,262.52
32	81.28	24½	11,113.00	23¾	10,772.81
33	83.82	25¾	11,679.99	25	11,339.80
34	86.36	27⅛	12,303.68	26⅜	11,963.49
35	88.90	28⅜	12,870.67	27¾	12,587.18
36	91.44	29¾	13,494.36	29⅛	13,210.87
37	93.98	31⅛	14,118.05	30⅜	13,777.86
38	96.52	32½	14,741.74	31¾	14,401.55
39	99.06	33⅞	15,365.43	33	14,968.54
40	101.60	35¼	15,989.12	34½	15,648.92
41	104.14	36⅞	16,726.20	36	16,329.31
42	106.68	38⅜	17,406.59	37½	17,009.70
43	109.22	40⅛	18,200.38	39¼	17,803.49
44	111.76	41¾	18,937.47	41	18,597.27
45	114.30	43½	19,731.25	42¾	19,391.05
46	116.84	45⅜	20,581.74	45	20,411.64
47	119.38	47¼	21,432.22	46⅞	21,262.12

TABLE 13.—HEIGHT AND WEIGHT TABLE FOR BOYS (Wood)

Height, in.	Yr.													
	5	6	7	8	9	10	11	12	13	14	15	16	17	18
39	35	36	37											
40	37	38	39											
41	39	40	41											
42	41	42	43	44										
43	43	44	45	46										
44	45	46	46	47										
45	47	47	48	48	49									
46	48	49	50	50	51									
47	..	51	52	52	53	54								
48	..	53	54	55	55	56	57							
49	..	55	56	57	58	58	59							
50	..	..	58	59	60	60	61	62						
51	..	..	60	61	62	63	64	65						
52	..	..	62	63	64	65	67	68						
53	..	..	..	66	67	68	69	70	71					
54	..	..	..	69	70	71	72	73	74					
55	..	..	..	..	73	74	75	76	77	78				
56	..	..	..	..	77	78	79	80	81	82				
57	..	..	..	..	..	81	82	83	84	85	86			
58	..	..	..	..	..	84	85	86	87	88	90	91		
59	..	..	..	..	..	87	88	89	90	92	94	96	97	
60	..	..	..	..	..	91	92	93	94	97	99	101	102	
61	..	..	..	..	..	..	95	97	99	102	104	106	108	110
62	..	..	..	..	..	..	100	102	104	106	109	111	113	116
63	..	..	..	..	..	..	105	107	109	111	114	115	117	119
64	..	..	..	..	..	..	...	113	115	117	118	119	120	122
65	..	..	..	..	..	..	...	...	120	122	123	124	125	126
66	..	..	..	..	..	..	...	...	125	126	127	128	129	130
67	..	..	..	..	..	..	...	...	130	131	132	133	134	135
68	..	..	..	..	..	..	...	...	134	135	136	137	138	139
69	..	..	..	..	..	..	...	...	138	139	140	141	142	143
70	..	..	..	..	..	..	...	...	...	142	144	145	146	147
71	..	..	..	..	..	..	...	...	...	147	149	150	151	152
72	..	..	..	..	..	..	...	...	...	152	154	155	156	157
73	..	..	..	..	..	..	...	...	...	157	159	160	161	162
74	..	..	..	..	..	..	...	...	...	162	164	165	166	167
75	..	..	..	..	..	..	...	...	...	...	169	170	171	172
76	..	..	..	..	..	..	...	...	...	...	174	175	176	177

conveniently be assumed as the standard with which weight may be compared. It is not so much the actual weight which is of importance, as the relationship of this to the normal weight for the height. Emerson and Manny[50] conclude from a study of available data that a deficiency of over 7 per cent underweight for the height indicates malnutrition, whereas 20 per cent overweight denotes obesity. Of course a child who is much below the average both in weight and height is abnormal, although the ratio of weight to height may be normal in his case. Emerson and Manny[51] also give tables of the optimum of weight for height. A helpful table is published by Faber[52] who recommends the adoption of a normal range rather than a single weight-height relationship. Attention may also be called to the study on height, weight and age in negro children by Royster and Hulvey.[53]

Even here a word of caution is to be uttered. There is so much variation in both weight and height, depending, among other factors, upon the

Table 14.—Height and Weight Table for Girls
(Wood)

Height, in.	Yr.													
	5	6	7	8	9	10	11	12	13	14	15	16	17	18
39	34	35	36											
40	36	37	38											
41	38	39	40											
42	40	41	42	43										
43	42	42	43	44										
44	44	45	45	46										
45	46	47	47	48	49									
46	48	48	49	50	51									
47	..	49	50	51	52	53								
48	..	51	52	53	54	55	56							
49	..	53	54	55	56	57	58							
50	..	..	56	57	58	59	60	61						
51	..	..	59	60	61	62	63	64						
52	..	..	62	63	64	65	66	67						
53	..	..	..	66	67	68	68	69	70					
54	..	..	..	68	69	70	71	72	73					
55	..	..	..	..	72	73	74	75	76	77				
56	..	..	..	..	76	77	78	79	80	81				
57	..	..	..	..	..	81	82	83	84	85	86			
58	..	..	..	..	..	85	86	87	88	89	90	91		
59	..	..	..	..	..	89	90	91	93	94	95	96	98	
60	..	..	..	..	..	..	94	95	97	99	100	102	104	106
61	..	..	..	..	..	..	99	101	102	104	106	108	109	111
62	..	..	..	..	..	..	104	106	107	109	111	113	114	115
63	..	..	..	..	..	..	109	111	112	113	115	117	118	119
64	..	..	..	..	..	..	...	115	117	118	119	120	121	122
65	..	..	..	..	..	..	...	117	119	120	122	123	124	125
66	..	..	..	..	..	..	...	119	121	122	124	126	127	128
67	..	..	..	..	..	..	...	...	124	126	127	128	129	130
68	..	..	..	..	..	..	...	...	126	128	130	132	133	134
69	..	..	..	..	..	..	...	...	129	131	133	135	136	137
70	..	..	..	..	..	..	...	...	...	134	136	138	139	140
71	..	..	..	..	..	..	...	...	...	138	140	142	143	144
72	..	..	..	..	..	..	...	...	...	...	145	147	148	149

racial and familial characteristics, constitution, social position, posture, activity, etc., that too much importance must not be attributed to the relationship, and especially to that between either of these and the age. Much has been written, too, upon the interrelationships of stem-length, sitting-height, vital capacity, weight, and the like, and various formulae and tables have been constructed to express these. (See Gray and Jacomb,[54] and Gray.[55]) It does not appear that for practical purposes these relationships are as yet superior to the commonly accepted one of height and weight.

Relation in Length of the Head, Trunk and Extremities.—In the newborn the length of the lower portion of the body, measured from the level of the iliac crest, is, according to Zeising,[56] about equal to that of the upper portion, while in adults it is 62 to 63 per cent of the total. The measurements of Taylor[57] on 250 new-born infants gave very similar results, 214 having a mid-point of the body at or above the navel. It is this which makes the infant's legs appear so short. Later the lower portion grows more rapidly than the upper, but not markedly so until puberty. In 500 children studied by Grover[58] the average length of the leg at birth was 43 per cent of the total length and at seven years 54 per cent. The head in the new-born, measured from the vertex to the larynx, is very long, about 25 per cent of the total body-length, against about 11 per cent in the adult (Hoffmann[59]). The proportionate length of the upper extremities does not alter materially with the increase in years. The relationships are shown in the accompanying diagram (Fig. 4). The influence of sex is somewhat apparent. According to Peckham[60] the length of the trunk of the girl is less than that of the boy until about the age of nine years, after which, until

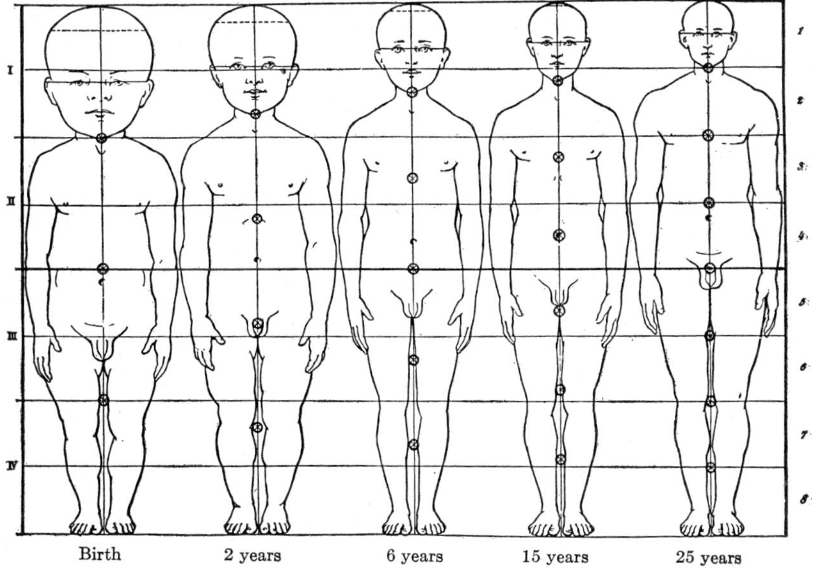

Fig. 4.—Growth-proportions at different life-periods. Showing the length of different portions of the body as compared with the head at different periods of life. At birth the body is 4 heads high, while in the adult it is 8 heads high. (*After Stratz, Der Körper des Kindes,* 1904, 64, *Fig.* 42.)

fifteen years, it is greater. On the other hand while the legs of the girl at nine years are longer, the boy much surpasses her later in length of leg. In fact girls increase very little in this respect after the age of fourteen or fifteen years, while boys grow both in legs and trunk.

General Surface.—By the age of two weeks the dark-red color of the skin of the body has changed to the rose-pink characteristic of infancy. Generally by the end of the first week or earlier any lanugo remaining begins to fall, together with a more or less extensive shedding of the epidermis, sometimes in small scales, sometimes in large flakes. This shedding lasts from two to three weeks. The sudoriparous glands are not very active in the first four weeks of life in healthy children. Very soon, however, they secrete well and the insensible and sensible perspiration is considerable, although free perspiration normally does not occur for several months. This subject is discussed fully in the papers of Levine, Wilson and Kelly.[61]

Head. Size and Shape.—The *circumference* at birth averages about 13 to $13\frac{3}{4}$ in. (33 to 35 cm.). The measurement in new-born girls is from 0.2 to 0.4 in. (0.5 to 1 cm.) less than in boys. Growth is at first rapid, but is very slow after the age of five years. Published statistics vary considerably, but a comparison of a number of investigations gives the following average figures of the circumference at birth, and of the increase:

TABLE 15.—CIRCUMFERENCE OF THE HEAD

Age.	Cm.	In.
Birth	33 to 35	13.0 to 13.8
6 months	42 to 45	16.5 to 17.7
1 year	45 to 46	17.7 to 18.1
2 years	47 to 48	18.5 to 18.9
3 years	48.5 to 50	19.1 to 19.7
4 years	50 to 52	19.7 to 20.5
5 years	52 to 53	20.5 to 20.9
Adult	53 to 55	20.9 to 21.7

As will be seen the growth in circumference is about 10 cm. (3.9 in.) during the first year, which is approximately ½ of the increase of the infant

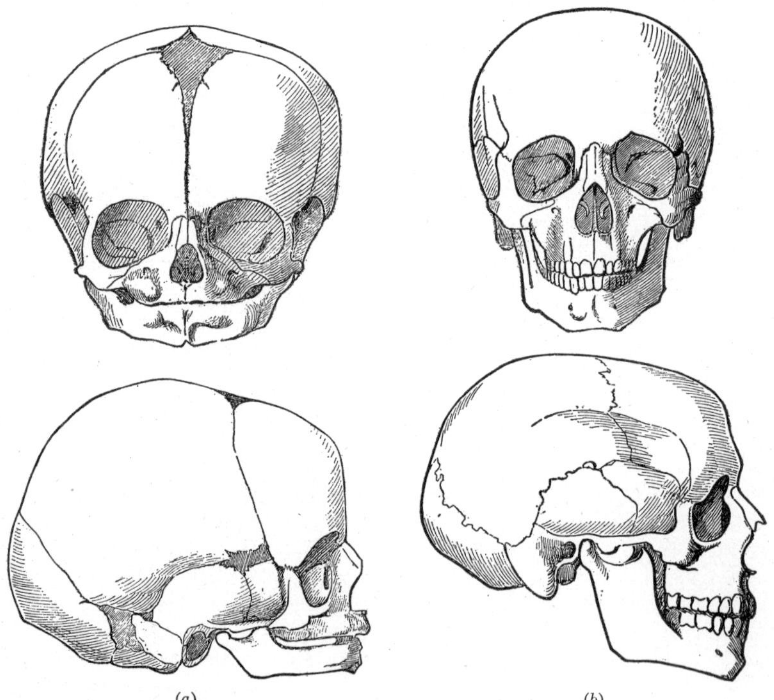

(a) (b)

Fig. 5.—Comparison of skulls. Of the infant (*a*) and of the adult (*b*). (*After Henke, Gerhardt's Handb. d. Kinderkr.*, 1877, *I*, 248; 249.)

in length. In the second year the increase is about 2 cm. (0.8 in.). Girls gradually fall behind to the amount of 1½ to 3 cm. (0.6 to 1.2 in.).

The *shape* differs decidedly in infants from that in adult life (Fig. 5). The facial portion is smaller than the cranial, the ratio in the new-born being 1:8 and in the adult 1:2 or 2½ (Froriep[62]). Its rate of growth is, however, more rapid (Weissenberg[63]). The caput succedaneum, *i. e.*, the swelling of the scalp resulting from pressure during labor, generally disappears by the tenth day or earlier. (See p. 222.)

Owing to the yielding nature of the bones and the ununited sutures the shape may be altered by long-continued pressure as by that during labor, or by the child lying too much upon the back or side, thus flattening the occiput or one of the parietal regions. This distortion is usually only of temporary duration.

Fontanelles.—The posterior fontanelle can be felt open until the age of six or eight weeks and sometimes until the third month. The anterior, of rhomboidal shape, increases in size according to the views of most observers until the ninth month, owing to the brain growing faster than the bones covering it. By the twelfth month it should be decidedly smaller. According to Kassowitz,[64] however, it should grow steadily smaller from the time of birth, and any increase in its size must be attributed to rickets. The fontanelle should be closed by the age of seventeen or eighteen months, yet even in normal children it sometimes closes earlier or later than this. However, closure should be accomplished by two years at the latest. There are great variations in the size of the anterior fontanelle at birth, and in the statements made regarding this. A diameter ranging from 2 to 2½ cm. (0.8 to 1 in.) between the parallel sides perhaps expresses the average.

Scalp.—Although the scalp at birth frequently shows only short, sparse hair it is often covered with a thick, rather dark, comparatively long growth, measuring from 1½ to 2 in. (3.8 to 5.1 cm.). This usually begins to fall at the end of the first week, finally leaving the head almost bald, although some hair persists much longer than this, and many infants retain a heavy growth for months. The new hair comes in only slowly, and is of firmer texture and generally lighter color. Unless precautions are taken a collection of oily scales very rapidly accumulates on the scalp.

Eyes.—The eyes at birth and in the first weeks of life are kept shut or half open and are largely devoid of expression. Their color is an indefinite gray-blue, except in negroes and very dark-skinned races, and this only later changes into the permanent hue of the iris, varying in different subjects. By the end of the first six months Schindler[65] found 70 per cent of normal infants blue-eyed, and even by the age of one year the pigmentation of the iris in those to be dark-eyed may not be complete. The eyes of atrophic infants become darker much earlier. The movements of the eyes are largely incoördinated. Tears are usually not shed until the age of three or four months.

Ears.—The meatus is not fully developed at birth, the portion finally osseous not becoming so until the fourth year. The direction of the meatus is inward and downward and the tympanic membrane is horizontal or inclined slightly upward. The tympanic cavity contains no air at birth but only swollen mucous membrane and mucus. The cavities of the middle ear and of the mastoid antrum have reached adult size by birth, but by five years when a large series of mastoid cells are present these are still only half the size of the adult's cells (Scammon[66]).

The **nose** of the new-born is relatively small and, as a whole, situated higher in the face than in adult life. The fat in the **cheeks** is comparatively well-developed and forms in each what is called the "sucking cushion." By a curious provision of Nature the fat here has less volatile fatty acids and a higher melting point than has other body-fat, and for this reason is the last to disappear in conditions of emaciation (Lehndorff[67]). Very rarely, as in the case reported by Neff and Billingsley,[68] the cushions may be hyperplastic. The **jaws** are small and in a rudimentary condition at birth. The angle of the ramus and body of the lower jaw is much more obtuse than later in life. During infancy the jaws grow considerably, but especially in later childhood they enlarge in order to permit the development of the permanent molar teeth.

Spine.—The spinal column of the new-born is of such flexibility that the existence of the natural curves of later life is doubtful. The sacro-coccygeal curve is present, it is true, but the remainder of the spine either forms one long continuation of this or is straight. Symington[69] has pointed out that the *neck*, as compared with the rest of the spinal column, is in reality relatively longer than in adult life, about equaling the lumbar portion. Its apparent shortness is due to the large amount of fat covering it and to the high position of the sternum. The curve in the neck, with the convexity forward, does not appear until the infant begins to hold its head erect, and never becomes fixed. Still later, with the learning to stand and walk, a similar curve forms in the lumbar region and one with the concavity forward in the dorsal region. The lumbar spine grows faster than the other portions until a little after puberty.

Thorax.—The chest in infancy is small as compared with the abdomen and with the thoracic development of later life. The combination of small chest, large abdomen, and high position of the narrow and insignificant shoulder-girdle, gives the trunk a peculiar barrel-shaped appearance. The *nipples* are small and are situated in the 4th interspace or over the 4th rib as in adult life.

The *ribs* are more horizontally placed than in adult life and the false ribs particularly project upward to a greater extent. The *diaphragm* extends somewhat higher, and the *sternum* is relatively smaller than in adult life. The upper border of the manubrium stands higher than later while the lower end of the sternum projects more sharply forward.

Whereas in adults the transverse diameter of the thorax is to the antero-posterior as 2:1 (Fetzer[70]) or 3:1 (Symington[69]), in the new-born the diameters (Eckerlein[71]) are nearly equal, the transverse being to the antero-posterior as 3:2. As a result the horizontal section of the thorax in early infancy appears nearly circular, while that of the adult is elliptical. The transverse diameter grows more rapidly than the other, and the adult shape of the chest is present to a large degree by the beginning of childhood.

There is considerable diversity in the estimates of different investigators regarding the circumference of the chest at birth taken at the height of the nipples, and the rate of growth in the first five years of life. Approximate figures, the average obtained from the statistics of a number of authors, read as follows:

TABLE 16.—GROWTH OF CHEST IN THE FIRST FIVE YEARS

Age.	Cm.	In.
Birth	32–33	12.6–13.0
6 months	41–42	16.1–16.5
1 year	44–46	17.3–18.1
2 years	45–48	17.7–18.9
3 years	50–51	19.7–20.1
4 years	52–53	20.5–20.9
5 years	54–56	21.3–22.0

In female children the circumference is from 0.5 to 1.5 cm. (0.2 to 0.6 in.) less than in male.

The difference in the rate of growth of the thorax in each sex after the age of five years is illustrated by Porter's[72] studies of over 34,000 measurements of school-children in St. Louis, Mo., and is shown in the following table:

Table 17.—Growth of Chest in Boys and Girls

Years.	Chest.			
	Boys.		Girls.	
	Cm.	In.	Cm.	In.
6	59.05	23.2	58.34	23.0
7	60.62	23.9	59.47	23.4
8	62.18	24.5	60.81	23.9
9	63.90	25.2	62.51	24.5
10	65.59	25.8	63.02	24.8
11	67.24	26.5	65.85	25.9
12	68.76	27.1	68.34	26.9
13	70.61	27.8	71.29	28.1
14	73.27	28.9	74.13	29.2
15	76.56	30.1	76.78	30.6
16	79.22	31.2	78.85	31.0
17	81.39	32.0	80.39	31.7
18	84.52	33.3	80.45	31.7

According to the observations of Monti[73] the average increase in circumference in the first year is 12 cm. (4.7 in.), in the second year 3 cm. (1.2 in.), and in the remaining years up to 12, 1.25 cm. (0.5 in.). There then occurs a sudden increase in the rate of growth to 4 cm. (1.57 in.) a year.

The comparison of the rate of growth in the circumference of the chest and of the head respectively is of great practical utility. The combination of the two tables already presented (pp. 16 and 18) gives the following results:

Table 18.—Comparison of Circumferences of the Head and Chest

	Head.		Chest.	
	Cm.	In.	Cm.	In.
Birth	33–35	13.0–13.8	32–33	12.6–13.0
6 months	42–45	16.5–17.7	41–42	16.1–16.5
1 year	45–46	17.7–18.1	44–46	17.3–18.1
2 years	47–48	18.5–18.9	45–48	17.7–18.9
3 years	48.5–50	19.1–19.7	50–51	19.7–20.1
4 years	50–52	19.7–20.5	52–53	20.5–20.9
5 years	52–53	20.5–20.8	54–56	21.3–22.0

Although there may be considerable variation within normal limits it is certainly a sign of feeble development when the circumference of the chest has not exceeded that of the head by the age of three years.

Abdomen.—The abdomen appears relatively large and prominent in infancy, this depending upon the large size of the liver, the great amount of subcutaneous fat present, and the small size of the pelvis and chest. Its circumference measures about the same as that of the chest up to two years after which period it is decidedly less. The stump of the *umbilical cord* remaining after birth gradually shrivels, exhibiting a small red area at its junction with the body. About the fourth to the sixth day the stump falls, leaving an ulcer which closes after five or six days. The umbilicus occupies nearly the central part of the body during the first two years. In adult life its distance above the soles is $\frac{3}{5}$ of the total length of the body.

Pelvis.—The pelvis in the infant is very small and more obliquely situated than later. The width of the body at the hips at all ages equals that of the shoulders in males, but is greater at all ages in females.

Limbs.—The bowing of the short *legs* present at birth (p. 2) persists until in the course of the second year. The tendency to hold the arms and legs in the fetal position with the feet dorsally flexed is exhibited more or less during the early months. Although infants are seemingly flat-footed, in reality the feet are shaped much as in adult life, the shortness and thickness seen especially in later infancy depending upon the large amount of fat in the subcutaneous tissue.

DIGESTIVE APPARATUS

Mouth.—The mouth in the early months is comparatively dry, with the tongue generally exhibiting a whitish coating. The jaws at birth will not meet. They are covered with gums of a pale-red color, and exhibit rather hard, narrow opposing ridges. No signs of the presence of teeth are visible.

Dentition.—The 20 *temporary teeth,* also called *deciduous, first,* or *milk* teeth, are at birth enclosed in dental follicles, and in alveoli in the jaw which are already osseous in nature. The crowns of the incisor teeth are even then entirely calcified, as are those of the other teeth to a considerable extent. The teeth and tooth-sacs are covered only by mucous membrane and sub-mucous connective tissue, and the alveoli are broad and allow of free growth. As calcification and elongation of the roots take place, the crowns are gradually forced onward in the direction of least resistance. Under this constant pressure outward the gums covering them atrophy, flatten and grow paler, and the teeth finally push through. Probably the only resistance offered has come from the sub-mucous tissue. Complete calcification of the fangs does not occur until the child is several years of age.

The germs of the *permanent* teeth, or *second* teeth, except the second and third molars, are already present in the jaws at birth, resting against the posterior wall of the dental sacs of the temporary teeth. The crowns of the anterior molars are calcified. In the other teeth of the set calcification begins at different periods between the first and the eighth year. Like the first set they increase in length, their eruption depending principally upon the calcification of the roots. Probably from insufficient supply of blood, occasioned by pressure of the advancing permanent teeth, the roots of the temporary set finally undergo absorption and the teeth drop out in much the same order as they came in.

Eruption of the Temporary Teeth (Fig. 6).—Many different statements have been published regarding the time of the eruption of the temporary teeth. The following table expresses a very generally accepted view. It will be noticed that the teeth erupt in distinct groups, with a pause between them:

Table 19.—Eruption of the Temporary Teeth

Group	Teeth / Pause	Age
First Group	2 lower central incisors	7 months
Pause	3 to 8 weeks.	Total 2.
Second Group	4 upper incisors	8 to 10 months
Pause	1 to 3 months.	Total 6.
Third Group	4 anterior molars and 2 lower lateral incisors	12 to 15 months
Pause	2 to 3 months.	Total 12.
Fourth Group	4 canines	18 to 24 months
Pause	2 to 4 months.	Total 16.
Fifth Group	4 posterior molars	20 to 30 months
		Total 20.

The upper and lower canines are popularly called the "eye-teeth" and the "stomach-teeth" respectively. In the third group the lower lateral incisors appear, according to many observers, before the molars, but there is no absolute rule for this. In fact the table represents only the most frequent order, and wide variations may occur within physiologic limits. The age of seven months may be considered the average time for the first tooth, yet any time not exceeding the first year may be called normal. From six to eight months is a very common range, and eruption at three or four months is not at all infrequent.

In perfectly normal states the eruption of the teeth is unattended by any symptoms whatever. The pathologic conditions which are believed to develop will be considered in the section upon Disorders of Dentition (p. 517).

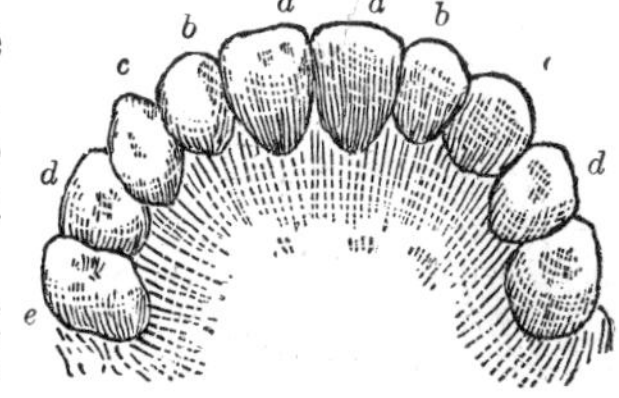

Fig. 6.—Diagram showing the temporary teeth. *a*, central incisors; *b*, lateral incisors; *c*, canines; *d*, anterior molars; *e*, posterior molars.

Eruption of the Permanent Teeth (Fig. 7).—The permanent teeth, or teeth of the second dentition, are 32 in number. The earliest to be cut are the first molars, which come in just posterior to the temporary second molars. They appear at about the age of six years and are consequently often called the "six-year-old molars." The other teeth erupt in much the same order as those of the temporary set. Although the order and dates of appearing are subject to considerable variation, the following table is a fair expression of them:

Table 20.—Eruption of the Permanent Teeth

	Years.
First molars	6
Central incisors	7
Lateral incisors	8
First bicuspids	9
Second bicuspids	10
Canines	11–13
Second molars	12–15
Third molars (Wisdom teeth)	17–25

The teeth of the lower jaw usually erupt somewhat before the corresponding ones of the upper jaw, the interval being often as much as several months. The permanent first molars are not a replacement but constitute 12 new

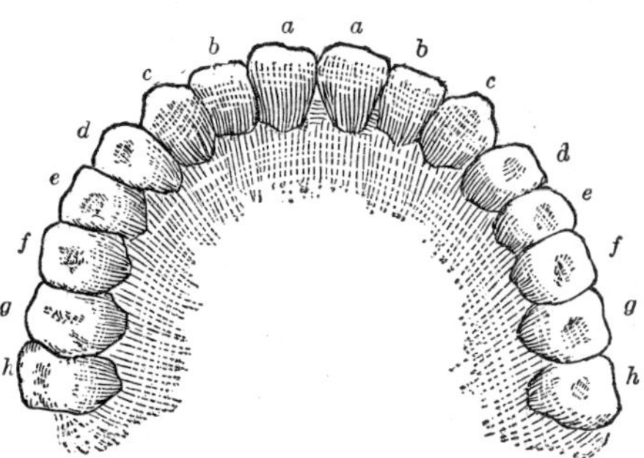

Fig. 7.—Diagram showing the permanent teeth. *a*, central incisors; *b*, lateral incisors; *c*, canines; *d*, first bicuspids; *e*, second bicuspids; *f*, first molars; *g*, second molars; *h*, third molars.

teeth additional to the original 20. The bicuspids take the place of the temporary molars. At about the age of six years the jaws contain all the teeth of both sets, visible or concealed, except the third permanent molars.

Salivary Glands.—The comparatively small amount of saliva secreted by the new-born accounts for the dryness of the mouth and the coating of the tongue. By the second month increase in the secretion begins and by the age of three or four months this is still further augmented and the child begins to "dribble." This increase takes place, as a rule, before the eruption of teeth, and appears to be in no way connected with it. Although according to the investigations of Korowin[74] and of Zweifel[75] ptyalin is present in the salivary glands at birth, any diastatic activity is inconsiderable until the increased secretion of saliva begins. Even then, since much of the fluid runs out of the mouth, its influence upon digestion is probably not great. As the first year advances the amount of saliva grows greater and by the age of one year its diastatic power is about as great as in adult life (Finizio[76]). The reaction remains fairly constantly neutral or alkaline. Urea is normally excreted in the saliva (Hench and Aldrich[77]) and an increase in the amount takes place when there is urea-retention in the blood. The determination of the salivary-urea may be used as an index of nonprotein nitrogen-retention, such as may occur in nephritis. The average normal amount in children is about 3.5 mg. per 100 cc. (Calvin and Isaacs[78]).

Esophagus.—The total length of the esophagus in the new-born, according to the statistics collected by Vierordt,[79] is about 10 cm. (3.9 in.) or, including the total distance from the teeth to the cardiac orifice, 17 cm. (6.7 in.). This latter distance at the age of three years is 30 cm. (11.8 in.) and in adult life 40 cm. (15.8 in.). The pseudo-valvular opening at the gastric end of the esophagus is stated by Gubaroff[80] to be imperfectly developed in infancy. This accounts in part for the greater ease with which vomiting occurs at this time of life.

Stomach.—The capacity of the stomach in infancy varies greatly and different observers have obtained dissimilar results. This is illustrated in the following table from which, however, an idea of the approximate size may be obtained:

TABLE 21.—CAPACITY OF THE STOMACH AT DIFFERENT PERIODS*

Age.	Fleischmann.[81]		Holt.[82]		Frolowsky.[83]		Pfaundler.[84]		Beneke.[85]	
	Cc.	Fl. oz.	Cc.	Fl. oz.	Cc.	Fl. oz.	Cc.	Fl. oz.	Cc.	Fl. oz.
Birth	...	...	36	1.2	...	...	...	...	35–43	1.2–1.5
1 week	46	1.6	...	....	50	1.7	...	...	....	....
2 weeks	72	2.4	44	1.5	70	2.4	...	...	153–160	5.2–5.4
1 month	80	2.7	59	2.0	112	3.8	90	3.0	....	....
2 months	140	4.7	100	3.37	158	5.3	100	3.4	....	....
3 months	...	...	133	4.50	167	5.6	110	3.7	....	....
4 months	...	...	148	5.00	178	6.4	125	4.2	....	....
6 months	...	...	176	5.75	...	...	160	5.4	....	....
9 months	...	...	...	....	253	8.6	225	7.6	....	....
1 year	...	...	263	8.9	...	...	290	9.8	....	....
2 years	...	...	...	....	...	...	...	...	740	25

* The original tables vary slightly from this, the data being for the number of weeks rather than of months. As the differences, however, are inconsiderable we have purposely distorted the figures a little to apply to the age in months.

Scammon and Doyle[86] in a careful clinical study on 323 infants found the physiologic gastric capacity on the first day of life equaling 7 Gm. (.24 fl. oz.), with a rapid increase to 81 Gm. (2.75 fl. oz.) by the tenth day. The maximum capacity was distinctly greater than these figures. Roughly we may estimate the capacity by adding at different periods 2 to the figure representing the age in months; 8 to 10 oz. being the maximum capacity for any infant. It depends, however, on the size of the child as much as or more than on the age alone. On the other hand, an infant not infrequently can digest, and requires, a larger amount of food than its age or size would indicate. This may well be because some of the liquid taken passes into the intestine before the meal is completed. Basing the dietetic requirements upon the estimated size of the stomach is consequently a procedure to be depended upon only with limitations. The capacity in artificially fed infants is somewhat greater than in those fed at the breast. The orifice of the pylorus measures 2 cm. (0.78 in.) in circumference in the new-born, according to Pfaundler.[87] The position of the stomach early in infancy had been generally considered to be nearly vertical or slightly oblique, and the form cylindrical; but the more recent investigations by Flesch and Péteri,[88] Smith,[89] and Pisek and Le Wald[90] showed that the organ changes its size and shape from time to time, depending upon the amount of food contained in it, that it is oftener horizontally situated rather than vertically, and that the pylorus generally occupies a comparatively high and anterior position. The amount of gastric secretion is large in infancy. The acidity of the gastric contents varies widely, depending upon the amount, concentration, time after ingestion, and character of the food or test-meal. The total acidity is greater with dilute than with concentrated foods of the same volume. When the hydrogen-ion concentration is high the buffer value is low, and the reverse is also true (Miles and Shohl[91]). In normal infants after a test-meal of 125 cc. of barley water Müller and Gutschmidt[92] obtained an average of free hydrochloric acid 9; combined 14.5 and total acidity 20.5. Izumita[93] discovered in infants, thirty-five minutes after a test-meal of 125 cc. of boiled wheat flour and cane sugar, free hydrochloric acid 0 to 18 and a total acidity of from 4 to 26. Since the free acid combines with such foods as milk it may not be discoverable until towards the end of digestion. Free acid may be present in the stomach of new-born infants who have never been fed (Hess[94]), and Griswold and Shohl[95] obtained a high acidity at this age (pH 2.5 to 2.6). Throughout infancy and childhood, however, most studies show that the total acidity and the free hydrochloric acid are less than in adults. Babbott, Johnston, Haskins and Shohl[96] found that with a milk test-meal the pH content in about 75 per cent of the readings was 3.9 to 4.6, the acidity increasing with the length of time after ingestion of the food. Bauer and Deutsch[97] believed lactic to be the predominant acid after ingestion of food in early infancy, and Heiman[98] found it in half the breast-fed infants examined. Others, however, have discovered it but seldom. Pepsin and rennin (which may not be distinct from pepsin) are present at all periods of life, even in the fetus. A fat-splitting ferment is also present, likewise in the fetus. Mucus occurs also, part of its function being to combine with acid.

Liver.—The liver at birth is hyperemic and large and its edge can be distinctly felt below the costal margin. To a great extent it covers the anterior surface of the stomach. It continues to be discoverable below the costal margin until about the age of five years, and, according to Zamkin[99] may extend downward as much as 3.5 cm. (1.36 in.) in healthy children up to the age of twelve years. The area of hepatic dulness is also greater in early life, the upper margin of this reaching the 4th rib. According to the statistics collected by Vierordt[100] its absolute weight averages 141.7 Gm. (5 oz.) in the male and 164 Gm. (5.8 oz.) in the female; *i. e.*, 4.5 per cent and 5.5 per cent of the body-weight, while in the adult it is but from 2.8 per cent to 3 per cent. The weight increases little or none during the first six months, and, in fact, diminishes slightly in the first weeks. Kowalski's[101] figures, however, do not corroborate this failure to increase in weight in the early months. Bile is secreted even before birth. The investigations of Jacubowitsch[102] indicate that the bile of the infant differs from that of the adult especially in the larger proportion of water and the smaller amount of biliary acids and of bile-salts present, and the consequent lesser power of digesting the fats. Among the numerous functions of the liver is a detoxifying effect on many alkaloidal, mineral and organic poisons. It also produces urea and uric acid; is able to deaminize amino-acids; forms dextrose even with substances, such as amino-acids and lactic acid, which are not carbohydrate in nature; stores glycogen; and produces bile and utilizes the bile pigments developed elsewhere in the body. It has to do with the fabrication of fibrinogen; in certain infections as part of the reticulo-endothelial system it destroys bacteria; is concerned with the oxidation of fatty-acids; and is involved in the manufacture of hemoglobin.

Bile is utilized in the metabolism and digestion of fat; has an effect on intestinal peristalsis; by its alkali-content takes part in maintaining the reaction of the intestinal contents; and accelerates the action of pancreatic lipase and slightly that of pancreatic amylase.

Pancreas.—The pancreas at birth weighs 3.5 Gm. (0.12 oz.) (Vierordt[103]), bearing about the same relation to the body-weight as in adult life. The ferments lipase, amylase and trypsin, as well as the internal secretion insulin, are present in the new-born and have been found, too, in the fetus.

Intestine.—The total length of the small intestine in the new-born would appear from Vierordt's[104] statistics to vary considerably, ranging from 2 to 3.5 meters (6.5 to 11.5 ft.). The large intestine according to the same authority measures from 0.42 to 0.48 meters (1.38 to 1.57 ft.). The relative length of the entire bowel as compared with that of the body is greater in children than in adults. The small intestine grows rapidly. Beneke[105] found it at birth 5¾ times the body-length, at two years about 6½ times, at seven years 5 times, and in adult life but about 4½ times. The length of the large intestine was about equal to that of the body, both in the new-born and in the adult. Robbin[106] observed that the relative length of the large intestine equaled from 80 to 130 per cent of the body-length in 91.3 per cent of 185 infants from birth to three years of age, and that of the small intestine equaled from 500 to 900 per cent of the body-length in 79.9 per cent of the cases. The sigmoid flexure is especially long in infants, being at birth, as stated by Treves,[107] almost equal to ½ the total length of the large intestine. It often forms a huge loop running up to the lower border of the liver. It is perhaps partly due to this great length that constipation occurs so frequently in infancy. During the first four months the sigmoid diminishes greatly in length, while the rest of the colon proportionately increases, the total length of the large intestine thus remaining unchanged. The vermiform appendix reaches its full length early in life. It is particularly prone to kinking in infancy and childhood, and is abundantly supplied with lymphoid tissue, both factors tending to the production of appendicitis. According to the conclusions of Gundobin[108] Peyer's patches are well developed, but less numerous in the new-born as compared with adults; the number of solitary follicles greater; Lieberkühn's follicles and the villi more abundant, and Brunner's glands numerous but not completely developed. The muscular strength of the intestine is comparatively feeble. The various ferments and hormones of the intestinal tract are present from birth.

DIGESTION IN INFANCY

(See also Digestive Apparatus, p. 20 and Absorption and Metabolism, p. 29)

The act of sucking has a pump-like quality. The base of the nipple is seized firmly by the infant's lips; the tongue is pressed against the nipple, making a longitudinal gutter in which this may lie and along which the milk is conducted backward; the soft palate and base of the tongue approach each other and shut off the posterior opening of the oral cavity from the nose. Then the cheeks sink in slightly, while the lower jaw is depressed, thus producing a partial vacuum, by means of which the milk is drawn from the breast or bottle. This type of suction is quite different from that seen in children two to three years old, where the action is by inspiration. The sucking cushions already referred to (see Cheeks p. 17) are supposed to prevent a too great collapse of the cheeks. To nurse satisfactorily the infant must be able to breathe easily through the nose, respiration through it not being interfered with by sucking, although it ceases momentarily during the act of swallowing.

The saliva plays but small part in digestion in early infancy. (See Salivary Glands, p. 21.) Later its diastatic action is of service in the case of infants receiving starch. Yet this action is not completed in the mouth, and, after the food is swallowed, should continue only for a short time as long as the gastric contents are alkaline or but faintly acid. On the other hand, Jackson[109] had children with total atresia of the esophagus spit saliva into a funnel connected with a gastrostomy tube, and noted that the nutrition, previously poor, immediately improved. He believes that saliva plays a much more important part in the nutritive processes of children than is generally realized.

The stomach is more of a simple receptacle in infancy than later in life. Some of the milk entering it passes immediately through the pylorus (Hess[110]); that remaining is promptly coagulated by the action of the rennin or by the hydrochloric acid present. Human milk forms small, loose curds, while cow's milk produces a much firmer, larger mass. This may be due to the greater percentage of casein present in cow's milk. The acidity of the gastric contents appears very soon after the ingestion of food, and steadily increases. (See Stomach, p. 22.) After the milk has been coagulated its solution by the pepsin begins, the hydrochloric acid now aiding in accomplishing this. Although there is some splitting of protein especially of that in breast-milk, yet much the greater portion of the coagulated milk passes out of the stomach of the infant but little affected in other respects by gastric digestion. There is no action exerted by the gastric secretion upon the carbohydrate, although the fat is acted upon to some extent by the lipase of the stomach.

The length of time during which the ingested food remains in the infant's stomach probably varies with the infant. A considerable portion of the milk leaves within one-half hour, the liquid portion containing the sugar and salts and the uncoagulated milk passing out first, and in the first month or two of life the organ may be empty in less than two hours. Later a somewhat longer time is required, but the average healthy breast-fed infant retains but little of the food in the stomach longer than at most two or two and one-half hours. This has been demonstrated radiologically by Levin and Barret,[111] Tobler and Bogen,[112] Flesch and Péteri,[88] Ladd,[113] Pisek and LeWald[90] and others. The onset of hunger-contractions was shown by Ginsburg, Tumpowsky and Carlson[114] to begin in two to three hours after the ingestion of food. It has been claimed, according to the experiments of Cannon[115] on animals, that the cardiac orifice closes automatically with a certain degree of normal acidity of the gastric contents. A number of investigations have been made upon the time for and the cause of the opening of the pylorus with regard to the influence of gastric acidity. The results are to a certain extent contradictory (Babbott, Johnston, Haskins and Shohl,[93] McClure, Reynolds and Schwartz,[116] Lockwood and Chamberlain,[117] Cowie and Lyons,[118] Theile[119]). It seems evident that some factor is concerned in addition to the reaction of the gastric and duodenal contents. The nature of the food taken influences the time it remains in the stomach. Human milk passes from it more rapidly than cow's milk. The greater the amount of casein, the longer is the retention of the food. Delay also depends to a large extent upon the amount of fat present (Tobler[120]). DeBuys and Henriques[121] demonstrated that the body-posture has much to do with the time for emptying, the rapidity being greatest in the right lateral position. The stomach is of little service in the absorption of food, only a small amount of the sugar and digested protein being taken up here; the fats, water, and salts practically not at all.

In the intestine the trypsin accomplishes the peptonizing of the milk not already acted upon in the stomach. Inasmuch as the saliva is present in such small amount in early infancy and the diastatic ferment of the pancreas is not secreted to any considerable extent in the 1st month, the power of digesting any starchy food at this period of life would be thought to be very limited. It must be stated, however, that investigations by Huebner[122] and others apparently prove that even infants of two months possess a positive power to digest starch; and clinical experience, as in the feeding of cases of pyloric stenosis, indicates a decided power of digestion at a very early age. The bile-salts in infancy in combination with the steapsin of the pancreas split the fat and permit of saponification and the forming of an emulsion. The secretion of the small intestine converts the various carbohydrates into the monosaccharides,—galactose, levulose and dextrose—and the protein-derivatives into amino-acids, in which form they are absorbed.

The peristalsis of infancy is less active than in later childhood or adult life, and the combination of this condition with the great relative length of the intestine probably gives the infant an especial ability to digest and absorb the large amount of milk taken. Independently of this, the infant possesses a very active power of absorption. This takes place principally from the small intestine, whence all the elements of the food can enter the system, the fat passing in practically only from this region. The large intestine can absorb all these elements, but to a very limited degree. The time of passage through the entire gastro-intestinal tract varies, according to Kahn,[123] from four to twenty hours, with an average of fifteen hours. Lesné, Binet and Paulin[124] by adding small amounts of carmine to the infant's feedings found the average time of passage to be ten hours at from one to two years, the duration being less in younger subjects and in the breast-fed.

Bacteria of the Gastro-intestinal Tract. **Mouth.**—A considerable number of species of bacteria appear in the mouth even very soon after birth and increases decidedly with the beginning of the taking of food. With the appearance of the teeth there is a further increase in the number of varieties. Among those oftenest found by Nobécourt and de Vicariis[125] are the bacillus lactis aerogenes, micrococcus candidans, bacillus coli, micrococcus pyogenes aureus and albus, and the streptococcus pyogenes and salivaris.

Stomach.—The number of bacteria normally found is limited, the hydrochloric acid having destroyed many of those swallowed with the food. Yet there are many contained within the masses of coagulated milk, which the acid cannot affect.

Intestine.—The healthy normal infant exhibits soon after birth a number of species of bacteria in this region, the meconium being sterile for only about twenty-four hours. The subject was originally investigated especially by Escherich[126] and later by Tissier,[127] Moro[128] and others. After breast-feeding commences the number of germs increases greatly although the varieties are not numerous. In general the most prominent bacteria in the intestinal tract in breast-fed infants are the bacillus bifidus, the bacillus acidophilus and to a less degree the bacillus coli and the bacillus lactis aërogenes. There are also sometimes present the bacillus perfringens, bacillus butyricus, micrococcus ovalis, various types of streptococci, staphylococci, bacillus proteus, bacillus subtilis, and certain others in smaller numbers. In breast-fed infants 25 or more per cent of the dried feces may consist of bacteria (Leschziner[129]) and in the artifically fed 40 per cent or more (Strassburger[130]). The upper part of the small intestine exhibits very few germs of any sort, chiefly the bacillus lactis aerogenes and the colon bacillus. The former is more abundant here than in any other portion of the intestinal canal. The lower part of the ileum and the colon contain an abundant growth of bacteria, the bacillus bifidus being the predominating germ. There are also present the bacillus acidophilus, the colon bacillus, the micrococcus ovalis, and a diminished number of the bacillus lactis aërogenes. The colon and rectum have a smaller number of living bacteria than is found in the cecum.

In artificially fed infants the variety of germs is greatly increased. The colon bacillus and intestinal cocci are the predominating micro-organisms, but the others mentioned are also present in large numbers. The colon bacillus and the bacillus lactis aërogenes are more numerous than in breast-fed children, and the bacillus aërogenes capsulatus is regularly found. In breast-fed infants the germs are largely fermentative (acid-forming, carbohydrate-splitting) and tend to be gram-positive, whereas in the bottle-fed they are especially those which are putrefactive (alkali-forming, putrefactive, protein-splitting) and tend to be gram-negative. The composition of the food, particularly its content of carbohydrate or of protein, and its acidity are largely instrumental in determining the nature of the flora. Lactose causes a rapid increase in the number of bacillus acidophilus. Bacterial souring of milk is effective because of the higher degree of acidity so produced rather than because of its content of micro-organisms. (Compare Knox and Ford,[131] Bahrdt and Beifeld,[132] Bosworth,[133] Kendall,[134] Bass,[135] Sisson,[136] Ford, Blackfan and Batchelor.[137])

Under pathologic conditions there may be an enormous increase in the number of the normal bacteria, and various others not native to the intestine are present; while at the same time germs which are normally present and harmless may possibly assume a special virulence and be productive of diseased conditions. Among those found are the bacillus proteus vulgaris, bacillus enteritidis, streptococcus enteritidis, bacillus pyocyaneus, and forms of the dysentery-bacillus.

Gases of the Digestive Tract.—The gas in the stomach is in part swallowed by the infant while nursing, and in part enters from the intestine. But little is produced by fermentation of the food, and a small quantity appears to be secreted by the gastric mucous membrane. In healthy children it consists of the elements of the atmospheric air only.

The gas in the intestine depends principally on the decomposition of the milk-sugar and consists of CO_2 and H. There are no foul-smelling gases in the intestine of breast-fed infants who are in a healthy condition.

Feces.—The first passages of the infant consist of the meconium. This is a tarry, dark, greenish-brown, almost odorless and faintly acid substance. It is sometimes passed before or during birth, and three to five times during the first two or three days of life. It contains cells from the intestine and the skin, minute hairs, fatty granules and globules, cellular detritus and intestinal mucus, together with biliary acids, coloring matter, cholesterin-crystals and other substances derived from the bile. The source of some of the elements is the amniotic liquid which the fetus has swallowed. Vierordt[138] estimates the total amount of meconium passed at 60 to 90 Gm. (2.12 to 3.17 oz.). Should the secretion of milk be delayed the meconium is replaced after two or three days by stools consisting of brownish or greenish mucus. With the secretion of breast milk the ordinary milk-feces of the infant appear. These are golden-yellow or canary-yellow in color, of salve-like consistence or of that of thin mush, and faintly acid in odor and reaction. With cow's milk the stools are alkaline, neutral or faintly acid, of a paler yellow color, have a more decided odor due to the decomposition of the protein, and are often firmer. Thoroughly digested breast-milk stools appear almost entirely homogenous (Fig. 8). A ratio of 3 to 1 between the fat and the protein produces an acid stool, while one of 1 to 1 makes the stool alkaline (Schlossmann[139]). Consequently an alkaline reaction of the stools of the bottle-fed infant is a natural result of a relatively high percentage of protein as compared with that of the fat. The acid reaction is commonly attributed to the lactic acid and the fatty acids present, but Bosworth[133] and his coworkers claimed that in healthy infants it was dependent upon the presence chiefly of formic and acetic acids, the latter being the cause of the acidity present in the healthy bottle-fed baby. This has been confirmed by Gerstley, Wang, Boyden and Wood,[140] who obtained also proprionic acid. Tisdall and Brown[141] found the pH of the stools of normal new-born infants varying from 4.7 to 5.1. An acidity as great as 4.6 was encountered only in severe diarrheal conditions in bottle-fed babies. Infants fed on protein milk, cow's milk dilution with added carbohydrate, or whole acid-containing milk with added carbohydrate, generally have stools more alkaline than pH 7.0. Numerous small whitish masses are very common in the stools of infants apparently entirely healthy and thriving; and this is especially true of those artificially fed. A brownish color may depend upon a relatively large proportion of protein. Mucus is frequently visibly present even in the stools of healthy breast-fed infants. It is not uncommon to find occult blood in stools passed during the first ten days of life. Bonar[142] believes this is due to the hyperemia set up by the beginning of digestion and bacterial invasion.

The number of evacuations is at first from 2 to 4 in twenty-four hours, and from about the sixth week to the age of two years from 1 to 3. The amount of fecal matter passed is estimated by Uffelmann[143] to be about 3 per cent of the milk taken, or, in the case of feeding with cow's milk, 4.3 per cent; averaging 3 Gm. per kilo (21 grains per lb.) of the body-weight. However, there is wide normal variation both in the number and in the weight of the stools.

The stools contain approximately 85 per cent of water. The greater part of the residue consists of cellular elements, mucus and bacteria. The milk taken is never wholly absorbed. Fat is always present in the feces, both as neutral fat and fatty acids, and as soaps from combination of these with the alkalies and alkaline earths. Any large amount of neutral fat indicates poor digestion. Holt, Courtney and Fales[144] found the fat of the dried feces to average 34.5 per cent and it was often even 50 per cent in breast-fed infants. In infants taking the ordinary modifications of cow's milk the average fat equalled 36.2 per cent. The sugar of the food is entirely absorbed. Protein is present only in very small amount in healthy infants. Knöpfelmacher[145] found that the greater portion of the nitrogen and phosphorus recovered from the feces of breast-fed infants is derived from the digestive secretions and not from the milk. About 8 per cent of the total protein ingested is lost in normal stools; more in diarrhea (Holt, Courtney and Fales[146]). From 8 to 10 per cent of the dried feces consists of mineral matter, chiefly calcium, derived partly from the food, partly secreted by the intestine. The proportion of mineral matter is higher in artificially fed infants. The small, whitish masses very frequently present in the bowel-movements of healthy, thriving children consist principally of fat or its derivatives and of epithelial cells. The yellow color is produced

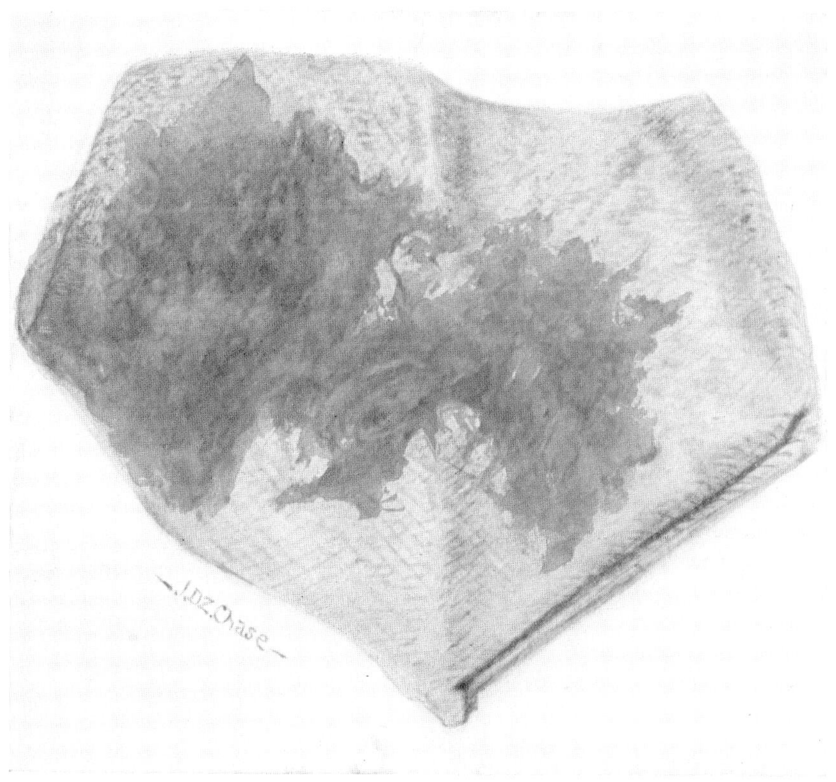

Fig. 8.—Thoroughly digested breast-milk stool.

by bilirubin, which is present unchanged in part. The pale greenish tint so frequently appearing in the stools of healthy children when or a short time after they are passed is the result of the oxidation of bilirubin to biliverdin. Such chemical combinations as phenol and skatol, which give the characteristic odor to the stools of adults, are not found in those of milk-fed infants. Various ferments are present in the feces, among them diastase, lactase, invertin, trypsin, rennin, a fat-splitting ferment, and others.

Under the microscope the bowel-movements of the infant exhibit fat-globules of various sizes; some molecular fat; needles of fatty acids; innumerable bacteria; cholesterin-plates; square and columnar epithelial cells; small round cells; some thin, granular, yellow, flake-like masses; lime-salts in crystalline form; and occasionally bilirubin-crystals, yeast-fungi and proteid matter.

The evacuations become a somewhat darker yellow as the infant grows older; and when the diet is more varied, and especially when the amount of milk is relatively diminished, they acquire more the characteristics of the stools of adults, both in color and odor. They are naturally soft, as a rule, and acid in reaction. It is only at about the age of two years that the stools become formed. This is, however, open to many exceptions, for even young infants may normally pass fully formed stools.

ABSORPTION AND METABOLISM OF THE FOOD

In addition to and summarizing some of the statements already made under Digestion (p. 24) a brief résumé may be given of the physiologic processes which attend and follow this, viewed from the standpoint of the food-elements rather than of the organs, and as applicable especially to infancy.

Water.—The large percentage of water in the milk indicates the need of the infant in that particular. Concentrated food is not so easily assimilated as a rule by healthy infants, even though the actual amount of solid matter ingested is not altered, and the work thrown upon the excretory organs is also increased if sufficient water is not ingested. The amount required is proportionately many times greater than in adult life. There is little need, however, of water given by itself when the diet is entirely liquid, since enough is obtained in the food; but for other reasons it is well to accustom an infant to it. Including that contained in the milk there are required per day in the first few months about 2.5 fl. oz. per pound (162.5 cc. per kg.) of body-weight, and after the first year about 1.75 fl. oz. per pound (114 cc. per kg.).

Fat.—The amount of fat in the food has a decided influence upon the time this remains in the stomach, the larger the amount, the slower being the discharge. This slow entrance into the small intestine permits of a readier digestion of it when it reaches this region. The fat is in no way affected by the saliva, but in the stomach the gastric lipase is able to break up a considerable portion of it. Comparatively little digestion of fat, however, occurs here, and no absorption at all. In the small intestine the fat is split by the pancreatic lipase in combination with the bile-salts and aided by the intestinal secretion, the fatty acids uniting with the alkalies and forming soaps, soluble and insoluble, and later an emulsion. It is in this form that the fat is absorbed by the small intestine, more than 90 per cent being utilized both in breast-fed and in normal bottle-fed infants. A resynthesis of neutral fat probably occurs in the cells of the intestinal wall. Very little is taken up by the large intestine. The absorption of fat in artificially fed infants can be modified by altering the proportion of the other elements of the food. Thus an addition of carbohydrate apparently increases the absorption of the fat and changes a soap-stool to one of a more normal acid character; and, on the other hand, an increase of the protein may similarly change a highly acid, loose stool into a firmer, more alkaline one. The fat appears to have little favorable influence upon the metabolism of protein, but is of importance in mineral metabolism, especially aiding in the absorption of calcium. About 35 per cent of the total caloric intake should be as fat. The fat in the stools may possibly be derived in part from the intestinal secretion and from decomposition of the carbohydrates; but probably much the largest portion is from the food.

Carbohydrate.—The only carbohydrate in milk is lactose; a disaccharide, resolvable into dextrose + galactose. In artificially fed infants the other disaccharides, saccharose (dextrose + levulose) and maltose (dextrose + dextrose), are often employed. Starch, too, a polysaccharide, is to be considered, and in older children cellulose. On the sugar the saliva has no action whatever, nor has the secretion of the pancreas unless maltose is employed, when there may be a slight reduction by the maltase. The starch is converted by the salivary, pancreatic and intestinal secretions into sugar; although some part of it is probably destroyed in infancy by bacterial action within the intestinal canal. The power of digesting starch rapidly increases with an increase of the quantity and strength of the amylolytic ferments. The invertin, maltase and lactase in the intestinal canal act respectively upon the saccharose, maltose, and lactose, reducing them to monosaccharides, in which form alone are they absorbable under ordinary conditions. Only when given in very large amounts do the disaccharides pass the normal intestinal mucous membrane. They then appear unchanged in the urine, with the exception of maltose, which may be broken up by the maltase of the blood and utilized. The monosaccharides are absorbed rapidly by the small intestine, especially in the upper part, and carried by the portal circulation to the liver where they are changed into glycogen. The large intestine also possesses to some extent the power of the reduction of the disaccharides and of absorption.

The different sugars are utilized by the infant to different degrees. All of them are fermentable, but lactose undergoes lactic acid fermentation, saccharose more readily alcoholic and less easily butyric acid fermentation, and maltose most easily butyric acid and next readily alcoholic fermentation. As compared to the other sugars, lactose is less fermentable by the various micro-organisms and yeasts of the intestinal tract. Lactose brings about a more favorable reaction in the intestinal tract for calcium absorption than do other sugars (Bergeim[147]). All the sugars in large amount have a tendency to loosen the bowels, but lactose to a less degree than maltose. It is stated by various authors, such as Hill,[148] Kahn,[149] and Feldmann,[150] that the normal infant can digest daily from 3.1 to 11 Gm. of lactose per kilogram of body weight; 7.2 Gm. of maltose and the same of saccharose. The tolerance is often greater than this. For example, Schick[151] found that 17 per cent of cane-sugar added to half milk was readily tolerated by newborn infants as a temporary substitute for human milk. It was even possible to add the 17 per cent of sugar to human milk, making the total sugar 24 per cent. Being the natural sugar of milk lactose should be easily digested and metabolized. Clinical experience shows this to be true. Gerstley, Wang and Wood[152] found that increasing the lactose in mixtures up to 12 per cent, a ratio to the protein of 4 to 1, actually decreased the amount of acid in the stools. There is evidence, too, that the feeding of lactose as compared with vegetable sugars produces tissues of less water-content, and consequently less subject to dehydration (Jarvis[153]).

The retention of the nitrogen of the protein is rendered more complete by the presence of carbohydrates. The carbohydrates would seem, too, when not in excess, to favor the absorption of fat, perhaps by preventing the formation of calcium and magnesium soaps. In excess they interfere with the fat-absorption by producing diarrhea, by which all the intestinal contents are rapidly removed from the body. In the stools the carbohydrates appear chiefly in the form of undigested starch, when this is given in unduly large amount to infants. Very little soluble carbohydrate is found. The gas in the intestine is dependent in part upon the decomposition of the carbohydrate by bacteria. This decomposition also aids in producing the acidity of the stools, which in general is in direct proportion to the amount of the carbohydrate ingested. The carbohydrate of the fetus is exhausted soon after birth, and acidosis may threaten. About 50 per cent of the total caloric intake should be as carbohydrate.

Protein.—The digestion of the protein takes place, as stated, partly in the stomach, under the influence of rennin, pepsin and hydrochloric acid, but chiefly in the intestine by the trypsin of the pancreas and the erepsin of the intestinal secretion. The action of this latter is upon the casein, peptones and albumoses, changing them into absorbable amino-acids. It would not appear to be a matter of indifference in what form the protein is present in the food. The value of the large percentage of whey in human milk may depend upon the fact that certain amino-acids are present in it in large amount, but in quite small quantity in the casein, and that those in the whey are necessary to growth. According to Osborne and Mendel[154] lactalbumin is a more efficient protein than casein, 9 per cent of the former being sufficient for growth, whereas from 15 to 18 per cent of the latter is necessary. Animal protein is for the most part completely absorbed (85 per cent); protein from legumes about 78 per cent and protein from vegetables about 83 per cent. The curds in the stools are composed of casein to a very limited extent; casein-curds being hard and tough and generally absent in the case of healthy infants, especially when boiled milk has been employed.

The needs of the infant in the matter of nitrogen derived from protein are not great. At least 1.5 Gm. of protein per kilogram of the body-weight (10.5 grains per lb.) is required daily to maintain a positive nitrogen balance, although it is claimed by some investigators that as little as 1.1 or even 0.6 Gm. are sufficient for this purpose. The maintenance of a positive nitrogen-balance, which can be taken to indicate that growth of nitrogenous tissue is occurring, does not depend solely upon the amount of protein ingested. While, as stated, the giving of carbohydrate in proper amount favors the retention of nitrogen, the fat has little if any favorable action, and in excess may act unfavorably. The approximate needs of protein when stated in terms of ounces of milk are about 1.5 to 2 fl. oz. per pound of the infant's weight (98 to 130 cc. per kilo). In human milk about 9 per cent of the calories are furnished as protein; in whole cow's milk about twice that.

It has also been claimed that whereas breast-fed infants receive but 1 or 1.5 per cent of protein, as contained in human milk, bottle-fed infants need 3 per cent or more (Holt and Fales[155]) on account of the fact that casein is the dominant protein of cow's milk, and that this substance is deficient in the necessary amino-acids required for growth. This in theory would seem to be correct, but it should be remembered that there is as yet no actual knowledge of the amounts of the amino-acids needed by the human infant, and that multitudes of infants in the past have thrived on the lower percentage of cow's milk protein.

Much has been written concerning the deleterious effects of protein when given in great excess over long periods of time. In the cases described by Benjamin[156] there were pallor, great atony, free perspiration and sometimes eczema, and Glanzmann[157] and Moll and Stransky[158] have emphasized the damage which may be produced by too long-continued use of large amounts of casein-milk. In an instance reported by Hoobler[159] a decidedly stuporous condition developed, whereas in cases recorded by Holt and Levene[160] there was continued fever. Newburgh, Falcon-Lesses and Johnston[161] have performed experiments which they believe demonstrate that excessive protein may cause renal damage, arteriosclerosis and other degenerative changes. While there seems to be no question that such results may follow it is not entirely clear that in some instances the apparent harmful effects of excessive protein may not have been due in reality to the lack of some of the other necessary ingredients of the diet.

In the older child the type of protein is not a matter of indifference. About $\frac{2}{3}$ of it should be animal in nature. Protein should never be considered simply as such. It is, after all, made up of its building stones, the amino-acids. Proper variation in the type of proteins ingested assures that there are furnished those amino-acids, such as lysin, tryosine, cystine and tryptophan, which are essential for growth and which the body cannot synthesize.

Mineral Matter.—The salts of human milk are readily absorbed from the small intestine, but to a negligible degree from other regions. The greater quantity of salts, except iron, in cow's milk as compared with human milk results in the amounts taken by the infant artificially fed being usually in excess of the needs unless the mixture be quite dilute. However, the forms in which these salts exist in human milk are more favorable to their absorption. Under normal conditions 40 per cent of the mineral of the ingested cow's milk is lost in the stools, chiefly as calcium phosphate. The presence of sufficient amounts of fat and sugar favors the retention of calcium probably by increased formation of acids;—intestinal acidity being favorable to calcium absorption. Any condition increasing intestinal alkalinity decreases the absorption of calcium. An excess of fat increases loss both of calcium and magnesium by the production of soaps in large amounts. There should be ingested at least 0.19 Gm. of calcium oxide for each kilogram of body-weight (Holt, Courtney and Fales[162]) and there should be about 4 Gm. of fat per kilogram (28 grains per lb.) to insure a proper metabolism of the calcium. Stearns[163] claims that in artificially fed infants there should be ingested daily about 40 mg. of calcium and 20 to 25 mg. of phosphorus per kilogram of body weight. In older children the requirements decrease, but a retention of less than 10 mg. of calcium and of phosphorus respectively is insufficient. Wang, Kern and Kaucher[164] in a study on 18 children found that when the calcium was above 32 mg. and the phosphorus above 79 mg. per kilogram per day a positive balance was obtained. There is a distinct relationship between the absorption of calcium and other minerals in that an excess of phosphorus, magnesium or potassium decreases the calcium assimilation. An excess of calcium also decreases phosphorus absorption due to the formation of an insoluble calcium phosphate. Calcium may be absorbed either from organic or inorganic combination; the part of it not retained being excreted in the urine or through the intestinal wall. Stearns[163] points out that about 98 per cent of the calcium retained is utilized in the formation of bone and the remainder is found in body-fluids; and that from 25 to 35 per cent of the total phosphorus in the body of new-born infants lies in tissues other than bone. It is considered that a retention-ratio of calcium to phosphorus of between 1.5 to 1 and 2 to 1 is normal for an infant;—a retention of less than 1.5 to 1 indicating more rapid growth of soft tissue than of bone. Sodium, potassium and magnesium are well absorbed from the small intestine, and excess eliminated through the urine and feces. The growing child needs about 4 to 5 Gm. of sodium chloride a day; about 2 to 3 of potassium oxide; about 0.3 to 0.5 of magnesium oxide (Potter[165]) and about 8 to 26 mg. of iron. According to Bunge[166] there is considerable iron storage in the liver at birth, and Büngeler and Schwartz[167] state that there is a storage of iron pigment by the reticulo-endothelial system, which begins after birth and reaches its height at the end of the second month of life. This reservoir is exhausted by eight to ten months of life.

FUNCTIONS OF FOOD-ELEMENTS

The following is a brief synopsis of much of what has preceded and of what will later follow concerning the relation of the elements of the food to their utilization in the body. The human body possesses an adjustability and an adaptability which can never be obtained by a mere machine. This is fortunate, because in disturbed intestinal and metabolic conditions abnormally balanced diets may become necessary; but this furnishes no warrant for employing such under normal conditions. The factor of safety in nutrition depends upon the metabolic adjustment whereby the body may form fat from protein and carbohydrate and carbohydrate from protein; and may probably utilize carbohydrate and fat as an aid in the synthesis of certain amino-acids, finally producing protein. A knowledge of the functions of the different food-elements is therefore absolutely necessary, because some of them are essential and others can be replaced only at the cost of undue gastro-intestinal work and metabolic activity.

Water.—The importance of fluid in the body is shown by the fact that it constitutes about 70 per cent of the muscular tissue and parenchymatous organs, from 15 to 30 per cent of the fatty tissue, and 80 per cent of the blood. The muscles contain about $\frac{1}{2}$ of the body-water; the skin about $\frac{1}{5}$; and the blood about $\frac{1}{13}$. Water in the body acts as a solvent and carrier of food-material and of excretory products; by vaporization from the lungs and skin it helps to regulate the temperature; and it controls osmotic pressure and the viscosity of the blood and other tissues.

Fat.—The chief purpose of the fat is to maintain body-heat or energy. It has also the secondary values of acting as a carrier of some of the vitamins and of affecting the absorption of minerals.

Carbohydrates.—These maintain body-heat and assist in the proper metabolism of fat, which might otherwise be incompletely burned and produce acetone-bodies. An important function of carbohydrates is the production of water in the process of their combustion.

Protein.—This element is essential to life and is concerned in the growth of new tissue and the replacement made necessary by wear and tear of the body-cells. It is especially dangerous in children to decrease the food-protein over long periods of time, inasmuch as true cellular growth cannot proceed without it. Protein should not, under usual circumstances, be employed as a major source of energy, since a considerably greater amount of work is involved in converting it to this purpose than in the case of fat and carbohydrate, and very little of it can be stored in a manner available for energy. (See also Allergy p. 484.)

Minerals.—These are concerned in the formation of the skeleton; the regulation of the acid-base balance of the body; the sustaining of osmotic pressure; the maintaining of normal excitability of the nervous and muscular tissues; and in such other processes as the control of weight, temperature and cardiac rate.

ENERGY METABOLISM

In various sections reference will again be made to the physiologic data obtained by metabolic studies as they apply practically. Most of the results are too technical for inclusion here and the reader who is further interested may consult other sources, such as the chapter on Energy Metabolism in the text-book of Morse and Talbot,[168] the monographs of Benedict and Talbot[169] and of Newburgh and Johnston,[170] and the article by Talbot[171] and other journal-articles on the subject.

Heat-production is measured either directly by means of a respiration-calorimeter, or indirectly by calculating the energy-value from either the oxygen consumed or the carbon dioxide produced. On account of its simplicity the indirect method has been adopted for general use.

The type of food being metabolized in the body may be estimated by determining the respiratory quotient, *i. e.* the volume of carbon dioxide eliminated divided by the volume of oxygen consumed. When carbohydrate alone is metabolized the respiratory quotient is 1, and when fat alone is oxidized it is 0.7. Protein as well as a mixed diet gives a respiratory quotient between 0.7 and 1, generally assumed as 0.82.

The term "basal metabolism" is commonly used to designate the heat-production measured when the subject is in complete muscular and mental relaxation, is without food for from twelve to eighteen hours, and is free from thermal influence. The basal heat production thus obtained may be expressed in terms of total calories per twenty-four hours, or calories per unit of body-weight, body-height, or body-surface. The basal metabolism of a child based on either weight or surface area increases from birth to about eighteen months of age, but from this period onward gradually falls throughout childhood. According to Talbot[172] the average basal metabolism of an infant at birth is about 50 calories per kilo of body weight per twenty-four hours. This value decreases steadily to about 30 calories for a child of thirteen years of age. An increase in basal metabolism during puberty has been found by several investigators (Topper and Mulier,[173] Göttche,[174] Lax and Petenyi,[175] Petereyi and Lax[176]).

The sick and inactive infant produces less heat than the healthy, lively one. Emaciated, active, crying infants have a basal metabolism above the average. It has been determined by Topper and Mulier[177] that older children who are overweight but otherwise normal usually have a normal metabolic rate, except for the tendency mentioned for it to be high in the prepuberty period. In children slightly underweight the basal metabolism is likewise usually normal, but decided malnutrition (over 25 per cent underweight) is frequently accompanied by definite lowering of the rate.

Activity is one of the greatest modifers of heat-production and accounts for the larger part of individual variation of energy requirement. According to Murlin, Conklin and Marsh[178] crying during 1 per cent of the time raises the metabolism about 1 per cent in infants. Talbot[179] states that in a very quiet infant 15 per cent may be added to the basal metabolism for activity; if normally active 25 per cent; and if extremely active 40 per cent. During sleep heat production is distinctly diminished (averaging about 15 per cent) (Wang and Kern[180]). In cretinism the basal metabolism may be as low as 40 per cent below the normal standard for the child. The specific dynamic action of foodstuffs (*i. e.*, the heat produced in the body which is not produced in a bomb calorimeter when the same amount is burned in it), is likewise a great modifier of heat-production. A large protein meal may increase the basal metabolism of a subject as much as 50 per cent. The peak usually occurs from two to four hours after the ingestion and the effect may last as long as ten hours. The specific dynamic action of carbohydrate is much less potent, about 10 per cent of basal, and it lasts only two to three hours; that of the fat is negligible. Specific dynamic action of a food should therefore not be confused with "utilizable" energy-value. The former increases the heat-production in the animal body, but the heat thus developed is not utilizable. On the contrary this extra heat lost by the subject must be supplied by giving additional food.

The utilizable energy-value derived from fat is 9.3 calories for each gram ingested; with 4.1 for carbohydrate and 4.1 for protein (Rubner[181]). From such studies and also from observation of the food consumed by average healthy infants and children the caloric (heat, energy) needs may be determined. The actual caloric requirements include, in addition to the basal heat-production, those for growth, for activity and for loss through excreta, and are about twice the basal value for the subject. Heubner's[182] figures, which he terms "energy-quotients," have often been taken as a guide. (See p. 93.) Although these are somewhat lower it is now generally considered that approximately 110 calories per kilogram (50 per pound) are needed in the first six months of life; by the end of the first year about 90 per kilogram (40 per pound), and by six years about 80 per kilogram (36 per pound) for boys and 75 (34 per pound) for girls. The adult standard of 48 per kilogram (22 per pound) is not reached until fifteen years or later. It cannot be emphasized too strongly that these figures are only average ones and that active and also underweight children may require more than the usual standard, and overweight and inactive children less.

ORGANS OF RESPIRATION

Upper Respiratory Passages.—The **nasal passages** in the infant are very narrow, and the **sinuses** for the most part not yet fully developed. In careful studies Davis[183] and Scammon[184] found the maxillary sinus present as an oval pocket at birth and pneumatization of the lateral ethmoidal mass usually complete. The sphenoidal sinus is very small in the first year, and the frontal sinus not present before the third year. The **larynx** is situated high in the neck, the lower border of the cricoid being opposite the upper border of the 5th cervical vertebra, instead of opposite the 7th as in adults. By puberty it has descended to the adult position and in boys increased much in size. The space between the vocal cords of the infant is extremely narrow. The bifurcation of the **trachea** is opposite the 3d dorsal vertebra in the new-born, but opposite the 4th in adults.

Lungs.—The lungs of the infant at term lie in a collapsed condition at the back of the thorax. After air enters them they are still small in volume as compared with adult life, and continue so throughout childhood. They weigh at birth about 24 Gm. (0.85 oz.), the relative weight being about the same as in adult life. The lower level during infancy is not quite so low in relationship to the ribs as it is in adult life (Gittings, Fetterolf and Mitchell[185]).

Respiration.—The type of respiration in the infant is generally described as abdominal. The careful experimental studies of Eckerlein,[186] however, showed that it is thoracic as well, neither type predominating constantly, but sometimes one and sometimes the other being evident. The respiration in infancy, and especially in the new-born, is very irregular, and the rate is much influenced by the slightest causes. At times quite long pauses take place. This irregularity is almost constantly present when the child is awake, and may occur even during sleep. The average rate in early life can be determined only approximately, and the estimations of investigators differ widely. By means of spirometer and plethysmograph Murphy and Thorpe[187] found that new-born infants had an average respiratory rate of 43 per minute (from 24 to 116), that the minute-volume of air was 721.4 cc. (from 433 to 1413), and that the mean tidal air was 16.7 cc. (from 10 to 27). The following table of the rate at different ages contains average figures only:

Table 22.—Rate of the Respiration per Minute

New-born	30 to 50.	Average about 35 to 40.
Balance of first year	25 to 35.	Average about 30.
One to two years	About 28.	
Three to four years	About 25.	
Four to five years	20 to 25.	
Adult life	16 to 18.	

The rate is from $\frac{1}{5}$ to $\frac{1}{4}$ less during sleep. Only with the beginning of childhood does the irregularity largely disappear, but even then the rate may be much increased by comparatively slight causes. It is not until the tenth year that the predominating costal type of breathing begins to develop in girls. The vital capacity is constantly greater in boys than in girls.

ORGANS OF CIRCULATION

Heart. **Size.**—The heart in the new-born weighs about 24 Gm. (0.85 oz.) according to the statistics of H. Vierordt[100] as compared with between 260 and 300 Gm. (9.17 and 10.58 oz.) in the adult. It is thus proportionately larger in the infant, equalling 0.76 per cent of the body-weight in the new-born and 0.46 per cent in the adult. After the first month the rate of increase is about the same for the heart and for the body respectively, except that at puberty there is a physiologic hypertrophy. The right ventricle is comparatively large and strong in early infancy, its walls being almost as thick as those of the left ventricle. From the second year onward, however, the muscle-mass of the right ventricle is not more than $\frac{1}{2}$ that of the left. The foramen ovale, situated at the lower posterior portion of the auricular septum, still exists at birth. From the anterior border of the inferior vena cava arises a thin membrane, the Eustachian valve, which during fetal life diverted the blood from this vessel through the foramen ovale into the left auricle (see p. 766). It gradually becomes closed entirely, generally prior to the twelfth week or earlier, but often not for some months.

Position.—The position of the heart is rather more horizontal in the infant. The relative dulness—which is the most important—begins in the first year at the 2d left interspace or, oftener, the 2d rib, extends to the right parasternal line, and reaches as far as from 1 to 2 cm. (0.4 to 0.8 in.) beyond the nipple line. The width at the position of the nipple is 6.6 to 8 cm. (2.6 to 3 in.). At the age of six years it reaches upward to the 2d intercostal space, to the right scarcely as far as the right parasternal line, and to the left to the nipple-line or slightly beyond. The greatest average breadth is about 10 cm. (4 in.). At twelve years the boundaries are the 3d rib, the right edge of the sternum and the left nipple-line. Its greatest breadth is 11.5 cm. (4.5 in.). The absolute dulness in the first year is bounded by the lower edge of the 3d rib, the left border of the sternum and the left nipple-line.

Apex.—The apex-beat in the first year is generally found in or oftener beyond the mammillary line, but quite frequently its position cannot be determined. After this period, although it may lie in various positions with regard to the mammillary line, it is oftenest outside of it up to the fourth year; on the line from this time up to the seventh year, and within it after the ninth year. It is nearly always in the 4th interspace in the first year, generally so in the second year, in the 4th and 5th interspaces from the third to the sixth years, and usually in the 5th interspace after the seventh year. The position of the apex is, however, subject to great variations within physiologic limits. A distance of 2 cm. (0.8 in.) outside the nipple line is to be looked upon, however, as a possible indication of enlargement or displacement.

Auscultation.—This shows all sounds to be loud, sharp, distinct, and more widely diffused than in adults. This is in part owing to the thinness of the chest wall. In infancy and up to the age of four or five years the second sound is weakest over the aortic cartilage and loudest over the pulmonary cartilage, but is everywhere weaker than the first sound of the heart. There is described a third heart-sound in normal children which is best heard with the ear alone and better in expiration. Its occurrence is prediastolic or middiastolic and its situation about the third or fourth rib between the sternum and the left mammillary line (Steinberg[188]).

Blood-vessels.—In the child these are relatively of somewhat greater capacity than in the adult. The pulmonary artery is decidedly larger than the ascending aorta, while in adult life they are of nearly the same size (Beneke[189]). The relative size of the heart as compared with the diameter of the ascending aorta is much less in children than in adults (Beneke). As a consequence of these two relations the general arterial tension is less than in adult life (see p. 38), and the blood-pressure in the lungs is greater than that of the general arterial system.

At the point where the pulmonary artery divides into its two main branches springs in the fetus the ductus arteriosus Botalli. Although the largest branch, this vessel is but a short trunk about ½ in. (1.3 cm.) in length at birth. It passes obliquely upward and joins the aorta just beyond the origin of the left subclavian artery. Since with the beginning of respiration the blood is diverted from the ductus arteriosus into the lungs, this canal closes prior to the second month, persisting only as a small fibrous cord in later life. (See also p. 766.) Among other vessels characteristic of antenatal life, and still present at birth, are the hypogastric arteries and their continuation, the umbilical. These are stout trunks arising from the internal iliac arteries and passing upward beside the bladder to and through the navel, whence, twisted around the umbilical vein, they reach the placenta. The distal portions of the arteries within the body of the child close completely in from two to five days after birth, forming fibrous bands, the anterior ligaments of the bladder. The proximal portions remain pervious for only a short distance from their origin, as the superior vesical arteries. The umbilical vein after entering the body from the navel passes upward along the free margin of the suspensory ligament of the liver. After giving off small branches to the hepatic substance, it divides in the transverse fissure into two main branches, the larger and shorter of which joins the portal vein. The other, the ductus venosus, continues along the posterior longitudinal fissure of the liver and joins the hepatic vein where this empties into the ascending cava. Both the umbilical vein and the ductus venosus close completely in from two to five days after birth, the part of the former within the body finally becoming the round ligament of the liver.

The activity of the circulation is greater in the child. K. Vierordt[190] estimates that the time elapsing from the moment the blood leaves the heart until it returns to it is in the new-born 12.1 seconds, at three years fifteen seconds, at fourteen years 18.6 seconds and in the adult 22.1 seconds.

The circulation during fetal life and the changes which take place at birth have so intimate a relation to congenital diseases of the heart that they will be described in connection with cardiac disorders (see p. 766).

Pulse.—Even in health the pulse tends to be somewhat irregular in force and frequency. It has been the general impression that this was true especially of infancy, but the electrocardiographic studies of Krumbhaar and Jenks[191] and of Seham[192] would indicate that arrhythmia is uncommon in infancy, but becomes increasingly frequent from the age of six years to puberty, 47 per cent of school-children showing an arrhythmia, according to Seham. Trifling causes, such as crying, nursing, or excitement or exercise of any other kind increase the pulse-rate from 20 to 40 beats per minute. It is often not easy to feel the radial pulse in the first months. The rate is less when the child is lying than when sitting, and sitting than when standing, and during early morning sleep may be 20 to 30 beats less than in the afternoon. There may be a familial tendency to rapid or slow pulse under normal conditions. The pulse-rate diminishes also with increasing age, but the figures of different observers vary much. An approximation would be expressed by the following:

Table 23.—Pulse-rate during Infancy and Childhood

Birth	130 to 150
First month	120 to 140
One to six months	About 130
Six to eight months	About 120
One to two years	110 to 120
Two to four years	90 to 110
Six to ten years	90 to 100
Ten to fourteen years	80 to 90

The rate is slightly greater in females except in the first few months.

Blood-pressure.—The blood-pressure is lower in children than in adults and exhibits little marked increase until near puberty, after which there is a somewhat abrupt rise. Extensive studies are reported by Judson and Nicholson[193] and by other American and European authors. An excellent review of the subject is given by Abt and Feingold.[194] The following figures are based on a compilation of a large number of data:

Table 24.—Blood-pressure in Normal Children

Age, years.	Systolic.	Diastolic.*
3–5	85–90	70
5–8	90–95	70
8–10	95–100	70–75
10–15	100–105	75–80

* Figures in mm. of mercury.

It is difficult and usually impossible to determine by the usual method blood-pressure under three years of age. Rucker and Connell[195] and Seitz and Becker,[196] employing the oscillatory method with an aneroid sphygmomanometer, found the mean systolic pressure in the new-born to be about 45 to 55 mm. and the diastolic about 40. The latter authors also state that at the end of the first week of life the systolic pressure is about 60 mm. and by the end of the first month 80. Wolff[197] found the systolic pressure rose gradually from about 60 mm. at birth to 74 at six months.

BLOOD

Blood. Amount, Specific Gravity and Volume.—Bakwin and Rivkin,[198] Lucas and Dearing[199] and others have estimated the blood-volume in infants by the vital-dye-method. The average from fifteen days to one year is about 10 per cent of the body-weight. In the new-born there is great variation with an average of 14.7 per cent. The specific gravity in the new-born is estimated by Lloyd Jones[200] to be highest at birth, equalling 1066, but by the end of the second week it has fallen rapidly and continues to decrease until the age of two or three years when it equals 1048 or 1050. The normal blood-concentration of the new-born, as demonstrated by Lust,[201] gave 22.3 per cent of dry substance during the period of from one to thirty days after birth, and 18 per cent from the age of one to ten months.

Hemoglobin.—The concentration of hemoglobin in the blood has been given, in most clinical work, in terms of percentage of normal. There are so many "standards" for normal that hopeless confusion has resulted. All modern work on hemoglobin is being expressed either in terms of grams of Hb per 100 cc. blood or in terms of the oxygen capacity per 100 cc. blood (1 Gm. per cent Hb = 1.34 cc. of O_2 per 100 cc.). The best average normal figure for adult male blood is 15.6 Gm. Hb. (20.9 vol. O_2 capacity) per 100 cc. of blood containing 5,400,000 erythrocytes per cubic millimeters. For more complete discussion see Peters and Van Slyke.[202]

It is well established by the work of Appleton[203] and Williamson[204] that hemoglobin in the blood of the new-born is extremely high at birth, over 150 per cent of normal (about 22 Gm. per cent Hb.). This falls steadily to a minimum at one year of about 75 per cent of normal (12 Gm. per cent Hb.) and then rises gradually to about 86 per cent of normal (13.4 Gm. per cent Hb.) by puberty (eleven to fifteen years).

There is no sex-difference in the hemoglobin concentration in children as there is in adults where the blood of males is 10 per cent higher than females. It is evident that any value for hemoglobin must be interpreted in terms of age. It is possible that this decline with subsequent rise is not entirely physiologic but that it can be controlled by diet.

Erythrocytes.—(See also page 1019 and Fig. 249.) The number of red blood-cells per c.mm. of blood reported in infancy varies so greatly that no satisfactory figures are available. Because of this the ratio of hemoglobin and cell count so valuable in adult hematology is at present of little value during the first few years of life. The erythrocyte count is relatively high in the new-born, often reaching 6 or 7 million per c.mm. A decrease in number begins after the second day. The diminished number continues to exist during the first year, and then there follows a gradual increase up to the age of from eight to twelve years, when the number normal for adults is attained. The average number of red blood-cells in early and later childhood is 4,000,000 to 4,500,000. Nucleated red blood-corpuscles (normoblasts) occur in the fetus and in small numbers during the early days of life, but after the first week their presence is unusual. The size of the red corpuscles varies very much in the new-born, pale corpuscles deprived of their hemoglobin (shadow-corpuscles) are present in considerable numbers, and poikilocytes may be seen. When the fragility is tested in normal children it is found that hemolysis begins in a 0.425 per cent sodium chloride solution and is complete in one of 0.325 per cent. Reticulated red cells, which normally appear in the adult's blood in the proportion of 0.5 to 2.0 per cent of the total red cells, are present in larger numbers in the new-born.

Leukocytes.—(See also p. 1020 and Fig. 249.) The leukocytes are present in relatively large numbers in the first days of life, equalling 16,000 to 20,000 or more to the c.mm., but diminishing to 12,000 or 13,000 by the age of two weeks. Little change occurs during the first year, but after this the number steadily falls, approximating 9500 at from one to six years, and 8000 at from six to fifteen years. There may be a very considerable variation within physiologic limits. The proportion among the different forms of leukocytes is very variable in infancy and childhood. At birth the polymorphonuclear neutrophiles constitute nearly 75 per cent with a predominance of younger forms, but within forty-eight hours the lymphocytes begin to increase in number. The proportion of lymphocytes and allied forms in infancy is approximately 50 to 60 per cent and that of polymorphonuclear neutrophiles 28 to 40 per cent. In adults they are 24 to 38 per cent and 62 to 70 per cent respectively. These proportions alter gradually, and by the age of 3 years they approach to, and by eight or ten years do not differ materially from, those of adult life. The number of eosinophiles is much more variable in the blood of infants and children, and may be considerably increased within normal limits even up to 6 per cent. In the first weeks of life a few myelocytes may be found and even later may occur in a large variety of pathologic conditions. A description of the different varieties of red and of white cells and their significance will be given under Diseases of the Blood. (See p. 1019.)

The following tabular arrangement shows in convenient form the hemoglobin and the approximate normal number of the formed elements of the blood and the variations with increasing age.

TABLE 25.—APPROXIMATE ELEMENTS OF NORMAL BLOOD

	Birth.	Second to third day.	Second week.	Three months to one year.	One to six years.	Puberty.
Hemoglobin, per cent of normal	150	135	110	75	80	85
Hemoglobin, Gm. per 100 cc	23	21	17	12	12.5	13
R.B.C. number per c.mm	6,000,000	5,000,000	4,500,000	4,500,000	4,500,000	5,000,000
W.B.C. number per c.mm	15,000–20,000	12,000–15,000	12,000–14,000	12,000	10,000–12,000	7,000–9,000
Polymorphonuclears, per cent	70–75	60–65	35–40	30–35	40–45	65–70
Lymphocytes, per cent	20–25	30–35	40–45	50–60	40–45	20–30
Large mononuclears and transitionals, per cent	4–8	5–10	10–12	8–12	3–5	3–5
Eosinophiles, per cent	5	5	4–6	2–3	2–3	1–2
Basophiles, per cent	0.5	0.5	0.5	0.5	0.5	0.5

Blood-platelets.—The normal number of platelets ranges from 300,000 to 450,000 to the c.mm. Even in the new-born these counts are usual, although the platelets may occasionally fall as low as 100,000.

Sanford, Gasteyer and Wyat[205] found that in normal new-born infants the high number of platelets and amounts of fibrinogen and prothrombin fall to normal adult values in a few days.

Bleeding-time.—The bleeding-time normally varies from one to three minutes, but in the new-born it may be prolonged. The method of determining the bleeding-time is described later (p. 149).

Coagulation-time.—This varies, according to the method used, from three to nine minutes, with an average of about five minutes. From the first to the fifth or even the tenth day of life the coagulation-time is normally somewhat prolonged. A delay of more than ten minutes indicates a pathologic prolongation. The method of determining the coagulation-time is described later (p. 149).

Iso-agglutinins and Iso-hemolysins.—Both iso-agglutinins and iso-hemolysins are present in the blood of even the youngest infant, thus making it advisable to type and match the blood in the selection of a donor for transfusion (Jones,[206] McQuarrie,[207] Happ and Zeiler[208]). DeBaisi,[209] however, claims that mothers may act as donors for their new-born infants without compatibility tests for agglutination and hemolysis. It would appear from the work of Smith[210] and Beradi[211] that the iso-agglutinins for the first ten days of life are the same as the mother's.

Blood-chemistry.—This has become an important factor in diagnosis, prognosis and treatment of such diseases and conditions as nephritis, diabetes, rickets, tetany, dehydration and acidosis. The accompanying table on p. 41 has been compiled from many sources and gives average figures. The blood-viscosity (Hess apparatus) is 4.5 to 5 as compared to water (Mikulowski and Chmielewska[212]). The total base (terms of cc. tenth normal) is 154 to 161; chloride 95 to 108; bicarbonate 19 to 27; undetermined acid 25 to 35 (Hamilton, Kajdi and Meeker[213]).

GENITO-URINARY SYSTEM

Organs.—The **kidneys** are distinctly lobulated and comparatively large at birth and generally extend lower than the crest of the ilium, espe-

TABLE 26.—BLOOD CONSTITUENTS*

	Infants, per cent.	Children, per cent.
Total protein (serum)	6.0–6.5	7.5–8.5
Albumin (serum)	....	4.3–6.5
Globulin (serum)	....	1.2–2.5
Fibrinogen (plasma)	....	0.3–0.6
N.P.N. (non-protein nitrogen)	20–40	20–40
Urea nitrogen	5–15	10–20
Urea	....	25–40
Ammonia nitrogen	0.1–0.2	0.1–0.2
Creatinine	0.5–2	1–2
Creatine + creatinine	....	5–8
Fats (total lipoids)	....	600–700
Cholesterol	80–125	140–170
Sugar	70–120	80–130
CO_2 content (serum) vol. per cent	45–65	45–65
CO_2 capacity (serum) vol. per cent	55–75	55–75
pH	7.3–7.5	7.3–7.5
Calcium (serum)	10–12	10–12
Calcium, diffusible	5–5.5	
Phosphorus, inorganic (serum)	4.5–5.5	4–5
Magnesium (serum)	2–3	2–3
Sulphates, inorganic (serum)	2.5–5	2.5–5
Potassium (serum)	18–22	18–22
Chlorides (as Cl) (serum)	300–365	300–365
Chlorides (as NaCl) (serum)	500–600	500–600
Lactic acid	10–20	10–20

* Figures given in mg. per 100 cc. of whole blood unless otherwise stated.

cially upon the right side. Their weight is estimated by H. Vierordt[100] at about 23 Gm. (0.81 oz.) or 0.75 per cent of the total body-weight, against 0.46 per cent in adult life. A few years after birth the kidneys assume the position occupied in later life. In the new-born section often reveals reddish-yellow streaks toward the apices of the papillae. These consist of deposits of urates in the tubules,—the uric acid infarcts described by Virchow.

The **bladder** in the infant is practically an abdominal organ, as the small pelvis is not capable of containing it. The **prepuce** has normally an extremely narrow orifice and is often more or less adherent to the glans. The cervix of the **uterus** is relatively long and the body small. The organ grows but little until puberty. It is more anteverted than in adult life. The **ovaries** lie in the abdominal cavity at birth and are relatively large (0.8 Gm. (12 grains)). (Adult 7.5 Gm. (0.25 oz.) H. Vierordt.[214]) The **testicles** are comparatively small (0.8 Gm. (12 grains)). They are generally found in the scrotum at birth. The **mammary glands** very frequently become somewhat swollen and begin to secrete a colostrum-like fluid (witch's milk) when the infant is three or four days old. This secretion is most abundant about the tenth day of life, and may continue for several weeks, but the total quantity is generally very small. This condition may be considered physiologic and occurs in about 80 per cent of infants of both sexes. It is due to the action of ovarian hormone that has traversed the placenta (Biddle[215]).

Urine. Amount.—Urine is, as a rule, present in the bladder at birth but in small quantity and little is secreted during the first 2 or 3 days. The average amount at the first passage is about 10 cc. (0.3 fl. oz.). The total daily quantity secreted in the first two days is inconstant, but is much less than later. As soon as the child begins to take fluid the secretion is much increased, and continues throughout childhood to be proportionately greater than in adult life. The amount is exceedingly variable, and the statements of different investigators differ widely. It is influenced by many causes, among them the amount of liquid ingested, the temperature of the air, and the state of the digestion or of the nervous system.

The following figures, based upon many estimations, are fairly representative approximations:

TABLE 27.—THE DAILY SECRETION OF URINE

Age.	Cc.	Fl. oz.
1st and 2d days	15–60	0.5– 2.0
3d to 10th day	100–300	3.4–10.1
10th day to 2 months	250–450	8.5–15.2
2 months to 1 year	400–500	13.5–16.9
1 to 3 years	500–600	16.9–20.3
3 to 5 years	600–700	20.3–23.7
5 to 8 years	650–1000	22.0–33.8
8 to 14 years	800–1400	27.0–47.3

Fuller details may be found in the writings of Martin and Ruge,[216] Cruse,[217] Herz,[218] Schiff,[219] Camerer,[220] Lesné and Merklen[221] and others.

Frequency of Micturition.—This varies from two or three up to six times in the first and second days of life. Quite commonly evacuation does not take place until more than twelve hours after birth, and often not until on the second or even the third day of life. After this excretion is very frequent during infancy, varying anywhere from five or six to even sometimes thirty or forty times in the twenty-four hours, the urine often being retained several hours during sleep. Engel[222] studied the frequency of micturition by an automatically registering electrical apparatus, and found it varying from ten to thirty times in twenty-four hours, with a normal average of twenty-five. After control of the bladder is obtained the frequency of urination varies from six to eight times in twenty-four hours.

Physical and Chemical Characteristics of the Urine.—The *specific gravity* during the first few days of life is relatively high (1012) (Martin and Ruge[216]) but after the ingestion of milk begins it rapidly falls to 1002–1006. When a mixed diet is commenced it gradually increases, and when the child is five or six years old it is about the same as in the adult. The specific gravity of the urine when the subject is recumbent is lower than when he has been standing or walking (Faerber and Demetriades[223]).

In *appearance* the secretion is at first highly colored and slightly turbid, owing to the concentration and to the presence of urates and mucus. Later, even during childhood, it is generally of a paler yellow than in adult life. Sometimes in infancy, particularly in the new-born, it stains the diaper a faintly reddish color through the decomposition of urates. The *reaction*, with the first passage decidedly acid, usually soon becomes neutral or alkaline; that of the morning urine being less acid than that of the afternoon. *Odor* is almost absent in infancy and even in childhood, unless the urine is high-colored. The ammoniacal odor often noted in the nursery usually is due to lack of care in changing the diapers, the urine decomposing after it has been passed. This is especially true if indigestion is present. (See p. 812.)

As regards the *chemical constituents* there is very little or no urea in the urine at birth. The proportion is much increased by the third day, but is still relatively low during infancy. Phosphates, chlorides and sulphates are also present in relatively small amounts. The proportions of all of these are increased when a mixed diet is commenced, but are still less than in adults. The amount of urea, however, as compared with the body-weight is greater in childhood than in adult life. Of the urinary nitrogen approximately 80 per cent is excreted as urea; 10 to 15 per cent as ammonium and the rest as uric acid, creatine and creatinine. The percentage of uric acid is especially large in the new-born, and, though diminishing after this, still remains throughout childhood in excess of that of adult life. The relation of uric acid to urea is 1:14 in the new-born and but about 1:70 in the adult. Creatine and creatinine are normal constituents, about 1 to 3 mg. of creatinine per kilogram of body weight being excreted daily by the new-born; about 20 mg. at two years of age and from 30 to 40 mg. in adult life.

The urine of healthy breast-fed infants usually contains no indican, but in those fed artificially it is generally present in small quantity. Older children on mixed diet exhibit indican to the same extent as do adults.

Albumin in small amount may very often be found in the urine of healthy new-born infants during the first ten days of life. Sugar likewise may occur, according to a number of investigators, the amount depending upon the quantity of sugar ingested (Greenthal[224]). Reuss[225] found glycocol a normal constituent in the new-born, and Ostrowski[226] observed urobilinuria frequently in healthy infants. Rennin and pepsin are said by Pechstein[227] to be always discoverable in the urine of children. Small amounts of the acetone-bodies are normally present (Veeder and Johnston[228]); and phenol is constantly found (Moore[229]). *Microscopically* nothing characteristic is noticed except that the presence of hyaline casts is not unusual in the case of young infants.

LYMPHATIC GLANDS

Entirely apart from the occurrence of infectious processes in the palpable glands, or even of the existence of the lymphatic diathesis, both of which are so common in children, the lymphatic glands are relatively numerous and well-developed in early life. Even in the new-born it is often possible to discover many by palpation, and as time passes the number and size of the glands soon increase.

THYMUS GLAND

The thymus gland is essentially an organ of early life. It is loosely attached to the sternum, but firmly to the pericardium. Its size is subject to great variation. According to Friedleben,[230] whose figures have been much quoted, the length from birth to the ninth month averages approximately 6.9 cm. (2.71 in.); from nine months to puberty 8.4 cm. (3.30 in.); and in adult life from 10 to 13 cm. (3.94 to 5.12 in.), the glandular tissue being then largely replaced by fat. It fills up much of the space in the lower anterior portion of the neck and behind the upper part of the sternum. Many studies have been made upon the weight of the thymus gland at different ages and with very varying results. The statistics of Friedleben are supported to a large extent by the extensive investigations of Hammar,[231] and the table on p. 44 gives the approximate figures based chiefly upon these two studies.

The results of other careful investigations have furnished decidedly lower figures than those given. Among these studies may be mentioned those of Bovaird and Nicoll,[232] Dudgeon,[233] Sokolow,[234] Vierordt[235] and Boyd.[236]

The general view appears to be that the thymus gland diminishes in size and weight as childhood passes. Hammar[231] opposes the older views and claims that the gland, though of lesser size after puberty, is not a transitory

TABLE 28.—WEIGHT OF THYMUS

Age.	Gm.	Oz.
Birth	14	0.5
6 months	20	0.7
5 years	22	0.8
10 years	26	0.9
15 years	35	1.2
25 years	3	0.1

organ but functions throughout life. Yamanoi[237] found more or less persistence of it in close to 26 per cent of 363 adult cadavers. It suffers a temporary loss of weight in the new-born, probably concomitant with the normal loss of body-weight, and in poorly nourished subjects the weight is diminished.

SUPRARENAL BODIES

The suprarenal bodies are relatively very large in infancy, weighing about as much as in adult life.

SPLEEN

The spleen weighs approximately 10 Gm. (0.35 oz.) at birth (Vierordt[238]). Its relative weight is slightly greater at this period than in adult life. (Adult 163 Gm. (5.75 oz.) Vierordt.) It can frequently be felt at or below the costal margin in early life, and in late childhood may still be palpable in some apparently normal children.

THYROID GLAND

The thyroid gland is comparatively large in infancy, weighing, according to the statistics of Vierordt,[239] 4.85 to 9.75 Gm. (0.17 to 0.34 oz.). This makes its size as compared with the body-weight 3 times as great as in adult life. The isthmus is small in children, but can be discovered by palpation if the subcutaneous fatty tissue of the neck is not too abundant at the point where the isthmus crosses the trachea below the cricoid cartilage. The lateral lobes, however, cannot be felt, and even a somewhat enlarged gland may be impossible of recognition during life.

TEMPERATURE

The temperature of the body at birth, taken in the rectum, is in the neighborhood of 37.8 C. (100.4 F.). It falls in an hour or two to about 36 C. (96.8 F.) but by the end of the first day of life rises to around 37.6 C. (99.7 F.). Throughout infancy a daily rise in temperature begins at 2 or 3 A. M., which gradually reaches its maximum in the early afternoon, to be followed by a fall which commences toward evening and continues until after midnight. The very extensive investigations of Jundell[240] upon over 3000 records showed that the daily fluctuation in the 2d half of the first week in perfectly healthy infants does not amount to more than 0.1 C. (0.18 F.), by one month averages about 0.25 C. (0.45 F.), and by six months equals 0.5 C. (0.9 F.). In early childhood the daily change equals nearly 1 C. (1.8 F.), which is somewhat greater than in adult life. The average temperature of childhood is rather higher than in adults, and elevations or depressions are more readily produced by slighter causes, such as exposure to external heat and cold. After the ingestion of nourishment infants show a brief fall of temperature, followed soon by a slight temporary rise above that existing before feeding (Demme[241]). The temperature during sleep is a little lower than when the infant is awake, and somewhat higher after exercise or crying. The axillary temperature in normal children is from 0.3 to 0.9 C. (0.54 to 1.6 F.) less than the rectal, and in sick children from 0.5 to 1.1 C. (0.9 to 2 F.). The rectal temperature is, of course, to be considered the representative one.

The cutaneous temperature may be taken by means of a thermocouple. In a monographic presentation of this condition in children Talbot[242] found the temperature of the skin of the trunk to be highest, next the face, and the extremities lowest. Usually the range was from 29.8 C. (84 F.) to 35.5 C. (95.9 F.), but there were great variations depending chiefly on external temperature and exercise.

NERVOUS SYSTEM

Brain.—The brain of the new-born is relatively very heavy, equalling about 380 Gm. (13.4 oz.) viz. 12 to 13 per cent of the body-weight, while in adults it is only around 2 per cent. Growth is rapid, especially in the first year, the weight increasing nearly 2½ times. After about the fifth year, however, the rate of increase in weight is very slow.

The following table, after Vierordt, shows the weight at different ages:

TABLE 29.—WEIGHT OF THE BRAIN AT DIFFERENT AGES

Age.	Male.		Female.	
	Gm.	Oz.	Gm.	Oz.
Birth	381	13.4	384	13.5
6 months	632	22.3	575	20.3
1 year	945	33.3	872	30.8
2 years	1025	36.2	961	34.0
5 years	1263	44.6	1221	43.1
10 years	1408	49.7	1284	45.3
25 years	1431	50.5	1224	43.2

The cerebellum is relatively smaller than the cerebrum as compared with adult life. The brain-substance is very soft at birth, and the grey matter is not sharply differentiated from the white. Although the convolutions are less evident than in adult life, they all become visible by the age of five weeks. The dura mater is adherent during the first and often also the second year. There is a greater amount of fluid in the subdural space than later in life.

Spinal Cord.—The spinal cord at birth is comparatively heavy, weighing 5.5 Gm. (0.19 oz.) or 0.18 per cent of the body-weight (Vierordt) against 0.06 per cent in adults. At birth it extends downward sometimes to the third lumbar vertebra, but in other cases only to the first, as in adults.

DEVELOPMENT OF MUSCULAR AND NERVOUS FUNCTIONS

For the first few weeks of life the infant lies very still wherever placed, unable to change its position, and sleeping most of the twenty-four hours. The action of the flexor muscles preponderates to some extent, and the hands are usually clinched much of the time, the head sunken forward, the back convex, and the forearms, thighs and legs flexed and drawn to the body. The head cannot be held erect, the alterations in the expression of the face are meaningless, and the apparent smile sometimes seen is not expressive of comfort. Any movements which occur are automatic or reflex. Sucking at the nipple, for instance, and the grasping by the hand of an object placed in it are done purely unconsciously. This automatic grasp of the new-born is so powerful that the child can sometimes be raised entirely from the bed before it relaxes. Soon a very distinct increase in general power takes place. The motions of the limbs become very active, but uncontrolled and still purposeless. In the second month the head can be held upright to some extent, and by the third or fourth month very well. By three months, or sometimes a little sooner, purposeful efforts at grasping objects begin, but without any idea whatever of distance being shown. By six months, although the motions are still largely impulsive, the child can make many well-directed movements and can grasp for and play with its toys. At this age it can sit supported very well, and unsupported to some extent, although frequently falling backward until nine or ten months old. The time when the infant is able to roll over varies greatly. A few can accomplish this by three months, but the majority not until much later.

At about six months the infant will often try to stand if held on its feet in the lap. At seven or eight months it makes attempts at creeping or at moving along the floor or bed in some other manner. Some children, however, never creep. When a year old, or sometimes even when nine or ten months, it will stand, holding to objects. Walking while supporting itself by the wall or by furniture begins soon after one year, the time for this, as for standing, varying greatly, and the power to walk without support is gained in a few months more. Falls are, of course, very frequent, and these are nearly always backward, bringing the child into a sitting position. This is due to the comparative weakness of the extensor muscles. The toes are always turned in when walking, and this condition is overcome only very gradually.

The time for the acquisition of muscular and nervous control of the passage of urine depends largely upon training. With special care it may sometimes be gained even by three or four months, at least during the day. Usually, however the control by day is not acquired until sometime in the second year. The age of two years is an extreme limit for children with whom any effort at instruction has been made. The same statements apply to the control of the fecal evacuations.

Reflex Action.—This is, for the most part, well-developed in the new-born, but subject to great variation. Many of its forms are entirely uncontrolled by the inhibitory influence which develops later; as, for instance, reflex evacuation of the bowels and the bladder. Some of the reflex movements which persist throughout life, as the plantar, Achilles, and patellar reflexes, are, on the whole, not so uniformly well-shown in the first and second years as later. Others, such as the cremasteric, corneal and pupillary reflexes, are claimed to be fully developed from birth. The abdominal reflex is present only irregularly, but becomes regularly positive by the second year. The lip-reflex is present in the new-born and gradually disappears with increasing age and Chvostek's facialis phenomenon is constantly present in the first month of life (Stevenson, Mitchell and Koch[243]). The investigations of Engstler[244] and of Leri[245] showed that the plantar reflex in the new-born is characterized by *dorsal* flexion of the toes (Babinski reflex). Gradually this condition changes, but it is not until the second year that plantar flexion is the rule. The existence of a typical Babinski phenomenon (isolated, slow, hyperextension of the big toe) is not universally accepted as present in infancy. Wolff[246] for example, claims that it occurs but rarely in the first six months of life, and that the reflex usually obtained is a dorsal extension of all the toes with or without fanning (see also p. 857). A reaction stated to be present during the first four to six months has been described by Moro[247] as an "embrace reflex." If the infant is placed on a table and this then forcibly struck on either side of him, his arms will be suddenly thrown out in the attitude of embrace, form an arc, and then approach each other with a slight trembling of the hands. Barkman's reflex[248] consisting of a contraction of the rectus muscle on the same side, following a stimulation of the skin just below one of the nipples, was found by Tsuji[249] in all of 103 children from two months to fifteen years of age.

DEVELOPMENT OF SPECIAL SENSES AND MENTAL POWERS

Sight.—In the first weeks the child probably cannot see, except to distinguish light from darkness, and will not wink when the finger is brought near the eye. The perception of light is decided and sometimes evidently unpleasant, since the infant closes its lids whenever the light is too bright. The eyes are expressionless and move slowly, and more or less of lack of coördination persists until the age of three months. The pupils react promptly to light at once after birth. Between the ages of three and six weeks the baby can fix its eyes upon objects, but even by the sixth day it may turn its face to the light. By seven weeks the reflex closing of the lids is well developed on the approach of an object close to the eyes. Colors probably cannot be distinguished until the age of a year and the ability increases very slowly with many children. Yellow, white, and red appear to be recognized before green and blue. In later childhood vision is unusually strong, and light can be endured better than in adult life. Hyperopia seems to be the normal condition in the new-born.

Hearing.—This is absent on the day of birth, due probably in part to the filling of the tympanic cavity by mucus and swollen mucous membrane, in part to the approximation of the walls of the meatus. In a few days, however, air enters the cavity and infants can then be awakened by loud noises. In the early months hearing is very acute and sleeping children are easily awakened by noise, and are especially sensitive to high and shrill tones. Infants of three months can generally determine the direction from which sound comes and may turn the head toward it.

Musical tones are sometimes recognized between the ages of one and two years, and a child of two years may distinctly prefer one tune to another and may possibly even know it by name. Very often, however, the ability to recognize tunes does not come until later in childhood, and sometimes never.

In later childhood the hearing is particularly acute, and very weak or very high tones are detected which an adult cannot hear at all.

Smell.—The sense of smell probably exists in the new-born, but is certainly weak, although infants born blind are said to be able to recognize milk by the odor. Except for the ability to differentiate pleasant from distinctly unpleasant odors, the sense of smell develops, on the whole, slowly, and is not fully acquired until later childhood.

Taste.—This is present at birth and the new-born can distinguish between agreeable and disagreeable substances, such as sweet and bitter. Although the sense of taste during infancy does not always appear very keen, many infants taking without objection medicine which is generally considered decidedly unpleasant, this probably depends on the fact that the taste for sweet is so remarkably developed that the infant often willingly takes anything to which sugar has been added in considerable quantity.

Touch.—This sense exists at birth, and the touching of the eyelashes, the lips or the hands promptly causes reflex movements. It is, however, much less strongly developed than later. In older children the tactile sensibility is very acute. That to *pain* is quite distinct in young infants, but comparatively weak if the area affected is small. Thus the pricking of the skin during a blood-examination or during vaccination frequently produces no crying.

The *temperature-sense* in general is probably present in the new-born, as is shown by the comfort a warm bath gives, and the crying produced by chilling of the surface. In the mouth the temperature-sense is active from birth, as evidenced by the refusal of many infants to take cold milk, while warm is readily accepted.

Mental Powers.—The infant at birth is largely in a vegetative state, and its mental powers are dormant. On the whole its sensations are probably pleasurable, or at least not disagreeable, and those which are unpleasant are evidenced by a cry. Hunger, pain, cold, lack of sleep and the like are expressed in this manner without the infant being actually conscious that anything ails it. In the second month it expresses pleasure by smiling, as when tickled; but smiles before this age are merely reflex, and often indicative of pain. It is not until five or six months that the average baby really laughs. In the third month there is distinct evidence of mind and thought. The first signs of memory are now witnessed, the child clearly recognizing its mother by smiling at her approach, or by ceasing to cry from hunger when preparations for nursing are witnessed. In the third or fourth month certain sounds especially awaken its attention and it is interested in bright and especially in moving objects. It also shows its mental activity by grasping after objects and by attempting, if it reaches them, to put them into its mouth. Before the age of six months the infant indicates by smiling its recognition of other known persons than the mother, and realizes the difference between strange and familiar places. When nine months old it will stretch out both hands intelligently, or will give its hand when told to do so, and enjoys a game of "peep-bo." It clearly understands many things even before it is able to speak any words itself. By the completion of the first year it has learned distinctly to indicate by expression of face and by gestures its likes and dislikes for the persons and acts of others.

In the second year the baby has some idea of numbers. Sensations of joy, anger, fear and the like are well-shown, but usually none of these makes more than a most transient impression. In fact, memory in infancy and early childhood is but weak. Later in childhood, however, it is at its highest point.

Speech.—All early sounds made by the child are impulsive. In the second month the child often begins to use certain tones of voice, frequently of a "cooing" character, to express comfort, but these are still automatic in nature. About the age of three or four months the infant commences to utter a few different vowel-sounds preceded by certain consonants, especially m and b; then d, p, n and j. These sounds are still not in any way imitative or even selected; but by the age of eight or ten months several such syllables are pronounced with some evidence of intent, and by the end of the first year "ma-ma," "pa-pa" or some similar words may be spoken intelligently. At eighteen months the infant can express by gestures and a few words many of its desires, and by two years it employs very short incomplete sentences of two or three words, using nouns and verbs. Qualifying words of speech are learned later. The time at which speech is first acquired is, however, open to great variation within entirely normal limits.

References

1. Jahrb. f. Kinderh., 1921, **96**, 32. 2. Arch. f. Gynäk. 1873, **5**, 547. 3. Nord. Med. Ark., 1875, **7**, No. 7, 8. 4. Dis. Inf. and Childh., 1911, 16. 5. Arch. f. Gynäk., 1896, **52**, 282. 6. Jahrb. f. Kinderh., 1893, **36**, 249; 1901, **53**, 381. 7. Upsala Läkaref Förh., 1882, **18**, 15. 8. Arch. Pediat., 1907, **24**, 321. 9. Med. Klin., 1907, **3**, 510. 10. Arch. f. Gynäk., 1913–14, **101**, 292. 11. Am. J. Dis. Child., 1923, **26**, 349. 12.

Arch. f. Gynäk., 1871, **2,** 52. 13. Sur l'homme et le dévelop. etc., 1836, **2,** 49. Ref. Fleischmann, Wien. Klinik., 1877, June and July. 14. Ueber regelm. Wägung der Neugenborenen., 1874. 15. Am. J. Dis. Child., 1918, **15,** 408. 16. Am. J. Dis. Child., 1919, **17,** 353. 17. Monatschr. f. Kinderh., 1910–11, **9,** 505. 18. Ztschr. f. Kinderh., 1910–11, **1,** 43. 19. Jahrb. f. Kinderh., 1914, **80,** 21. 20. Am. J. Obst., 1915, **71,** 526. 21. Am. J. Dis. Child., 1922, **24,** 497. 22. Pediatria, 1923, **31,** 709. 23. Carnegie Inst. of Wash., 1915, Pub. No. 233, 10; 11. 24. Boston M. and S. J., 1887, **116,** 157. 25. Wien. Klinik., 1877, June & July. 26. J.A.M.A., 1922, **78,** 1865. 27. Am. J. Obst. and Gynec., 1929, **18,** 863. 28. Jahrb. f. Kinderh., 1896, **41,** 312. 29. Inaug. Dissert. Greifswald, 1903; Ref. Arch. f. Kinderh., 1904, **39,** 207. 30. Ztschr. f. Kinderh. Orig., 1916, **14,** 149, 31. Boston M. and S. J., 1923, **189,** 349. 32. Children's Bureau U. S. Dept. Labor. Community Child Welfare, 1921, Ser. 2, Bureau Pub. No. 84. 33. 8th Ann. Rep. Mass. State Bd. Health, 1877, 275. 34. Tr. Acad. Sc. St. Louis, 1894, **6,** No. 12, 312. 35. 6th Ann. Rep. State Bd. Health Wisconsin, 1881, 28. 36. Griffith, N. Y. Med. J., 1917, **106,** 823. 37. Am. J. Dis. Child., 1919, **18,** 20. 38. Period. in Gewicht, etc., Copenhagen, 1886; Ref. Vierordt's Daten u. Tabell., 1906, 25. 39. Am. J. Physiol., 1920, **52,** 121. 40. Lehrb. d. Sänglingskr., 1921, 190; 232. 41. Lehrb. d. Kinderh., 1911, **1,** 8. 42. Am. J. Dis. Child., 1914, **8,** 321. 43. Bull. soc. de pédiat. de Paris, 1906, Feb., 53. 44. Brit. M. J., 1911, **1,** 1423. 45. Jahrb. f. Kinderh., 1895, **40,** 84. 46. Am. J. Dis. Child., 1918, **16,** 359. 47. J.A.M.A., 1927, **88,** 908. 48. Child Health Organiz., 1920. 49. Am. J. Dis. Child., 1921, **22,** 265. 50. Arch. Pediat., 1920, **37,** 468. 51. Arch. Pediat., 1929, **46,** 382. 52. Am. J. Dis. Child., 1929, **38,** 758. 53. Am. J. Dis. Child., 1929, **38,** 1223. 54. Am. J. Dis. Child., 1921, **22,** 265. 55. Am. J. Dis. Child., 1922, **23,** 406. 56. Nova Acta Acad. Caes. Leop. Carol. natur. curios., 1858, **26,** 2; 783. Ref. Vierordt. Daten u. Tabell., 1906, **30,** 31. 57. Am. J. Dis. Child., 1919, **17,** 353. 58. Arch. Pediat., 1915, **32,** 473. 59. Ref. Vierordt Daten u. Tabell., 1906, 15. 60. 6th Ann. Rep. Wisconsin State Bd. Health, 1881, 60. 61. Am. J. Dis. Child., 1929, **37,** 791; 1930, **39,** 917. 62. Die Characteristik des Kopf. nach dem Entwickelungsgesetze desselb. Berl., 1845; Ref. Henke, Gerhardt's Handb. d. Kinderkr., 1887, **1,** 250. 63. Jahrb. f. Kinderh., 1908, **68,** 316. 64. Verhandl. d. deutsche Gesellsch. f. Kinderh., 1885. 65. Ztschr. f. Kinderh., 1919, **19,** 153. 66. Am. J. Dis. Child., 1927, **33,** 356. 67. Jahrb. f. Kinderh., 1907, **66,** 286. 68. Am. J. Dis. Child., 1930, **40,** 813. 69. Anat. of the Child, 1887. 70. Ueber d. Einfluss. d. Militardienstes auf. d. Korperentwickelung, 1879, 198; Ref. Vierordt's Daten u. Tabell., 1906, 98. 71. Ztschr. f. Geburtsh. u. Gynäk., 1890, **19,** 120. 72. Tr. Acad. Sc. St. Louis, VI, No. 12, 354. 73. Kinderh. in Einzeld., 1899, **1,** 565. 74. Centralbl. f. d. med. Wissensch., 1873, **11,** 261. 75. Unters. ü. d. Verdaungsapparat d. Neugeboren, 1874. 76. Rev. d'hyg. et de méd. inf., 1909, **82,** 24. 77. J.A.M.A., 1922, **79,** 1409. 78. Am. J. Dis. Child., 1929, **29,** 70. 79. Daten u. Tabell., 1906, 112. 80. Arch. f. Anat. u. Entwickelungsgeschichte, 1886, 395. 81. Klin. d. Pädiat., 1875, **1,** 17. 82. Arch. Pediat., 1890, **7,** 963. 83. St. Petersburg Dissert., 1876. Ref. Vierordt Daten u. Tabell., 1906, 115. 84. Wien. klin. Wchnschr., 1897, **10,** 964. 85. Deutsche med. Wchnschr., 1880, **6,** 448. 86. Am. J. Dis. Child., 1920, **20,** 516. 87. Ueber Magencapacität, etc. Bibliotheca medica., 1898, 35. 88. Ztschr. f. Kinderh. Orig., 1911, **2,** 263. 89. Arch. Pediat., 1914, **31,** 784. 90. Am. J. Dis. Child., 1913, **6,** 232. 91. Am. J. Dis. Child., 1927, **34,** 429. 92. Arch. f. Kinderh., 1928, **84,** 250. 93. Jahrb. f. Kinderh., 1930, **129,** 319. 94. Am. J. Dis. Child., 1913, **6,** 264. 95. Am. J. Dis. Child., 1925, **30,** 541. 96. Am. J. Dis. Child., 1923, **26,** 475. 97. Jahrb. f. Kinderh., 1898, **48,** 220. 98. Arch. Pediat., 1910, **27,** 648. 99. Arch. Pediat., 1926, **43,** 169. 100. Arch. f. Anat. u. Entwickelungsgeschichte, 1890; Suppl. Band. 62. 101. St. Petersburg Dissert., 1900, 21; Ref. Morse and Talbot Dis. of Nutrit. and Inf. Feed., 1920, 16. 102. Jahrb. f. Kinderh., 1886, **24,** 377. 103. Daten u. Tabell., 1906, 44. 104. Daten u. Tabell., 1906, 117. 105. Deutsche med. Wchnschr., 1880, **6,** 433. 106. Am. J. Dis. Child., 1920, **19,** 370. 107. Hunterian Lectures, 1885, 10. 108. Jahrb. f. Kinderh., 1892, **33,** 439. 109. Arch. Pediat., 1923, **40,** 324. 110. Am. J. Dis. Child., 1914, **7,** 428. 111. Presse méd., 1906, **14,** 503. 112. Monatschr. f. Kinderh., 1908, **7,** 12. 113. Am. J. Dis. Child., 1913, **5,** 345. 114. J.A.M.A., 1915, **64,** 1822. 115. Am. J. Physiol., 1908, **23,** 105. 116. Arch. Int. Med., 1920, **26,** 410. 117. Arch. Int. Med., 1923, **32,** 71. 118. Am. J. Dis. Child., 1911, **2,** 252. 119. Ztschr. f. Kinderh. Orig., 1917, **15,** 318. 120. Ergebn. d. inn. Med. u. Kinderh., 1908, **1,** 514. 121. Am. J. Dis. Child., 1918, **15,** 190. 122. Berl. klin. Wchnschr., 1895, **32,** 201. 123. Ztschr. f. Kinderh., 1921, **29,** 321. 124. Arch. de. méd. d. enf., 1920, **23,** 449. 125. Arch. gén. de méd., 1905, **196,** 3201. 126. Darmbakterien des Säuglings., 1886. 127. Compt. rend. soc. de biol., 1899, **6,** 943; 13th Internat. Med. Cong., 1900; Méd. de l'enf., 208. 128. Jahrb. f. Kinderh., 1905, **61,** 687; 870. 129. Deutsche Aerzte-Ztg., 1903, **5,** 385. 130. Ztschr. f. klin. Med., 1902, **46,** 433. 131. Bull. Johns Hopkins Hosp., 1915, **26,** 27. 132. Jahrb. f. Kinderh., 1910, **72;** Ergänzungsh., 71. 133. Am. J. Dis. Child., 1922, **23,** 323. 134. Wisconsin M. J., 1913, **12,** 1. 135. South. M. J., 1923, **16,** 1. 136. Am. J. Dis. Child., 1917, **13,** 117. 137. Am. J. Dis. Child., 1917, **14,** 354. 138. Gerhardt's Handb. d. Krankh., 1877, **1,** 118. 139. Centralbl. f. Kinderh., 1906, **11,** 237. 140. Am. J. Dis. Child., 1928, **35,** 580. 141. Am. J. Dis. Child., 1924, **27,** 312. 142. Am. J. Dis. Child.,

1918, **36,** 725. 143. Deutsch. Arch. f. klin. Med., 1881, **28,** 442. 144. Am. J. Dis. Child., 1919, **17,** 241; 423. 145. Jahrb. f. Kinderh., 1900, **52,** 545. 146. Am. J. Dis. Child., 1915, **9,** 213. 147. J. Biol. Chem., 1916, **70,** 35. 148. Boston M. and S. J., 1918, **179,** 1. 149. Jahrb. f. Kinderh., 1921, **94,** 15. 150. Ztschr. f. Kinderh., 1921, **28,** 325. 151. Ztschr. f. Kinderh., 1918, **17,** 1; 1920, **27,** 57. 152. J.A.M.A., 1930, **95,** 1233. 153. Am. J. Dis. Child., 1930, **40,** 993. 154. J. Biol. Chem., 1924, **59,** 339. 155. Am. J. Dis. Child., 1921, **22,** 371. 156. Ztschr. f. Kinderh. Orig., 1914, **10,** 185. 157. Jahrb. f. Kinderh., 1915, **72,** 251. 158. Jahrb. f. Kinderh., 1922, **100,** 3. 159. Am. J. Dis. Child., 1915, **10,** 153. 160. Am. J. Dis. Child., 1912, **4,** 266. 161. Am. J. M. Sc., 1930, **179,** 305. 162. Am. J. Dis. Child., 1920, **19,** 97. 163. Am. J. Dis. Child., 1931, **42,** 749. 164. Am. J. Dis. Child., 1930, **39,** 768. 165. Arch. Pediat., 1928, **45,** 633. 166. Lehrb. d. phys. u. path. Chemie., 1894, 99. 167. München. med. Wchnschr., 1927, **74,** 1822. 168. Dis. Nutrition and Inf. Feed., 1930. 169. Carnegie Inst. Washington, 1914, Pub. No. 201; 1915, Pub. No. 233. 170. Exchange of Energy Betw. Man and Environment, 1930. 171. Am. J. Dis. Child., 1914, **8,** 1. 172. Am. J. Dis. Child., 1921, **21,** 519. 173. Am. J. Dis. Child., 1929, **38,** 299. 174. Monatschr. f. Kinderh., 1926, **32,** 22. 175. Monatschr. f. Kinderh., 1927, **36,** 381. 176. Monatschr. f. Kinderh., 1927, **36,** 385. 177. J.A.M.A., 1929, **92,** 1903. 178. Am. J. Dis. Child., 1925, **29,** 1. 179. Physiol. Rev., 1925, **5,** 477. 180. Am. J. Dis. Child., 1928, **36,** 83. 181. Ztschr. f. Biol., 1885, **21,** 377. 182. Jahrb. f. Kinderh., 1910, **72,** 121; Lehrb. d. Kinderh., 1911, **1,** 50. 183. Development and Anatomy of Nasal Accessory Sinuses in Man, 1914; Ann. Otol. Rhin. and Laryng., 1929, **27,** 940. 184. Am. J. Dis. Child., 1927, **33,** 356. 185. Am. J. Dis. Child., 1916, **12,** 579. 186. Ztschr. f. Geburtsh. u. Gynäk., 1890, **19,** 120. 187. J. Clin. Investigation, 1931, **10,** 545. 188. Ztschr. f. Kinderh., 1925, **40,** 620. 189. Daten u. Tabell., 1906, 171. 190. Gerhardt's Handb. d. Kinderkr., 1888, **1,** 107. 191. Heart, 1917, **6,** 189. 192. Am. J. Dis. Child., 1921, **21,** 247. 193. Am. J. Dis. Child., 1914, **8,** 257. 194. Am. J. Dis. Child., 1930, **40,** 1285. 195. Am. J. Dis. Child., 1924, **27,** 6. 196. Zentralbl. f. Gynäk., 1920, **44,** 1338. 197. Arch. Pediat., 1930, **47,** 165. 198. Am. J. Dis. Child., 1924, **27,** 340. 199. Am. J. Dis. Child., 1921, **21,** 96. 200. J. Physiol. 1887, **8,** 4; 1891, **12,** 299. 201. Jahrb. f. Kinderh., 1911, **73,** 85. 202. Quant. Clin. Chem., 1931. 203. J. Biol. Chem., 1918, **34,** 369. 204. Arch. Int. Med., 1916, **18,** 505. 205. Am. J. Dis. Child., 1932, **43,** 58. 206. Am. J. Dis. Child., 1921, **22,** 586; 598. 207. Bull. Johns Hopkins Hosp., 1923, **34,** 51. 208. J.A.M.A., 1924, **82,** 227. 209. J.A.M.A., 1923, **81,** 1776. 210. Am. J. Dis. Child., 1928, **36,** 54. 211. Pediatria., 1929, **36,** 250. 212. Acta pädiat., 1928, **8,** 185. 213. Am. J. Dis. Child., 1929, **38,** 314. 214. Daten u. Tabell., 1893, 29. 215. J.A.M.A., 1929, **92,** 943. 216. Ztschr. f. Geburtsh. u. Frauenkr., 1876, **1,** 279. 217. Jahrb. f. Kinderh., 1877, **11,** 393. 218. Wien med. Wchnschr., 1888, **38,** 1510. 219. Jahrb. f. Kinderh., 1893, **35,** 21. 220. Würtemb. Correspondbl., 1876, **46,** No. 11. 221. Rev. mens. des mal. de l'enf., 1901, **19,** 61. 222. Deutsche med. Wchnschr., 1914, **40,** 1960. 223. Monatschr. f. Kinderh., 1927, **35,** 346. 224. Am. J. Dis. Child., 1920, **20,** 556. 225. Ztschr. f. Kinderh. Orig., 1911–12, **3,** 12; 286. 226. Przeglad lekarski, 1912, No. 17; Ref. Monatschr. f. Kinderh. Referat., 1913, **12,** 172. 227. Ztschr. f. Kinderh. Orig., 1911, **1,** 357. 228. Am. J. Dis. Child., 1916, **11,** 291. 229. Am. J. Dis. Child., 1917, **13,** 15. 230. Die Physiol. der Thymusdrüse, 1858. 231. Ergebn. d. Anat. u. Entwickelungesch, 1909, **19,** 253. Endocrinology, 1921, **5,** 543. 232. Arch. Pediat., 1906, **23,** 641. 233. Path. Soc. Tr. London, 1904, **55,** 151. 234. Jahrb. f. Kinderh., 1923, **103,** 157. 235. Daten u. Tabell., 1906, 44. 236. Am. J. Dis. Child., 1927, **33,** 867. 237. Schweiz. med. Wchnschr., 1921, **51,** 557. 238. Daten u. Tabell., 1906, 29. 239. Daten u. Tabell., 1906, 43. 240. Jahrb. f. Kinderh., 1904, **59,** 521. 241. 14th med. Bericht. über d. Thätigheit Jennersch. Kindersp. in Bern., 1877, 7. Ref. Daten u. Tabell., 1906, 364. 242. Am. J. Dis. Child., 1931, **42,** 965. 243. Am. J. Dis. Child., 1927, **34,** 425. 244. Wien. klin. Wchnschr., 1905, **18,** 567. 245. Gaz. des malad. inf., 1903, **5,** 277. 246. Am. J. Dis. Child., 1930, **39,** 1176. 247. München. med. Wchnschr., 1918, **40,** 1147. 248. Acta med. Scandinav., 1923, **58,** 364. 249. J. Pediat., (Tokyo) 1925, 1612; Ref. Am. J. Dis. Child., 1930, **39,** 882.

CHAPTER II

HYGIENE

Prenatal Hygiene.—The health and manner of life of the prospective mother may exercise enormous influence upon the well-being of the future child. Constitutional diseases such as syphilis, and all acute or chronic maladies affecting her require treatment. The general hygiene must be overseen, and especially must the amount and nature of amusements and of exercise taken be carefully supervised. Thus the diet must be generous, well-balanced, and digestible and contain sufficient vitamins; the dress one which does not constrict; the condition of the breasts and nipples carefully attended to before the birth of the child; violent or sudden movements avoided; sufficient outdoor life obtained; the condition of the kidneys carefully watched; the nervous system maintained in a quiet state, and, in general, the hygienic instructions followed which are better detailed in works upon obstetrics.

First Care of the New-born.—In from five to ten minutes after birth, as soon as pulsation has ceased in the cord, a ligature of sterilized surgeon's silk is applied about 1½ in. (3.8 cm.) from the abdomen, and the cord then cut. (For further dressing of the cord, see p. 55.) The child is then wrapped in a soft and warmed blanket and laid in some warm and safe place for a short time until its toilet can be commenced. When ready for this the nurse seats herself on a low chair beside the baby's bath-tub, taking the child, still in its blanket, into her lap, and having the vessels of hot and cool water, the bath-thermometer, and other required articles close at hand. All draughts should be cut off by the use of a screen and by closing doors and windows, and the bathing done before an open fire or other source of heat, unless the weather is very warm. The eyes also should be protected against bright lights. The surface of the body is now rubbed with white petrolatum or olive oil to soften the vernix caseosa, particular attention being given to all the creases and folds in the skin. Next the eyes are washed with a saturated solution of boric acid in boiled water squeezed into them from absorbent cotton after separating the lids. Should the mother have had a suspicious vaginal discharge, a few drops of a 1 per cent solution of nitrate of silver should be instilled with a dropper, and these washed out later by normal salt solution; and it is, indeed, a safer plan to use this or to instill a 5 to 10 per cent solution of argyrol or other organic silver compound in every case. The interior of the nostrils is now gently cleansed, as far as possible, with absorbent cotton, and the mouth *very* gently with absorbent cotton wrapped around the nurse's finger or, better, around a slender wooden applicator, and moistened with warm sterilized water. So important is it that the mouth-washing be done gently that many pediatrists insist, with much reason, that it should not be done at all; since the slightest trauma of the mucous membrane produces an area ready to develop stomatitis. The face is washed with warm water applied with a sponge or wash-cloth, but without soap, and is then dried with a soft towel. The scalp is next soaped, washed and dried. The toilet of the head being now completed, the rest of the body is rubbed with soap and water, and the baby then placed in the tub filled with water at 100 F. (37.8 C.), kept there for a minute or two, and finally removed to the nurse's lap, where it is wrapped in a fresh flannel blanket, or in the flannel apron which it is advisable she should wear. Here it is patted thoroughly dry with soft towels, particular attention being given to all the folds and creases of the body, these parts being finally powdered slightly with an unscented talcum powder. The child is then dressed and placed in its bed. Should it seem chilled, as shown by blueness and coldness of the extremities and nose, it should have hot bottles put about it, using great caution against burning it. During the toilet it is important to keep the temperature of the bath uniform by adding hot water as required.

In the case of premature or weakly children it is best to omit general bathing entirely until the vitality has become greater, and to substitute rubbing every two or three days with warm oil or petrolatum. (See p. 214.)

Certain matters appertaining to the child's toilet must be considered more in detail:

Bathing.—Succeeding baths resemble the first, except that the preliminary oiling is omitted. In place of the tub-bath, however, only a daily sponging is given until the cord has separated, in order that the dryness of its dressing shall not be disturbed. Throughout infancy and childhood the bath is given daily, either as soon as the child wakens in the morning or before the daily nap, but never soon after eating. The duration of immersion varies from one or two to five minutes, enough water being used to cover to the neck when the baby is in a semi-reclining position. The nurse, sitting on the right side of the infant, holds it in the tub by grasping its left shoulder and arm with her left hand, thus supporting its head and back on her left forearm. In some cases the reaction after the bath is unsatisfactory. It is then better to employ sponging only.

The temperature of 100 F. (37.8 C.) of the first full bath may be diminished gradually, until, when the age of six months or a year has been attained, it is from 90 to 95 F. (32.2 to 35 C.) in winter, or 85 to 90 F. (29.4 to 32.2 C.) in hot summer weather, the reaction of the child always being the guide. In the second year the temperature may be from 85 to 90 F. (29.4 to 32.2 C.), according to the effect on the child. After the fourth year the morning bath may be from 75 to 80 F. (23.9 to 26.7 C.) given as a sponge, shower, or tub-bath, with the duration brief, the room warm, and the drying vigorous. In this way it is generally a useful tonic. The temperature of the water should always be determined by a bath thermometer; not guessed at, as is too often the case.

The *bath-tub* is commonly of painted or, better, enameled metal, oval in shape. For the sake of greater convenience to the nurse or mother it may be placed upon a low stand when the bath is given. A very convenient tub is a folding one of rubber, but it is not as easily kept clean.

The *baby's basket* is employed to contain many of the articles commonly used in the toilet. It holds soap, hair-brushes, sponges, powder, and the like, and a certain amount of clothing. A *wash-cloth* is best suited for applying soap. It should be very soft, of flannel, diaper-cloth, or cotton stockinet. All folds and hollows of the surface should be thoroughly washed, but no effort made to cleanse the auditory canal.

For the removal of the soap a *sponge* is to be preferred, as water can be more easily squeezed from it upon the body. It should be of fine texture and free from all silicious particles. The sponge and wash-cloth may be kept in the pockets of the baby's basket, but only after they have been thoroughly dried.

The *soap* employed should be unirritating and free from excess of alkali. Some of the unmedicated superfatted soaps are serviceable. Imported castile soap is an old favorite. All soap must be used cautiously, lest the skin become irritated.

Towels should be soft and absorbent. Well-washed and, preferably, old diaper-cloth constitutes one of the best materials. Later in life Turkish towelling is excellent. Young infants should be patted dry and then rubbed with the palm of the hand. Later, more vigorous drying with the towel may be employed. As the skin of the infant is extremely sensitive, dusting it with some absorbent *powder* after bathing is advisable, especially in all the folds and hollows. For this purpose talcum or starch is useful. The addition of any perfume is unnecessary and not advisable. Occasionally the application of a very small amount of petrolatum is advantageous if the skin seems too dry. Some nurses systematically employ oiling for all infants, but in our opinion powder is to be preferred.

Local Toilets.—The *eyes* of the young infant should be washed daily with boric acid solution during the first days of life. They should be carefully protected against excess of light on account of the sensitiveness to it which exists especially in the new-born and even into the second month of life and longer. Later in infancy and childhood care must still be taken that the child does not injure its eyes by light too intense, insufficient, or badly placed, and the possibility of errors of refraction existing must be borne in mind, lest serious trouble arise. The *mouth* of the young infant may be very gently washed once or twice a day, with absorbent cotton wrapped around the little finger or a wooden toothpick or applicator and moistened with sterilized water, but this should be done with the greatest caution, inasmuch as the mucous membrane of the mouth in infancy is extremely sensitive. The advisability of omitting the mouth-washing entirely has already been alluded to (p. 51).

After the first *teeth* appear, the mouth should be washed and the teeth themselves rubbed with a moistened cloth morning and evening. When most of the temporary set are cut, a small tooth-brush of softened bristles is to be preferred to the cloth. Occasionally is required the use of a carbonate of lime tooth-powder on the brush, or even of powdered pumice-stone applied with a match-stick, if stains appear on the teeth. As early as possible older children should be taught to use the toothbrush, and to draw floss-silk between the teeth after each meal. All decay, even of the first set, must be watched for, and the services of a dentist obtained at once, since not only are the carious teeth unsightly, but they cause toothache, occasion indigestion, and even interfere with the eruption of the second set in the proper position. It is especially to be remembered that the permanent anterior molars may appear and even decay, the mother meantime mistaking them for the teeth of the primary set. (See Dentition, p. 20.)

The *scalp* should be soaped daily for some months at the time of the general bath. After the age of six months, however, it is not desirable to use soap so frequently, lest the hair be made dry and brittle. In childhood soap must be used occasionally, and water daily, even with the longer hair of girls. The first brush employed should be of camel's hair. Later, when the hair grows coarser, a stiffer brush is required, in order to remove all scaliness. Combs should be used always with great care, and only for parting the hair. In infancy they are not needed. Hair should be trimmed frequently, and even in the case of girls be kept short until well into early childhood.

The *nails* of the fingers should be cut often even in young infants, and be kept clean with a soft nail-brush. The toe-nails should never have the corners rounded off, lest ingrowing follow.

In addition to the daily general bath, the region of the *anus* and *genitals* should be washed with water, without soap, after every movement of the bowels during infancy. If there is much irritation of the skin, starch-water may be substituted with advantage. Daily, too, the prepuce ought to be fully retracted and the glans cleansed carefully with soap and water. Adhesions between the prepuce and glans are very common. These are usually readily broken by "stripping," if this procedure is done early (see Adherent Prepuce, p. 844). The labia majora should be separated at the morning-bath and the vulva washed carefully, the direction of the washing being *toward* the anus in order to avoid as far as possible the forcing of feces into the vagina.

CLOTHING*

The interest in the clothing of infancy is made manifest by the fact that Publication No. 62 of the U. S. Dept. of Agriculture lists 1184 publications on the subject.

The great requisites are softness, lightness, warmth, looseness, and simplicity. With the exception of the diapers, garments made of wool or partly woolen stuff are usually recommended for use next to the skin; yet in hot summer weather wool is often very irritating, and this is true at all seasons in the case of many infants. Under these circumstances materials such as linen-mesh, silk, or cotton, are to be selected. As a result of careful studies Faber and Hadden[1] recommend knitted cotton as both more absorbent and warmer than is wool, linen or silk. The superiority of cotton is also supported by the investigations of Snelling and Brown.[2] The weight of the garments must, of course, vary with the season, but it is important even in winter not to have these of such a weight that perspiration is readily produced. Extra warmth is easily obtained by the use of sacks and the like, which can readily be slipped on or off as required. More children are dressed too warmly than the reverse. It should be borne in mind that the indoor temperature in most households and buildings in the winter is about 70 F., and that the clothing must be designed to suit this. When the child goes out-of-doors extra outer clothing should then be worn. The underclothing should cover the whole body except the head and the hands in order to prevent sudden chilling after perspiration. There should be no pressure which can be avoided. All petticoats should be suspended from the shoulders, and should be simple in construction, fastening with but a few buttons or with a narrow ribbon. Infant's clothes are procurable which can be fastened by tapes and safety pins making buttons unnecessary. The old-fashioned "pinning blanket" is to be condemned.

First Clothing for Infancy.—Considering the garments more in detail, and modified by what has just been said about material, those which may be recommended for infancy are as follows:

1. An *abdominal band*, which is of flannel, and is wrapped about the abdomen next to the skin. It holds the dressing of the cord in place. After the falling of the cord the wearing of any band by healthy infants may be omitted entirely, but it is generally advised to replace the flannel band by a knitted circular one of wool or of wool and silk, which is pinned to the diaper and supported by shoulder straps.
2. A *diaper*, which should be of cotton or linen diaper-cloth or, still better, of cotton stockinet. A small diaper-square may be placed within the outside diaper in such a position that it will receive the urine and feces. This greatly lessens the thickness and consequent heating. A rubber or other impervious cover should never be employed except temporarily in traveling. The diapers should be changed as soon as found to be wet by urine, and should never be used again until after they have been washed. If these precautions are not observed chafing is liable to result. No soda should be employed in washing them.
3. High crocheted or knitted *socks* of silk or woollen yarn.
4. A loose *shirt*, long sleeved and extending below over the band, with the opening the whole length of the front and fastened by small flat buttons, or overlapping well in front and secured by tape. This may be made of all

* Fuller details concerning the clothing, the layette, etc., may be found in the Griffith's "The Care of the Baby," published by W. B. Saunders Co., Phila.

wool, wool and cotton, wool and silk, or cotton, and should be of thickness varying with the season.

5. A sleeveless *petticoat* of white flannel throughout, or a flannel skirt attached to a loose cambric waist, fastened at the back or over the shoulders with flat buttons, and extending not more than from 6 to 10 in. (15 to 25 cm.) below the feet. The prevailing fashion makes the skirt shorter than this even in the early months, but the longer one is better from a hygienic point of view. In warm weather the flannel petticoat may be discarded.

6. A *slip* or *dress* of nainsook or lawn, loose, with long sleeves, and opening at the back like the petticoat and of the same length, or only a trifle longer.

A once popular costume known by various proprietary names is similar to that described except that the knitted, close-fitting shirt is replaced by a long loose garment very similar to, and almost as long as, the petticoat described, but with long sleeves. This shirt, the petticoat and the slip may be fitted together, one within the other, and then all three slipped on at once, thus saving considerable turning of the baby back and forth while being dressed. This style is suitable only for long clothing, as the short clothing of later infancy allows too much air to enter under the loose inner shirt.

Besides the garments mentioned the infant needs a *shawl* or a *shoulder blanket* of flannel, to be used as a protection when taken out of the room. Sometimes a thin, knitted worsted *sack* is useful if the room happens to be cooler than usual. This allows for movement of the arms. A flannelette *wrapper* is also often serviceable to put on before the child has its bath. For wear out-of-doors there is required for winter a warm long *cloak* and a warm *hood.* In hot summer weather only a cambric or silk cap is required.

At night the child should be dressed in a fresh diaper, band and shirt, and then have put on a long, roomy *nightgown* of flannel, canton flannel, or stockinet, closing with a drawing string at the bottom. In summer it may be of muslin, and need not be fastened below. No socks are required at night.

Dressing the Cord.—Before the clothes are put on for the first time the stump of the umbilical cord must be dressed. It is dried as far as possible, powdered with bismuth, boric acid, or a mixture of salicylic acid and starch and wrapped thickly in antiseptic absorbent cotton. It is then laid against the abdomen, a thin compress put over the navel, and the binder applied. The wrappings of the cord should not be changed until the cord falls, provided there is no evidence of putrefaction. The greatest care should be taken to prevent the soiling or wetting of the dressing. The ulcer remaining after the separation of the cord should be dressed with powdered boric acid applied on a pad of absorbent cotton.

Method of Dressing.—After the morning bathing and drying, the nurse, still holding the infant lying on its back in her lap, puts the band about it, or, if this is a knitted one, slips it on over the feet. The diaper is next placed under the buttocks and the ends brought around in front and fastened with a large safety pin to each other and to the tab of the band. Neither band nor diaper must ever be so tight that the hand cannot readily be slipped between it and the skin. The socks are then drawn on. The petticoat is next adjusted inside of the dress, and the two slipped on together over the feet. The baby is now laid upon its abdomen and these garments buttoned. After the child is old enough to sit alone they may conveniently be slipped on over the head. In very hot weather the baby need wear only the diaper and band.

Short Clothes.—At about the age of six months, the choice of the time depending upon the season of the year, the infant is put into *short* *clothes.* Its costume then consists of a band, diaper, shirt, petticoats and slip similar to those described, except that the skirts reach only nearly to the ankle, and that it is very customary now to make the flannel petticoat always with a muslin waist and to have a second white petticoat over this. In addition, the child requires *stockings* and *shoes.* The stockings should be white, in order to avoid any action of irritating dyes, and made of silk, woollen or partly woollen goods, or, in hot weather, of cotton. They should always be long enough to reach to the diaper, to which they may be pinned, and should be loose and with broad toes, in order to prevent undue constriction of the feet.

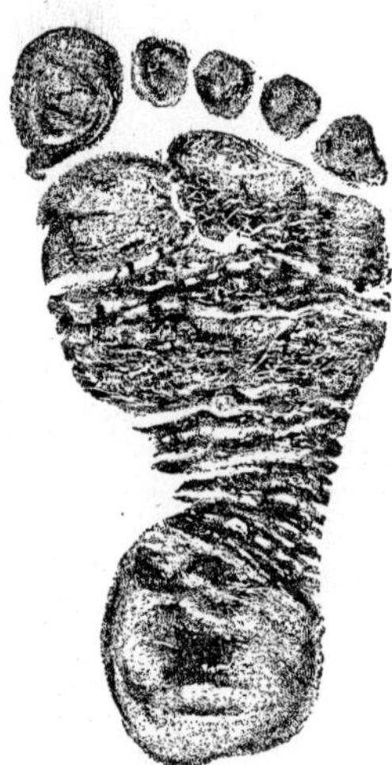

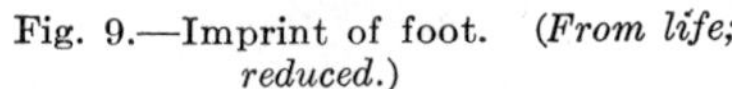

Fig. 9.—Imprint of foot. (*From life; reduced.*)

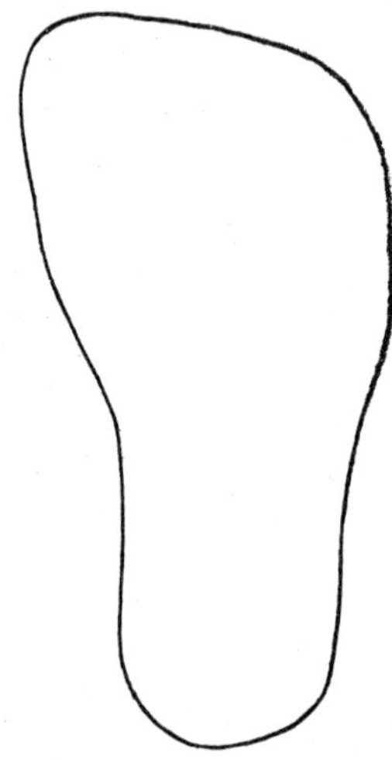

Fig. 10.—Outline of sole of shoe to cover Fig. 9.

As the child becomes more active there is often great difficulty in keeping the diaper from falling off. Careful pinning to the band will obviate this, or the infant may wear *diaper-suspenders,* or a small light waist to which both diaper and stockings can be attached, the latter by means of elastics or tapes.

The first foot-covering may be moccasins of kid, chamois-leather or felt. When the child begins to stand and creep true shoes are required. These may be of soft kid, with soles of kid or thin leather. From the beginning they should be rights and lefts, conformed to the natural shape of the foot and with broad toes and without heels (Figs. 9 and 10).

The clothes for the night are the same as in earlier infancy. For use out-of-doors the coat must be shorter after the child has learned to walk, and warm knitted or Jersey *leggings* are useful in winter.

In addition to the articles mentioned the infant now needs quilted *bibs* to catch the overflowing saliva. Later, a serviceable article is a *creeping apron.* This should be large and roomy, opening at the back but closed at the bottom, except for the apertures, fastening just below the knee, forming an exit for the leg. *Rompers* may be used in place of the apron.

Clothing of Childhood.—At two years of age, or less, when the diaper can be dispensed with, the clothes of *childhood* replace those of infancy. The binder is abandoned, if it has been worn hitherto, and the clothing should consist of the following articles:

1. An *undershirt,* long-sleeved and high-necked, of material as before and of thickness varying with the time of year, but never too heavy.

2. *Drawers*, close-fitting merino for winter, looser and of muslin for hot summer weather. These longer drawers are not now fashionable, but much safer for winter weather.

3. *Stockings*, long at all seasons. It is not desirable to dress little children in short stockings and drawers, leaving the legs bare.

4. A white *muslin skirt* without a waist.

5. A loose, high-necked, sleeveless *waist* provided with buttons, to which the stocking-supporters, drawers, and skirt can be attached. If desired, the white skirt can be made attached to a waist of its own, but this offers no advantage and adds an unnecessary layer over the trunk.

6. A *flannel skirt* with muslin waist, to be worn in winter.

7. A *dress*, which commonly indicates by its type the sex of the wearer.

8. *Shoes*, which, after walking begins, should have the sole somewhat flexible, but not too thin; and be $\frac{1}{2}$ in. longer than the foot, and $\frac{1}{4}$ in. wider at the toe than at the heel. When the child is two to three years old the posterior part of the sole should be slightly thicker—*i. e.*, with a "spring"—but should have no true heel until the age of seven or eight years.

The clothes for the night consist of a *shirt* and *night-drawers*, the latter having closed feet if the child sleeps restlessly and displaces the bed-clothes. The material may be cotton-flannel or stockinet for winter, and muslin or thin cotton for summer. Only in later childhood does the girl begin to use a night-gown and the boy a night-shirt; or pajamas may be worn by either sex. When out of doors the hood should be worn in cold winter weather until the age of two years at least. Warm coats, leather leggings, rubber overshoes and the like are to be used as requirements demand.

At about two years or earlier some distinction of sex is made in the style of the clothing, and by three or four years the boy assumes the ordinary clothes for his sex.

Sun-suits are very popular during the summer time and allow the exposure of a large area of the body to the sun's rays. The value of this is discussed in the section on Heliotherapy (p. 204). Sun-suits consist of trousers to which is attached a net waist or straps going over the shoulders.

SLEEP

Hours for Sleeping.—A healthy infant in the first few weeks of life sleeps nearly all the time; in all from nineteen to twenty-one hours, rousing only when being nursed, washed and dressed, or when hungry or uncomfortable. As it grows it requires less and less sleep, and at two months will often lie awake quietly for an hour or so at a time, and show a tendency to some regularity in the hours of sleeping. By the age of six months, sixteen to eighteen hours are required daily; by one year, fourteen to sixteen hours; at two to three years, twelve or thirteen hours; at four to five years, eleven or twelve hours; at twelve to thirteen years, nine or ten hours. Sleep during infancy is always easily disturbed by light, noise, and handling. In children it is deeper. From the beginning the healthy child should be taught to sleep at regular times, and to be put to sleep in proper ways. Walking the floor, rocking, singing to sleep, and the like, are entirely unnecessary. They establish the child in a bad habit, and make a slave of the mother. If the infant is certainly well, it should be put in its bed at the time for sleep and left alone in the room. If it wakes in the night it must not be taken from its bed unless it is time to nurse it, or the diaper requires changing. Knowing no other method it will soon content itself with this. Allowing a child to go to sleep while nursing at the breast or bottle and before it has finished should be prevented as far as possible. Before the age of three or four months the baby is made ready for bed at 5.30 to 6 P. M., and should rouse but once or twice during the night. During the day it may sleep at first all it will, but must be wakened for feeding when this is due. This is a matter of importance, as otherwise there can be no regularity in the feeding hours. After this age it may be put to bed at from 6 to 7 P. M., be wakened at 9 or 10 for feeding, as long as this is required, and be trained, as soon as possible, to sleep without further rousing until 6 or 7 A. M. It will now be awake for longer periods in the day time, and by the age of six months or earlier will content itself with a nap in the morning of from one and one-half to two hours or more, and perhaps a shorter one in the afternoon. The nap in the day should be of regular length, and the child not allowed to sleep over the time for feeding. At the age of from one to two years the afternoon nap may be omitted, unless the child seems to require it; the morning nap lasting usually one and one-half to two hours. After two years the morning nap may be shortened to one or one and one-half hours. The child should continue to take it up to the age of four years, if possible. Children of four years should go to bed at 8 P. M. or earlier, and the time be gradually changed to not later than 9 P. M. by the age of ten to twelve years.

When the infant begins to take a regular morning nap, it is best that it should be undressed for it, and be put to bed as though it were night. Often the morning dressing may conveniently be delayed until after the nap, and the morning bath then given. The hour for the morning nap will depend partly on the disposition of the child, and partly on the season of the year. A portion of the day should be selected which will not interfere with the daily outing. A certain degree of latitude is therefore to be allowed in the fixing of the time and in the necessary duration of the day-time sleep. Sometimes it is better to transfer it to the early afternoon. The two great desiderata sought for are, first, regularity, and, second, the obtaining of the long quiet sleep at night.

When asleep, the child may assume any position most comfortable to it. In the case of young infants the necessity of the position being changed from time to time must not be forgotten. (See Disorders of Sleep, p. 886.)

Place to Sleep.—The infant should not sleep in the bed with its mother. There is danger of her overlying it, to say nothing of the constant temptation to nurse the child too often. It is liable, too, to receive too little fresh air, as a result of getting its head under the bed-clothes. The first bed generally used is the *bassinet*. This is made of enamelled wicker or wood, with high sides, lined, best unprovided with curtains, and with or without a hood at one end. It should be high enough above the floor to escape the draughts. It is preferable to the crib for the early months of life, as it gives the child more support and keeps it warmer. At the age of eight or nine months and up to that of five years a *crib* is used. This should have sides which let down on hinges or slides and are high enough to prevent the child falling out, and be provided with a woven-wire mattress. A very serviceable device, especially for sleeping out-of-doors in summer, is the screened nursery crib.

The *bedding* for the bassinet and crib is the same. There should be, namely, a thin, hair-mattress, a rubber cloth, in the case of infants, to go over this, and a doubled sheet. Sometimes a quilted bed-cover may be put under the sheet to increase the warmth in winter time. The pillow should be small; a soft, thin, feather pillow with a linen pillowslip. A curled-hair pillow may be substituted in summer if desired.

The *coverings* of the child when in bed should consist of a muslin sheet, as many light blankets as needed, and a light spread. A down quilt is an advantage in winter. Owing to the restless sleep of so many children, some form of bed-clothes-fastener is desirable. A great many children are covered far too warmly at night, with the result that sleep is rendered restless, free perspiration occurs and cold is very easily taken.

It is theoretically better that the infant from the beginning sleep in a separate room from its mother, under the care of a competent nurse. Often this cannot be arranged for many reasons. After the age of a year, it certainly should have, if possible, a separate room at night. Older children are preferably placed in individual beds.

AIRING, EXERCISE, AMUSEMENTS, AND TRAINING

Airing.—With regard to airing, no absolute rule can be formulated. At two weeks of age the nurse may take the infant into another room of a somewhat cooler temperature, proper protection being given by dressing it in its out-door clothing. Before this age it should not be exposed to a temperature of less than 70 F. (21.11 C.). By one month it may be taken into the open air for ten or twenty minutes, and longer on subsequent visits, until finally it is out of doors two or three hours or more daily. This applies to the spring and autumn, if the temperature is not lower than 60 F. (15.55, C.), but in warm summer weather it may go out even at an earlier age, while in midwinter it should not do so until it is three or four months old or possibly even later. In place of this it may have its daily airing in a room, the windows of which have been open for a short time, but closed just before the child enters it. Later, when used to the outer air, the windows may be left open during its presence. When possible, autumn babies should be gotten out of doors before the winter sets in. If this cannot be managed, the use of the room with open windows may often be advantageously continued until spring. The important matter is that the infant shall become accustomed *gradually* to the cool air, and that as soon as possible it shall have an abundance of fresh out-door air.

It is a mistake to take an infant out every day no matter what the weather. Very damp, windy, or intensely cold days are to be avoided and the airing in the room with open windows employed instead. A temperature of 20 F. (6.66 C.) is an indication that the infant had better stay in the house. Always the condition of the hands and feet and the color of the face are to be watched, and the airing stopped if the infant shows the least chilliness.

Although the bed is usually a better place, there is no reason why a child may not sleep out of doors in the day-time in warm weather, or even in cold if the temperature is above freezing and the child well protected and carefully watched. Some children invariably fall asleep when taken out. In the night-time, however, the child should sleep in a room where it can be under better supervision. This does not mean that the room should not have fresh air in abundance.

The first going out should be in the nurse's arms, as this gives greater protection and warmth. After the age of three or four months, depending upon the season, a perambulator should be used. This should have a sunshade or hood which is lined with some dark color, such as green or brown, to avoid injury to the eyes by the reflected or transmitted light. The infant should recline in the coach, but after the age of seven or eight months may sit supported a portion of the time, care being taken that the back does not become fatigued.

Exercise.—After the first two weeks of life the infant begins to move its arms and legs freely. It can be assisted in this by having the clothing loose and not too long. At two weeks it should be exercised by being systematically carried about in the arms several times a day, lying on a pillow in order to give support to the spine. At the age of one month the pillow may be discarded. At three or four months the infant may be seated upright in the nurse's arm with her hand supporting its back. It should not be supported invariably on the right or the left arm or lateral curvature of the spine is liable to develop. This carrying about by the nurse is a matter of vital importance. Infants who lie too much in their cribs do not thrive as they should. At about six months of age it may be propped with pillows in a sitting position, but only for a little while at a time. From the age of three or four months on the child may be placed at times upon a thick blanket or mattress, spread upon the floor or elsewhere, securely out of draughts. Here it can make all movements of which it is capable, and has also a good chance later to creep as soon as it is able. The great likelihood of the existence of draughts upon the floor, especially in cold weather, must never be forgotten. Children who have learned to creep or walk will take all the exercise they need. The baby should take its own time to learn to walk, and no appliances to aid it in this are advisable. The legs should be carefully watched for evidence of bowing. (For the age for creeping and walking, see p. 46.) The perambulator or some form of baby-coach must still be used for most of the airing until the age of two and one-half or even three years, the child being allowed to walk when it desires, but for not too long at a time, lest fatigue ensue or the arch of the foot be overstrained.

Various different forms of exercise will be advisable as the child grows older, in order to bring into play different muscles of the body and to preserve symmetry in development. Little restraint need now be imposed unless the child is delicate, or is of the nervous and excitable nature which disposes it to exercise to the point of exhaustion. All out-door sports should be encouraged for both sexes. The tricycle and similar apparatus can be used early, and later the bicycle. Swimming, skating, riding, tennis, and the like are all excellent. Jumping rope is harmless unless overdone. In winter, especially in cities, it is often difficult to obtain sufficient exercise. Dancing and work in a gymnasium now become the best substitutes.

Training and Amusements.—Teaching the control of the bowels and bladder should be commenced early, certainly by the age of three months. If the infant is systematically supported on a receptacle at the time when the evacuation of the bowels is found most likely to occur, generally after a meal, much may be gained. The control of the bladder is more difficult to acquire, but even before the end of the first year some infants can be taught it, at least during the waking hours. Patience and perseverance are required, and punishment at any age is out of the question.

Amusements begin early, and those may gradually be added which educate the mind to a certain extent. Yet the training of the mind must always hold a secondary place, lest overstimulation of it result. In fact all amusements which cause much excitement are to be avoided, and this is especially true just before bed-time, or insomnia will be a natural result. By the age of five or six months a rattle or a rubber doll will be enjoyed. Later more toys are needed for the house, and others to be used out of doors. Mental and moral training can soon be commenced by using judgment in the selection of the amusements. Thus the constant providing of new toys teaches a child discontent, lack of valuation and lack of care of those which it possesses, as well as lack of neatness. Pernicious, too, is the constant effort of the mother to amuse the child, since it should be taught to amuse itself. Many toys may be chosen which instruct, such as picture-books, Noah's arks, picture-blocks, and, later, lettered blocks.

The inculcating of obedience, unselfishness, absence of self-consciousness, fearlessness, and general kindliness to all created things can hardly be commenced too early. There is no hurry about teaching a child to talk, but the use of "baby-talk" in addressing it is always to be avoided.

Girls and boys should play together and at the same games as long as disposed. They have a natural disposition to do this until the age of nine or ten years is reached, unless they have been taught to do differently. Yet a careful, unobserved supervision should early be kept over the play, since sexual innocence in early years is by no means so common as is often assumed.

Sex-education.—This is largely a duty of the parents, the physician instructing them and helping to solve unusual difficulties. Children will often obtain incorrect and vicious information upon such matters from unreliable and secret sources unless it is given to them truthfully and sympathetically by their elders. Furthermore the sex impulse cannot be ignored, and the problem must be met. Formal speeches and lectures have a greater value for older children than for younger ones, and would not be so necessary if the subject of sex instruction had been earlier properly taught. The natural questions which arise in connection with parts of the body and their functions must be answered simply and without embarrassment, and there should be avoided creating in the mind of the child a sense of shame or evil connected with them. As the child becomes older the relation of the sexes must be discussed frankly and the manner and means of reproduction explained. Instruction concerning reproduction in plants and lower animals leads naturally to the simple elucidation of similar matters in the human. High ideals of sexual purity must be put before the young for their own sake, and not simply be insisted upon because of fear and custom alone. The whole subject of sex must be accepted as a natural one, but not discussed too frequently. Publications such as those by de Schweinitz,[3] Dickerson[4] and Hood[5] are of value to parents in the consideration of this subject.

School-life.—Most important is it that the mental powers shall not be forced. Precocity is not desirable. The kindergarten is excellent for young children, and much instruction is gained in this way. Yet even this is sometimes too stimulating. There is nothing gained in having a child learn to read before the age of six years. Even at this period the hours spent in school are generally far too long. From three to four hours daily from the age of six or seven up to that of ten years are quite enough. Ocular defects, lateral curvature of the spine, loss of appetite, poor general health and nervous irritability are common results of improper school life.

As to the fittings of the school-room, the chairs employed should be low enough to allow the feet to rest comfortably on the floor, and should be so constructed that they support the *lower* part of the back. The desks must not be high, or the child's eyes are brought too close to its work and the spine is liable to be distorted when he writes. The light must be so disposed that there is no glare in front, and that trying cross-lights are avoided. There should be at least 300 cu. ft. (8.49 cubic meters) of air space for each individual, and, in addition, the air should be constantly and completely changed by ventilation several times an hour.

Open Air Schools.—For children who have positive tuberculin reactions and who have been exposed to tuberculosis—*i. e.*, the so-called "pretuberculous group"—open air schools have been established in some communities. They have been developed also for well children. Some are primitive and consist only of a roof with supports but no walls. Others are more carefully constructed, the open air feature being secured by numerous windows. In cold weather not every child reacts well to such an environment, and it remains to be shown conclusively that it decreases in them the incidence of respiratory infections. There should by all means be provision for heating such school rooms in severe cold weather, and great care and supervision should be exercised in regulating the routine of the school and the type of clothing worn by the children.

NURSERY

Day-nursery.—Inasmuch as the baby spends so much of its time in the nursery, the *position* of this in the house is of the greatest importance. It should be selected with reference to winter rather than summer, since the child will be out of doors so much of the time in the latter season. It ought to be, if possible, the brightest, airiest room in the house. The preferable exposure is south, or, if this is not obtainable, east rather than west on account of the morning sun. A corner-room with south and west windows is ideal. The windows should not extend to the floor, since the children readily take cold as a result of getting too close to them. Other things being equal, the nursery should be on the top floor, if this is not directly under the roof, as it is more out of the way here. It should have at least 500 cu. ft. (14.16 cubic meters), and preferably 1000 cu. ft. (28.32 cubic meters) of *air space* for every person occupying it, and in addition should be properly ventilated by a constant and abundant supply of fresh air. Window-ventilation of some form accomplishes this fairly well yet with some danger of draughts. Probably the best of all ventilation, in houses not especially built to secure it in other ways, is obtained by an open fireplace with a fire burning. Sometimes it is safer to ventilate from an adjoining room. In addition to the constant ventilation the room should be aired thoroughly with wide-open windows once or twice a day at times when it is unoccupied.

Draughts upon the floor nearly always exist in cold weather even when the windows are closed, the air being chilled by the cold panes. Double sashes will prevent this to a great degree, but in very cold weather it is better to keep the child away from the windows and even off the floor.

In the line of *heating* probably nothing equals a hot-air furnace, especially if the air comes from over hot-water pipes, as it is easily controlled and supplies fresh warmed air from without. A fireplace, or a properly constructed coal stove, is effective in the same way, but gives an uneven heat and is less manageable. Gas-stoves or oil-stoves should never be used unless provided with smoke-pipes connected with the chimney. For the rapid heating of the room before the bath electric heaters are best. Steam and hot water radiators, though serviceable heating apparatus, afford no ventilation whatever. Steam heat is liable to make the air too dry and some apparatus to avoid this may be advisable. A shallow pan of water placed on the radiator is a simple but not very effective means of accomplishing the result.

All hot registers, fireplaces and the like, and all lights, should be so guarded that a child cannot possibly burn itself. A couple of thermometers should be placed in different parts of the nursery, one of them near the floor, since it is in here that so much of the time is passed. The temperature of the room should be as uniform as possible at from 66 to 70 F. (18.9 to 21.1 C.).

The *furnishings* of the nursery may be attractive, yet simple and arranged with a view to cleanliness. The floor should be well-made, the cracks stopped, and the whole may be painted or varnished, but not with a slippery finish. Carpeting in the form of one or several rugs is required. These should not be tacked down. The walls and ceiling are best painted. If paper is used it should contain no poisonous coloring matter. Windows should have no heavy curtains. They should be fitted with bars and the doorway or top of the stairs with a swinging or sliding gate. The furniture of the nursery is better if not upholstered. Chairs with projecting rockers and furniture with sharp corners are to be avoided. Among the equipment is the "nursery-chair" on which the infant is placed when it is to empty its bladder or bowels, and only then. Portable screens are very useful. A nursery refrigerator is a great convenience.

The nursery must be kept scrupulously clean and neat. No wet diapers are to be kept hanging about, and no empty nursing bottles or empty dishes left in it. A stationary washstand may be in the room, but the trapping must be perfect to prevent the entrance of sewer-gas.

Night-nursery.—Although a room especially for the night is not an essential, yet it is a great convenience when there are several small children in the family. The requirements for the sleeping room are the same whether this separate room or the day-nursery be used, and the infant should sleep here whether at night or during its daily naps unless the latter are taken out of doors. The heating and ventilation are provided as in the day-nursery, and the room for infants ought to be thoroughly aired and then warmed again after each occasion on which it is used. There must always be some arrangement for heating the infant's food at night, such as an alcohol-stove or small gas or electric heater. The temperature of the room should be about 65 or 70 F. (18.3 or 21.1 C.) during the early weeks and later from 50 to 65 F. (10 to 18.3 C.). A window can be partly open as a rule, but it is not wise to have it widely open during very cold weather. Light ought not to burn all night. If it is necessary to have this on occasions, a small wax night-light or a candle is excellent. Nothing equals electric light, as it consumes none of the oxygen. Small shaded electric lamps can be purchased. If oil-lamps are used for lighting before the child is put to bed they must be out of harm's way where they cannot be upset. The beds must be carefully placed out of the way of draughts. The use of folding screens is an aid to this end. If the child is bathed and dressed in the night-nursery the temperature of the room should be elevated to 70 F. (21.1 C.) before the toilet begins.

Sick-room.—In the case of ordinary slight ailments no special room is required, one of the nurseries being generally employed; but in more serious illnesses, or where special quiet is demanded, the room selected should be away from sources of disturbance. Numerous bottles of medicine should not be allowed to stand about. They are unsightly, and there is danger of giving the wrong drug. Ventilation is very important, yet sometimes difficult to obtain satisfactorily and with safety in certain diseases. Sometimes it is necessary to ventilate entirely from an adjoining room where the air is kept fresh and warmed.

The special requirements of the sick-room for infectious diseases will be described in considering that subject. (See Infectious Diseases, p. 250.)

NURSES

The Nurse-maid.—Two of the greatest requisites in a nurse-maid are intelligence and docility. Consequently the nurse-maid should be preferably in middle life, but better young than old. The old nurse-maids are commonly so opinionated that their methods, generally bad ones, cannot be changed. There are, of course, exceptions to this. The maid should be neat, strong, healthy and of loving and patient disposition. No matter how faithful and efficient she may seem, no mother, even the inexperienced, dare give up her own constant supervision.

The Graduate Nurse.—The nurse trained specially for the care of infants and children during illness will be of the greatest service to the patient, the family, and the physician, if with a proper knowledge of nursing she combines a special recognition of the responsibilities and relationships which the nursing of a sick child creates. A few of the qualifications required may be passed in review:

1. The nurse should be accustomed to and have a fondness for little children, since the care of a sick child is most exacting. Without this special fondness and native fitness she should not undertake nursing of this sort.

2. She should be quick to recognize and prompt to report important symptoms. This requires careful training and inborn acuteness of observation, combined with good judgement.

3. She should be quiet, gentle, firm, resourceful, and comforting. The influence of such a nurse upon the mental state of a nervous infant and nervous mother is often most remarkable.

4. The nurse must carry out the physician's directions implicitly and without criticism before the family; yet know when emergency justifies and compels a failure to do this. Unless she has this quality her actions are too much those of an automaton.

5. She must not be imposed upon by the family. No nurse can do good work who is exhausted by unrelieved nursing of a fretful, ill infant. As families are prone to forget this, the physician should see to the matter.

6. On the other hand, the nurse should be willing and helpful, and consider less her rights and privileges than she does the comfort and recovery of the sick child. Since the installing of a nurse in the house necessarily adds to the responsibilities, expenses and cares of the manager of the household the nurse should avoid in every way possible making herself a burden.

References

1. Arch. Pediat., 1926, **43**, 283. 2. Am. J. Dis. Child., 1930, **39**, 9. 3. Growing Up, 1930. 4. So Youth May Know, 1930. 5. For Girls and the Mothers of Girls, 1914.

CHAPTER III

BREAST-FEEDING

Advantages.—The general superiority of breast-feeding can hardly be questioned. Many of the older statistics (see Mortality, p. 172) showed that the average probability of death in the first year in artificially fed infants as compared with the breast-fed was in the ratio of 4 or 5:1. In the studies of Rose[1] upon 164,000 individuals and of Hoefer and Hardy[2] upon 383 children it was claimed that deleterious effects of earlier bottle-feeding could be detected in later childhood and even in adult life. The older results must, however, be accepted with a certain reserve in the light of the improvement in recent years in the matter of artificial feeding. Faber and Sutton,[3] for instance, in a careful study showed that in their own cases artificially fed babies did better than the breast-fed after the first three or four months. This apparently would indicate that in the mothers under their observation the secretion became insufficient in quantity or quality, with the result of a falling off in the gain of weight and an increased occurrence of infections. The conclusions properly drawn were that under ideal conditions of climate, hygiene and medical care weaning could be done safely at the end of the first quarter year, and that it should be entertained if the infant ceased to show continuance of health and gain in weight.

Ability of Mothers to Nurse.—The long-continued propaganda for artificial feeding, especially with proprietary foods, had in the course of years the natural sequence that breast-feeding in many localities became comparatively uncommon, or at least continued for a very short time. We have reviewed the subject rather extensively elsewhere.[4;5] Conditions vary greatly with the locality. In Japan and Greenland breast-feeding has been the rule, and was with the Eskimos of Alaska before the present closer contact with the whites. In many cities of America and Europe only a small proportion of infants are nursed more than a few months. Much of the apparent inability is probably due to unwillingness and to a lack of teaching of the importance and benefits of breast-feeding. Experience in private practice or in clinics, such as that of Jaschke,[6] Manning,[7] Dietrich,[8] and Sedgewick,[9] where special effort had been made to increase the percentage of nursing infants, prove conclusively what can be accomplished in this respect. Nevertheless the frequency of maternal nursing is far from what could be desired; and it is undoubtedly true that the nervously organized mother of the upper classes often is unable to nurse her infant in spite of her strong desire to do so. Yet in numerous cases it is the ill-considered advice of the nurse, or still oftener of the physician, which is the cause of early weaning or of failure to nurse at all. Indeed the causes which are assigned for the failure are often of the most trivial nature. Many a woman whose breast-milk has been slowly diminishing, or has ceased entirely for a day or two, will still be able to nurse if given proper treatment and encouragement. So, too, the failure of the secretion to appear in the first few days after parturition is no reason for abandoning her efforts, inasmuch as it is not at all infrequent to have the full secretion delayed for a number of days. A scanty supply of milk is no excuse for immediate weaning, since even the small amount, helped out by artificial feeding, is better for the baby than no breast milk at all. Again, the apparent fact that the milk disagrees with the infant should be regarded with suspicion, especially in the early weeks after birth, inasmuch as it often happens that when the mother has resumed her ordinary method of life, both the quantity and the quality of the secretion will change in a satisfactory manner.

Probably one of the chief causes for the early disappearance of the secretion is the failure to obtain a satisfactory emptying of the breast. This is especially liable to occur when the infant is weakly and grows easily fatigued by sucking. Another cause often assigned for failure to nurse is painful fissuring of the nipples. This is a real problem, but generally can be solved with care and patience. In addition in the poorest classes is the very real difficulty that nursing women are often obliged to go to work. This frequently necessitates early weaning. It is a matter which can best be dealt with from a civic point of view, aid being given to mothers in these circumstances.

Preparation of the Prospective Mother.—In view of the importance of breast-feeding the preparation of the prospective mother for this is of great importance. The general hygiene has already been considered (p. 51). If the nipples are retracted nipple-protectors may be worn. Useful, too, to develop the nipples is gentle traction by the fingers, or, still better in some cases, by the application of the breast-pump several times daily. Neither procedure, however, should be practised until the last four weeks of pregnancy. The nipples may be hardened by applying twice a day equal parts of glycerine, tannic acid and water, or a saturated solution of boric acid in equal parts of alcohol and water.

Hygiene of the Nursing Mother.—The care of the nipples during the period of lactation is even more important than before the birth of the child. After nursing they should at once be washed and dried gently and then smeared with a little sweet oil or petrolatum. If they become excoriated or fissured the application of a small amount of a bismuth-ointment (equal parts of bismuth and ol. ricini) or of compound tincture of benzoin is often efficacious. If boric acid solution is used it must be thoroughly washed away with sterile (boiled) water before nursing, inasmuch as it could possibly cause poisoning of the infant. Sometimes an initial soreness will pass away entirely in a few weeks. In other cases, where the pain of nursing is intense, the use of a nipple-shield must be tried. Great care must be observed to keep this scrupulously clean. It has been suggested (Moll[10]) that fissures are largely due to faulty position of the nipple in the infant's mouth. The nipple should be vertical in the mouth from the overhanging breast. A useful dressing for pendulous breasts is described by DeBuys.[11]

During the first few days after childbirth the nursing mother should eat rather cautiously, taking small quantities of easily assimilable food frequently, lest overfeeding produce indigestion. There is no need, however, for any great restriction of diet. Toward the end of the first week she may have meat and later may, as a rule, eat plentifully of any nutritious, digestible food. In addition to this, milk, cocoa, or some other light liquid nourishment should be taken at bed-time and possibly between meals, but never if this decreases appetite for other food. The ingestion of excessive amounts of milk, such as 2 or 3 quarts a day, should be avoided, as this will usually cause indigestion in the nursing mother, or, if tolerated, will result in gain in her weight without influencing the breast-milk. Milk, in fact, is not an absolutely necessary food for the nursing mother, as well shown by Appleton.[12] Green vegetables should be given every day because of their vitamin-content and their value as roughage. The cereals used should be preferably of a cooked variety, and it is often of advantage to give them twice a day. Weak tea and coffee are permissible. The healthy mother needs no stimulants. Delicate mothers are sometimes much benefited by one of the malt liquors, but strong alcoholic drinks are inadvisable. Smoking in moderation cannot be said to be harmful.

A proper amount of exercise in the open air, taken with regularity, favors greatly the production of a nourishing milk. Walking is beneficial and golfing, tennis and swimming need not be prohibited as a rule, provided they do not result in fatigue. Late hours should be avoided and plenty of rest and sleep obtained. All causes of nervous excitement and of worry should be carefully shunned.

Rules for Nursing.—The infant should be put to the breast after it has been washed and dressed, and as soon as the mother is sufficiently rested to allow it. It lies upon its left side to nurse from the right breast, and *vice versa*, its head being supported by the arm of the mother, who rests upon her side or is propped up slightly in bed. When the mother is able to sit up she should lean slightly forward while nursing, partly supporting and steadying the breast with the fingers of one hand, in order to keep its weight from pressing against the infant's nose and interfering with its breathing. If the milk flows too freely it may be restrained by slightly compressing the base of the nipple with the finger and thumb. One breast should be sufficient for one nursing. The giving of both breasts is inadvisable, unless a scanty secretion makes it necessary. A good secretion is stimulated by a thorough emptying of the breast, and the giving of both of them is liable to leave neither empty. An infant should nurse for not more than fifteen or twenty minutes, and should not be allowed to go to sleep until it has finished its meal. At the end of the nursing the baby should be held erect or over the shoulder for a few seconds to allow it to eruct any swallowed air. It should then be kept quiet and for a time on its right side or abdomen to facilitate gastric drainage. Many infants are uniformly contented with a shorter period, because they have nursed with vigorous rapidity; others stop nursing in a few minutes because of feebleness or because the breast is empty; others from habit, or from an insufficient milk-supply, wish to nurse longer. The weighing of the infant before and after nursing will determine the amount of milk ingested. (See p. 69.)

Intervals.—During the first two days but little secretion of any kind is in the breast, the needs of the infant are slight, and it is not necessary to nurse the child oftener than from 4 to 6 times in the twenty-four hours. The employment of some substitute such as a solution of sugar or a weak condensed or dried milk preparation is generally unnecessary, but water should be given freely. If there is no milk by the third day feeding with a weak substitute-mixture must be commenced while efforts at nursing are still continued. Only in exceptional cases, as in prematurity or where the infant seems particularly hungry, is earlier feeding required. As has been pointed out elsewhere (p. 4) no real benefit is gained by feeding an infant with breast-milk of another woman from the first day of birth. From the beginning the greatest regularity should be observed in the times for nursing, keeping in mind, too, that at night both mother and child should have as much undisturbed sleep as possible. The duration of intervals between feedings has been a subject of much discussion. The fact that the healthy, breast-fed infant empties its stomach often within one hour after nursing, and practically always in not more than two or two and one-half hours (see p. 25) is an indication that an interval as long as four hours, as recommended by many, may be too great, and that the shorter intervals, which have so long been in vogue, should not be too rapidly abandoned. There can be no absolute rule applying to all infants, although there should be regular intervals for each individual. Whether the infant is fed every three hours or every four he will probably receive the same amount of food in the twenty-four hours. One advantage of the shorter interval is the possibility of earlier cessation of night feedings, since a greater number of them can be given during the day. In the case of a hearty infant taking a large amount of food at each nursing the intervals will necessarily be longer. A more delicate infant with less appetite, or one with a limited gastric capacity, will need more frequent feedings. The following statements can therefore apply only in a general way, being viewed as average figures for average babies:—After the first two days, in which the infant is fed only every four to six hours, the intervals between nursing, *i. e.*, the *beginning* of each nursing, should be of three hours duration up to 9 or 10 P. M., with 2 nursings later in the night. After one month of age only 1 late night nursing is usually required, and after three months this may be omitted unless the infant wakens for it. By five months the intervals of the day may be of three or preferably four hours duration, depending upon the case, and nursing after 10 P. M. should not be needed. The determining of the exact hours of the day for the nursings will depend in part on the time the infant regularly wakens in the morning, which is usually 6 or 7 A. M., and in part upon the hours of its regular daytime naps. The child should be awakened for its food when the appointed time comes during the daytime and at the 9 or 10 P. M. feeding. This will soon train it to waken of its own accord at the proper time. During the night it may sleep as long as it will, the hours for nursing being movable ones.

Amount of Food.—This can be determined with even less fixity than in the case of the intervals, owing to the very different demands of different infants. It also varies from time to time in the same infant, and often surprisingly so at different nursings. If an unusually large amount is ingested at one nursing the child will naturally require less at the next, or perhaps refuse it altogether. This occurrence need, therefore, be no cause for alarm in the case of a healthy infant. The important consideration is that a sufficient total quantity of breast-milk be taken in the twenty-four hours. Reference to the table upon page 73 will show what may be regarded as the average amount taken at each nursing and during the whole day. In any event the greater part of the milk is ingested in the first five minutes of nursing, as pointed out by Feer.[13] Smith and Merritt[14] found that from 40 to 60 per cent of the milk was obtained in the first two minutes and from 60 to 85 per cent in the first four minutes; while after eight minutes very few babies received any milk.

Causes Making Nursing Inadvisable or Impossible.—Many causes may render nursing impossible or harmful. (See p. 78.) Pregnancy is one of the chief of these, the milk becoming insufficient or indigestible, or disappearing entirely. The return of menstruation is often regarded by mothers as a necessary cause for weaning. This is a mistake. The milk may be entirely unchanged, or temporarily and only slightly altered. It is true that such an occurrence sometimes heralds a permanent cessation of secretion, but there is no need by weaning to anticipate this. The development of an acute brief illness may necessitate a temporary cessation, this depending altogether on the individual case. The effect upon the mother is that to be considered; and the decision should not be made hastily. If it is determined to give breast-feeding under these circumstances every precaution should be taken, such as the wearing of a mask and the like, to prevent infection being carried to the baby, or milk may be expressed or pumped and then boiled before it is administered. If diphtheria is the disease present preventive serotherapy may be employed. The occurrence of a long-continued illness, such as typhoid fever, generally prohibits nursing, as the milk is liable to be poor and the strain on the mother too great. The presence of healed tuberculosis is a contraindication, chiefly because the drain upon the mother is too severe. A woman with active tuberculosis, especially of the lungs, must not nurse, both for her own sake and on account of the danger of infecting the infant through the close contact. Sepsis, nephritis, puerperal eclampsia, diabetes, insanity, and frequently repeated epileptic seizures are contraindications. Other chronic illnesses or the existence of a delicate state of health may make nursing inadvisable, both because of the harmful effect upon the mother and because the milk is liable to be of poor quality. However important breast-feeding may be for the infant, the mother's health should be the first consideration. One must be sure, however, that nursing will almost certainly be harmful to her. It is true that the strain often does cause loss of weight and strength in an anemic or neurotic mother; but it is generally a condition which can be tolerated without any permanent harm, certainly for a time, at least, and the effort at nursing ought to be made. Syphilis existing in the mother is generally no contraindication to her nursing, since the child is usually syphilitic, even though it appears healthy and without manifestations of the disease. In a certain number of cases, however, the infant may escape being syphilitic when the mother is diseased. Within its limitations the Wassermann reaction of the infant's blood may be depended upon to settle the status, and if this is negative it is better that the infant be not nursed. On the other hand, the mother of the syphilitic infant is always already infected, and even though in a latent stage and with a negative Wassermann reaction she may nurse her infant without danger to herself. (See Syphilis, p. 427.) Mastitis prohibits nursing from the diseased breast as long as the suppuration continues. Retraction of the nipple which cannot be overcome, and fissures which will not heal, causing unbearable pain, often make the continuance of nursing impossible. Sometimes a nipple-shield will overcome the difficulty, and in any case thorough trial of nursing should be made before this is abandoned. Sheets[15] reports a case of congenital occlusion of the lacteal openings of the nipples in which puncture through the nipples allowed nursing to be established. The secretion of milk on which the infant persistently does not thrive makes weaning imperative. There exists, however, a far too great readiness on the part of physicians to advise weaning under these circumstances, without sufficiently long-continued efforts to remove the difficulty.

On the part of the infant nursing may be temporarily or permanently interfered with by severe rhinitis, cleft palate or conditions of great debility. The last is seen especially in premature infants, or those with congenital asthenia from other causes, the baby being too weak to suck properly. In this event the breast-milk must be fed from a dropper or a Breck feeder until the child becomes stronger.

Signs That Breast-feeding Is Not Satisfactory.—The breast-milk may be insufficient in quantity; the child may for various reasons fail to get enough of the contents of the breast; or the milk may be inferior in quality. Not every breast-milk is suitable for the infant even when sufficiently abundant. It is important to determine as promptly as possible whether nursing is satisfactory, as otherwise valuable time may be lost and damage done. The normal infant shows a steady gain in weight. This does not mean, however, that the gain must be regular and unbroken from day to day, for such is by no means the rule; nor does it indicate that a gain which is not quite up to the normal figures necessitates a change in diet. A baby who is receiving a supply of milk deficient in quality or quantity falls constantly behind in its weight-curve and in its appearance of well-being; is liable to become hungry too soon, to cry much of the time when or before nursing is properly over, to sleep very little, and often to have too few bowel-movements in the twenty-four hours. The matter can be determined with certainty by weighing the baby. (See p. 67.) Sometimes a weight-curve which has been entirely satisfactory perhaps for some months makes a decided deviation from the normal during one or two weeks, yet without there being any other noticeable disturbance in the condition of the child. This is very liable to mean that the maternal secretion is unsuitable. In other cases the milk clearly produces symptoms of indigestion. Actual vomiting should not occur in the normal infant, unless as a result of its being disturbed in some way. It may not infrequently be on account of indigestion having developed, either from the milk being too abundant or too rich in some respect. For the same reason the stools may be too frequent or not well digested, and the occurrence of colic is a very common evidence of indigestion. If with these symptoms the baby is still thriving normally in other respects, there can be no thought of weaning, although an effort at a modification of the secretion (p. 81), or of some of the details of the method of feeding should be made, and treatment for the indigestion given. Sometimes, if the failure to gain has been of but short duration, the giving of a purgative such as castor oil, or the temporary cessation of breast-feeding for a day or two, the milk being meantime pumped or expressed, will permit the infant to resume nursing, and a normal gain in weight may be hoped for. Again, a child may fail to gain on account of the existence of some disease other than a digestive one, and a careful study of the case must be made for some concealed ailment before concluding that the breast-milk is unsatisfactory. The special symptoms produced by an excess of the different elements of food are very unlikely to occur in the breast-fed infant, unless a very high percentage of fat is present. Idiosyncrasy to breast-milk has been described by a few authors (Sztark;[16] Kreutzer and Mendilaharzu[17]). In these cases there occurs fetid diarrhea, colic and vomiting follow breast-feeding, and there is a cessation of these symptoms when other food is substituted. Hypodermic injections of from 1 to 5 cc. (0.03 to 0.17 fl. oz.) of mother's milk repeated 2 or 3 times are said to desensitize the infant and allow the continuance of breast-feedings without digestive disturbance. (See also Allergy, p. 484.)

MIXED FEEDING

Many women, even although healthy, secrete only enough milk to nourish their infants in part. In other cases the mother's milk may be sufficient, but her health is suffering and an addition to the breast milk is required. Where only a small amount of supplementary food is needed one of the dry or evaporated milks or newer infant's foods may be given temporarily; but soon, or at once if the supply of breast-milk is very small, a milk-mixture should be supplied of a strength to accord with the digestion, the gain in weight, and the caloric needs of the infant. It is a wise procedure to make this at first somewhat weaker than the actual demands, and to increase its strength when tolerance for the new food is established. The artificial food may be a *substitute* feeding, replacing entirely certain of the nursings, or it may be given as a *supplemental* (or *complemental*) feeding in the form of a small bottle after or before each nursing. The giving of substitute feedings, without immediate nursing preceding, is extremely liable to hasten complete disappearance of the breast-milk, since frequent emptying of the breasts constitutes their best stimulation. From this point of view the supplemental feedings before or after each nursing seem to be preferred. The amount to be provided in each supplemental feeding depends upon the quantity of breast-milk taken by the infant. (See p. 73.) In the meantime, since the meager secretion of milk may be only temporary, every effort should be made to improve the mother's health, correct faults in her daily routine, and remove, as far as possible, sources of anxiety or other psychic causes which decrease the secretion of milk. Pumping or expressing the milk from the breasts may be required if the infant does not empty them satisfactorily.

When the mother's health demands the obtaining for her of increased leisure and freedom, the giving the infant 1 or 2 substitute feedings may be tried safely after the age of two or three months, provided that the total number of daily nursings remains not less than 5 in twenty-four hours. Sometimes for the sake of this increased freedom, the breast-milk, if abundant, may be pumped or expressed, kept on ice, and given to the infant from a bottle at the proper time. In the same way, for the purpose of accustoming the infant to the bottle, water, plain or sweetened, may be given. For the water itself there is no need, however, if the breast milk is abundant, inasmuch as the percentage of water in milk is large.

WEANING

Whenever possible weaning should be done gradually. At first only one bottle is given daily, using a food weaker than the needs actually demand, and gradually increasing the strength of it until one sufficiently nourishing is found to be well tolerated. In a few days another breast-feeding should be omitted and two feedings of milk-mixture given. This process is continued until the infant is entirely on artificial food. The causes which make weaning necessary have already been discussed (p. 68). In addition to these the absolute refusal of the child to take anything but the breast may require it. This is a very real and not infrequent factor in cases where the mother's milk is not entirely sufficient. It is sometimes necessary to withdraw the breast absolutely and almost starve the child for several days before it will take its artificial nourishment. This can often be avoided by teaching the breast-fed child, early in life, to suck water from a bottle, or to take one bottle-feeding a day. When, however, the emergency arises, the bottle should be offered to the child in the mother's absence, as the infant is more prone to be content with it under these circumstances.

The question arises as to when weaning should be carried out in the average case. It has already been stated (p. 64) that after three months artificial feeding can usually be successfully instituted if necessary, and even before this if imperative. When nursing is entirely satisfactory there seems no good reason for terminating it before six months or perhaps eight months of age. To nurse longer than eight months offers no advantage and may even be deleterious to the infant unless other foods are given in addition. There prevails a false notion that conception cannot occur in a nursing mother, and this accounts for certain instances of long-continued breast-feeding. Weaning should not be done in hot weather if it can be avoided.

FEEDING BY A WET-NURSE

Advantages.—The milk of a wet-nurse is beyond question generally the best substitute for mother's milk. Many infants have been saved by wet-nursing who would unquestionably have perished if artificial feeding had been continued. This is particularly true of marantic infants with serious digestive disturbances. It is a mistake often made to defer the employment of a wet-nurse until it becomes a last resort.

The Wet-nurse's Baby.—There is no objection to having the wet-nurse take her own baby with her into her new position. In fact, she is less liable to be anxious about it, and this conduces to the maintenance of her milk supply. If this is not done the employer should see to it that the infant is well cared for. There are instances when the opportunity for nursing both the foster-child and the wet-nurse's own infant may be an advantage, the latter perhaps being partly bottle-fed. On the other hand there should be maintained a very careful supervision of the wet-nurse, since, if she has milk sufficient for only one child, it is naturally her own to whom she will give the preference.

Selection of a Wet-nurse.—The wet-nurse selected should be strong, between twenty and thirty years of age, of quiet disposition, and not nervous. Other things being equal, her general health should be good, although delicate looking wet-nurses not infrequently supply excellent milk. Particularly she should be not anemic, not too fat, and free from any evidence of syphilis or tuberculosis, or of parasitic or infectious disease of the skin. The presence of a positive tuberculin-reaction is, of itself, not a contraindication to her employment. A Wassermann test should be made; but, conversely, a syphilitic foster-baby should not nurse from a healthy wet-nurse, although the expressed milk may be fed from a bottle. The nipples must be prominent enough to be grasped easily by the child and be free from fissures. The mammae should be firm and hard before nursing and should become flabby to some extent when emptied. If they do not, their size and shape before nursing probably depend on their containing more fat than glandular tissue. The best test, however, of the amount of secretion is the weighing of the infant before and after nursing, since the appearance of the breast is so often deceptive. The weighing should be done after each nursing for a day or more and repeated later if necessary.

The nurse's baby should by preference be some weeks old in order to show that the milk has been nutritious, and that a condition of equilibrium has been reached. If her child is healthy and well-nourished it is an indication that the milk will probably agree with the foster-child. There is no necessity of having the nurse's own child and her foster-child of very nearly the same age, inasmuch as there is comparatively little change in a woman's milk after the first month.

When practicable the nurse's milk may well be analyzed before she is employed, although this is not important. Should her milk not seem sufficiently abundant during the first days after she is engaged, one must not at once despair of her, for the scantiness may be remediable by hygienic treatment, or may be merely the result of nervous impressions such as excitement from assuming the new position, worry at weaning her child, and the like.

The moral character of the wet-nurse has no effect whatever upon the child; that is to say, traits of character are not transmitted with the food. It is similarly a matter of indifference whether her color is white or black. Yet her character cannot be entirely disregarded for other reasons. If she is intemperate, vicious and irresponsible, an infant cannot be safely entrusted to her charge, however normal her milk-secretion may be. A wet-nurse who is a primipara should certainly not be rejected because she is unmarried. If she has had more than one illegitimate child she is probably depraved in other respects and should not be trusted.

Hygiene of the Wet-nurse.—The rules for the diet and hygiene of the wet-nurse are those already given for the nursing mother (p. 65). Yet it is important to remember that the diet of the household is perhaps not that to which the nurse has been accustomed, and that no sudden change to a richer and more delicate diet should be made, lest some alteration in the character or quantity of the milk due to indigestion or other causes result. It is important, too, that a woman who has followed an active working life be not forced to sit about and do nothing. Such a course is sure to affect her milk. She should as far as possible do the kind of work, eat the sort of food, and in general live the life to which she has been accustomed.

Breast-milk Dairy.—It is difficult at times to procure a wet-nurse. This becomes a problem not only in institutions where large amounts of human milk could be used to advantage but in private practice as well, since the presence of a wet-nurse in the household is often not an unmitigated blessing. Among others Talbot,[18] Hoobler[19] and Chapin[20] describe their solution of this matter. Mothers come to stations where their milk is extracted under supervision and pooled, or nurses go to homes and collect this milk. Such a breast-milk dairy can be successfully operated without financial loss as the milk can be sold at from 10 to 30 cents an ounce. By this strict supervision contamination and dilution are avoided. Tampering with breast-milk can be determined by examining its content in protein and chlorides, which if too low indicates dilution with water, and if too high the addition of cow's milk (Talbot[21]). Emerson[22] has suggested drying human milk to preserve it. Others have tried freezing it and keeping for long periods of time in this manner. If there is any question as to the existence of such diseases as syphilis or tuberculosis in the women supplying the milk, it should be boiled.

HUMAN MILK

Quantity.—The quantity secreted depends largely upon the demands of the infant. Consequently there is less milk supplied in the early period of infancy than later. There is great and surprising variation in the amounts at each nursing which often cannot be correlated with the satisfaction shown by the child. Some seem to thrive on a smaller amount than do others, this depending on the strength of the milk and such other factors as the activity of the infant. The following table based on that of Feer,[23] compiled from a number of sources, represents only average figures:

TABLE 30.—SECRETION OF BREAST MILK

Age.	Average amount taken daily.		Average amount at each nursing.	
	Gm.	Fl. oz.	Gm.	Fl. oz.
First week	310	10.5	66	2.2
Second week	558	18.9	90	3.0
Third week	601	20.3	97	3.3
Fourth week	666	22.5	111	3.7
5 to 8 weeks	725–818	24.5–27.6	125–141	4.2–4.8
9 to 12 weeks	800–832	27.0–28.1	138–146	4.7–4.9
13 to 16 weeks	847–879	28.6–29.7	154–157	5.2–5.3
17 to 20 weeks	842–922	28.5–31.2	153–174	5.2–5.9

During the first few days the amount is small varying from 10 to 40 cc. (0.34 to 1.3 fl. oz.). The figures which have been given show only the amounts taken by the infant, but the breasts upon stimulation are capable of secreting large quantities. Instances are cited by Rommel,[24] Laurentius,[25] Brodsky,[26] Kollmann[27] and others in which quantities as high as 5400 cc. (5.7 quarts) were secreted in a single day, and in Brodsky's case there was a total secretion of 1193 liters (1260 qts.) in three hundred thirty-nine days.

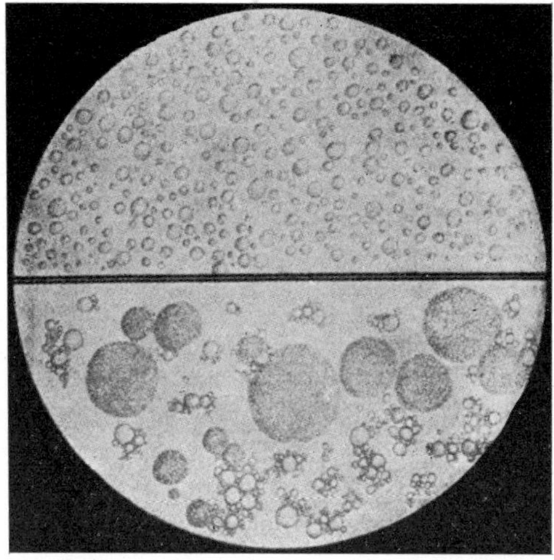

Fig. 11.—Milk and colostrum. Upper half human milk; lower colostrum. Magnified. (*Thiemich, Feer's Lehrbuch der Kinderheilkunde*, 1914, 6.)

Colostrum.—The secretion occurring during the first three or four days after the birth of the child, and to some extent before its birth, is called "colostrum." It differs from milk not only to some degree in chemical composition, but in the presence of the "colostrum corpuscles." These are cells probably of lymphoid nature as Czerny[28] believes, or derived in part from the "mast" cells (Unger[29]). They are 4 or 5 times larger than the average leukocyte, are phagocytic, contain a nucleus, are filled with fat-globules, and are at first very numerous (Fig. 11). They persist in constantly decreasing numbers until the end of the second week. A longer continuation indicates that the milk is not in a healthy state. The corpuscles reappear also when nursing is intermitted for a day or two, or when the breasts are not sufficiently emptied. Any breast-milk in which colostrum-corpuscles are present in decided numbers is liable to disagree with the infant. In addition to the corpuscles and fat-globules, mononuclear and polymorphonuclear leukocytes may be found. The fat-globules of colostrum are very unequal in size.

Most investigators agree that the colostrum of the first few days before milk begins to be secreted is richer in protein and salts and poorer in sugar and fat than the fully-developed milk. The results from analyses made by different investigators, given approximately, show a percentage range of fat 3.25 to 4; protein 1.75 to 3; lactose 5.25 to 6.5; ash 0.2 to 0.4; total solids about 12 and water about 87. The color of colostrum is deep lemon-yellow due to the presence of the corpuscles, the reaction decidedly alkaline, and the specific gravity 1.040 to 1.060. It is coagulated firmly by heat and by acids. The excess of protein and of salts is perhaps the cause of the slightly laxative action which colostrum is believed to possess. The fat of colostrum is richer in oleic acid than is that of human milk (Engel[30]); and according to Bauer[31] the protein is of the nature of a direct transudate, in contradistinction to that of fully developed milk, and is analogous to that found in blood-serum. The mineral matter differs from that of milk in that magnesium and phosphorus are in relatively greater amounts and possibly the calcium also, while the proportion of sodium is smaller.

Composition of Human Milk.—Human milk, like that of other animals, is an emulsion consisting chiefly of water, containing suspended or dissolved in it certain amounts of fat, sugar, protein and salts. It is the product of actual secretion by the breast, the epithelial cells not undergoing destruction in the process of its formation. It is not a transudate, although to a limited extent substances, such as certain drugs, may simply pass through the gland and be excreted in the milk. It begins to be secreted by about the third day after birth, or sometimes later, the characteristics of colostrum being still present to some extent during the first two weeks after childbirth. It is of a bluish-white color and has a slightly sweetish taste and an amphoteric or faintly alkaline reaction with litmus paper. Kerley, Gieschen and Myers[32] have shown that with phenolphthalein it is always faintly acid. The white color is not due solely to the existence of fat in emulsion, but probably also to the presence of casein and calcium phosphate, since it is to be seen as well in fat-free milk. The specific gravity averages about 1.030 to 1.031 with a normal range of 1028 to 1034. In contrast to cow's milk only slight coagulation is caused by acid, and none by rennet except in the presence of acid, and then not firmly. The casein is changed to paracasein under the influence of rennet. Under the microscope are found crowded oil-globules varying in size (Fig. 11). In addition to these are a limited number of leukocytes and a very large number of extremely minute particles consisting of casein.

Numerous and careful analyses of the composition of milk have been made. There is necessarily a considerable variation among individual women and those of different races and conditions of life, and even of the same woman at different times of the day. (Compare Czerny and Keller.[33]) For an approximate analysis of average human milk the following may be assumed as a working guide:

Table 31.—Average Composition of Human Milk

	Per cent.
Fat	3.5– 4.0
Sugar	6.5– 7.0
Protein	0.1– 1.5
Ash	0.2
Water	87.0–88.0
Total solids	12.0–13.0

There are also present in small amounts certain nitrogenous substances not of the protein class; citric acid; and a number of other bodies little understood.

THE DIFFERENT CONSTITUENTS OF MILK AND THEIR NORMAL VARIATIONS

Fat.—The fat in milk is in the form of many globules of size varying from 0.0033 to 0.01 mm. in diameter, and in number averaging 1,026,000 to the c.mm. (Bouchut[34]). According to Holt[35] the fat is very similar to the neutral fat of the blood-serum. The globules form an emulsion with the milk-plasma. It is disputed whether they are surrounded by a distinct albuminous membrane which prevents their coalition. Abderhalden and Voltz[36] maintain its existence but believe it is not casein but perhaps a mixture of different proteins. Chemically the fat consists principally of the oleate, myristate, palmatate and stearate of glycerole, the first being especially abundant. The others, as well as the volatile acids—butyric, capric, caproic and caprylic—are present in small amount as compared with cow's milk (Ruppel[37]); *viz.*, 2.5 per cent of the total fat in human milk; 27 per cent in cow's milk. The proportion of the total fat in the milk is capable of great variation, more than that of any other constituent. The percentages may certainly range from 2 up to 5 or even more in milk which may yet be called healthful for practical purposes. Not infrequently these limits are much exceeded, the percentage dropping occasionally to 1.5 or even less, while in one instance one of us observed it exceed 11 in milk otherwise normal. There has even been noted a decided variation in the percentages of fat dependent upon the time of day (Denis and Talbot[38]).

Sugar.—The sugar present in human milk is identical with, or closely allied to, the lactose occurring in cow's milk. Its proportion is less liable to vary than that of fat and protein, and is fairly fixed at from 6.5 to 7 per cent in healthy milk, although variations decidedly below or above these figures sometimes occur.

Protein.—The total protein-matter, as studied by later and more accurate methods, may be given as from 1 to 2 per cent within entirely normal limits, and with a decided capability of variation from these figures. A percentage of 3.5 or even more is not uncommon and is sometimes digested well. Two principal protein bodies are uniformly recognized: casein and lactalbumin. There exists in addition the protein substance frequently described by some writers as "lactoglobulin," which seems to be identical with that of the blood-serum, and still others have been reported. Wroblewski[39] described one rich in sulphur which he called "opalisin." Nuclein and lactoprotein are also reported. For practical purposes, however, only the first two need be considered. One of the principal characteristics of human milk as compared with cow's milk is the relatively large quantity of lactalbumin. The results obtained by different investigators are by no means uniform, but there is a general agreement that in human milk the percentage of lactalbumin as compared with that of casein is greater than obtains in cow's milk. (See Lehmann,[40] Konig,[41] Ciccarelli.[42]) Average figures would probably give the combined lactalbumin and lactoglobulin 39 to 44 per cent; casein 41 per cent; residual nitrogen 15 to 20 per cent (Talbot[43]). It is the lactalbumin which contains certain essential growth-promoting amino-acids not present in casein.

The casein is a nucleoalbumin which is held in suspension in the milk-plasma through the action of the calcium phosphate. It is believed that it is not entirely identical with the casein of cow's milk, being not so readily coagulated by acids, salts or rennet, and the coagulum formed being fine and loose, and dissolving readily in an excess of acid. On the other hand, it has been claimed that this depends upon the diverse percentages present in the two forms of milk and the relative difference in the amounts of lactalbumin and of salts. Whereas in cow's milk it is present as a calcium caseinate, in human milk it probably acts as a potassium caseinate. Inasmuch as the coagulation of casein is favored by soluble calcium salts and retarded by the salts of the alkalies, it may well be that the small amount of calcium and of casein and the larger amounts of sodium and potassium in human milk is the cause of the production in it of small and finely divided curds by the action of rennin (Bosworth[44]). Whatever the chemical differences, if any, may be, the work of Bordet,[45] Wassermann[46] and others, has shown from a biological standpoint that dissimilarities do exist between the caseins of different mammalian milks. The experiments have demonstrated that, whereas the blood-serum of animals sensitized to one mammalian milk will react with the protein of the milk of this species, it will not do so with that of other species.

The lactalbumin is in solution in the milk. It is allied to or identical with serum-albumin.

Nonprotein Nitrogen.—In addition to the nitrogenous bodies described as protein, there are others classified as "nonprotein nitrogen," or "residual nitrogen." They constitute approximately from 15 to 20 per cent of the total nitrogen of the milk. They consist in large part of urea, but other substances have also been described.

Mineral Matter.—The salts of milk are a somewhat complex substance. A series of analyses of Holt, Courtney and Fales[47] of milk of the middle portion of lactation gave the following results:

Table 32.—Percentages of Mineral Matter in Human Milk

Calcium oxide	0.0458
Magnesium oxide	0.0074
Phosphoric oxide	0.0345
Sodium oxide	0.0132
Potassium oxide	0.0609
Chlorine	0.0358
Total ash	0.2069

The amounts of these ingredients vary much in different milks, as well as in the fore-milk and the last milk of a single nursing. The total quantity of mineral matter in human milk is likewise subject to decided variation within normal limits, from 0.15 to 0.25 per cent being a not unusual range. Human milk as compared with that of the cow is poorer in calcium and in phosphorus but possesses a larger amount of iron. In neither milk is there sufficient iron for the infant's needs, but this is a matter of no consequence, since the iron stored in the liver supplies the deficiency for the first eight or ten months of life. The phosphorus in human milk is to a great extent in a different state from that contained in cow's milk. It exists largely in organic combination and is believed to be chiefly in the form of lecithin and nucleone, both of which are in small amount in cow's milk. It is claimed by Dorlencourt and Calugareanu-Nandris[48] that feeding large amounts of iron to women increases the secretion of their milk. About 77 per cent of the phosphorus in human milk is in organic combination, against about 27 per cent in cow's milk. Most of the mineral matter of the milk is in solution except the calcium phosphate. Burhans and Smith[49] found the salts of the milk varying somewhat in the race, the calcium and organic phosphorus being decreased in negroes and the chlorides increased. Other mineral salts may perhaps occur in milk other than those mentioned in the usual analyses. Zondek and Bandmann[50] found 3 times as much copper as in cow's milk. Changes in the proportions of the mineral constituents may be produced by the long-continued use by the mother of a defective diet (Courtney[51]). Sisson and Denis[52] state also that decided variations in certain substances, such as chlorine, are frequent in the milk of mentally unstable women.

Citric Acid.—This is present in an average amount of 0.05 per cent (Scheibe[53]).

Ferments.—The following ferments have been reported as present in human milk: Amylase, lipase, a proteolytic ferment, a glycolytic ferment, superoxidase, peroxidase, reductase, one which decomposes salol and one which coagulates fibrin. With some of these the apparent results may be due in reality to the action of bacteria present in the milk. In any event it remains to be proven that they have any great importance.

Protective and Other Bodies.—It has been claimed by Moro[54] and others that the blood-serum of breast-fed infants has a bactericidal power greater than that of the bottle-fed. It has also been thought that immunizing substances in breast-milk may be utilized by the infant. For example diphtheria antitoxin is found in the milk of immunized animals. However, there is here a species-difference, and the investigations of Kuttner and Ratner[55] make it appear probable that in the human infant the transmission of diphtheria antitoxin is chiefly through the placenta. Very likely this is true of other antibodies, agglutinins, and the like.

Vitamins.—Vitamins are present in human milk, but may be lacking if the mother's diet is deficient over a long period of time. This is especially true of vitamin B (Macy, Outhouse, Long and Graham[56]). It can be shown, too, experimentally that breast-milk is not strongly antirachitic. Adding cod liver oil to the mother's diet does little to increase the antirachitic value of her milk, but exposing her to ultra-violet irradiation is helpful in this respect. (See p. 454.)

Caloric Value.—This may be assumed to be about 20 to 22 calories to the ounce; (30 cc.); but it varies, depending upon the strength of the milk and particularly its fat-content.

Action and Function of the Different Constituents of Human Milk.—The functions of water, fat, carbohydrate, protein and minerals of milk have been described in Digestion and the Absorption and Metabolism of the food. (See pp. 24; 29.)

Bacteria in Milk.—Healthy human milk generally contains a few bacteria. These make their way in through the nipple. Consequently the first milk drawn by the child when nursing is that in which they are contained and the remaining is generally sterile. The principal germs found are the staphylococcus albus and, less commonly, aureus. For practical purposes human milk may be considered germ-free. When the mammary gland is suppurating the number of germs is necessarily much increased. This may also sometimes be true where the woman is subject to sepsis. Certain pathogenic germs, as those of tuberculosis and typhoid fever, may very exceptionally occur in the milk of women suffering from these diseases. Wang and Coonley[57] in 450 examinations of the milk of 28 tuberculous women found tubercle bacilli in no instance with 1 possible exception. Uhlenhuth and Mulzer[58] inoculating rabbits with milk from syphilitic women were able to produce in them the lesions of syphilis.

Blood in Milk.—Hemorrhage from the nipple may occur when there is fissuring of the nipple, in acute and chronic mastitis, in tumor or trauma of the breast, and as a form of vicarious menstruation. Occasionally it seems to be physiologic due to congestion following delivery. The subject is discussed by Abt.[59]

Characteristics and Effects of Poor Milk.—Owing either to the individual peculiarity of the baby, or to faults in the quality of the milk, some infants fail to digest the maternal secretion but thrive on that of a wet-nurse; or the milk which disagrees with one infant suits another perfectly. An analysis of the milk may show in what the fault in composition consists, but more important is the character of the symptoms produced. One of the faults of the milk is that of being too rich in both fat and protein; the percentage of sugar not varying materially in the milk of different women. This over-rich milk is oftenest observed in the case of women who are taking too little exercise, eating too freely, and digesting well. The infant exhibits the various symptoms of indigestion and often loses weight. Less often the fat is increased while the protein remains normal in amount. Sour vomiting and curds in the stools are then liable to result. Much more frequently, however, a poor milk is secreted containing either a low, or oftener a high, percentage of protein and a very low percentage of fat. Poor milk of this sort is frequently scanty in quantity and is seen oftenest in neurotic, debilitated, anemic, over-worked, or over-anxious women. The infants do not thrive and may be constipated and exhibit no symptoms of indigestion whatever, or may sometimes suffer (if the protein is in large amount) from intestinal indigestion with colic and loose stools, often brownish and offensive. Vomiting is not a frequent symptom. The attempts to be made to modify defective breast-milk are described elsewhere. (P. 80.)

Examination of the Breast-milk.—There are several indications that milk is being secreted in sufficient *quantity*. If the breasts fill up well and become hard and round between the nursings; if the infant nurses from but one breast and is satisfied by that, and if it does not require more than twenty minutes to complete its nursing, the probability is that the milk secreted is abundant. On the other hand, if the breast remains soft and flabby; if the child nurses much too long and seems dissatisfied, or will nurse but a few minutes and then refuse to make further efforts; if it cries much, yet seems to have no colic or other disease; and if it does not gain in weight, yet has no illness to account for this, the milk is probably insufficient in quantity or perhaps poor in quality. It should also be emphasized that human milk even when of good quality always appears less opaque and more bluish-white than cow's milk.

As a rule there is no necessity for the chemical examination of the milk, the condition of the infant and the amount taken constituting the important criteria.

The quantity taken by the infant in nursing may be ascertained by weighing the baby before and after feedings—the difference in the weight in ounces being approximately equivalent to the number of ounces of breast-milk ingested. It is, however, the total daily amount of milk taken which is of importance, not that at a single weighing. The percentage of fat may be determined by the Babcock test and the protein by the precipitation method of Bogg.[60]

Conditions Altering the Character of the Milk. (See also p. 77.) (*a*) **Period of Lactation.**—This is a factor of no special importance. Earlier studies, such as those of Schlossmann[61] showed a slight decrease in the protein and mineral matter as lactation advanced, the fat altering but little. Later investigations as by Holt, Courtney and Fales[62] and Poole[63] revealed no material alteration, even with long-continued nursing, and Birk[64] reports an instance of a wet-nurse with very little variation from normal in her milk after supplying it for nearly three years.

(*b*) **Intervals of Nursing and Time at the Breast.**—Most studies have shown that the longer the intervals between nursing the more watery does the milk become. It is apparently the fat which is increased by shortening the nursing intervals. At the end of the nursing the milk is richer in fat than at the beginning, and according to Macy, Nims, Brown and Hunscher,[65] it is also richer in protein, casein-nitrogen, total solids and phosphorus. Calcium is diminished in the last portion of the milk (Stransky[66]).

(*c*) **Number of Pregnancies and Age of Mother.**—The differences between the milk of women at different ages and between that of primiparae and multiparae are neither material nor constant, the health of the mothers being much more important than any differences discoverable by analysis.

(*d*) **Pregnancy.**—This generally diminishes the quantity of the milk and affects its quality, the amount of fat especially being reduced, and the milk sometimes approaching the character of colostrum-milk. In other cases the milk remains abundant and of good quality, and the infant could safely be kept upon the breast; but this is not the rule, and on the mother's account the child should be weaned.

(*e*) **Menstruation.**—No certain alteration of the milk follows if menstruation reappears. In some cases the percentage of fat is diminished and that of the protein and of the sugar increased, or the general health of the infant may exceptionally be acutely disturbed. In most instances the milk is entirely unaffected, or, perhaps, at most only during the first day or two of menstruation. Often the menses appear but once and do not return until lactation is normally over. The greatest caution, therefore, should be exercised lest weaning be hasty and unnecessary. If acute symptoms develop the child could be fed artificially for the first few days while menstruation lasts. (See also Causes Making Nursing Inadvisable or Impossible p. 68.)

(*f*) **Diet.**—Diet exercises some influence upon the character of the milk secreted. The total solids may be diminished by insufficient nourishment of the woman or by an excessive amount of fluid intake by her. An abundant and rich diet, if well digested, given to women previously under-fed, may increase the total solids as well as the quantity of milk. In some cases an unnecessarily great caloric intake such as milk or as other food, merely increases the woman's adipose tissue without affecting the milk. A diet deficient in vitamins may result in the production of milk also faulty in this respect. Certain vegetables with strong taste and odor may communicate these to the milk. The relation of allergy to breast-milk will be discussed elsewhere. (P. 485.)

(*g*) **Exercise.**—This, too, influences the character of the milk decidedly. Deficient exercise combined with a healthy appetite is liable to increase the percentages of protein and of fat; a proper amount of exercise to decrease an excess, if the woman has been too inactive; excessive exercise, with consequent fatigue, to increase the protein.

(*h*) **Mental and Nervous Influences.**—The effect of these is greater than perhaps from any other cause. It not infrequently happens that fright, anger, sorrow, or other great emotion will quickly so affect the milk that the infant is made ill by it, or the secretion may be permanently arrested. More prolonged nervous influences, such as worry, fatigue and the like, affect quality and quantity. What the changes are is not certainly known nor what causes them.

(*i*) **Illnesses.**—A good state of the general health is often a prerequisite to the secretion of good and abundant milk. In other cases the milk continues unaffected in spite of the mother being delicate and frail. This is often at the expense of the mother. Acute temporary ailments have but little effect upon the milk. In more severe febrile diseases the amount of milk may be much diminished and the percentage of fat decreased and that of the protein increased.

(*j*) **Drugs.**—These may be divided into those claimed to influence the secretion of milk and those which are excreted by the mammary glands with the milk. The former will be referred to again in considering the modification of breast-milk (see below). Of the latter it may be said that, contrary to the opinion among the laity, few drugs pass into the milk to any considerable extent, and the occurrence is so irregular and uncertain that efforts at medication of the child by way of the breast-milk would be unsatisfactory.

Alcohol imbibed in very large amounts may appear only in traces in the milk or, in rare instances taken in this way may produce serious illness in the infant. *Atropine, hyoscine and colchicine* pass directly into cow's milk in small amounts, and probably do so as well into human milk. *Opium* taken by the mother very rarely has any effect on the child. Yet, as cases are on record where dangerous action has occurred, it is best to administer it cautiously and in doses smaller than usual. *Iodine* given to the mother in the form of iodides or applied as iodoform in a dressing passes readily into the milk. *Bromine* does so to some extent and occasionally in a way to produce a marked bromide eruption (Knowles,[67] Van der Bogert,[68] Boone[69]). *Mercury* has practically no effect. It passes to the child only in small amount and after prolonged administration to the mother. *Nicotine* occasionally passes into the milk, but only in cases of excessive smoking. *Chloral* has, as a rule, no influence. Any effect appears only in weakly children who are nursed within an hour after the ingestion of the drug by the mother. *Arsenic, antimony, hexamethylenamine, antipyrine, caffeine,* and *phenacetin* pass into the milk to a limited extent. In the form of arsephenamine arsenic appears to have a decided effect on the child in some instances. *Quinine* has little if any influence on the infant as a rule, and only when given to the mother on an empty stomach, and when the child is still in its first half-year. *Lead* and *iron* enter the milk to some extent. *Salicylic acid* in its different combinations affects it very decidedly. The *mineral* and *vegetable acids* have no effect upon it. The *saline purgatives* occasionally pass into it to some degree, while the *vegetable purgatives,* as senna, aloes, rhubarb, and cascara, as a rule do not (Gow[70]). *Chloroform* and *ether* appear to be without influence, with rare exceptions.

Modification of Breast-milk.—An effort may be made in various ways to modify the secretion in quantity or quality and thus to avoid the abandoning of nursing.

Quantity.—A threatened drying up of the secretion may often be prevented by seeing that the breast is thoroughly emptied at each nursing. There is no better stimulant to increase secretion than this. Before abandoning breast-feeding on account of a refusal of a weakly infant to nurse, the effort should be made to empty the breast artificially and then to feed the milk. This is nearly always necessary in premature infants. Pumping can be employed but is frequently very unsatisfactory with the ordinary apparatus. Abt's[71] electric breast pump we have found very satisfactory. A water-suction pump is also successful (Moll[72]). Better than the use of the ordinary breast pump is the expression of the milk. To accomplish this the breast should be taken between the thumb above and the fingers beneath. The thumb is then pressed downward toward the fingers, and at the same time carried forward to the base of the nipple, and finally a forward pull given, which makes the milk flow from the nipple.[73] The taking of an abundant amount of liquid in some form is often an aid, with due caution that this does not merely increase the quantity while diminishing the total solids in a breast-milk already poor in quality. Milk and cocoa, however, have no advantage over other fluids, so far as quantity is concerned; and in the case of a woman already well-nourished, may merely result in making her unduly fat. Malt liquors seem to have an influence in increasing the quantity in some cases and may be used for this purpose, with caution that no addiction to alcohol is established. In all undernourished women a generous diet should be given and overwork avoided. In women of a nervous temperament the life should be as quiet as possible, all exciting influences avoided, and rest at night be undisturbed, the care of the infant at this time being delegated to the nurse, and, if it seems best, the night-feedings being of artificial food or of milk previously expressed from the breast and kept on ice. With all nursing women the routine previously recommended (p. 65) should be followed. Among other methods which are advised to increase the secretion are gentle daily massage of the breasts, faradization, and the administration of galactagogues. Regarding the last there is no certain evidence that any of these are of value. Experiments upon animals by some investigators appear to show such power in the administration of corpus luteum, placenta, whole pituitary or its posterior lobe, the suprarenal glands, or in the auto-injection of human milk, but the results claimed have not been definitely established. Any benefit obtained would appear to be from a temporary stimulation, liable to be followed by a decrease. Pilocarpine, cotton-seed, anise, and other drugs have been tried, but there is little evidence in their favor. Several authors claim that irradiation with ultra-violet light increases milk production. It may be said in this connection that the ingestion or injection of atropine may diminish the quantity of milk secreted.

Quality.—In the very few instances in which the milk in general appears too rich to be suitable, the condition can often be remedied by insisting upon a more active life with abundant exercise, and by reducing the amount of food taken. Lengthening the interval between the nursings and diminishing the total solids ingested may be of avail. The excess of *protein* so common in defective breast-milk in neurotic women can sometimes be remedied by increasing the amount of exercise up to a healthful feeling of fatigue, and by taking measures to relieve the nervous condition. If, however, the exercise goes beyond this point, the percentage of protein may be increased. An excessive percentage of *fat* can be lessened, with the protein, in the over-fed and idle women referred to by reducing the total amount of food ingested and increasing the exercise. It is also reduced by lengthening the nursing intervals. When the amount of fat is deficient usually little can be accomplished except in the starvation cases, where an abundant diet and a diminution of work may increase the fat-percentage with that of the protein and the total secretion. Alteration of the diet has little effect upon the secretion of fat in women already well-nourished and exercising sufficiently. A diet high in vitamins, especially in vitamin A, is said to increase the fat content and perhaps the vitamin content as well. The amount of *sugar* in the milk cannot be influenced with any certainty. (For discussion of measures to increase the antirachitic value of breast-milk see p. 454.)

References

1. Deutsche Monatschr. f. Zahnh., 1905, **23,** 3. Ref. Verhandl. der deutsche. Gesellsch. f. Gynäk., 1907, **12,** 829. 2. J.A.M.A., 1929, **92,** 615. 3. Am. J. Dis. Child., 1930, **40,** 1163. 4. Griffith, New York M. J., 1909, **90,** 1097. J.A.M.A., 1912, **59,** 1874. 5, Mitchell, J.A.M.A., 1916, **66,** 1690. 6. Med. Klin., 1908, **4,** 257. 7. Arch. Pediat., 1920. **37,** 214. 8. J.A.M.A., 1922, **79,** 268. 9. Am. J. Dis. Child., 1921, **21,** 455. 10. Med. Klin., 1922, **18,** 403. 11. Am. J. Dis. Child., 1927, **33,** 732. 12. Am. J. Dis. Child., 1929, **37,** 284. 13. Jahrb. f. Kinderh., 1896, **42,** 225. 14. Am. J. Dis. Child., 1922, **24,** 413. 15. J.A.M.A., 1920, **80,** 551. 16. Arch. de méd. d. enf., 1921, **24,** 555. 17. Semana méd., 1922, **2,** 242. 18. J.A.M.A., 1911, **56,** 1715. Boston M. and S. J., 1913, **169,** 760. 19. Tr. Am. Pediat. Soc., 1924, **36,** 55. 20. J.A.M.A., 1923, **81,** 200. 21. Boston M. and S. J., 1927, **196,** 653. 22. J.A.M.A., 1922, **78,** 641. 23. Jahrb. f. Kinderh., 1896, **42,** 195; 1902, **56,** 421. München. med. Wchnschr., 1905, **52,** 444. 25. Arch. f. Kinderh., 1911, **56,** 275. 26. Arch. f. Kinderh., 1914, **73,** 166. 27. Arch. f. Kinderh., 1927, **80,** 81. 28. Henoch's Festschrift, 1890, 194. 29. Virchows Arch. f. path. Anat.,

1898, **151,** 159. 30. Sommerfeld's Handb. d. Milchkunde., 1909, 810; Ref. Morse and Talbot, Dis. Nutrit. and Inf. Feed., 1915, 96. 31. Deutsche med. Wchnschr., 1909, **35,** 1657. 32. New York M. Rec., 1903, **64,** 201. 33. Des Kindes Ernährung, Ernährungstörungen und Ernährungstherapie, 1906, **1,** 416. 34. Gaz. d. hop., 1878, **51,** 66; 75. 35. Am. J. Dis. Child., 1931, **42,** 726. 36. Ztschr. f. phys. Chem., 1909, **59,** 13. 37. Ztschr. f. Biol., 1895, **31,** 1. 38. Am. J. Dis. Child., 1919, **18,** 93. 39. Ztschr. f. phys. Chem., 1898–99, **26,** 308. 40. Arch. f. d. ges. Physiol., 1894, **56,** 577. 41. Chem. d. menschl. Nahrungs-u. Genussmittel., 1903, 110. 42. Pediatria., 1908, **6,** 912. 43. Am. J. Dis. Child., 1914, **7,** 445. 44. Am. J. Dis. Child., 1921, **22,** 193. 45. Ann. Inst. Pasteur, 1899, **13,** 225. 46. Verhandl. 18; Cong. inn. Med., 1900, 501. 47. Am. J. Dis. Child., 1915, **10,** 229. 48. Nourrisson, 1929, **17,** 227. 49. Am. J. Dis. Child., 1923, **26,** 303. 50. Klin. Wchnschr., 1931, **10,** 1528. 51. Am. J. Dis. Child., 1923, **26,** 534. 52. Am. J. Dis. Child., 1921, **21,** 389. Ref. Morse and Talbot, Dis. Nutrit. and Inf. Feed., 1920, 122. 54. Jahrb. f. Kinderh., 1902, **55,** 396. 55. Am. J. Dis. Child., 1923, **25,** 413. 56. J. Biol. Chem., 1927, **73,** 189. 57. J.A.M.A., 1917, **69,** 531. 58. Deutsche med. Wchnschr., 1913, **39,** 879. 59. Arch. Pediat., 1923, **40,** 719. 60. Bull. Johns Hopkins Hosp., 1906, **17,** 342. 61. Arch. f. Kinderh., 1900, **30,** 288. 62. Am. J. Dis. Child., 1915, **10,** 233. 63. Arch. Pediat., 1930, **47,** 698. 64. Monatschr. f. Kinderh., 1923, **25,** 30. 65. Am. J. Dis. Child., 1931, **42,** 569. 66. Ztschr. f. Kinderh., 1926, **40,** 671. 67. New York M. J., 1909, **89,** 586. 68. Am. J. Dis. Child., 1921, **21,** 167. 69. Canad. M.A.J., 1922, **12,** 570. 70. Practitioner, 1893, **50,** 168. 71. J.A.M.A., 1923, **81,** 391. 72. Wien. med. Wchnschr., 1929, **79,** 1185. 73. U. S. Dept. Labor, Children's Bureau; Care of Child. Series, No. 5, Publ. 83.

CHAPTER IV

ARTIFICIAL FEEDING IN THE FIRST YEAR

The nourishment of an infant with anything other than the secretion of the human breast is properly termed "artificial feeding" or "substitute feeding." A food cannot be constructed which is exactly similar to human milk nor one that can be looked upon as a standard. Fortunately the digestion and metabolism of the healthy infant possess an adaptability which makes this unnecessary. These facts should lead to caution in the interpretation of results obtained, since an infant may maintain a reasonable state of nutrition even though its diet be not properly balanced. The aim, however, should be optimum nutrition. It must always be remembered that the baby is an individual, to whom general rules can apply only in a general way.

COW'S MILK

The milk of various animals has at times been used for infant feeding in different countries, from necessity or because of theoretical advantages. That from the ass, goat, sheep, buffalo, sow and mare has been employed, but for practical purposes the milk of the cow is the only one which can generally be made use of in most civilized countries, and any greater nearness in composition of other milks to human milk is of no special advantage, since all require *modification,* as by dilution or the addition of sugar, cream, water, etc., or in other ways, before they should be used.

Goat's Milk.—The milk of the goat has been employed when cow's milk is not obtainable. Its percentage-composition according to several analyses is approximately fat 4, carbohydrate 4.5, protein 4. It is therefore largely similar to cow's milk (see Table 33, p. 84), but its fatty-acid content is greater. While the goat is little subject to tuberculosis it is a vector of undulant fever, and its milk should be pasteurized or boiled. Goat's milk offers no special advantage over cow's milk except in cases of hypersensitiveness to the latter. Severe anemia has repeatedly been reported in young infants fed upon goat's milk. The cause of this is unknown, but it apparently does not depend upon deficiency of iron, and it has been suggested that the fatty-acids so abundant in this milk in some way affect the bone-marrow (see Brouwer;[1] Kirsch, Hoffer and Kirsch;[2] Blühdorn;[3] Calvin[4]). It is often difficult to obtain clean, fresh goat's milk. A proprietary canned goat's milk is on the market.*

Characteristics of Cow's Milk.—The color of cow's milk is more yellowish-white than that of human milk. When absolutely fresh and obtained with proper care it possesses an indefinite, slightly sweetish taste and is practically without odor. The specific gravity ranges within normal limits from 1.028 to 1.033, with an average of 1.032. The reaction with litmus is faintly acid or amphoteric. With phenolphthalein it is always acid, and to a greater degree than human milk. The fat-globules vary greatly in size, the larger ones decidedly predominating. They are generally considered to be less numerous than in human milk, and the emulsion consequently not so fine. Holt,[5] however, claims that there is practically no difference in the microscopic appearance of the two milks. Coagulation occurs readily by acid and by rennin, the resultant curd being firm and tough. When a certain degree of acidity is reached the milk will coagulate when heated. According to Bosworth and Van Slyke[6] the casein exists in cow's milk in the form of calcium caseinate. Bosworth[7] further maintains that the casein of human milk probably exists in the form of potassium caseinate and that it is this fact, despite the essential similarity of the two caseins in other respects, that accounts for the poorer coagulation in human milk. The smaller amount of casein present in human milk is also a factor in making a softer curd.

Effect of Heat on Milk.—Raising the milk to 50 C. (122 F.) produces a slight skin upon the surface, which becomes greater if the milk be boiled. This is due largely to a partial coagulation and drying of the casein, while fat may be contained in it also. Insoluble calcium salts, too, are present and by their adhering to the container a considerable amount of them may be lost. A temperature of 75 C. (167 F.) partially precipitates the lactalbumin, and prolonged boiling does this entirely. Heating up to or near the boiling point gives rise to the characteristic odor of boiled milk, partly by the production of a sulphur-compound from the lactalbumin, and a brownish tint is developed by the boiling if prolonged, dependent upon the caramelization of the sugar. The cream, too, rises imperfectly or not at all in milk which has been heated for half an hour to a temperature of 65 C. (149 F.) (Rosenau[8]), owing to the effect upon the emulsion of the fat globules. The rising of the cream is prevented to some extent even at a temperature of 145 F. (63 C.) and the action of the rennin is also interfered with, the curd which forms being softer and more flocculent. If the milk is boiled the process of coagulation by rennin is even more disturbed. Brennemann[9] has shown that boiled milk forms softer curds in the human stomach as well as in the test tube. Digestion of casein by trypsin is better in heated than in raw milk. Among other changes produced by heat are the driving off of the carbonic dioxide, oxygen, nitrogen and iodine; a precipitation of the phosphates of the alkaline earths and of part of the citric acid; a diminution in the organic phosphorus and the hydrogen-ion concentration; and a destruction to some degree of the ferments, the alexins and the bactericidal properties of the milk. Few changes, however, occur except at a temperature of over 65 C. (149 F.). A large number of bacteria of different sorts are destroyed at this temperature or even at 60 C. (140 F.), although the peptonizing bacteria of the spore-bearing class and many acid-producing germs are more resistant (see p. 86). The heating of the milk for a

* Meyenberg "Alpure" Goat's milk, Salinas, California.

brief time to the temperature of boiling or even higher has little if any effect on the fat-soluble vitamin A. The water-soluble vitamins are more easily inhibited or destroyed by heat.

Effect of Freezing.—Freezing would appear to produce a separation of the oil-globules, but other action is uncertain. If long-continued it has been claimed to have a very decided influence upon the chemical composition. Such freezing as may ordinarily be encountered in the household employment of milk does not usually have any harmful effect upon infants receiving it, although sometimes constipation, vomiting or diarrhea may be produced.

Caloric Value.—This naturally varies greatly with the differences in the composition of cow's milk. The range of figures is from 614 to 724 calories per liter (581 to 685 cal. per qt.). For clinical purposes it can be estimated at about 20 calories per fluid ounce (30 cc.).

Examination of Cow's Milk.—There is so little variation in the amount of protein, sugar and salts in mixed herd-milk that for practical purposes these may be taken as fixed amounts, and only tests made for the specific gravity, the reaction, the variation of the fat, and the presence of bacteria and adulterants. Variations in the specific gravity may indicate that the milk has been tampered with. The removal of cream from the milk increases the specific gravity and the addition of water lowers it. The reaction is tested by litmus paper or other indicators. Strongly alkaline milk has probably been adulterated. The amount of fat can best be measured by the Babcock test. It may sometimes be necessary to examine for the presence of such preservatives as boric acid, salicylic acid and formaldehyde. A microscopic examination will demonstrate pus and foreign contaminating substances, and filtering will show the presence of dirt.

Composition of Cow's Milk.—The milk of healthy cows may vary widely, depending upon peculiarities of the individual and of the breed, the character of the food, the period of lactation, the amount of milk which has been drawn from the udder, the time of day, and other factors. Even the mixed milk of a herd is subject to variations. The difference is particularly evident in the fat, that of the other ingredients, especially the sugar and mineral matter, being but slight. As a result of the conditions mentioned the published analyses of the chemical composition of cow's milk vary considerably. The following table gives an approximate average analysis:

TABLE 33.—AVERAGE COMPOSITION OF COW'S MILK

	Per cent
Water	86.0–88.0
Total solids	12.0–14.0
Fat	3.5– 4.0
Sugar	4.5
Protein	3.5– 3.75
Salts	0.7

Nature and Normal Variation of the Constituents of Cow's Milk.—(See also Human Milk, p. 75, for fuller description of the differences.)

Fat.—The fat, as stated, is by far the most variable element. Percentages run in round numbers all the way from 2 to over 6 in different cows and in different breeds, but in the individual cow are relatively constant. The herd-milk of Jersey and Guernsey cattle is from 1 to 1.5 per cent richer in fat than is average cow's milk; while the sugar and protein are also somewhat in excess. Holsteins and Ayrshires produce a milk slightly poorer than the average in fat. The amount of fat depends also upon the food given and the general treatment and health of the animal.

It much resembles in composition the fat of human milk, olein and palmitin predominating, but the volatile fatty acids being relatively more abundant and the amount of oleic acid less.

Sugar.—The sugar may range in individual cows from 3.5 to 5.5 per cent in round numbers, but in mixed herd-milk the variation is inconsiderable. The nature of the food has but little influence upon it. The sugar is lactose, and is generally believed to be identical with or closely allied to that of human milk.

Protein.—The protein may range from 2.5 to 4.5 per cent in different healthy cows, but in mixed herd-milk is fairly uniform, the variation being not over 0.5 per cent. The percentage of 4, formerly commonly accepted, is generally not equaled. That of 3.5 to 3.75 more fairly represents the standard. The protein consists of casein, lactalbumin, and small amounts of lactoglobulin, as in human milk but in different proportions. There is also an alcohol-soluble protein. The results obtained by investigators vary, but the usual ratio of casein to lactalbumin may be assumed as about 6:1. The casein coagulates more readily by acids and by rennin than does that of human milk and possibly differs chemically from it, and certainly biologically. One of the most important differences between human and cow's milk is in the amino-acid composition. It is probable that the amino-acids in human milk are in better relative amounts and proportions for the growth of the human infant than in cow's milk. Hijikata[10] found the amino-acids lysine, arginine, guanine, adenine, choline and histidine in cow's milk.

Mineral Matter.—The mineral matter varies according to different analyses, and is influenced to some extent by the food. The analysis of Söldner is compared in the following table with that of Bunge for human milk, showing the contrasts of the relative percentages. The figures are those quoted by Hammarsten.[11]

Table 34.—Percentages of Mineral Matter of Cow's Milk and of Human Milk

	Cow's milk, Söldner.	Human milk, Bunge.
Potassium oxide	0.172	0.0703
Sodium oxide	0.051	0.0257
Calcium oxide	0.198	0.0343
Magnesium oxide	0.02	0.0065
Ferric oxide	0.00035[12]	0.0006
Phosphoric oxide	0.182	0.0469
Chlorine	0.098	0.0445

The mineral matter of cow's milk differs from that of human milk chiefly in the much larger total amount present; in the greater proportion of phosphorus, calcium, potassium and magnesium; and in the smaller quantity of iron. Part of the calcium is combined with the casein; the rest is united with phosphoric acid to form phosphates, which hold the casein in suspension in the milk. Milk contains also copper, manganese and iodine. The content of the last can be increased by feedings whereas an increased ingestion of calcium, phosphorus, iron, copper, or manganese has no such result.

The difference in the salt-content of human milk and cow's milk may account in great part for any difficulty in the digestion of the latter. Phosphates and calcium caseinate act as buffers; *i. e.*, as substances which are capable of uniting with acid or alkali without undergoing a change in chemical reaction. As Marriott and Davidson[13] maintain, cow's milk, by reason of its higher calcium and phosphorus content and its consequent higher buffer-value, can neutralize a considerable portion of the acid of the gastric juice. This acid has important functions to perform, and any decided reduction in the amount of it may be associated with digestive disturbance.

Ferments, Extractive Matter, Etc.—Cow's milk differs further from human milk in the presence in it of a much larger percentage of citric acid (cow's milk 0.2 per cent; human milk 0.05) and a much smaller amount of lecithin and of nucleone. The citric acid content of the milk is variable and is affected by the ration. A number of ferments are to be found. Other characteristics of human milk are, however, absent from that of the cow. (See p. 74.) Raw cow's milk under certain conditions has a bactericidal action which causes a decrease in bacterial content on standing.

The digestion and absorption of fat, carbohydrate, protein and minerals and their functions have been discussed in Chapter I, pp. 24; 29.

Vitamins.—The milk of pasture-fed cows is richer in vitamins than is that of those on dry fodder. A number of investigations, such as those of Osborne and Mendel,[14] and of Daniels, Byfield and Loughlin,[15] have shown that vitamin B may be diminished or lacking, and the same is true of vitamin C (Hess, Unger and Supplee[16]). The antirachitic factor in milk can be increased by feeding the cows irradiated yeast (Hess, Lewis, MacLeod and Thomas[17]).

Bacteria in Cow's Milk.—All cow's milk, as ordinarily supplied, contains numerous bacteria. Even when first drawn from the udder this is the case, although it is true that by far the greatest number of bacteria are found in the first part of the milk, the last portion being nearly free. In addition to the germs within the udder, direct contamination occurs through the dust of the stable, dust from the cow's udder and belly, contaminating cow-manure, the hands of the milker, and, most especially, unclean utensils; and, inasmuch as milk forms one of the best of culture-media, the multiplication of these is extremely rapid and the number of varieties great. The average market-milk when pasteurized should not contain more than 50,000 bacteria to the cubic centimeter when delivered to the consumer. This is the standard adopted by some cities, others allowing a greater number. Many communities do not allow the sale of any raw milk unless certified or inspected. When raw market milk is examined it may contain from 50,000 to 1,000,000 bacteria to the cubic centimeter depending on the time of year, but the latter figure is the upper limit which should be permitted. Older figures often showed as high as 10,000,000 or more, a number greater than found in city sewage (Rosenau[18]). The varieties which may be present are very numerous, depending upon the surrounding sources of contamination. Those derived from the udder are forms of staphylococcus and streptococcus and the pseudodiphtheria bacillus. Those entering in other ways may be classified into *nonpathogenic* and *pathogenic*.

Of the *nonpathogenic* the most frequent are the lactic acid-producing bacteria, developing lactic acid by acting upon the sugar. Prominent among these are the streptococcus lacticus, the bacillus lactis acidi and, less frequently, the bacillus lactis aërogenes. These germs enter the milk during milking or afterward, at the same time with others, some of them often later disappearing through the production of an acidity which is unsuited to their growth. A second class is the butyric acid group, breaking up the sugar and fat and producing butyric acid. A third group is composed of the proteolytic bacteria which, usually after coagulating the milk, may cause a breaking up of the protein. Many of these are also capable of producing lactic acid, as for instance the bacillus coli, which is the one of this group most commonly present. The bacillus proteus, bacillus alkaligenes and certain other germs belong to the proteolytic class. Numerous other organisms may occur, among them pyogenic germs derived from a diseased udder, bacteria giving rise to various discolorations of the milk, or others which give it a bitter or other unpleasant taste. The germs of the lactic acid group do not themselves appear to be harmful, since the acid produced serves to check the growth within the intestine of the proteolytic bacteria. The aim, however, should be to have present as few germs of any kind as is possible.

A large variety of *pathogenic* germs has been found at times in milk, and epidemics have repeatedly been traced to this source. Infection through milk is true especially of typhoid fever, scarlet fever and diphtheria. Epidemics of septic sore throat have been produced in the same way. Tubercle bacilli of the bovine type may also be found in cow's milk, although generally only if the udder is tuberculous, and the milk may likewise be contaminated from various outside sources by the human type of bacillus. Among other pathogenic germs occasionally occurring in milk, and in some instances producing disease in infants and children, are those of cholera, dysentery, undulant fever and anthrax.

The number of bacteria in cream is greater than in milk, even when this is obtained by centrifuging and with all precautions against contamination.

Many of the forms of lactic acid-producing bacteria and most of the nonspore-bearing pathogenic ones are killed by heating even to a temperature of 140 F. (60 C.). The tubercle-bacillus is more resistant but is destroyed when heated to 155 F. (68.3 C.) for thirty minutes. Rosenau[19] found it no longer infectious when heated to 140 F. (60 C.) for two minutes. The butyric-acid bacilli and the spore-bearing proteolytic germs require a higher temperature, and even that of boiling does not destroy their spores. Some of the toxins produced by bacteria are heat-stable.

Freezing does not kill the harmful bacteria. The lactic acid organisms do not grow at low temperatures whereas proteolytic bacteria do. Putrefaction may, therefore, take place even though curdling does not occur.

Pus in Milk.—All cow's milk contains a few leukocytes. As a result of extended studies, Bergey[20] and Stokes[21] concluded that the presence of more than 10 leukocytes per field of a $\frac{1}{12}$ immersion lens, obtained by centrifuging 10 cc. of milk, constitutes pus, especially when the cells are grouped in small masses and accompanied by chains of streptococci. There is, however, a very great range in the number of cells found in milk from healthy cattle, and the determination of the presence of pus by numbers alone is unsatisfactory (Lewis[22]).

Cream.—Cream is to all intents merely a super-fatted milk, and, strictly speaking, any milk containing more than 4 per cent of fat should be called cream. As the percentages of fat increase those of sugar, protein, and mineral matter diminish. The following table represents approximate averages based upon the figures given by a number of investigators:

TABLE 35.—PERCENTAGES OF FAT, SUGAR AND PROTEIN IN CREAMS OF DIFFERENT STRENGTHS

Per cent cream.	Fat.	Carbohydrate.	Protein.
32	32	3.40	2.5
20	20	3.90	2.9
16	16	4.20	3.05
12	12	4.30	3.20
10	10	4.40	3.30
7	7	4.45	3.40

For practical purposes these slight diminutions of carbohydrate and protein may be disregarded in infant feeding. Cream is obtained either by skimming or dipping, being then called "gravity" cream, or by the use of the separator and then entitled "centrifuged" or "separator" cream. Practically all the cream sold on the market is separator cream. By this process it may be made of almost any strength desired up to 30 or even 40 per cent or more of fat.

Top-milk.—This is the term applied to any number of the upper ounces of the milk in a milk-jar after having stood several hours, irrespective of whether all or part of the cream layer is removed or even some also of the portion below this. To obtain top-milk a quart of milk, as soon after milking as possible, is strained into one of the ordinary quart milk-bottles, closed, cooled, and then kept on ice or in ice-water for six hours or longer. In dairy-milk delivered in jars or bottles the cream has usually already risen, and there is no need for it to stand longer if the cream-layer is sharply defined. To obtain top-milk one may employ syphoning or pouring, but the best method is to use the 1 oz. dipper especially devised for the purpose by Chapin[23] and purchasable through druggists, and to dip off as many ounces as desired.

Top-milk (Layer Milk) has the advantage over cream in economy when a mixture is desired the fat percentage of which exceeds that of the protein. It has the disadvantage that there is some variation in the actual fat-strength of the different layers according to different authors. This is, however, a minor matter. The average fat-strength of the different layers may be seen in Table 37. The figures apply to milk containing approximately 4 per cent of fat. With richer milk showing 5 per cent all that is necessary is to remove and discard the top 2 oz. and then to proceed with the dipping as though this had not been done.

It should again be said in this connection (see p. 83) that the employment of pasteurization or boiling before the cream layer separates interferes with the proper rising of the cream and makes the strength of top-milk very uncertain.

Skimmed Milk, Bottom Milk, Fat-free Milk.—The milk remaining after any of the cream has been removed by dipping is denominated skimmed milk or bottom milk. Its percentages of sugar and of protein are slightly higher than, but for practical purposes the same as, those of whole milk. The entire milk below the cream layer contains about 1 per cent of fat; the lowest portion of the milk-jar decidedly less; but milk practically fat-free can be obtained only by use of the separator. A comparison of the relative strengths of the different elements in whole milk, skimmed milk and fat-free milk, as given by Morse and Talbot,[24] may be seen in the following table:

Table 36.—Comparison of Whole Milk, Skimmed Milk and Fat-free Milk

	Fat, per cent.	Sugar, per cent.	Protein, per cent.
Whole milk	4.0	4.5	3.50
Skimmed milk	1.0	5.0	3.55
Fat-free milk	0.25	5.0	3.65

The relative strength of the fat, sugar and protein in the different layers of milk may be seen in the table on p. 89. For the sake of ease in calculation the figures have been distorted slightly, the sugar becoming 4, instead of 4.5 per cent, and the protein 4, instead of the more accurate range of 3.50 to 3.75 per cent, while the fat of the upper 16 oz. has been made 8, instead of the more correct 7 to 7.50 per cent. The differences are, however, insignificant for practical purposes, and the great convenience of the approximate ratio justifies the alteration. (See p. 92.)

TABLE 37.—PERCENTAGE-STRENGTHS OF TOP-MILK AND SKIMMED MILK LAYERS

Milk obtained from a quart of 4 per cent milk by dipping, as previously described (p. 88), gives:

	Fat, per cent.	Protein and sugar, per cent.	Approximate ratio.
Upper 2 oz.	24.0	4	6 to 1
Upper 4 oz.	20.0	4	5 to 1
Upper 6 oz.	16.0	4	4 to 1
Upper 8 oz.	12.0	4	3 to 1
Upper 10 oz.	10.0	4	2.5 to 1
Upper 16 oz.	8.0	4	2 to 1
Upper 20 oz.	6.0	4	1.5 to 1
Upper 24 oz.	5.0	4	1.25 to 1
Upper 32 oz. (whole-milk)	4.0	4	1 to 1
Lower 30 oz.	3.0	4	0.75 to 1
Lower 28 oz.	2.0	4	0.50 to 1
Lower 16 oz.	1.0	4	0.25 to 1
Lower 8 oz.	0.5	4	0.0 to 1

Requirements of Good Milk.—There are certain requisites which must be insisted upon in order to make cow's milk a safe and satisfactory food. First of all it must be clean. Cleanliness with regard to contamination by bacteria is important. There should be an absence of pathogenic germs and but a small number of those of other sorts. The milk should be tampered with in no way, as by the addition of preservatives, the removal of any of the cream, or the addition of water. Much of that furnished is very decidedly over twenty-four hours old before it is used. If it has been pasteurized it should be distinctly stated on the bottle that this has been done. An unusually low bacterial count in milk not known to have been produced with especial care suggests the employment either of chemical preservatives or of heat. The milk should be kept constantly at a temperature not over 45 F. (7.2 C.) from the time it is bottled until it is prepared for use, and the time of transportation should be as brief as possible. Uniformity in strength is necessary, with conformity to the analytical standards of normal milk, and it should consequently contain at least 3.5 per cent of fat. If the cow's milk varies materially it may be impossible to modify it in a way which will agree with the child to whom it is fed. If it is from cows which are ill its quality becomes impaired, or it may become decidedly harmful to the infant. Consequently mixed herd-milk is to be preferred to that from a single cow, as less liable to exhibit sudden alterations in character.

Certified Milk.—The evident lack in ordinary dairies of the fulfillment of any such regulations as those just mentioned led to the establishment in various cities of Milk-Commissions, which in 1907 associated themselves as the American Association of Medical Milk-Commissions. The purpose of a milk-commission is to prescribe rules and regulations for dairies with which a contract is to be made, and to determine by inspection that the prescribed requirements and agreements are fulfilled. Personal systematic inspection of the dairy is made from time to time by members of the Commission, and repeated examinations of the buildings and the cows conducted by the Commission's veterinarian, and of the milk by its chemists and bacteriologists. To dairies the product of which fulfills the requirements a certificate is given to that effect, and such milk is properly called "certified milk." Some Commissions also allow a second grade called "inspected" milk. It was formerly insisted that certified milk be raw, but a small amount of that sold now is pasteurized. Its bacterial count before the use of any heat must be under 10,000 to the cubic centimeter.

Certified milk usually and rightly sells at an increased price, since the cost of its production is necessarily increased. With sufficient ordinary care, however, a great improvement in the quality of ordinary market-milk can be made without any material increase in the expense.

GENERAL PRINCIPLES OF SUBSTITUTE FEEDING

Comparison of Human and Bovine Milk.—Before proceeding to the study of the preparation of milk-mixtures, we may conveniently place before us in tabular form the contrasts between human and bovine milk which have already been considered. The figures are approximate ones:

Table 38.—Principal Contrasts of Average Bovine and Human Milk

	Cow's milk.	Human milk.
Specific gravity	1032	1030–31
Color	White	Bluish-white
Bacteria	Always present	Practically none
Coagulation by rennet and acid	Readily and produces firm curds	Less easy and produces soft, flocculent precipitate
Reaction to litmus	Generally acid	Alkaline or amphoteric
Fat	4 per cent; containing more volatile fatty acids	3.5–4 per cent; containing less volatile and more oleic acid
Sugar	4.5 per cent	7 per cent
Total protein	3.75 per cent	1–1.50 per cent
Total lactalbumin	0.3 per cent[25]	0.5 per cent[25]
Total casein	3.0 per cent[25]	1.2 per cent[25]
Mineral matter	0.7 per cent	0.2 per cent
Total solids	12–14 per cent	12–13 per cent
Water	86–88 per cent	87–88 per cent

Modification of Milk.—In adapting cow's milk to infant feeding it is usually *modified* in some way. Any element taken from or added to milk modifies it, even the addition of water or the application of heat. The objects sought in various types of modification are as follows: Prevention of the development of bacteria or their destruction or reduction in number; prevention of the formation of large, tough curds; alteration in reaction; change in the amount of protein or alteration of it by peptonization or the employment of casein or of whey; alteration in salt-content; alteration in the amount of fat; alteration of the amount and type of sugar. While some or all of these changes may be demanded at times, in the average healthy infant the modification need not be as extensive as these requirements would indicate. In the following pages will be described the methods of modifying cow's milk for infant feeding.

The Calculation of the Milk-formulae.—There would appear to be 4 different points of view from which we could approach the preparation of an infant's bottle mixture. All these are, it will be noticed, methods of *calculation.*

In the *first* are studied the proportional, or percentage, amounts of the basic ingredients, such as fat, sugar and protein, with regard to the quantity of each which is the optimum in the food for the individual case, and the influence which any one of them may have upon the digestion and absorption of another. The formula is then worked out from the proportions thus determined. This has been called the *Percentage Method*, a name which has been greatly misapprehended and misunderstood, and which is in reality a misnomer.

The *second* basis of food preparation is calculated upon the caloric needs of the infant, regardless, at least theoretically, of the relative digestibility and utilizability of the different ultimate constituents. This has been called the *Caloric Method*, likewise a misconception, because other considerations have always to be taken into account.

In the *third*, the *Method of Pirquet*, the food-preparations are calculated on a relationship between the sitting-height, the normal weight, and the extent of the absorbing surface of the intestine. The system is complicated and but little used in this country at the present time.

The *fourth* method bases the nature and quantity of the food upon the assumed need of the infant for different absolute amounts of fat, carbohydrate, and protein respectively, without regard to the percentage relationship, but estimating the total amount of these present in a definite quantity of whole milk, and determining how much whole milk, *i. e.*, how much of these basic ingredients, is necessary for the feeding of an infant of a definite weight. This might properly be called the *Method Calculated from the Absolute Food-weight Requirements.* Inasmuch as by this method whole milk is usually employed, diluted in various proportions, this has often been called the Simple Dilution Method. This, too, is a misnomer, inasmuch as quite generally, beside the usual dilution with water, a carbohydrate in the form of some sugar is added in definite percentage amount, and because also whole milk dilutions can equally well be used in the percentage method for the production of certain formulae. The process, therefore, becomes no longer a simple dilution.

As a matter of fact, knowledge involving features of at least three of the so-called "methods" is necessary, and no one of them can scientifically be used alone. The estimation by percentages involves a final reduction to absolute quantities of sugar and milk, whether whole, top or skimmed. The estimation of the calories of the food is often an essential in determining whether or not this is of sufficient caloric strength to supply energy-needs of the infant, but is useful in no other way. The thinking in actual quantities of the basic ingredients involves, if for instance sugar has been added, a determining of the amount of this already present and the necessary percentage to be added to raise the carbohydrate content to 6 or 7 per cent, if this chances to be the figure desired.

Percentage-feeding.—This method is, like the others, one of *thinking*, not of feeding; one in which the food mixture is built up from its basic elements to obtain any composition desired. It is one of great flexibility and is especially useful in cases of children with disturbed digestion or with any degree of intolerance for certain of the food ingredients. Many pediatrists employ it chiefly to ascertain the percentage of each of the constituents of the food-mixture which is being given, thus checking up the actual amounts which have been calculated as necessary for the food requirement. These amounts should, of course, be known as well as their relationship to each other. Biedert[26] emphasized its importance in a general way; and, still earlier, Cumming[27] had given a clear exposition of it. Rotch[28] brought the matter into prominence. In constructing an infant's food-formula one may employ whole milk, cream, top milk, or skimmed milk, depending upon the percentages desired, as well as water or a cereal decoction as a diluent, and the addition of sugar in some form. When the method first came into popularity whole milk and cream dilutions were solely employed and a method of calculation was published by Baner.[29] Later it was found to be more convenient and economical to do away with purchased cream and to use "layer-milk" as shown in Tables 39 and 40, these being a modification of a milk card previously published by one of us.[30] The slight alterations made in the figures have already been noted (p. 88). We must bear in mind, as previously stated, that milk which has been pasteurized does not separate readily into layers of definite fat-strength.

TABLE 39.—AUTHOR'S MILK CARD*

Table giving approximate percentage-strengths of different layers of milk.

	Per cent fat.	Per cent protein and sugar.	Ratio.
Upper 2 oz.	24	4	6 to 1
Upper 4 oz.	20	4	5 to 1
Upper 6 oz.	16	4	4 to 1
Upper 8 oz.	12	4	3 to 1
Upper 10 oz.	10	4	2.5 to 1
Upper 16 oz.	8	4	2 to 1
Upper 20 oz.	6	4	1.5 to 1
Upper 24 oz.	5	4	1.25 to 1
Upper 32 oz. whole milk	4	4	1 to 1
Lower 30 oz.	3	4	.75 to 1
Lower 28 oz.	2	4	.50 to 1
Lower 16 oz.	1	4	.25 to 1
Lower 8 oz.	0.5	4	.0 to 1

To find the amount of any layer of milk to be used to give percentages desired

Equation:

$$\frac{\text{Total amount of food} \times \text{percentage of fat desired}}{\text{Fat-strength of layer of milk used}} = \text{Amount of this milk in the mixture.}$$

1. Select from the "Layers of Milk" Table the milk which possesses the desired ratio of fat to protein.

2. Substitute in the equation.

3. As the sugar-percentage has been reduced equally with that of the protein, add sufficient sugar to raise to the desired percentage.

Example: 20-oz. mixture desired. Percentages desired = Fat 3, Sugar 6, Protein 1. Use upper 8 oz. (fat 12 per cent, protein 4 per cent, *viz.:* 3:1). Then $\frac{20 \times 3}{12} = 5$ oz. of upper 8 oz. with 15 oz. of water in the 20-oz. mixture. The protein necessarily becomes 1 per cent, and the sugar likewise. The mixture already containing 1 per cent of sugar, add 5 per cent of 20 oz., *i. e.*, 1 oz. of sugar to increase this to the 6 per cent desired.

To Determine the Percentages Present in Any Milk-mixture Already in Use

$$\frac{\text{Quantity of substance used (milk, cream, or skimmed milk)} \times \text{its percentage-strength}}{\text{Total quantity of food}} = \text{Percentage of element (F., S. or P.) in the mixture.}$$

Example: The mother has mixed: Upper 8 oz.; 6 oz.—Lower 8 oz.; 3 oz.—Milk-sugar 3 level tablespoonfuls.—Water 27 oz. Total quantity = 36 oz. The upper 8 oz. contains 12 per cent fat (see Table). Both top and bottom milk contain 4 per cent protein and sugar. Three tablespoonfuls sugar = approximately 1 oz. The fat of the lower 8 oz. may be ignored. Then $\frac{6 \times 12}{36} = 2 =$ Fat percentage from the top-milk. $\frac{3 \times 0}{36} = 0 =$ Fat-percentage from the bottom milk. $\frac{9 \times 4}{36} = 1 =$ Protein and sugar percentages from combined top and bottom milk. The 1 oz. additional sugar divided by 36 = approximately 3 per cent sugar added. There being already 1 per cent sugar derived from the milk, the total sugar = 4 per cent.

* These cards may be obtained from Edward Pennock, 3602 Woodland Ave., Phila.

The method of calculation of a 20 oz. formula of any desired strength is exemplified in Table 39 in which an imaginary formula is given—not at all a usually desirable one. The percentage strength in this table and in the next have been made to accord with Table 37 p. 89.

A little consideration of Table 39, will show many ways of simplifying the preparation of the food. Thus a mixture containing 3 per cent of fat and 2 per cent of protein may be made equally well either by adding 10 oz. of the upper 20 to 10 oz. of water or by mixing 5 oz. of the upper 8 oz. with 5 oz. of the lower 8 and 10 oz. of water.

It can readily be seen that a mixture of any desired amount may be obtained by a simple multiplication of the amounts of milk, water and sugar given in Table 40, p. 93. Thus if a 30 oz. mixture is to be made the multiplication factor would be 1.5. It is understood that the percentage-method does not give absolutely accurate figures since milk, the original ingredient, is not itself uniform in composition.

Those who wish to avoid all calculation as far as possible may have recourse to the figures given in Table 40. This is based on the percentage strengths as given in Table 37. Fraley's formula has been used for the determination of the calories. (See p. 94.)

The difference in fat percentage between the lower 16 and the lower 20 oz. is so slight that the latter may be used to replace the former in case one is using but a single quart of milk.

To Ascertain the Percentages Contained in Any Milk-mixture.—It is often of the greatest value to be able to determine readily just what the percentage of the elements may be in a mixture which one finds is being given to the child. The method of doing this is illustrated in the example in Table 39, p. 92, which is an example merely, not a formula recommended. If a

TABLE 40.—AUTHOR'S MILK-CARD (Reverse Side)

Showing amount of different layers to be used for the preparation of various percentage-mixtures, and the caloric values of the mixtures. Ready method for selecting amounts employed in making various 20-oz. milk-mixtures, and the caloric values resulting.

Percentages desired of.			Lower 8 oz.	Lower 16 oz.	Lower 28 oz.	Whole milk.	Upper 24 oz.	Upper 20 oz.	Upper 16 oz.	Upper 10 oz.	Upper 8 oz.	Water oz.	Sugar oz.	Caloric value of mixture.	Calories per oz.
Fat.	Sugar.	Protein.													
0.5	5	1	...	..	5	....	..	..	..	..	..	15	0.8	175	8.75
0.5	6	2	...	10	..	....	..	..	..	..	..	10	0.8	225	11.25
1	6	1	...	..	..	5	..	..	..	..	..	15	1	225	11.25
1	6	1.5	2.5	..	..	5	..	..	..	..	..	12.5	0.9	237.5	11.88
1	6	2	...	..	10	....	..	..	..	..	..	10	0.8	250	12.5
0.75	6	3	...	15	..	....	..	..	..	..	..	5	0.6	275	13.75
1	6	4	...	20	..	....	..	..	..	..	..	0	0.4	300	15
1.5	6	1	...	..	..	....	..	5	..	..	..	15	1	250	12.5
1.5	6	1.5	...	..	..	7.5	..	..	..	..	..	12.5	0.9	262.5	13.13
2	6	1	...	..	..	....	..	..	5	..	..	15	1	275	13.75
2	6	1.5	2.5	..	..	....	..	..	5	..	..	12.5	0.9	287.5	14.38
2	6	2	...	..	..	10	..	..	..	..	..	10	0.8	300	15
2.5	6	1.5	2.5	..	..	....	..	..	..	5	..	12.5	0.9	312.5	15.63
2.5	6	2	...	..	..	....	10	..	..	..	..	10	0.8	325	16.25
2.5	6	2.5	...	..	..	12.5	..	..	..	..	..	7.5	0.7	337.5	16.88
3	6	1	...	..	..	....	..	..	..	..	5	15	1	325	16.25
3	6	1.5	2.5	..	..	....	..	..	..	..	5	12.5	0.9	337.5	16.88
3	6	2	...	..	..	....	..	10	..	..	..	10	0.8	350	17.5
3	6	3	...	..	..	15	..	..	..	..	..	5	0.4	375	18.75
4	4	4	...	..	..	20	..	..	..	..	..	0	...	400	20

If 1.3 is used as a multiple to obtain the number of calories to the ounce (see p. 94), the figures vary somewhat from those in the last column of Table 40, but the difference is immaterial.

cereal decoction, as of barley water, has been used instead of the 27 oz. of plain water the carbohydrate content has, of course, been slightly increased thereby. The amount may be calculated by the same equation as follows:

$$\frac{27 \text{ (oz. barley water)} \times 1.2 \text{ (\% starch in barley water)}}{36} = 0.9\% \text{ starch (carbohydrate)}$$

The Caloric Method.—This is, likewise, a method of calculation. It is based upon the estimated calories required by the average infant at different ages, irrespective of how much of each of the different basic ingredients of the food may be needed or how well it may be tolerated. The studies were made by Heubner[31] on a few breast-fed infants. The total daily caloric needs divided by the weight of the infant gave the "Energy Quotient," *i. e.*, the number of calories required per kilogram of the body-weight. The commonly adopted standard for the Energy Quotients is as follows:

Age.	Calories per kilogram.	Calories per pound.
First three months	100	45
Second three months	90	40
Third three months	80	35
Fourth three months	70	30

For bottle-fed infants the need is often greater than this to the extent of 5 to 10 calories per pound or 10 to 20 per kilogram; and our experience has been that infants thus fed show an increased rate in growth and, it is believed, a better retention of nitrogen (Nelson[32]). This greater need is especially true of premature and emaciated infants. To attempt, therefore, to select for the infant a food based solely on its caloric strength would be a grave error, more especially, too, since the caloric needs are at best only approximations. The system is, however, very valuable as a check to determine quickly whether a food is of proper caloric strength.

The caloric value of many milk-mixtures can be calculated with great simplicity, since each ounce of whole milk represents approximately 20 calories and each ounce of sugar 120 calories. When water is used as the diluent no further calculation is necessary. (The caloric value of other foods is given on p. 130.) For example if the mixture consists of 30 oz. of milk, 10 of water, and 1 of sugar its caloric value is 720.

$$(30 \times 20 = 600, + 1 \times 120 = 120. \quad \text{Total } 720).$$

If the infant taking this mixture weighs 15 lb. he is receiving 48 calories per pound ($720 \div 15 = 48$).

If the percentages of a mixture are known the formula proposed by Fraley[33] may be employed. This in brief is $(2F + S + P) \times 1\frac{1}{4}Q = C)$ or, in detail, twice the fat-percentage, plus the sugar-percentage, plus the protein-percentage, multiplied by one and a quarter times the total quantity of food-mixture given in the day, equals the total number of calories furnished by the day's food. Supposing, for example, a milk-mixture contains fat, 3 per cent; sugar, 6 per cent; protein, 2 per cent; 6 bottles of 6 oz. each administered; *i. e.*, 36 oz. in the twenty-four hours. Substituting these figures the formula will read

$$(2 \times 3 + 6 + 2) \times (1\tfrac{1}{4} \times 36) = 14 \times 45 = 630 \text{ calories}.$$

Further experience has shown that this formula gives a total caloric value which is a trifle low, and a more accurate result can be obtained by using the modification suggested by Holt and Howland.[34] In the form of an equation this reads: $(2F + S + P) \times 1.3 =$ No. of calories in 1 fl. oz. of the food. The result thus obtained multiplied by the total number of ounces of food used during the day gives the caloric value of the day's food.

When the metric system is employed calculation of calories is as follows: One Gm. of fat furnishes in the economy 9.3 calories, and 1 Gm. of protein and of carbohydrate each 4.1 calories. Then supposing an infant is receiving a liter of a food-mixture containing fat 3 per cent; sugar, 6 per cent and protein 1.5 per cent, if we multiply 1000 Gm. by each of these figures we obtain as present in the food:

Fat $= 1000 \times 0.03 = 30$ Gm.
Sugar $= 1000 \times 0.06 = 60$ Gm.
Protein $= 1000 \times 0.015 = 15$ Gm.

If now we multiply each of these amounts by the number of calories which 1 Gm. produces, we obtain:

Fat	$= 30 \times 9.3 =$	279.0 calories
Sugar	$= 60 \times 4.1 =$	246.0 calories
Protein	$= 15 \times 4.1 =$	61.5 calories
Total in 1 liter of food	=	586.5 calories

The Pirquet Method.—So much interest was aroused in Pirquet's system of nutrition, that a brief synopsis of it seems necessary. It was intended for the feeding of older children as well as for infants. The premises upon which the author based his system may be stated briefly as follows: It was believed by him that the sitting height bears a very close relationship to the normal body-weight. From this has been formulated a law, according to which the cube-root of 10 times the weight in grams approximately equals the sitting height in centimeters. This may be expressed by the equation (Pelidisi):

$$\frac{\sqrt[3]{10 \text{ weight}}}{\text{sitting height}} = 1 = \frac{100}{100}.$$

If the weight is greater than the average, the ratio will be more than $\frac{100}{100}$; if it is less the ratio will be less than $\frac{100}{100}$. By this formula Pirquet judged whether the actual weight of an individual corresponds to the weight normal for his sitting height. The term *Pelidisi* has been coined out of the initials of the constituents: P standing for *pondus*, the body-weight in grams; Pe recalling the fact that it is not simple weight but *pondus decies*, 10 times the weight; Li indicating that the weight must be converted into a linear function by taking the cube-root of it; Di meaning "division" and Si "sitting height."

The calculation of food-values in calories was objected to by him, chiefly because it does not allow for the portion of the food ingested which is unavailable for heat-production, and a physiologic unit is used instead called the *nem* (Nahrungs-Einheit-Milch), which is the nutritive, combustible value of 1 Gm. of average human milk. This milk-unit is employed as a metric unit, and is combined with the Latin prefixes for metric fractions (a decinem meaning, for instance, one-tenth of a nem, etc.) and with the Greek prefixes for multiples of the unit (a dekanem meaning 10 nems). Tables are available which give the nem-value of food-stuffs. The protein and the fat should be kept each within from 10 to 20 per cent of the total intake. It was found that when fat was difficult to obtain the difference could be made up with sugar without apparent injury, but this substitution is not advocated except when necessary. Pirquet accepted Henning's work, which is said to show that the length of the intestinal canal is, on an average, 10 times the sitting height, and believes that the square of the sitting height may be taken as a *symbol* of the absorbing surface of the intestinal tract, which stands in true relation to the intake of food. By observing a large number of individuals, data were secured as to the amount of food, calculated in decinems, which is ingested per square centimeter of absorbing intestinal surface as calculated from the sitting height; or, to use another coined word, how many *decinemsiqua* are ingested (*siqua* being the word which represents the square of the sitting height). The maximum amount of food which a normal individual can digest within twenty-four hours is about 10 decinems per square centimeter of the square of the sitting height (*i. e.*, 10 decinemsiqua). The minimum amount of combustible material to maintain the body-weight in a condition of absolute quiet is 3 decinemsiqua. The *aequum* is the amount of food required to maintain weight under a given condition of activity. The optimum amount of food in children is greater than the aequum because at this period additional food must be ingested to insure growth. Usually 1 decinemsiqua is added to the aequum for this purpose.

An example may be cited: A boy of eleven years with a sitting height of 70 cm. has an absorbing surface of 70 by 70 or 4900 sq. cm. The maximum that he could digest would be 10 decinems per square centimeter or 4900 nems. The minimum, if he stays in bed without moving at all, would be 3 decinemsiqua; *i. e.*, 4900 by $\frac{3}{10}$ or 1470 nems. Though he sits in school for some hours, he is likely to be very active during the rest of the day. Therefore, 3 decinemsiqua more than the minimum are added to maintain his weight; *i. e.*, 6 decinemsiqua per day. In order to provide for growth and gain we must give 1 decinemsiqua more, or 7 decinemsiqua in all ($\frac{7}{10}$ of 4900, or 3360), which is his optimum allowance.

This system of calculating nutritional standards and food-values undoubtedly served a most useful purpose in the feeding of large groups of individuals under certain conditions. It is, however, decidedly complicated, and there seems to be little advantage in adopting it. Perhaps the most important criticism of Pirquet's system is that the assumption is quite certainly incorrect that sitting height and absorbing surface of the intestinal tract and food requirements stand in close relation to each other. The reader who wishes to learn more of the system should consult the publications of Pirquet,[35] Carter[36] and Faber.[37]

Method Calculated from the Absolute Food-weight Requirements.—This method is based upon the knowledge of the actual amounts of the basic ingredients, fat, carbohydrate and protein, needed by the average normal infant per kilogram or per pound of its body-weight (see p. 31), rather than upon the relative known percentages of the mixture. It has often been called the Simple Dilution method, but this is not an appropriate title, inasmuch as the food practically always has a definite percentage of sugar added to it and is consequently not a simple dilution; and because, too, simple dilution indicates a method of feeding and not a method of calculating. It has been found, however, that whole milk contains the necessary elements in suitable amounts and proportions, and that the giving of 1.5 fl. oz. of it to the pound of body-weight was sufficient to supply all the needs in the first month of life in the matter of fat and protein, and 1.75 to 2 fl. oz. per pound after this period, the added sugar making up the deficiency in carbohydrate. There should be 0.1 oz. of sugar added for each pound of body-weight. From a clinical point of view it was observed that the average healthy infant can well digest and assimilate the whole milk dilutions, even though the amount of protein is greater than the actual need for this substance. Metabolism experiments also have demonstrated that an increased retention of nitrogen occurs when such dilutions are given. Theoretically it may be said that, while we have no exact knowledge of the needs of the infant in this respect, cow's milk protein should perhaps be given in greater amount than that found in breast-milk, since the former probably contains less of the amino-acids necessary for growth.

A simple method of calculating the ingredients of a mixture derived according to the method is as follows:

1. *To Obtain the Number of Ounces to Be Given at Each Feeding.*—Add the figure 2 to the figure representing the age in months.

2. *To Obtain the Total Number of Ounces for Twenty-four Hours.*—Multiply the number of ounces to be given at each feeding by the number of feedings to be given in twenty-four hours (see Table 41).

3. *To Obtain the Number of Ounces of Whole Milk to Be Used.*—Multiply the weight in pounds by 1.5 in the first month of life and thereafter by 1.75 to 2.

4. *To Obtain the Number of Ounces of Diluent.*—Subtract the number of ounces of milk to be used from the total number of ounces for twenty-four hours.

5. *To Obtain the Number of Ounces of Sugar to Be Added.*—Multiply the weight in pounds by 0.1.

Example.—Suppose that a mixture is to be calculated for an infant of two months of age whose weight is 9 lb.

1. 2 (age in months) + 2 = 4 (number ounces each feeding).

2. 4 (number ounces each feeding) × 7 (number feedings in twenty-four hours) = 28 (total number ounces in twenty-four hours).

3. 9 (weight in pounds) × 1.75 (number ounces milk per pound) = 15.75 (approximately 16, the number ounces milk to be used in the mixture).

4. 28 (total number ounces in mixture) − 16 (number ounces milk) = 12 (number ounces diluent).

5. 9 (weight in pounds) × 0.1 (number ounces sugar per pound) = 0.9 (approximately 1 oz. sugar to be added to mixture).

The percentages in this mixture can easily be calculated by employing the equation previously given (Table 39) as follows:

$$\frac{\text{16 (number ounces milk)} \times \text{4 (per cent of fat, carbohydrate and protein in the whole milk)}}{\text{28 (total number ounces in mixture)}} = \text{2.3 (per cent fat, carbohydrate and protein).}$$

$$\frac{\text{1 (number ounces sugar)} \times \text{100 (per cent carbohydrate in sugar)}}{\text{28 (total number ounces in mixture)}} = \text{3.6 (per cent carbohydrate from added sugar).}$$

The mixture then has approximately 2.3 per cent fat, 6 per cent carbohydrate and 2.3 per cent protein. When whole milk without added diluent is given it is no longer necessary to use sugar, although it may, if desired, be added to make a total of 6 per cent.

The caloric value is obtained by multiplying 16 (number ounces of milk) by 20 (caloric value of each ounce) = 320, to which figure is added 120, the caloric value of the 1 oz. of added sugar, making a total of 440. The infant is, therefore, receiving approximately 50 calories per pound (440 ÷ 9).

There are certain limitations and objections to the making of mixtures from diluted whole milk with a sugar addition. The method is intended primarily for the average normal healthy infant with good digestion. Some will require more milk than in the calculations given; others can only take less. Some can take only a small quantity at each feeding and require that the figure 1 replace 2 to be added to that for the age to give the number of ounces at a feeding. Some infants, however, suffer from disturbed digestion in which there is more or less intolerance for the fat of cow's milk. In such cases, or for other reasons, the food-preparation may be more readily constructed by the estimation of the diminished percentage of fat which it is thought that the infant can properly digest, and then employing a dilution of one of the lower layers of milk with its lower fat percentage, and finally adding the required percentage of carbohydrate to furnish sufficient calories for the infant's needs. In other cases it may be desired to have the fat percentage exceed that of the protein, as it does in human milk; and in such an event one of the upper layers of the milk must be employed instead of whole milk. It is the opinion of many pediatrists that in healthy infants carbohydrate does not properly replace fat, and that a fairly large amount of this latter element should be given if it can be digested. It is also to be remembered that the protein needs of the infant are small (p. 31) and that it may not be advisable to utilize an excess of protein merely to produce calories which can more easily be obtained from the carbohydrate or the fat (p. 33). While, therefore, although the average healthy infant can thrive upon milk dilutions with a high percentage of protein, the optimum food would appear to be one in which there is a normal fat-protein ratio, and this often applies with certainty to infants whose health is disturbed.

The Quantity of Food and the Frequency of Feeding.—The quantity of the milk-mixture to be given varies, of course, with the age. The frequency of feeding, too, the hours for this and the relation of feeding to sleep, are governed by the principles which control breast-feeding (p. 66). The following table gives an approximation of the frequency and the amounts at different ages, the quantity being gradually increased as the age advances:

TABLE 41.—INTERVALS AND AMOUNTS OF ARTIFICIAL FEEDING

Age.	Intervals of feeding, hours.	Number of feedings in twenty-four hours.	Amount at each feeding, ounces.
1 to 4 weeks	2½–3	7–8	1– 3
1 to 5 months	3–4	6–7	3– 7
Over 5 months	4	5–6	7–10

The number of feedings to be given during the night in the first year is discussed under Breast-feeding (p. 67).

There is, of course, much latitude to be allowed in using the table, dependent upon the digestion and the demands of the child. Regularity is important, but the amount taken at a feeding and the number of feedings in the twenty-four hours vary greatly with the case. An infant always hungry may need to exceed the amount for its age or to be fed at shorter intervals; another taking large feedings may need longer intervals. It is important, too, to be guided considerably by the weight. An unusually large child may require more than the age calls for, while a small marantic infant may be able to take only much less. There can be no fixed rule. In general, a healthy infant may have all the food it will take at the feeding-time, provided it can retain and digest it; but care should be observed that an unusually large appetite is not dependent upon the giving of too weak a formula.

Further Details for Milk-modification.—With the differences between cow's milk and human milk in view (pp. 74 and 84), we may take up the method to be employed to eliminate these as far as is necessary.

Altering the Reaction.—With proper milk this is hardly necessary in the case of the average well infant. Formerly it was customary to add lime-water or some other alkali. The chief value of this was to prevent the formation of large, tough curds, which, as will be explained later, is better done by heating the milk. At the present time it is a wide-spread practice to add acids of various sorts. The reasons for this as given by Marriott and Davidson[13] are that cow's milk, by virtue of its higher protein, calcium and phosphorus content, and its consequent higher buffer-value compared to breast-milk, can neutralize a considerable portion of the acid of the gastric juice, and that the optimum condition for the action of enzymes in the stomach and duodenum may be thereby disturbed. Furthermore the acid, if added in sufficient amount, is destructive to bacteria. Many of the acid-milks bring this mixture only to an acidity of pH 4 or 5, but, in order to have a decided bactericidal effect a pH of 3.5 or thereabouts is necessary. The preparation of acid-milks will be detailed later (p. 104), but it should be stated here that, while the theory of their use is correct, and while they have a place in the feeding of the sick infant, an extended experience has convinced us that the average normal infant does as well on mixtures to which neither acids nor alkalis are added.

Preventing the Formation of Firm Casein-coagula.—The addition of lime-water (25 per cent of the mixture) or sodium citrate (1 grain for each ounce of milk) will accomplish this. The addition of a cereal diluent such as barley water is another method which acts mechanically like a colloid, and peptonizing is still another procedure. By far the simplest and best method is boiling the milk for three minutes, or otherwise heating it as is done in the commercial preparation of evaporated or dried milks.

Altering the Proportions of the Milk-elements.—This may be accomplished in different ways according to the needs of the case and the preference

TABLE 42.—PREPARATIONS CHIEFLY OF MALTOSE AND DEXTRIN*

	Water, per cent.	Protein, per cent.	Maltose, per cent.	Dextrin, per cent.	Ash, per cent.	Mineral matter, added per cent, and other additions.
Amaizo corn syrup......	23.3	.....	23.6	30.9	0.7	Dextrose 15.0 per cent; sucrose 6.5 per cent
Borcherdt's malt sugar..	1.95	4.4	87.4	4.35	1.9	
Karo corn-syrup, red label.	25.4	.....	22.0	36.0	0.2	Sucrose 9.0 per cent; dextrose 7.4 per cent
Loeflund's food maltose..	.....	.....	40.0	59.7	0.3	....
Mead's dextrimaltose, No. 1................	5.0	.....	51.0	42.0	....	2.0 per cent sodium chloride
Mead's dextrimaltose, No. 2................	5.0	.....	52.0	43.0	....	....
Mead's dextrimaltose, No. 3.	5.0	.....	51.0	41.0	....	3.0 per cent potassium bicarbonate
Maltzymose............	22.1	1.61	67.2	6.95	2.0	....
SMACO maltose with lactose and dextrin.	2.0	.....	35.0	32.0	0.5	Lactose 30 per cent as hydrate
SMACO maltose and dextrin..............	2.0	.....	50.0	47.0	0.5	....
Squibb's vitavose.......	3.0	15.0.	38.0	20.0	4.0	Plus malto-dextrose 20 per cent
Staley's syrup..........	25.0	.....	....	38.6	0.59	Maltose and dextrose combined 33.1 per cent; sucrose 4.0 per cent

* Analyses from manufacturer's list or from reports of the Committee on Foods of the American Medical Association.

of the physician. In the normal healthy infant the proportions of fat and of protein may be reduced by the simple dilution of whole milk as already described (pp. 91; 96). This is liable, however, to give an amount of protein which is either higher than the actual needs or of fat which is lower than the optimum. (See p. 31.) While, therefore, the average healthy infant can well utilize the milk dilutions with a high protein content, if it is desired to give a food in which the percentage of protein is lower than that of the fat, one of the top-milk mixtures may be employed. (See pp. 89 and 92.)

To practically all mixtures carbohydrate should be added in such amounts that it may properly balance the fat and the protein and serve also to raise the caloric value of the food. The digestibility of the various sugars has already been described (p. 30). Practically considered it seems to make little difference whether cane sugar, milk sugar or one of the malt sugar preparations is employed. The approximate measurement of the sugars by tablespoonfuls is as follows:—Lactose 3 level tablespoonfuls to the ounce; maltose-dextrin preparations 4 level tablespoonfuls to the ounce; saccharose 2 level tablespoonfuls to the ounce. Theoretically lactose is preferable since it is biologically and chemically similar to the sugar of breast-milk, and tends to produce a more optimum acidity in the intestinal tract. There are available a number of preparations of maltose-dextrin sugars consisting of mixtures of maltose (varying from 40 to 85 per cent) and of dextrin (varying from 10 to 60 per cent). We have omitted certain of these, which, although practically only dextrinized cereals, are largely advertised to the laity as "Infant Foods."

There are several liquid malt extracts such as Borcherdt's, Maltine, Kepler's, Burrough's, Lilly's, Loeflund's, Parke-Davis, Denver, and Hoff's which, while not ordinarily employed as additions to milk, may be used for this purpose. They may be given also for their diastatic and vitamin content as they contain especially the vitamin B complex. These extracts vary in composition, but have approximately 40 to 60 per cent maltose and 5 to 15 per cent dextrin. In some of them dextrose is present varying from 12 to 15 per cent and the percentage of protein material is only about 4 or 5 per cent.

The various malt-soup preparations will be referred to later (Chapter V, p. 113). There is no question that sugar is one of the most digestible elements in milk, and while it usually is added to make the total percentage in the mixture about 5 to 7, it can be employed in much greater concentration (Chapter I, p. 30).

Starch.—Starch is a useful carbohydrate in those cases where a high percentage of the latter is required. There is, however, no reason to give barley-water or other amylaceous decoctions as a routine measure. While young infants can digest starch it is not required in the diet of the healthy child until about the age of five months, by which time a cooked cereal fed with a spoon answers the purpose.

Sterilization.—The effect of heat upon milk has already been described (p. 83). The chief practical advantage of subjecting it to boiling (212 F. (100 C.)) is that this, or other forms of heating to this temperature or higher, as in commercial evaporation or drying, prevents the formation of large, tough curds in the stomach and thus makes the milk more digestible. The effect upon bacteria has already been considered (see pp. 83; 86). Any inhibition of vitamins brought about by heating is unimportant inasmuch as these should be given in some form in addition to the milk mixture (pp. 123; 133).

Pasteurization.—This term had its origin in the employment by Pasteur of a temperature of less than 100 C. (212 F.) for the preservation of wine. As applied to milk it consists of subjecting it to a temperature of less than boiling, one of from 140 to 165 F. (60 to 73.9 C.) being ordinarily recommended, and the heat maintained for from thirty to sixty minutes. The lower the temperature the longer the time pasteurization should continue. It produces little if any change in the milk chemically, but the pathogenic bacteria are killed as well as many of the nonpathogenic ones. After pasteurization the milk should be cooled rapidly and kept cold in order to inhibit subsequent bacterial growth. Home-pasteurization need seldom be carried out since the process is not often required. The best apparatus for the purpose is the Freeman[38] pasteurizer. Commercial pasteurization is today so closely guarded by the Health Authorities in most communities that a grade of pasteurized milk may be obtained which is safe under most conditions for infant feeding. Usually all milk sold is pasteurized, and so required by law with the exception of certified and inspected milk (p. 89).

Electrical Treatment.—This will destroy certain pathogenic bacteria but the method has not been employed to any extent.

Laboratory-modification of Milk.—Through the efforts of Dr. T. W. Rotch,[39] ably seconded by Mr. G. E. Gordon the principle of the "Milk Laboratory" was evolved, and one such established in Boston in 1891 by the Walker-Gordon Laboratory Company. Similar laboratories have since been organized in other cities of the United States and in London. The physician merely writes a prescription calling for the various proportions of the milk elements he wishes, the total number of bottles, the amount of food for each, the nature of the diluent, and any other requirement desired. If the food is to be pasteurized or sterilized, a starchy addition to be dextrinized, fermentation by lactic acid bacilli to be produced, or any other change made, this is specified in the prescription. The price of laboratory modified milk is necessarily high and for this reason, as well as on account of the frequent inaccessibility of a laboratory, home-modification is that which must oftenest be adopted. In fact, comparatively little prescription milk appears to be in use at the present time.

Home-modification of Milk.—From the foregoing discussion it can be seen that the calculation of the desired formula is in reality a simple process. Having decided on the amounts of milk, sugar and diluent to be used the physician must give the mother or nurse clear, concise, and preferably written directions. It is of advantage to employ printed slips.

Articles Required in Preparing the Food. *Bottles.*—These should be of well-annealed glass to prevent breaking when exposed to heat. They may be of any shape desired, but are best narrow and cylindrical, since they occupy less space when of this form, and fit better in the bottle rack. The mouths of the bottles should be rather wide, rendering cleansing easier. The bottles must be perfectly smooth within, without angles or depressions which can collect milk. A series of markings pressed into the glass indicate the number of ounces of contained fluid. There should be enough bottles provided to permit of all the food for twenty-four hours being prepared at one time.

Nipples.—These are preferably of black rubber and of conical or slightly bulbous shape. The openings should be large enough to allow the milk to drop easily when the filled bottle is inverted, but not to run from it in a stream. If the holes are not of sufficient size they may be enlarged with a red-hot needle. As the nipple gets worn by use it collapses too easily and the holes grow too large. Special forms of nipples to "ventilate" the bottle are not to be recommended, as it is difficult to keep them clean. Too long a nipple is liable to press upon the palate and produce ulceration.

Cream-dipper.—Should it be desired to employ any of the layer milks previously discussed (p. 88) the Chapin dipper may well be used (p. 88).

Sugar-measure.—The most convenient method of measuring the sugar is to employ the Chapin dipper, recommended for dipping layer milks. While holding 1 oz. of milk, it gives somewhat more than ½ oz. (Av.) of milk-sugar. This fact must be impressed upon the mother. Another way is to employ a tablespoon, but this is less satisfactory, as the variation in size is so great. Still another method is to place 1 oz. of sugar, as determined by weighing it, in a small paste-board box, level it, and then cut off the box at the line of the sugar. If tablespoonfuls are to be employed, the level one is better, inasmuch as the rounded tablespoonful gives more variation. Whatever method is used, the sugar should be poured into the measure until it is over-filled; the holder tapped sharply once or twice on the table, not more, and the excess of sugar removed with a case-knife.

Too long tapping settles the sugar to too great an extent. Cane-sugar is heavier, and maltose-dextrin preparations lighter, than lactose. Should it be desired to substitute one of them for lactose, it may be roughly estimated that 1 oz. of lactose equals 3 level tablespoonfuls or $1\frac{1}{2}$ dipperfuls; 1 oz. of a maltose-dextrin, 4 level tablespoonfuls or 2 dipperfuls; and 1 oz. of saccharose, 2 level tablespoonfuls or 1 dipperful. (For weight of tablespoonfuls and dipperfuls of sugar and cereal-flours see also p. 112.)

Glass Graduate; etc.—A graduate holding 8 fl. oz., with the first ounce divided into drams, is a great convenience in measuring the amounts of fluid required. One of the graduated nursing bottles may, it is true, be used instead, but these are not so accurately marked.

In addition are required some sterilized unabsorbent cotton to make the stoppers for the bottles, or cork or rubber stoppers; pulverized boric acid; a bowl or pitcher in which to mix the food; a covered vessel to hold the nipples; a glass funnel; a bottle brush; a bottle rack; and a bottle warmer.

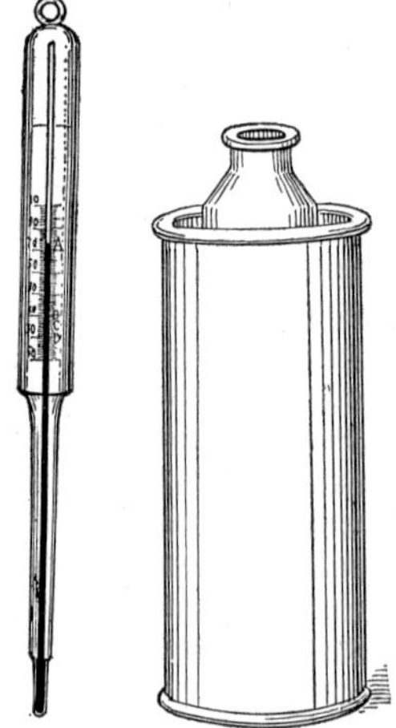

Fig. 12.—Milk-bottle, heating tin, and thermometer.

Regarding the ingredients required, the best milk possible is to be obtained, running close to 4 per cent butter-fat. Certified milk (p. 89) should be used if it can be afforded; if not, a good grade of pasteurized market milk may be bought. In many cities there is sold a milk termed "AA." This is no cleaner or better than the so-called "A" milk but contains a higher percentage of fat,—too high, in fact, for infant feeding. Milk-sugar should be purchased at least a pound at a time, as it is cheaper in this way. The fact that it is frequently impure is not to be forgotten.

Preparing and Giving the Food.—The entire mixture for the day should be made at one time. As soon as the milk is delivered it should be put into the refrigerator, and the cover of the milk-bottle not removed until it is time to make the mixture. The top of the bottle should then be wiped off with a clean cloth or absorbent cotton wet with a boric-acid solution. If whole milk is to be used it should be poured into a pitcher or graduate and back into the bottle, repeating this process several times in order to mix it thoroughly. If a top-milk mixture is required dipping should be done before the milk-jar is shaken. Next the amount of water for the day's food should be brought to a boil in a saucepan, the required number of ounces of milk added, and the whole again boiled for from three to five minutes, with constant stirring. After removal of the mixture from the stove, but while it is still warm, the requisite amount of sugar is added and finally enough water to replace that lost by evaporation during the boiling.

The feeding bottles for the day are now filled through the funnel, the openings wiped dry and stoppered, and the bottles put in the bottle rack and cooled rapidly in running water, and then put in the coolest part of the refrigerator until they are to be used.

When about to feed the infant the bottles should be warmed in the bottle warmer (Fig. 12), a thermometer placed in the bottle, not in the warmer, recording the temperature, which should be from 98 to 100 F. (36.7 to 37.8 C.). The nipple is then removed from the boric acid solution, dipped for a moment in boiling water, and applied to the neck of the bottle. Holding the bottle upside down the milk should drop from it rapidly. The infant should be held in the lap while it is being fed, and the bottle withdrawn from time to time to allow air to enter it, as otherwise the nipple is liable to collapse. After the feeding the infant should be held erect for a few seconds to allow swallowed air to be brought up. The infant should be able to empty the bottle in from ten to twenty minutes. Any milk left over must be thrown away at once.

After feeding the bottles should be washed with a solution of borax or of washing soda, scrubbed with a bottle brush and finally filled with a solution of borax and stoppered with cotton or a cork. Just before filling with the food all the bottles for the day should be emptied, washed, and boiled for five minutes. The funnel, graduate and other utensils needed should, if possible, be boiled each day with the bottles. The nipples immediately after use should be scrubbed thoroughly both inside and outside, turning them inside out for this purpose. They are then kept in a boric acid solution.

Concentrated Feeding.—Concentrated foods of different types are often employed in infant-feeding. A number of these are mentioned elsewhere, among them the Czerny-Kleinschmidt butter-flour mixture (p. 115), thick cereal-gruels (p. 112), lactic acid milks (p. 104), the egg-pudding food of Moll and Stransky and others (p. 114) and Keller's malt-soup (p. 113). Finkelstein's casein-milk (p. 108) is also to be considered as a concentrated food, especially when twice the usual amount of curds is added, as well as sometimes 10 per cent or more of sugar, as is done on occasions. Foods of even higher caloric value have been recommended, and under certain conditions are serviceable. Helmreich and Schick[40] have used a mixture approximately twice the caloric value of milk, which is denominated *Dubo*. This consists of whole milk to which has been added 17 per cent of sugar, the two being mixed and boiled for one minute. In a later publication Schick[41] recommends the addition to breast-milk of from 8.5 to 17 per cent of saccharose. He found this especially useful in premature infants in whom it is difficult to obtain the required calories from the amount of ordinary breast-milk which they can be made to ingest. In the absence of breast-milk, whole cow's milk with sugar may be tried, often with good results.

The *indications* for concentrated feeding are in complementing breast-feedings; in vomiting of a nervous type or due to pyloric stenosis and pylorospasm or to pertussis; in malnutrition without definite digestive disturbance; in anorexia of nervous or other origin or due to infections; in increased intracranial pressure; or in prematurity or other conditions where, from feebleness or other cause, there is difficulty in obtaining the ingestion of a sufficient number of calories. This form of feeding is sometimes of value in the exudative diathesis and in eczema of the moist type. The high caloric value of these foods makes it possible to give them in small quantity and at infrequent intervals, and the tolerance of the digestive tract for them is often great. They should be regarded as temporary foods, only to be used when there are distinct indications, and to be discontinued after a few weeks. They are usually contraindicated in hot weather and where there is evidence of indigestion. When they are employed, the fluid intake may be kept up by the administration of water between feedings, unless it is desired to use the diminished amount of water as a therapeutic measure, as in pleural effusion, enuresis, edema or increased intracranial pressure.

Whey.—This consists of milk from which the casein has been removed by the use of rennet although the lactalbumin remains. The amount of fat is diminished very greatly, being entangled in the curd which the rennet produces. Whey is prepared as follows: Into a quart of warm, fresh milk, heated to 100 F. (37.8 C.) are stirred 2 teaspoonfuls of liquid rennet or of essence of pepsin. After coagulation has taken place the milk is placed in the cold for about one-half hour, the curd then broken up with a fork in order to liberate the whey, and the latter strained through cheese-cloth or muslin without pressure. There will be obtained from 1 to 1½ pints of whey. The finer-meshed and thicker the cloth the more fat will be removed by it. When it is desired to produce a whey containing very little fat, a fat-free, separator milk or the milk from a quart jar after the cream has been removed should be employed. Failure to coagulate firmly indicates that not enough rennet was used or that the milk had been boiled previously or was too cold. If whey is to be mixed later with milk or cream, the rennin remaining in it must be destroyed by heating it for some time to a temperature of 140 F. (60 C.) or over (pasteurizing), otherwise the casein of the cream will coagulate. If it is heated to 167 F. (75 C.) coagulation of the lactalbumin begins. Various analyses of whey have been made. The average of many of them, according to the figures of König,[42] is as follows: Fat 0.32 per cent; sugar 4.83; whey-protein 0.85; salts 0.64; water 93.36. Later analyses have given the whey-protein as high as 1.0 per cent.

Whey-cream Mixtures.—Whey was for many years a favorite food for cases of weak digestion, either given for a brief period, alone except for the addition of cane-sugar, or combined with small amounts of cream. Later, with increasing confidence in the digestibility of casein, the use of whey has been neglected and even condemned, on the ground that the whey-protein was injurious in many cases of digestive disturbance. Although the need for whey-combinations is comparatively infrequent, yet there are numerous instances especially in early infancy when they are of undoubted benefit. In fact, the whey is the element which contains the bulk of the necessary amino-acids, the casein being very deficient in these. If it is desired to construct a whey-cream mixture in which the percentage of fat shall be high and that of casein very low richer creams must be employed, following the percentage calculations in Table 39.

Peptonized Milk.—For infants with feeble digestion the pancreatizing of the milk before it enters the alimentary canal was formerly much used and was sometimes of benefit. This is usually accomplished by the action on the milk of the trypsin derived from the pancreatic juice of the pig, which partially digests the casein before it is ingested and prevents the formation of tough coagula. As the pancreatic extract requires the presence of an alkali in order to act, it is commonly sold combined with bicarbonate of soda, in the form of a powder in individual glass tubes. The pancreatizing is accomplished by dissolving the contents of 1 tube in 2 oz. of cool water and adding to 1 pint of cool milk; and then allowing the vessel containing the mixture to stand in hot water of a temperature of not over 115 F. (46 C.), *i. e.*, as warm as the finger can bear without discomfort. It may remain here for twenty or thirty minutes, or a shorter time if the slightest bitter taste is discovered, and is then quickly cooled and kept on ice, or, better, heated quickly to boiling. The temperature of boiling destroys the trypsin and prevents further peptonization, thus avoiding the development of the bitter taste. In this connection it is interesting to note that Bessau, Rosenbaum and Liechtentritt[43] have shown by repeated experiments that if the peptonizing is done by pepsin instead of pancreatin, the length of time that the milk remains in the stomach is shortened by 25 per cent.

Acid-milks.—The reasons for the use of buttermilk and other lactic acid milks are detailed in another place (p. 105). Theoretically they assist in the maintenance of optimum acidity for digestion, mineral absorption and enzyme-action. Perhaps more important is the fact that all of them are so prepared that they allow small, fine curd-formation, and that they have a high caloric value. The acid-milks are widely employed for the feeding of both well and sick infants. (See p. 106.) There are several powdered lactic acid milks which are so prepared by the manufacturers that they may be diluted with water in the proportion of about 1 level tablespoonful of the powder to 2 oz. of water and are then ready for use. (Table 16, p. 117.)

Buttermilk.—The term "buttermilk" is properly applied to the milk which remains after the butter-fat has been removed by churning. Its employment for the feeding of infants with delicate digestion, for many years widely followed in Holland, appears to have been first urged upon the profession by Ballot[44] in 1865. Renewed attention was directed to it by the writings of de Jager,[45] Salge,[46] Teixeira de Mattos,[47] and, later, by many others. The composition of buttermilk varies according to different published analyses, and depends to some extent upon whether made from whole sweet milk, sweet cream, or sour cream. By all methods the fat-percentage is low, that of the protein rather high, and that of the sugar more or less reduced. The approximate percentage analysis is fat, 0.5–1.0; sugar, 0.3–4.0; protein 2.5–4.0. Buttermilk is always distinctly acid from the development in it of lactic acid and contains usually about 0.5 per cent of this. The caloric value is between 300 and 400 calories per liter (284 and 379 per quart), being little if any stronger than skimmed milk. Ordinary commercial buttermilk is hardly fit for use in infant-feeding, as it is liable to be contaminated by undesirable germs. It is best made carefully at home in the following manner: A quart or more of either whole milk or skimmed milk, as fresh and clean as possible, is pasteurized and placed in a clean vessel. After the addition of a culture of lactic-acid bacilli it is allowed to stand for eighteen to twenty-four hours at a temperature of about 100 F. (37.8 C.) until softly curdled. The Bulgarian bacillus cultures have been most often employed, but other lactic acid germs may be used, including the bacillus acidophilus (see p. 106). Since there are a number of cultures on the market, many of which have little value for the purpose, an active variety should be selected. An ounce or two of the buttermilk of the day before may be transferred to the quart of milk instead of using the pure culture, but this should not be continued for more than a week without a fresh start with a pure lactic acid bacillus culture, since contamination with other organisms may take place. If whole milk has been used it is then churned energetically for twenty to thirty minutes in a small glass churn, the butter removed, and the buttermilk kept on ice until wanted. If skimmed milk was employed the curd may simply be beaten with a fork and rubbed through a fine sieve in order to break it up. Prepared from whole milk without churning its final percentage is similar to that of the milk employed. With skimmed milk the fat percentage is naturally reduced. The living lactic-acid germs present are considered serviceable in some digestive disturbances where it is desired to destroy by their growth the proteolytic bacteria. When only the chemical action of the buttermilk is desired, boiling will destroy the germs. Boiling, however, curdles the casein into large masses, unless vigorous stirring is used to prevent this.

Buttermilk-mixture.—To increase the strength of buttermilk the usual custom is to add wheat-flour and cane-sugar. The preparation may be made in the following manner, somewhat after the proportions recommended by Teixeira de Mattos.[47] One level tablespoonful ($\frac{1}{4}$ oz.) of wheat, rice or other flour is rubbed into a paste with 6 to 8 oz. of a quart of buttermilk, and $4\frac{1}{2}$ level tablespoonfuls ($2\frac{1}{4}$ oz.) of granulated sugar are added. This is then mixed with the remainder of the quart and the whole boiled for twenty-five minutes, with constant stirring. If it is desired to preserve the germs alive, the flour and sugar are boiled in the 8 oz. of buttermilk in a double boiler, and then when cool added to the remaining buttermilk. The advantages of the buttermilk-mixture depend upon its acid content, its relatively high caloric value (560 to 660 calories per quart (592 to 697 per liter)), and its fine curd formation.

Lactic-acid Milk.—Lactic-acid milk is a term which might conveniently be limited usually to whole milks prepared in some manner other than by churning, yet containing lactic acid. Whole milk buttermilk should properly be inserted here. Koumiss and Matzoon are of this class in that they contain lactic acid.

Marriott[48] advocated for athreptic infants the use of undiluted lactic acid milk to which corn-syrup had been added. The lactic-acid milk is prepared as in the making of buttermilk. The corn-syrup used is an ordinary commercial variety. Forty-five volumes of the syrup may be mixed with 55 volumes of water, this mixture containing about 50 per cent carbohydrate. This thinned syrup in the quantity desired is added to the lactic-acid milk, and after slight agitation of the mixture by stirring it is put into the refrigerator until it is to be used. It is advisable to begin with a mixture of equal parts of whole lactic-acid milk and fat-free lactic-acid milk or, in the case of infants convalescing from diarrhea, fat-free lactic-acid milk alone. The proportion of whole lactic-acid milk is then increased until no skimmed milk is being used. The addition of the syrup is then begun, 3 per cent of carbohydrate being added at first; and if no diarrhea occurs the percentage of carbohydrate is gradually increased up to 10 per cent or over, *i. e.*, from 1 to 3 oz. of corn syrup may be used to the quart. The number of ounces of the mixture used should be approximately the same as if any other milk were being employed.

Another form of lactic-acid milk is that recommended by Shaw and Williams[49] in which the lactic acid is produced by spontaneous souring. Fresh whole milk is poured into a bowl, covered with cheese-cloth and allowed to sour for two days in a warm room until it thickens like junket. It is then churned in a small glass butter-churn for several minutes. A heaping tablespoonful of sugar and one of flour for each quart of milk are added and the whole boiled for five minutes while stirring. This acid milk is used without dilution. Hamburger[50] had previously stated that milk which had been spontaneously soured by the heat of summer could be utilized by mixing with flour and sugar and then boiling.

Acidophilus-milk.—This has of recent years become a very popular form of lactic-acid milk, both for infants and older subjects. In its preparation fermentation is produced by the bacillus acidophilus in place of the bacillus Bulgaricus. This organism, which was isolated both by Moro[51] and Finkelstein,[52] is a normal inhabitant of the intestinal tract of man. In health and in the absence of intestinal putrefaction it is found in large numbers in the stools, and may be increased by feeding milk or lactose (Hull and Rettger[53]). If it is desired rapidly to transform the intestinal flora so that the bacillus acidophilus predominates, milk which has been fermented with the organism may be fed. The ingestion of tablets or broth-cultures of the organism is not very effective; certainly not to the same extent as the feeding of acidophilus-milk itself, since this contains so many more viable organisms. (See p. 105.) The preparation of acidophilus-milk is described by Rettger and Cheplin[54] as follows: Cow's milk is sterilized by boiling. A liter (1.056 quarts) of milk should be heated for from about twenty-two to twenty-four minutes. After cooling to at least 37 C. (98.6 F.) it is inoculated with pure strains of bacillus acidophilus, and is then kept at a temperature of 35–37 C. (95–986. F.) for twenty-four hours. Viable milk-cultures are used as the inoculum, at least 10 cc. of which are transferred for each liter of milk treated (0.3 fl. oz. per quart).

Acidophilus-milk may be used in infancy in the same conditions in which lactic-acid milk, prepared in other ways, would be employed. It is also serviceable in correcting constipation and in the treatment of colitis. Feeding acidophilus-milk is a valuable adjunct in the treatment of typhoid fever (Torrey[55]) and a trial of it is indicated in chronic intestinal indigestion.

Lactic-acid Milk U.S.P.—For the sake of distinguishing clearly, this term may be applied to the food described by Marriott and Davidson[56] which possesses distinct advantages. As later modified by Marriott[57] the preparation is as follows: Cow's milk is boiled for five minutes, thoroughly cooled, and the skin removed. U.S.P. lactic acid is now dropped in slowly while stirring, in the proportion of $\frac{3}{4}$ dram (3 cc.) to each pint (473 cc.) of milk. This milk keeps well even if not refrigerated. It is claimed that dilution of the milk is not usually necessary even in new-born or premature infants. Corn-syrup is added to the mixture, using 1 fl. oz. to the day's mixture for infants up to two weeks of age and from $1\frac{1}{2}$–2 oz. for older infants. If equal amounts of water and the syrup are mixed with the acid, such a solution may be added directly to the milk without the formation of large curds. Nelson[58] found that infants fed with undiluted whole cow's milk with lactic acid added, retained more calcium and phosphorus, had a higher blood phosphorus than infants receiving diluted milk, and exhibited the blood calcium at the high limit of normal.

When evaporated milk is used the following simple method is described by Marriott[57]: 3 oz. (89 cc.) of corn-syrup are mixed with some water, about 1 teaspoonful (5 cc.) of U.S.P. lactic acid is added and the whole is made up by adding water to a volume of 1 pint (473 cc.). This pint of stock solution is added to an equal volume of evaporated milk.

Hydrochloric-acid Milk.—Faber[59] who has studied the pH of the gastric contents also believes in the addition of acid to milk-mixtures. Twenty-five cc. (0.84 fl. oz.) of tenth-normal hydrochloric acid are added to each 100 cc. (3.38 fl. oz.) of milk used. The milk is boiled before the addition of the acid. Mixtures with fairly high fat-percentages are necessary to obtain the best results. Marriott and Davidson[60] prefer lactic acid because it is an organic acid, believing that hydrochloric acid can be added safely only in limited amounts, inasmuch as it is an inorganic acid and must be eliminated. This throws a strain on the acid-base regulating mechanism and leads to an acidosis. Greene[62] claims that hydrochloric acid in the amounts used may in small infants cause the appearance of casts and red blood cells in the urine. According to Faber[61] organic as well as inorganic acids deflect metabolism from the normal, and for this reason acid-milks of any type should not be used routinely, but only on specific indication.

Vinegar-milk.—Dunham[63] recommends the employment of vinegar instead of other acids for making an acid-milk, as a rule adding 1 oz. of vinegar to each 15 oz. of cow's milk. This gives a pH of about 4.2.

Lemon-juice Milk.—Hess and Matzner[64] have found that the addition of lemon juice to milk in the proportion of about $\frac{3}{4}$ oz. (22 cc.) to the quart of milk will reduce the buffer-action in the same manner as the addition of lactic acid. The pH of the mixture will vary from about 5.54 to 5.30; the latter figure when diluted milk is used instead of whole milk. The lemon-juice is added to the diluent and then stirred into the milk, or it may be added drop by drop to the undiluted milk. The amount of lemon-juice employed is also sufficient to act as an antiscorbutic. If desired the yolk of one egg may be added to the quart of mixture, in this way furnishing the antirachitic factor and iron. Lemon-juice milk may also be made with evaporated milk, using 1 teaspoonful of lemon-juice for each ounce of the milk.

Citric-acid Milk.—Gonce and Templeton[65] recommend an acid-milk prepared as follows: 4 Gm. (60 grains) of dehydrated citric acid is added to a quart of milk which has been boiled for five minutes and cooled to room temperature. It is not necessary to add the citric acid slowly.

Casein-milk.—(Eiweiss-milk. Protein-milk. Albumin-milk.) Although not a translation of the German title "Eiweissmilch," applied by Finkelstein and Meyer,[66] the title "Casein-milk" would appear to express well the nature of the food. The percentage-composition averages approximately, fat, 2.5; lactose 1.5; protein 3.0; salts 0.5. The caloric value is about 450 per liter (426 per quart). A little saccharin may be used for sweetening if necessary. The formula was based on the belief that the sugar and the salts of the food are the most dangerous elements in many diseased conditions. By diminishing the amounts of these the fat is rendered more easily digestible. Later, after the digestion of the infant has improved, the percentage of sugar is raised by the addition of a maltose-dextrin combination. Although the truth of the original theories which led to the production of casein-milk has repeatedly been disproved, and so admitted by Finkelstein, the fact remains that the preparation is one of very great value, particularly in many diarrheal disturbances in infancy.

The preparation of casein-milk is rather difficult and requires close attention to details: One quart of whole-milk is heated to about 100 F. (37.8 C.), ½ oz. of liquid rennet or essence of pepsin added, and the milk then allowed to stand at this temperature in a water-bath for half an hour, by which time it will have been curdled. The mass is then put upon a fine cloth and the whey strained off without pressing, about an hour being allowed for this. The curd is then rubbed through a very fine wire sieve, using the bowl of a spoon to do the rubbing, 1 pint of water being used in the process; and this sieving repeated 4 or 5 times, using the same water and later adding if necessary enough to preserve the original volume. To the pint thus obtained 1 pint of buttermilk is added. The whole is then sterilized by boiling vigorously, and constantly stirring during the process in order to prevent clumping.

Owing to the difficulty in preparing casein-milk various commercial substitutes are used. These are prepared by mixing in the proportion of 1 oz. (about 3½ tablespoonfuls) to 11 oz. of warm water, by which the formula of the original casein-milk as recommended by Finkelstein is approximately obtained. Table 43 shows the relative compositions of these preparations.

TABLE 43.—ANALYSES OF COMMERCIAL CASEIN MILKS AND CASEIN PREPARATIONS[1]

	Protein, per cent.	Fat, per cent.	Lactose, per cent.	Salts, per cent.	Ash, per cent.	Moisture, per cent.	Lactic acid, per cent.
Hoos's albumin milk	38.5	30.2	21.5	......	5.0	2.0	3.0
Mead-Johnson's powdered protein milk	39.0	26.5	24.0	......	6.0	1.5	3.0
Merrell-Soule powdered protein milk	37.0	27.0	23.0	......	9.25	3.0	3.0
Merrell-Soule powdered boilable protein milk	38.0	28.0	25.0	......	6.0	3.0	0.75
Casec	88.0	2.0	....	......	4.5	5.5	
Larosan	88.7	2.3	....	......	4.0	5.0	
Protolac	83.65	0.6	....	3.23+	....	4.85	

[1] Analyses from Manufacturer's statement or from reports of Committee on Foods of the A.M.A.

The last three substances in the table represent the composition of certain soluble casein-flours. The addition of approximately ⅓ oz. (about 4 level tablespoonfuls) of any of these to each 32 oz. of the mixture would raise the protein percentage approximately 1 per cent.

REFERENCES

1. Jahrb. f. Kinderh., 1923, **102,** 257; **103,** 51. 2. Wien. klin. Wchnschr., 1924, **37,** 568. 3. München. med. Wchnschr., 1922, **69,** 1220. 4. Arch. Pediat., 1921, **38,** 584. 5. Am. J. Dis. Child., 1931, **42,** 726. 6. Am. J. Dis. Child., 1914, **7,** 298. J. Biol. Chem., 1913, **14,** 203. 7. Am. J. Dis. Child., 1921, **22,** 193; 613. 8. Hygienic Laboratory Bulletin, 1912, No. 56, 648. 9. Arch. Pediat., 1917, **34,** 81. 10. J. Biol. Chem., 1922, **51,** 165. 11. Phys. Chem., 4th Ed., 1904, pp. 455; 460. 12. Ztschr. f. Biol., 1874, **10,** 309. 13. Am. J. Dis. Child., 1923, **26,** 542. 14. J. Biol. Chem., 1918, **34,** 537. 15. Am. J. Dis. Child., 1919, **18,** 546. 16. J. Biol. Chem., 1920, **45,** 229. 17. J.A.M.A., 1931, **97,** 370. 18. Hygienic Laboratory Bulletin, 1912, No. 56, 429. 19. Hygienic Laboratory Bulletin, 1912, No. 56, 684. 20. Dept. Agric. Pa. Bull., No. 125. 21. Ann. Rep. Health Dept. Baltimore, 1898; Ref. No. 21, Bergey. 22. Am. J. Dis. Child., 1913, **6,** 225. 23. New York M. J., 1899, **70,** 657. 24. Dis. Nutrit. and Inf. Feed., 1920, 230. 25. Arch. f. d. ges. Physiol., 1894, **56,** 577. 26. Untersuch. u. d. chem. Unterschiede d. Menschen-u. Kuhmilch, Inaug. Dissert., Giessen, 1869. 27. Am. J. M. Sc., 1858, **36,** 25; Food for Babies, 1859. 28. Brit. M. J., 1902, Sept. 6, p. 653. 29. New York M. J., 1898, Mar. 12, p. 345. 30. Griffith, J.A.M.A., 1918, **71,** 441. 31. Ztschr. f. diat. u. physikal. Therapie, 1901, **5,** 13. 32. Am. J. Dis. Child., 1930, **39,** 701. 33. Arch. Pediat., 1912, **29,** 123. 34. Dis. of Child., 1916, p. 181. 35. System der Ernährung, 1917; An Outline of the Pirquet System of Nutrition, 1922. 36. J.A.M.A., 1921, **78,** 1541. 37. Am. J. Dis. Child., 1923, **25,** 339. 38. Med. Rec., 1892, **42,** 8; Arch. Pediat., 1896, **13,** 595; J.A.M.A., 1907, **49,** 1740. 39. Arch. Pediat., 1893, **10,** 97. 40. Ztschr. f. Kinderh., 1921, **30,** 121; 147; 363. 41. Arch. Pediat., 1925, **42,** 397. 42. Chemie der menschlichen Nahrungs-u. Genussmittel, 1903, **1,** 389. 43. Jahrb. f. Kinderh., 1921, **95,** 123. 44. Nederl. tijdschr. v. Geneesk., 1865, **2,** 402. 45. Nederl. tijdschr. v. Geneesk., 1895, **31,** 679. 46. Jahrb. f. Kinderh., 1901, **54,** 681. 47. Jahrb. f. Kinderh., 1902, **55,** 1. 48. J.A.M.A., 1919, **73,** 1173. 49. Arch. Pediat., 1922, **39,** 516. 50. München. med. Wchnschr., 1919, **16,** 557. 51. Wien. klin. Wchnschr., 1900, **14,** 114. 52. Deutsche med. Wchnschr., 1900, **26,** 263. 53. J. Bact., 1917, **2,** 47. 54. Arch. Int. Med., 1922, **29,** 357. 55. J. Infect. Dis., 1915, **16,** 72. 56. J.A.M.A., 1923, **81,** 2007. 57. J.A.M.A., 1927, **89,** 862. 58. Am. J. Dis. Child., 1931, **31,** 1090. 59. Am. J. Dis. Child., 1923, **26,** 401. 60. Am. J. Dis. Child., 1923, **26,** 542. 61. Am. J. Dis. Child., 1926, **31,** 395. 62. Am. J. Dis. Child., 1928, **35,** 38. 63. Am. J. Dis. Child., 1925, **29,** 200. 64. J.A.M.A., 1924, **82,** 1604. 65. Am. J. Dis. Child., 1930, **39,** 265. 66. Berl. klin. Wchnschr., 1910, **47,** 1165. Jahrb. f. Kinderh., 1910, **71,** 525. München. med. Wchnschr., 1911, **58,** 340.

CHAPTER V

FOODS OTHER THAN MILK. SPECIAL NAMED MIXTURES. PROPRIETARY FOODS

In the present chapter will be considered merely the character and uses of certain foods, independently of any special age-limit for their employment.

PROTEIN-FOODS

It happens constantly that some animal substance other than milk is needed as a temporary substitute during illness in the first year; or as a more permanent article of diet then or after this period. The following may be mentioned:

Albumen-water.—This consists of the white of one egg stirred in enough cool water to make 8 oz., and strained if necessary. It is an excellent temporary substitute for milk in acute cases of failure of digestion, but a very weak one, containing about 1.3 per cent protein. The possibility of it being directly absorbed as a foreign protein when intestinal disturbance is present is not to be forgotten. A sensitization to egg might be produced in this way. Albumen-water may be given cool or slightly warm, with or without sugar or with a pinch of salt, and from a glass or a bottle according to the taste and fancy of the infant. It may be flavored with a few drops of lemon or orange juice or with whiskey.

Fresh Beef-juice.—This may best be prepared in either of two methods:

1. Season with salt and very slightly broil a piece of steak free from fat, then cut it into small pieces and express the juice with a meat-press. A lemon-squeezer may be used instead, but this method is more wasteful. A pound of beef will make about 2 or 3 fl. oz. of juice. The juice must be kept on ice until needed. It may then be warmed slightly or given cold with a spoon. Some infants prefer it with the addition of sugar.

2. A pound of minced steak is put into 6 or 8 oz. of water, salted slightly, and allowed to stand on ice over night. It is then squeezed out well with the meat-press, or is strained through muslin by twisting tightly. Juice thus obtained is somewhat thinner and weaker than by the first method, but is decidedly larger in quantity.

By ten months of age beef-juice may constitute a part of the daily food for a healthy infant, if so desired, 2 or 3 tablespoonfuls being allowed daily. The caloric value is about 8 to the ounce. The opinion that beef juice is high in iron content is not supported by the facts, inasmuch as this is considerably less than in equivalent portions of several of the vegetables, as well as in other proteins such as egg-yolk (see Anemia, p. 1025). Beef-juice is a proper article of diet, however, because of its amino-acid content. It should not be employed as an exclusive diet, but may be alternated with albumen-water or cereal decoctions in cases where it is desired to avoid milk for a time.

Minced Underdone Beef.—A thick piece of underdone steak, as free from fat and connective tissue as possible, is scraped, grated, or minced very fine; pounded to a pulp in a mortar, and seasoned with salt. For infants it may now be rubbed up with a little water to the consistency of thick cream and fed from a spoon, giving 3 or 4 teaspoonfuls in the course of the day.

Scraped beef is a very concentrated form of nitrogenous food, sometimes useful even in subjects less than one year of age. In the second year 1 or 2 tablespoonfuls without water may be given daily. (See p. 125.) We have more than once seen tape-worm develop from the use of raw beef given in this way, but the danger may be avoided entirely by the slight broiling referred to.

Meat-broths.—Foods of this class are of practically no value as actual nourishment, if of the class of "clear broth." They are sometimes of benefit during the first year as a temporary substitute for milk-mixtures, and in the second year may be one of the ordinary articles of diet. Broths should not be given in amounts which by mere bulk impair the appetite for other and more nutritious foods. The principles and method of preparation are the same for all, and the following description for making beef-broth applies to the others: 1 lb. of lean meat is cut into small pieces, and these, together with portions of the cracked bones, put into 1 pint of cold water. This is heated very slowly, allowing it to simmer for three or four hours and replacing the water as it evaporates; and is then strained, cooled and the fat removed. The strainer used should be coarse enough to allow of the finely divided muscle-fiber passing through, as this increases the nutritive value very decidedly. The addition of a cereal flour also adds to the value as a food.

Beef-tea.—This may be prepared as follows: (1) Scrape or cut fine 1 lb. of lean meat and place it with some bone in 1 pint of cold water in a jar. Let it stand in the cold for one hour, stirring occasionally. Then heat the jar in a saucepan of water at not over 167 F. (75 C.) for another hour, stirring occasionally. It should then be raised to the boiling point for a moment, strained, cooled and the fat removed. Warm slightly and season before giving it. In place of straining, the liquid may be simply poured off.

To this should be added the additional liquid obtained by firmly pressing the pieces of meat which remain. (2) Another more rapid method is the following: Place the pound of meat in ½ pint of boiling water. Keep this gently warm for ten minutes; strain; cool rapidly and remove the fat.

Beef-tea is distinguished from beef-broth particularly by the considerable amount of gelatin contained in the latter. This is derived from the prolonged boiling of the bones and of the connective tissue. Beef-tea has little nutritive value, about 3 calories to the ounce, and practically none at all if sufficient heat has been used to coagulate the protein, and if this has been removed by straining.

Gelatin.—Commercial gelatin has approximately 86 per cent protein and contains practically no fat or sugar. There are about 4 level tablespoonfuls of gelatin to the ounce (28 Gm.; containing 24 Gm. of protein and equal to 98 calories), and this amount may be added to the day's mixture. The gelatin is soaked for a short time in cold water and then dissolved in ½ pint of boiling water. It was a popular addition to milk-mixtures in former years and its mechanical action is quite similar to that of cereal decoctions. Chemically it is an incomplete protein and is lacking in certain of the amino-acids, and consequently it should always be given with other proteins.

Soy-bean Flour.—This substance may be properly classed among protein-foods serviceable for temporary use when, for any reason, the protein of milk is not desired. According to Ruhräh[1] the flour contains over 44 per cent of protein. A combination of it with olive oil, barley flour, sodium chloride and calcium carbonate was designed by Hill and Stuart[2] to give, when mixed with water, percentages of fat 2.8, carbohydrate 4 and protein 4.2. The food has been put on the market commercially under the name of Sobee and is further mentioned in the table on p. 120.

AMYLACEOUS FOODS

The employment of starchy food in the first year has repeatedly been referred to (see pp. 93; 105; etc.). Although the power of digesting it is present in early infancy, there is no need for the administration of starch to the healthy, normal, artificially fed infant during the early part of the first year. Its addition to the diet by the age of five or six months is usually advantageous in order to accustom the child to it. In the case of illness, however, weak or stronger amylaceous additions or substitutions are often of the greatest value, and this is particularly true when there is difficulty in the digestion of sugar. Starch is also useful to prevent the casein from forming tough coagula.

The Weight of Various Carbohydrate Substances.—In the making of amylaceous decoctions in the home, measuring by bulk is usually the only method which can be employed; but for better knowledge it is necessary to know the weight also, in order to estimate the percentages obtained. Tablespoons are the measure oftenest used, but as these vary so much in size, it is better to employ the Chapin dipper (p. 88) or other ounce-measure. We have made a series of weighings, with the results shown in the table on p. 112.

The figures can be only average ones, especially as regards the weight of the tablespoonful. Barley and oat flours are slightly lighter, and rice and wheat flours slightly heavier than the figures given. In measuring, the tablespoon or the dipper should be filled from a smaller spoon, tapped sharply 2 or 3 times, and the excess scraped off with a case-knife. Too much tapping settles the contents too greatly. Casein-flour is included in the table as a convenience.

Table 44.—Approximate Weights of Grains, Flours and Sugars (Measured by Tablespoon and by Fl.-oz. Dipper)

One level tablespoonful of barley or other flour weighs about $\frac{1}{4}$ oz. Av.
One level dipper of barley or other flour weighs about $\frac{1}{2}$ oz. Av.
One level tablespoonful of Bermuda arrowroot weighs about $\frac{2}{5}$ oz. Av.
One level dipper of Bermuda arrowroot weighs about $\frac{4}{5}$ oz. Av.
One level tablespoonful of pearl barley weighs about $\frac{1}{2}$ oz. Av.
One level dipper of pearl barley weighs about $\frac{3}{4}$ oz. Av.
One level tablespoonful of rice weighs about $\frac{1}{2}$ oz. Av.
One level dipper of rice weighs about $\frac{4}{5}$ oz. Av.
One level tablespoonful of rolled oats weighs about $\frac{1}{6}$ oz. Av.
One level dipper of rolled oats weighs about $\frac{1}{3}$ oz. Av.
One level tablespoonful of lactose weighs about $\frac{1}{3}$ oz. Av.
One level dipper of lactose weighs about $\frac{3}{4}$ oz. Av.
One level tablespoonful of dextrin-maltose weighs about $\frac{1}{4}$ oz. Av.
One level dipper of dextrin-maltose weighs about $\frac{1}{2}$ oz. Av.
One level tablespoonful of saccharose weighs about $\frac{1}{2}$ oz. Av.
One level dipper of saccharose weighs about 1 oz. Av.
One level tablespoonful of casein-flour weighs about $\frac{1}{4}$ oz. Av.
One level dipper of casein-flour weighs about $\frac{1}{2}$ oz. Av.

Amylaceous Gruels. Porridges and Decoctions.—There is little difference in the strength of the various cereal preparations, the usual one for the porridges being about 4 level tablespoonfuls to the pint. If in any greater strength they should have prolonged cooking in a double boiler. The composition of all the amylaceous preparations, with slight variations, may be calculated on the basis that 1 level tablespoon ($\frac{1}{4}$ oz.) to the quart of water yields a protein percentage of about 0.12, and of carbohydrate about 0.6. The fat and mineral content may be ignored for practical purposes. For those who fear vitamin deficiency a valuable preparation has been suggested by Tisdall, Drake and Brown.[3] This is now on the market under the name of Mead's cereal. It consists of wheat flour, oatmeal, corn meal, wheat germ, bone meal, dried brewers' yeast, and alfalfa, and is irradiated by ultraviolet rays and contains vitamins A, B_1, B_2, E, and the antirachitic factor. Its percentage composition is fat 3, carbohydrate 71.8, and protein 15; and it is rich in calcium, iron, phosphorus and copper. Most of the whole wheat cereals such as Ralston's Food, Wheatena, Pettijohn's and the like, contain vitamin B complex.

Various thinner starchy decoctions fill a useful place for different purposes:

Barley-water may be most conveniently made from barley-flour, 1 level tablespoonful being cooked slowly for fifteen minutes in 1 pint of water, strained, and any water evaporated then replaced. Its nutritive value is little, but it is an excellent temporary substitute for milk in cases of acute indigestion. It is also often used as a diluent for milk-mixtures. It should be made fresh every day and kept on ice.

Oatmeal-water may be made by putting 2 level tablespoonfuls of oatmeal into 1 pint of water and letting it simmer for two hours or more, replacing the water as it evaporates, and finally straining. It may be employed as a diluent for milk-mixtures. It is distinctly laxative in many children, and in many cases disagrees decidedly.

Farina-water may be made and used in the same way as barley-water, but it produces a somewhat thicker decoction.

Rice-water is of the same strength as barley-water, using 1 tablespoonful of the flour or 2 of washed rice to the pint. It is supposed to have a constipating effect.

Arrowroot-water, although not a cereal substance, is useful under the same conditions as is barley-water, and is made in the same manner, but using $1\frac{1}{2}$ level tablespoonfuls to the pint. Both it and rice-water consist almost entirely of starch and are poor in proteins.

Malt-soup.—The preparation was first made and urged by Liebig,[4] but was later modified by Keller[5] and came rapidly into prominence as a serviceable form of nourishment for a certain class of sick infants. Its value rests on the fact that a large percentage of unconverted starch, together with maltose and dextrin, is present in the food. The method of preparation as commonly advised is as follows:

1. $1\frac{3}{4}$ oz. Av. ($6\frac{1}{2}$ level tablespoonfuls) of wheat-flour are mixed with 11 fl. oz. of cold cow's milk and rubbed through a sieve.
2. $2\frac{1}{2}$ fl. oz. of malt-soup extract are added to 22 fl. oz. of warm water.

The two are then added one to the other and the whole heated slowly to boiling, with constant stirring, and enough water finally added to replace that which has evaporated. The malt-soup extract should contain 7 grains of carbonate of potash to the fluidounce, the object of this being to alkalinize it and thus to limit its diastatic action, and also, according to Keller, to prevent the development of any acidosis in the infant. The caloric value of this mixture is about 625 calories per quart (660 per liter). Most of the malt-soup extracts on the market already contain the alkali; but any which are nondiastatic may be used if potassium carbonate is added in the amount mentioned. The formula given produces percentages of approximately fat 1.33, carbohydrate 11.4, protein 1.58, varying somewhat with the preparation of malt-soup extract used. It is not, however, necessary to use these amounts, and malt-soup may be prepared in various strengths.

Liquid and powdered malt-soup extracts, the latter with or without the addition of wheat-flour, may be obtained on the market. The dry, powdered forms are convenient to prepare, especially those to which flour has been added. The following table contains analyses of both liquid and dry malt soup extracts, the figures given being those of the manufacturers.

TABLE 45.—MALT SOUP PREPARATIONS

	Water, per cent.	Protein, per cent.	Maltose, per cent.	Dextrin, per cent.	Starch, per cent.	Ash, per cent.	Mineral matter added, per cent.
Borcherdt's malt soup extract	21.79	6.4	57.57	11.7	....	2.54	1.1 potassium carbon.
Borcherdt's dri-malt soup extract	3.8	8.66	71.1	13.5	....	2.94	1.1 potassium carbon.
Borcherdt's dri-malt soup extract with wheat flour	2.3	8.2	46.8	9.4	31.1	2.2	....
Loeflund's malt soup stock	22.3	3.73	54.26	17.6	....	2.11	....
Mead's dry malt soup stock with wheat flour	5.0	....	47.0		46.5	....	1.0 potassium bicarb.

Flour-ball.—Flour-ball was formerly much employed as an addition to milk when a cereal was required. It is made by tying a pound of flour tightly in a bag and boiling for ten hours. When cold it is taken from the bag and completely dried with heat. The outer coating is then removed, and the remaining inner portion grated. One or 2 teaspoonfuls are added to each bottle. The advantage claimed for it was that the flour was partially dextrinized and thus rendered more soluble, requiring less cooking. Flour-ball in a prepared state may be obtained on the market under the trade name of Florena.

SPECIAL MIXTURES CHIEFLY WITH PERSONAL NAMES

There have been recommended a very large number of special mixtures to which are often attached the names of physicians first describing them. A few of these are mentioned below on account of the frequency with which the names are, or have been, met with in medical literature, not because of a desire especially to advocate them here. A further description of some of them will be found in the second edition of this book or in the references given below. Few of them have been employed to any extent in the United States, and some are now entirely out of vogue. Modern scientific pediatrics is opposed to the use of any one preparation as a routine feeding. Rather must the mixture be modified to meet the needs of the case. Powers[6] states that the analyses of many of the special mixtures used in infant feeding showed that they differed chiefly in the concentration or in the amount of dilution. Some of the preparations have indeed been manufactured and sold commercially, and would be more properly included in the next section.

Among the foods little employed at present are Backhaus'[7] Milk, Biedert's[8] Cream-Mixtures, Feer's[9] Milk-Preparation, Friedenthal's[10] Milk, Gärtner's[11] Mother-Milk, Hesse-Pfund[12] Infant's Food, Lehndorff and Zak's[13] Dialyzed Milk, Meig's[14] Gelatin-Food, Monti's[15] Whey-Milk, Schloss'[16] Modified Milk, Steffen's[17] Veal-Broth and Milk, Szekely's[18] Casein-Free Milk, Vigier's[19] Humanized Milk, Voltmer-Lahrmann's[20] Pancreatized Milk, von Dungern's[21] Renneted Milk.

Homogenization of Milk.—This has been employed in the production of a number of infant foods. The milk is minutely divided under high pressure. The fat-globules are thus rendered exceedingly small and the cream will no longer rise. Homogenized olive oil added to fat-free milk has been used by Ladd.[22] Homogenization is also employed in the making of synthetic milks. (See p. 116.)

Almond-meal Milk.—Almonds have been used in the preparation of some proprietary foods. As a home-made preparation Chapin[23] tried a combination of 100 Gm. (3.52 oz.) of finely ground almonds, covered with 200 cc. (6.76 fl. oz.) of water, allowing this to stand on ice over night, and then pressing out the liquid and adding 300 cc. (10.14 fl. oz.) more water. The percentage-composition of the food obtained equals fat 7.02, carbohydrate 1.2, protein 4.4, ash 0.55, water 86.74. A very similar preparation has been used with success by Raudnitz.[24] Moll[25] likewise employed almond-meal, combining it with whey. He has used it extensively and successfully as a temporary food in acute dyspeptic conditions, when it was desired to eliminate casein entirely. The whey is prepared by adding 4 to 5 Gm. (61.6 to 77.0 grains) of calcium lactate to 1 liter (33.8 oz.) of milk, boiling and filtering, and then adding from 3 to 5 per cent of rice-flour or corn-meal, and cane-sugar as desired up to 10 per cent. The almond-meal is made by soaking 150 Gm. (5.29 oz.) of almonds in cold water for from twelve to twenty-four hours, then grinding them in a mill with the gradual addition of 1 liter (33.8 oz.) of water and straining through a cloth. Equal parts of this and of the whey-preparation are mixed and boiled for five minutes. The prepared food contains percentages of fat 2.95, sugar 6.50, starch 1.5–2.5, protein 1.85, ash 0.45.

Sunflower-seed Milk.—Ribadeau-Dumas, Mathieu and Willemin[26] used sunflower seeds as a source of protein. Sodium chloride was added and it was found necessary to add also fruit juices, malt, and cod liver oil to the diet to make up for the deficiency of vitamins. No milk is employed in the usual mixture.

Poppy-seed Milk.—L. O. Finkelstein[27] employed a decoction of poppy seed with flour and sugar added. This may be mixed with buttermilk if desired.

Egg-pudding Diets.—Moll and Stransky[28] advise for cases of disordered digestion, spasmophilia, and diarrheal disease in infants over three months of age a so-called "milk-free pudding," which is free from casein, although containing whey. It is prepared as follows: 80 Gm. (2.7 oz.) of a finely bolted flour, 1 Gm. (15.4 grains) of salt, and ½ Gm. (7.7 grains) of baking soda are stirred in 200 Gm. (6.76 fl. oz.) of water. The yolk of an egg is then mixed with 40 Gm. (1.41 oz.) of sugar and added to the mixture. The white of an egg is now beaten into a snow and stirred in with the rest. The whole is next put into a pudding-dish which has been greased with butter and powdered with flour, and is cooked in a water-bath for one-half hour. When the child is to be fed, the pudding is rubbed through a sieve and mixed thoroughly with an equal part of whey. The caloric value of the food is about 750 calories per liter (709 per quart). Another food of this class, that devised by Stoeltzner,[29] consists of 10 Gm. (.35 oz.) of corn-flour and 0.5 liter (16.9 oz.) of water made into a gruel. To this are added 0.5 liter (16.9 oz.) of fresh milk and 60 Gm. (2.1 oz.) of sugar. The mixture is boiled and a beaten egg stirred into it. It is claimed that this egg-soup is useful in weak and premature infants.

Czerny-Kleinschmidt Butter-flour Mixture.—The use of this food was originally reported by Czerny and Kleinschmidt.[30] We[31] have employed it with success, as have many others. The boiled butter raises the fat percentage of the mixture, but the total volatile fatty-acid content is relatively low. In the actual process of preparation 20 Gm. (2½ level tablespoonfuls) of butter are placed in a pan and heated over a gentle fire until foaming takes place, and until any odor of volatile fatty acids present shall have disappeared. This requires from three to five minutes. Twenty Gm. (2½ level tablespoonfuls) of fine wheat-flour are then added and the mixture again boiled over a gentle fire with constant stirring until the mass becomes thin and of a brownish color (four or five minutes). Now 300 Gm. (10 fl. oz.) of warm water and 15 Gm. (1½ level tablespoonfuls) of sugar are added. The whole is again boiled and rubbed through a fine sieve. This may conveniently be called the "stock solution." For use it is mixed with the desired amount of previously boiled, cooled milk, and the whole kept cold until needed. The addition of salt is not necessary, as this is contained in the butter. For children under 3000 Gm. (6.6 lb.) in weight ⅓ milk is added to ⅔ of the butter-flour stock. For those of 3000 Gm. (6.6 lb.) or over ⅖ of milk and ⅗ of butter-flour stock are employed. Not more than 200 Gm. to the kilogram of body-weight (*i. e.*, about 3 fl. oz. to the pound) should be given daily, and usually smaller amounts than this are required, owing to the high caloric value of the food. The strength of the food may be diminished by reducing the amounts of butter, flour, or sugar, but in any manipulation the amounts of butter and flour should remain equal. The percentages and caloric value of butter-flour as usually employed follow:

	Fat, per cent.	Carbohydrate, per cent.	Protein, per cent.	Cal. per oz.
⅔ stock, ⅓ milk	4.6	8.2	1.5	24.6
⅗ stock, ⅖ milk	4.6	7.8	1.7	24.3

Butter-flour mixtures should not be used in advanced stages of malnutrition or when fever and diarrhea are present. Premature infants do well on it, but the amounts of butter and flour should be reduced to 15 Gm. each (about 2 level tablespoonfuls).

Many modifications of the butter-flour mixture have been recommended, among them more concentrated forms which Moro[32] uses and to which no water is added. One of these, for example, consists of 1 liter (about a quart) of whole milk, 30 Gm. (4 level tablespoonfuls) of flour, 50 Gm. (6 level tablespoonfuls) of butter and 70 Gm. (7 level tablespoonfuls) of sugar, and has approximately 9 per cent fat, 14 per cent carbohydrate, 4 per cent protein and 46.8 calories per ounce. Others have employed the boiled butter, adding it to skimmed milk with or without flour. In our own experience, the addition of flour is to be preferred.

Synthetic Milks.—The best known of these is that designed by Gerstenberger[33] and his colleagues. This, under the title of *Synthetic Milk Adapted* (*S.M.A.*) is a combination of various vegetable and animal fats, including cod liver oil, resulting in a fat very similar to that of human milk. Skimmed milk is used as the protein constituent and lactose as the added sugar, and salts in the correct amounts are included. The whole is mixed and homogenized. The food is often useful, especially for premature or very young infants, or infants with malnutrition where human milk is not available. It is contraindicated in diarrhea. The food has become a commercial one. A number of other synthetic milks have been put on the market, among them Recolac and Similac. The percentage composition of those which have been mentioned here will be found in Table 49, p. 120.

PROPRIETARY (COMMERCIAL; PATENTED) FOODS

By the title "proprietary" or "patented" food is here indicated a food of this nature directly advertised to the *laity*, usually with what must be considered extravagant claims for its value. There are numerous preparations on the market advertised to the medical profession solely, and consisting entirely of starch or of some form of sugar, or largely of protein, or containing special ingredients and not claiming to be anything else. These foods are, of course, *proprietary*, but not in the sense in which the term is commonly employed and as used here; and since they are advertised only to physicians, and consequently are not liable to be given by a mother without advice, there can be no possible objection to their employment.

The so common and wide-spread employment of the proprietary infant-foods is probably one of the most pernicious factors of the time in the feeding of infants, as indeed it has been for years. It is not because the composition of these foods is necessarily faulty which renders them so harmful, although this is frequently the case, but it is the manner in which they are freely advertised to the laity and freely used by mothers without consultation with their physicians. It is frequently only after an infant becomes ill, having taken a large variety of the foods for weeks or months, that the advice of the physician is asked about the propriety of their use. In other cases physicians themselves are largely responsible for this state of affairs, as they are prone to yield too readily to the temptation to prescribe the foods without due consideration.

The proprietary foods are for the most part unreliable and unnecessary. It is true that many infants have done well upon commercial foods, but they would almost certainly have grown as satisfactorily if a proper milk-modification had been given. There can be nothing of advantage in a proprietary food which cannot be equally incorporated in a home-made modification, and at much less expense. When such a food is employed the physician should be fully cognizant of its composition.

The number of proprietary foods which are now or have been on the market is vast; and it would be a waste of time and space to attempt to consider them all. The analytical tables which follow are given in order to show how closely, or oftener how remotely, they resemble human milk in composition.

The various proprietary foods may be classified as follows:

I. *Condensed Milks.*—These consist of whole or skimmed milk condensed by evaporating, and often with the addition of cane-sugar.

II. *Malted or Dextrinized Foods.*—The basis of these is starch which has been completely converted. To some of them milk has been added in the process of manufacture. A few have still other additions.

III. *Amylaceous Foods.*—These are composed entirely or partly of unconverted starch. Quite commonly it is recommended that they be mixed with milk. Milk and milk-sugar have been added in the process of manufacture of some of them.

IV. *Miscellaneous Foods.*—Infant-foods often with milk as a basis with the addition of other substances than, or in addition to, starch or sugar. They are incompletely or not at all dextrinized.

V. *Protein-foods.*—These consist of commercial foods claimed to be especially rich in protein. They are not primarily intended for use in infancy, but are often of temporary benefit.

VI. *Commercial Vegetable Foods.*—These likewise are proprietary preparations, but are not designed to be the sole food for infants. They often serve very useful purposes.

I. Condensed Milks.—These, including dried milk, evaporated milk and evaporated cream, are made by evaporating the milk by heat to a greater or less degree and then sealing it in cans. All of them need dilution with water before they can be employed.

They may be divided into:

1. Dried Milk.—There are various preparations of this upon the market sold under different names. Some of them are made from whole milk; others from skimmed milk, and some have a lactic acid addition. Dried milk has been used quite extensively in infant-feeding, and generally is well tolerated by infants over six weeks of age. It is especially valuable when good, clean cow's milk cannot be obtained; *e. g.*, when travelling. Much of the vitamin content may be retained in dried milk (see p. 135). Studies by Dick and Dick,[34] Hucker and Hucker,[35] Gibben and von Pourtales,[36] and others have shown that, while dried milk is not sterile, such

TABLE 46.—ANALYSES OF DRIED MILKS

Dried milks.	Water, per cent.	Fat, per cent.	Protein, per cent.	Lactose, per cent.	Dextrose, per cent.	Mineral matter, per cent.
Human milk	87–88	3.5–4	1–1.5	....	....	0.20
Dried milks						
Alacta (Mead)	1.5	12.0	33.0	46.5	....	7.0
Dryco (all Dryco irradiated with ultra-violet light)	3.0	12.0	32.0	46.0	....	7.0
Glaxo	2.5	20.0	26.0	46.0	....	5.5
Klim	1.5	28.0	26.74	38.0	....	5.8
Mammala	5.0	12.0	24.0	54.0	....	5.0
Mead's powdered milk	1.5	28.0	26.8	37.7	....	6.0
Mead's powdered lactic milk	1.5	27.2	26.0	36.3	....	6.0
Mead's powdered lactic milk with 29.5 per cent dextri-maltose added	1.5	19.15	18.3	25.5	29.5	4.25
Merrell-Soule powdered lactic milk	3.0	28.0	26.0	33.0	....	6.0
Merrell-Soule skimmed lactic milk (Akrelac)	3.0	1.0	36.0	47.8	....	8.0
Merrell-Soule powdered skimmed milk	2.8	1.0	36.5	51.8	....	7.9
SMACO powdered skim milk	2.0	2.0	35.5	51.0	....	8.0

pathogenic germs as streptococci, dysentery bacilli and tubercle bacilli have been destroyed. In preparation for feeding the powdered milk is mixed with a little cold water to make a paste. The remainder of the water is then added while warm and the mixture is thoroughly stirred and shaken. Each bottle should be made separately just before use. When given to quite young infants the strength of the mixture should not be more than 1 teaspoonful to two ounces of water in the case of the heavier dried milks, as Klim, or half this amount in the case of the lighter dried milks, as Dryco. This may be increased later but should never be given in more than 4 times the strength mentioned. Almost any dried milk, to correspond approximately to whole milk should be given in the proportion of 1 ounce of dried milk by weight to 8 ounces of water. The total amount of each feeding varies, of course, according to the age. A number of authors have described a "dried-milk fever." This is evidently due only to the lack of fluid intake and does not occur when sufficient liquid is given. Table 46 gives an analysis of dried milks in which the figures are either those of the manufacturer or of the Committee on Foods of the American Medical Association.

2. Evaporated (Condensed) Milks.—Evaporated milks are now very widely employed. About 60 per cent of the water is removed by evaporation in a partial vacuum. The various brands are more or less of the same composition, approximate percentage-content being of water 68, fat 10, lactose 12, protein 8, ash 2. The law requires that they shall not contain less than 7.8 per cent of fat and 25.5 per cent of total milk solids. Certain changes take place in the process of manufacture. The fat globules are broken up into smaller particles, the casein is altered so that finer curd formation takes place with acid or rennin, and there are slight alterations in the mineral constituents. There is only moderate diminution in the vitamin content. While not sterile the important pathogenic germs have been killed. The study of Jeans and Sterns[37] showed that there was satisfactory retention of nitrogen, calcium and phosphorus when evaporated milk was fed. There is no doubt that clinically many babies do well on them, but they can hardly be considered preferable to good fresh milk.

In the sweetened condensed milks the composition is similar, but with approximately 40 per cent added saccharose.

II. Dextrinized (Malted) Foods.—The basis of these, often called also Liebig's Foods, is starch usually derived from wheat-flour or barley-

TABLE 47.—ANALYSES OF DEXTRINIZED FOODS*

	Water.	Fat.	Protein.	Soluble carbohydrates.	Mineral matter.	Remarks.
Human milk	87–88	3.5–4	1–1.5	6.5–7	0.20	...
Dextrinized foods.						
Liebe's soluble food	22.34	Trace	6.47	68.80	1.71	An extract of malt made from wheat.
Mellin's food	5.62	0.16	10.35	79.57	4.30	Wheat, malted barley and bicarbonate of potash.
Laibose	6.00	17.00	18.00	55.00	4.00	A combination of whole-milk with dextrinized wheat.

* Analyses those of the manufacturers or from Blauberg-Archive für Hygiene, 1897, 30, 125.

flour which has been entirely converted into soluble carbohydrates, generally by the action of the diastase of a malt-extract. These carbohydrates consist of dextrin and maltose and intermediate substances. The foods should not give the iodine reaction for unconverted starch. Other maltose-dextrin preparations, as well as the malt-soups, not advertised to the laity as Infant's Foods, will be found discussed elsewhere (pp. 99; 113); and some of the more complicated commercial malted foods are mentioned under Miscellaneous Foods in Table 49, p. 120.

Among some "Infant's Foods" which are practically only dextrinized cereal preparations are those shown on p. 118.

III. Amylaceous Foods.—All of these contain unconverted starch in larger or smaller amount. In some of them malt-extract, pancreatic extract or some form of sugar has been added; but in none of them, according to the analyses, is the starch entirely transformed. In the case of many of them it is admitted to be present and the food is intended to be added to milk-mixtures. In others the food is recommended without any statement regarding the presence of starch, or even with the claim that none exists in it. The accompanying table gives published analyses of a number of starch-containing foods which have been placed on the market from time to time.

IV. Miscellaneous Foods.—In this class are placed a number of foods in the composition of which other substances than starch or sugar have been used, or which in some way do not properly belong to any of the previous classes. In some the proportion of cream is increased either by direct addition of this or by removal of a part of the protein, and, the food being afterward condensed, the title of condensed cream might with propriety be employed. Some are malted or peptonized; in some unconverted starch is present, and the food might be placed among the amylaceous preparations were it not for the addition of other substances. Table 49 gives published analyses of some of them.

V. Proteid or Nitrogenous Foods.—These form a mixed group in all of which the nitrogenous element is claimed to be high as compared with other ingredients. They are not intended to be permanent substitutes for human milk and some

TABLE 48.—ANALYSES OF AMYLACEOUS FOODS*

	Water.	Fat.	Protein.	Total carbohydrates.	Insoluble carbohydrates.	Soluble carbohydrates.	Mineral matter.	Remarks.
Human milk	87–88	3.5–4	1–1.5	6.5–7	.....	6.5–7	0.20	....
Amylaceous foods								
Allenbury's malted food	6.50	1.00	9.20	82.80	.....	.....	0.50	Wheat-flour and malt. Contains unconverted starch.
Benger's food	11.29	1.10	10.43	76.20	66.30	9.90	0.96	Wheat-flour and pancreatic extract. The large amount of starch becomes for the most part converted when the food is prepared for use.
Dennos	6.80	1.00	9.70	79.80	61.10	18.70	2.00	A partially dextrinized whole-wheat flour, to which are added small amounts of cane-sugar, dextrin and sodium chloride.
Imperial Granum	10.57	1.32	19.37	67.30	51.88	15.42	1.13	A baked wheat flour.
Mead's cereal	7.00	3.00	15.00	71.80	.....	.....	....	Rich in calcium, phosphorus, iron and copper and in vitamins A, B, E & G.
Neave's food	5.03	1.70	13.20	80.40	74.27	4.71	1.09	Practically all starch.
Nestle's milk food	2.50	6.50	14.65	74.35	14.00	60.35	2.00	A condensed milk with baked wheat-flour and cane-sugar.
Robinson's patent barley	10.10	0.90	5.10	82.00	.....	.....	1.90	Merely barley flour.
Savory and Moore's food	5.34	1.06	10.79	81.90	54.09	27.81	0.91	Wheat-flour and malt. Much grape and cane-sugar added.

* Analyses are those of manufacturers or from Cautley, Sutherland's System of Diet and Dietetics 1908, 217, or Hutchison's Food and Dietetics 1917, 468.

TABLE 49.—ANALYSES OF MISCELLANEOUS FOODS*

	Water.	Fat.	Protein.	Total carbo-hydrates.	Insoluble carbo-hydrates.	Soluble carbo-hydrates.	Mineral matter.	Remarks.
Human milk	87–88	3.5–4	1–1.5	.....	.....	6.5–7	0.20	....
Miscellaneous foods								
Allenbury's food, No. 1	5.70	14.00	9.70	66.85	.....	66.85	3.75	Desiccated milk; excess casein removed; vegetable-albumin, milk-sugar and cream added.
Allenbury's food, No. 2	3.90	12.30	9.20	72.10	.....	72.10	3.50	Like No. 1, but with addition of some malted flour.
Eskay's albumenized food	1.70	3.52	6.70	87.02	31.20	55.82	0.99	A milk sugar with cereals and inorganic salts.
Frame food diet	5.00	1.20	13.40	79.40	.....	.....	1.00	Baked flour; cane-sugar; extract of bran. Rich in protein and unaltered starch.
Lactogen	2.00	25.00	16.20	.....	.....	53.30	3.50	Cow's milk dried with added milk-fat and lactose.
Liebig's Malto-leguminose mit Zucker	8.44	1.37	20.34	65.10	48.19	16.91	2.97	Leguminous flour partly malted.
Protein S.M.A. acidulated	2.00	22.00	35.00	28.00	.....	.....	6.00	Prepared as in S.M.A. but with proportions very similar to protein-milk. It is, however, higher in percentage of protein. Contains also fresh lemon-juice.
Recolac	1.00	27.00	16.00	53.00	......	53.00	3.00	Butter-fat replaced by mixture of vegetable and animal fats, including cod liver oil. Dextrin and maltose added. Casein reduced and changed to potassium caseinate.
Similac	3.00	27.10	12.50	.....	.....	54.40	3.20	Contains sodium, potassium and calcium caseinates, lactalbumin and vegetable fats.
SMACO maltose with lactose and dextrin.	2.00	.....	.....	97.00	......	97.0	0.50	Maltose 35.0 per cent; dextrins 32.0 per cent; lactose 30.0 per cent.
S.M.A.	1.00	28.00	10.00	59.00	.....	.....	2.00	Combination of various animal and vegetable fats with skimmed milk, lactose and salts. Homogenized.
Sobee	3.18	22.50	33.20	32.61	.....	.....	8.50	A combination of Soy bean flour with olive oil, barley flour and salts.
Horlick's malted milk	3.06	8.78	16.35	67.95	.....	.....	3.86	Milk; barley and wheat malted.

* Analyses are those of the manufacturers or from the reports of the Committee on Foods of the American Medical Association.

of them fill a useful place. They may be divided into (1) beef-extracts, (2) beef-juices, (3) peptonized meat preparations, (4) other proteid foods.

1. The Commercial Beef-extracts.—These, although popularly supposed to be highly nourishing from the amount of protein contained, possess in reality but a small percentage of this, while the extractive matter and salts are present in large amounts. They are prepared under the influence of water, heat and pressure. Some of the muscle-fiber which remains is added and the liquid then evaporated. Only those in which the fiber has been thus used contain an amount of protein worth considering. A table of analyses of a number of them published by Hutchison[38] shows a total percentage of soluble protein varying in round numbers from 3 to 33 per cent. As only small quantities are customarily given, or could, indeed, be tolerated on account of the excess of mineral matter and extractives, the amount of protein received by the infant is in reality trifling; given in doses of a few drops, as is often done, either alone or in addition to the milk in the bottle.

2. Beef-juices.—These consist of expressed juice or serum of the beef. According to analyses of a number of the commercial preparations, as published by Hutchison,[39] the percentage of coagulable protein varies from 17 per cent to 0.3 per cent, nearly all of those in his list containing not over 5 per cent. Although some of them are richer in protein than is freshly prepared beef-juice, yet, as in the case of the beef-extracts, the salts and extractive matter are generally present in too large an amount to permit of the giving them in sufficient quantity to be of real benefit. Our preference has always been decidedly for the freshly prepared beef-juice (p. 110).

3. Beef-powders and Peptonized Beef-preparations.—Some of these are extensively employed for temporary use in infant-feeding and infant-therapeutics. Prominent among them are a number whose nitrogenous value is slight and whose percentage in alcohol is high. On account of their comparatively pleasant taste they may be used in place of other alcoholic stimulants in infancy and childhood. The following analyses are given by Harrington.[40]

TABLE 50.—ALCOHOLIC STRENGTHS OF LIQUID BEEF-PREPARATIONS

	Alcohol by volume, per cent.	Total solids, per cent.
Liquid peptonoids	23.03	14.91
Panopeptone	18.95	17.90
Nutritive liquid peptone	14.81	15.20
Hemaboloids	15.81	6.36

4. Other Proteid Foods.—Among other preparations the following may be mentioned:

Somatose.—A meat-powder completely peptonized and containing over 80 per cent of protein (Neumann[41]). Another form, Milk-somatose, is derived from milk and contains about 70 per cent of protein (Neumann). Somatose is useful as an addition to milk.

Dry Peptonoids.[42]—This contains 40 per cent of protein, the remainder of its nutritive value depending entirely on carbohydrates (51.5 per cent).

Plasmon represents in powdered form 75 to 80 per cent of albumin derived from milk, with the addition of 5 to 7 per cent of carbonate and bicarbonate of soda. It is in reality an alkali-casein (Laves[43]).

Sanatogen (Street[44]).—This is a preparation containing about 90 per cent of casein, with sodium-glycerophosphate and a small amount of unidentified nitrogenous compound. It would appear to possess no advantage over the very much cheaper commercial casein.

Certain other high-protein foods have already been mentioned in connection with the preparation of casein-milk (p. 108).

VI. Vegetable Foods.—There may be mentioned here a number of vegetable preparations on the market. Spinach is available in a powdered form (Spintrate) which is said to be rich in vitamins A, B, and G and to contain iron, calcium and phosphorus. This may be added to milk without cooking. There are several other commercial preparations of vegetables canned or preserved in glass containers (Certifoods, Gerber's, Van Camp's, Clapp's), cooked and made into a puree, and designed especially for feeding infants and children. It is stated that these are rich in vitamins and in minerals, especially iron and phosphorus. Although expensive these preparations are convenient and satisfactory, but they are no better than properly cooked home products.

References

1. Arch. Pediat., 1909, **26**, 496; Am. J. M. Sc., 1915, **150**, 502. 2. J.A.M.A., 1929, **93**, 985. 3. Am. J. Dis. Child., 1930, **40**, 791. 4. Suppe für Säuglinge, 1865. 5. Malzsuppe, eine Nahrung f. Magendarmkranke Säuglinge, 1898. 6. Am. J. Dis. Child., 1925, **30**, 453. 7. Berl. klin. Wchnschr., 1895, **32**, 561; 589. 8. Die Kinderernährung im Säuglingsalter, 1900, 189. 9. Jahrb. f. Kinderh., 1913, **78**, 1. 10. Zentralbl. f. Physiol., 1910, **24**, 687. 11. Wien. med. Wchnschr., 1894, **44**, 1870. 12. Arch. f. Kinderh., 1898, **24**, 226; 1903, **36**, 407. 13. Wien. med. Wchnschr., 1910, **60**, 1930. 14. Dis. of Child., 1877, 332. 15. Kinderheilk., 1899, **1**, 158. 16. Ueber Säuglingsernährung, 1912. 17. Jahrb. f. Kinderh., 1895, **40**, 421. 18. Wien. med. Wchnschr., 1905, **18**, 341. 19. Soc. de therap., 1893, Jan. 25; Ref. Marfan, Traité de l'allaitement, 1903, 439. 20. Pfaundler u. Schlossmann, Handb. d. Kinderh., 1906, **1**, 1311. 21. München. med. Wchnschr., 1900, **47**, 1661. 22. Trans. Am. Ped. Soc., 1915, **27**, 117. 23. Arch. Pediat., 1919, **36**, 28. 24. Prag. med. Wchnschr., 1914, **39**, 13. 25. Monatschr. f. Kinderh., 1923, **26**, 250. 26. Nourrisson, 1930, **18**, 161; 209. 27. Ztschr. f. Kinderh., 1929, **48**, 552. 28. Jahrb. f. Kinderh., 1922, **100**, 3. 29. Deutsche med. Wchnschr., 1930, **56**, 4. 30. Jahrb. f. Kinderh., 1918, **87**, 1. 31. Griffith and Mitchell, New York M. J., 1921, **114**, 137. 32. Monatschr. f. Kinderh., 1920, **18**, 97. 33. Am. J. Dis. Child., 1915, **10**, 249; 1919, **17**, 1. 34. Am. J. Dis. Child., 1927, **34**, 1040. 35. Am. J. Dis. Child., 1929, **38**, 310. 36. Am. J. Dis. Child., 1931, **41**, 1100. 37. Am. J. Dis. Child., 1931, **42**, 708. 38. Food and Dietetics, 1917, 96. 39. Food & Dietetics, 1917, 100. 40. Boston M. and S. J., 1903, **148**, 283. 41. München. med. Wchnschr., 1898, **45**, 72. 42. Advertisement, J.A.M.A., 1914, **63**, 183. 43. München. med. Wchnschr., 1900, **47**, 1339. 44. J.A.M.A., 1914, **63**, 1831.

CHAPTER VI

GENERAL CONSIDERATION OF THE DIETARY FOR INFANTS AND CHILDREN

DIET IN THE FIRST SIX MONTHS

In this chapter is discussed the feeding in general of average, well infants and children. The quantity of the various foods will differ in individual children, depending particularly on their activity. Even in presumably well subjects the ability to digest certain foods will vary. The experiments of Davis[1] are interesting in that they seemed to demonstrate that even young infants were able to select their own foods from a list of simple natural ones, and in quantities sufficient to maintain themselves with optimum digestion and good nutrition.

In the first six months of life a suitable milk-mixture constitutes the basis of the diet if breast-milk is not available. Orange juice should be started by three months of age in the breast-fed infant, and even earlier in the artificially fed, beginning with 1 teaspoonful a day and shortly increasing this until 1.5 to 2 oz. are given daily by six or eight months of age. It may be taken diluted with an ounce or so of water, and unsweetened unless the orange juice is sour, at any time of the day that is convenient. It is not necessary, as formerly thought, to give it at least an hour before or after a feeding, although this is preferable and seems to agree better with many babies. Orange juice is rich in vitamin C and possesses also a fair amount of the vitamin B complex. This is of importance in view of the practice among some pediatrists of adding to the infant's diet substances in which vitamin B is present. Various other concentrated preparations containing vitamin B are available, such as yeast or cereal germ, and certain maltose-dextrin combinations are claimed to be rich in it or to have had it added. It has seemed to us unnecessary to use in the young infant's diet any other form of this vitamin than is found in milk and orange juice. Even heating the milk does not entirely inhibit the action of the vitamin B present in it. Later when the coarser cereals, vegetables, and other foods are added to the diet, any deficiency in vitamin B is still less likely to occur. (See Vitamins, p. 135.)

Cod liver oil may well be given to both breast-fed and artificially fed infants, beginning at one month of age and continuing until at least the beginning of the third year. Ten to 15 drops is an initial daily dose, rapidly increased to 1 teaspoonful three times a day by the fourth month of life. Irradiated ergosterol (viosterol) may be combined with the cod liver oil. (See Prophylaxis of Rickets, p. 454.) It must be remembered that viosterol contains only vitamin D, and that it does not replace cod liver oil, which is rich in both A and D.

By five months of age spoon-feeding of a well-cooked, bran-free cereal porridge, such as cream of wheat or farina may be started, and from a daily amount of 1 teaspoonful may be increased to a tablespoonful or more. The porridge should be cooked for thirty minutes over a flame, or for one or preferably two hours in a double boiler, a small amount of salt being added. It is better not to use sugar either now or later in childhood, although there is no actual objection to a small amount of it, except that the child will later always demand it. The cereal should be somewhat thinned by pouring over it some of the milk-mixture or, in the case of the breast-fed infant, a little boiled and diluted milk. There is no physiologic reason for giving in the first six to eight months any other foods than those mentioned, nor can long clinical observation demonstrate any necessity at this period for the employment of vegetables, eggs, meat or other foods. The mere fact that some babies can digest such foods does not argue for their use, but only demonstrates the great adaptability and flexibility of the infant's digestive and metabolic functions.

Further details as to the feeding-intervals and the like have been discussed in Chapters III and IV.

DIET IN THE SECOND SIX MONTHS

By eight, or, at most, ten months of age the milk may generally be undiluted. By the time a quart of whole milk is given daily, other foods must be depended on to increase the caloric intake. In fact, as a rule at no time in normal infancy and childhood should much more than a quart of milk be allowed in the ration. By eight to ten months vegetables, beef juice, and other forms of starch than the cereals may be included in the diet. The vegetables contain iron, which has been deficient in the other foods allowed before this time, unless beef-juice has been given earlier, and this mineral is needed since in the latter half of the first year the iron stored in the body is becoming exhausted. Such vegetables as spinach and carrots are best, and they should be well-cooked, or, better, steamed in order to conserve the salts, and then rubbed through a fine sieve. Canned vegetables may be employed if desired. (See p. 122.) Beef-juice, which is not so rich as the vegetables in iron, should be freshly prepared (see p. 110) since the commercial extracts are not proper substitutes. It may be given from a spoon or poured over the starchy vegetable. It is better to continue with the bran-free cereal porridges, such as farina and cream of wheat, although the coarser cereals may be serviceable in constipated infants. Rice and macaroni are useful and, less frequently, baked potato. Stale bread, toast, or zwieback, given dry or moistened with milk, may be allowed occasionally. Four feedings a day are usually sufficient, not counting the orange juice. At each of these 8 oz. of milk is offered in addition to any other food. Any new food should be given in small amounts until the digestive capacity of the individual infant is ascertained, and only one new food started at a time. A suggested schedule for an infant of ten to twelve months follows:

Table 51.—Diet from Ten to Twelve Months

6 A. M.	8 oz. of milk.
7 A. M.	2 oz. of orange juice.
10 A. M.	2 to 3 tablespoonfuls of cereal porridge; 8 oz. of milk.
2 P. M.	three days a week, 1 to 2 tablespoonfuls of beef-juice; four days a week, 1 to 2 tablespoonfuls of green vegetable; every day, a starchy vegetable; every day, 8 oz. of milk.
6 P. M.	8 oz. of milk; small piece of toast or zwieback moistened with warm milk.

It should be said of this and of the succeeding schedules that they are suggestive merely, since circumstances may make alterations necessary. It often occurs that at the first and last feedings, at which milk alone is taken, the infant may require 9 or 10 oz. of this, whereas at the other feedings some of it may be refused. The total daily ration of not over 1 quart can readily be adjusted. The time of the feedings, too, may need changing, but the interval of approximately four hours should be preserved.

DIET FROM TWELVE TO EIGHTEEN MONTHS

The diet just described for an infant of ten months of age is considered by many pediatrists as unnecessarily varied until after the first year. In any event some further amplification of it should be made by the age of twelve months. Certainly by this time, even more than previously, it may be necessary to give less than 8 oz. of milk at the heavier feedings and perhaps more at the lighter, but a total of 24 to 32 oz. is sufficient. A part of the milk ration may be used on the cereal porridges. Caution must be observed lest the infant take an over-supply of milk instead of the more concentrated solid foods. Weaning from the bottle may be started and the milk given from a cup. The milk may be taken whole except in the not infrequent case of infants who tolerate it better if it is slightly diluted. It should be boiled as in the first year. Four meals a day are given as before, not counting the orange juice. The cereals may be increased in quantity and perhaps allowed twice a day, and the coarser ones may now be employed, such as Wheatena, Ralston's, Pettijohn's, Mead's, and oatmeal. These may, at first, be strained, but soon the sieve should be made coarser and then abandoned. Stewed fruits such as cooked prunes, dried apricots, peaches and apples may be eaten, pressed through a rather fine sieve before serving. The orange juice should be continued daily. In addition to spinach and carrots may be given beet-tops, asparagus tips, peas, and string beans finely divided by sieving. Beef-juice is continued and egg may be cautiously tried. Egg-yolk is a very valuable source of iron as well as of calcium, phosphorus and of all vitamins but C. If broth is employed it should be well thickened with vegetable pulp and rice or barley and should have the finely divided meat fiber remaining in it. Otherwise its caloric value is very low and it should not replace other food.

There have been numerous proposed schedules printed varying with the preference of the writers. The differences in some respect will depend upon the time when sleep during the day seems to be most desired by the child, and a good deal, too, upon the household arrangements. In the following schedule "A" is arranged upon the supposition that the infant needs a feeding before the morning nap, while "B" puts the sleep in the afternoon.

Table 52.—Diet from Twelve to Eighteen Months

A

6 A. M. or on waking	Orange juice.
7.30 A. M.	Breakfast: 2 to 3 tablespoonfuls of cereal; 6 to 8 oz. milk.
10.30–11 A. M.	8 oz. of milk before the morning sleep.
2 P. M.	Dinner: three to four days a week, 2 tablespoonfuls of beef-juice; two to three days a week, ½ to 1 soft boiled or poached egg; every day 2 tablespoonfuls green vegetable and the same amount of starchy vegetable; 8 oz. of milk or a thick broth.
5.30–6 P. M.	Supper: 1 to 2 tablespoonfuls of cereal porridge or a slice of toast or zwieback; stewed fruit three times a week or more; 6 to 8 oz. of milk.

B

6 A. M. or waking	Orange juice.
7.30 A. M.	Breakfast: 2 to 3 tablespoonfuls of cereal; 6 to 8 oz. milk.
12 Noon	Dinner: three to four days a week, 2 tablespoonfuls beef-juice; two to three days a week, ½ to 1 soft boiled or poached egg; every day 2 tablespoonfuls green vegetable and the same amount of starchy vegetable; 8 oz. of milk or a thick broth.
3.30–4 P. M.	8 oz. of milk after the nap, with 2 to 3 tablespoonfuls of cereal.
5.30–6 P. M.	Supper: 1 to 2 tablespoonfuls of cereal or a slice of toast or zwieback; stewed fruit three times a week or more; 6 to 8 oz. of milk.

With either of these it may be necessary to give a feeding at 9 or 10 P. M. through a portion, at least, of the period, but in that event it may be best to curtail slightly the amount of milk allowed during the day time so that the total daily quantity is not over 32 ounces. Junket, tapioca, rice-pudding, and similar desserts may be added to the dinner if desired. With regard to any possible household objection to breakfast as early as 7.30 A. M. it is to be remembered that the cereal porridges which require long cooking can be prepared on the previous afternoon and kept warm over night.

DIET FROM EIGHTEEN MONTHS TO TWO YEARS

At eighteen months of age some few changes in quantity and variety of food should be made. It is frequently found that a 3 meal-a-day schedule is more satisfactory than one with a lighter 4th feeding of milk in the mid-morning or mid-afternoon. Large, active infants may require this, but many will be more willing to take solid foods if only 24 oz. of milk are allowed. The milk should still be boiled, and certainly by this time it should be drunk largely from a cup, although there can be no objection to one bottle-feeding a day, especially in the evening. Part of the milk may occasionally be given as junket. Such meats as chicken, lamb, beef, or fish should be added to the diet. The chicken and fish should be well cooked, but the lamb chops and beef should be somewhat underdone. The meat should be finely minced or scraped, and be started in amounts of a teaspoonful, gradually increasing to a tablespoonful or more. Simple desserts, not too sweet, may be given, such as tapioca-pudding, rice-pudding, bread-pudding, cornstarch or a baked apple. Vanilla ice-cream, if not too rich, may occasionally be allowed for dessert. Crackers may be eaten at meal time, but not between. Butter may be used on zwieback, toast, and stale bread, or in the vegetables. At first about a rounded teaspoonful of butter daily should be allowed and this gradually increased to 2 to 3 teaspoonfuls. Measuring the daily ration in the morning will avoid using an excess. Well-cooked vegetables such as asparagus-tips, stewed celery, and string beans and peas may be eaten, put through a sieve as before. The eggs may be given soft boiled, poached or as a custard. A diet list follows:

Table 53.—Diet from Eighteen Months to Two Years

Breakfast (7–8 a. m.)	8 oz. of milk; 2 tablespoonfuls of a cereal porridge varied from time to time; a soft-boiled or poached egg; orange juice or orange; strip of crisp bacon; bread and butter.
Noon meal (12–1 p. m.)	8 oz. of milk; soup or broth 3 to 4 oz.; 1 to 2 tablespoonfuls of green vegetables with butter; 2 tablespoonfuls of potato, hominy grits, macaroni or rice; 1 tablespoonful of meat; 1 tablespoonful of dessert.
Evening meal (6 p. m.)	8 oz. of milk; 2 tablespoonfuls cereal or pudding; stewed fruit; bread and butter.

Again it should be stated that this diet list is only a suggestion, as are the hours for meals. If a feeding of milk is regularly given in the middle of the morning the dinner may well be arranged for 2 p. m. and 6 oz. of broth thickened with vegetable pulp, rice and barley, may replace the milk at that time. Many children do not well tolerate eggs given daily. Foods other than those suggested are unnecessary and the dietary need not be a monotonous one if varied from time to time in the porridges, meats and vegetables allowed.

DIET FROM TWO TO FIVE YEARS

Meat which is merely cut up, not scraped or minced, is now added to the list. Once a day is usually sufficiently often for it until the child is about five years old. Stewed fruit in greater quantities can be used, and many fresh fruits if ripe are excellent, such as peaches, grapes, raspberries, bananas if thoroughly over-ripe. Strawberries may be tried but very cautiously and only if sweet and quite ripe. Lima beans and tomatoes and salsify may be added to the list of vegetables. Fresh, pure milk should be given, but need not be boiled, and a total of 24 oz. should be sufficient. Cream need never be used. Cereals should be of the home-cooked variety, and the ready-to-serve kind avoided as a steady diet. If the child finds the prescribed supper insufficient eggs may occasionally be given in addition, but in this event should not be allowed for breakfast on such days.

The meals, up to about the age of two and one-half years, are best taken in the nursery, but after this time the child may well sit at the family table in its high chair, or at a small table close by, provided it never be given articles of food not suited to its age. Three meals a day are sufficient under usual conditions, with the heaviest one at mid-day, and nothing should be given between them. If circumstances necessitate a long interval between meals, an orange or a cracker may be allowed, but it is preferable not to give milk. (See Anorexia p. 559.) Any increase of diet should be made cautiously and only one new article at a time. During very hot weather it may, indeed, be better to return to a diet suitable for a younger child. The amounts of food given must necessarily vary and depend, as previously stated, upon individual digestion and activity. The schedule otherwise is much the same as that for the eighteen months to two years period. After the age of three years there may be a steady, but gradual, increase in the variety of the dietary.

DIET AFTER FIVE YEARS

After five years there may be a rather liberal allowance of food, and it is unnecessary, and perhaps better not, to be too specific in prescribing amounts of food to be taken by the average well child. The following schedule is a helpful one for the early period after five years to about the age of six or seven years. By this age the diet may be largely similar to that really suitable for adults, although close supervision must still be maintained.

Table 54.—Diet after Five Years

Foods Permitted

Meats—Broiled beefsteak, lamb, chops and chicken; roasted or boiled beef, mutton, lamb, chicken, turkey; broiled or boiled fish; liver; oysters; occasionally veal.

Eggs—Soft-boiled, poached, scrambled, omelette, hard-boiled.

Cereal Foods—Light and not too fresh wheat and occasionally Graham bread; toast; zwieback; plain unsweetened crackers, as oatmeal, soda, water, etc.; hominy grits; wheaten grits; corn-meal; barley; rice; oatmeal; macaroni; cream of wheat; farina; Pettijohn's; Ralston's; Wheatena; occasionally some of the ready-to-serve breakfast foods.

Soups—Vegetable soups and meat broths of nearly any kind.

Vegetables—White potatoes; boiled onions; spinach; peas; carrots; asparagus-tips; string and other beans; lettuce; tomatoes; stewed celery; young beets; cabbage; arrowroot; tapioca; squash, and cauliflower.

Fruits—Nearly all if stewed and slightly sweetened. Of raw fruits (used moderately) peaches are one of the best; ripe bananas; pears well ripened; grapes; oranges; apples (baked, sauce or raw); raspberries; strawberries, and blackberries. Give only small amounts of berries and stop if they disagree.

Desserts—Light puddings, as rice pudding, bread pudding, plain custards; jelly; junket; ice cream; light cake.

Foods to Be Avoided or Used Cautiously

Hot bread; hot rolls; ready to serve cereals; ham; sausage; pork; salt fish; corned beef; kidney; goose; all fried foods; raw onions; radishes; cucumbers; baked beans; egg plant; corn; nuts; pastry; salads; pickles; pineapple; watermelon; tea; coffee; pies; soda water; preserved fruit; candy (except occasionally pure fruit drops, peppermint wafers, chocolate).

In regard to the prohibition of certain foods it should be stated that sometimes this is made too rigid. After the age of 5 years many children may be allowed, on occasion at least, a rather varied diet. Some of the older diet lists advised for children prohibited a number of articles of food which are both acceptable and digestible by the average child. For example, the skins of certain grapes are certainly not as indigestible as other articles of diet allowed. We have never seen any real harm come about by the eating of the seeds of grapes in older children. The ready-to-serve cereals, while perhaps not as nutritious as some of the cooked varieties, are perfectly proper articles of diet and some of them are of rather high caloric value and have a rather high vitamin and mineral content.

General Directions

Not more than a pint and a half of milk in the twenty-four hours (3 glasses, one with each meal). Do not use cream.

Three meals a day with nothing between.

Measure out 3 rounded teaspoonfuls of butter in the morning. See that only this quantity is taken in the twenty-four hours. Use butter on toast, in cereal porridge, and on vegetables.

Some meat, including fish, daily at the mid-day meal, and perhaps twice a day.

Green vegetables such as spinach, beets, asparagus, string beans or peas once a day, finely divided but not put through a sieve, may be given twice a day as required.

Cooked cereal porridge once a day. A white vegetable or cereal food (as macaroni) once or twice a day.

Egg four times a week.

Breakfast—Milk, cereal, egg, bread and butter, cocoa in place of milk, orange or other fruit.

Mid-day meal—Soup or broth, meat or fish, potato, rice or macaroni, green vegetables, toast, milk in a simple dessert or on cereal, bread and butter.

Evening meal—Milk, pudding, toast, custard, junket, prune-juice and pulp or stewed fruit, bread and butter.

In older children meat and vegetables twice a day.

Some time between the ages of five and ten years the child will begin to take the regular dinner with the family in the evening. This will modify the dietary to some extent.

AMOUNT OF FOOD-ELEMENTS AND NUMBER OF CALORIES REQUIRED AFTER THE FIRST YEAR

A knowledge of the percentage-composition and caloric value of the foods given after the first year is less often required than in infancy, but still frequently serviceable. This is particularly true when indigestion of some form develops, or when the question of over-feeding or under-feeding arises. The caloric needs of children after the age of one year have received considerable attention. The matter is reviewed by Locke,[2] as also by Knox,[3] based upon studies by Camerer,[4] Sommerfeld,[5] and others. Benedict and Talbot[6] have given a number of figures for basal metabolism. McCann[7] has reviewed the subject of calorimetry and mentioned the caloric requirements of children, and Holt and Fales[8] have summarized in a critical way the work done on the food-requirements for this period of life. The total amounts of the different ingredients necessary vary decidedly, this depending in part upon the fact that the food-elements are to a considerable extent interchangeable. Thus if, for instance, a larger amount of fat is given the total quantity of food required is less, on account of the greater caloric value of this. The average amounts given by Sommerfeld, based upon various collected estimations, are shown in the following table:

TABLE 55.—DAILY QUANTITY OF THE DIFFERENT FOOD-ELEMENTS REQUIRED

Age, years.	Protein, Gm.	Fat, Gm.	Carbohydrates, Gm.
2–4	40–64	32–62	110–205
5–7	50–58	30–43	145–197
8–10	60–88	30–70	220–250
10–11	68–86	44–85	211–270

In round numbers he places the needs as:

From two to four years, protein 50 Gm. (1.76 oz. Av.), fat 50 Gm. (1.76 oz. Av.), carbohydrates 140 Gm. (4.94 oz. Av.).
From five to eight years, protein 80 Gm. (2.82 oz. Av.), fat 65 Gm. (2.29 oz. Av.), carbohydrates 220 Gm. (7.76 oz. Av.).
From eight to twelve years, protein 85 Gm. (3 oz. Av.), fat 80 Gm. (2.82 oz. Av.), carbohydrates 275 Gm. (9.70 oz. Av.).

The actual amount of food needed increases steadily as the child grows older, but the relative amount as compared with the body-weight, *i. e.*, the energy-quotient, decreases steadily. This is dependent in part upon the diminished ratio between the surface and the body-weight, and in part upon the relatively more rapid growth in the younger subjects. Taking the weight as our guide, the caloric requirements for the first year have already been detailed (p. 94). For the age of two years and upward, as determined by Camerer,[4] they may be seen in Table 56, as given by Sommerfeld.[5] All but the protein may be varied, but this should be approximately the amount given in the table. About 30 per cent of the food should be of animal origin, and about 50 per cent of the protein should be of this nature, the rest being of vegetable derivation (Camerer). An examination of the table shows that the protein should be from 20 to 25 per cent of the total diet excluding water.

This percentage of protein in Camerer's estimations is slightly greater than the very commonly adopted ratio of protein 15, carbohydrate 61, and fat 24, which is favored by E. Müller.[9] Holt and Fales obtained very similar figures, based on a summary of the work on food-requirements done by others and on their own studies of the diets taken by over 100 normal healthy children of both sexes from one to sixteen years of age. They emphasize the fact already pointed out by others, that in calculating the

TABLE 56.—DAILY TOTAL AMOUNT OF FOOD-ELEMENTS IN GRAMS, AND OF THE CALORIES, PER KILOGRAM OF BODY-WEIGHT

Age in years.	Sex.	Total food, Gm.	Water, Gm.	Protein, Gm.	Fat, Gm.	Carbohydrates, Gm.	Calories per kilogram of body-weight.
2–4	Each	93.1	75.3	3.6	3.1	9.2	75.3
5–7	Girls	84.4	67.4	3.0	1.9	10.7	69.0
	Boys	84.3	66.6	3.5	2.5	10.9	76.6
7–10	Girls	75.5	59.0	2.7	1.3	9.9	59.2
	Boys	70.8	55.5	2.8	1.3	10.4	61.0
10–14	Girls	54.0	41.4	2.1	1.4	8.4	51.4
	Boys	56.1	44.4	2.5	1.0	7.7	47.3

total caloric needs there must be considered the requirements for basal metabolism, for growth, for food lost in excreta, and for muscular activity. The average for the first 3 factors is nearly uniform for children of the same weight living under similar conditions. The requirement for activity varies widely with different individuals. The total caloric needs of individuals of both sexes during adolescence exceed the requirements of the adult of moderate activity by nearly 1000 calories. The results of the studies by Holt and Fales,[8] which are satisfactory for the average case, are shown in the following table.

TABLE 57.—CALORIC, PROTEIN, FAT AND CARBOHYDRATE REQUIREMENTS OF CHILDREN

	At one year, average per kilo.	By six years, and throughout growth-period, average per kilo.	Per cent of total calories.	Remarks.
Total calories	100	Boys 80 Girls 76	..	Adult standard of 48 calories per kilo is rapidly approached after fifteen years.
Protein	4.0 Gm.	2.6 Gm.	15	⅔ of protein is animal. ⅓ of protein is vegetable.
Fat	4.0 Gm.	3.0 Gm.	35	
Carbohydrate	12.0 Gm.	10.0 Gm.	50	½ of carbohydrate is sugar. ½ of carbohydrate is starch.

The figures of Bartlett[10] and others differ from those commonly accepted, the claim being that in children over two years 0.6 to 1.0 Gm. of protein per kilo of body-weight may be sufficient.

9

TABLE 58.—PERCENTAGE-COMPOSITION AND CALORIC EQUIVALENTS OF VARIOUS FOODS

Food material.	Protein, per cent.	Fat, per cent.	Carbo-hydrate, per cent.	Ash, per cent.	Calories per avoirdu-pois, oz.	Calories per kilogram or liter.
Milk Foods:						
Cow's milk (average)	3.3	4.0	5.0	0.7	20	719
Skimmed milk; commercial fat-free	3.4	0.3	5.1	0.7	11	375
Skimmed milk; after removal of gravity cream	3.3	1.0	5.0	0.7	13	429
Buttermilk	3.0	0.5	4.8	0.7	10	364
Whey	1.0	0.3	5.0	0.7	8	276
Butter	1.0	85.0	.....	3.0	225	7949
Meats:						
Beef, lean ribs	19.6	12.0	.....	1.0	54	1918
Beef, lean round	21.3	7.9	.....	1.1	46	1609
Beef, roasted, A.P.	22.3	28.6	.....	1.3	101	3572
Beef-steak: round, cooked, fat removed, A.P.	27.6	7.7	.....	1.8	53	1852
Beef-steak, loin broiled	23.5	20.4	.....	1.2	81	2866
Beef-juice	4.9	0.6	.....	1.5	7	254
Beef-liver	20.4	4.5	1.7	1.6	38	1334
Mutton, leg, lean	19.8	12.4	.....	1.1	56	1962
Lamb-chop, broiled	21.7	29.9	.....	1.3	104	3671
Fish, halibut	18.6	5.2	.....	1.0	35	1246
Fish, mackerel	18.7	7.1	.....	1.2	40	1422
Bacon, smoked, lean	15.5	42.6	.....	11.0	130	4597
Fowl	19.3	16.3	.....	1.0	65	2304
Capon, cooked	27.0	11.5	.....	1.3	61	2172
Turkey	21.1	22.9	.....	1.0	85	2998
Turkey, roast	27.8	18.4	.....	1.2	81	2855
Eggs:						
Eggs, white boiled	12.3	0.2	.....	0.6	16	551
Eggs, yolk boiled	15.7	33.3	.....	1.1	107	3759
Sugar and Starch:						
Cane-sugar, granulated	....	....	100.0	....	116	4101
Milk-sugar	....	....	....	....	116	4101
Arrowroot	....	....	97.5	0.2	113	4002
Cornstarch	....	....	90.0	....	105	3693
Sago	9.0	0.4	78.1	0.3	102	3605
Tapioca	0.4	0.1	88.0	0.1	103	3638
Cereals:						
Barley, pearled	8.5	1.1	77.8	0.1	103	3638
Barley-flour	10.5	2.2	72.8	2.6	103	3616
Oatmeal	16.1	7.2	67.5	1.9	116	4101
Oats, various preparations	16.3	7.3	66.8	1.7	116	4090
Rice	8.0	0.3	79.0	0.4	102	3594
Wheat, cracked	11.1	1.7	75.5	1.6	105	3715
Wheat-flour (average)	11.4	1.0	75.1	0.5	103	3638
Wheat, whole, flour	13.8	1.9	71.9	0.9	105	3693
Wheat, farina	11.0	1.4	76.3	0.4	105	3715
Wheat, macaroni	13.4	0.9	74.1	1.3	104	3671
Wheat-bread, average	9.2	1.3	53.1	1.1	76	2679
Whole-wheat bread	9.7	0.9	49.7	1.3	71	2513
Bread, graham	8.9	1.8	52.1	1.5	76	2668
Wheat bread, toast	11.5	1.6	61.2	1.7	89	3131
Zwieback	9.8	9.9	73.5	1.0	123	4343
Rolls (average)	8.9	4.1	56.7	1.1	87	3075
Corn-meal	8.4	4.7	74.0	1.3	108	3814
Corn-bread	7.9	4.7	46.3	2.2	75	2657
Corn-hominy	8.3	0.6	79.0	0.3	103	3638
Crackers, various average	10.7	8.8	71.9	1.8	119	4200
Vegetables:						
Asparagus, A.P.	1.8	0.2	3.3	0.7	7	231
Beans, lima	7.1	0.7	22.0	1.7	36	1257
Beans, string	2.3	0.3	7.4	0.8	12	430
Beets	1.6	0.1	9.7	1.1	13	474
Carrots	1.1	0.4	9.3	1.0	13	463
Celery	1.11	0.1	3.3	1.0	5	187
Lettuce	1.2	0.3	2.9	0.9	6	198
Onions	1.6	0.3	9.9	0.6	14	496
Peas	7.0	0.5	16.9	1.0	29	1025
Potatoes	2.2	0.1	18.4	1.0	24	848
Potatoes, sweet	1.8	0.7	27.4	1.1	36	1257
Spinach	2.1	0.3	3.2	2.1	7	243
Squash	1.4	0.5	9.0	0.8	13	474
Fruits:						
Apples	0.4	0.5	14.2	0.3	18	639
Blackberries	1.3	1.0	10.9	0.5	17	595
Dates, pressed	2.1	2.8	78.4	1.3	101	3561
Figs, pressed	4.3	0.3	74.2	2.4	92	3252
Grapes	1.3	1.6	19.2	0.5	28	992
Oranges	0.8	0.2	11.6	0.5	15	529
Peaches	0.7	0.1	9.4	0.4	12	419
Pears	0.6	0.5	14.1	0.4	18	650
Prunes, dried	2.1	....	73.3	2.3	88	3087
Raspberries, red	1.0	....	12.6	0.6	16	562

Table 59.—Composition and Caloric Value of Definite Portions of Food Prepared for Use*

Foodstuff.	Quantity.	Protein.		Fats.		Carbohydrates.		Total calories.
		Gm.	Calories.	Gm.	Calories.	Gm.	Calories.	
Meats:								
Beef-juice	1 fl. oz.	1.47	6.02	0.18	1.67	0	0	8
Scraped beef	1 round. tbsp. (20 Gm.)	4.18	17.15	2.12	19.72	0	0	37
Beef-steak	1 round. tbsp. (20 Gm.)	4.7	19.28	4.08	37.94	0	0	57
Roast-beef (lean)	1 round. tbsp. (10 Gm.)	2.33	9.57	0.16	1.54	0	0	11
Fish, such as bluefish	1 round. tbsp. (20 Gm.)	5.18	21.24	0.09	8.38	0	0	30
Lamb chop	1 round. tbsp. (15 Gm.)	3.25	13.35	4.48	41.71	0	0	56
Chicken	1 round. tbsp. (10 Gm.)	2.7	11.07	1.15	10.7	0	0	22
Bacon	1 slice	3.15	12.9	19.44	180.8	0	0	194
Soups:								
Beef soup	1 fl. oz.	1.32	5.4	0.12	1.12	0.33	1.35	8
Bouillon (canned)	1 fl. oz.	0.66	2.72	0.03	0.27	0.06	0.25	3
Chicken soup (canned)	1 fl. oz.	3.15	12.92	0.24	2.22	0.72	2.95	18
Consomme (canned)	1 fl. oz.	0.75	3.07	0	0	0.12	0.5	4
Tomato soup (canned)	1 fl. oz.	0.54	2.22	0.33	3.07	1.68	6.9	12
Vegetable soup (canned)	1 fl. oz.	0.87	3.57	0	0	0.15	0.62	4
Pea soup (canned)	1 fl. oz.	1.08	4.42	0.21	1.95	2.28	9.35	16
Dairy products and eggs:								
Butter	1 ball; or 1 round. tsp.	0.15	0.6	12.75	118.6	0	0	119
Milk, whole, 4–5–3.3	1 fl. oz.	0.99	3.99	1.2	11.16	1.5	6.15	21
Cream, gravity, 16–4.2–3.03	1 fl. oz.	0.91	3.75	4.8	44.64	1.2	5.1	53
Sk. milk, gravity, 1–5–3.3	1 fl. oz.	0.99	3.99	0.3	2.79	1.5	6.15	13
Sk. milk, commercial, 0.3–5.1–3.4	1 fl. oz.	1.02	4.18	0.09	3.84	1.53	6.27	11
American cheese	1 cu. in.	5.7	23.6	7.18	66.7	0.06	2.0	91
Hen's egg	1	6.60	27.1	6.00	55.8	0	0	83
Hen's egg, white	1	4.16	17.1	0.06	0.6	0	0	18
Hen's egg, yolk	1	2.89	11.8	5.99	55.7	0	0	68
Omelette { 3 tbsp. milk; 3 eggs; 1 h. tsp. butter }	½	9.80	40.2	14.01	130.3	1.55	6.4	177
Vegetables:								
Beans, baked (home made)	1 h. tbsp.	3.61	14.8	4.25	39.57	10.95	44.87	99
Beans, baked (canned)	1 h. tbsp.	2.65	10.87	0.96	8.93	7.51	30.8	50
Butter beans	1 h. tbsp.	0.94	3.90	0.06	0.55	2.9	11.9	16
Lima beans	1 h. tbsp.	3.20	13.1	0.27	2.5	11.8	48.4	64
String beans	1 h. tbsp.	0.24	1.0	0.33	3.05	0.57	2.35	6
Beets	1 h. tbsp.	0.8	3.3	0.03	0.35	2.59	10.6	14
Beet tops	1 h. tbsp.	1.10	4.5	1.70	15.8	1.6	6.55	27
Cabbage	1 h. tbsp.	0.20	0.83	0.03	0.3	0.13	0.53	2
Carrots	1 h. tbsp.	0.18	0.73	0.05	0.53	1.13	4.63	6
Celery, creamed	1 h. tbsp.	0.47	1.93	1.66	15.43	1.15	4.73	22
Celery, uncooked	1 small stalk	0.17	0.7	0.02	0.17	0.48	1.97	3
Dandelion greens	1 h. tbsp.	1.19	4.9	0.50	4.7	5.33	21.9	30
Peas, green	1 h. tbsp.	2.05	8.43	1.04	9.7	4.38	18.37	36
Potato, Baked	Medium sized	3.77	15.5	0.20	1.9	32.07	131.5	149
	⅓ med. size or 1 h. tbsp.	1.26	5.17	0.66	0.63	10.69	43.83	50
Potato, Boiled	⅓ med. size or 1 h. tbsp.	1.28	5.13	0.05	0.47	10.45	42.83	48
Potato, Creamed	1 h. tbsp.	0.90	3.70	1.29	12.02	4.77	19.55	35
Potato, Mashed or creamed	1 h. tbsp.	1.30	5.35	1.50	13.95	8.90	36.5	56
Squash	1 h. tbsp.	0.68	2.80	0.41	3.80	6.8	27.9	34
Spinach	1 h. tbsp.	1.05	4.3	2.05	19.05	1.3	5.35	28
Tomato, canned	1 h. tbsp.	0.42	1.7	0.7	0.65	1.4	0.7	8
Tomato, uncooked	1 slice, ¼ of med. size	0.6	2.45	0.1	0.92	2.0	8.2	12
Turnips	1 h. tbsp.	0.22	0.9	0.04	0.35	0.45	1.85	3

* Tbsp. = Tablespoonful—H. Tbsp. = Heaping Tablespoonful.—Tsp. = Teaspoonful. Home made soups give amounts about as those in the table; cream-soups also, plus the value of the milk and flour added. The figures for cereals are for these boiled and without the addition of milk or sugar. Other cereals not mentioned (such as cream of wheat, Ralston's, wheatena and Pettijohn's) may be calculated as for oatmeal. In all the puddings and in practically all the cakes egg is present. For exact ingredients see Locke's "Food Values."

Table 59.—Composition and Caloric Value of Definite Portions of Food Prepared for Use.*—(*Continued*)

Foodstuff.	Quantity.	Protein.		Fats.		Carbohydrates.		Total calories.
		Gm.	Calories.	Gm.	Calories.	Gm.	Calories.	
Fruits:								
Apple	Average size	0.45	1.8	0.45	4.2	16.20	66.4	72
Orange	Average size	1.5	6.2	0.25	2.3	21.25	87.1	96
Peach	Average size	0.64	2.6	0.13	1.2	9.86	40.4	44
Pear	Average size	0.78	3.2	0.62	5.8	19.81	81.2	90
Plum	Average size	0.32	1.3	0	0	6.69	27.4	29
Raspberries	1 h. tbsp.	0.37	1.1	0	0	3.44	14.1	15
Strawberries	1 h. tbsp.	0.25	1.02	0.15	1.4	1.85	7.57	10
Dates	1	0.16	0.65	0.2	1.93	5.86	24.03	27
Figs	1	0.84	3.44	0.058	0.54	14.47	59.28	63
Raisins	1	0.057	0.23	0.07	0.7	1.71	7.02	8
Apple, baked, 3 tbsp. to apple	1 h. tbsp.	0.2	0.83	0.19	1.8	9.77	40.03	43
Apple-sauce	1 h. tbsp.	0.08	0.33	0.33	3.1	15.5	63.6	67
Apricot, stewed	1 h. tbsp.	0.71	2.9	0.49	4.53	18.22	74.7	82
Jelly, currant	1 h. tbsp.	0.36	1.5	0	0	27.16	111.4	113
Prunes, stewed	1 prune + juice	0.25	1.02	0.05	0.47	11.15	45.72	47
Rhubarb, stewed	1 h. tbsp.	0.2	0.8	0.14	2.2	16.2	66.4	69
Banana	Average size	1.3	5.33	0.6	5.58	22.0	90.7	101
Breadstuffs:								
Corn bread	3 × 2 × ¾ in.	3.08	12.6	1.83	17.0	18.06	74.1	104
Rye bread	3½ × 3 × ½ in.	3.51	14.4	0.23	2.1	20.74	85.0	102
Cinnamon buns	1	4.23	17.3	3.24	30.1	26.59	109.0	156
Graham bread	3¾ × 2¾ × ½ in.	3.29	13.5	0.67	6.2	19.28	79.1	99
Rolls, French	1	3.32	13.6	0.98	9.1	21.72	89.1	112
Rolls, Vienna	1	3.83	15.7	0.99	9.2	25.43	104.3	129
Baker's wheat bread	3½ × 3 × ½ in.	2.76	11.3	0.39	3.6	15.93	65.3	80
Whole-wheat bread	3½ × 3½ × ½ in.	4.07	16.7	0.38	3.5	20.87	85.6	106
Zwieback	3½ × 2 × ½ in.	1.47	6.0	1.49	13.9	11.03	4.52	65
Butter cracker	2 in. diam.	1.10	4.5	0.85	7.9	7.11	29.2	42
Graham cracker	3 in. sq.	0.80	3.3	0.75	7.0	5.9	24.2	34
Saltine	2 in. sq.	0.32	1.3	0.38	3.5	2.06	8.4	13
Soda cracker	3 in. sq.	0.59	2.4	0.55	5.1	4.38	17.7	25
Cereals:								
Farina	1 h. tbsp.	0.82	3.4	0.10	1.0	5.72	23.5	28
Hominy	1 h. tbsp.	1.10	4.5	0.10	0.95	8.9	36.5	42
Macaroni	1 h. tbsp.	1.5	6.15	0.75	7.0	7.9	32.4	45
Oatmeal	1 h. tbsp.	1.4	5.75	0.25	2.35	5.75	23.6	32
Rice	1 h. tbsp.	2.8	11.5	0.10	0.9	24.4	100.0	112
Desserts:								
Gingerbread	2 × 3 × 1 in.	3.48	14.3	5.4	50.2	38.1	156.2	221
Sponge cake	2 × 3½ × ½ in.	1.45	6.0	2.46	22.9	15.16	62.2	91
Apple pie	⅙ pie	3.91	16.0	12.35	114.9	53.93	221.1	352
Bread pudding	1 h. tbsp.	2.76	11.3	2.69	22.3	19.24	78.9	224
Chocolate pudding	1 h. tbsp.	2.49	10.25	3.95	36.75	13.91	57.05	54
Baked custard	1 h. tbsp.	3.65	15.0	3.71	34.4	10.25	42.05	92
Snow pudding	1 h. tbsp.	2.26	9.25	0.01	0.15	5.86	24.05	33
Tapioca pudding	1 h. tbsp.	1.93	7.93	2.04	18.9	7.42	30.4	57
Blanc mange	1 h. tbsp.	2.38	9.75	2.45	22.85	8.41	34.5	67
Floating Island	1 h. tbsp.	2.49	10.23	2.54	23.63	4.5	18.47	52
Ice cream	1 h. tbsp.	2.6	10.7	5.08	47.25	8.86	36.35	94
Spanish cream	1 h. tbsp.	5.85	24.0	3.68	34.25	10.62	43.55	102
Ginger snap	2¼ in.	0.33	1.4	0.43	4.0	3.8	15.6	21
Ladyfingers	4 in.	1.76	7.2	1.0	9.3	14.12	57.9	74
Molasses cookies	4 × 3 in.	1.44	5.9	1.74	16.2	15.14	62.1	84
Sugar cookies	3 in.	0.77	3.2	1.12	10.4	8.05	33.0	47
Honey	1 tbsp.	0.12	0.5	0.0	0.0	24.36	100.0	101
Sugar, granulated	1 h. tbsp.	0.0	0.0	0.0	0.0	30.0	123.0	123
Maple syrup	1 tbsp.	0.0	0.0	0.0	0.0	21.4	87.9	88
Gelatin	1 tbsp.	8	32.8	0.0	0.0	0.0	0.0	33

As regards the fat of the diet, the studies of Holt, Courtney and Fales[11] show that vegetable fats, such as nut-butter and corn-oil, are well assimilated in early childhood, and that to a certain extent they can well replace the more expensive animal butter-fat derived from the milk. There must not, however, be a complete substitution, since the vegetable fats are deficient in fat-soluble vitamin A (see p. 134). Sherman and Hawley[12] found from an experimental study that children from three to fourteen years of age required a diet containing about 1000 Gm. (33.81 fl. oz.) of milk daily, to provide the best storage of calcium; but 24 oz. seems to be a satisfactory amount according to most clinicians.

In closing this discussion of the food-requirements of childhood, it must be emphasized that the estimations of different writers vary widely, and that at most they are largely theoretical. The practical conclusion must be that, with good health and good digestion, the amount of food given must vary with the child and depend upon its rate of growth whatever its theoretical demands may be.

PERCENTAGE-COMPOSITION AND CALORIC VALUE OF VARIOUS FOODS IN INFANCY AND CHILDHOOD

In Table 58 may be found the percentage-composition and caloric value of a number of dietary articles likely to be employed in infancy and childhood. They are taken, with a few exceptions, from the "Constitution of American Food-materials" by Atwater and Bryant,[13] and practically all later authors have followed these analyses. The edible portion of the food is that referred to in nearly all instances, and always unless otherwise mentioned, when the letters "A.P." (as purchased) are appended, as by the authors. All foods are raw unless otherwise stated. The equivalents of the caloric values for kilograms are inserted in addition to the avoirdupois estimations of Atwater and Bryant. The caloric values are given in round numbers. In the measuring of milk and other liquids, as expressed in ounces, since 1 pint of water weighs practically 1 lb. avoirdupois, the difference between the fluid ounce and the ounce avoirdupois is slight enough to be disregarded, both as to percentage-composition and caloric value.

Caloric Value of Cooked Foods.—The caloric estimation of cooked articles of diet can be only approximate, depending upon the manner in which the cooking is done. This applies with especial force to the porridges, since the proportions of water and of cereal substance vary greatly according to the recipe employed. Table 59 (p. 131) is one which we have adapted and rearranged from the long and useful lists given by Locke[14] and by Rose.[15] For further details regarding the method of preparation the reader is referred to these books upon the subject.

VITAMINS

(Accessory Food Factors)

Funk, in suggesting the name vitamins, proposed it only as a temporary one until their true nature was discovered, and it is now known that they are not amines. In fact, Funk[16] stated that the substance protective against beriberi was not a protein. However, the term "vitamins" has been justified by use and is more convenient than that of "accessory food factors." A very large amount of literature on the subject has accumulated since the description by Funk.[17] Previous work by Eijkman,[18] Hopkins[19] (whose studies began in 1906), and others had suggested the presence and necessity of these food-elements. The reader may be referred especially to the reviews by Sherman and Smith,[20] McCollum and Simmonds,[21] and Funk.[22] While the exact chemical nature of the vitamins is unknown, it is certain that they are essential for normal nutrition, and that the lack of them results in deficiency diseases, often called "avitaminoses," although in just what manner they act is still undetermined. These conditions are characterized by certain alterations in body-tissue and function, some of which will be mentioned in this section and others in more detail in the chapters on Rickets

(p. 442) and Scurvy (p. 457). Reference to the vitamins has also been made in various sections, as in those on Human Milk (p. 77), Cow's Milk (p. 86), and Diet (p. 123). While the several vitamins are distinct in some of their effects and will be considered individually, they have certain interrelations. The lack of all of them during the period of growth leads to a stunting of this. There is some experimental evidence that when animals are fed increased amounts of vitamin A and D the need for vitamin B is increased.

Many of the studies on vitamins have been made on such animals as rats, guinea-pigs and monkeys. While in most instances the results of these can be considered applicable to the human, this is not always the case and difference between species may cause variation in effect. Vitamins have created a wide interest, and there has been the usual tendency to ascribe to a newly-discovered and imperfectly-studied fact more than its fair share of importance, and also prematurely to employ theories in the treatment of obscure maladies. The average American diet has been supposed by a number of authors to be deficient in the quantity of certain vitamins if not lacking entirely. This is difficult to prove, inasmuch as the quantitative vitamin needs of the human are not known. It is only under extreme conditions, as in famine or severe and prolonged gastrointestinal diseases with faulty absorption, that clear-cut symptoms of beriberi or xerophthalmia develop. To determine whether less obvious symptoms, such as failure to gain, predisposition to infection and the like, are due to partial vitamin deficiency is another matter. Too many complicating factors enter into the picture.

Several distinct varieties of vitamins are recognized and may now be described in some detail.

The fat-soluble **vitamin A** (*antixerophthalmic, anti-infective vitamin*) is present in certain animal fats, such as those of eggs and butter, but it is found to a much greater extent in cod-liver oil and other fish-liver oils as those of the halibut. It is not present in vegetable fats. It exists also in green leafy vegetables such as spinach and cabbage, and in peas, but is usually absent in roots and tubers, except those with yellow pigment such as carrot and turnip. The yellow plant-pigment, carotin, is the precursor of vitamin A, the conversion probably taking place in the liver. Those margarines which are churned in milk contain it. It is not destroyed or lessened by the application of heat unless this is long continued. Storage of this vitamin in the body can occur. If it is absent for a time from the diet of the experimental animal, xerophthalmia with xerosis of the conjunctiva and keratomalacia will develop as the most striking symptom, and the same conditions may arise in the human infant deprived of the vitamin (Bloch,[23] Ross,[24] Mori,[25] Wilson and DuBois,[26] Schwartz,[27] Weech[28]). Xerosis of other tissues may occur and lead to dryness and desquamation of the skin and mucous membranes. In fact the specific morbid process produced by a deficiency in vitamin A is a widespread replacement of normal epithelium by stratified keratinizing epithelium (Wolbach and Howe[29]). Spence[30] found as an early symptom desquamation from the urinary tract, and it is stated that in rats the appearance of cornified epithelial cells in the vaginal secretion is the earliest manifestation. Night-blindness (hemeralopia) may be an early symptom according to Holm.[31] In the rat a deficiency of vitamin A leads to infections in the ears, sinuses, tongue, and other parts of the body. In monkeys colitis develops. It may be that these infections occur because of the lack of an intact epithelium, as described above, which allows entrance of bacteria. Bloch[32] and others claim that this anti-infective property of vitamin A is also active in man, but entirely convincing proof of this is lacking. Vitamin A is necessary for growth and reproduction, and deprivation of it is said also to cause diminution in the fibrinogen of the blood.

The water-soluble **vitamin B**, which formerly was thought to be a single factor or substance, is now known to consist of at least 2 vitamins and may consequently be termed the vitamin B-complex. Vegetables such as cabbages, tomatoes, turnips, spinach, onions, beets, potatoes, carrots and beans, are dietary sources of this food-factor, as are the glandular organs of animals (kidney, liver, pancreas), milk, eggs, and the germ of cereal grains. In yeast it is especially abundant. Milk, both human and cow's, may be deficient in vitamin B-complex according to some investigators (Macy and coworkers[33]). Refined (milled) flour has most of the vitamin removed.

One of the 2 substances in vitamin B-complex is the heat-labile vitamin B_1 also called vitamin F and known as the antineuritic or antiberiberi vitamin; the other is the relatively heat-stable vitamin B_2, or G, or the antipellagric vitamin. Foods so far as studied may differ in their content of B_1 and B_2. For example, cereal grains are rich in B_1, poor in B_2; cow's milk and green leafy vegetables contain more B_2 than B_1; bananas are rich in B_2, deficient in B_1. It should be stated further that the terminology of vitamins is again somewhat confused by the fact that B_2 or G is sometimes denominated the P.P. (Pellagra-Preventing) factor, and that a few authors, apparently believing that there are 3 substances, employ the term B_1 for the antineuritic factor, B_2 for the growth-promoting, and G for the antipellagric. As usually considered, however, absence of B_1 (F) or the antineuritic factor leads to polyneuritis, anorexia, loss of weight, anemia, nervousness and spasticity. In this connection it may be mentioned in passing that Matsumura[34] and his coworkers claim that absence of this vitamin merely predisposes to polyneuritis, or beriberi, and that the principal etiologic factor is a gram-negative motile bacillus (beriberi bacillus). The symptoms described as occurring in fowls and other experimental animals have been observed in the human infant also (Andrews;[35] Moore and Brodie[36]). Lactation seems to be favorably affected by an abundant supply of vitamin B_1. Basal metabolism is lowered by deficiency of it (von Árvay[37]). Pediatrists often suggest that extracts of it as contained in preparations of yeast, cereal germs and rice polishings be given to infants and children. (See p. 123.) Storage of this vitamin in the body is poor. In some instances intake may be sufficient but disorders of the gastrointestinal tract, such as celiac disease, result in deficient retention of it. If B_2, or G, the antipellagric factor, is absent from the diet of rats, there occur loss of weight, irritation of mucous membranes, lethargy, bloody diarrhea and a state of skin and tissues resembling human pellagra, and the presumption is that this disease is produced in the same manner.

The water-soluble **vitamin C** (*antiscorbutic vitamin*) occurs in certain common fruits and vegetables. Oranges, lemons, grape-fruits, and, to a lesser extent, apples and bananas, are sources of supply, and the berries have a large content. Tomatoes, either raw or canned, are particularly rich in it, and most of the green vegetables such as lettuce, string beans, and cabbage will yield a fair amount. While less is present in roots and tubers, yet young carrots, onions, turnips and potatoes have been found to possess sufficient to be protective. Egg-yolk contains a limited quantity, if any, while the amount in milk is dependent on the fodder of the cow, as previously stated. Commercial canning preserves the amount in vegetables to a considerable degree. Cereal grains and legumes contain little vitamin C, or none at all according to some authorities. The body can store this vitamin to a limited extent. It is relatively easily destroyed by heat and drying if long continued, but it is possible to dry food such as milk at high temperature for short periods without destroying the vitamin. Deprivation of it in animals and man leads to the production of scurvy (p. 457), and partial lack to such symptoms as anorexia and loss of weight without the classic symptoms of this disease. Less certain is the effect of deprivation on the resistance to infections. Decalcification of teeth and caries are part of the symptomatology of deprivation of vitamin C.

Vitamin D is the antirachitic factor. This is present in large amount in codliver and certain other fishliver oils; to a lesser extent in butter and in milk. It is found in the small unsaponifiable fraction of codliver oil, and this fact is taken advantage of in making concentrates. Egg-yolk contains the antirachitic vitamin and so does liver, but in vegetables there is practically none of it. It is not easily destroyed by heat. The body can store it to a certain extent. It is different from the fat-soluble A in that the latter may be destroyed by oxidation. Ergosterol may be called the parent substance or precursor of vitamin D, since ergosterol becomes antirachitic upon properly applied ultra-violet irradiation. Many substances may be rendered antirachitic by this means. The effect on the body of sunlight or ultra-violet irradiation from an artificial source is due to the activation of ergosterol in the skin. Absence or partial deprivation of vitamin D leads to disturbance of the metabolism of calcium and phosphorus and the development of rickets (p. 443) and other calcium faults, such as dental caries and poorly calcified teeth. Growth is also interfered with, and muscles and probably all other body-tissues suffer. Feeding enormously excessive amounts of the vitamin in the form of irradiated ergosterol may cause calcium deposition in blood-vessels, kidneys and other structures.

Vitamin E (Substance X) is also called the *reproductive* or *antisterility vitamin*. It is found in wheat-embryo, fresh lettuce, oats and yellow corn. Animal fats such as codliver oil contain practically none of it and there is little in milk. Some is present in other animal tissues. Its storage in the body is limited. Its absence in experimental animals causes failure of placental function with death of the fetus, and in the male degeneration of germinal epithelium.

From the knowledge which has been gained concerning vitamins certain practical applications may be deduced: (*a*) When it is consistent with digestibility, food should be cooked rapidly at a high temperature rather than by prolonged heating; (*b*) If milk is cooked any length of time this should be done in a double boiler to prevent oxidation; (*c*) Alkali should not be added to foods until after they have been heated; (*d*) An infant on a diet consisting largely of cow's milk, even if this be raw and fresh, should be protected by the administration of vitamin-containing substances such as orange juice and codliver oil. The emphasis should be upon the employment of a balanced diet of fresh natural vitamin-containing foodstuffs rather than upon the giving of vitamin preparations. There is no objection to the use of vitamin-concentrates when they are indicated, and a therapeutic trial may be given them; but they do not take the place of a proper ration and should not be employed as an isolated method of treatment.

In Table 60 will be given a list containing with others most of the foods mentioned in this chapter with their vitamin content. Much work remains to be done in this matter and the table shows only approximate amounts. There exists considerable confusion concerning the so-called "vitamin units" and the quantitative needs for the several vitamins. The Vitamin Committee to Suggest Standards for the Eleventh United States Pharmacopoeia[38] has recommended that vitamin A be so standardized that 1 unit shall equal 0.001 mg. of the preparation of carotin which is in the National Institute of Medical Research in London; that 1 unit of vitamin D shall represent 1 mg. of the solution of irradiated ergosterol in the same institution; that 1 unit of vitamin B_1 shall be equivalent to 10 mg. of the

TABLE 60.—VITAMIN CONTENT OF FOODS*

Type of food.	Value as source of vitamins.				
	A.	B.	C.	D.	E.
Breads:					
Graham bread	XX	XXX	---	---	XXX
Rye bread	XX	XXX	---	---	
Wheat, whole	XX	XX	---	---	XXX
Wheat, white	X	XX	---	---	
Zwieback		XX	---		
Cakes:					
Pound cake	XXX	XXX	---		XXX
Sponge cake	X	X	---		X
White cake	X	X	---		
Cereals:					
Barley, pearl	XX	XXX	---		XX
Corn flakes	XX	XXXX			
Corn meal, cooked	XX	XXXX	---		
Cream of Wheat, cooked		XXX	---		
Farina, cooked		XXX	---		
Macaroni, cooked	---	---	---		
Oats, rolled, cooked	XX	XXXX	---		XXX
Puffed Rice	---	---	---		
Puffed Wheat	---	XXX	---		XXX
Rice, cooked	---	---	---	---	---
Tapioca	---	XXX			XX
Shredded Wheat	X	XXXX			XXX
Wheatena, raw	X	XXXX	---		
Hominy grits	---		---		
Cheeses:					
American	XXXX	XXX	---		
Cottage Cheese	XX	XXX			
Cream Cheese	XXX	XX			
Swiss Cheese	XX	---			
Cookies:					
Lady fingers	XX	X	---		X
Molasses cookies	---	---	---		
Oatmeal cookies	X	XX	---		
Vanilla wafers	---	---	---		
Eggs:					
Whole	XXXX	XXX	---	XXX	XX
White	---	---	---	---	---
Yolk	XXXX	XXX	---	XXX	XXX
Fats:					
Butter	XXX			X	X
Cod liver oil	XXXX	---	---	XXXX	
Cottonseed oil	X	---	---	---	X
Oleomargarine	XX	---	---		XX
Olive oil	X	---	---	---	X
Fish:					
Oyster, raw	X	XX	XX		
Halibut, cooked	XX	XX			
Mackerel, raw	XX	XX			
Salmon, canned	XX	XX			
Flour:					
Arrowroot					
Barley	XX	XXX	---	---	XXX
Corn starch	---	---	---	---	---
Graham	XX	XXX	---		
Rye	---	XX	---		
Soy-bean meal					
Wheat, patent	---	XX	---	---	---
Wheat, whole	XX	XXXX	---	---	XXX

* From Bradley (Tables of Food Values, 1931). X = small amount of vitamin; XX = fair source of vitamin; XXX = a good source of vitamin; XXXX = an excellent source of vitamin. Blank space = evidence as to vitamin content insufficient. --- = absence of vitamin.

TABLE 60.—VITAMIN CONTENT OF FOODS.—(*Continued*)

Type of food.	Value as source of vitamins.				
	A.	B.	C.	D.	E.
Fruit:					
Apple	XXX	XXX	XX		
Apple, sauce	XX	XX	---		
Apricots, canned	XXX	XXX	XXX		
Apricots, dried					
Bananas	XX	XXX	XXX		
Cantaloupe	XXXX	XXXX	XXXX		
Grapefruit	XX	XXX	XXXX	---	
Grapes	XX	XXX	XX		
Lemon juice	XX	XXX	XXXX		
Orange juice	XX	XXX	XXXX		
Peaches, fresh	XX	XX	XXX		
Peaches, dried	XX	XX			
Prunes	XXX	XXX	---		
Prunes, stewed	XXX	XXX	---		
Raspberries			XXXX		
Rhubarb, cooked			XXXX		
Strawberries	XX	XXX	XXXX		
Grape juice	X	XX	---		
Meats:					
Kidneys, cooked	XXX	XXX	---		
Liver	XXXX	XXXX	XX	XX	XXX
Steak, cooked	X	XX	---		
Lamb chops, broiled					
Bacon, cooked	X	XX			
Ham, boiled	X	XX	---		
Chicken, broiled	---	---	---		
Chicken, creamed	X	X			
Sweetbreads, beef	XXXX	XXXX	X		
Milks:					
Buttermilk	XXX	XXX	XX		
Milk, condensed, sweet	XXXX	XXX		XXX	
Milk, condensed, unsweetened	XXXX	XXX		XXX	
Milk, whole	XXXX	XXX	XX	XX	XX
Cocoa	XXXX	XXX	XX	XX	XX
Puddings:					
Cup custard	XXX	XX	---		XX
Rice with milk	X	X	---		---
Bread	XX	XX	---		X
Vegetable Soups:					
Quite similar to vegetables					
Vegetables:					
Asparagus, canned and fresh		XXXX			
Beans, lima, fresh	XX	XXX	X	---	XX
Beans, string	XXX	XXX	XXX		
Beets, cooked	XX	XX	---		
Beet greens, cooked	XXX	XX	X	---	XX
Cabbage	X	XXX	XXXX	---	
Carrots	XXXX	XXX	XXXX		
Cauliflower	XX	XXX	XX		
Celery	XX	XXX	XXXX		XX
Corn	XX	XXX	---	---	XX
Lettuce	XXXX	XXX	XXXX	XX	XXXX
Onions, escalloped	XX	XX	XXX	---	---
Peas, canned and green	XXX	XXX	XXX	---	XX
Potatoes, cooked	XX	XXX	XX	---	
Spinach	XXXX	XXXX	XXX	XX	XXX
Squash, creamed	XXX	XX	XX		
Tomatoes, canned and fresh	XX	XX	XXXX		

vitamin prepared in the Medical Laboratory, Batavia, Java; and that 1 unit of vitamin C shall correspond to 0.1 cc. of fresh juice of the lemon.

Vitamin Preparations.—Cod liver oil and irradiated ergosterol (viosterol), although sold by many different commercial firms, are not to be classified as proprietary remedies, but there are many other preparations especially of the vitamin B complex which are sold under trade names. There are available concentrated forms of cod liver oil and other fish liver oils which contain vitamins A and D. Several of the cod liver oils have irradiated ergosterol added to them. Those products accepted by the Council on Pharmacy and Chemistry of the American Medical Association may be considered reliable.

References

1. Am. J. Dis. Child., 1928, **36,** 651. 2. Boston M. and S. J., 1913, **169,** 702. 3. J.A.M.A., 1916, **67,** 432. 4. Der Stoffwechsel des Kindes, 1896. 5. Pfaundler und Schlossmann, Handb. d. Kinderh., 1906, **1,** 401. 6. Carnegie Inst. Washington, Publ., 302, 1921. 7. Medicine, 1924, **3,** 1. 8. Am. J. Dis. Child., 1921, **21,** 1; 1921, **22,** 371; 1922, **23,** 471; 1922, **24,** 44; 1922, **24,** 311. 9. Pfaundler und Schlossmann Handb. d. Kinderh., 1923, **1,** 425. 10. Am. J. Dis. Child., 1926, **32,** 641. 11. Am. J. Dis. Child., 1919, **18,** 157. 12. J. Biol. Chem., 1922, **53,** 375. 13. U. S. Dept. Agric. Office of Exper. Station Bull., 28; Revis. Edit., 1906. 14. Food Values, 1916. 15. A Lab. Handb. for Dietetics, 1917, 3d Edit. 1930; Feeding the Family, 1917. 16. Lancet, 1911, **2,** 1266; J. Physiol., 1911–12, **43,** 395. 17. J. State Med., 1912, **20,** 341. 18. Arch. f. path. Anat. u. Physiol., 1896, **148,** 523. 19. J. Physiol., 1912, **44,** 425. 20. The Vitamins, 1931, 2d edit. 21. The Newer Knowledge of Nutrition, 1930, 4th Edit. 22. The Vitamins; transl. by Dubin from 2d German edit., 1922. 23. Jahrb. f. Kinderh., 1919, **89,** 405; Am. J. Dis. Child., 1924, **27,** 139; 1931, **42,** 263. 24. Am. J. Dis. Child., 1921, **22,** 232. 25. Quoted by McCollum, J.A.M.A., 1923, **81,** 894. 26. Am. J. Dis. Child., 1923, **26,** 431. 27. J.A.M.A., 1925, **85,** 2025. 28. Am. J. Dis. Child., 1930, **39,** 1153. 29. J. Exper. Med., 1925, **42,** 753. 30. Arch. Dis. Childhood., 1931, **6,** 17. 31. Am. J. Physiol., 1925, **73,** 79. 32. Am. J. Dis. Child., 1931, **42,** 263. 33. J. Biol. Chem., 1927, **73,** 189; 203. 34. J.A.M.A., 1929, **92,** 1325. 35. Phillipine J. Sc., Sec. Trop. Med., 1912, **7,** 67. 36. Am. J. Dis. Child., 1927, **34,** 53. 37. Biochem. Ztschr., 1928, **192,** 369. 38. Personal Communication, Vitamin Committee to Suggest Standards for Eleventh U. S. Pharmacopoeia.

CHAPTER VII

CHARACTERISTICS OF DISEASE IN INFANCY AND CHILDHOOD

The diseases of early life vary decidedly from those occurring later. Not only are the causes often different, but the reaction of the growing tissues in early years is not the same as in adult life. Anatomic and physiologic distinctions also exist. There is consequently seen a tendency to the development of certain diseases in infancy and childhood, and an immunity toward others. The susceptibility of the incompletely developed nervous system is very great, often masking the real nature of the disorder. Trifling factors thus produce general symptoms which are, or appear to be, severe out of all proportion to their causes, similar agencies acting in adults giving rise to no symptoms of moment. The initial effect of deleterious influences is often unusually marked in early life, and the development of symptoms very rapid and apparently severe; while, on the other hand, the recuperative power is great, and convalescence is speedy. Various causes render the examination of a sick child difficult. There are also marked peculiarities at this period in the reaction of the system to certain drugs, some of the materia medica being unusually well-tolerated, and others not at all so.

After early childhood is passed, and particularly after the age of seven or eight years, the peculiarities of disease incident to the age of the patient are less marked.

ETIOLOGY

Among the causes predisposing to the development of certain disorders in children direct or indirect *inheritance* plays an important rôle. Syphilis is congenitally transmitted, as probably are very occasionally such of the acute infectious diseases as typhoid fever, scarlatina, and some others, and not infrequently variola. Tuberculosis existing in the parents certainly predisposes to its development in the offspring, but the disease itself is rarely transmitted, and many cases of apparently hereditary predisposition are in reality instances of exposure. Rheumatism and gout exert a similar predisposing influence, as do various nervous disorders, such as epilepsy, insanity, a neuropathic tendency, and some of the muscular dystrophies and diseases of the spinal cord. Some of these maladies may not actually show themselves until childhood is past, although the seeds of them are present in the system. *Sex* influences the occurrence of certain diseases, such as the preponderance of pyloric stenosis and hemophilia in males, and of pyelitis and chorea in females. Of importance, too, is the existence of various *diatheses* (see p. 480) manifesting themselves at birth or later, to which the occurrence of certain symptoms seen in early life is to be attributed.

To be mentioned also is the etiologic influence upon the diseases of the infant of the various *morbid conditions incident to fetal life and to birth*, which will be referred to again (p. 170). Maternal impressions have frequently been considered a powerful factor in the production of some of these, but positive proof of any causal relationship is entirely unsatisfactory.

Imperfect feeding and hygiene are among the most active causes of disease in infancy and childhood. As a result arise the many forms of disturbed digestion and their consequences; such constitutional conditions as rickets and scurvy; the disordered states of the respiratory apparatus so common in children; and the diseases which depend upon lack of proper care of the nervous system. The influence of *school-life* is responsible for many nervous ailments, affections of the eyes, deformity of the spine, disturbance of the general health, and acute respiratory disorders developing from exposure to infection.

Infection, indeed, has unusual etiologic power in children, the great majority of cases of acute infectious diseases being witnessed at this period. This is partly due to a greater degree of susceptibility; partly to a much greater opportunity of exposure; and partly to the fact that most adults have already become immune through earlier occurrence of these affections.

GENERAL METHODS OF EXAMINATION AND DIAGNOSIS

There are a few respects in which the study of disease in infancy and childhood is easier than in adult life. Existence having been of shorter duration, there is generally a shorter history to be obtained. There are fewer complicating conditions, at least in the acute affections, and fewer previous bad habits of living to be taken into account.

On the whole, however, the subject presents many and varied difficulties. Many affections exhibit in childhood symptoms different from those of adult life, and the significance of even the same symptom often differs; while there are also many diseases which are almost or entirely peculiar to early life. Again, the infant cannot, without speech, describe its symptoms, and the older child often cannot be trusted to give an accurate account. The inability to control the patient presents another difficulty, and the constant crying of an infant may render a satisfactory examination impossible. Considerable skill, patience and tact are therefore required.

Obtaining the History.—As a sequence to what has been said, dependence must be placed on the gathering of a careful and complete clinical history from the mother or nurse. Those particularly interested in hospital records may consult the article by Hoyer and Mitchell.[1] In infancy there is, of course, no history obtainable from the patient, and even up to the age of six or seven years, the child either refuses to answer questions on account of timidity, or makes replies which are not dependable. The presence of pain, for instance, may be denied when it really exists, or maintained when not existing, and the localization by the patient is very misleading, pain in the chest being perhaps referred to the throat or abdomen, and so on. There should be some definite order followed in the procuring of the history from the attendant. Considerable latitude is, of course, allowable, dependent upon the nature of the ailment; yet, in general, the first point should be a brief statement of the present complaint limited to a few words; next, the past clinical history of the patient; third, the detailed account of the present illness; and, last, the family history. To reverse this order renders the asking of numerous useless questions unavoidable.

After eliciting very briefly the chief symptoms from which the child seems to be suffering, it is often well to allow the mother to give as full an account as possible of the case, in her own way and undisturbed by interruptions, unless these become necessary. Ordinarily the history may best be heard in the presence of the child, who, meanwhile, is growing accustomed to the physician's presence, and who, unknown to itself, is at the same time under the quiet observation of the physician's eye. Yet there are numerous exceptions to this. If the mother's mind is distracted by the child's crying, she will be unable to answer questions satisfactorily. So, too, if an older child is seen listening too intently to the story about itself, it may readily be affected injuriously, and in this event the history should be obtained in another room. While, as a rule, the mother's opinions are of little value, her statements of *what she has noticed* must be listened to and weighed with care; since by her constant association with the child, and by her natural anxiety, her powers of observation have sometimes become very keen, and she is rendered peculiarly able to detect even slight changes from the ordinary condition of health. After the mother has finished her account, she should be subjected to careful questioning, much, or all, of the child's life being passed in review. Leading questions must be avoided, for the suggestions which these offer are very liable to lead to erroneous statements.

Previous History.—In the case of infants this should date from birth; and this applies with equal truth to many older subjects. Among the data concerning which information will be sought are the existence of prematurity; of asphyxia following birth; the nature of the labor; the process of dentition; the time when sitting and walking were begun; the birth-weight and the subsequent alterations; the frequency of micturition; the degree of perspiration; the character of the sleep; the existence of mouth-breathing; the state of the bowels; the condition of general nutrition and the time when any change in this was seen; the condition of the nervous symptoms in general; and the psychic development, often best shown by the degree of interest taken and the ability to understand and to talk. Particular attention must be paid to the minutest details of the different methods of feeding which have been employed and to the effects of these; whether weaning has taken place, and, if so, why. The statement, for instance, that the baby had been fed on modified milk is not sufficient. The *proportions* of milk, water and the like should be ascertained. Especial care must be given, too, to discovering the date, nature, mode of onset and duration of all previous illnesses. This is often a matter of some difficulty, and may require careful, patient questioning.

Present Illness.—We can next take up the illness from which the child is now suffering. The exact date of onset and the sequence of the symptoms are important, and may require time and skill to elicit. At least the mother is generally able to say at what date she considered the child to have been entirely well. A detailed description of the past symptoms is to be sought for. The nature of the questions varies, of course, with the case. The degree and persistence of fever is important, although the history in this respect is of little value unless the thermometer has been used. The state of the general nervous system should be reviewed to discover, for instance, the occurrence of restlessness, crying, sleeplessness, drowsiness, coughing, twitching or pain; the degree of apparent exhaustion or prostration, as indicated by the previous desire of the patient to be in bed or out, and the presence or absence of a desire to play with toys; the position in bed; and the like. In digestive disorders an account should be obtained of the mode of onset and the nature of the food at the time; the history of vomiting or diarrhea and the number of daily occurrences of these; the character of the vomitus or the stools; and the state of the appetite.

Family History.—The nature of the questions now to be asked will naturally depend upon what has already been learned. They should include the clinical history of other children of the family, the parents, and often of other direct or indirect antecedents when the existence of a possible inheritance is involved. Among the matters which need to be investigated are the general health of the family and antecedents; the occurrence in them of tuberculosis, nervous disorders, rheumatism, gout, insanity, alcoholism; the number of children living or dead and the causes of death. The question of parental syphilis must usually be approached with caution. In place of direct questions information may be gained, for instance, regarding the occurrence of numerous miscarriages, the history of maternal cutaneous eruptions, and the like.

Method of Examining the Child.—Now follows the direct examination of the child,—an examination which, as stated, has been all this while quietly going on to a certain extent. Very young infants take no notice of the physician's presence. Older children, however, often have much fear of strangers, and perhaps, from previous experience or suggestion, especially of physicians. A quick glance at the patient on entering the room, or the manner in which a word of cheery greeting is received, will frequently reveal something of the personal characteristics in this respect. It is often a good plan to seem to ignore absolutely a somewhat irritable or timid child. It then quite commonly happens that, fear being allayed and a certain degree of pique created, the child itself makes the advances, whereupon the most friendly relations between the doctor and patient may soon be established. Avoidance of all hurry, and the use of gentle words and actions, often aid in rendering a child willing to submit quietly to an examination. Sometimes this can be made to appear a game which the physician is playing with his little patient.

In the case of many children whose timidity seems too great to be overcome, and especially with those who have been spoiled by indulgent parents, and who seem to resent in an ugly spirit the physician's presence, nothing whatever is gained by delay, and it is best to proceed quietly, gently, yet firmly with the examination, regardless of any objections made. Many such children, observing that the physician goes on with his work in spite of protest, learn the uselessness of this and behave better at future visits. Very often the difficulty is with the mother rather than with the child.

A sincere love for children, a quick recognition of a child's peculiarities of disposition, a ready adaptability to meet them, and above all, continued experience rapidly lessen the difficulties in the study of disease in early life. Fortunately, practice enables a physician to make an examination of many unruly children almost as satisfactorily as of those who are quiet and docile.

Order of Procedure.—This depends somewhat on circumstances, and the greatest flexibility in the plan is to be allowed. Those examinations are first made either which arouse least objection or which are most important. If the child is sleeping, or often if it is lying awake in its bed, a superficial inspection of it may be made. Such a time may be favorable for feeling the radial pulse and for the palpation of the abdomen; for should the infant begin to cry satisfactory examination of the abdomen is rarely possible. Next, the temperature should be taken before prolonged crying can have increased it. Following this, the general inspection should be completed. Should crying or coughing occur the character of these may be noted.

The physical examination of the thorax may next be carried on, auscultation being practised first, if the child is quiet, since this often causes less alarm and less tendency to cry than percussion does. At some time during quiet the reflexes may be tested. Last of all the mouth and throat must be inspected, and frequently the nose, eyes, and ears. The urine should be obtained for examination, and in many instances the investigation is not complete without a study of the blood and of the cavities of the thorax, abdomen, or spinal canal for the presence of fluid and the character of this. Special cases require a radiologic and bacteriologic study.

Some of these methods will now receive consideration in fuller detail. The clinical significance of the observations made will be considered in the chapter upon Symptomatology (p. 155).

Inspection.—This furnishes often greater results than any other method for arriving at a diagnosis. It is the first examination to be made, and begins, although at a distance, as soon as the physician comes into the presence of the patient. After a general inspection made of the child while asleep or awake, it should, when possible, be undressed, wrapped in a warm blanket and laid on the mother's lap or on the bed. When a condition of exhaustion, low bodily temperature, the presence of pain on movement, the existence of diseases of the upper respiratory tract, or other cause renders complete undressing undesirable, the body must be uncovered and examined part by part throughout before the study is ended. Unless the child is thus undressed very valuable data would be undiscovered; such as differences in the form and degree of motion of the two sides of the chest; the position of a visible apex-beat; the presence of epigastric or episternal pulsation or retraction; the occurrence of important eruptions of the skin; distention of the abdomen or of the abdominal veins; visible peristalsis; beading of the ribs; etc. In addition to these matters inspection must take cognizance of the state of the general nutrition; the physiognomy; the color of the face and lips; the shape of the head; the condition of the fontanelle and of the eyes; the shape of the abdomen; visible glandular enlargement; the position of the body in bed; the shape and movements of the limbs; the condition of the genitals; the character of the sleep; the degree of restlessness or of apathy; the method of nursing; the existence of nasal or oral discharge; the character of the cough and cry, and of the stools, urine and vomited matter. The rate and rhythm of the respiration are to be determined; the occurrence of mouth-breathing noted, as well as the existence of thoracic rattling which can be heard at a distance; and the presence of dyspnea and its degree and method of manifestation are to be studied. The character of respiration and its regularity may be observed well by watching the movement of the thorax and abdomen while the child is asleep. Nothing can be determined if the child is at all excited.

Special inspection of the *ears* is often required, and should be practised in all doubtful cases where there is unexplained fever, pain, restlessness or stupor. Examination of the *eyes* sometimes gives valuable information. The presence of conjunctivitis is to be noted and of swelling and discoloration of the lids. The use of the ophthalmoscope is possible even in very young children, and important conditions of the eye-ground may often be discovered. Inspection of the *nose* with the mirror and speculum can be carried out in docile children. That of the anterior nares may reveal the presence of nasal diphtheria, so often unsuspected.

Inspection of the *mouth* and *throat* should always be made as a matter of routine at the first visit, and the possibility of subsequent development of disease here always kept in mind. The condition of the tongue, gums and teeth can often be seen if the patient is crying. For a more thorough inspection of the mouth in infancy, the fingers, previously well washed, may be pushed gently in between the gums at one or both sides of the mouth. This, or the pressing of the chin downward will be enough to open the mouth, and to allow a visual examination of it to be made easily. To view the pharynx satisfactorily demands quickness and a certain degree of dexterity. A tongue-depressor is required, and for this nothing answers better in family practice than a teaspoon with a smooth handle free from sharp irregularities. Serviceable here or for office use are the wooden depressors made for this purpose, and in occasional cases, where considerable force is required, a strong metal depressor with the extremity curved slightly downward.

The infant or young child should be seated in the mother's lap, facing a window and with the back of its head against her right arm or shoulder. Its hands should be held, or better still, a blanket or shawl be wrapped about the arms and body close under the chin. All preparations are to be made before the physician approaches the child. In this way much less fright is occasioned. He now stands slightly to the mother's right side and in front, places one hand upon the child's head in order that he may steady it and turn it in any direction desired, and with the other hand introduces the depressor, utilizing a moment when the child opens its mouth to speak or cry or to make some remonstrance. With older children who have learned to keep the mouth tightly shut, the depressor can readily be worked in from the side, or the nostrils compressed for a moment to make the mouth open. Every movement must be gentle and without hurry, yet quickly carried out. As soon as the depressor is in the mouth, it is pushed slowly backward. When it reaches the base of the tongue the child gags and necessarily opens its mouth widely, the soft palate rising, and the tongue sinking. At this moment a rapid yet complete inspection of the fauces can be made. All this procedure may and should be accomplished in a few seconds. The only exception to this is in the case of young infants. Here the reflex gagging is less well-developed, and forcible depression of the tongue is required. It is in such cases that the metal depressor is serviceable.

In the case of older, vigorous, and very obstreperous children who struggle violently, a somewhat different plan of holding is required. The mother or nurse seats herself facing the light, with the child in her lap and its back against her body. Wrapping her knees about its feet and legs she grasps its left hand in her right and its right in her left and draws them to her. This movement crosses the child's arms over its chest and draws its head against the mother's breast, thus rendering the patient powerless. When the physician wishes to have both of his hands free for the treatment of the throat, a modification of this method can be adopted. This consists in the mother holding the child's legs between her knees as before, with its arms extended laterally above her elbows while she clasps her hands on the top of its head. In this way the head is controlled as well as the legs and arms.

Occasionally timid little children, who have learned to fear a depressor, will tolerate the physician's little finger, previously well cleansed, pressed for a moment against the base of the tongue. The possibility of having the finger bitten must not be forgotten. Some children will themselves depress the tongue with their own finger. Under certain circumstances, as, for instance, in cases of extreme weakness, it is often best to omit the examination of the throat unless there are symptoms pointing to some trouble there. This is true especially of laryngospastic children, in whom a dangerous spasm of the larynx may readily be produced by the examination.

The inspection of the *larynx* in infancy and childhood is often important, but frequently difficult to accomplish.

Palpation.—In palpating a young child it is important to avoid causing alarm. The hand of the physician should be warm and every touch light. When the child is asleep it is well to attempt to feel the pulse or to palpate the abdomen. To examine the pulse the warm fingers may be applied very lightly over the radial artery, and the physician's hand should readily follow, without restraining, any movements of the hand of the patient. If the child is awake its attention may often be diverted by toys. If it becomes alarmed observations of the pulse are rendered worthless. In infants under six months it is often impossible to feel the radial pulse. In such cases it may be counted at the fontanelle. With similar precautions the rate of respiration may be determined by placing the hand upon the abdomen.

To palpate the abdomen satisfactorily its walls must be relaxed. During sleep, or when the child is being diverted in some way, is the time to be preferred. The flat of the warm hand should be laid carefully upon the skin under the clothing. Light palpation is employed first, in order not to awaken resistance of the abdominal walls. Local tenderness and any unusual resistance may be discovered. The edge of the liver or of an enlarged spleen or any superficially situated tumors may be detected. Now deeper palpation may be attempted. If this causes resistance and the child cries, the hand may sink a little deeper every time a breath is taken, and, by maintaining the advantage thus gained, even conditions deep-seated within the abdomen may sometimes be discovered. The value of bimanual palpation is not to be overlooked. Sometimes rectal examination may aid greatly a simultaneous palpation of the abdomen with the other hand. When a child continues to scream violently and continuously, abdominal palpation is generally unsatisfactory. At times by keeping the hand in position, and diverting the child, an opportunity to palpate may after all be obtained; yet often the examination is best made under anesthesia.

In palpating the chest, one seeks for the position of the apex-beat, differences in the expansion of portions of the thorax, the presence of the rachitic rosary or other bony alterations, bulging or retraction of any region, precordial thrill, and the fremitus communicated by bronchial ronchi and less frequently by the voice. Sometimes bimanual palpation in an intercostal space may detect fluctuation in cases of pleural effusion. Palpation is a most important means of diagnosis in cases of retropharyngeal abscess as also of adenoid vegetations in little children. In either condition the finger introduced through the mouth will render the diagnosis easy.

Percussion.—This must always be lightly performed and not continued long enough to produce fatigue or undue annoyance. Heavy percussion not only is the cause of discomfort but defeats its object, since the chest-walls of the child are so thin that a heavy blow causes a general reverberation and conceals the dulness of a small spot which would otherwise have become apparent. The finger used as a pleximeter should be firmly applied, but the percussion should be done gently and with but one finger, and with a movement of the finger only or the slightest action of the wrist. Direct percussion with the tip of the middle finger tapping the chest-wall often gives the best results. The feeling of resistance is as important as the hearing of dulness. Crying causes no real difficulty, as the tapping can be done at the moment the child stops to draw breath. When there is not crying, percussion should always be made during both inspiration and expiration. In percussing the back or the axillae, the child may sit, or, in the case of infants, may be held upright in the nurse's arms with its head looking over her shoulder. In either case, however, its position must be straight; not with one arm much higher than the other, or with the spine at all twisted. A faulty position will give untrustworthy results. Indeed, a chest much deformed from spinal disease often cannot be percussed with satisfactory results. A child too ill to be kept in a sitting position may be placed flat on its abdomen. This position may sometimes conveniently be made use of in less feeble patients, since it is one to which healthy infants are accustomed in being dressed. For the examination of the front of the chest the child may conveniently be laid on its back in bed.

Percussion is not as satisfactory in children as in adults, owing to the smaller and more resilient chest and to the variety of sounds produced. It is extremely easy entirely to overlook small areas of consolidation. Even considerable pleural effusion may give no very dull sound. On the other hand, one may perhaps find areas of apparent dulness with which there are neither symptoms nor other physical signs to correspond, and which have no pathologic significance, so far as can be discovered. This is especially true for the apices, as has been pointed out clearly by Hamill[2] and by Mielke.[3] Among other peculiarities of percussion in healthy children is the loud, full note obtained over the whole chest, which would be called tympanitic in adults. A cracked-pot sound is often easily obtainable even in perfectly healthy children who are crying, or sometimes even in those entirely quiet (see also p. 161).

These difficulties and causes of uncertainty in no way militate against the importance of a careful percussion of every chest in which disease is suspected, since this examination, combined with experience in disease in children, will often be of the greatest possible service.

Percussion of the abdomen reveals the presence of unusual gaseous distention, free fluid, enlargement of organs, morbid growths, or inflammatory processes (p. 161).

Auscultation.—Auscultation of the lungs in children, and especially in infants, may often be done with the ear applied directly to the chest or with only a thin unstarched garment between. This method is suitable when we are seeking for the scattered coarse râles of a bronchitis, or for large areas of bronchial or of feeble breathing; but for the more exact localization of sounds, or the discovery of lesions in doubtful cases, a stethoscope is indispensable. Yet in all such, both the mediate and immediate method should be followed, for it sometimes happens that sounds undiscovered by the one will be revealed by the other. Either the disc double stethoscope or that with the ordinary bell-piece may be employed, according to the preference of the examiner. Children often dislike greatly not only the appearance of the instrument, but also the sensation of the hard, cold bell-piece pressed against the skin. The first difficulty can be overcome by allowing the child to handle or play with the stethoscope before it is used; the second by warming the part which is to touch the chest, or by having it covered with a soft rubber ring or surrounded by a rubber cup. The bell must be small in order to make it adapt itself well to the surface of a child at all thin. The use of the soft rubber referred to is an aid here. The posterior part of the chest should usually be examined first since this often may be done before the infant discovers what is going on, but all parts must eventually be carefully studied, never forgetting the axillae. The child may be seated or held in the arms for the examination of the back. Infants, or older children too ill to sit up, should lie on the abdomen. The lateral portions of the chest are best examined while the child is sitting or held; the front is best examined while it is lying in bed. The patient must never be so low that the position of the physician is made uncomfortable through stooping, as otherwise the congestion produced interferes with exact hearing and accurate results cannot be obtained.

Crying does not interfere materially with auscultation of the lungs, if the ear is at all practised, since inspiration can be listened for when the child draws breath between cries, unless there are noisy laryngeal sounds attending it. In fact, crying is often advantageous in making inspiration deeper, and it is frequently only during crying that vocal resonance can be properly studied in infancy. Increase of vocal resonance may sometimes be determined by observing the closeness of the râles to the ear in a certain locality. Crying disturbs considerably the auscultation of the heart-sounds. They can then be heard well only when the child inspires. If there is no crying, the rapidity of the cardiac action may be determined by the stethoscope over the apex, in cases where the pulsations at the wrist cannot be counted readily. The irregularity in respiration, especially present in infants, is to be borne in mind, as the very long pauses which occur might deceive the unwary into believing that respiration was inaudible.

Among some of the peculiarities of auscultation in childhood, the loudness and harshness of the respiratory murmur is to be mentioned, a condition denominated "puerile" and considered pathologic when present in adults. In infancy, however, respiration is superficial and feeble. The ease with which the heart-sounds can be heard at the back, and in fact all over the thorax, even when there is no consolidated pulmonary tissue intervening, and with which râles and even bronchial respiration produced in one lung can sometimes be heard in the other is to be noted, as is also the facile transmission through the lungs, especially to the apices, of sounds produced in the upper respiratory tract. It is especially, too, in children that respiration approaching a bronchial character is heard under the clavicles and in the interscapular spaces close to the spine, particularly on the right side, yet without possessing pathologic significance.

The results of auscultation in pneumonia in early life often present important differences from those obtained in adults. This is so true that the diagnosis of this disease must often rest upon the symptoms rather than on the physical signs. The lateness of the development of physical signs is often characteristic, for the attack may sometimes nearly run its course before any signs whatever can be detected. This is perhaps especially true in bronchopneumonia, in which disease the smallness of scattered patches may produce no characteristic alteration of the respiratory murmur. (See p. 161.)

Temperature-taking.—The applying of the hand to the skin to determine the existence or nonexistence of fever is entirely untrustworthy. High temperature, it is true, can often be detected by the hand resting upon the body under the clothing, but the method has repeatedly led to grave mistakes. The use of the clinical thermometer is the only means to be relied upon. The instrument should remain in place a little longer than the "one minute" or "half-minute" would indicate as necessary. The only absolutely accurate procedure, however, consists in leaving it in position until the maximum temperature is reached, watching the mercury meanwhile to determine this. The dislike of most small children for temperature-taking is often too great to permit of employing this plan, and a little experimenting with a quick self-registering thermometer will show with approximate correctness how long is generally required to reach the maximum.

In well-trained children of four years the thermometer may be placed in the mouth, although there is even then some danger of having it bitten. In younger subjects the rectum is the only proper place. Records obtained in the axillae are untrustworthy for various reasons. It must be remembered, too, that the oral and rectal temperatures, which should be about the same, and each of which gives the correct readings, are at least a degree higher than the axillary, even when this has been accurately ascertained. The employment of the groin or the popliteal space for temperature-taking is to be condemned since the record is seldom dependable.

The bulb of the thermometer should be oiled slightly and pushed into the rectum until well out of sight, the infant meantime lying in any position comfortable to it. The nurse should then keep the tip of her finger upon the end of the instrument. There is no necessity of restraining the infant's legs, and it may be allowed without danger to kick all it desires if the hand merely guards the thermometer. It is better that the rectum be empty of feces, but this is not an essential. Only when the thermometer in the rectum produces pain and straining, as in some cases of diarrheal disturbance, should the axilla be used for obtaining the record. The time for taking the temperature should not be after a hard attack of crying, as the height of it may be increased. For the same reason, crying during the observation should be prevented, if possible, by diverting the child.

Examination of the Urine.—The obtaining of the urine is often a matter of some little difficulty in infancy. In the case of male infants it may be procured by applying a condom over the penis, or a small bottle with a sufficiently wide neck which may be held in place by bandages or adhesive strips extending to the waist. For female infants the neck of the bottle may be passed through an oblong piece of adhesive plaster, firmly attached there in a way to prevent leaking, and the plaster then applied over the vulva and perineum; or a glass cup, such as is used to hold seed in bird cages, may be kept in place over the vulva by the pressure of the diaper. In some cases it may suffice to put a large wad of absorbent cotton inside of the diaper, examine the cotton at frequent intervals, and express the urine as soon as possible after it is passed. This method is not so satisfactory since it interferes with microscopic examination. A better procedure is to allow the infant to lie upon a small, circular, rubber air cushion with the opening in the center and a small pus-basin placed beneath this. The surrounding portion of the bed is then built up with pillows to the level of the cushion, and the infant, without a diaper, lies here until the urine is passed into the basin. A simpler plan is to allow the infant without a diaper to lie for a time upon a rubber cloth. In hospital practice a metabolism-bed may be used. Children a year old, or sometimes less, may be put at frequent intervals on a chamber in the hope of procuring urine in this way. Urination is most likely to occur at the time of nursing or taking fluid. In the event that none of these methods succeeds, a small silk catheter, No. 9 or 10 French scale or No. 4 American scale, may be employed. Except in very young infants, and sometimes even in these, the instrument can be passed without difficulty. The greatest precautions must be taken against infection, and the method employed only when the obtaining of uncontaminated urine is necessary, as in cases of suspected pyelitis in female infants.

Blood and Blood-pressure.—The examination of the blood is accomplished as in adult life, testing the hemoglobin-percentage, the number of and changes in the erythrocytes and leukocytes, and in some cases the coagulability, fragility of the corpuscles, specific gravity, and any chemical alterations which may be present. The blood-pressure, too, is estimated as in adults, with such modifications of the apparatus as the small size of the patient often demands. The study of the blood-chemistry (p. 40) may well be left to the laboratory expert, but some of the procedures to be described are readily performed by the clinician. The *coagulation-time* (Sabrazes' method[4]) may be determined by testing the 2d or 3d drop of blood obtained on pricking the finger or ear. A capillary glass tube of 3 or 4 in. (7.6 or 10.2 cm.) in length is filled with the blood, and at intervals of thirty seconds a small section is scratched with a file and broken between the fingers. Coagulation is complete when a long worm-like coagulum is obtained. The normal time for coagulation is three or four minutes. Another simple method is given by Rodda.[5] The heel of the infant is punctured, and the 2d drop of blood allowed to flow into a clean watch-glass, having a diameter of 2.5 in. (6.37 cm.), in which has been placed a No. 6 lead shot. A second watch-glass is inverted over the first, and the watch-glasses are gently tilted every thirty seconds until the shot is firmly embedded in the clot. The average coagulation-time by this method is seven minutes.

The *bleeding-time* is determined by the method of Duke.[6] A deep puncture is made in the lobe of the ear, and at intervals of thirty seconds the drops are taken up on a piece of filter-paper without allowing the paper to touch the skin. Normally the bleeding will stop in about one to three minutes.

In testing for *increase of fragility* (*i. e.*, decreased resistence) of the red blood-cells, the method of Ribierre[7] modified by Giffin and Sanford[8] is simple and satisfactory for clinical purposes. It requires, however, considerable experience and dexterity and is best referred to a clinical laboratory. Normally hemolysis (laking) begins in from 0.42 per cent to 0.3 per cent sodium chloride solution, and is complete in 0.36 to 0.32 per cent. Patients with increased fragility show laking with stronger solutions than do those with normal blood.

Blood Matching.—Matching to determine suitability of blood for transfusion may be performed as follows: Three cc. of blood is obtained by venous puncture from the donor and, the same amount from the recipient; or even a smaller amount with a capillary tube from the finger or the ear lobe. One to 2 drops of the recipient's blood is placed in a test-tube half full of 0.9 per cent sodium chloride solution and the tube gently shaken to secure suspension of the cells. The remainder is allowed to clot, or, better still, centrifuged in order to obtain the serum. Both these procedures are repeated with the donor's blood. One drop of the donor's serum is placed on a glass slide and to it is added 1 drop of the suspension of the recipient's cells, a cover glass then being applied. It is preferable to use a hanging-drop slide and to seal the edges of the cover glass with vaseline. On another slide is placed a drop of the recipient's serum with a drop of the suspension of the donor's cells. These slides are observed under the microscope at once, and again after an hour. If no agglutination has taken place on either slide transfusion may safely be performed. In an emergency and when donors are difficult to obtain blood may be used in which the serum of the recipient does not agglutinate the cells of the donor, even though the serum of the donor agglutinates those of the recipient. In this connection it may be mentioned that the red blood cells of persons whose blood is in group IV (the universal donors) will not be agglutinated by any serum.

Cutaneous Sensibility and Muscle-power.—The study of both of these is often important. In the case of the first the pain-sense may be tested by means of a needle, but unseen by the child or it will be impossible to determine whether the drawing away of the limb is the result of pain or of fear. The presence of a paralytic or pseudo-paralytic condition is often easily discovered by simple inspection. In other cases one may offer an infant a toy or other object and observe whether this can be grasped by either hand, the other being meanwhile restrained; or one may put the arm or leg in a position which is an uncomfortable one and see whether the infant can move it back; or test the power of moving after sticking with a needle.

The Reflexes.—The knee-jerks may be tested when the child is sitting, diverted, on its mother's lap. A good plan is to support the foot or to encircle the thigh above the knee with one hand. Any jerk which occurs can be felt as well as seen. The knee-jerk can not always be elicited easily, sometimes owing to the flabbiness and weakness of the muscles, sometimes to the absence of relaxation on the part of the child. The existence of ankle-clonus and of the Babinski and other reflexes of the lower extremities should be investigated, and sometimes those of other parts of the body as well. The matter will be referred to again in the section upon Nervous Diseases (p. 857). The reflexes under normal conditions in early infancy have already been referred to (p. 46).

Puncture of Serous Cavities.—In very many diseases a diagnosis cannot be made without the puncture of the pleural, pericardial or peritoneal cavity, or of the spinal canal, cisterna, or cerebral ventricles. For most punctures in early life a small glass syringe and a needle of about 18 gauge are suitable, or at times a smaller needle for young infants. The usual antiseptic surgical technique should be closely followed and the instruments should always be tested before use. Even local anesthesia by cocaine or its derivatives is seldom required, and the discomfort of freezing by ethyl chloride is greater and longer continued than that of the puncture. Previous sedative treatment may be helpful, even by morphine if necessary.

Puncture of Pleural Cavity.—The nurse should hold the child firmly in a sitting position with its arms drawn forward and the healthy side of the chest pressed against her in such a manner that any sudden movement will not break the needle. The site chosen for puncture is that where the physical signs are most suggestive, especially where the dulness is greatest, but avoiding the cardiac or hepatic regions. Other things being equal, the posterior axillary line in the 7th interspace may be selected. With the sterilized finger pressed firmly upon the upper border of the rib, the needle attached to the syringe is introduced just above this as a guide, thus avoiding both the rib and the blood-vessels running beneath it. A depth of $\frac{1}{2}$ to 1 in. (1.27 to 2.54 cm.) is sufficient. Too short a puncture fails to penetrate the chest-wall and any plastic exudate present; too deep a one may pass through the fluid and enter the lung. The syringe must always be held lightly during the whole process, in order to avoid danger of snapping the needle if the child moves, and the puncture done quickly but carefully. Traction on the piston may be followed by the appearance of fluid, but sufficient time must be allowed, since a purulent effusion often flows very slowly. Should nothing be found at the first puncture in cases where the presence of pus seems probable, a second or a third should be made immediately in other regions, and if these are unsuccessful the puncture repeated in a few days.

Puncture of Pericardium.—The needle used should preferably be smaller than that commonly employed for the pleural cavity or for lumbar puncture, although if thick pus is encountered one with as great a gauge as 18 may be necessary. When inserted the needle is attached to the syringe. There are several points recommended for aspiration, which will avoid opening the pleura or wounding the internal mammary artery or the heart. The usual selection is the 5th left intercostal space 1 in. (2.54 cm.) from the edge of the sternum. If the 4th space is used the needle should be inserted at a distance of about 2 in. (5.1 cm.) from the sternal border. In small infants the distance from the sternum should be less. The 5th right interspace close to the sternum may also be chosen. If the pericardium is approached through the epigastrium, the needle is entered opposite the 7th left costal cartilage or in the mid-line just below the ensiform cartilage, and, with the patient in the recumbent position, is then pointed upward and to the left and pushed through the diaphragm. The outermost limit of cardiac dulness to the left is preferred by some authors as the point of selection for aspiration. In a large effusion the pericardial sac may be in actual contact with the posterior thoracic wall and puncture may be performed here. Puncture should never be made over a place where there is a friction rub.

Lumbar Puncture.—(See p. 859.) For the obtaining of spinal fluid a needle of about 18 gauge is best, although one of lesser caliber such as a hypodermic needle may be necessary in very young infants because of the small space between the vertebrae. The child either sits with the body bent forward and firmly held in this position, or lies on its right side (Fig. 13) turned partially upon the abdomen with a small pillow beneath this. The knees and shoulders are then drawn well forward and firmly held by an assistant. In this position the spines and laminae of the vertebrae become more widely separated from each other. An imaginary transverse line at the level of the crests of the ilia crosses the spinal column at the 4th lumbar vertebra. The needle, unattached to the syringe, is now introduced either in the 3d or the 4th interspace. It should be inserted in the median line and in a direction almost perpendicular to the spinal column. It is only in older children that a slightly upward tilt is needed. At a depth varying from 1 to 2 in. (2.5 to 5 cm.) it enters the subarachnoid space below the termination of the spinal cord. As a rule the fluid begins to drop at once, or sometimes, if the pressure is high, even to spurt. If it is purulent in nature, it may be necessary to attach the syringe, and to use a slight suction to start the flow; but after this the syringe should be removed and the exudate allowed to escape unaided. Sometimes raising the head and shoulders slightly will suffice. The fluid should be received in a sterilized test-tube to allow of making cultures. A specially devised manometer may be serviceably employed to measure the degree of intraspinal pressure present. At times a dry tap results, even in cases of undoubted meningitis. This may be due to the failure of the needle to enter the canal, to its being plugged with fibrin, to the thick character of the fluid, or to the fact that the inflammatory process has shut off the brain and the upper portion of the cord from the parts below. If the needle is introduced too far it will impinge on the opposite wall of the spinal canal. This accident does no harm except the wounding of small blood-vessels, as a result of which the fluid which appears is at first bloody, and may continue to be so if there has been much hemorrhage.

The child must be prevented from sudden movement and the needle held loosely to avoid the danger of breaking it in the spinal canal;—an accident which we have seen happen through neglect of these precautions, and when too slender a needle had been employed. Lumbar puncture is generally entirely without danger, although deaths have followed the procedure. The pulse should, therefore, be watched carefully, and no effort made to withdraw all the fluid possible, lest the degree of intracranial pressure be too violently disturbed. If tumor of the brain is suspected only sufficient fluid should be withdrawn for diagnostic purposes, since any great reduction of intracranial pressure under such conditions may be dangerous.

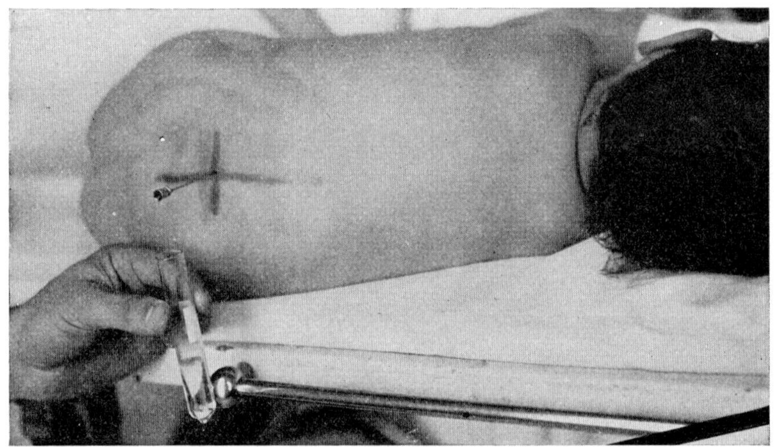

Fig. 13.—Lumbar puncture. The lines indicate the vertebral column and the transverse line between the crests of the ilia. Puncture is done at the crossing of these.

Ventricular Puncture.—The patient is placed on the back and the head is firmly held. When the fontanelle is open trephining is not necessary. The region of the fontanelle is shaved, and the skin rendered antiseptic by the usual methods. A spinal puncture-needle of No. 18 gauge or smaller is inserted, with the stylet in place, through the right lateral angle of the fontanelle, and pointed parallel to the axis of the body or a little inward. This position is selected in order to avoid any possible injury to the speech-centers. The depth to which the needle must go to obtain fluid varies with the degree of distention of the ventricles. In an infant the undistended ventricle lies 2 to 3 cm. (0.78 to 1.18 in.) from the surface of the skull. It is a good plan to insert the needle 1 cm. (0.39 in.) at a time, withdrawing the stylet at each stop to see whether fluid can be obtained. Serum may be injected in smaller amounts than that of cerebrospinal fluid removed, or dye may be introduced for the purpose of diagnosing hydrocephalus (see p. 948).

Cisterna-puncture.—The technique of this procedure is described by Ayer.[9] Some modification is necessary for infants and children (Mitchell and Reilly[10]). The patient is placed on the right side, with the neck slightly flexed toward the chest and the head and back kept in alignment, so that there is no scoliosis or torsion. A needle of 18 gauge or less with a short bevel is employed. The thumb of the left hand is placed on the first bony point encountered below the occipital protuberance (the spine of the axis) and the needle, held in the right hand, is inserted in the midline just above the thumb. The needle is pushed forward and upward in such a way that the point is directed toward the glabella. The distance from skin to cisterna magna is about 2.25 to 3.5 cm. (0.88 to 1.38 in.) depending upon the age and size of the child. It is probably well to have a guard on the needle about 2.5 cm. (0.97 in.) from its point, increasing this distance to 3.5 cm. in older children. When the cistern is entered there is a decidedly greater "give," or sensation of entering a cavity, than is experienced in lumbar puncture. Ayer states that it is a good practice to aim the needle a little higher than the external auditory meatus, and if it strikes the occiput to depress the point just enough to pass the dura at its uppermost attachment to the foramen magnum. We have employed this procedure very frequently. Only on one occasion have we seen any serious consequences from it and the extensive statistics of Ayer[11] and Ebaugh[12] show its harmlessness if properly performed.

Radioscopy.—Of recent years the use of the roentgen-ray for purposes of diagnosis has been constantly becoming more important. By its employment may be discovered the outlines of the heart and its actual size, the existence of areas of pneumonia or of tuberculosis, the presence of enlarged tracheobronchial lymph-nodes, the outlines of the thymus gland, the presence of pleural effusion and collapse of the lung, the size and position of the liver, alteration in the position of the gastro-enteric tract, and other physiologic and pathologic conditions. Advantage may be taken of it in studying bony deformities in rickets, and also in watching the changes as the disease improves. Scurvy will show characteristic subperiosteal hemorrhages and other alterations. Intracranial lesions may be demonstrated—pituitary tumors or enlargement shown by increase in size of the sella turcica; hydrocephalus after air has been injected into the subarachnoid space. Ureteral catheterization and the injection of opaque solutions with subsequent radioscopic study may be performed in early life. The bladder may be studied after opaque solutions have been injected into it, and the urinary tract visualized after the intravenous injection of such iodine-containing substances as iopax and skiodan (p. 814). A very serviceable purpose of the fluoroscope is the observation of the movements of the heart, lungs and stomach, and, with the aid of barium, the rapidity of the emptying of the last-mentioned organ and of the intestine. It is invaluable in the diagnosis of opaque and also nonopaque foreign bodies in the lungs. In the esophagus atresia and foreign bodies and their location may be demonstrated by observing the progress downwards of barium in suspension or in capsule. Lipiodol, a vegetable oil containing 0.54 Gm. of iodine to the cc., introduced into radiology by Sicard and Forestier[13] may be injected into the bronchi through a special type of tracheotomy tube, and a roentgen-ray picture taken after this clearly outlines the bronchial tree, cavities, and the like. Armand-Delille and Gelson[14] injected lipiodol after puncturing the crico-thyroid membrane, and Iglauer[15] injected it through an intubation-tube, thus avoiding an incision in the neck. A catheter inserted through the mouth into the trachea may likewise be used for this purpose. In older patients the lipiodol may be made to enter the trachea by the "passive method" in which the swallowing reflex is first abolished by local anesthetization (Ochsner[16]). The drug has also been given by intraspinous and cisternal injection to aid in the localization of tumors and blocks in the spinal canal, but it may cause local inflammatory and degenerative changes in the cord and meninges if allowed to remain. Iodipin, containing 40 per cent of iodine in a vegetable oil, may be employed in the same manner, or bromipin, a brominized oil, may be used, or iodochlorol, an oily solution of iodine and chlorine, or skiagenol, a 20 per cent solution of iodine. The gall-bladder may be visualized by the oral or intravenous administration of sodium tetrabromphenolphthalein (see p. 659).

Great care is needed in the interpretation of roentgen-ray pictures, especially those of the chest in children. An extensive knowledge of the findings in the normal chest is necessary, otherwise too much stress will be placed upon shadows which have little significance. An excellent paper upon this phase of the subject is that of Pancoast, Dunham and Baetjer,[17] and Bigler's[18] contributions are very helpful. The pediatrist should familiarize himself with interpretation by examination of the pictures and consultation with the roentgenologist, working in conjunction with him and allowing him the benefit of the clinical history and diagnosis. Many unnecessary roentgen-ray pictures are taken because of lack of care in clinical diagnosis. The roentgen-ray is often simply an accessory to diagnosis. In other cases it is the only possible way of making or confirming it.

Glucose-tolerance.—This is best tested in the manner described by Janney and Isaacson.[19] A solution is prepared of 1.75 Gm. (27 grains) of glucose in 2.5 cc. of water, and this amount is given for each kilogram (2.2 lb.) of body-weight. The patient fasts from 7 P. M. until the test is completed. An estimation of the blood-sugar is determined early in the morning and the solution of glucose is then administered. A second determination is made in one hour, and a third in two hours more. The normal maximum concentration of blood-sugar should be reached in approximately one hour and should not be over 150 mg. per 100 cc., and the original figure should be regained by the third examination. Infants have a somewhat greater tolerance than have older children and adults. McLean and Sullivan[20] found in children of from one to three years of age that the average amount of sugar in the blood three or four hours after a light meal was 96 mg. per 100 cc.; in one hour after the ingestion of the glucose 128 mg., in two hours 113 mg.

Electrical Examination.—This is of great value in many instances of nervous disease for the determination of the extent and nature of paralyses of different sorts, and the reaction characteristic of a spasmophilic state. To obtain the reactions satisfactorily it is sometimes necessary to give an anesthetic. The subject is referred to later (p. 858).

Encephalography (*Ventriculography*).—The injection of air into the spinal subarachnoid space for more effective roentgenologic study of the brain was first performed by Dandy.[21] By lumbar puncture 5 to 10 cc. of spinal fluid is removed and an equal quantity of air injected, this replacement continuing until the fluid is practically completely drained; usually about 60 to 120 cc. of air being injected. A 3-way stop-cock may be employed attached by pieces of rubber tubing to the needle and to the syringe, although this is not necessary. The patient may be in a sitting position with the head bent slightly forward or may be lying on the side. It is advised by some authors that the manometer's reading be kept below 20 mm. of mercury. If bloody fluid is obtained or if there develop signs of increased intracranial pressure the injection should be stopped. It is not necessary to filter, heat, or sterilize the air. Reaction to the procedure not infrequently develops, and there may be headache, fever, and occasionally collapse during the injection, and aseptic meningeal irritation. Death has occurred when large brain-tumors have existed, and the presence of these contraindicates the procedure. In acute encephalitis we have seen air injections temporarily increase the severity and frequency of convulsions. By encephalography may be diagnosed the presence of cerebral atrophy, and of dilitation or blocking of the ventricles and the subarachnoid space, and occasionally early adhesions may be broken up.

REFERENCES

1. Methods and Problems of Medical Education 14th Ser., The Rockefeller Foundation, 1929. 2. Arch. Pediat., 1907, **24,** 92. 3. Berl. klin. Wchnschr., 1914, **51,** 1218. 4. Ref. Stitt, Pract. Bact., 1923, 307. 5. Am. J. Dis. Child., 1920, **19,** 269. 6. J.A.M.A., 1910, **55,** 1185. 7. Thèse de Paris, 1903, 104. 8. J. Lab. and Clin. Med., 1919, **4,** 465. 9. Arch. Neurol. and Psychiat., 1920, **4,** 529. 10. Am. J. Med. Sc., 1922, **164,** 66. 11. J.A.M.A., 1923, **81,** 358. 12. J.A.M.A., 1925, **85,** 184. 13. Bull. et mém. soc. méd. d. hôp. de Paris, 1922, **46,** 463. 14. Am. J. Dis. Child., 1924, **28,** 527. 15. J.A.M.A., 1926, **86,** 1879; 1931, **97,** 1517. 16. J.A.M.A., 1929, **93,** 188. 17. Am. Rev. Tuberc., 1922–23, **6,** 338. 18. Am. J. Dis. Child., 1929, **38,** 978; 1166; 1930, **39,** 91. 19. J.A.M.A., 1918, **70,** 1131. 20. Am. J. Dis. Child., 1928, **37,** 1146. 21. Ann. Surg., 1918, **68,** 5.

CHAPTER VIII

SYMPTOMATOLOGY AND DIAGNOSIS

THE characteristics of appearance and development present in health have already been considered in discussing Anatomy and Physiology. Some of the symptoms pertaining to diseased states in early life and the significance of these may now be reviewed briefly. A more complete description of many of them will be found under the headings of the individual diseases.

SIGNIFICANCE OF SYMPTOMS

Position and Movements.—A child with a commencing illness attended by pain or fever usually no longer exhibits the quiet, motionless sleep of health, but tosses from side to side. When awake, too, this restlessness is in like manner increased, the patient wishing to be taken from bed, put back, rocked, or carried about, indicating the excited state of its nervous system. On the other hand at the beginning of an infectious disease and sometimes in digestive disturbances it will often lie unusually still, sleeping constantly, the evidence apparently of the toxic state existing. All movements are slow in debilitated conditions, and a child exhausted profoundly may lie for hours without motion, with its face directed upward instead of to one side, as it commonly is in health. The same position and the lack of motion are seen in coma from any cause.

Restlessness in infancy, especially during sleep, with an unusual tendency to kick the covers away, is an early symptom of rickets. Restless sleep may also depend upon hunger, pain, nervousness, great fatigue, noises or light in the room, or unusual excitement before going to bed. Later, restlessness at night may accompany certain forms of chronic gastroenteric indigestion. An intense degree of restlessness, called "jactation," may occur in some respiratory diseases, especially those of the larynx; in acidosis with air-hunger; severe chorea; great cerebral anemia, and sometimes in severe attacks of infectious disease including sepsis.

Orthopnea may attend diseases of the respiratory apparatus or of the heart, the child resting comfortably only when propped up in bed or when held upright in the nurse's arms with its head against her shoulder. Sleeping with the head thrown back and the mouth open is often the result of obstruction by adenoid growths. A rocking of the head from side to side on the pillow may be observed in infants with rickets, sometimes in meningitis or headache, and is frequently an expression of an intensely nervous state. Keeping the head bent backward is seen in basilar meningitis of different forms, and to a less degree in headache. A fixity of the head and neck also attends cervical caries or torticollis, the head in the latter condition being usually turned to one side. Boring the head into the pillow may indicate meningeal disturbance. Lack of power to hold it erect denotes great general weakness, or may be an evidence of congenital or acquired torticollis, of idiocy, or of some other nervous disorder, such as, in later childhood, advancing Friedreich's ataxia. Inability to walk may be the result of idiocy, of actual paralysis, or of a pseudoparalysis dependent upon syphilis or, oftener, rachitis. Failure to move one or more limbs properly may denote paralysis, or merely the pseudoparalysis of rickets or syphilis referred to, or may depend upon congenital dislocation of the hip-joint, or indicate that motion is avoided because painful, as in infantile scurvy, or be due to the existence of a spastic rigidity or to an ataxic condition. Lying upon one side sometimes occurs in pleural effusion of that side. Lying with the head retracted, the back hollowed, the knees and elbows flexed and the arms crossed over the chest—the so-called "gun-hammer position" (*en chien de fusil*)—is frequently a symptom of meningitis. Lying upon the abdomen may indicate abdominal pain, but with many children it is only a habit.

Often an infant will repeatedly put the hands fretfully to the head when there is headache, to the mouth when pain exists there, or to the ear when earache is present. In the last condition the side of the head is frequently held pressed against the pillow or the mother's breast. Pulling at the ear accompanied by fretfulness may, however, be only a nervous habit in a child suffering from rachitis or other debilitating disease. Rubbing or picking at the nose indicates coryza or gastro-enteric disturbance, or is a neurotic habit merely. It is not a special indication of the presence of intestinal parasites. Pulling at the throat sometimes occurs when there is much dyspnea. The violent irregular alternate flexion and extension of the limbs upon the trunk, and of the trunk itself, accompanied by clinching of the hands and the characteristic cry, denote the pain of colic. The keeping of the thumbs drawn into the palms and the toes flexed or rigidly extended often indicates impending convulsions, or tetany. At the same time it is to be borne in mind that every very young infant has a tendency to keep the thumbs thus inverted much of the time. Rigidity of the limbs may occur, as in meningitis, cerebral paralysis, and spinal caries. More or less extensive tonic spasm may be seen in tetanus and meningitis. Irregular, jerking, incoördinate movements in older children occur in chorea. Clonic, to-and-fro movements with unconsciousness are characteristic of convulsions, while true ataxic movements are seen in Friedreich's ataxia and allied conditions. Tremor is rarely observed in children, except as a result of chorea, some organic nervous disease especially encephalitis, or of such weakness as develops after fever. The shaking of a true rigor is uncommon in early childhood and infancy, being replaced by coldness, pallor, drowsiness, unusual quiet, or a convulsion.

Surface of the Body.—A yellowish tint of the cutaneous surface and of the sclera is seen in icterus. In well-nourished infants there is, however, normally a sufficient deposit of fat under the conjunctiva to give a slightly yellowish tint. The yellowish discoloration of carotinemia involves particularly the palms, soles and the nasolabial folds, the sclera escaping. Flushing of the face is common in fever, and is also often observed in chronic gastro-intestinal indigestion of older children, and from the action of belladonna. Slight eczema or chapping of the cheeks simulates flushing to some extent. The rosy tint natural to many healthy children is not to be forgotten. A flush which comes and goes slowly, on the face or on a part of it, or on the trunk when exposed to the irritation of the air, is a characteristic symptom frequently present in meningitis. The broad red line which develops after drawing the finger over the abdomen in cases of meningitis (*tache cérébrale*) is of the same nature. This symptom is, however, not pathognomonic but only suggestive of this disease. Very marked blueness of the whole face, the fingers and toes, and the mucous membrane of the mouth is present in congenital cardiac affections, less often in the intense dyspnea arising in laryngeal stenosis, and sometimes in severe pneumonia. A slightly bluish tint of the lips and cheeks is of common occurrence in cases of post-natal affections of the heart. A slaty-gray cyanosis may develop in toxic, dehydrated enteric cases. The red flush present on the cheeks in many cases of pneumonia quite commonly has a bluish tint to it. Moderate distention of the veins running over the scalp and at the root of the nose occurs in debilitated children, but especially in rickets. The veins of the scalp are also much distended in hydrocephalus. Great distention of the veins of the face and neck attends any decided degree of dyspnea. Dilatation of the veins over the abdomen and lower part of the thorax is witnessed in cases of malignant abdominal growth or sometimes of tuberculous peritonitis. A faintly purplish tint of and under the eyelids and above the mouth is often seen in infants with debility or even with any slight disturbance of health. In very many children, however, a tint of this sort or, still oftener, a shadow under the eyes is an individual peculiarity, the health in general being unaffected.

Marked pallor of the skin accompanies nausea, anemia of any sort, rickets, chronic diarrhea, chronic suppurative processes, nephritis, some severe cases of pneumonia, and frequently heart disease. Very little can be estimated about anemia, however, by the appearance of the skin. The color of the mucous membranes furnishes a much better index. Combined with coldness, pallor may replace in the infant the chill of adult life. An earthy color is frequently observed in severe chronic diarrhea and a brownish-yellow color of the skin, especially of the projecting portions of the face, in congenital syphilis. A marbled appearance of the surface of the body is often present in debilitated infants with feeble circulation. This becomes particularly noticeable if the skin is unduly cold. The various eruptions of the exanthematous fevers are oftenest witnessed in children, since these diseases are far commonest at this age. Infants show an especial tendency to inflammations of the skin, such as miliaria, eczema and forms of erythema. Profuse sweating, especially of the head, is an early symptom of rickets. When general over the body it is very frequently the result of an undue amount of clothing. Coldness of the extremities is present in weakly babies with poor circulation and in infants suffering from colic. Clubbing of the fingers and toes occurs in congenital cardiac disease and in chronic affections of the lungs and pleura. A shining red appearance of the palms and soles in young infants is a symptom of inherited syphilis, while peeling of the skin in older children, seen especially about the fingers, suggests convalescence from scarlet fever. It occurs also in acrodynia.

Edema of the skin, especially of the face and feet, may indicate nephritis or valvular disease of the heart, or may be an evidence of severe malnutrition and feeble circulation. Angioneurotic edema sometimes occurs in children. A localized asymmetrical atrophy of the muscles points to poliomyelitis or neuritis, while an undue development, especially of the calves, may indicate pseudohypertrophic muscular dystrophy. Local swellings of the joints are observed in all forms of arthritis, and the swelling about the joints and of the shafts of the long bones in scurvy is not to be forgotten. Curvature of the spine of various forms may be dependent upon disease of the vertebrae, old pleurisy, unequal length of the limbs, rickets, or faulty positions in being carried or in sitting. General wasting in infancy, with the skin in loose wrinkles and folds, is oftenest the result of insufficient nourishment, of persistent diarrhea or vomiting, of chronic intestinal indigestion, or less often of tuberculosis or congenital syphilis.

Face and Expression.—The mouth is open during sleep in cases of adenoid and tonsillar hypertrophy, or when the nose is obstructed by secretion. Chewing movements may occur when there is indigestion or inflammation of the mouth. A general puffiness of the whole face, with redness of the eyes, is often present during pertussis or measles. Puffiness is also witnessed in the edema of advanced marantic conditions, and especially about the eyes in nephritis. A pale circle about the mouth accompanies nausea.

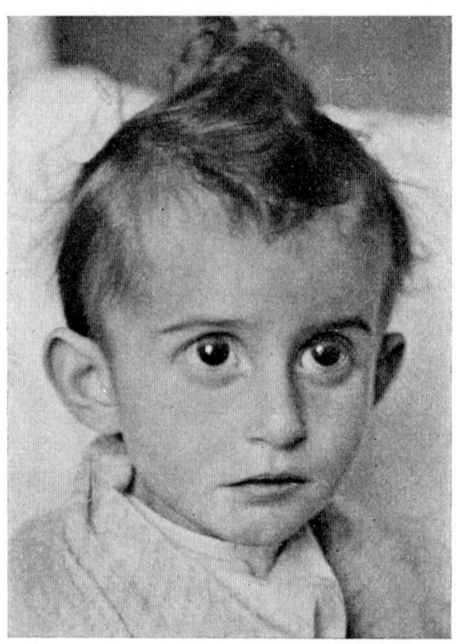

Fig. 14.—Sunken tissue about the eyes. Child of nineteen months in the Children's Medical Ward of the Hospital of the University of Pennsylvania. Chronic intestinal indigestion with troublesome vomiting, mucus in stools, and loss of weight. Improved.

Pain is shown during sleep by contortions of the face of various sorts. Thus there is sometimes an expression of pain with contraction of the brows in headache, while the smiling of very young infants during sleep often signifies abdominal pain. Discharge from the nose occurs in coryza, and is often, also, one of the first symptoms of nasal diphtheria, in which case it is likely to be bloody. The "snuffles" of new-born infants suggest congenital syphilis. In older children persistently reddened eyelids, combined with a swollen upper lip, wide nostrils, thick nasal discharge, muddy complexion, and enlarged cervical lymphatic glands, may indicate the existence of the lymphatic-exudative diathesis with tuberculosis, a combination to which the title "scrofulosis" was formerly applied. Moving of the alae with every inspiration, often accompanied by an anxious expression of the face is observed in dyspnea, most commonly from pneumonia or from stenosing affections of the larynx. Occasional movement of the alae is, however, of frequent occurrence in healthy infants. A flattened, somewhat sunken bridge of the nose is characteristic of congenital syphilis, but by itself is not sufficient to warrant this diagnosis. In atrophic conditions in infancy, when the fat has largely disappeared or there has been great loss of fluid through diarrheal discharge, the face becomes lined in a marvelous manner, especially when the child cries, suggesting the features of a very old man. The most prominent of these lines is that called the "nasal," extending from the alae of the nose and running in a half circle around the corners of the mouth. Other special lines have been described but have little importance.

In severe acute disease, atrophic states, or when there is pain or indigestion, the eyes may be only partially closed during sleep. Twitching of the lids and crossing or rolling upward or outward of the eyes indicates impending convulsions. The eyes in hydrocephalus are depressed downward, with the lower part of the iris covered by the lower lid and the sclera above the iris visible. After a severe acute attack of diarrhea or vomiting the tissues about the eyes shrink, leaving them peculiarly large and staring (Fig. 14). The pupils are dilated or unequal, or sometimes contracted in meningitis or other intracranial disorder. Nystagmus may often be seen under these conditions, but may be a congenital disturbance, or a purely functional one combined with spasmus nutans or gyrospasm. Strabismus, too, is frequently an attendant of intracranial disease, but is equally well a congenital defect. Keeping the eyes shut or turned from the light or buried in the pillow indicates photophobia from conjunctivitis, keratitis, or headache dependent oftenest on meningitis. A film-like appearance of the cornea develops in children who are moribund. Ulcers on the cornea often occur in syphilitic or tuberculous children. Tubercle of the choroid, choked discs, and other important intraocular conditions may be discovered by ophthalmoscopic examination.

Head and Neck.—Various alterations of the head appear, some of which add to the altered expression of the face. In chronic hydrocephalus the head is globular, the forehead overhangs, and the face appears small. In rickets the head has in general a square or oblong form, with the top flattened and the frontal and parietal eminences unusually large. The face looks small and is given a somewhat square appearance through the widening of the lower jaw. The head is proportionately large in premature infants. Asymmetrical heads are due to the pressure by forceps or oftenest to the existence of rickets, the lying too much on one side producing the deformity in the latter case. Faulty position may, however, produce the deformity even when rickets does not exist. Flattening of the occiput may be due to pressure, the result of the rachitic infant lying too constantly upon its back. Asymmetrical, microcephalic, and other deformed states of the head may be found in idiocy. Spots of thin membrane-like bone (craniotabes) may occur in the occipital region of infants in the early months of life. The fontanelle is unduly prominent and tense in hyperemia of the brain from any cause, meningitis, tumor, and chronic hydrocephalus. It is much enlarged with the sutures open in the last disease, as it is to a less extent in rickets. It is depressed in debilitated conditions or after profuse diarrhea, and especially in collapse. Not infrequently the bones of the skull overlap under these circumstances. The fontanelle closes very early in microcephalus and late in rickets. A systolic murmur is sometimes audible in the neighborhood of the anterior fontanelle, especially in cases of rickets, but may sometimes be heard in healthy children. Tenderness over the tragus and over the mastoid may indicate otitis and mastoiditis. Swelling of the occipital and superficial cervical glands is often the result of inflammation of the scalp; while that of the glands below the body of the jaw commonly depends upon affections of the pharynx and nasopharynx. A fluctuating swelling in the neck may be due to abscess of the glands or sometimes to a retropharyngeal abscess pointing here. The hair is worn from the back of the scalp in cases in which there is much rocking of the head, as in rickets.

Mouth and Throat.—Blueness of the lips has already been alluded to (p. 157). Fissuring around the mouth may be a symptom of congenital syphilis. Ulceration at the angles of the mouth (*perlèche*) may be observed. (See p. 517.) Herpes is seen as an accompaniment of some of the febrile diseases especially pneumonia and meningococcic meningitis, or oftener developing independently of these. Grinding of the teeth occurs especially in children with cerebral disease or suffering from convulsions, but also in those with slight digestive disturbance, and in some cases it seems to be only an insignificant although disagreeable habit. It has nothing specifically to do with infestation by intestinal parasites. Notching of the permanent upper incisor teeth is seen in congenital syphilis. The mucous membrane of the mouth may exhibit mucous patches in syphilis, and is one of the earliest sites for the appearance of the eruptions of some of the infectious fevers. A hemorrhagic swollen condition of the gums is seen in infantile scurvy. The tongue is coated in most disorders of digestion, but in some instances is bright-red and smooth. It is coated in many fevers; bright-red with prominent papillae ("strawberry tongue") in scarlatina; thick and protruding in cretinism; furrowed and dry in Mongolism; worm-eaten in appearance in the so-called "geographical tongue"; cyanotic in congenital heart-disease and slightly so in pertussis, and may, like the rest of the mucous membrane of the mouth, exhibit the lesions of some of the forms of stomatitis. In children with severe cough, and especially with pertussis, who have cut the lower incisor teeth ulceration of the fraenulum linguae is not infrequent.

Cleft palate is a congenital defect, while perforations are generally the result of congenital syphilis. High arching of the palate may attend some forms of idiocy, but may also be present in children with normal mental condition. It is not infrequently associated with deviation of the septum and the presence of adenoids.

Thorax.—The chest in rickets is small and exhibits the rachitic rosary in front and bulging of the ribs behind, with marked depression in the lateral regions. On horizontal section this gives the well-known "violin-shape." A horizontal depression beneath the nipples is also characteristic of rickets, especially where there has been much disturbance of the respiratory apparatus, and may be well-marked in obstruction by adenoid growths. A typical pigeon-breast is due often to obstruction to respiration by adenoids. This and other very great deformities of the thorax may be the result of curvature of the spine. A very unusual prominence of the precordium occurs in cardiac hypertrophy in heart-disease in children. Diminished expansion of one side with lack of movement of the intercostal spaces is dependent upon pleural effusion of that side, adhesions from a former pleurisy, or, to a lesser degree, upon pneumonic consolidation. Contraction of one side results from old pleural adhesions. Bulging of the intercostal spaces, with lack of movement, occurs in large pleural effusions; yet effusion may sometimes be present and the interspaces still move. Decided dyspnea from any cause produces in children great retraction of the interspaces with each inspiration. The degree of retraction of the epigastrium and of all the lower portion of the thorax, with tugging of the sternocleidomastoid muscles, and sinking of the episternal notch, is often remarkable at this time of life. It may occur with intrathoracic lesions, but is generally greatest in cases of stenosis of the larynx. Yet a considerable amount of moving of the epigastrium combined with lower thoracic retraction is a normal accompaniment of respiration in healthy infants, and still more so in rachitic subjects. Displacement of the heart's apex by pleural effusion is to be noted. Dulness over the manubrium of the sternum or between the scapulae may indicate the presence of greatly enlarged bronchial glands. In infancy the substernal dulness may be produced by the thymus gland. Other regions of dulness of small size may be occasioned by old pleural thickening, encysted empyema, areas of collapsed lung, or small pneumonic patches. More extensive dulness may be due to pleural effusion, pneumonia, or widespread pulmonary collapse.

An unusually deep tympanitic percussion note or a Skodaic tympany may indicate in children the presence of pneumonic consolidation. It may persist throughout nearly the whole attack. A cracked-pot sound is especially often heard in advancing or receding pneumonia, although it is often, too, present in healthy lungs. Localized ringing râles of unusual loudness and nearness to the ear frequently signify pneumonic consolidation. Feeble respiration over one side of the chest may indicate pulmonary collapse or pleural effusion. It may in some instances, however, be the only discoverable evidence of pneumonia. This has repeatedly led to the erroneous supposition that that side was affected on which the loudest respiration was heard. In other cases of pneumonia a slight harshness of respiration is the only physical sign. Another interesting feature is the frequency with which numerous râles occur in bronchitis in children as compared with adult life. Bronchial respiration generally denotes consolidation, but only when accompanied by other symptoms. As already stated it may often be heard through a pleural effusion, and is normally present to a certain extent in certain parts of the lungs. (See p. 147.) In the supraspinous fossæ it may at times be a sign of enlarged bronchial glands.

The various cardiac murmurs heard offer nothing peculiar in childhood, except that the characteristics of those of congenital disease of the heart are to be borne in mind, as well as the frequent occurrence of accidental murmurs. These will be referred to in considering Diseases of the Heart (pp. 378, 802). A very distinct precordial thrill occurring in a young infant points strongly to congenital heart disease.

Abdomen.—Unusual gaseous distention of the abdomen is a common symptom of rickets as also of colic. It is likewise present in wasting disease due to chronic digestive disorders, is a constant attendant upon idiopathic dilatation of the colon and upon some forms of indigestion in the later years of early childhood and is often a serious symptom in pneumonia. Great flatulent distention with much tenderness may occur in peritonitis, and to a less degree in inflammatory diseases of the intestine. Distention by liquid is noticed in tuberculous peritonitis and in abdominal dropsy from cardiac, renal and, more rarely, hepatic disease. Irregular distention by solid masses occurs in tuberculous peritonitis, fecal accumulation, enlargement of the liver and spleen, morbid growths, intussusception, and in localized inflammatory processes. Marked retraction of the abdomen is seen in cholera infantum, in meningitis, especially of the tuberculous variety, and in many exhausting diseases. Absence of movement during respiration may be due to inflammation or to paralysis of the abdominal walls. The outlines of the stomach and of the coils of intestine may often be detected in atrophic children with distention and great thinning of the abdominal walls. Quite active peristalsis is noticeable in cases of pyloric stenosis and of intestinal obstruction.

Method of Sucking and Swallowing.—Sucking may be almost impossible when the nares are occluded, as by severe acute coryza, congenital syphilis, or unusual adenoid growth, since the infant cannot breathe while the mouth is closed on the nipple. Harelip or cleft palate likewise interferes with sucking on account of the inability to produce the necessary vacuum in the oral cavity. Refusal to nurse after making a short effort may indicate soreness of the mouth, or may denote that little or no milk is obtained from the breast. Swallowing with a noisy gulping sound and with a grimace or a cry of pain occurs in soreness of the throat. Sucking for a moment and then stopping to breathe attends pneumonia, while entire refusal to suck may accompany extreme weakness or coma. It is an unfavorable sign. Inability to swallow, even when fed by a dropper or spoon, is seen in tetanus, eclampsia, stricture of the esophagus, and in children extremely ill from exhausting diseases. Choking over the food, with difficulty in swallowing, occurs in severe cases of retropharyngeal abscess. Regurgitation through the nose indicates pharyngeal paralysis, oftenest after diphtheria.

Respiration.—Acceleration of breathing is very common in children, and the rate is out of all proportion to that which similar causes would occasion in adults. It is seen in fever and, very markedly, in pneumonia, and is constantly present to a variable degree in rickets, even when there is no catarrhal disturbance of the respiratory apparatus. The increase in the respiratory rate for each degree of temperature is approximately the same as in adult life, *i. e.*, about $2\frac{1}{2}$:1, with the rate of increase slightly greater than this in infancy and slightly less in later childhood (M. Solis-Cohen[1]). Any excitement will accelerate respiration greatly in infancy. Dyspnea, *i. e.*, *labored* breathing,—which may or may not be rapid as well,—may occur in any condition which interferes with proper aeration of the blood. It is most typically seen in stenosis of the larynx from diphtheria, sometimes in retropharyngeal abscess, and in cases of foreign body in the trachea or bronchus. It may occur also in pneumonia, pleurisy, diseases of the heart, severe anemia, uremia and acidosis. In this last the type may be that of a deep, sighing "air-hunger," often designated "hyperpnea." In moderate dyspnea the inspiration is labored, prolonged and noisy; but in bad cases the expiration has the same character as well. Sometimes the rhythm of the respiration is altered, and instead of the inspiration being the louder and longer, with the pause following expiration, the latter is the louder and more accentuated and the pause follows a short inspiration. This is oftenest seen in pneumonia. It may, however, sometimes occur in healthy infants if excited. A catch in the respiration is frequently observed in abdominal or thoracic pain. It is witnessed very characteristically in pneumonia and pleurisy, in which the inspiration is short, and "catchy," and is followed by a moaning expiration, the so-called "expiratory moan." Snoring at night points strongly in children to occlusion of the nasopharynx by adenoid vegetations. A curious spluttering, gurgling respiration is heard in retropharyngeal abscess. The natural great irregularity of the respiration in young children, and especially in infancy, is much increased in cerebral affections. This greater irregularity may also sometimes be seen in painful affections, especially of the chest. Sighing, with unusual intermissions in the respiration, is a common symptom of meningitis, yet it may at times occur in healthy infants. A respiration approaching the Cheyne-Stokes type is frequently observed in early life in disorders of the brain, even though only functional in character. Although commonly of grave import, it is by no means so much so in infancy as in adult life. Great slowing of the respiration may take place in cerebral diseases, as in coma. It also occurs in narcosis from opium. Frequent yawning may indicate serious failure of the circulation or sometimes impending syncope.

Vital Capacity.—The vital capacity as measured by the spirometer is diminished in heart-disease in proportion to the degree of respiratory embarrassment dependent upon loss of compensation. There is temporary reduction of it in acute bronchitis; very great in pneumonia; temporary immediately after an attack of asthma; and none at all in tuberculosis unless there is extensive involvement of the lung. Dyspnea on exertion is much more marked when reduced vital capacity results from cardiac disease than when it is caused by disease of the lungs.

Pulse.—The first examination of a child's pulse-rate is inconclusive, owing to the not infrequent familial or individual deviation from the average. The pulse becomes more rapid during fever, following exercise, accompanying debility, anemia, exhaustion or other causes, and especially, in early life, under the slightest excitement. This last is so true that any conclusions are almost impossible when an infant is awake, unless entire placidity is obtained. Other things being equal, and all undue excitement being removed, the increase for each degree of temperature is not as great as in adult life, and the younger the child, the less is the relative augmentation, the increase for 1 F. being about 4 beats of the pulse during infancy (Solis-Cohen[1]) instead of 10 beats as in adults. The relationship of the rate of the pulse to that of the respiration, which is normally 4:1 in adults is altered somewhat in infancy, being then about 3:1. The irregularity of the pulse natural to young children (see p. 37) becomes intensified in many affections of the brain, and to a less degree in pericarditis and chorea. It is unusually rapid in scarlatina, independent of the severity of the attack. There may be slowing of the pulse in many disorders of the brain, due to a stimulation of the vagus; in jaundice, produced in the same way by the action of the bile; in decreased metabolism; during convalescence from acute febrile diseases; produced reflexly through pressure upon the eyeball or the abdomen; and sometimes in nephritis and other conditions with increased arterial tension; while during the course of many cases of typhoid fever the pulse is slower than would be expected. The "trip-hammer" pulse of aortic regurgitation occurs in childhood as in adults; the capillary pulse of this disease may be readily obtained in the finger-nails or in the lips, and the pulsus paradoxus is found in adhesive exo-pericarditis.

Temperature.—Most important in this connection is the ease with which abnormal alteration of temperature takes place in early life. High elevation may result from slight causes, such as constipation or even excitement. Moro[2] found that 22 out of 25 children experimented upon showed elevation of the rectal temperature after vigorous exercise. Temporary fever is not uncommon in the new-born. (See p. 246.) More or less irregular elevation may be seen in children with moderate debility, especially during convalescence from an acute disease. The variations in the course of a febrile temperature, including the difference between morning fall and evening rise, are liable to be greater in children than in adult life, and the thermolabile condition of certain children must not be forgotten. In fact in some children, especially those of a highly neurotic nature, the temperature is persistently elevated during at least a part of the day, even with the child at rest, without this possessing any significance. Very high temperature may attend the infectious fevers, some of the cases of milk-poisoning, and the heat-exhaustion occurring in very hot weather. High fever of short duration is borne, as a rule, better in childhood than in adult life.

Depression of temperature occurs after the crisis in such diseases as pneumonia; and in severe diarrheal diseases, collapse, hemorrhage, sclerema neonatorum, congenital heart disease, premature birth, and in very many cases where insufficient nourishment is taken or assimilated. In all weakly children the temperature is readily depressed by external cold. Interesting studies on the cutaneous temperature of children are reported by Talbot and his associates.[3]

Cry.—The observation of the cry constitutes one of the most important methods of diagnosis in infants. A healthy, comfortable and contented infant does not cry. A cry of any sort always has a meaning, even though it indicates nothing more than some slight dissatisfaction. Persistent violent crying, rather fretful than sharp, is often due to hunger. It is unappeasable by anything except the giving of food, when it ceases at once and permanently. Sometimes a cry of this nature is in reality dependent on thirst, especially if there has been severe diarrhea. A similarly continuous cry, but more high-pitched and piercing, attends persistent severe pain, most commonly earache. The offering of food quiets it only momentarily if at all. Pain of a less severe nature, the existence of the intense itching of eczema, the pain from the pricking by a pin concealed in the clothing, the presence of a wet diaper, and many other sources of discomfort produce obstinate crying, but of a less piercing and violent character. The cry of colic is very violent but more or less paroxysmal, a momentary pause being followed by a sudden renewal without discernible reason; it is attended by the movements of the body already described as characteristic (p. 156). The giving of food may quiet it for a time, the warm milk lulling the pain, but it soon returns as bad as before. It may cease suddenly after the expulsion of gas from the stomach or bowel. A similar cry sometimes attends the passage of gravel or may be observed in intussusception. A sudden acute pain, such as results from a fall or other slight accident or the touching of some tender part, produces violent but temporary crying, soon appeased. Crying just before, with, or after the evacuation of the bowels indicates intestinal pain, or sometimes pain at the anal opening. Crying may also attend the passage of urine and may denote pain in the bladder or the irritation of scalded areas by the secretion.

A weak, peevish, fretful cry, sometimes almost constant, is heard in many conditions attended by much debility. Under such circumstances speaking to or even looking at the child may start the cry. A louder but fretful cry in a healthy child, often attended by rubbing of the eyes with the fists, indicates sleepiness. An almost inaudible cry occurs in severe stenosis of the larynx and in cases of great exhaustion. Puckering the face into the position for crying, but absolutely without sound resulting, is seen in these conditions when extreme, as also after tracheotomy or intubation. The absence of crying is also witnessed in comatose states. There is likewise very little crying accompanying decided dyspnea, such as attends severe pneumonia or pleural effusion, on account of the lack of breath for it. The cry of pneumonia is suppressed and short, and the expiratory moan described in considering Respiration is often heard (p. 162). Yet children with pneumonia sometimes cry loudly if the dyspnea is trifling. As a rule, however, loud crying indicates that there is little wrong with the lungs. Hoarseness of the cry is heard in laryngitis, and a hoarse, whimpering, and somewhat nasal cry occurs in congenital syphilis. A nasal cry is present also in coryza of other nature. A characteristic "brazen" cry is heard in spasmodic croup. Crying is usually unattended by the production of tears until about the third month. After this age crying without tears indicates a condition of dangerous debility. A sudden shriek at intervals, without ordinary crying, uttered by a child in a stuporous state, suggests tuberculous meningitis ("hydrencephalic cry"). Sudden crying out at night may, however, be produced by the night-pains of disease of the bones. After infancy is passed violent, unappeasable crying, with which a child suddenly starts from sleep, is indicative of night-terrors. In later infancy and childhood the cry of anger is often witnessed. It is loud, violent, without any piercing character, unattended by any evidence of pain, and generally associated with some evident reason for wrath. The infant while crying from this cause often stiffens itself all over, or throws its head backward; while the older child may stamp its feet, throw itself upon the floor, and even beat its head against the floor or wall. Finally, there is the very common and very deceptive cry occurring in infants who have in various ways not been well trained, which is merely an expression of discontent with their condition, although without anger or pain. A baby, for instance, wakens from sleep and cries violently. As soon, however, as it is taken up by the nurse its crying ceases, and smiles replace the tears.

Cough.—A short suppressed cough followed by a facial expression of pain is heard in pneumonia and pleurisy; a peculiar barking, brazen cough in spasmodic croup or the early stage of laryngeal diphtheria; a tight hoarse cough in laryngitis and tracheitis. Long, hard paroxysms of dry cough sometimes causing pain in the chest occur in the early stages of severe bronchitis, and a loose rattling cough in bronchitis after secretion is established. The long paroxysms of rapid, short expiratory efforts, continuing until suffocation seems impending and followed by a crowing inspiration, are characteristic of pertussis. In this disease mucus is often driven from the mouth. A very similar cough may occur in enlargement of the bronchial glands, yet not often accompanied by a whoop. It may be particularly troublesome at night, as is likewise the cough in pertussis. A peculiarly severe, ringing, brazen cough, in some respects resembling that of croup but often paroxysmal, is sometimes caused by the existence of glandular or other tumors or abscesses within the thorax, or the presence of a foreign body in the air-passages. An annoying "tickling," hacking cough occurs in pharyngitis, especially when the uvula is elongated. When the pharyngitis is severe the cough causes pain in the throat. A hard dry cough, often severe, is heard in passive congestion of the lungs produced by disease of the heart. Indigestion is sometimes attended by a hacking cough, the so-called "stomach cough." Asthma has a short dry cough, not paroxysmal. A "habit cough" may persist after the exciting cause of cough has ceased to exist.

Voluntary expectoration of *sputum* following cough does not, as a rule, take place in any disease until six or seven years of age. Sputum for examination must be obtained by introducing an elastic catheter or a pledget of cotton or cloth on an applicator to the base of the tongue. This occasions coughing, whereupon the sputum may be aspirated by the catheter or caught on the cloth.

Pain.—Pain, either subjective in origin or produced by handling, is of the most varied form and significance in early life. It has already been discussed to some extent under different headings. The determination of the seat of pain in infants and young children is often very difficult. Frequently tenderness can be ascertained by handling various parts, and observing whether a cry or a grimace is produced. Children under five years seldom locate pain exactly in attempting to describe it. Pain in the *head* is very common. It may indicate the onset of fever, whether this be of short or of more prolonged duration, being a frequent early symptom of typhoid fever and still oftener of meningitis. It is common in intracranial tumor. In other cases it is dependent upon coryza, anemia, dyspepsia, eyestrain, otitis, fatigue, excessive mental work at school, migraine, dental caries, nephritis or heart-disease. Pain referred to the *mouth* may indicate stomatitis of various sorts, or toothache. In the *throat* it may attend many forms of inflammation there. Pain in the *neck* may be due to inflammation of the lymphatic glands, mumps, tonsillitis, or the tenderness of the muscles in torticollis. It may also be a symptom of caries or of basilar meningitis, especially when the pain is increased by motion. Pain in the *thorax* depends most frequently upon pleurisy and pneumonia. It may then be present only during cough. Occasionally pain in one side is produced by herpes zoster. Heart-disease is sometimes attended by severe attacks of precordial pain. Tenderness of the chest on grasping the child under the arms to lift it may occur in pleurisy, and also in rickets. The symptom may be deceptive, as the pain can be in reality located in some other part of the body, which the lifting has disturbed. Pain in the *abdomen* depends upon digestive disturbances, peritonitis, appendicitis, or intussusception, and is not uncommonly a symptom of spinal caries. In the form of "umbilical colic" (p. 577) it is most frequently of nervous origin. Inflammatory affections of the chest quite frequently produce a pain which is referred to the abdomen. Pain with stiffness on moving the *back* strongly suggests caries of the spine. In the *limbs* it may depend upon rheumatism or other form of arthritis, or on poliomyelitis, but in infancy is far oftener a symptom of scurvy. It becomes particularly evident when the child is handled. Pain is liable to attend inflammatory affections of the bones, among which may be mentioned periostitis and osteomyelitis. The existence of undiscovered fractures in infancy is a fruitful and puzzling source of severe pain. Hip-joint disease occasions pain which is referred to the thigh, or, commonly, to the knee. Caries of the spine may produce pain in the lower limbs. An unusual degree of local or general hyperesthesia is not uncommon in different nervous disorders.

Breath.—A rancid, butyric-acid odor may be present on the breath of infants suffering from the vomiting of gastric indigestion. Acute febrile conditions or acute indigestion may produce that of acetone, or give rise to other odors of an unpleasant character. In ozena, ulcerative stomatitis, the accumulation of secretion in the tonsils, and the sputum from pulmonary abscess and from bronchiectatic cavities the odor may be very offensive, while in gangrene of the lung and in noma the sickening odor is almost unbearable. A stercoraceous breath is exceptionally noticed in intestinal obstruction.

Vomiting.—Vomiting is a symptom so frequent in early life and due to such varied causes that it will receive independent consideration later (p. 552). In this connection a few of its diagnostic indications may be mentioned. Simple regurgitation, without effort, of food which is little if any changed, occurs in the case of healthy infants who have taken more milk than they can comfortably hold, or who have been carelessly handled after feeding. True vomiting is accompanied by more effort and by evidences of nausea, such as pallor of the face and perspiration. It is very common at the beginning of acute febrile diseases in early life. When acute and of brief duration, accompanied by nausea and coated tongue, and perhaps followed by diarrhea, it is generally the sign of acute gastro-intestinal disturbance. Very obstinate vomiting, frequently with much mucus, occurs in chronic gastric indigestion and gastritis in infancy and in cases of stenosis of the pylorus. Vomiting may be the evidence of a toxic state, as seen, for instance, in uremia and in acute milk-poisoning. If repeated frequently for days, and attended by retracted abdomen, headache, moderate fever, and some degree of constipation, it is very suggestive of meningitis, or, in the absence of fever, of brain-tumor. Recurrent vomiting is a disorder not to be forgotten. Vomiting is common after violent paroxysms of coughing, especially in pertussis and severe bronchitis. Very intractable vomiting with distention of the abdomen and some degree of constipation occurs in peritonitis. When obstinate constipation is combined with obstinate vomiting, the existence of obstruction of the bowels, sometimes congenital, may be suspected.

Finally, the extreme ease with which vomiting is brought about in infants and in children must be borne in mind. This is especially true when once the tendency to it has been developed. Thus in many infants slight moving of the body after a meal is sufficient to cause vomiting. The mere taste of the food may occasion vomiting, both in infants and older children, everything being ejected the taste of which is not liked. This is probably the reason why nourishment given to infants by gavage may be retained, when that entering the mouth in the usual way may be vomited. Many children seem able to vomit at will if anything displeases them.

Bowel-movements.—Alteration of the character of the feces is common in disease in infancy. A large amount of white, lumpy material in the stools, especially of bottle-fed infants, generally indicates too large an amount of fat in the food. Mucus appears very readily in the stools of infants. It may have no significance whatever, or may indicate merely a catarrhal process, but in large amount and accompanied by fever and straining suggests an inflammatory condition. It is generally present in considerable quantity after the administration of a purgative, such as castor oil. Blood in the passages may denote a purely local process, such as fissure, hemorrhoids, congestion or constipation. Mixed with mucus and attended by straining efforts it may be the evidence of enterocolitis or intussusception; and when in larger amount, without mucus, may be one of the symptoms of purpura haemorrhagica, severe ulceration or rectal polypi. Black stools suggest the existence of hemorrhage in the upper intestinal tract. A pea-green color is often physiologic, but the presence of dark-green slimy masses is very frequent in intestinal indigestion and in enterocolitis. Putty-colored stools may be due to deficiency in the secretion of bile, but oftener in infancy white or grey, formed or unformed stools are seen in those who are taking much more butter-fat than they can digest. Hard, scybalous masses coated with mucus occur in older children with forms of intestinal indigestion of a chronic nature. Intestinal parasites of different sorts or their ova may frequently be discovered.

The *odor* of the stools during disease varies. In cholera infantum the passages are nearly odorless; in other forms of diarrhea in infancy they may be sour-smelling and irritating to the adjacent skin, have a peculiar "mousey" odor, or may be very offensive, the difference depending upon whether indigestion of carbohydrate or of protein is present. The giving of such substances as beef-juice and egg-water often produces exceedingly unpleasant odors. The action of certain drugs and food upon the *color* of the passages is to be remembered; iron producing a black, and bismuth a greenish-black hue, and such substances as hematoxylin and krameria, formerly much in use, a reddish color. Infants fed upon a high carbohydrate-diet, such as malt-soup or buttermilk-mixtures, exhibit smooth, brownish stools. A fuller discussion of the character of the feces in disease will be given later (p. 578).

The *number* of passages varies greatly; and in estimating the importance of this matter, the character and amount of the food taken must be considered carefully. Constipation in infancy is sometimes a sign of a very thorough digestion which leaves little waste-material to pass; in other cases it may depend on the great length of the sigmoid flexure in early life; in others upon impaired general health; and in still others, when combined with a failure to gain in weight, it may be caused by insufficient nourishment. On the other hand, an undue number of movements, unless diarrheal in character, may be merely a natural method of getting rid of an excess of nourishment. Frequent, diarrheal stools may be due to inflammatory conditions of the mucous membrane, or tuberculous or other ulceration; toxic influences, as in the infectious fevers; local irritation such as by improper articles of food; or reflex causes, as seen in diarrhea after surface-chilling.

Urine. (See also p. 806.)—*Retention of urine* may be dependent upon the pain which urination causes, as in vulvitis, inflammation of the prepuce or glans, or the existence of very acid urine. Sometimes it is the result of obstruction, as in cases of calculus in the urethra, very narrow foreskin, malformations of the urinary tract, or stone in the bladder. *Suppression* or very *great diminution* in the amount of urine may attend acute nephritis, acute fever, profuse diarrhea, severe vomiting, renal calculus, and sometimes intestinal obstruction. *Great increase* in the amount of urine occurs in diabetes, diabetes insipidus, after crisis in fever, after attacks of abdominal pain or of convulsions, and in some forms of chronic Bright's disease. *Albuminuria* is occasionally physiologic. It occurs also in Bright's disease, in severe cardiac affections, in many febrile states, sometimes in scurvy, and from the admixture of pus or blood. In old specimens of urine it may depend upon the growth of bacteria. *Blood* in the urine, unless in very small amount, makes it appear smoky, muddy or bright-red in color. It may occur in Bright's disease, scurvy, in some grave cases of infectious fevers, purpura, stone in the bladder, and especially in stone in the kidney. Often the presence of blood manifests itself most noticeably by a stain on the diaper. Sometimes the altered color is due to hemoglobin and not to the presence of corpuscles. This is true of infectious hemoglobinuria of the new-born. A paroxysmal hemoglobinuria is occasionally seen in older children. The urine is of an orange-yellow color in jaundice, and the ingestion of beets will sometimes produce a reddish tint. Uric acid sand may appear on the diaper of infants, while in other cases an excess of urates makes the urine of infants milky in color. Pus in the urine is found in inflammation of any part of the urinary tract, as pyelitis, cystitis or urethritis. It also results from contamination by the discharge in vulvovaginitis.

Blood.—The significance of the alterations of the blood in disease can best be discussed elsewhere (see p. 1019).

Serous Cavities.—By the puncture of the pleural cavity the existence of effusion is made known and the character of the fluid determined. The diagnosis between pneumonic consolidation and pleural effusion often hinges upon the result of this procedure. By lumbar puncture the existence of forms of meningitis can be positively determined in most cases. The diagnosis of the nature of an abdominal disorder may, in like manner, be aided by the employment of puncture in some instances.

The appearance and character of the fluid obtained by the puncture of serous cavities, including the kind of formed elements present in it, is shown by microscopic and chemical examination. The presence and nature of any bacteria found must receive careful consideration. The matter can better be studied in another connection (see Puncture of Serous Cavities, p. 150 and Pleurisy, pp. 755–759).

Mental and Nervous Symptoms.—Incidental reference has already been made to various diseased states of the nervous system. What follows is by way of addition or recapitulation. Further discussion will be found in the section upon Nervous Diseases (p. 856).

Various forms of mental defect are to be recognized. The mother often wrongly supposes that the child's failure to take notice, walk, or talk is due respectively to defective sight or hearing, paralysis of the legs, or tongue-tie. To determine whether failure to notice objects at the proper age is due to idiocy or to blindness is often a matter of difficulty. An ophthalmoscopic examination may settle the question. Slowness in learning to speak, when not dependent upon imbecility, can be the result of defective hearing or of a general slowness of development caused by ill-health. Often, too, it seems to be merely a peculiarity of the individual, irrespective of other conditions, and need then cause no anxiety. A marked tendency to allow the saliva to dribble out of the mouth is a characteristic of the idiotic state. A condition of confusional insanity, almost maniacal at times, may develop after fevers, especially typhoid. Simple anger becomes so uncontrollable in many children that it occasionally seems almost maniacal. Delirium is a frequent attendant on high temperature in children, and does not necessarily indicate the existence of any serious condition. It may occur even in infancy, although at this age convulsions tend to replace it. Convulsions, indeed, are very prone to develop in early life. They may be due to many causes, often of the most trivial nature. Pneumonia and all the infectious fevers, especially scarlatina, may be ushered in by them, and even high temperature from other sources is likely to produce them in some subjects. Spasmophilia is a peculiarly frequent predisposing cause. They may result, too, from peripheral irritation of various sorts, particularly of the gastro-enteric tract, and from diseases of the brain, and uremia. Occurring in the new-born they are frequently the sign of intracranial trauma or disease.

Hysteria may be witnessed even in early childhood, and the presence of malingering is often to be recognized. In fact, the power of imagination is so great in childhood that pains are very liable to be complained of if the suggestion of pain is made to the child. Aphasia in children has not the grave import nor the diagnostic value of the symptom in later life. It sometimes occurs temporarily after typhoid fever.

Psychic and nervous symptoms are much more easily evoked in early than in adult life. Great restlessness or excessive talking during sleep, somnambulism, and such semi-delirious states as in night-terrors are readily produced by such slight causes as temporary fever, indigestion and overexertion. Extreme excitement, with crying, may be due to disease or may be dependent only upon accidental causes. Great irritability is evidence of an unhealthy state. Sometimes it may be due to incipient chorea or some insidious disease, or merely be the result of indigestion or malaise; but in other instances it points strongly to the beginning of meningitis, especially the tuberculous form. Indifference to surrounding objects and the ceasing to play with toys denotes a serious affection of health. It may depend upon great weakness or upon intracranial disorder. An unusual desire to go to bed, or an unwillingness to get up at the usual time may be a distinctly suspicious indication. Stuporous and comatose states with the attendant symptoms occur in actual organic disease of the brain, or may be the result only of severe functional disturbance of it. Thus the condition of "pseudohydrocephalus," very closely resembling meningitis, may develop as an attendant upon great weakness, especially after severe diarrhea. Absence of the patellar reflex may occur in poliomyelitis, the muscular dystrophies, diphtheritic and other neuritic paralyses and in Friedreich's ataxia. Prolonged rest in bed and great weakness may diminish it. Increase of it may be a symptom of cerebral palsy, Pott's disease, and of some forms of cerebellar disease, or may oftener be without serious import.

References

1. Arch. Pediat., 1905, **22,** 915. 2. Monatschr. f. Kinderh., 1917, **14,** 214. 3. Am. J. Dis. Child., 1931, **42,** 965.

CHAPTER IX

MORBIDITY AND MORTALITY

TENDENCY TO DISEASE IN INFANCY AND CHILDHOOD

THE greatest tendency to disease exists in the first year of life, and especially in the new-born; the least at the age of from ten to fifteen years. There is besides (p. 139) a predisposition to certain diseases during infancy and childhood as contrasted with adult life, and a comparative freedom from others. There is a difference, too, in the susceptibility to particular diseases at the various periods of early life. Thus in the new-born exists a group of affections, almost characteristic, which are due either, first, to disease or defects of development persisting from fetal life, or, secondly, to injuries or disease arising at or shortly after birth. In the first class are the malformations and congenital disorders, as of the heart, intestines and brain; the forms of imperfect development visible to the eye; and the inherited affections, especially syphilis. There is also the congenital asthenia with which many infants are born. While this asthenia is a common result of prematurity, it may occur independently of it. In the second group are the injuries resulting from parturition, notably the paralysis dependent upon meningeal hemorrhage or injury of the brain or nerves; hemorrhage into other viscera; various dislocations and fractures; and injuries connected with the surface of the body, such as cephalhematoma. In this group, too, are a number of diseases largely peculiar to the new-born, including atelectasis, pyloric stenosis, certain types of pneumonia and icterus, forms of septic infection, ophthalmia of the new-born, etc.

From the end of the first three or four weeks of infancy up to the end of the *first year* of life the prevailing diseases are those of the digestive apparatus, over one-half of them belonging to this category and being oftenest the result of artificial feeding. The nervous system is also unusually sensitive, and convulsive disorders are prone to occur. The general feebleness of the young infant and its deficient power of reaction render it less able to resist cold, excessive heat, and other debilitating influences. Respiratory diseases are very common, pneumonia being often of the catarrhal form and frequently fatal. Scurvy is seen especially at this time, as are the earlier manifestations of rickets. Affections of the thymus gland are to be noted. Acute infectious diseases are not so prone to occur, with the exception of pertussis and the septic infections, and to a less extent measles. Diseases of the skin are common, thrush is a frequent affection, and tuberculosis is often encountered, usually as a general tuberculous infection. Inflammation of the lymph-nodes, either simple or tuberculous, begins to be frequent at this age, particularly of the internal nodes. Intussusception is more common than later and spasmophilia becomes frequent after the age of six months.

In the *second year* of life the respiratory diseases remain frequent, while the digestive disorders are on the whole less so and less fatal than earlier. Spasmophilic manifestations continue to be at their height up to eighteen months of age, and convulsions still occur readily from the slightest causes. Meningitis is common, rachitis extremely so, and pyelitis often seen. Diseases of the lymph nodes, especially in connection with other disorders, continue with a frequency characteristic of early life. Adenoid growths of the nasopharynx and hypertrophy of the tonsils become common. In this period, too, begins the marked predisposition to acute infectious fevers, especially diphtheria. Throughout the first two years of life acquired affections of the heart are very unusual and rheumatism rare. Tuberculosis shows itself as peritonitis, adenitis, meningitis, tuberculous bronchopneumonia, and very often as a widespread general tuberculous infection. Typhoid fever is relatively uncommon, and its symptoms often obscure.

During *early childhood; i. e.*, from the age of two to that of six years, certain forms of digestive disturbances are common, particularly disorders of the stomach and small intestine. Diarrhea is less troublesome than in infancy. More or less malnutrition is of great frequency, often dependent upon mild digestive disorders. The occurrence of tonsillitis, pharyngitis and various forms of stomatitis increases. Respiratory affections are very common, and spasmodic croup becomes one of the terrors of the household. Rheumatism and acquired affections of the heart are occasionally observed. The tendency to the acute infectious diseases appears to be approaching its height. Appendicitis, rare under the age of two or three years, begins to be often observed.

In *later childhood; i. e.*, after the age of six years, chorea, rheumatism, disorders of the heart and diseased conditions of the tonsillar tissue are common. Dependent upon school-life are to be noted, functional neuroses, myopia, scoliosis, headache, anemia, and the like. The infectious diseases continue extremely frequent. Meningitis is of common occurrence, and various psychoses appear as puberty is approached.

Chronic affections of the kidney, with the exception of pyelitis, are comparatively infrequent during the whole of infancy and childhood. Acute nephritis may readily attend the infectious diseases, and often in infancy is associated with severe diarrheal disturbances. Diseases of the bones and joints, generally tuberculous, are frequent in all periods of early life, although less so in infancy than in childhood. Disease of the brain-substance is rare except when secondary to meningeal disturbance, and that of the spinal cord, nerves, and muscles likewise: the exceptions being poliomyelitis, which is common in infancy and early childhood; the neuritis following diphtheria; the transverse myelitis resulting from spinal caries; and the muscular dystrophies and certain systemic nervous affections which are characteristic of childhood.

Season has an influence on morbidity, poliomyelitis and asthma being more prevalent in autumn; spasmophilia more so in winter; and contagious diseases less likely to be epidemic in summer. *Sex* likewise plays a part, as seen in the greater frequency of pyloric stenosis, spasmophilia and congenital heart disease in males, and of pyelitis, rheumatic fever and primary peritonitis in females. Hemophilia occurs only in males. *Race* is a factor in some conditions. Thus the negro seldom suffers from pyloric stenosis, while sickle-cell anemia is confined to that race. The *birth-order*, or place in the family, seems to be a predisposing factor at times, the first-born being apparently more subject to developmental anomalies, including congenital heart-disease and pyloric stenosis.

FETAL MORTALITY. STILL AND PREMATURE BIRTHS

Fetal mortality, including miscarriages and still-births, shows a high percentage of the total number of conceptions. The proportion of miscarriages to pregnancies is variously estimated at from 1:7 to 1:4 (Ballantyne[1]). The statistics of the relationship of still-births to total births vary from 1.3 to 5.9 per cent in different countries (Ruppin,[2] Chambrelent,[3] U. S. Census,[4] Howard,[5] Drake[6]), the figure given by Bailey[7] of 3.5 at the Cornell Maternity Clinic in N. Y. probably representing the average. Stuart[8] found that of 650 infant deaths occurring in Boston during the first year 264 were still-births. In Holland Sanders[9] found that of 1807 still-births at term 1087 were boys.

Premature birth is also a frequent cause of death during infancy. (See Prematurity, p. 210.)

MORTALITY IN INFANCY AND CHILDHOOD

Mortality Especially in the First Year.—In older studies, such as those of Erőss[10] in 1895, Westergaard[11] in 1901, Holt and Babbitt[12] in 1915, Mitchell[13] in 1920, and Reuben[14] in 1922 the death-rate in the first year was about 18 to 20 per cent,* this constituting about 25 to 30 per cent of the total number of deaths for all ages. In the figures given by Holt and Babbitt 33 per cent of the deaths in the first year occurred in the first month, in Mitchell's figures 39 per cent, and in those of Bolt,[15] based on the reports of the Census Bureau, approximately 50 per cent. Bolt states that the decline in infant mortality had taken place almost entirely after one month of age. Statistics given by Rich[16] and Baker[17] for America show a diminishing infantile death-rate in recent years, as do the publications of the American Child Health Association,[18] according to which the rate declined from 9.8 per cent in 1917 to 6.22 per cent in 1930 in the Birth Registration Area, while in some localities it has been as low as 4 or 5 per cent. European statistics in general are in support of this, Schlossmann,[19] for example, stating that from 1913 to 1925 the rate in Düsseldorf fell from 11.36 to 9.68 per cent.

The influences of *crowding* and *bad hygiene* are linked to the factors of *economic* and *educational status* and are very positive. Hers[20] and others found the mortality higher in *large families*, but Vercoe[21] has observed no deterioration in the average child accompanying successive pregnancies, even in very large families, and the cause must be considered as associated with the defective hygiene, and insufficient nourishment. Some studies indicate that the rate is higher in *cities* than in rural districts, but this is not constantly found, except as dependent upon crowding, bad hygiene, and the like.

The influence of *artificial feeding* on mortality in the first year is very striking according to older statistics. This is well shown by the study of Woodbury,[22] who in 22,422 live-born infants in 8 cities in the United States found that the mortality among the artificially fed infants was from 3 to 4 times as high as among the breast-fed. With greater care this proportion decreases. (See p. 64.)

Geographical distribution apparently has an influence on the mortality-rate, but this probably depends largely upon the varying economic and educational status.

Season has a decided bearing, both the hottest and the coldest seasons being attended by a higher mortality. In hot weather there is the direct influence of heat upon the infant, as well as the favoring of bacterial growth in poorly handled milk; in cold weather the incidence of respiratory infections increases greatly.

Sex exerts some influence. During the ten-year period, 1915 to 1924, Bakwin[23] found from 130 to 134 deaths in white male infants under one year of age as compared with 100 deaths in white females, the contemporaneous proportion of males to females born being 106:100. By four years of age the mortality of the sexes is about equal.

It is difficult to determine the influence of *race* apart from attendant climatic and hygienic conditions. All studies in the United States show a high infant mortality in negroes, and some statistics indicate that within the white race it is greatest in the first year in the Italians, Bohemians, and Hungarians. However, in the first month of life, as the Census Reports

* This refers to the number of deaths in infants under one year of age compared with the total number of live births.

studied by Bolt[15] indicate, the death-rate of the children of Polish and Hungarian mothers is significantly lower than in the children of native American mothers.

Causes of Death at Different Ages.—Of cases dying in the *first month* of life prenatal causes, such as acute or chronic diseases of the mother, account for probably from 60 to 75 per cent (Mitchell;[13] Stuart[8]). Death incident to birth and occurring shortly after it is very frequent, depending oftenest upon intracranial trauma or hemorrhage, as claimed by Wolcott,[24] Schwartz,[25] Crothers,[26] and others; Wolcott finding hemorrhage in about ½ the cases. In 800 necropsies of infants dying in the first month Cruickshank[27] found the three most frequent causes of death to be: (1) conditions produced by birth-asphyxia, atelectasis, birth-injury or prematurity 67.5 per cent; (2) infections 29.75 per cent; (3) gross developmental defects 2.75 per cent. On the other hand, of 650 deaths in infants reported by Stuart[8] 122 were caused by malformations and 99 by congenital defects.

In the *first year* as a whole, various statistics show that about 30 per cent or more of the deaths are due to diseases of the digestive system, and that respiratory diseases (pneumonia and bronchitis) account for from 10 to 15 per cent. Convulsions, often listed as the cause, are usually terminal or symptomatic phenomena, and the term debility, or inanition, is difficult to evaluate when given in statistics as the cause of death. These two conditions, convulsions and debility, may be claimed as roughly accounting each for about 10 or 15 per cent of deaths in this period. Hereditary syphilis is more fatal in the first year than at any other time, and tuberculosis is almost as common a cause of death as later. With the exception of erysipelas, pertussis and measles, the number of deaths from the acute infectious disorders is generally less than later, but only owing to their smaller incidence, since they have a relatively unfavorable prognosis at this period.

In the *second year* the mortality is less, being only about ⅕ as great as in the first year (Abbott[28]). Gastrointestinal diseases and respiratory affections are the most prominent causes, the latter gradually increasing in importance and the former decreasing. Infectious diseases begin to play a more prominent part and the deaths from tuberculosis are numerous.

In *early childhood* (two to six years) deaths are chiefly due to the acute infectious diseases or their complications. In *later childhood* (six to twelve years), while the mortality is lower than at any other period of life, the principal causes of death are still the infectious disorders, although respiratory diseases and tuberculosis are common factors, diarrheal disorders being much less important. Acquired disease of the heart becomes important only in later childhood.

In the study made by the White House Conference[29] from the figures for the Registration Areas of the U. S. for 1926, 1927 and 1928 it was found that, if communicable diseases are classified according to the greatest number of deaths in the different age-groups, the order for the chief diseases in the group under one year is: Bronchopneumonia, lobar pneumonia, influenza (all forms), whooping cough, syphilis, measles, and tuberculosis (all forms). In the group of from one to four years the order is: Bronchopneumonia, diphtheria, lobar pneumonia, influenza (all forms), measles, whooping cough, and tuberculosis (all forms). For the age-group of five to nine years, the order is: Diphtheria, tuberculosis (all forms), lobar pneumonia, influenza (all forms), bronchopneumonia, measles, and scarlet fever. For that of from ten to fourteen years, the order is: Tuberculosis (all forms), lobar pneumonia, influenza (all forms), typhoid fever, diphtheria, bronchopneumonia, tetanus, scarlet fever, poliomyelitis, measles, and meningococcus meningitis. For the age-group of from fifteen to nineteen years, the order is: Tuberculosis (all forms), lobar pneumonia, influenza (all forms), typhoid fever, bronchopneumonia, meningitis, malaria, measles, syphilis, scarlet fever, poliomyelitis, and diphtheria.

Epstein[30] reviewed 1000 necropsies in children from birth up to the age of thirteen years. Taking the group as a whole, pneumonia, based on the pathologic findings, was the most frequent cause of death. Tuberculosis was second; and in order of frequency there followed septicemia, congenital malformations, intoxications, purulent meningitis, contagious diseases, acquired heart disease, marasmus, and peritonitis, while many other conditions played a subordinate part.

Sudden Death.—Death occurring suddenly and unexpectedly is not infrequent, especially in the first two years of life, but the cause is often very obscure. In some instances the child has appeared in perfect health; in others the death occurred during some debilitating disease, yet without any discoverable reason for the sudden ending. Sometimes there had been some easily overlooked symptoms, which would probably have made the diagnosis possible and accounted for the death had a physician been in attendance. In some cases a necropsy reveals the cause, but in many it does not. The feeble resisting power of infancy and the great excitability of the nervous system are the principal reasons for predisposition to sudden death at this age (Griffith[31]).

Respiratory disorders are generally considered the most prominent factor. Coryza in the new-born may rarely be the cause through what has been described as "aspiration of the tongue" (Bouchut[32]). Death in the same way is stated occasionally to occur in young infants with pertussis. Asphyxia from over-lying probably does not happen so frequently as once supposed. Enlargement of the uvula has been designated a cause of fatal closure of the glottis, but the occurrence of the accident seems doubtful. Spasm of the glottis is perhaps one of the most frequent apparent causes; certainly so in those infants who had seemed to be in perfect health. This laryngospasm depends in some cases, at least, upon spasmophilia, while in others it is likely that the laryngospasm was only apparent, and the death is associated with lymphatism, and really caused by a sudden cardiac failure. Thus it seems probable that the sudden death assigned to enlarged thymus gland is not in fact connected with this, but with the lymphatism of which the thymus enlargement is but a symptom. (See Diseases of the Thymus Gland, p. 1074; Lymphatic Diathesis, p. 482.) At least the fact remains that an enlarged thymus gland, hypertrophy of lymphoid tissue, and petechial hemorrhages may be the only findings at necropsy.

A rapidly developing bronchopneumonia, especially in the new-born, may sometimes kill with apparent suddenness, the attendants having noticed no symptoms. In other exceptional cases there may occur what appears to be a sudden paralysis of the respiratory center, the patient dying suddenly, or developing increasingly rapid difficult respiration and dying in a few hours. We have seen this condition occasionally (see p. 232).

Sudden death is of comparatively frequent occurrence in atrophic infants or those prematurely born. Thus it often happens that an infant, ill for days or weeks with unchanged evidences of debility, will unexpectedly be found dead in bed, without there having been any alteration in symptoms. Necropsy often shows no lesions whatever, or may reveal atelectasis, to which very young debilitated infants are greatly predisposed. In many other instances of atelectasis, however, the process comes on much more gradually and with evident symptoms. In some cases of marantic states the death may be due to the depressing effect of chilling, or to a fall of body-temperature without discoverable cause.

Death with hyperpyrexia is often very unexpected in children who have been perfectly well or only moderately ailing but a few hours before. This may be seen in heat-stroke in infants, in malignant eruptive fevers, acute sepsis, and, still more frequently, in pneumonia in early life. Rarely sudden fatal asphyxia may result from the rupture of a caseous bronchial gland or of a retropharyngeal abscess into the respiratory tract. In other cases death is due to pressure of intrathoracic growths, abscesses, or enlarged glands upon the pneumogastric nerve. The aspiration of food into the windpipe after vomiting has been assigned as a cause. It probably occurs much less often than has been supposed, and only in infants so weak that the ability to cough has almost disappeared. Instances of asphyxia from the entrance of ascarides into the larynx have been reported, but in most of these it is probable that the worms entered the respiratory tract after death. Edema of the glottis is also an occasional cause.

Sudden death from heart-failure is not infrequently seen in convalescence after diphtheria. It may also occur in debilitated states or in respiratory diseases, especially pleural effusion, following too sudden a movement, improper position, or excitement. The same sudden cessation of the heart's action may take place in acute nephritis on account of the strain of increased arterial tension. Sudden stopping of the heart may occur in chronic valvular disease or as a result of distant nervous influences. It is probable that the sudden death which has occasionally followed quick movement or excitement in apparently healthy children, such, for instance, as the tossing of the child into the air, or which has occurred after exploratory puncture of the pleura, the giving of a hypodermic injection, or the administration of an anesthetic, has been in reality caused by inhibition of the heart's action in subjects with lymphatism.

Convulsions are a very common immediate cause of sudden death in children already ill or in those in whom no disease has been detected. Congenital syphilis is a not infrequent cause, even in infants who appear perfectly healthy (Fournier[33]).

Various malformations and accidents not already mentioned may also produce it. Among these are perforation of the intestine, entrance of foreign bodies into the respiratory passages, strangulated hernia, and hemorrhages from or into the intestinal tract or other parts of the body. Particularly in the new-born may be noted injuries from forceps and hemorrhages into the suprarenal body and cranial cavity.

References

1. Dis. of the Fetus., 1892, **1,** 8. 2. Schmidt's Jahrb., 1902, **273,** 233. 3. Nourrisson, 1920, **8,** 321. 4. Vital Statistics, **2,** 142. 5. Am. J. Hyg., 1921, **1,** 197. 6. A Study of Infant Mortality in Cincinnati, 1925. 7. Am. J. Obst. and Gynec., 1926, **12,** 817. 8. New England J. Med., 1931, **204,** 149. 9. Geneesk. Gids., 1927, **5,** 1101; 1129; Abst. in Am. J. Dis. Child., 1928, **36,** 175. 10. Ztschr. f. Hyg., 1895, **19,** 371. 11. Die Lehre von der Mortalität und Morbidität, 1901; Ref. Pfaundler und Schlossmann's Handb. d. Kinderh., 1906, **1,** 1; 279. 12. J.A.M.A., 1915, **64,** 287. 13. Arch. Pediat., 1920, **37,** 151. 14. New York M. J., 1922, **116,** 462. 15. Causes and Prevention of Neonatal Mortality U. S. Dept. Labor, 1929. 16. Arch. Pediat., 1905, **22,** 762. 17. 15th Intern. Cong. on Hyg. and Demography, 1912; III; 3; pt. 1, 139. 18. Statistical Rep. of Inf. Mort. for 1917, 1921, 1922, 1927, 1928, 1929, 1930. 19. Klin. Wchnschr., 1927, **6,** 1248. 20. Nederl. tijdschr. f. Geneesk., 1920, **64,** 371. 21. Lancet, 1922, **1,** 758. 22. Am. J. Hyg., 1922, **11,** 668. 23. Human Biol., 1929, **1,** 90. 24. Am. J. Dis. Child., 1921, **21,** 488. 25. München. med. Wchnschr., 1922, **69,** 1110. 26. Arch. Pediat., 1923, **40,** 266. 27. Med. Res. Council Rep., 1930, **145,** 12. 28. J. Mass. Assoc. Boards of Health, 1898, Dec. 29. Communic. Dis. Control, Sec. 2, Pub. Health Serv. and Administrat., 1931, 10. 30. Am. J. Dis. Child., 1931, **41,** 1363. 31. Am. Med., 1903, **5,** 989. 32. Mal. des nouveau-nés., 1885, 279. 33. La sem. méd., 1901, **21,** 20.

CHAPTER X

THE THERAPEUTICS OF INFANCY AND CHILDHOOD

Therapeutics in infancy and childhood possesses a few characteristics which sometimes render the subject easier and more satisfactory than in later years. All the tendencies of life are toward recovery, and the system generally responds well to remedial measures. Drugs when given should be in sufficient strength to do good, but never to do harm, and they should not be administered at all unless distinctly indicated. Under-dosing is futile; over-dosing harmful. To the latter there exists a wide-spread tendency among physicians. In the large majority of cases little medicine of any sort is required, and the careful attention to hygiene and diet is sufficient, with possibly such slight aiding of nature as the giving of a laxative, a diuretic, a warm bath, rest in bed, and the like.

Despite what has just been said the therapeutics of childhood for the most part presents many difficulties to the inexperienced. These depend chiefly on the fact that the child does not react toward remedial measures merely as a small-sized man would do, but has in many respects its own susceptibilities. Some methods of treatment influence the system more powerfully than in adult life; others, useful in adults, are not so in childhood. The difficulty in administering medicines to many children is another factor. Numerous children, as a result of whim, or of the unpleasant taste or smell of a medicine, refuse this altogether. The giving of it may do harm through the struggling which arises, or may be always followed by vomiting. The taste of this same medicine may be not at all disagreeable to another child.

The therapeutics of early life may be divided into (A) *Administration of medicines by the mouth,* (B) *Dietetic treatment,* (C) *Treatment other than by drugs by the mouth.* The order mentioned by no means indicates their relative importance. The older method of measuring by apothecaries' weights and measures will be chiefly referred to here, not as preferable, but because it is at the present time much the most familiar, and because there seems to be no practical advantage in writing prescriptions in the metric system and ordering the administration of the medicine in drops or teaspoonfuls. Metric equivalents are given in the parentheses whenever this seems best. A fluiddram is equivalent to practically 4 cc., a fluidounce to 30 cc., a grain to 65.0 milligrams, and a dram (apothecary) by weight to nearly 4 Gm. We are usually obliged in family-practice to regard a teaspoonful as equaling 1 fluiddram and a tablespoonful as the equivalent of $\frac{1}{2}$ a fluidounce; although the great variation in the size of spoons renders this inaccurate. A small glass graduate should always be recommended. A teaspoonful is approximately 5 cc. and a tablespoonful 15 cc.

A. ADMINISTRATION OF MEDICINES BY THE MOUTH

1. Method of Giving Medicine.—In this, as in all forms of medical treatment in early life, we must as far as possible avoid the occasioning of fright, pain, or great excitement of any sort. Previous good training by the parents will have rendered the administration of medicines much easier. The physician, on his part, must see first, that the doses are small; second, that the taste is as pleasant as it can be made; and third, and most important, that the giving of any drug is really necessary. It is often impossible to conceal a disagreeable taste and in such an event force may become necessary. Whether this shall be employed, or the treatment by drugs foregone, depends upon the needs of the case. Judgment must be exercised, remembering, as stated, that the harm from the fear and excitement may much exceed the good which the medicine might do. This scarcely applies to the cases of less severe ailments in vigorous children, when the refusal depends merely on ill-temper or obstinacy.

Where medicine has to be administered by force, the child should be wrapped as for the examination of the throat (p. 144) and held by an attendant, and the nostrils compressed for a moment, or, with infants, the chin pressed backward and downward. Generally the mouth opens and the spoon may be inserted to the back of the tongue, emptied, and slowly withdrawn. There is difficulty in swallowing if the spoon is not removed. Often an infant who spits out the greater part of a teaspoonful of medicine will take it very nicely if it is given in divided portions. Sometimes it may well be administered from a larger spoon, as there is less danger of spilling it should the child struggle.

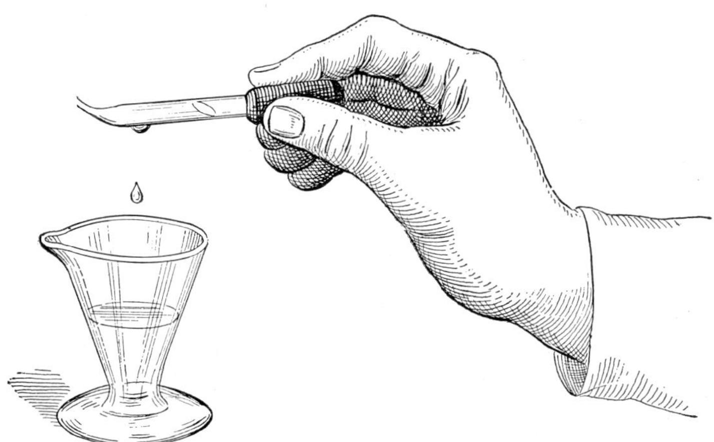

Fig. 15.—Medicine-dropper. Showing the correct method of dropping from the thicker portion of the tube.

The attendants should be told that, in cases where medicine must be given, it is better to waste little time in pleading and in argument, but to use firmness and decision from the very beginning. The child must in no case be deceived regarding the character of the medicine, as its confidence is lost thereby, and the giving of the next dose will be only the harder. For the same reason a disagreeable medicine should never be surreptitiously mixed with the food. In stuporous, delirious, or greatly exhausted conditions liquid medicine may be administered with a medicine dropper while the child is on its back. This should be inserted between the cheek and the teeth to prevent its being bitten. Nauseating remedies should not be given upon an empty stomach when this can be avoided.

In the ordering of quite small doses, or in the prescribing of powerful drugs, the physician must carefully remember the difference between the minim and the drop of many solutions, particularly of alcoholic ones, such as tinctures; and that the size of the drop also varies with the mouth of the bottle or with the dropper from which it is obtained. Consequently it is best to reckon the dose in minims rather than drops. For this purpose a minim-glass should be used; or, if drops are ordered, the attendant should be told exactly the method of dropping to be employed. The small, sharply-pointed medicine-droppers furnish a drop scarcely more than half the size of one obtained from the edge of the bottle-mouth. A curved dropper should be used, and the drop should fall from the thicker portion (Fig. 15). It is important, too, to recognize the differences in the sizes of spoons; which makes it safer to measure as a dram or a half ounce in an accurately graduated medicine-glass the "teaspoonful" or "tablespoonful" doses prescribed. (See p. 176.) Mothers and nurses should be cautioned against attempting to measure half a teaspoonful with a teaspoon. The shape of the bowl of the spoon makes this impossible. To obtain half a teaspoonful, 1 teaspoonful of the medicine should be mixed with 1 teaspoonful of water, and the child given a teaspoonful of the mixture. Similarly a 5-minim glass may be made to measure 1 minim by adding to the 5 minims of the medicine 20 minims of water and giving 5 minims of the mixture.

Unless really necessary those medicaments should not be used which cause unpleasant secondary effects, sometimes worse than the disease itself. Those, too, are to be avoided, when possible, which are almost uniformly disliked by children; and the individual fancy of the patient should be studied as well. Much can be done to disguise unpleasant tastes to a certain extent. As a rule, infants and children like sweetened mixtures, and syrups, saccharin or glycerine may be used for sweetening. Among the serviceable syrups for this purpose, especially for older children, are those of ginger, raspberry (rubus idaeus), chocolate, orange-flower, wild cherry, vanilla, and lemon. For infants the simple syrup of the Pharmacopoeia is to be preferred. The aromatic waters are well-liked, such as peppermint, spearmint, cinnamon, and orange-flower. For infants spearmint water (aqua menthae viridis) is to be preferred to peppermint (aqua menthae piperitae) since the taste of the latter is somewhat sharp. The elixir aromaticus and the elixir glycyrrhizae (elixir adjuvans) are very serviceable for disguising an unpleasant taste in the case of older children. They contain, however, about 25 per cent of alcohol and are not suitable for employment in full strength in the case of young subjects. Bitter medicines are generally disliked by children, but infants often appear to find them not unpleasant, especially if an abundance of sweetening is added. In this point there is the greatest individual difference seen. In some instances the bitter taste appears to make the infant vomit promptly. Nearly all liquid medicines may be sweetened and diluted with water when given. Instruction on this point should be included in the directions upon the label on the bottle. An exception exists where sugar may disagree with the digestion; in the case of oils or emulsions; or where the addition of water makes the larger bulk still more difficult of administration.

The taking of a sip of sweetened water, milk, sweetened lemon-juice or orange juice, or the sucking a mint-drop or chocolate immediately before medicine is given dulls the sense of taste to some extent. Another sip immediately after aids in covering the unpleasant taste. The mother should be instructed that the employment of sweets in this way is to be confined to the occasions of giving medicine. Quinine may be disguised to a certain extent by licorice, or still better by syrup of yerba santa or syrup of chocolate. A nearly tasteless preparation such as quinine ethyl carbonate (aristochin) may replace it to a considerable extent. Castor oil may be given in emulsion with an aromatic water; floated on ice water, lemon juice, sarsaparilla or whiskey and water; or stirred in hot milk. By the last method it is rendered nearly tasteless. The child must, of course, not be told that it is milk. In the case of infants it may be administered warmed in the spoon to make it less thick. Many infants vomit it, and to these it should not be given at all. Others do not appear to dislike it in the least. There are some serviceable tasteless preparations on the market. To older children it is generally distasteful unless disguised. Cod liver oil is often taken readily by young children and infants. It may be given plain or in an emulsion flavored with mint or chocolate, or combined with a syrupy malt extract.

Drugs in powdered form, if comparatively tasteless and small in amount, may be placed directly upon the tongue, and washed down with a sip of water or milk. It is still better to have them combined with sugar when prepared. Powders of larger size may be mixed with a teaspoonful of jam, preserves, scraped apple, or the like, if there is no contra-indication. Entirely tasteless powders may conveniently be given on milk-toast or bread-and-milk and not be perceived at all.

Little children cannot take pills. Those of three or four years of age, if well trained, will swallow them readily if they are small. If the substance is bitter it should be sugar-coated, or the drug enclosed in capsules. The pill may be conveniently offered in a small portion of jam or of preserved or fresh fruit. The rule already expressed still holds good; that no deception is allowable, and that the child should always be told that it is "medicine."

2. Dosage.—Various posometric tables have been constructed for use in childhood, and various methods proposed for the calculation of the proportionate doses as compared with those of adults. No fixed rule, however, can be entirely accurate. This is both because the relative susceptibility to different drugs varies greatly at this time of life, and because one cannot be guided either by age or by size alone. The rule of Clarke makes the weight of the child the numerator and 150 pounds the denominator, the resulting fraction being the portion of the adult dose to be employed. However, a child of six months weighing no more than a child of one month may need a decidedly larger dose than its weight would indicate. The rule of Young, which adds 12 to the age and divides the age by the result, ignores entirely the elements of size and weight. In practice, both age and weight must be considered. For the average child, Young's rule is a very convenient one down to the age of two years. Earlier than this the dosage may be based partly upon the age and partly upon the weight. The following table of proportionate dosage may be employed as a guide, but in a general way only. (See next section.)

TABLE 61.—PROPORTIONAL DOSES

Adult	1
18 years	$\frac{3}{4}+$
12 years	$\frac{1}{2}$
8–10 years	$\frac{2}{5}$
6 years	$\frac{1}{3}$
4 years	$\frac{1}{4}$
3 years	$\frac{1}{5}$
2 years	$\frac{1}{7}$
1 year	$\frac{1}{10}$
9 months	$\frac{1}{15}$ or $\frac{2}{3}$ dose for 1 year
6 months	$\frac{1}{20}$ or $\frac{1}{2}$ dose for 1 year
Birth to 3 months	$\frac{1}{30}$ or $\frac{1}{3}$ dose for 1 year

3. Susceptibility to Certain Drugs.—Here it is necessary to mention only a very few drugs to which either children are very susceptible or which are remarkably well tolerated by them. Prominent in this connection are the opiates, which in the first two to three months of life must be given with great caution. This is especially true of infants in debilitated or stuporous conditions. After the age of three months the susceptibility diminishes, although still present to some extent. Inasmuch as the individual reaction to opiates varies greatly, the initial dose should always be small, and caution given to the attendants to watch for any over-action. The average doses for one year will be found in Table 62. Nothing said here is intended to discourage the employment of opiates in early life, since they are frequently invaluable remedies.

Table 62.—Table of Dosage at the Age of One Year

		Gm.
Acetanilid	$\frac{1}{4}$–$\frac{1}{2}$ gr.	0.016 0.032
Acetyl salicylic acid	$\frac{1}{4}$–1 gr.	0.016 – 0.065
Aconite, tincture	$\frac{1}{8}$–$\frac{1}{4}$ m.	0.008 – 0.016
Adrenaline (1:1000 solution)	2–4 m.	0.123 – 0.246
Alcohol: brandy	5–30 m.	0.31 – 1.86
champagne	1–3 dr.	3.7 –11.1
gin	10–60 m.	0.62 – 3.7
port wine	10–60 m.	0.62 – 3.7
sherry	10–60 m.	0.62 – 3.7
whisky	5–30 m.	0.31 – 1.85
Ammonia: acetate, liquor	15 m.	0.92
aromatic spirits	2–5 m.	0.123 – 0.31
carbonate	$\frac{1}{2}$–1 gr.	0.032 – 0.065
chloride	1–2 gr.	0.065 – 0.13
Antipyrine	$\frac{1}{4}$–1 gr.	0.016 – 0.065
Arsenic, Fowler's solution	$\frac{1}{4}$–1 m.	0.015 – 0.062
Asafetida, milk	15–60 m.	0.92 – 3.7
Aspirin (See Acetyl salicylic acid)		
Atropine	$\frac{1}{2000}$–$\frac{1}{1000}$ gr.	0.000032– 0.000065
Belladonna, tincture	$\frac{1}{2}$–2 m.	0.031 – 0.123
Bismuth: salicylate	1–2 gr.	0.065 – 0.13
subcarbonate	5–8 gr.	0.324 – 0.518
subgallate	2–4 gr.	0.13 – 0.259
subnitrate	5–8 gr.	0.324 – 0.518
Brandy (See Alcohol)		
Bromides, sodium and potassium	1–4 gr.	0.065 – 0.259
Bromoform	1–2 m.	0.062 – 0.123
Caffeine citrate	$\frac{1}{4}$–$\frac{1}{2}$ gr.	0.016 – 0.032
Caffeine sodio-benzoate (hypodermically)	$\frac{1}{4}$–$\frac{1}{2}$ gr.	0.016 – 0.032
Calcium chloride	1–2 gr.	0.065 – 0.13
Calcium gluconate	2 gr.	0.13
Calcium lactate	2 gr.	0.13
Calomel (See Mercury)		
Camphor (hypodermically in oil)	$\frac{1}{5}$–$\frac{1}{2}$ gr.	0.013 – 0.032
Cascara, fluid extract	1–4 m.	0.062 – 0.246
Castor oil	30–60 m.	1.85 – 3.7
Chalk-mixture	15–60 m.	0.92 – 3.7
Champagne (See Alcohol)		
Chloral hydrate	$\frac{1}{2}$–2 gr.	0.032 – 0.13
Chloroform, spirits	2 m.	0.123
Codeine (See Opium)		
Cod liver oil	15–60 m.	0.92 – 3.7
Creosote carbonate	1.5 gr.	0.097
Digitalis, infusion	5–30 m.	0.31 – 1.85
Digitalis, powdered	$\frac{1}{5}$ gr.	0.013
Digitalis, tincture	$\frac{1}{4}$–2 m.	0.015 – 0.123
Ephedrine	$\frac{1}{8}$–$\frac{1}{2}$ gr.	0.008 – 0.032
Gin (See Alcohol)		
Ginger, tincture	1–5 m.	0.062 – 0.31
Hexamethylenamine	$\frac{1}{4}$–$\frac{1}{2}$ gr.	0.016 – 0.032
Hydrochloric acid, dilute	1–2 m.	0.062 – 0.123
Ipecacuanha: powdered	$\frac{1}{8}$–$\frac{1}{4}$ gr.	0.008 – 0.016
syrup	3–8 m.	0.185 – 0.493
syrup (as emetic)	60 m.	3.7
Iron: carbonate, mass	$\frac{1}{2}$–1 gr.	0.032 – 0.065
carbonate, saccharated	$\frac{1}{4}$–1 gr.	0.016 – 0.065
citrate	$\frac{1}{4}$–1 gr.	0.016 – 0.065
chloride, tincture	$\frac{1}{2}$–1 m.	0.031 – 0.062
iodide, syrup	1–5 m.	0.062 – 0.31
lactate	$\frac{1}{4}$–1 gr.	0.016 – 0.065
pyrophosphate	$\frac{1}{4}$–1 gr.	0.016 – 0.065
reduced	$\frac{1}{4}$–$\frac{1}{2}$ gr.	0.016 – 0.032

TABLE 62.—TABLE OF DOSAGE AT THE AGE OF ONE YEAR (*Concluded*)

			Gm.
Laudanum (See Opium)			
Luminal (See Phenobarbital)			
Magnesia	citrate, solution	1–4 dr.	3.7 –14.8
	milk	1–2 dr.	3.7 – 7.4
	oxide	5–30 gr.	0.324 – 1.94
	sulphate	3–10 gr.	0.194 – 0.65
Mercury	calomel	$\frac{1}{4}$–1 gr.	0.016 – 0.065
	calomel, divided doses (as purgative)	$\frac{1}{2}$–1 gr.	0.032 – 0.065
	with chalk (gray powder)	1–2 gr.	0.065 – 0.13
Morphine (See Opium)			
Nitre, sweet spirits of		2–6 m.	0.123 – 0.370
Nux vomica, tincture		1–2 m.	0.062 – 0.123
Opium	codeine, sulphate	$\frac{1}{100}$–$\frac{1}{50}$ gr.	0.0006 – 0.0013
	deodorized tincture	$\frac{1}{4}$–$\frac{1}{2}$ m.	0.015 – 0.031
	Dover's powder	$\frac{1}{8}$–$\frac{1}{2}$ gr.	0.008 – 0.032
	laudanum	$\frac{1}{8}$–$\frac{1}{2}$ m.	0.008 – 0.031
	morphine, sulphate	$\frac{1}{150}$–$\frac{1}{100}$ gr.	0.0004 – 0.0006
	paregoric (camphorated tincture)	3–10 m.	0.185 – 0.62
Phenacetin (acetphenetidin)		$\frac{1}{4}$–1 gr.	0.016 – 0.065
Phenobarbital		$\frac{1}{16}$–$\frac{1}{8}$ gr.	0.004 – 0.008
Phenolphthalein		$\frac{1}{2}$–1 gr.	0.032 – 0.065
Phenyl salicylate		$\frac{1}{2}$–1 gr.	0.032 – 0.065
Quinine, sulphate		$\frac{1}{2}$–1 gr.	0.032 – 0.065
Rhubarb, aromatic syrup		15–30 m.	0.92 – 1.85
Salicylic acid (See Sodium)			
Salol (See Phenyl salicylate)			
Santonin		$\frac{1}{4}$–$\frac{1}{2}$ gr.	0.016 – 0.032
Senna, syrup		15–30 m.	0.92 – 1.85
Sodium	bicarbonate	1–2 gr.	0.065 – 0.13
	phosphate	5–20 gr.	0.324 – 1.3
	salicylate	$\frac{1}{2}$–2 gr.	0.032 – 0.13
	sulphate	3–10	0.194 – 0.65
Squills, syrup		3–10 m.	0.185 – 0.62
Strophanthus, tincture		$\frac{1}{4}$–2 m.	0.015 – 0.123
Strychnine, sulphate		$\frac{1}{500}$–$\frac{1}{200}$ gr.	0.00013 – 0.0003
Terpene hydrate		$\frac{1}{4}$–$\frac{1}{2}$ gr.	0.016 – 0.032
Veronal (barbital)		1–3 gr.	0.065 – 0.194
Whisky (See Alcohol)			

At the other end of the scale is belladonna and its alkaloid, for which the tolerance is usually remarkably great in early life, and even in the early weeks. Frequently a much larger dose may be required in childhood than the average adult could bear comfortably. There is a great difference, however, in the individual reaction, and the initial dose should be tentative, and the attendants informed of the possible effects. Cocaine is a dangerous remedy in early life. Carbolic acid preparations applied locally may readily produce poisoning in infancy. The dose of calomel and castor oil is proportionately much larger than in adult life; quinine is borne in exceptionally large amount; and the coal tar derivatives, such as antipyrine and phenacetin, when used only in fever-free conditions, may need to be administered in proportionately large doses. Nitroglycerin may be taken in a dose as large as for an adult, and ipecacuanha may often be safely administered to a child in an amount which would cause vomiting in the average adult. The individual susceptibility to it varies greatly.

4. Approximate Average Dosage of Different Drugs.—Every medicine must be tried tentatively with every child needing it, and the amount to be given must vary not only with the susceptibility but with the necessity. Urgent cases need vigorous treatment. The table on pp.

180 and 181 of approximate dosage for a child of one year of age may be of service as a partial guide. The doses in metric equivalents are in the second column.

B. DIETETIC TREATMENT

In this connection will be considered only a few general rules for the diet in acute diseases, not specifically gastro-intestinal in nature. Fuller details are found in various other sections, as in the discussion of Infant Feeding and especially under the captions of the individual diseases.

In many of the febrile diseases vomiting is the first symptom. When this is active, little or no effort should be made to give nourishment. So, too, the dislike for food often seen in acute febrile disorders need be no cause of alarm. It is a natural result of the impaired digestive power always attendant, and nourishment should not be urged. If the symptom, however, is prolonged, or when exhaustion is threatening from lack of food, the physician must feed sufficiently, although cautiously. It may even be necessary to employ gavage or nasal feeding. Curiously, in some cases of obstinate vomiting in infants, food given by gavage, immediately following lavage, will be retained when swallowed nourishment is not. (See Gavage, p. 201, Nasal Feeding, p. 202.) A sick child may usually have water as often and as much as it desires. It is chiefly when the water appears to excite vomiting that the amount must be restricted. Thirst is very intense in the febrile disorders, and it has been the misguided practice of many of the laity to limit the amount of water. This is both dangerous and cruel. The water should be cool, but not cold. Sometimes, for older children, a carbonated water is to be preferred. Orange juice with a moderate amount of sugar added may be well taken and is useful on account of its caloric value and carbohydrate content. Nursing infants with fever should have water given from a spoon or bottle, since, if allowed to quench their thirst by nursing, they may readily over-feed themselves. On the other hand, it sometimes happens, where the giving of nourishment is important, that the existence of thirst may be taken advantage of in older children, and the child induced to drink cool milk if water is withheld; or water may be given as a reward after the milk is taken.

Great regularity should exist in the feeding of sick children. Liquid nourishment should be given preferably every three hours; or sometimes every one or two hours or oftener when very little is taken at a time. The impairment of the digestive power present in acute febrile disorders, not themselves of digestive origin, often makes it advisable that the food be weakened and especially that the fat be reduced. Infants who have been receiving a modified milk-mixture should have this made less strong, and children who have been on solid food require a liquid diet. Of all forms of liquid diet for older children that oftenest serviceable is milk, which should be diluted and may often be alkalinized with lime-water with advantage. Where milk is disliked by or, as in some digestive disorders, disagrees with the child we may employ such foods as egg-water or raw egg-white given in other ways, beef-juice, commercial peptonized beef-preparations, and broths thickened with starchy food. Clear broths, though appetizing, have little nutritive value. Jellies do not nourish to any extent, but well-made ice-cream is often a valuable food in selected cases for children who have lost appetite and need feeding. It should be given, however, rather as a reward, and not made a constant article of diet, as its sweetness is liable to cause or increase indigestion.

In long-continued illnesses often one of the greatest problems is to maintain the state of the general nutrition in a satisfactory manner. We have repeatedly seen children whose chief ailment after some illness was that they had been, and still were, greatly underfed. In some cases it may be necessary to attempt the administration of food in the form of nutrient suppositories or enemata. As a rule these are unsatisfactory at this time of life.

C. TREATMENT OTHER THAN BY DRUGS BY THE MOUTH

1. Hypodermic Medication by Drugs.—This holds a minor place in the therapeutics of infancy and childhood on account of the pain and fright produced. It is, however, too much neglected, since under many circumstances it is invaluable; as when a rapid absorption of a medicine is required, where the rebellion against swallowing medicine is excessive, or where it is important that the stomach be spared as much as possible. Morphine hypodermically may arrest convulsions or exhausting diarrhea. As in the case of adults a hypodermic dose should be, as a rule, considerably less than that given by the mouth. For sudden cardiac depression medication is far better given in this way, and for respiratory failure hypodermic injections of atropine are largely employed.

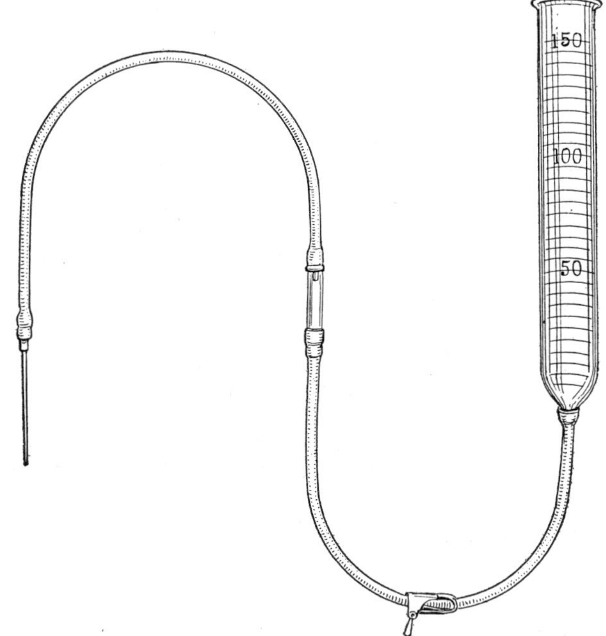

Fig. 16.—Apparatus for hypodermoclysis. The receptacle may be covered with hot cloths if necessary to maintain the heat.

2. Hypodermoclysis.—The injection of large amounts of sterilized normal saline solution (0.9 per cent) under the skin, is invaluable in some states of exhaustion or where there has been great loss of fluid from the tissues as a result of diarrhea, vomiting or hemorrhage. Distilled water should be employed in making the solution. Solutions of glucose (5 per cent) are sometimes to be preferred because they cause no retention of chlorides, possess a nutritive and diuretic value, and combat ketosis. The fluid is contained in a glass funnel, or in a bottle or other vessel with an opening at the bottom (Fig. 16). To this a rubber tube is attached with a hypodermic needle of fairly large caliber on the other end. All should be carefully sterilized before using. The needle may be introduced into any region with abundant loose areolar tissue, as in the flank, below the scapulae, or the lateral parts of the abdomen. The fluid should be warmed to about 100 F. (37.8 C.) before use. It may be allowed to flow by gravity from a vessel suspended about 2 ft. (61 cm.) above the patient, or be given slowly with a large hypodermic syringe. Heat should be maintained about the suspended vessel by the application of warm cloths or hot water bottles, since from one-half to one hour may be required to complete the injection. From 1 to 8 oz. (30 to 240 cc.) may be given in the early weeks of life, the amount varying with the weight of the patient. The injection may be made once daily, or oftener if need be. A solution of bicarbonate of soda may be given by hypodermoclysis in cases of severe acidosis. Inasmuch as it is impossible to sterilize this without transforming the bicarbonate into the irritating carbonate, the solution may be prepared as follows: Bring a liter (33⅓ fl. oz.) of distilled water to the boiling point. Remove from the flame. Add immediately 30 grains (1.9) of sodium bicarbonate (C.P.) taken directly from the center of the original container and weighed in a sterilized vessel. Cool the solution to a temperature of 100 F. (37.8 C.) and use what is required at once. Even when prepared in this way there is no certainty, however, that it will not prove very irritating, and it is better to administer the solution intravenously. (See p. 198.)

3. Intraperitoneal Injections.—As emphasized by Blackfan and Maxcy,[1] saline solutions may often be advantageously injected into the peritoneal cavity. A large amount of fluid may be given in this manner; it is all retained and quickly absorbed; the injections may be frequently repeated,—as often as every eight hours if necessary; there is little discomfort to the patient. Substances other than saline solution, such as 2 to 3 per cent sodium bicarbonate (Epstein[2]) or 6 per cent glucose (McLean and Lang[3]) have been given into the peritoneal cavity. A certain amount of reaction (sterile inflammation) in the peritoneum occurs even with saline solution (Denzer and Anderson[4]) and this is increased when more irritating solutions are employed.

Shohl[5] has recommended a method for the preparation of glucose solution for intraperitoneal injection. He[6] has also described one for the production of a solution of bicarbonate of soda for this purpose. They may be regarded as reliable, but require considerable technical skill and are best prepared in a laboratory. Grulee and Sanford[7] and Schwentker[8] have also published procedures for the production of glucose solution for intraperitoneal use. Intraperitoneal injections of diphtheria-antitoxin have been recommended (Platou[9]). Neoarsphenamin has been injected by Rosenberg[10] into the peritoneal cavity of the experimental animal, and in 1 human case with good results, and further experiments by Grulee, Sanford and Waldo[11] showed this to be safe. Citrated or defibrinated blood may be administered in the same way (see p. 200), as may iron (5 cc. of colloidal iron as ferric hydroxide) (Grulee and Sanford[12]).

The technic of intraperitoneal injection is as follows: After first ascertaining that the bladder is empty and that there is no very decided abdominal distention, the abdomen is painted with tincture of iodine. The solution to be injected, at a temperature of 100 F. (37.8 C.) is now put into a sterile glass container which is graduated. The bottom of this vessel is connected by a rubber tube with a needle of 18 gauge having a point beveled at 45 degrees. A large syringe may also be used. The skin of the abdomen in the midline, or on either side of the rectus muscle, about ⅓ of the way from the umbilicus to the pubis, is elevated between the thumb and forefinger of the left hand. The right hand plunges the needle, with the solution flowing from it, through the abdominal wall. The needle should be pointed in an upward direction and should be inserted just through the abdominal wall, the thickness of which will differ with the individual case. An elevation of the glass container of 2 or 3 ft. (62 or 92 cm.) above the abdomen will be sufficient to cause the proper rapidity of flow of the solution. When slight abdominal distention occurs the needle is withdrawn and a sterile dressing applied. The amount of fluid injected varies with the case but will be from 3 to 10 oz. (90 to 300 cc.) or more.

4. Suppositories and Enemata.—These constitute a useful method of giving medicines. Quinine may be conveniently administered by suppository, using at least double the oral dose. Suppositories of gluten or of glycerine of small size are serviceable for the relief of constipation, as is often the simple soap-suppository or "soap-stick." Chloral and bromide of potash are to be administered by enema in cases of convulsions, and the salicylates may also be employed in this way in rheumatic conditions. Somewhat larger doses of the drugs are necessary than when given by mouth, but the size of the injection should not be large or it will not be retained. From 1 to 3 oz. (30 to 90) is sufficient, a convenient and bland vehicle being mucilage of acacia or thick starch-water. Sulphate of magnesia in a dosage of 2 oz. (57) in 6 to 10 oz. (177 to 296) of water may be administered by rectum for its dehydrating effect on the tissues of the body, including the brain and the subarachnoid spaces. (See also Intravenous Injections, p. 198.) Fischer[13] has for several years employed hypertonic salt-solution in this way. The enema is conveniently given by the ordinary infant bulb syringe, the fluid being warmed slightly and injected slowly. After the injection the nates must be kept pressed together, or the nurse's thumb held over the anus for a considerable time, to prevent the expulsion of the fluid. Astringent enemata were formerly much employed, as of tannic acid and of nitrate of silver. They must always be weak, especially the latter, or irritation and straining are produced. About $\frac{1}{8}$ grain (0.008) of the silver salt or 1 to 2 grains (0.065 to 0.13) of tannic acid to 1 oz. (30) of water are sufficient, and even this strength is not always well tolerated. The injection of nitrate of silver should be followed by that of a solution of common salt. Suspensions of bismuth are frequently serviceable in cases of irritation of the lower intestinal mucous membrane, using 1 dram (3.9) of the subcarbonate to 4 or 5 oz. (118 or 148) of mucilage of acacia. When medicated enemata are to be employed the bowel should first be unloaded by an ordinary enema. For this purpose, or whenever local treatment of constipation is desired, a small injection of 1 fluidram (3.7) of glycerine, undiluted or mixed with from 1 to 2 oz. (30 to 60) of water often suffices; or a larger one of normal salt-solution or of soapy water may be given, allowing the child to receive as much as it can comfortably hold. When there are hardened fecal masses present an enema of from 1 to 2 oz. (30 to 60) or more of warm cotton-seed oil is very serviceable. This should be retained for some hours, or perhaps over night, and then followed by an injection of soapy water. Nutrient enemata are of very little service for infants, as they are seldom retained if given frequently enough to be of any possible service. They are sometimes of value in older children. The administration of a 5 per cent solution of glucose in this way has become popular. Although it has been denied that it can be absorbed to any extent from the lower bowel, it seems to do good clinically and can be shown to raise blood sugar especially when there is hypoglycemia. Arsenical preparations, such as neosalvarsan, may be given by rectal injection, using about one and a half times the intravenous dose of the drugs. The reports on the efficacy of this method of treatment of syphilis are conflicting. Arsenic is certainly absorbed from the lower bowel, as it has been found in the urine when given in this manner (Modigliani and Castana[14]) but the effect on clinical symptoms is variable.

5. Irrigation of the Intestine.—In some diseased conditions thorough irrigation of the entire colon is serviceable. The child should be laid on its back on a bed or table, with its hips slightly elevated and its thighs flexed on its abdomen. The bed should be protected by a large rubber sheet, so arranged that it will carry off the water into a receptacle beneath. The injection should be given from a fountain-syringe or glass funnel and tube at an elevation of about 2 ft. (62 cm.) above the child. A hard-rubber nozzle may be used, a small roller-bandage being wrapped about this to act as a plug when pressed against the anus (Fig. 17). A nozzle of this sort allows of the firm pressing of the nates about it, in order to prevent the expelling of the fluid. There is no advantage offered by the employment of the so-called "high injection"; *i. e.*, the inserting of an oiled rubber-catheter for a considerable distance into the bowel and the injection of the

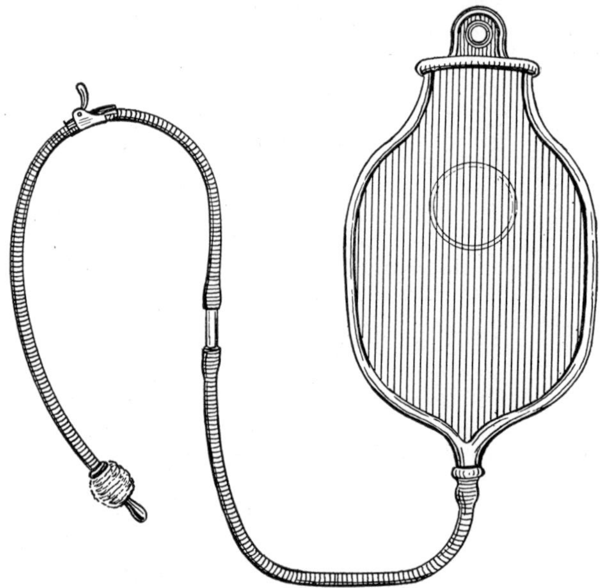

Fig. 17.—Fountain-syringe for intestinal irrigation. A roller-bandage wrapped around the nozzle checks the expulsion of the liquid.

fluid from a fountain-syringe through this. If the fluid of any injection is not expelled promptly, there is only one other direction in which it can pass, namely, toward the cecum; and it will do this whatever method of administration is followed.

The injection should be given slowly and with occasional stopping of the flow by squeezing or clamping the tube, in order to accustom the bowel to the pressure. There is no fear of over-distention occurring, if the bag of the syringe is not too greatly elevated. The infant will now and then expel the fluid with force at the sides of the nozzle, but the injection should be continued until a gallon (3785) or more has been used, or until the fluid expelled shows little, if any, fecal matter. The colon will hold a surprisingly large amount. A pint (473) may be introduced and retained without distention at the age of six months, and 1 to 2 pints (473 to 946) or more at the age of two years. After the injection is completed the syringe should be removed and the liquid allowed to escape.

The temperature of the fluid should generally be about 95 to 100 F. (35 to 37.8 C.) or somewhat less. In some instances slightly cooler injections of 75 to 90 F. (23.9 to 32.2 C.) are better, as where severe local inflammation exists, or where there is high fever, since the reduction of the body-temperature can be accomplished very satisfactorily in this way. Cool injections must not be used in greatly debilitated infants with low body-temperature or where collapse is impending. The fluid employed for irrigation may be simply water, or better, a normal salt-solution (0.9 per cent) *i. e.*, about 1 teaspoonful of table-salt to the pint. Where there is much local inflammation irrigation with starch-water (1 teaspoonful to the pint, boiled) is often very serviceable. If the starch-water is too thick or grows too cool while passing through the tube, it may jelly and cease flowing. Weak antiseptic solutions are also recommended.

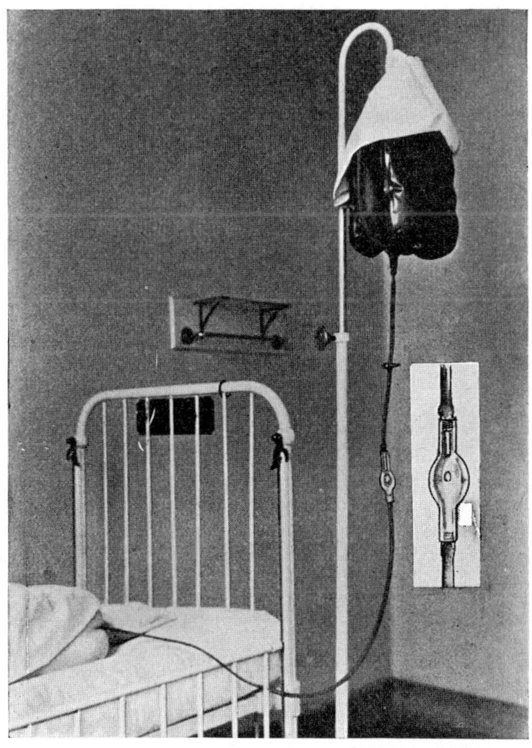

Fig. 18.—Apparatus for the drop-method of enteroclysis. The rapidity of the flow is controlled by a screw-clamp. Hot water-bags surround the vessel containing the liquid. (*a*) Larger view of the dropper-apparatus.

6. Enteroclysis.—In some cases of wasting disease or of collapse a pint (473), more or less, according to tolerance, of warm normal salt-solution may be introduced and allowed to remain (enteroclysis), the syringe being removed and the nates pressed together, the purpose being to have as much as possible absorbed into the general circulation. A favorite plan is the "drop-method" (Fig. 18) by which the catheter is kept in place for some hours, passing the fluid in the form of drops at the rate of about 20 per minute.

7. Inhalations.—These are very useful in the therapeutics of early life. They may consist of water-vapor alone or modified, or of other substances in the form of vapor or spray. For the giving of a spray the steam-atomizer (Fig. 19) is very serviceable. The small glass vessel in front of the boiler may be filled with water or lime-water, or with solutions containing benzoin, small amounts of turpentine, or eucalyptus.

Water-vapor may be produced abundantly by the slaking of lime in the room, or by repeatedly plunging red-hot iron—such as flat-irons, stove-lids and the like—or hot bricks or stones into tubs containing only small amounts of water. It is impossible, however, to keep a large room satisfactorily filled with steam in this way and the use of a croup-tent is strongly to be recommended (Fig. 19). This may be improvised by placing a large opened umbrella over the patient and draping blankets over this. A better plan is to fasten poles, such as broom-handles, upright at each corner of the crib, and to connect the tops of these by cord. Blankets may be thrown over the framework thus constructed, so that they fall down well about it. An "A" shaped opening is left near the head of the patient, and through this the vapor from a croup-kettle or vaporizer is

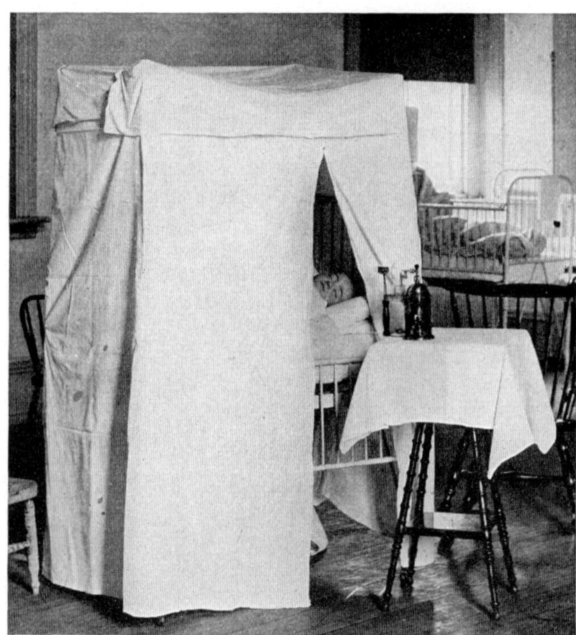

Fig. 19.—Croup-tent. Steam-atomizer on the table.

conducted. The end of the spout should be close to or just within the door of the tent, but not close enough to give too great heat or to permit the child to strike it, and not pointed towards the face. The croup-kettle sold provided with an alcohol lamp is not to be recommended on account of the danger from fire, and a small electric stove for heating the kettle, or an electric vaporizer, is better.

8. Inunctions.—Inunctions are much used for the local treatment of various conditions, and sometimes to obtain general absorption of a drug. Mercury is conveniently administered in this way, a small amount of the official ointment or the oleate being rubbed into the axillae or groins. A favorite plan in the case of infants is to apply it over the abdomen on a flannel binder. Salicylic acid, especially in the form of salicylate of methyl, is readily absorbed by the skin. There is some danger, however, of its local application producing severe constitutional symptoms (Zumbroich[15]). Cod liver oil has been much used by inunction. Its odor is extremely unpleasant when employed in this manner and it is questionable whether it offers any advantage over other oils.

9. Applications to the Nose and Throat.—**Gargles** cannot generally be used before the age of six or seven years, as the child is liable to swallow or reject them. **Painting the throat and nose** evokes resistance in nearly all cases, but is sometimes imperative, and is often easier than the use of the spray. The method of procedure has already been given in describing the examination of the throat. In the treatment of the throat, substances should be selected which do no harm if swallowed. The application should be made quickly but effectively, using a large camel's-hair brush mounted on a stick, or better, cotton wrapped firmly about a wooden or a stout aluminum applicator. Painting the mucous membrane of the nose with medicated petrolatum is often very serviceable, and is usually a much easier method of treatment than the use of the atomizer unless the patient is docile. A small camel's-hair brush or cotton applicator is required, and the procedure should be very gently carried out. In place of this in the case of infants the patient may be placed on its back upon the knees of the nurse, with its head hanging well backward and downward, and liquid petrolatum, medicated if desired, dropped into each nostril with a blunt-tipped medicine-dropper. In this position gravity takes the fluid to the upper part of the nostrils.

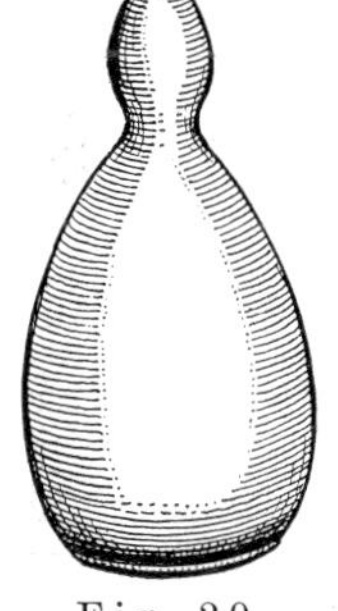

Fig. 20.—Olive-tipped soft rubber syringe for nasal douching.

The hand-atomizer may be employed for **spraying the nose or throat.** For oily solutions an apparatus should be chosen which gives a strong spray in a short time and without too much labor. Some are very unsatisfactory. Liquid petrolatum is much used, medicated in various ways as by camphor, menthol, etc. Aqueous sprays are serviceable for cleansing. For this purpose liquor sodii boratis compositus (Dobell's solution) or other weak alkaline-aromatic solution is serviceable. Peroxide of hydrogen is also much employed. A preparation of this should be selected which is not acid, and the dilution should be at least 1:4 for treatment of the nose.

Syringing the nose is sometimes required. For this purpose the best syringe is one entirely of soft rubber (Fig. 20) holding about $1\frac{1}{2}$ fl. oz. (44), or a fountain-syringe may be employed with a soft rubber nozzle. The child when debilitated should lie upon the side, the syringe being applied to the upper nostril and the injection continued until the liquid comes clear from the lower nostril. The head and body are then turned to the other side, and the syringing done through the second nostril. The danger that spraying or syringing will force material into the Eustachian tube, or into the sinuses in older children, is a real one; and care and gentleness are required with the avoidance of much pressure. In cases where the child is strong it may be allowed to sit, having the head a little forward.

Syringing the throat is carried out in much the same way, the child sitting upright or lying upon its side. In the case of either the nose or throat only mild, harmless solutions should be employed, such as normal salt-solution or a weak one of boric acid.

Insufflation of medicine in powdered form upon the mucous membrane of the nose and pharynx finds some place in the therapeutics of children, especially in such diseases as pertussis and diphtheria. The powder may be blown in with an insufflator. The application of drugs in this way to the larynx of infants and young children is in our experience difficult and unsatisfactory, certainly requires special training or skill, and is liable to produce severe laryngeal spasm.

10. Counter-irritants.—Treatment of this sort is particularly valuable in children. There is good physiologic reason for its use in pain, as it has been shown that afferent cutaneous impulses have a close relation to the mechanism of visceral pain (Weiss and Davis[16]). The delicacy of the skin in most cases is such that care must be taken to avoid too great irritation.

Blisters are not suitable for infants and are not without danger of serious injury to the skin even in childhood.

Mustard-plasters or poultices are very serviceable in such conditions as bronchitis and pharyngitis. Their strength should depend largely upon the age of the patient. In infancy 1 part of mustard to 5 or 6 of flour or flaxseed meal is sufficient. For older children 1 of mustard to 3 or 4 of flour will answer. The mustard and flour are mixed dry and then stirred with hot water. The paste is then spread between two layers of thin muslin or linen and applied. It is left on a sufficient time to redden the skin thoroughly, yet not long enough to blister. The time varies with the individual, and the skin should be inspected frequently. The plaster may be applied every day or several times a day according to the effect upon the skin and the requirements of the case. Mustard mixed with white of egg and glycerine instead of with water is less liable to irritate. The application of mustard in the form of baths or packs is considered later (p. 193).

Pepper-plasters and nutmeg-plasters were formerly favorites and are sometimes useful. Lard or mutton-suet is spread upon a piece of muslin and liberally dusted with black pepper or powdered nutmeg. The plaster should be worn continuously, until sufficient irritation is produced.

Friction with turpentine and oil, oil of amber, soap-liniment, camphorated oil and the like is often used in bronchitis, adenitis, and other inflammations. The substance should be rubbed on with the hand or with a small piece of flannel until the skin is slightly reddened. In the case of many infants it seems impossible to produce satisfactory counter-irritation in this way, and the mustard-plaster is then to be preferred.

The spice-bag is an old-fashioned but excellent application for colic in early infancy. Equal parts of ground ginger, cloves, cinnamon, and allspice are mixed and put into a small square flannel bag and spread evenly. The bag is then quilted to keep the powder in place. Before applying it should be wet with hot alcohol-and-water. The same bag may be used repeatedly until it begins to lose strength too greatly.

Turpentine-stupes are serviceable in abdominal pain or tympanites. A piece of flannel is wrung out in very hot water and sprinkled evenly with turpentine, about half a teaspoonful being used for each square foot of flannel, or rather less for infants. It is then applied and covered with oiled silk and a dry cloth. Its action must be watched lest too much irritation result.

Dry cups are occasionally useful in cases of severe bronchitis, bronchopneumonia, nephritis, or passive congestion of the lungs from cardiac disease. Their action is more powerful than that of friction or mustard-plasters.

11. Hydrotherapy.—The employment of water as a remedial measure, applied to the surface of the body in general or to portions of it, is one of the most important of therapeutic agents in infancy and childhood. Yet one of the greatest principles attaching to it is that hydrotherapy is not intended solely or even chiefly for the reduction of temperature. It serves many useful purposes in afebrile states; while when employed for patients with fever its favorable action is to be measured not so much by the degree of the reduction of temperature as by the other good effects produced. Hydrotherapy is often a harmful measure when used, as it too frequently is, with the apparent determination on the part of the physician to reduce the temperature of the body at any cost. Fever is only a symptom and, unless unduly high or prolonged, not one which does harm.

General baths may be divided into (*a*) sponge-baths, (*b*) tub-baths, (*c*) shower-baths, (*d*) sheet-baths, (*e*) vapor-baths, (*f*) medicated baths. Of the *local baths* may be mentioned (*g*) foot-baths, (*h*) compresses and fomentations. Baths may also be classified according to the temperature of the water. A convenient approximate classification is into: (1) Cold bath (40 to 70 F.) (4.4 to 21.1 C.); (2) Cool bath (70 to 80 F.) (21.1 to 26.7 C.); (3) Tepid bath (80 to 90 F.) (26.7 to 32.2 C.); (4) Graduated bath (85 to 90 F.) (29.4 to 32.2 C.) reduced; (5) Warm bath (90 to 100 F.) (32.3 to 37.8 C.); (6) Hot bath (100 to 105 F.) (37.8 to 40.6 C.).

(*a*) The **sponge-bath** with *warm* water should be employed daily in nearly every case of illness. The child should be undressed completely and laid between blankets. The sponging should be done with care and without exposure, one part of the body being thus washed and dried before another is approached. *Cool* or *tepid* sponging is of great value for the reduction of temperature, and is often in early life as serviceable as is the whole bath in the case of adults. There is not the same need of the precaution alluded to against exposure of the body, since reduction of the temperature is the object in view. The sponging should be continued for from five to fifteen minutes, avoiding the production of decided cyanosis or long-continued depression of the pulse-strength. Some degree of pallor and of lessening of the force of the pulse is a frequent result, and considerable judgement is required to determine whether or not the bath is doing harm. Some children with fever do not bear cool sponging or even tepid sponging at all well.

(*b*) The **warm tub-bath** is an excellent measure in depressed conditions in the eruptive fevers marked by a retrocession of the eruption. Through its action the cardiac strength improves and the rash consequently reappears. It is also a useful antipyretic measure at the beginning of nearly any acute febrile disease, and is often serviceable in reducing temperature in continued fevers when a cooler bath is not well borne. It is a diaphoretic in cases of nephritis, is an excellent sedative in great nervous excitement, and reduces the temperature and relieves the dyspnea of bronchopneumonia. Care must be taken to avoid exposure. The room should be warm, the child kept in the bath from five to ten minutes, according to the effect, and wrapped in blankets with little drying as soon as removed from the water. In most cases of fever in infants and early childhood it is much to be preferred to sponging.

The **hot tub-bath** is a powerful stimulant, serviceable in cases of severe exhaustion or collapse, or when the vital powers are failing and atelectasis developing, as in cases of premature birth or of bronchopneumonia in weakly infants. The temperature of the water should be 100 F. (37.8 C.) to not over 105 F. (40.6 C.) *determined by the thermometer*, and the infant should be immersed for not more than three minutes. Occasionally the procedure seems to do more harm than good, and to hasten a fatal ending which was inevitable. In other cases, however, the good results are surprising and justify any risk which may attend the measure.

The **tepid tub-bath** and the **graduated tub-bath** are useful antipyretic measures where sponging or the warm bath fails. In the graduated bath the water is 90 F. (32.2 C.) at the start and is gradually cooled down to 80 F. (26.7 C.) or sometimes less. Most older children bear bathing of this sort well, and the measure is very serviceable in continued fevers, and often fatigues the patient less than sponging. Many children however, are not benefited, and some do not tolerate baths of this temperature. One should, therefore, not persist with bathing merely because fever continues. The child should be in the water from five to ten minutes, being vigorously rubbed meanwhile, and carefully watched against too great depression.

In very hot weather, when an infant appears to be exhausted by the continued heat, it is sometimes of advantage to give several tepid tub-baths daily for their bracing and cooling effect.

The **cool and cold tub-baths** are not often needed in childhood except in cases of very great hyperpyrexia, such as develops in sunstroke and sometimes in pneumonia and the eruptive fevers. In giving cold baths under these conditions the temperature of the child must be constantly watched and the bath stopped some time before apyrexia is reached.

(*c*) The **shower-bath or affusion,** is an excellent tonic and stimulant for somewhat delicate children. The child should stand in a tub of warm water in a warm room. The cooler water may then be applied from an ordinary shower-apparatus, or may be poured over the head and trunk from a pitcher or squeezed from a large sponge. The duration of the affusion should be brief, a minute or less being sufficient, followed by brisk rubbing with a Turkish towel. The water may be tepid, cool, or cold, according to the strength of the child and the degree or reaction which follows. If this latter is not satisfactory, warmer water should be used or the shower-bath not employed at all.

(*d*) The **sheet-bath, or wet pack,** may be either hot or cold. To apply a *cold pack* a rubber cloth is put over the bed and a sheet, previously wrung out in cold water, laid upon it. The child is now stripped, placed upon and enveloped, except the head, in the sheet, and, outside of this, in a blanket. It is often advisable to leave the feet out and to put a hot water bag to them. The child may receive a second pack in fifteen or twenty minutes, or may be left in the first for an hour or more if it has fallen asleep. When removed from the pack it should be wrapped in a warm, dry blanket.

The cold pack applied in this way is useful for quieting nervousness and often for reducing moderate fever. When a more decided antipyretic action is desired it is necessary to renew the pack every five minutes several times in succession, sometimes using ice water, but only if the temperature of the body is excessively high. It is often more convenient to substitute cloths dipped in ice water for the sheet, since these may more easily be removed, remoistened and replaced. The wrapping in the blanket may be omitted in these cases. A cold cloth must always be kept to the head.

The *hot pack, or blanket-bath,* is given by covering the child with towels wrung out in hot water, or wrapping it in a blanket similarly treated; and then enveloping in several dry blankets. The pack may be renewed in half an hour. The hot pack is often serviceable for producing free perspiration in cases of nephritis.

(*e*) The **vapor-bath** is employed to cause profuse perspiration in nephritis. The bed is well covered by a blanket and the child is stripped and laid upon this. Other blankets are then thrown over the child, reaching beyond the feet and nearly or quite to the floor, but kept away from the body by half barrel-hoops, a chair in the bed, or some other support (Fig. 21) except where they are tucked in closely about the neck. Into the air-space thus formed about the child vapor is now conducted from a croup-kettle. The process is continued from fifteen to thirty minutes if the child tolerates it well. Care must be taken that the vapor does not play directly against the body, since unconscious children have repeatedly been severely burned in this way. In the absence of a croup-kettle, vapor may be produced beneath the bed by slaking lime, or by hot iron dropped into water, the vapor being given an opening through which it can rise and surround the child.

The *hot-air bath* is applied in a similar manner and for the same purpose, dry hot air from an alcohol lamp or small gas-stove being conducted under the covers by a metal pipe (Fig. 21). An electric heater may be used or several electric light globes. With any procedure every precaution must be taken against the igniting of the bedclothing, and sheets must never be used instead of woollen blankets.

(*f*) **Medicated baths** are of much service in childhood. The *warm* or *hot mustard tub-bath* is a powerful stimulant in cases of cardiac failure or where for any reason it is desired to bring the blood to the surface of the body. Often the good results obtained are surprising. Mustard is added to the water in the proportion of 1 oz. (28) (4 level tablespoonfuls) to 1 gallon (3785) of water. The duration of immersion should be ten minutes, or less if the skin has become well reddened or if the bath is not well borne. The development of a sensation of tingling produced by the mustard-water on the nurse's arms is also an indication to remove the child. The

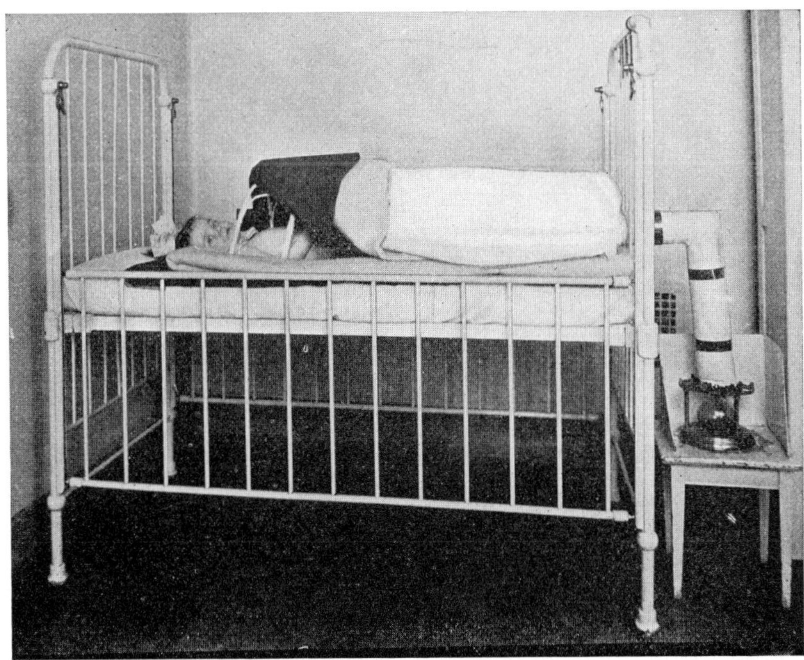

Fig. 21.—Apparatus for giving a hot-air bath. Rubber sheet and outer blanket turned back to show the supporting hoops above the child. Covered metal pipe conducts the hot air beneath the coverings at the foot of the bed.

mustard-pack is a convenient and useful application in cases oi prostration or collapse where the physician fears the greater disturbance of the tub-bath. The child is stripped as for the ordinary pack, laid upon a blanket, and covered, except the head, with a cloth dipped in hot mustard-water, slightly stronger than that used for the tub-bath. The blanket is then wrapped around the body, and tucked in well around the neck in order to keep the vapor from the eyes. The pack may continue for ten minutes or more according to the degree of redness of the skin which it produces. A very efficient method of applying a powerful mustard-pack is recommended by Heubner.[17] We have occasionally seen it produce surprising results in patients apparently almost moribund. Heubner advises the mixing of "2 handfuls of mustard-flour to a liter of warm water, and stirring thoroughly until the odor of the mustard has become distinctly irritating to the nose and eyes. A cloth is now dipped in the mustard-water, wrung out slightly, and wrapped completely about the patient up to the neck, and a blanket wrapped outside of this. The child remains in the pack ten minutes, and is then washed quickly and thoroughly with warm water, and re-enveloped in a fresh pack of simple warm water, where it remains two to three hours."

The *starch-bath* may be made of the strength of ½ cupful of boiled starch to every 4 gallons (15,142) of water. If the starch has already jellied it may be reheated, or pressed through moistened cheese-cloth. This bath is useful in some affections of the skin. Starch-water for washing the skin may be made in the same way.

The *soda-bath* consists of a solution of 1 tablespoonful of carbonate of soda (washing soda) to every 4 gallons (15,142) of water. It is used for the same purposes as the starch-bath, and is often combined with it by dissolving the soda in the starch-water.

Salt-baths have been much used as a tonic treatment for debilitated children, particularly those with rickets. Rock-salt, coarse table-salt, or preferably dried sea-salt may be dissolved in water in the proportion of 4 oz. (113) (10 level tablespoonfuls) to 1 gallon (3785) of water. The child may be washed with or immersed in this after having had the soap-suds of the ordinary washing removed with plain water. The duration of immersion depends on the temperature of the water and the condition of the case in general. Doubtless salt-baths, if sufficiently cool, do good, but whether this is in any way due to the presence of the salt is questionable.

The *bran-bath* is made by putting 1 lb. (454) (about 3 pints) or more of bran into a thin muslin bag and boiling this in water for a quarter of an hour. This water is then added to that of the bath until the whole is slightly milky in appearance. Bran-baths have been employed in many irritated conditions of the skin in infants and children.

The *sulphur-bath*, used sometimes in chronic rheumatic disorders and in some affections of the skin, is made by dissolving 20 grains (1.3) of potassium sulphide in each gallon (3785) of water employed. It cannot be given in a metal tub.

Disinfecting baths are now seldom employed after recovery from infectious diseases. They may consist of a 2 per cent solution of carbolic acid for older children, or of liquor sodae chlorinatae, diluted to the strength of 6 fl. oz. (177) to 1 gallon (3785) of water. A solution of corrosive sublimate of the strength of 1:10,000 may be used instead.

Various *mineral springs* furnish whole medicated baths useful in many affections, notably those of Nauheim for the treatment of cardiac diseases, and various hot sulphur springs for rheumatic conditions. Modifications of the Nauheim baths may be given at home.

(*g*) Of the **local baths** the *foot-bath* is one of the most serviceable for older children. It is generally given in the form of the hot mustard foot-bath, of the strength of 1 oz. (28) (4 level tablespoonfuls) of mustard to 1 gallon (3785) of water. Care must be observed that the room is warm and the bed-clothes also. The child, dressed in its night-clothes, sits on the edge of the bed, well wrapped with blankets, including the thighs, while the feet and legs are in the tub of mustard-water. After five or ten minutes the feet are rapidly dried and wrapped in a warmed blanket, and the child put to bed. Exposure is avoided even more completely if the tub is in the bed under the covers, while the child lies with the knees drawn up and the feet in the mustard-water.

(*h*) **Compresses and fomentations** constitute what may be called local forms of baths. *Cold compresses* consist of thin cloth, folded into several layers, dipped in ice water, wrung out and laid on the affected part. They must be light, not wet enough to drip, and changed every few minutes. They are serviceable in inflammation of the eyes, sprains, etc. *Hot com-*

presses, or *fomentations*, are made of flannel in several layers, which has been wrung out in water as hot as can be borne. This wringing is conveniently done by dropping the wet flannel into a dry towel and then thoroughly twisting this. The nurse then tests the flannel against her cheek, applies it quickly to the part, and covers it with oil-silk and then with dry flannel or a dry towel. It should be renewed in an hour, or less if it is desired to maintain decided heat.

(*i*) **Poultices.**—The poultice is intended to furnish a wet dressing which will retain heat longer than a fomentation. It is commonly composed of flaxseed-meal, but other substances may be used instead, such as cornmeal, bread, starch, slippery elm, etc., according to circumstances. The *flaxseed-poultice* is made by stirring ground flaxseed into a small quantity of water nearly or quite boiling, until it is of the consistency of hot mush, too thick to flow. This is spread upon a thick piece of cotton or linen cloth, the edges folded over slightly, and the whole covered with cheese-cloth, gauze, or a thin old pocket handkerchief. The nurse should test it against her cheek to see that it is not too hot, apply it, cover it with oiled-silk or paraffin-paper, and enclose with a bandage. It should be renewed every few hours if the heat is to be maintained. The *slippery-elm-poultice* and the *corn-meal-poultice* are prepared in the same way, from ground elm-bark or from cornmeal. They have no special advantages over the flaxseed-poultice. The *bread-and-milk poultice* is popular and easily prepared. Stale bread crumb is stirred into hot milk until the proper consistency is attained. It is then spread as described. Any of these poultices are applicable to many cases of local inflammation when there is no open wound. In the latter case an antiseptic fomentation is generally preferred.

In many cases of pain and tenderness, as in some abdominal affections, where a flaxseed-poultice would be too heavy, a *bran-poultice* may be substituted. A flannel bag is partly filled with bran, thoroughly wet with boiling water, wrung out in a towel, and applied. In place of this a *hop-poultice* may be prepared in the same way. Neither of these is as popular as formerly. The *mustard-poultice* has been described in considering counter-irritants. The *jacket-poultice* and the *cotton jacket*, the latter if properly made acting somewhat like a poultice, are apparently going more and more out of vogue.

12. Dry Cold.—This may be applied by coils of small lead or rubber tubing, fitted to the affected part, and through which cold water is conducted (Leiter's coils). A more convenient method, however, is the employment of ice-bags. Applied to the head an ice-bag is often of benefit for reducing temperature in febrile diseases; applied over the abdomen it is even more effective for this purpose. It often gives relief from the pain of pleurisy or cardiac disease. Ice is also useful applied below the angle of the jaw in cases of tonsillitis. The bags employed should, however, be of thin rubber. The long sausage-shaped bag of thick rubber generally sold for application to the neck is not serviceable. The ice-bag used in any region of the body should never be quite filled or it cannot adapt itself well. The local employment of ice must be watched very carefully, and is more suitable for older children than for young infants. In the latter it may cause dangerous depression. It is often best to insert one or more layers of thin cloth between the bag and the skin to prevent harmful action upon the latter. The experience of Zondek[18] upon rabbits showed that cooling of the surface of the head produced a prompt and very decided fall of the temperature within the brain, even as much as 2.4 C. (4.4 F.). This should make us cautious in the employment of the treatment.

13. Dry Heat.—This is useful particularly for the relief of pain and for the treatment of chronic articular affections. In acute painful conditions, such as otitis; for the relief of shock or collapse; and for low temperature in marantic or premature infants the employment of hot water-bags or bottles constitutes an excellent therapeutic procedure. For chronic articular inflammation dry heat may be applied by baking in a special apparatus made for the purpose, or by the use of radiant heat from a group of electric lamps. With all infants and in unconscious states at any age precautions must be carefully taken against burning the patient.

14. Blood-letting.—Venesection is rarely indicated in infancy and early childhood and seldom in older children. There are exceptional cases of uremia or of acute distention of the right side of the heart where it does good. Local blood-letting by wet cups should rarely be employed except in strong subjects in later childhood. Leeching may occasionally be serviceable in dilatation of the right side of the heart, uremia, otitis, meningitis, and pneumonia in strong children.

15. Vaccine-, Serum-, and Protein-therapy.—This method of treatment has come of recent years into great prominence, but, like all new methods, has been over-rated, while possessing undoubted value in some conditions. A great deal depends upon the care with which the microörganisms are secured and the vaccines prepared. In most instances autogenous vaccines are to be preferred to stock ones. Some bacteriologists have recommended that vaccines be prepared only from those bacteria to which the patient shows a cutaneous reaction following intradermal injection. The subject of the oral administration of vaccines is a controversial one. Vaccine-treatment consists in the hypodermic administration of a suspension of dead bacteria. As a prophylactic measure for typhoid fever it appears certainly to have established its position, and for the treatment of the attack it is possibly of value. In most of the streptococcic infections the usefulness of vaccines is doubtful. Sometimes they seem to do good in erysipelas, and the treatment is well worth trying. Staphylococcic infections offer a better field, especially in suppurative processes in the skin. The value of vaccine in pertussis is still under discussion, and it must be stated that the efficacy of the treatment has at least not been proven. The same may be said regarding the employment of gonococcus-vaccine in vulvovaginitis, and of that of the colon bacillus in pyelitis. In all these disorders instances are on record of decided improvement following their use; while other investigators have failed to accomplish any good whatever.

The serviceableness of diphtheria antitoxin is beyond question, as appears to be that of the toxin-antitoxin and toxoid preventive treatment of this disease and of tetanus antitoxin as a prophylactic measure. The same is true also of the serum-treatment for cerebrospinal fever; and that for some forms of pneumonia is encouraging. Tuberculin has not maintained the position once hoped for it, and is a remedy by no means without danger. The serum-treatment of scarlet fever in selected cases (see Scarlet Fever, p. 266) seems to be becoming established, and also the prevention of the disease by toxin injections.

Of considerable interest is the use of foreign protein-substances given by mouth, subcutaneously or intravenously for their nonspecific effect. In certain hemorrhagic conditions the injection of a foreign protein, or even of human serum or of blood itself, appears to be distinctly beneficial in controlling the bleeding. It has been claimed by some writers that much of the value of any vaccine or serum is due to nonspecific reaction, but experience and theory do not permit the employment of nonspecific measures when specific measures are available. Especially is this true in the case of such diseases as diphtheria and meningococcic meningitis. A great variety of substances have been used to produce nonspecific reaction, among them bacteria such as colon bacilli, typhoid bacilli; Coley's fluid; horse-serum and antidiphtheritic serum; boiled milk; and secondary proteoses and peptone. Usually these are given subcutaneously or, in smaller doses, intravenously; but a few, such as peptone, have been tried by mouth. It is to be noted that the conditions which are treated by nonspecific therapy are, as a rule, those which are difficult to cure and for which specific measures are not available or are of little value. Good results have been claimed and undoubtedly have followed at times this treatment in asthma, eczema, typhoid fever, various acute and chronic cutaneous diseases, psychoses, encephalitis, chronic suppuration, arthritis, ocular infection, anemia, malnutrition, gastro-intestinal disturbances, influenza, pneumonia, scarlet fever, streptococcic infections, etc. It is necessary, in order to obtain results, that a certain amount of reaction should occur after the injections. This reaction is shown by chill, fever, increased pulse, and malaise. The mechanism by which nonspecific therapy acts is a matter of discussion. By some investigators it is supposed to be closely allied to anaphylaxis. In some manner the body-defences are stimulated and antibody-formation is increased, leukocytosis occurs, and there is an increase of the fibrinogen in the plasma and of globulin in the blood. The theories have been reviewed by Petersen[19] and Miller.[20]

Mention should be made of the prophylaxis and treatment of such diseases as scarlet fever, measles, chicken-pox, mumps and poliomyelitis by the injection of human convalescent serum. This will be discussed under the individual diseases.

16. Intravenous Injections.—The superficial veins, such as those at the bend of the elbow, the external jugular, and those of the scalp and at the ankle, may be employed, and even when they are small and collapsed may be entered, by those who are expert, by means of a needle without the necessity of cutting down upon them. The longitudinal sinus at the position of the fontanelle may be used as recommended by Marfan[21] and studied by Tobler[22] and others. In puncturing the sinus an 18 gauge needle which has a bevel of 45 degrees is used. The posterior angle of the fontanelle is entered in the mid-line, with the needle at an angle with the head of about 35 degrees and pointed backward.

Substances cannot be injected into the longitudinal sinus with entire impunity. It is easy to transfix its wall if the patient moves, and the injected material may enter the subarachnoid space or be forced into the brain-tissue. We have seen 3 instances of this when arsenical preparations were employed. Unilateral convulsions resulted in all, and 2 of the infants died. At necropsy obtained in 1 of these cases there was distinct necrosis of one cerebral hemisphere. In order to prevent movement of the needle various apparatus have been designed by Helmholz,[23] Goldbloom[24] and Ratner.[25] Ratner's apparatus consists of a small block perforated so that a needle of any caliber may be used, and beveled so that the sinus may be entered at an acute angle. Before the injection of any fluid into the sinus, one should be sure that the needle is within it, as shown by the successful aspiration of blood into the syringe. While less employed than formerly for this purpose, blood for the Wassermann reaction or for blood-culture may be obtained from the longitudinal sinus. It is usually true, as claimed by Brown and Smith,[26] that transfixing the sinus with a needle does not cause internal bleeding, but this is not always the case as we have seen demonstrated at necropsy.

Intravenous injections of various substances are employed in many conditions. In dehydration, shock, and after hemorrhage there may be injected 0.9 per cent sodium chloride solution, or 5.0 per cent glucose solution, or the two may be combined. In the dehydration due to diarrhea the foregoing solutions and other special ones have been used (see p. 581). In hemorrhage and shock solutions of gelatin or of acacia are again being tried (Keith[27]), although blood-transfusion is certainly preferable (see p. 199). Sodium bicarbonate in 4 to 5 per cent solution may be given intravenously in acidosis (see p. 490 and p. 590). In tetany calcium gluconate may be given in 1 per cent solution, the preferable diluent for this being 5 per cent glucose solution. The amount of these solutions used for the various purposes mentioned depends upon several factors but should be approximately 20 cc. per kg. (0.31 fl. oz. per pound) of body-weight.

A number of sera and antitoxins, such as diphtheria antitoxin, antimeningococcic serum, antistreptococcic and antierysipelas sera and poliomyelitis serum may be given intravenously according to indications (see these diseases). Among other solutions and chemicals given intravenously may be mentioned tryparsamide and various other arsenicals in the treatment of syphilis and trypanosomiasis (see p. 439); 0.5 per cent gentian violet (5 mg. of the drug per kilogram of body-weight) in septicemia due to the staphylococcus and the green-producing streptococci; 1.0 per cent acriflavine (5 mg. of the drug per kilogram of body-weight) in that dependent upon gram-negative micro-organisms and in malignant endocarditis; 0.5 to 1.0 per cent mercurochrome (5 mg. of the drug per kilogram of body-weight) in septicemia due to hemolytic streptococci, and in erysipelas, pyelitis and other infections; quinine hydrochloride 10 grains (0.65) in 100 cc. of salt solution in severe malaria.

The employment of intravenous injections of sodium chloride, magnesium sulphate or glucose has proved of value in certain conditions in which there is increase in intracranial pressure (Fischer,[28] Weed and McKibbon,[29] Haden,[30] Fay[31]). The action is a dehydrating one on the tissues of the body including the brain and the ventricles, and the injections would be indicated in edema of the brain, uremia and intracranial injuries. They have been of use in our hands in combating the increase of intracranial pressure occurring in serous meningitis, in acute infections, in uremia, in the acute stages of encephalitis, and in purulent meningitis. Their effect is usually manifest within a few hours, and may be maintained over a long period by daily repetition of the injections. They are contraindicated in the presence of shock and such symptoms as subnormal temperature and rapid and increasing pulse-rate. Sodium chloride may be used in 15 per cent solution, glucose in 25 to 40 per cent solution, and magnesium sulphate in 2 per cent solution. They should be administered slowly, at body-temperature; taking about ten minutes to give 15 or 20 cc. (0.507 or 0.676 fl. oz.) of the solution, and the blood-pressure carefully observed during the injection. The amount will depend upon the condition and the age of the patient as well as the results obtained, but in general will vary from 50 to 150 cc. (1.7 to 5.0 fl. oz.).

Reactions may occur in intravenous therapy due to the effect of the drug or substance injected or of the water used in making the solution. The water should be freshly distilled 2 or preferably 3 times in an all-glass still. The solution should be at body-temperature; never more than 25 cc. (0.8 oz.) injected per minute and in some cases, as noted above, and especially when hypertonic solutions are used, much more slowly than this. Hyman and Hirschfeld[32] describe a method whereby fluids can be given intravenously over a period of many hours and Titus and Dodds[33] an apparatus for regulating the flow and temperature of the solutions. Matas[34] had previously recommended a simple method for slow intravenous injections.

17. Intraspinal and Intracranial Therapy.—Various sera are used intraspinally, such as antimeningococcic, antipneumococcic, antistreptococcic, antitetanic and influenzal. Convalescent serum may be so introduced in poliomyelitis. In some diseases, such as chorea (Goodman[35]), so-called "auto-sera" have been given, the blood serum obtained by bleeding the patient being injected into the spinal canal. These matters will be discussed more fully under their respective headings. In meningitis, especially of the tuberculous variety, numerous antiseptics have been employed for intraspinal injection but without avail. For spinal anesthesia a 25 per cent sterile solution of magnesium sulphate in the dose of 0.09 cc. per kilogram of body-weight (0.00136 oz. (0.65 minums) per pound) should be used; or cocaine (0.5 to 1.0 per cent) or its derivatives may be given. The employment of either substance is best in the hands of an expert. Besides the treatment of meningitis by the intraspinal or intracranial route the method may be employed for other purposes, such as the treatment of syphilis. (See p. 438.)

The techniques for the performance of lumbar puncture, ventricular puncture and cisterna puncture have been described elsewhere (pp. 151; 152). Whether used for diagnosis or treatment, the method of entering the subarachnoid space is the same. If, after drainage, serum is to be injected it should always be first warmed to about 100 F. (37.8 C.) and an amount administered smaller than that of fluid removed. The serum should enter slowly, about ten minutes being consumed in giving 15 cc. (0.5 fl. oz.), and the patient's condition closely observed during the process; symptoms such as great restlessness and feeble pulse, with slowing of the rate, being indications of too great an increase in cerebrospinal pressure and necessitating the cessation of introduction of the serum. In certain cases where the fluid is very thick it is of advantage to wash out the subarachnoid space either by introducing 5 or 10 cc. (0.17 or 0.33 fl. oz.) of normal saline solution and allowing it to flow out again, or by inserting one needle into the cisterna and another into the lumbar region and washing from above downward.

18. Transfusion of Blood.—In considering the indications for transfusion it is helpful to remember that a hemoglobin of 40 per cent is sufficient to carry on oxidation in a person at rest. It is believed that most of the newly injected red blood cells disappear after four to seven days, but some investigators, as W. Ashby,[36] claim a much longer time. Transfusion has been found useful in hemorrhage, purpura, shock, toxemias, infections, anemias, malnutrition, and other conditions. In toxic states, such as those following burns, it appears to be helpful to perform exsanguination transfusions, in which blood is removed from the patient before it is replaced by the donor's blood (Robertson[37]). The transfusion may be accomplished directly into the vein from the circulation of the individual furnishing the blood, or the blood may be aspirated into a glass syringe and then promptly injected into one of the large veins of the child, such as the median cephalic, median basilic, external jugular, popliteal, or femoral, or the longitudinal sinus. Either procedure requires technical skill, the first especially so. The simplest method is the employment of a citrated blood, using 1 part of a fresh sterilized 2 per cent solution of sodium citrate and 9 parts of blood. This prevents coagulation. With any method the blood of the donor must be typed and matched with the patient's blood (see p. 149). This is true also even for new-born infants (see p. 40). The donor should be free from syphilis; should not have taken drugs, especially iodides, arsenic, mercury and salicylates, for at least three days before the transfusion; and preferably should have fasted several hours. Reactions consisting of fever, chill, dyspnea, embarrassed circulation and urticaria occur in about 1 or 2 per cent of cases. The mechanism of these is unknown, but they are considered by some authors as allergic or anaphylactic in nature. Fever in the patient, unless very high, need not be considered a contraindication, since reactions are not more common in febrile than in afebrile states. The amount of blood to be injected varies with the indications and the condition of the patient. Ordinarily from 1 to 2½ fl. oz. (30 to 75) of blood may be injected at the age of six months or less, 3 to 4 fl. oz. (89 to 118) at one year, and 4 to 6 fl. oz. (118 to 177) at two or three years. Krahulik and Koch[38] recommend the following formula:

$$\frac{\text{Weight}}{\text{Weight} + 40} \times 500 = \text{number of cc. of blood to be transfused.}$$

The amount of blood necessary to increase the red blood cells of the patient about 1,000,000 per cubic millimeter is approximately 15 cc. (0.5 oz.) per kilogram (0.23 fl. oz. (6.8 cc.) per pound) (Halbertsma[39]). In some cases of anemia and malnutrition repeated small transfusions seem to have a more beneficial effect than single large ones.

Dunievitz and Bruckman[40] report the intracardiac injection of whole (uncitrated) blood in a new-born infant, giving 40 and later 85 cc. (1.35 and 2.89 fl. oz.) through a No. 19 gauge needle inserted in the fourth interspace about 2½ cm. (1 in.). to the left of the sternal border. Sidbury[41] employed the umbilical vein for transfusion in the new-born, this vessel being patent up to the fourth day of life. A small amount of saline solution was first introduced to determine that the vein was still open. Shaw[42] employed the venous spaces of the penis as an avenue for transfusion. Moore and Dennis[43] highly recommend subcutaneous injections of blood, typing and matching being unnecessary. There may be given 50 cc. (1.7 oz.) per kilogram of body-weight (0.77 fl. oz. (22 cc.) per pound).

19. Intraperitoneal Transfusion.—As shown by Siperstein and Sansby[44] citrated blood may be injected into the peritoneal cavity and act as a true transfusion, with entrance of red blood cells into the circulation (Ruh and McClelland[45]). Florey and Witts,[46] Opitz and Metis,[47] and others prefer defibrinated blood. Hill, Smith and Cross[48] have successfully combined intraperitoneal transfusion with intraperitoneal saline injections, simply introducing the required amount of blood during the saline injection and through the originally inserted needle. Blood given intraperitoneally should be matched (p. 149) as for intravenous transfusion, and the amounts injected the same as those mentioned for it. The technique is similar to that for other intraperitoneal injections (see p. 184). Intraperitoneal transfusion is serviceable particularly in the anemias and in malnutrition. When urgently needed blood should be given by intravenous injection rather than by the intraperitoneal or the subcutaneous route. In marked toxic states and extreme malnutrition the blood does not appear to be so well absorbed from the peritoneal cavity. We have seen necropsies in children dying several days after the injection where blood was still present. This has been noted too by McKhann[49] and Floyd.[50]

20. Lavage.—Very frequently obstinate acute or chronic vomiting will be made to cease by lavage, after the administration of drugs has failed entirely. A stomach-tube is employed, composed of a soft rubber catheter, No. 13 or 14 American scale, connected by a piece of thin glass-tube to a section of soft rubber tubing, the other end of which is attached to a funnel of hard rubber or glass. The infant sits in the lap of the mother while the nurse introduces the end of the catheter moistened with water or glycerin (Fig. 22) into the mouth and gently but quickly passes it backward into the pharynx and downward into the stomach. A slight resistance is felt as the tube reaches the beginning of the esophagus. The finger of the left hand, placed upon the tongue, may be used as a depressor and a guide. There is very little danger of the tube entering the larynx, but should it do so violent coughing and cessation of breathing will demonstrate the fact.

About 10 in. (25 cm.) of the catheter should be inserted, measuring from the gums. The funnel is then raised slightly to permit gas to escape and the solution is then poured into it and allowed to find its way into the stomach. Pinching the tube between the finger and thumb and sliding these along it toward the mouth is sometimes needed to start the flow.

After from 4 to 8 fl. oz. (118 to 237) have been given the funnel is lowered as far as possible, in order to syphon out the gastric contents into a basin. The tube is then pinched to prevent air from entering, the funnel raised, and more fluid poured in. This is repeated several times until from a pint to a quart (473 to 946) of fluid has been employed and the washings come away clear of curds or mucus.

The solution ordinarily used is a warm (100 to 110 F.) (37.8 to 43.3 C.) normal saline solution (0.9 per cent), simple boiled water, or, where there is much mucus, an alkaline solution containing 1 per cent of bicarbonate of soda. The procedure may be performed daily until no longer needed.

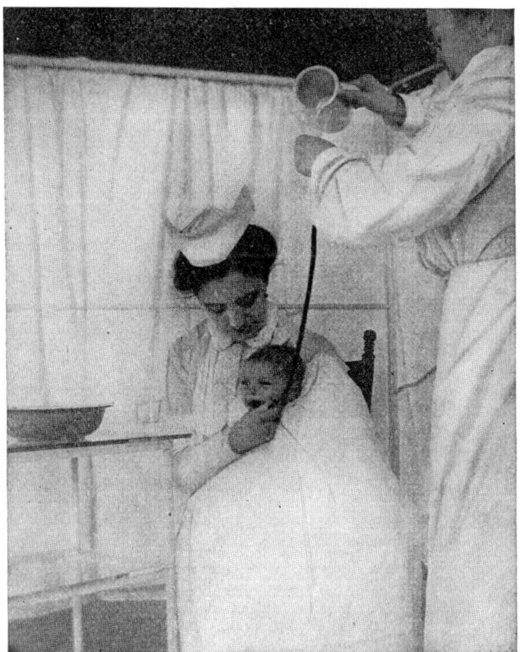

Fig. 22.—The performance of lavage of the stomach.

21. Gavage.—The forced feeding of infants is so closely connected with lavage that it may well be described in this connection. After the stomach has been washed, the tube may be left in position and the child fed through it. The funnel should be held elevated for a moment before the food is poured into it, in order to permit gases to escape from the stomach. Instead of sitting, the child should be flat upon its back, as it is less likely to regurgitate when in this position. For the same reason it must be kept entirely quiet after the gavage. In older subjects it may be necessary to use a mouth-gag to keep the tube or the finger from being bitten. When the tube is about to be withdrawn it should be pinched tightly to prevent food from dropping from it into the pharynx, as this is liable to induce vomiting. The last part of the withdrawal should also be done very quickly. Should vomiting immediately occur a second gavage may sometimes be given at once with advantage.

Gavage is very easy to perform and is extremely useful in the case of infants who are unwilling or unable to take sufficient nourishment, or in those where vomiting is troublesome. In the latter case lavage should precede each gavage; in the former lavage is not necessary. It is of frequent observation that food given by gavage will often be retained much better than when swallowed. Cases where extreme anorexia threatens life may often be fed with success by gavage. The food may sometimes be thoroughly peptonized with advantage. Sometimes it must be weak on account of an impaired digestive power; in other cases, where the trouble is the refusal to take nourishment in the ordinary way, it may often be given rather stronger and in larger amount than usual, since the intervals of feeding are longer. Children may be fed in this way 3 or 4 times a day, or occasionally more frequently. In some cases where the sole cause is unwillingness to take food, it is not necessary for the tube actually to enter the esophagus, and a short piece of tubing may be passed merely through the mouth to the pharynx and the liquid introduced from a funnel or syringe through this.

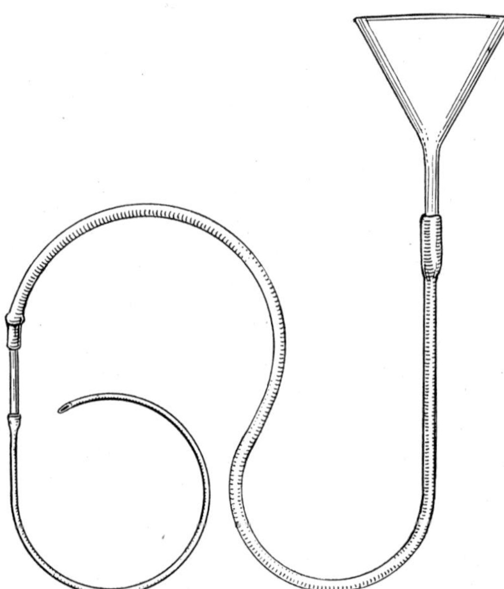

Fig. 23.—Funnel and tube for nasal feeding.

22. Nasal Feeding.—In older children who close the jaws tightly and where a mouth-gag would be required to permit of inserting a tube into the esophagus, as also after intubation, it is better to feed through the nose. The procedure is similar to that described for gavage, except that a smaller tube is required, No. 8 or 10 American scale (Fig. 23).

23. Anesthesia.—Little can be said in this connection which does not apply to adults as well. As a rule anesthetics are well borne in early life. There is a possible danger of sudden death in cases of lymphatism. Ether is by all odds the safest anesthetic and the one usually to be preferred. The excitement and resistance which it occasions may be avoided by beginning the anesthetization with ethyl chloride, which, however, is a more dangerous anesthetic if depended on solely, particularly in infancy. Nitrous oxide may be used in the same way, or alone for short operations in older children, but is not so safe for infants. Ether is generally to be avoided in diseases of the lungs and in nephritis. Whether ether or chloroform is selected, the vapor should be administered slowly and with the admixture of plenty of air; and this applies with especial force to chloroform.

24. Psychotherapy.—The enormous importance of this form of therapeutics in early life is too frequently overlooked. It requires, however, more extensive discussion than can be given it in this connection and it will be considered more fully later under Diseases of the Nervous System.

25. Mechanotherapy.—**Massage,** even when carried out in a very simple and unscientific manner, and in a way which any mother can do, occupies a valuable place in the therapeutics of infancy. The rubbing of the body with the flat of the hand, lubricated with sweet oil, cold cream, or cocoa butter, is an excellent procedure in feeble circulation, malnutrition, anemia, and paralytic conditions. Still better is it to encircle the arm or leg of the infant with the well-greased thumb and forefinger, and to push up and down the limb with the exercise of considerable pressure. More effective is a gentle kneading of the muscles done by a trained masseuse. The procedure usually soon becomes very soothing and agreeable to the patient. Care must always be taken to avoid undue exposure of the body lest chilling result. In older children a more systematic massage, given by one experienced in the method, is often useful, especially so in paralytic or pseudo-paralytic states, faulty habits of sitting or walking, lateral curvature of the spine, and the like. Abdominal massage is frequently one of the best remedies for obstinate chronic constipation.

Resisted movements may be used either alone or combined with massage. They are serviceable, for instance, in some cases of paralysis and of diseases of the heart and for the training of any especially weak muscles.

For children sufficiently old **gymnastic exercises** are of great value, conducted by a trained observer and selected to meet the needs of the individual case. Even without such an advantage, a series of exercises can be chosen by the physician and supervised by an intelligent mother or nurse in the patient's home. These may be used to overcome the results of faulty habits of standing, sitting or walking; distortions of the chest following rachitis or pleurisy; or deformities acquired in other ways. It is necessary, of course, to know the action of the different muscles and to outline special exercises to bring these into play. Exercises under water are used in certain forms of paralysis, especially that following poliomyelitis. The reader may be referred to treatises upon exercise and orthopedic surgery.

In the class of mechanical therapeutics is, of course, to be placed the application of **mechanical apparatus** of different sorts, as those used in the treatment of hip-joint disease, the paralysis of poliomyelitis, and the like. This is eminently in the domain of orthopedic surgery. Merely to be mentioned here is the use of mechanical support in combination with muscle-training for lordosis and faulty position of other sorts, with consequent enteroptosis, constipation, poor digestion and similar conditions. The subject has been instructively discussed by Talbot and Brown.[51]

Rest, with or without isolation, is often most important. Thus in chorea, many cases of cardiac disease, epilepsy, and hysteria it is by far the most important part of the treatment. The fact is always to be remembered that nervous, active children are constantly liable to take by far too much exercise. In such cases systematic enforced rest during a portion of the day is to be enjoined. Many functional nervous disturbances may be aided by recumbent rest for an hour in the middle of the day. That the child sleep at this time is an advantage, but need not be insisted upon. If he is wakeful or restless, he may be allowed to look at a picture-book or to have some not too exciting story read to him.

Electricity properly applied is a useful form of mechanotherapy in paralytic conditions and in some other affections. The fright which the application may cause often interferes largely with the benefit which might be expected. Only the weakest current should be employed at first, and never one of sufficient strength to cause pain. Indeed, the first application may well be that of the wet sponges alone, the battery being in action but unconnected. The current to be chosen depends upon the nature of the disease. As a mere matter of muscle-exercise the faradic is indicated.

26. Roentgenotherapy.—The value of this as a therapeutic method has been constantly coming into increasing prominence. Although its field is as yet limited, it has established its importance in such conditions as some forms of splenic hypertrophy, notably chronic leukemia; enlargement of the thyroid and thymus glands; cervical and tracheobronchial adenitis; inflammations; and in eczema, tinea tonsurans, nevi and other affections of the skin. The subject has become so specialized and the treatment requires so much judgment and experience that it cannot be given further consideration here.

27. Heliotherapy.—There is value in the sun's rays, or in rays produced by an artificial source, of which advantage may be taken in the treatment of disease. It is not always certain which rays of the sun's spectrum or the spectrum produced by artificial means are operative in producing the various effects. In certain conditions, such as rickets, spasmophilia, and other faults of mineral metabolism it is the short ultraviolet rays which are effective, since they produce an increase of calcium and phosphorus in the blood and a retention of these in the body. In other conditions the infrared or heat rays are beneficial. Further effects claimed to be brought about by the action of sunlight which are particularly attributed to the effect of the ultraviolet rays are an elevation of the bactericidal power of the blood, an augmentation of the percentages of red blood cells and reticulocytes, a stimulation in the production of lymphocytes and of young (or single-lobed nucleated) polymorphonuclear cells, and an increase in the number of eosinophiles and of platelets (Sanford,[52] Ilhan,[53] Dorne[54]). It should be stated, however, that stimulation of red blood-cell and reticulocyte formation cannot be found by all investigators; Hoeffel and Lyons,[55] for example, who studied the matter carefully, not finding any such effect. It would certainly appear that, while there should be no controversy concerning the effect on the retention of calcium and phosphorus in the body and the increase of these minerals in the blood, the other results of heliotherapy on the blood are uncertain. When used in the treatment of anemia it should be only an adjunct to other forms of therapy. It also seems evident that in the studies on the effect of heliotherapy and of ultraviolet light, the question of dosage used in the different experiments has confused the results.

Among other results claimed is an augmentation in the blood-sugar after irradiation, although this finding has not been consistent. It would appear from the work of Fries and Topper[56] that there is no appreciable effect of ultraviolet light on basal metabolism in children, and little effect on blood pressure. The excretion of sulphates and chlorides is said to be increased. In local infections there is apparently a bactericidal action.

At the beginning of exposure there may be an elevation of temperature, as also of the rate of both respiration and pulse, these soon striking an equilibrium.

Excessive light treatment produces an irritation of the skin and in some patients chronic dermatitis. Insomnia and irritability are brought about. Further results of an undue amount of irradiation concerning which there is a difference of opinion may be mentioned. Loss of weight is one of these, but this is not always evident in clinical practice and Hess and Smith[57] could not demonstrate it experimentally in animals, nor could they find degeneration of the glands of internal secretion which others have stated to be an effect Diminished bactericidal power of the blood is not accepted as a result by all authors, nor is the destruction of red blood cells and the production of leukopenia as claimed by Mayerson and Laurens.[58]

Children must be exposed only gradually to the rays of the sun or the lamp, in order to avoid burns of the skin and the nervous irritation and insomnia which occasionally occur. Continued irregularities of temperature and of pulse are indications of intolerance to treatment. Some clinicians believe that those patients whose skin does not pigment receive little good from heliotherapy. Others, however, have insisted that the melanin pigment is protective and that excessive tanning should be avoided. Our own view is that, while the degree of pigmentation is not entirely proportionate to the good effect obtained, it is desirable to secure it. When a moderate amount has developed, a few days' rest should be taken and heliotherapy again started. In other words, neither marked pigmentation nor constant erythema is to be desired. The program of exposure may be as follows when the direct sun's rays are to be employed: On the first day the exposure is made of the feet, and consists of from 1 to 3 periods, each lasting from three to five minutes, with intervals of at least an hour if several periods are employed. On the second day there are from 2 to 3 periods, an hour apart, of five to ten minutes applied to the feet, and of three to five minutes for the legs. On the third day there are two or three periods, with intervals of an hour, of ten to fifteen minutes to the feet, five to ten minutes to the legs and three to five minutes to the thighs. In this manner the exposures are increased, until by the end of the first month the patient can remain in the sunlight, practically totally exposed, from three to five hours a day, and by the third month he can remain from five to eight hours.

When season and other conditions permit, the sun's rays are to be preferred to artificial sources of light. In certain localities, particularly where the humidity is not excessive and winds or moving air can be prevented, heliotherapy can be carried out during the winter season. It should be remembered that ordinary window glass filters out the short ultraviolet rays. Certain special glasses (Corning glass, Helioglass, Vitaglass, Celoglass) will transmit these rays to some extent. While these glasses become less efficient after prolonged use they will, as shown by Wyman, Drinker and Mackenzie[59] and others, transmit sufficient of the sun's ultraviolet rays to cause healing in rickets, to elevate the blood calcium and phosphorus, and to tan the skin. In the winter time there are fewer short ultraviolet rays in the sun's spectrum. In very hot climates there is an undue proportion of heat rays in comparison to ultraviolet ones (Frawley[60]). Smoke, dust and, to a lesser extent, moisture filter out the ultraviolet rays, and they also cannot penetrate clothing which is heavy and dark in color.

Artificial sources of light are the carbon arc lamp, the mercury vapor lamp, and the tungsten-filament lamp (see Coblentz[61]). The first of these may be made to approach the solar spectrum more closely than the second but it does not emit so great a quantity of the short ultraviolet rays; the third is a weaker source of all rays. Great care must be taken in treatment by these lamps, and especially with the mercury vapor lamp when it is new. Only a half-minute exposure at a distance of 120 cm. (3.9 ft.) should be given at first and this increased gradually by half-minute increments every day or every other day, and the distance decreased to 75 cm. (2.46 ft.). Four or five minutes daily or 3 times a week is sufficient exposure with a strong mercury vapor lamp, but with the carbon arc lamp it may be increased to thirty minutes or longer especially at greater distances than 90 cm. (2.9 ft.). So-called "cored carbons" should be used and the lamp should take 20 amperes at an arc voltage of about 50. A twin arc lamp may take 10 to 15 amperes, *i. e.*, may be attached to the usual lighting circuit. Groups of patients may be treated with the larger carbon arc lamps. The eyes should always be protected by dark glasses when the mercury vapor or the carbon arc lamps are used.

Heliotherapy is specific in the treatment of rickets (p. 454) and spasmophilia (p. 874). In tuberculosis it is particularly valuable in the forms affecting lymph-nodes, bones, peritoneum and intestine (see these); in active pulmonary tuberculosis it must be employed with caution. It may at times be helpful in eczema and other cutaneous conditions, including the tuberculous disorders and pyodermia. It is employed by many physicians as a general tonic and for the treatment of recurrent respiratory infections and catarrhal conditions, but its value in these is problematical. In controlled clinical experiments little effect has been found (Mackay,[62] Barenberg and Lewis,[63] Colebrooke[64]). Secondary anemia is another condition in which heliotherapy seems to do good, although, as previously mentioned, this is denied by some authors. The irradiation of pregnant women is advocated by certain clinicians. (See p. 454.) Patients with active heart-disease and nephritis should be treated by heliotherapy cautiously if at all. In renal rickets the use of ultraviolet light does little good (see p. 827) but in celiac rickets it is helpful. (See p. 611.)

There are several methods for determining the intensity of artificial sources of ultraviolet light. These are respectively the zinc sulphide (Clark[65]); the acetone methylene-blue (Webster, Hill and Eidenow[66]); the erythema unit (Rost and Keller[67]); and the oxalic acid uranyl sulphate (Anderson and Robinson[68]).

28. Climatotherapy.—It is a matter of everyday experience that the cure or relief of many diseased conditions will be accomplished more surely and promptly by change of climate than in any other way. Children with subacute bronchitis often react quickly to such a procedure. Asthma, pertussis, chronic or recurring rheumatism, chronic nephritis, tuberculosis, anemia, a debilitated state of the general or the nervous system, and slow convalescence from many acute diseases are all aided by it. The choice of locality is to be made carefully. A fuller discussion is out of place in this connection, and reference may be made to works upon Climatology. Here it may be said only that many of the good effects of change of climate can be obtained by a more careful regulation of the hygiene at home, particularly in the matter of obtaining sufficient fresh air in the living rooms, both by day and by night, a life largely in the open air, and the guarding against overheating from too great warmth of the clothing.

References

1. Am. J. Dis. Child., 1918, **15,** 19. 2. Arch. Pediat., 1920, **37,** 656. 3. Am. J. Dis. Child., 1920, **19,** 359. 4. Am. J. Dis. Child., 1921, **21,** 565. 5. Am. J. Dis. Child., 1929, **38,** 943. 6. Am. J. Dis. Child., 1929, **38,** 927. 7. Am. J. Dis. Child., 1928, **36,** 445. 8. Am. J. Dis. Child., 1930, **40,** 533. 9. Arch. Pediat., 1923, **40,** 575. 10. J.A.M.A., 1924, **82,** 682. 11. Am. J. Dis. Child., 1928, **35,** 47. 12. Am. J. Dis. Child., 1931, **41,** 53. 13. Edema and Nephritis, 1921. 14. Pediatria, 1923, **31, 258;** 324. 15. Monatschr. f. Kinderh., 1918, **15,** 167. 16. Am. J. M. Sc., 1928, 176; 517. 17. Lehrb. d. Kinderh., 1911, **2,** 269. 18. Ztschr. f. phys. u. diät. Therap., 1922, **25,** 84. 19. Protein Therapy and Nonspecific Resistance, 1922. 20. Medicine, 1927, **6,** 513. 21. Ref. Blechmann, Nourrisson, 1914, **2,** 150. 22. Monatschr. f. Kinderh., 1915, **13,** 384. 23. Am. J. Dis. Child., 1915, **10,** 194. 24. Am. J. Dis. Child., 1920, **19,** 229. 25. Am. J. Dis. Child., 1921, **21,** 199. 26. Am. J. Dis. Child., 1917, **13,** 501. 27. J.A.M.A., 1929, **93,** 1517. 28. Edema, 1910, 129. 29. Am. J. Physiol., 1919, **48,** 512. 30. J.A.M.A., 1919, **73,** 983. 31. J.A.M.A., 1923, **80,** 1445; 1924, **82,** 766; 1925, **84,** 1261. 32. J.A.M.A., 1931, **96,** 1221. 33. J.A.M.A., 1928, **91,** 471. 34. Ann. Surg., 1924, **79,** 643. 35. Arch. Pediat., 1916, **33,** 649. 36. J. Exper. Med., 1919, **29,** 267. 37. Arch. Surg., 1924, **9,** 1. 38. Am. J. Dis. Child., 1930, **39,** 34. 39. Am. J. Dis. Child., 1922, **24,** 269. 40. Arch. Pediat.,

1925, **43,** 139. 41. Am. J. Dis. Child., 1923, **25,** 290. 42. J.A.M.A., 1928, **90,** 446. 43. Northwest. Med., 1928, **27,** 140. 44. Am. J. Dis. Child., 1923, **25,** 107; 202; J.A.M.A., 1923, **80,** 1763. 45. Ohio State M. J., 1923, **19,** 780. 46. Lancet, 1928, **1,** 1323. 47. Jahrb. f. Kinderh., 1924, **107,** 269. 48. Arch. Pediat., 1926, **43,** 186. 49. Boston M. and S. J., 1926, **195,** 1241. 50. Am. J. Dis. Child., 1929, **37,** 1007. 51. Am. J. Dis. Child., 1920, **20,** 168; 1921, **21,** 347. 52. Am. J. Dis. Child., 1929, **37,** 1187. 53. Arch. f. Kinderh., 1928, **83,** 270. 54. Arch. Physiol. Therap., 1929, **10,** 296. 55. Am. J. Dis. Child., 1930, **40,** 484. 56. Am. J. Dis. Child., 1927, **34,** 159; 166. 57. Am. J. Dis. Child., 1931, **41,** 775. 58. Am. J. Physiol., 1928, **86,** 1. 59. Am. J. Dis. Child., 1930, **39,** 969. 60. Am. J. Dis. Child., 1931, **41,** 751. 61. J.A.M.A., 1930, **95,** 411. 62. Arch. Dis. Childhood, 1927, **2,** 231. 63. J.A.M.A., 1928, **90,** 504. 64. J.A.M.A., 1929, **93,** 1395. 65. Am. J. Hyg., 1929, **9,** 646. 66. Lancet, 1924, **1,** 745. 67. Bestrahlung mit Quarzlampe, etc., quoted by Gerstenberger and Hartman, J.A.M.A., 1929, **92,** 367. 68. J. Am. Chem. Soc., 1925, **47,** 718.

DIVISION II

DISEASES

SECTION I

DISEASES OF THE NEW-BORN

Monsters and similar malformations arise during *embryonal* life, that is, through the first two lunar months. They are the products of defective development rather than of disease and are better considered in works on teratology. Treatment of the ovaries with roentgen-ray during early pregnancy may result in the production of monsters. Certain of the diseases of the *fetus; i. e.*, developing during the last eight lunar months of intra-uterine life, continue as diseases of the new-born, since the pathology is the same for both periods. Others, however, seem incompatible with the continuance of life outside the uterus. Any grouping of Diseases of the New-born is at best artificial and incomplete. In the following pages, are discussed chiefly (1) some of those diseases of fetal life which are, at times, capable of continuing in the living child at birth, and (2) certain affections which are peculiarly liable to be acquired by the new-born child or are witnessed only at this time. There are excluded from this section or mentioned only briefly (1) numerous diseases of the new-born which are more conveniently treated of later, (2) diseases limited to fetal life and not seen in the living infant, and (3) most instances of defective embryonal development.

In hospitals it is essential that identification of the new-born baby be certain. The several methods employed will be merely mentioned here: (1) Writing the infant's name on its chest with indelible pencil, (2) the name on tape or adhesive plaster attached to the body, (3) bracelets or necklaces containing the name on lettered beads, (4) thumb prints or foot prints.

CHAPTER I

PREMATURE INFANTS

Etiology.—In general it may be assumed that a birth-weight of less than 2500 Gm. (5.5 lb.) or a length under 45 cm. (17.7 in.) is an indication that the infant is premature, the criterion of length being more reliable than that of weight. After the thirty-eighth week of intra-uterine life the infant can no longer be called premature, inasmuch as it is then perfectly developed to all intents. The statistics given for the frequency of premature birth usually emanate from institutions and range from 5 to 25 per cent. According to Bolt[1] the yearly death-rate from prematurity in the United States Birth Registration Area varied in the years from 1915 to 1926 from 1.7 to 1.8 per cent, the total neonatal mortality (deaths under one month of age) during this period ranging from about 6.5 to 10 per cent.

Among the causes of premature birth are especially conditions affecting the mother, such as syphilis; acute infections and febrile disorders; such chronic conditions as nephritis, tuberculosis and heart disease; trauma, violent exercise, and fright, shock or pain; malpositions of the uterus, placenta praevia and premature separation of the placenta; and endocrine disturbances. The percentage of prematurity depending upon syphilis varies statistically from about 12 (Baumm[2]) to 3 per cent (Capper[3]). In Capper's study of 437 premature births over 50 per cent were in the first-born and 15 per cent in twins or triplets. Malformation of the fetus is another cause.

Characteristics at Different Periods of Intra-uterine Life.—A brief description may be given of the characteristics of the infant born prematurely after different periods of intra-uterine life which are compatible with at least temporary viability. The lengths and weights of the body are those given by Ballantyne.[4] The months are calendar months:

At twenty-four weeks (five and one-half months), the fetus measures from 28 to 34 cm. (11 to 13.4 in.) in length and weighs 676 Gm. (1.49 lb.). There is a large amount of lanugo, the skin is wrinkled and the vernix caseosa is present. The eyebrows and lashes are evident. The deposit of subcutaneous fat has only just commenced. The testicles have descended to the internal inguinal ring. The eyelids have become separated.

At the close of twenty-eight weeks (six and one-half months), the fetus measures about 38 cm. (15 in.) in length and averages a weight of 1170 Gm. (2.58 lb.). The whole body, except the palms and soles, is covered with lanugo and the vernix caseosa is present. The hair on the head is about 0.5 cm. (0.2 in.) in length. The skin is dull-reddish and somewhat wrinkled. There is little subcutaneous fat. The pupillary membrane which had previously covered the pupil has commenced to disappear. Meconium is found in the intestine. The testicles have nearly or quite descended. (Figs. 24 and 25.)

At the age of thirty-two weeks (seven and one-half months) the fetus measures from 39 to 41 cm. (15.4 to 16.1 in.) and weighs 1571 Gm. (3.46 lb.). The lanugo has diminished on the body and the hair increased on the scalp. The skin is still dark-red and wrinkled, although the subcutaneous fat has increased. The nails are harder and horizontal, but do not project beyond the ends of the fingers. The pupillary membrane has disappeared. The testicles have fully descended. The infant is very feeble, of low body-temperature, hardly opens the eyes, and cannot suck.

At the age of thirty-six weeks (eight and one-half months), the fetus measures 42 to 44 cm. (16.5 to 17.3 in.) and weighs 1942 Gm. (4.28 lb.). The subcutaneous fat has very decidedly increased and the wrinkling of the skin is much less, while the face is more rounded. The lanugo has largely disappeared. The deep-red color of the skin is now found only on the genitals. The hair on the scalp is over 1 cm. (0.39 in.) in length. The nails do not reach the finger-tips.

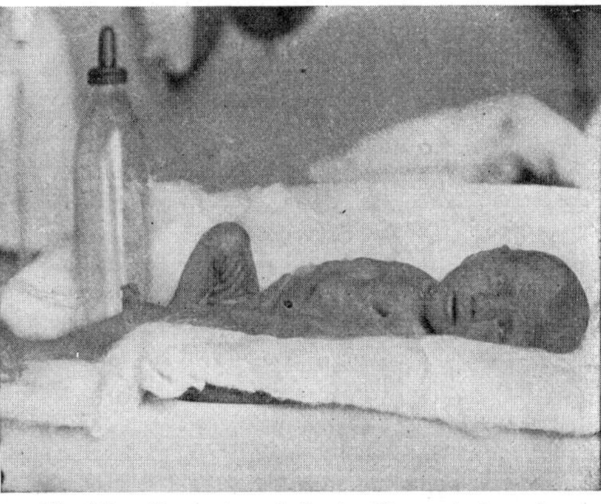

Fig. 24.—Premature infant. Born at six and one-half to seven months; weight on admission to the Children's Hospital of Philadelphia when ten days old 2 lb., 8 oz. (227). The size of the infant can be estimated by comparison with the 8-oz. nursing-bottle.

General Symptoms.—The general symptoms characteristic of prematurity vary with the duration of the period of intra-uterine life. In typical cases the cry is feeble and infrequent; the body-temperature is low and maintained at the normal only with difficulty; the infant moves its limbs but little and lies most of the time in an inactive, torpid state; there is a great tendency to recurring atelectasis and consequent cyanosis; the skin is often icteric and red, or pale, or cyanotic; the respiration is markedly irregular, feeble and intermittent; the power to suck is often absent, and swallowing is slow. Inasmuch as the infant was born before its natural time, all the organs are in an imperfectly developed condition. Yet, as mentioned by Ylppo[5] and Herz[6] the mortality depends largely upon pathologic lesions, such as intracranial hemorrhage due to trauma incident to birth, rather than upon the imperfect development. Necropsy studies by Hess and Chamberlain,[7] Clein[8] and others show that the most frequent cause of death is usually intracranial hemorrhage, with atelectasis next in order, and with such infections as pneumonia, otitis media and the like not uncommon causes. In 62 necropsies on premature infants at the Cincinnati General Hospital intracranial hemorrhage was found in 31 and atelectasis in 25. Congenital anomalies and malformations occur in about 2 or 3 per cent of the cases.

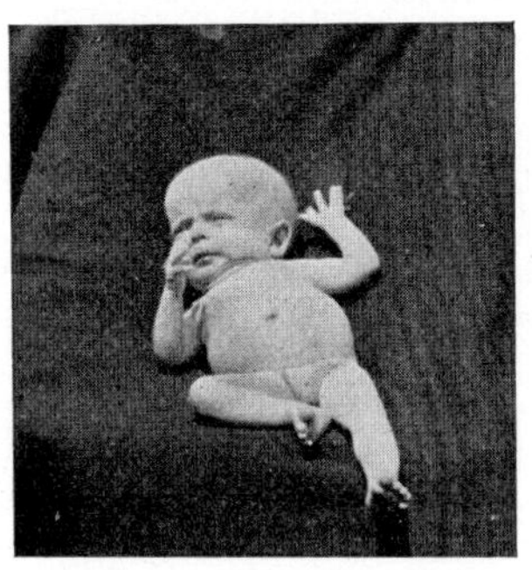

Fig. 25.—Premature infant. Same case as in Fig. 24. Now aged six months. Weight 7 lb., 10 oz.

Course and Prognosis (See also p. 170).—Even with successful treatment the progress is slow; repeated relapses into atelectasis are prone to occur; convulsions and pneumonia are liable to develop; the danger of infection is decided; the digestion is often feeble; a toxic condition often develops; there is constant difficulty in maintaining the body-temperature, and the occurrence of any chilling may be followed by fatal results; the gain in weight is slow; and internal hemorrhage takes place readily, sometimes in the suprarenal bodies and especially, as stated, within the cranium, generally from the meninges. A number of observations, such as those by Looft,[9] Capper,[3] Herz[6] and Ranke[10] demonstrate that mental and nervous disorders may develop in later childhood, a cerebral hemorrhage at birth being supposedly largely responsible for this. In Capper's series of 437 premature infants 5 per cent developed epilepsy, 5 per cent cerebral spastic paralysis and 7 per cent idiocy or imbecility. Looft stated that 24 per cent of 129 premature infants showed subnormal mental development varying from mild inferiority to idiocy. Sunde[11] in a group of 559 premature infants who had reached the ages of six to twenty-one years found 5.7 per cent mentally defective. According to Capper,[3] too, even without such serious defects premature infants are liable to be slow in talking, backward in school, and psychopathic or neuropathic. In contrast to these statements is the interesting study of Mohr and Bartelme[12] who found by intelligence tests that the later mental development in premature children showed no inferiority to those born at full term. Our own opinion is that if actual organic injury is escaped, the later development of premature infants both physically and mentally is as satisfactory as those born at full term, although there may be for a few years, and sometimes as long as five or six, some retardation. The mental and physical status should be judged upon the basis of the degree of prematurity, the greater this is the slower being the development. Among the striking features which may persist for one or more years are the relatively large size of the head (megacephalus) and the exophthalmos. The initial relative loss of weight in premature infants is greater than in the normal new-born (see p. 4). After a few months, anemia, rickets and spasmophilic manifestations are prone to appear. Bunge[13] showed that in the full-term, new-born animal there is considerable iron storage in the liver. In the premature infant, however, there is but a small amount of it, since the deposition in the liver takes place only in the latter part of fetal life. The question of iron pigment in the reticulo-endothelial system after birth is unsettled; Bungeler and Schwartz[14] finding it present in both premature and full term infants, while Lichtenstein[15] claimed a negative balance in premature infants, indicating a functional insufficiency of the hemopoietic system. It has been shown by Givens and Macy[16] and by Schmitz[17] that calcium is deposited in the fetus chiefly in the last few months of intra-uterine life. This necessitates an insufficiency in the prematurely born, and partly accounts for the frequent and early development of rickets and spasmophilia. There is also a low calcium retention in the premature (Hamilton[18]).

The immediate prognosis depends upon several factors such as the skill and promptness of the care given, the type of feeding, and the age of the infant. The total mortality is usually estimated to be 50 per cent or more, but such figures mean little because of the variability of the factors mentioned. Reference may be made, among other observations, to the statistics of Potel[19] which give viability based upon age; to those of Ostrčil,[20] based upon length; and to the studies of Hess and Chamberlain[7] and Ranke[10] based upon weight. Summarized these investigations show that, as regards age, an infant born at the end of twenty-four weeks usually dies within a few hours; at the close of twenty-eight weeks recovery occurs in about 50 per cent of the cases (Fig. 25); and that at the end of thirty-seven weeks the majority of infants will live. The figures show, too, the inaccuracy of the widespread belief that the seven-months infant is more likely to survive than one born at eight months. Rare instances are on record of survival at earlier than the sixth fetal month. In Ostrčil's investigations, based upon the length,—a better criterion than weight,—the chances of living were 21 per cent in infants of 40 cm. (15.8 in.) and these increase gradually up to 58 per cent at 47 cm. (18.5 in.). As regards weight, infants of less than 1000 Gm. (2.2 lb.) practically never live, although there are some remarkable instances of viability reported, such as those of Mansell[21] (510 Gm.) (18 oz.), Pulford and Blevins[22] (680 Gm.) (24 oz.), and Bonnaire[23] (820 Gm.) (28.8 oz.). We have seen a premature infant survive whose weight on its third day was 624 Gm. (22 oz.). The mortality is greatest in the first two or three days after birth. Cook[24] found that if an infant survived the first twenty-four hours, its chances were doubled and that after three days, the mortality dropped to about 15 per cent. However, the total mortality is likely to be increased by infection, such as pneumonia and the like, developing somewhat later, as well as by the rickets, anemia and spasmophilic manifestations which occur at a still later period. Thus Levy[25] in a series of 403 premature infants found the greatest mortality in the third week.

Treatment.—The principles involved in treatment are the maintenance of body-temperature, proper feeding, and avoidance of infection. The accomplishment of the first of these is by some form of an *incubator*, in which the attempt is made to maintain the temperature at a fixed degree

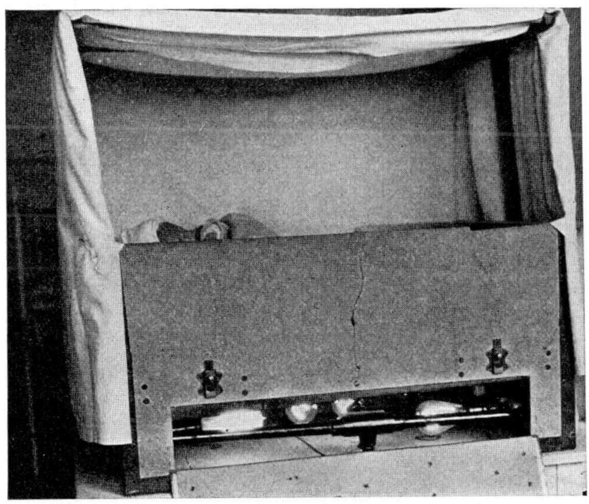

Fig. 26.—Bed for premature infant. Iron framework covered with asbestos-board. Cover thrown back. Door open at bottom showing electric lamps.

and to supply warm, fresh, moist air. One of the best of these is the Hess[26] bed and its modifications. A still better plan, when possible, is to have a room in which the temperature can be maintained at 85 to 90 F. (29.4 to 32.2 C.) and fresh warmed air constantly supplied. In an emergency a lined clothes basket or an infant's metal bath-tub may be employed; the infant wrapped in cotton and then in a blanket, and finally placed in the tub with a thick layer of cotton beneath and above it, covering it completely except the face. Hot water-bottles are then placed in the cotton close to but not touching the infant, or an electric warming pad may be employed. A serviceable device which we have used, and which can be readily and inexpensively made, consists of an asbestos box having an upper and lower compartment with perforations between the two. In the upper is a mattress and in the lower is installed a series of electric lamps, any desired number of which may be turned on to produce the required heat (Fig. 26). In all of these so-called "incubators" a thermometer at the side of the infant is used to ascertain the temperature. Under any conditions it is usually found that the temperature should range from 85 to 95 F. (29.4 to 35 C.) and the relative humidity be from about 60 to 65. If special apparatus is not available to increase humidity, wet cloths may be spread on the radiators and changed as they dry, or several basins of water allowed to evaporate slowly. Yaglou, Drinker and Blackfan[27] found in a study of the influence of air conditions on the growth and development of premature infants that the following were successful: A ventilation rate of 25 air changes per hour; an air movement of 15 ft. a minute; a relative humidity of 65 per cent; and an environmental temperature varying from 100 to 76 F. (37.8 to 24.4 C.) depending upon the general condition of the infant and its body-weight. The aim should be to keep the baby's temperature steady, and irregular rises and falls are an indication that it is not doing well. The difficulty of maintaining a steady temperature is well illustrated by the continuous temperature records taken by Tyson and Burt,[28] who later[29] described an automatic recording temperature-controller, with which the control of heat supply is based directly on the infant's axillary temperature and is automatically turned on or off. Transportation of the infant from one place to another must be done with great care. Hess[30] describes an electrically heated bag for this purpose, which can even be attached to the current of an automobile battery or to that of a Pullman car. Whatever sort of heating bed may be used, the infant should wear no clothing whatever, but be wrapped and covered with raw cotton in the manner already described. A diaper, or an extra layer of absorbent cotton, should be laid under the nates. In changing this, and, in fact, under all circumstances, the child must be handled or exposed as little as possible. No one with a respiratory infection must be allowed near the child. Unless strong enough to nurse from the breast, it is not necessary to remove it from the receptacle even for feeding, but a frequent change of position in bed is important. Bathing should not be employed at all, unless it be hot baths as needed for the relief of atelectasis. Once a day the child may be rubbed all over with warm sweet oil. After an evacuation of the bowels or bladder the nates may be cleansed with cotton and warm oil. The infant's rectal temperature should be taken every few hours, and an effort made to keep it at over 98 F. (36.7 C.) and as steady as possible. When it is found that the temperature is maintained without artificial heating, this may be gradually abandoned, and the child dressed in the ordinary manner.

The best food by all odds is suitable breast-milk. The infant should nurse from the breast when its strength permits, or, if not, the milk may be pumped and given with a medicine dropper or the so-called "Breck feeder." At first the milk may be somewhat diluted or, if necessary, breast-milk may be reinforced by the addition of from 5 to 15 per cent or more of saccharose. (See Concentrated Food, p. 103.) Gavage sometimes causes less disturbance than allowing the infant to swallow. Hoffa[31] advised keeping the stomach tube constantly in place. When mother's milk is not available, breast milk from other sources should be used when obtainable. (See Wet Nurses, p. 71.) A large variety of artificial foods have been employed, such as the milk-mixtures, whey-mixtures, buttermilk and other acid milks, peptonized milks and the like. Since the amount of food which can be ingested is often small, concentrated foods such as butter-flour mixtures or the so-called "Dubo," may sometimes be given successfully (p. 103). Some of the synthetic milks which have a relatively high caloric value and digestibility are quite satisfactory (see p. 116). Hill[32] recommends a formula consisting of 3 parts of breast milk and 1 part of evaporated milk. Regarding the quantity of food and the frequency of its administration there can be no absolute rule. The basal metabolism and the caloric needs of premature infants have been studied by a number of authors, among whom should be mentioned Talbot, Sisson, Moriarty and Dalrymple,[33] and Murlin and Marsh.[34] Talbot and his associates found the basal metabolism to be low because there is a very small amount of active heat-forming tissue; Murlin and Marsh that on the basis of body-surface the basal metabolism was low, but on that of weight it was slightly higher than for full-term infants. There is, too, a low blood sugar, which in some cases persists for three or four months (van Creveld[35]). A large excess in caloric intake over basal metabolism is, however, necessary because of the relatively greater amount of growth essential in these babies, and because, too, of the greater body surface as compared with the body weight. Yet there is no need to furnish food of high caloric value in the first week or two, and in the first two or three days only a sugar-solution need be given. Later the daily requirement is probably from 110 to 130 calories per kilogram (50 to 59 per lb.). The frequency of feeding must be based upon the amount which the infant can take and retain. At first this may be only 2 or 3 drams (7 to 11), and feedings must then be given every one to two hours. It is in such cases that the more concentrated feeding may be necessary. When stools are loose and frequent we have had success by adding one of the casein-flour preparations to breast-milk or reinforcing with it the artificial food (see p. 108).

The treatment of the premature infant is in other respects symptomatic. The relief of atelectasis and cyanosis is to be obtained by reflex stimulation, as by plunging into a hot bath of 100 to 105 F. (37.8 to 40.6 C.), preferably containing mustard, in order to produce crying. The inhalation of oxygen or of oxygen and carbon dioxide is often of service, and a retort of the gas should be close at hand for immediate use when required. Infection is to be very carefully avoided, especially by great attention to the care of the navel, and the employment of sterile water for any washing necessary. In the after-care of premature infants it is well to remember the tendency to anemia and rickets, and both of these conditions should be treated prophylactically. Iron may be administered as ferric citrate, $\frac{1}{4}$ grain (.016) a day dissolved in orange-juice, or as syrup of ferrous iodide, 5 to 10 minims (.31 to .62) a day, and iron-containing foods given as early as digestion permits. Cod liver oil should be started early and viosterol as well. The former may be in doses of 5 to 10 minims (.31 to .62) and increased to 2 drams (7) or more daily, the latter should at first be given in doses of 15 to 40 minims (.93 to 2.5) daily and this large dose later decreased. Exposure to sunlight and ultraviolet light from an artificial source should also be used as early as safe. Even vigorous treatment may fail to prevent rickets entirely.

References

1. Causes and Prevention of Neonatal Mortality, U. S. Dept. Labor, 1929. 2. Zentralb. f. Gynäk., 1923, **47,** 1624. 3. Am. J. Dis. Child., 1928, **35,** 262; 443. 4. Antenatal Path. and Hyg., 1902, 77. 5. Ztschr. f. Kinderh., 1919, **20,** 212. 6. Monatschr. f. Kinderh., 1929, **45,** 1. 7. Am. J. Dis. Child., 1927, **34,** 571. 8. Am. J. Dis. Child., 1929, **37,** 751. 9. Acta paediat., 1927, **7,** 15. 10. Acta paediat., 1929, **9,** 46. 11. Acta obst. et gynec. Scandinav., 1930, **9,** 477. 12. Am. J. Dis. Child., 1930, **40,** 1000. 13. Lehr. d. phys. u. path. Chemie., 1894, 99. 14. München. med. Wchnschr., 1927, **74,** 1822. 15. Acta paediat., 1921, **1,** 194. 16. J. Biol. Chem., 1922, **50,** 34. 17. Arch. f. Gynäk., 1923, **121,** 1. 18. Am. J. Dis. Child., 1920, **20,** 316. 19. Thèse de Paris, 1895. 20. Monatschr. f. Geburtsh. u. Gynäk., 1905, **22,** 45. 21. Brit. M. J., 1902, **1,** 773. 22. Am. J. Dis. Child., 1928, **36,** 797. 23. Bull. soc. de méd. légale de France, 1912, Ref. Arch. f. Kinderh., 1913, **59,** 213. 24. Arch. Pediat., 1921, **38,** 201. 25. Jahrb. f. Kinderh., 1928, **121,** 41. 26. Feeding and Nutritional Disorders in Infancy and Childhood, 1925, 517. 27. Am. Soc. Heating and Ventilating J., Sect. Heating, Piping and Air Conditioning Eng., 1930, **2,** 605. 28. Am. J. Dis. Child., 1929, **38,** 944. 29. Am. J. Dis. Child., 1930, **39,** 321. 30. J.A.M.A., 1928, **90,** 541. 31. Arch. f. Kinderh., 1922, **72,** 6. 32. Am. J. Dis. Child., 1930, **40,** 59. 33. Am. J. Dis. Child., 1922, **24,** 95. 34. Proc. Soc. Exper. Biol. and Med., 1922, **19,** 431; Am. J. Dis. Child., 1925, **30,** 310. 35. Am. J. Dis. Child., 1929, **38,** 912.

CHAPTER II

SEPSIS IN THE NEW-BORN

Many of the septic infections of the new-born exhibit such special features or localizations that there will be described here only general septic infection.

Etiology and Pathologic Anatomy.—The incidence of sepsis is less than formerly. In rare instances it may take place before birth, the fetus then generally being born dead. The cause in such cases is probably the penetration of bacteria through the placenta, the mother herself being ill, often with sepsis. In some instances, the infection is through the amniotic fluid, the primary lesion then being a pneumonia. It may develop through injuries received during or after birth, as through abrasions of the skin, or by the entrance of septic matter derived from discharges of the mother into the mouth, rectum or vagina of the infant. Infection may be from an inflamed breast of the mother. Operations performed on the new-born, such, for instance, as circumcision, the opening of a cephalhematoma, or the incision of the frænulum linguae may serve as portals of entry. In the great majority of instances, however, infection starts at the umbilicus, beginning oftenest before complete separation of the cord, and is first manifested by an umbilical arteritis (see p. 238). The fact that the umbilical wound has healed is no proof that infection of the umbilical vessels does not exist. A large variety of bacteria, especially streptococci and staphylococci, are capable of acting as the infective agent.

Beginning at the portal of entry, wherever this may be, the infection may either remain local or become more general, there occurring in the new-born but little protecting lymphadenitis to prevent this. General septic infection may occasionally take place when the portal of entry is not discoverable. If the sepsis is local only, there may be produced phlegmonous inflammation of various parts of the body involved, as mammitis, omphalitis, etc.; and in cases of aspiration of septic fluid, pneumonia.

In infants still-born or dying very shortly after birth, the subjects of intra-uterine infection, there are found macerated skin, petechiae on the surface of the body and on the serous membranes, bloody or serous effusion into the serous cavities, and smaller or larger extravasations of blood into, and fatty degeneration of, the internal organs. In those acquiring the disease somewhat later the findings are much the same, and there are also various lesions of different organs, depending upon the localization of the septic process. Among the more common lesions are pneumonia, pleurisy, and involvement of the bones and joints, kidney and digestive apparatus.

Symptoms and Diagnosis.—The symptoms usually appear either immediately after birth or at some time within the first ten days. They vary greatly, depending upon the seat of the lesions. As a rule, however, in general septic infection there is great and characteristic depression of strength with rapid loss of weight and entire anorexia. Fever is irregular. It is generally present at the onset and frequently high, but may be absent throughout and the temperature is often subnormal toward the end. Severe diarrhea is a common symptom; vomiting may occur; icterus is frequent and often intense, or the skin may be of a pale-gray tint, and septic erythemata are frequently observed. The pulse is rapid and weak, the respiration irregular; sometimes deep and rapid. The occurrence of small or larger hemorrhages in different parts of the body is a common and characteristic symptom. The child looks ill, is usually apathetic or somnolent, has a feeble cry and sometimes develops the evidences of collapse. Various nervous symptoms may be seen, among them tossing, rolling of the head, hypertonic states, twitching of the muscles, tremor, and sometimes convulsions. The urine generally contains albumin. Enlargement of the spleen may be present. The coagulation-time of the blood is increased; leukocytosis may or may not exist. Blood-cultures may reveal septic germs, making the diagnosis positive.

When the disease is prolonged the symptoms may be masked, the principal one being a rapid, continuous loss of weight, until finally the development of some local septic process makes the condition clear. Naturally in many instances the character of the symptoms is modified by the development of those of localized involvement as well.

Course and Prognosis.—Some cases run a rapid course, ending fatally in from one to three days. Others last for weeks; but in all the prognosis is very unfavorable. The mildest and more slowly progressing cases may occasionally recover. The earlier the infection occurs and the more wide-spread the lesions, the worse the prognosis.

Treatment.—This consists principally in prophylaxis. Every possible source of infection should be removed. Should the mother be suffering from puerperal fever, the child must be separated from her. All injuries and wounds must be carefully treated. The umbilicus should receive special attention. When the disease has developed, stimulating and supporting measures should be carried out; dehydration should be treated by the administration of fluids in various ways (not intraperitoneally); and surgical drainage employed as local conditions indicate. Polyvalent streptococcus serum may be used intravenously or intramuscularly, and blood transfusions may be helpful stimulating measures.

CHAPTER III

ACUTE FATTY DEGENERATION OF THE NEW-BORN

(Buhl's Disease)

THIS condition was first described by Buhl[1] in 1861. Cases have since been reported by Hecker,[2] Runge,[3] Lucksch,[4] and Elizalde and Puente.[5] While it is described here separately, it should, in all probability, be considered as a form of sepsis. Those who classify it as a distinct disease have variously ascribed it to the effect of ether given to the mother, to defective oxygenation of the fetus, and to prolonged asphyxia of the infant. The **pathologic anatomy** in general consists of a marked tendency to hemorrhages, often icterus, and widespread parenchymatous inflammation and fatty degeneration. The **symptoms** are much the same as those of sepsis, with a special disposition to cyanosis and hemorrhage, although external bleeding may be absent. Icterus develops if the infant lives long enough, and the hemorrhagic symptoms tend to disappear after the fifth or sixth day. The disease may last but a few hours before the fatal ending and it rarely continues as long as two weeks. A positive **diagnosis** can be made only by the discovery after death of the very marked and widespread fatty degeneration. The **prognosis** is entirely unfavorable. The **treatment** would be similar to that for sepsis.

REFERENCES

1. Ref. Runge, Klinik. d. Geburtsh., 1861, **1,** 296. 2. Arch. f. Gynäk., 1876, **10,** 537. 3. Krankh. d. ersten Lebenst., 1893, 162. 4. Prag. med. Wchnschr., 1913, **38,** 167. 5. Rev. di la Assoc. Med. Argentina, 1921, **34,** 10.

CHAPTER IV

ACUTE INFECTIOUS HEMOGLOBINEMIA OF THE NEW-BORN

(Winckel's Disease; Haemoglobinuria neonatorum; Cyanosis afebrilis icterica perniciosa cum haemoglobinuria; etc.)

Although Winckel[1] recognized the existence of hemoglobinuria as a symptom in an epidemic affecting 23 children in the Lying-in Hospital of Dresden, yet an earlier epidemic in which 10 children were attacked was well described by Bigelow[2] in 1875. A condition probably the same had already been reported by Parrot[3] and by Charrin[4] in 1873, and still earlier by Pollak[5] in 1871. Cases have also been described by Ljwow[6] and Feldman.[7]

The affection is a rare one. It occurs generally in institutions and in an epidemic form. That it is an infection seems certain, but the nature of this is unknown. Bacteria are usually not discovered in the organs at necropsy. The **pathologic anatomy** consists of punctate hemorrhages in most of the internal organs, sometimes with fatty degeneration, especially in the liver and heart-muscle. The spleen is much enlarged and dark colored. The renal cortex is thickened and brownish, and exhibits small hemorrhages. The pyramids are blackish-brown and show narrow, black streaks converging towards the papillae, these being due to the deposit of hemoglobin in the canals. The umbilical vessels are usually normal. The **symptoms** begin on the fourth to eighth day of life with restlessness, anorexia, prostration and intense cyanosis and icterus. The temperature is rarely elevated, and may be subnormal. The urine is pale-brown and voided frequently in small amounts with straining, and contains hemoglobin, granular casts, renal epithelium and albumin, but no bile or biliary acids. The stools vary in color from dark-green to yellowish or brown. A thick, syrupy fluid of a blackish-brown color exudes from the incised skin. The blood shows leukocytosis, numerous granules, and a great diminution in the number but increase in the size of the red blood-cells, many of which are pale in color. Collapse develops with great rapidity and convulsions are liable to terminate the case. Recovery is occasionally observed. The **diagnosis** from Buhl's disease rests upon the presence of hemoglobinuria and the occurrence in epidemics. The **treatment** can be only symptomatic and similar to that described for sepsis.

References

1. Deutsch. med. Wchnschr., 1879, **5**, 303. 2. Boston M. and S. J., 1875, **15**, 277. 3. Arch. de phys. norm. et path., 1873, 512. 4. Thèse de Paris, 1873. 5. Wien. med. Presse., 1871, 457. 6. Medicinskoje Obosrenje, 1893, No. 14; Ref. Jahrb. f. Kinderh., 1894, **38**, 497. 7. Brit. J. Child. Dis., 1927, **24**, 113.

CHAPTER V

HEMORRHAGE IN THE NEW-BORN

Hemorrhage at this early period of life is more common than in later childhood. Ritter found it in 1.46 per cent of 13,000 infants and Townsend[2] in 0.44 per cent of 7225 births, Abt[3] estimates its incidence as from 1 to 500 or 700 in institution-infants, and Wilson[4] reported it in 1.3 per cent of 3364 new-born infants. In the figures just quoted there is some confusion. Townsend[2] and Wilson[4] evidently included intracranial hemorrhage in their figures, but this does not seem to be the case in Abt's[3] estimate, and Ritter[1] discusses chiefly visible hemorrhages. According to recent knowledge intracranial hemorrhage is a more frequent occurrence than certain older studies would indicate, and this will be discussed in a subsequent section (see pp. 916; 935).

Etiology.—Hemorrhages are more common in the first two weeks of life and in institutions. In certain instances they may be the result of trauma or accident, as in hematoma of the scalp (p. 221) or of the sternocleidomastoid muscle (p. 222), and in some cases of umbilical bleeding (p. 239). Various visceral hemorrhages, especially within the cranium, seem to depend on prolonged and difficult labor (pp. 916; 935). Prematurity predisposes to hemorrhage in early life (p. 211); sepsis (p. 216) is another cause; and congenital syphilis is a factor in some cases (Hess;[5] Pontoppidan;[6] Wilson[4]). Special hemorrhage-producing bacteria have occasionally been described (Schloss and Commiskey[7]). In many cases the cause is not clear. It has been thought that the resistance of the blood-vessel walls is weakened in some way. Ylppo,[8] for example, observed that the skin of new-born infants, especially if premature, easily developed subcutaneous hemorrhage upon the application of negative pressure with a suction cup. Prolonged coagulation-time may be found at times but not consistently (Schloss and Commiskey[7]), and hemorrhages may occur even when the coagulation-time is normal (p. 40). In other cases it has been claimed that the prothrombin, the antithrombin, or the fibrinogen factor is at fault (Lucas[9] et al.; McCollum[10]).

Townsend[2] applied the term "*hemorrhagic disease of the new-born*" to the occurrence of hemorrhages of unknown etiology simultaneously in many parts of the body. It was earlier described by Minot,[11] is observed frequently, and has been the subject of much consideration. It has no connection with hemophilia (p. 1035). Moore and Brodie[12] report what must be an unusual instance in which avitaminosis of the mother during pregnancy appeared to be the cause of the hemorrhage. McCollum[10] also thinks that avitaminosis may be a factor, and Kuglemass and Tritsch[13] report a case in which, by modifying the diet of the mother, hemorrhage in the 6th offspring was apparently prevented, although it had occurred in the 5 preceding infants.

In summarizing the etiology of hemorrhage in the new-born it seems evident that in certain instances hemorrhage may occur purely from the factor of trauma without there being any underlying or constitutional fault. In other cases there is a hemorrhagic tendency and bleeding occurs without any unusual trauma or injury. Perhaps, too, trauma is operative at times in combination with some defect of the blood, the exact nature of which is not clearly understood.

Locality of the Lesions.—Various and usually multiple regions of the body are affected, and some of these occurrences will be described under separate headings, such as melena (p. 220); and hemorrhage within the cranium (pp. 915; 916; 935), into the suprarenal capsule (p. 1083), from the genito-urinary tract (pp. 809, 854), into the spinal cord (p. 962), and at the umbilicus (p. 239). Bleeding may take place into the abdominal cavity and into the peritoneum or the abdominal organs,—in some cases then being due to trauma, the hemorrhages in that event usually being large and single; in some to sepsis; and in some occurring independently of these causes. In 49 infants with abdominal hemorrhage Lundqvist[14] found 5 in the liver-substance, 14 beneath the liver-capsule, 18 in the suprarenals, 12 intraperitoneal and 1 from a ruptured spleen. Others, such as Bonnaire and Durante[15] and Genell,[16] have also reported cases of hemorrhage into and from the liver. Other regions to be mentioned are the lungs and pleura, thymus gland, nose, ears, eyes, and skin.

Symptoms and **Diagnosis.**—The *traumatic* hemorrhages as a rule reveal themselves promptly, except those of the abdominal and thoracic viscera, where no symptoms at all may appear until, perhaps, a sudden collapse occurs followed promptly by death. Those of a *spontaneous* nature manifest themselves generally by visible bleeding in several regions of the body. Inasmuch as infants tolerate loss of blood very badly, a comparatively small hemorrhage may readily produce weakness of pulse, great depression of strength and loss of weight. Anemia is a natural result. The temperature may be elevated, but is often subnormal. Icterus is a common symptom. Diagnosis is difficult only in the cases where the hemorrhage is concealed, and it must be remembered that visible may be combined with internal bleeding.

Prognosis and Course.—These depend much on the cause, on the amount of blood lost, and on the duration of the process. The mortality was formerly high, varying from about 60 to 80 per cent (Ritter,[1] Townsend[2]), but in recent years, with improved methods of treatment, it has improved. If death takes place it is usually in the first week of life.

Treatment.—Attempt should be made to determine the cause of the hemorrhage, *i. e.*, whether it is dependent upon syphilis, trauma, sepsis, or the like. Local measures to arrest bleeding, such as compression, adrenalin, silver nitrate and astringents, are indicated in certain cases. Cold must be applied cautiously because of its depressing effect. Adrenalin hypodermatically (1 to 4 minims (0.062 to 0.248) of a 1:1000 solution) has been recommended but seems to have little action. Calcium chloride or lactate in amounts of 20 to 40 grains (1.3 to 2.6) in twenty-four hours in divided doses has been employed, although theoretically it can be expected to do little good, since the calcium-content of the blood of the new-born is usually high (Lucas[9]). The best therapeutic measure is whole blood given intravenously or intramuscularly or by other routes such as into the umbilical vein (p. 200). Intraperitoneal injections had better not be given in the first ten days of life. Should human blood not be available, horse-serum or rabbit-serum may be given. Fluid injections also may be indicated.

MELAENA NEONATORUM

This term may be employed to describe cases which are quite dissimilar in origin and nature, but which show the characteristic symptoms, *i. e.*, the discharge of black, altered blood (μέλαινα: black) from the intestines or, by vomiting, from the stomach. The condition was first described by Ebart[17] in 1723. In *Melaena spuria* the blood enters the infant's stomach or intestines from outside sources, as from a hemorrhage from the mouth, nose or lungs, from a wound in the nipple of the nurse, or from the swallowing of maternal blood during labor. In *Melaena vera*, which is the form about to be considered, it comes from the effusion of blood into the stomach or intestines. Even the cases of the latter group may again be divided into the *symptomatic*, in which other manifestations, often hemorrhagic, of a constitutional disease are present, and the *idiopathic*, in which the melena is the only symptom observed, and there is no evidence of a general hemorrhagic condition.

Melena is a comparatively uncommon disorder, occurring about once in every 1000 or 2000 births, according to different estimations (Gerhardt-Seifert[18]). In Ritter's[1] 190 cases of hemorrhage 39 occurred from the intestine, 28 from the mouth, and 20 from the stomach.

The **etiology** is not clearly understood, and certainly varies with the case. Lesions of the mucous membrane or of the deeper vessels of the gastro-enteric canal are prominent causes, but the method of their production is far from clear. Often they are the result of congestion, which may itself be brought about in various ways incident to birth, such as prolonged asphyxia, violent efforts at extracting the child or at its resuscitation, compression of the umbilical cord, congenital diseases of the heart, congenital syphilitic hepatitis, and the like. In some cases there are duodenal ulcers (p. 625) or other intestinal ulceration. Meckel's diverticulitis may produce melena, ulceration may be in the esophagus (Müller[19]), or dilated veins in the esophagus may rupture (Vorpahl[20]). The three causes last mentioned are oftener the producers of later hemorrhage than of true melaena neonatorum. Often the blood makes its way into the intestine without any discoverable lesion of the mucous membrane, and the condition appears to be part of the hemorrhagic disease referred to.

The **pathologic conditions** consist of any causative factor such as ulceration, syphilis, sepsis or the like; evidences of anemia; and tarry blood in the intestinal tract. The first of the **symptoms** is hemorrhage, which begins from the second to the fourth day after birth, and appears as black or blackish-red material from the bowel or, less often, in the vomitus. The amount lost is usually sufficiently large rapidly to produce anemia, prostration and finally collapse. There is no abdominal pain, and fever is absent or transitory. Bleeding lasts seldom more than two to three days, and in the cases which survive recovery is generally rapid, except for the anemia.

The **prognosis** is grave in untreated cases, older statistics such as those of Silbermann[21] giving over 50 per cent mortality. In idiopathic melaena vera the mortality is usually considerably less, and especially when the bleeding is from the bowel alone (10 per cent, Vassmer[22]). The cause and amount of the bleeding and the promptness and character of the treatment are influential factors.

The **treatment** in general is that described for hemorrhage in the new-born (p. 220). In addition cold applications to the abdomen may be tried, but are likely to be too depressing; calcium lactate, tincture of ferric chloride, and gelatine have been used by mouth, the last freely in 5 to 10 per cent solution. Starvation until the hemorrhage has been arrested has been advocated, but seems too dangerous, and nutrition should be maintained by breast milk, sugar solutions or whey.

CEPHALHEMATOMA

This is a form of hemorrhage in the new-born producing a fluctuating swelling situated between the bones of the skull and the overlying tissues (*cephalhaematoma externum*). Rarely the blood is effused within the skull between the bone and the dura mater (*cephalhaematoma internum*) or externally below the aponeurosis (*cephalhaematoma subaponeurotica*). The description which follows applies to cephalhaematoma externum. It is not common, occurring in about 0.5 per cent of deliveries. Only in very rare instances does it develop later than the first few days after birth. Males are more frequently affected; trauma seems often to be the cause;

it is more common in prolonged vertex-presentations and more frequent in the children of primaparae (Meyer,[23] 34 of 40 cases). Yet trauma is not the only factor, since it may occur in premature infants, or after an easy labor, or may be part of a general hemorrhagic disorder of the new-born. Asphyxia favors its production. The chief **symptom** is the swelling, discovered about two or three days after birth, but having begun earlier, and increasing in size for six to eight days. It is then tense, fluctuating, cannot be reduced by pressure, rarely pulsates, and does not increase in size with crying. It is most frequently situated over the right parietal bone. In 127 cases Henning[24] found it here in 57 and over the left parietal in 37. Being subperiosteal in situation it does not pass over the fontanelle or beyond the suture-lines of the bone involved. Should it apparently pass over the suture it is because it is a double hematoma. After existing two or three days a ridge of ossifying tissue begins to form around the periphery. This gradually widens, the tumor softens and grows smaller, and a feeling suggesting crepitation can often be perceived. The effused blood is absorbed in two or three months, the bony wall persisting a longer time. The **prognosis** is entirely favorable, unless the cephalhematoma is only part of a general hemorrhagic disorder, or unless suppuration develops, which is exceptional. In **diagnosis** there could be confusion with *caput succedaneum* during the first few days of life. This condition consists of an edematous swelling of the connective tissue of that portion of the scalp which has been presenting through the patulous os uteri, and is the result of the obstruction to the circulation at the periphery and the absence of pressure over the swollen region. The fact that it disappears in a few days, and the absence of fluctuation and of the development of any marginal wall, serve to distinguish it from cephalhematoma. Subaponeurotic cephalhematoma is distinguished by the absence of a boundary wall and of limitation by the sutures. *Meningocele* and *encephalocele* (p. 914) resemble cephalhematoma to some extent, but they may exhibit pulsation, are influenced by respiration and by crying, are to some extent reducible, often with the production of convulsions, and correspond in position to a suture or the fontanelle. *Abscess of the scalp* is attended by heat, tenderness, and discoloration of the skin, with constitutional symptoms. A *telangioma* resembles a hematoma but slightly. There is no bony wall nor fluctuation; while crying makes it larger and pressure somewhat smaller and the skin is discolored.

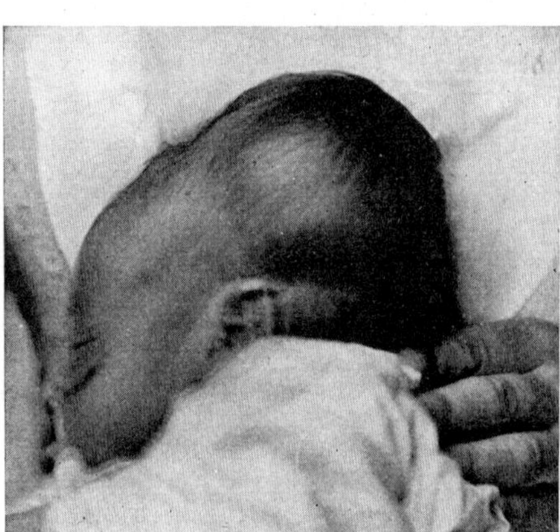

Fig. 27.—Cephalhematoma.

The best **treatment,** as a rule, appears to be a wholly expectant one. The child should be so placed that no injury to the hematoma can occur, and recovery entrusted to time. No applications are required and incision should not be performed unless suppuration develops.

HEMATOMA OF THE STERNOCLEIDOMASTOID MUSCLE

This is of rare occurrence and is usually the result of traction in breech-presentations, but it may also be produced by forceps in vertex-presentations, or may occur without discoverable cause. The tumor is small, having a diameter not over 1½ in. (3.8 cm.). It is at first tender and soft, but later the tenderness disappears and hardness develops as cicatrical changes take place. It is usually situated on the right side (31 of 38 cases reported by Henoch[25]). Although dating from birth it may not become apparent until the age of two weeks or later. The head may or may not be drawn to the affected side and the chin turned toward the other. The **prognosis** is nearly always good, the swelling disappearing after a few months. It is probable, however, that congenital torticollis may be produced in this way (p. 986). No **treatment** is required at first, although later massage and passive movements of the head may be beneficial.

References

1. Oesterreich. Jahrb. f. Pädiatrik., 1871, **1**, 129. 2. Boston M. and S. J., 1891, **125**, 218; Arch. Pediat., 1894, **11**, 559. 3. J.A.M.A., 1903, **40**, 284. 4. Arch. Pediat., 1905, **22**, 43. 5. Arch. Pediat., 1904, **21**, 598. 6. Hospitalstidende, 1906, **59**, 626; Ref. Brit. J. Child. Dis., 1916, **13**, 308. 7. Am. J. Dis. Child., 1911, **1**, 276; 1912, **3**, 216. 8. Ztschr. f. Kinderh., 1924, **38**, 32. 9. Am. J. Dis. Child., 1921, **22**, 525. 10. Canadian M. A. J., 1928, **18**, 550. 11. Am. J. Med. Sc., 1852, **24**, 310. 12. Am. J. Dis. Child., 1927, **34**, 53. 13. J.A.M.A., 1929, **92**, 531. 14. Acta obst. et gynec. Scandinav., 1930, **9**, 331. 15. L'Obstetrique, 1911, **4**, 825. 16. Acta obst. et gynec. Scandinav., 1930, **9**, 180. 17. Widerhofer, Gerhardt's Handb. d. Kinderkr., 4, **2**, 408. 18. Lehrb. d. Kinderh., 1897, 71. 19. Ztschr. f. Kinderh., 1921, **30**, 234. 20. Arch. f. Gynäk., 1912, 96, 377. 21. Jahrb. f. Kinderh., 1877, **11**, 378. 22. Arch. f. Gynäk., 1909, **89**, 275. 23. Hospitalstidende, 1877, **4**, 585; 616. 24. Gerhardt's Handb. d. Kinderkr., **2**, 49. 25. Vorlesungen über Kinderkrankheiten, 1895, 35.

CHAPTER VI

ICTERUS IN THE NEW-BORN

Icterus is of very frequent occurrence in the new-born. It may conveniently be divide into (1) symptomatic, and (2) idiopathic icterus.

1. *Symptomatic icterus* depends upon sepsis and such rare conditions as infectious hemoglobinemia, acute fatty degeneration of the new-born, syphilitic hepatitis, congenital cirrhosis of the liver and congenital obliteration of the bile-ducts. These, with the exception of the last, are discussed elsewhere. In symptomatic icterus the discoloration of the skin is generally very decided, and there are other symptoms of the causative disease evident. The urine often shows the presence of bile, and, in obstructive jaundice, the feces often the absence of it.

2. In *idiopathic icterus* in the new-born there is present no discoverable congenital or acquired anatomical defect which can produce jaundice by obstruction. In this class are to be placed the cases of congenital hemolytic icterus and familial icterus (see p. 663). The great majority of cases, however, constitute a very common form to which the application of the title icterus neonatorum is usually limited.

CONGENITAL OBLITERATION OF THE BILE-DUCTS

(Congenital Biliary Cirrhosis)

This is a rare condition of which, however, Holmes[1] in 1916 estimated that nearly 120 cases had been reported, and probably 50 or 60 have since been added. Ladd[2] reported 20 cases occurring in the Children's Hospital and the Infant's Hospital, Boston. We have seen several cases, 3 confirmed by necropsy and 2 of these published by one of us.[3] Congenital biliary cirrhosis, although described at times as a distinct affection, seems to be, as claimed by Rolleston and Hayne,[4] Skormin[5] and others, of the same nature as obliteration of the bile-ducts.

Etiology and Pathology.—The condition appears to be a congenital malformation, the ducts at one stage of their embryologic development being solid cords (Ylppö[6]). It has never been proven that syphilis is a factor. It has been suggested that a prenatal inflammatory obliteration of the ducts may take place. There is liable to be a familial tendency. In some cases partial patency is present at birth and total obliteration develops later; in some the ducts, common, hepatic and cystic, are fibrous cords; in others the common duct is obliterated with dilatation above; in still others narrowing of all the ducts and obstruction by plugs of inspissated bile and epithelium occur (Ladd[2]). Partial obliteration not becoming complete would explain certain cases of severe congenital jaundice reported by Arkwright,[7] Weber[8] and Pearson.[9] The gall-bladder may be absent or distended. The liver is usually the seat of hypertrophic cirrhosis, but the blood-vessels are seldom involved. The spleen is enlarged.

Symptoms.—The principal symptom is icterus, which is present at birth or develops within the first week or occasionally later. The color is intense and often of a greenish hue. The occurrence of acholic stools is also of importance. Sometimes ordinary yellow movements are present at first, to be replaced later by the characteristic appearance. The passage of green feces does not, of course, necessarily indicate the presence of bile. The urine is intensely bile-stained; fever is not a symptom; but vomiting is liable to occur. Hemorrhages from the umbilical cord and into different parts of the body are a very characteristic symptom yet not pathognomonic. Emaciation develops if the case is at all prolonged. A direct van den Bergh reaction will be found. In a case studied by Wallgren[10] the infant was able to absorb fat in spite of atresia of the common bile-duct.

Course and Prognosis.—The outcome is necessarily fatal in the cases in which complete organic obliteration of all the ducts finally occurs. Death takes place in convulsions or stupor, generally only after several weeks or even months, although sometimes the child dies in the first week of the disease. Perhaps the longest duration of life recorded was in a child dying at seven and one half months reported by Nobecomb and Janet.[11]

Treatment.—The only treatment is operative, and this may not avail on account of the complicating biliary cirrhosis present. Yet Ladd has shown that it may be undertaken successfully in many cases in which either the gall-bladder or the common duct has a patent connection with the liver.

ICTERUS NEONATORUM

Etiology and Pathogenesis.—Careful observations would probably show that icterus is present to a slight degree in almost all new-born infants. In the literature the incidence is variously stated, ranging from 10 per cent (Möbius[12]) to 84 per cent (Cruse[13]). Boys are oftener affected than girls; first-born infants oftener than later ones; and premature, light-weight, or atelectatic ones oftener than others.

A large amount of investigation has been conducted in the attempt to discover the cause of the condition. The various theories fall respectively into the classes of hepatogenous and hematogenous. As shown by Hirsch,[14] Ylppö,[15] Schiff and Faerber,[16] Cserna and Liebmann,[17] Meyer and Adler,[18] Mitchell,[19] Goldbloom and Gottlieb[20] and others, there is an increase in bilirubin of the blood of new-born infants, which is greater when visible icterus is present. An indirect van den Bergh reaction may be obtained, suggesting extrahepatic or hemolytic jaundice. Many studies have shown, too, that the new-born infant has a polycythemia for a brief period, and this has been attributed by Goldbloom and Gottlieb[21] to the relative oxygen unsaturation of the fetus. The condition disappears after birth, and, as there is no longer any need for the large number of red cells, excessive destruction of them takes place. Whether there is any increased fragility of the red cells or any hemolysin present has been a matter of controversy. It has been maintained also (Ylppö) that the liver is functionally immature and unable to dispose of the large amount of bile pigment, jaundice consequently resulting.

Numerous other views have been expressed, some of which may be mentioned here. Birch-Hirschfeld,[22] for example, believes that there is a compression of the larger biliary ducts by an edema of Glisson's capsule, and Silbermann[23] attributes the jaundice to a compression of the biliary capillaries, the result of the congestion of the blood-vessels brought about by the products of the increased blood destruction. Quincke[24] and Kondo[25] believe that the hyperbilirubinemia is in part at least due to absorption from the intestine of meconium-bilirubin; DeLuca[26] and Glaser[27] that in some cases disintegration of extravasated blood from intracranial hemorrhage may be a contributory factor. For further discussion of the subject the reviews of van Crevald[28] and of Mitchell[29] may be consulted.

At least this may be said:—that there is no question of the increased blood destruction after birth and that more recent studies show that bile pigment may be formed from this by the reticulo-endothelial system. This would be in essence then a nonobstructive or hemolytic form of icterus, and this seems to be the most likely explanation of icterus neonatorum. As Barron[29] points out, the two factors regarded by Rich[30] as necessary for the production of true nonobstructive jaundice are present,—namely, increased red-cell destruction and insufficient liver-cell function. Perhaps confusion arises due to the employment of the terms "hematogenous" and "hepatogenous," since the liver would be concerned even in the matter of increased blood destruction because of its inability to dispose of the excessive bilirubin.

Pathologic Anatomy.—Inasmuch as the condition is not a fatal one, necropsies are performed only on those infants who have died from other causes. The only characteristic finding is widespread icterus of skin, subcutaneous connective tissue, lining of arteries, and most of the serous membranes and exudates. The tissues of the brain, spinal cord, spleen, kidneys and liver are only slightly discolored, if at all. Sometimes infarcts of biliary coloring matter have been found in the kidneys and brain.

Symptoms.—The icterus begins oftenest on the second or third day of life; the skin being the part most discolored in varying degrees of intensity, although the sclera is usually involved, as are the mucous membranes. The urine is generally free from bile-pigment by the ordinary tests, and the stools unaltered in character. The pulse, respiration and temperature are unaffected, and the liver and spleen are slightly if at all enlarged. There is little if any influence on general health, although in infants with marked icterus there may occur an unusual tendency to sleep, as well as a greater loss of weight and a slower regain of it than in nonicteric ones. According to Greuter[31] there is often a prolongation of coagulation-time of the blood, which disappears by the ninth day even if icterus is still present.

The duration of icterus neonatorum is about three or four days in the milder cases, but may be as long as two weeks.

Diagnosis.—The distinction is to be made between icterus neonatorum and the various forms of symptomatic icterus. This is to be done in part by the presence of other symptoms in the latter condition. Then, too, in symptomatic icterus the urine is more liable to be visibly discolored by the bile-pigment. In cases of decided obstructive jaundice the stools show an absence of bile. A very slight degree of discoloration of the skin speaks rather for icterus neonatorum, while a late development of it indicates some other cause. Yet an early diagnosis is often impossible. This is especially true in slight cases of catarrhal icterus due to duodenal catarrh, and still more in the instances in which icterus neonatorum happens to be combined with other diseases of the new-born, such, for instance, as sepsis. Congenital obliteration of the bile-ducts gives rise to an intense icterus developing very promptly after birth and persisting. Certain severe cases of icterus in the new-born, including the familial type, will be discussed later. (See p. 662.) Such infants are distinctly ill, and the icterus is accompanied by other signs, sometimes of a hemorrhagic nature.

Treatment.—Nothing is indicated, and nothing can be done, for the average case. A number of methods have been proposed for the prevention of the condition by the treatment of the pregnant mother, but these seem to be quite unnecessary.

References

1. Am. J. Dis. Child., 1916, **11,** 405. 2. J.A.M.A., 1928, **91,** 1082. 3. Griffith, Arch. Pediat., 1905, **22,** 257; 1908, **25,** 174. 4. Brit. M. J., 1901, **1,** 758. 5. Jahrb. f. Kinderh., 1902, **56,** 203. 6. Ztschr. f. Kinderh., 1913, **9,** 208. 7. Edinburgh M. J., 1902, **54,** 156. 8. Edinburgh M. J., 1903, **56,** 111. 9. Underwood's Dis. Child., 1842, 9th Ed. 101. 10. Acta paediat., 1926, **6,** 123. 11. Arch. de méd. d. enf., 1922, **25,** 90. 12. Ref. Hilgenberg, Monatschr. f. Geburtsh. u. Gynäk., 1925, **68,** 326. 13. Arch. f. Kinderh., 1880, **1,** 353. 14. Ztschr. f. Kinderh., 1913, **9,** 198. 15. Ztschr. f. Kinderh., 1913, **9,** 208. 16. Jahrb. f. Kinderh., 1922, **97,** 245. 17. Klin. Wchnschr., 1923, **2,** 122. 18. Zentralbl. f. Gynäk., 1924, **48,** 1514. 19. Am. J. Dis. Child., 1928, **36,** 486. 20. Am. J. Dis. Child., 1929, **38,** 57. 21. J. Clin. Investig., 1930, **9,** 139. 22. Gerhardt's Handb. d. Kinderkr., 4, **2,** 691. 23. Jahrb. f. Kinderh., 1887, **26,** 252. 24. Arch. f. exper. Path. u. Pharmakol., 1885, **19,** 34. 25. J. Pediat., Tokyo, 1926, 1745; abst. Am. J. Dis. Child., 1927, **33,** 816. 26. Semana med., 1921, **2,** 635. 27. Am. J. Dis. Child., 1928, **36,** 195. 28. Am. J. Dis. Child., 1925, **30,** 240. 29. Medicine, 1931, **10,** 77. 30. Physiol. Rev., 1925, **5,** 182. 31. Ztschr. f. Kinderh., 1923, **35,** 210.

CHAPTER VII

ANEMIA OF THE NEW-BORN

(Primary Anemia of the New-born; Congenital Anemia)

Ecklin[1] reported the first clinical case although the possibility of the condition existing had previously been suggested. Pasachoff and Wilson[2] found 28 cases mentioned in the literature, but Abt[3] accepts less than 15 of those reported in detail as belonging in the present category. We have seen only 3 cases. No **cause** for symptomatic anemia, such as hemorrhage, can be discovered. The parents have usually been normal and labor has been at full-term and uneventful. The fault seems to be either a congenital defect of the erythrogenic system or some obscure toxic effect on it. At necropsy there have been found hemosiderosis of the liver and spleen; the myeloid reaction usual in anemia in the bone marrow, liver and spleen; and evidences of anemia of the body, and perhaps icterus. Marked pallor noticed about the first or second week of life and often mild icterus are the only **symptoms** and, if recovery follows, there are no sequels, the blood returning to normal after four or five months or longer. The hemoglobin is found to be from 20 to 50 per cent, the red cells as low as 1,000,000, and leukocytosis may or may not be present. In the red cells there are varying degrees of achromia, anisocytosis and poikilocytosis, and normoblasts may be found. There are also immature white cells, but not in much greater number than normal for the age of the patient. The coagulation-time, the platelet-count, the bleeding-time, and the fragility of the red cells are usually normal, although the last two may be increased. In

Abt's[3] case phagocytic mononuclear leukocytes were found in the circulating blood. The **prognosis** is good, only a few of the reported cases failing to recover. In **diagnosis** there should be excluded all conditions and diseases which could cause symptomatic or secondary anemia and the normal peculiarities of the blood in early life should be remembered (p. 38). The **treatment,** if any is needed, consists in medication with iron and, in severe cases, injections of blood.

References

1. Monatschr. f. Kinderh., 1919, **15,** 425. 2. Am. J. Dis. Child., 1931, **42,** 111. 3. Am. J. Dis. Child., 1932, **43,** 337.

CHAPTER VIII

ASPHYXIA NEONATORUM

The term "Asphyxia" as applied to the new-born indicates a condition in which respiratory movements are either absent or insufficient, although the heart's action continues.

Etiology.—The disease may either be (A) of *intra-uterine* or (B) of *extra-uterine* origin, the latter being much less frequent. The distinction depends on whether or not the circulation through the placenta has been interfered with.

(*A*) Intra-uterine Asphyxia.—This develops before or during birth. According to Henderson[1] the natural stimulus initiating breathing in the normal infant at birth is the carbon dioxide produced in its own body. Among maternal causes which are operative by preventing the initiation of pulmonary respiration may be mentioned excessive uterine contraction, unduly prolonged labor, uterine hemorrhage, and severe complicating illness or the death of the mother. On the side of the child are such factors as detachment of the placenta, compression of the brain interfering with the action of the heart, and compression of the umbilical cord. Efforts at intra-uterine respiration may occur as a result of the undue stimulation of the respiratory centers. It has been denied by some that such efforts are sufficient to cause aspiration of amniotic fluid, but the careful studies of Duvoir,[2] and Farber and Sweet[3] prove that this occurs. In cases, however, where the asphyxia has developed slowly the respiratory centers have sustained a paralyzing effect, and efforts at breathing have not taken place.

It is evident that the likelihood of the occurrence of intra-uterine asphyxia must increase with the duration of labor, especially of its second stage. The statistics of Veit[4] show very strikingly that the mortality from asphyxia after a second stage of four hours or more was over 3 times as great as when it had lasted but one hour.

(*B*) Extra-uterine Asphyxia (*Atelectasis pulmonum*).—This form is less frequent unless there be included asphyxia the result of intracranial hemorrhage. The child is born without any evidence of asphyxia, but develops it soon after birth from some of the numerous causes which interfere with the gaseous interchange. Among these may be mentioned obstruction to the access of air, as by unruptured membranes, or by maternal discharges in the infant's air-passages; malformation of the diaphragm; intra-uterine pneumonia or pleural effusion interfering later with the action of the lungs; malformation of the lungs; severe injuries to the brain and intracranial hemorrhage, which afterward affect the action of the respiratory centers; malformation of the heart, which renders the carrying of oxygenated blood impossible; etc. Premature birth is a very potent cause of extra-uterine asphyxia, the active factor being the general feebleness of the child, the weakness or imperfect development of the respiratory nerve-centers, or a similar condition of the muscles and bones of the chest-wall or of the lungs preventing satisfactory pulmonary or thoracic expansion.

Pathologic Anatomy.—The lesions found are those characteristic of suffocation and consist of congestive and hemorrhagic changes. In addition there may be discovered other lesions, such as intracranial hemorrhage and the like.

If the child has made attempts at inspiration while still in the uterus, mucus, bloody amniotic fluid or meconium may be found in the respiratory passages. Pulmonary congestion and atelectatic changes of various degrees will be present.

Symptoms. (*A*) Intra-uterine Asphyxia.—In asphyxia of intra-uterine origin certain symptoms, such as retardation, weakness or inaudibility of the fetal heart-sounds discoverable before birth, make the diagnosis very probable. A suspicious symptom is the discharge from the maternal vagina of meconium which has just been passed by the infant, as a result of the increased intestinal peristalsis that asphyxia produces. Sometimes, too, intra-uterine efforts at respiration may occasionally be detected by the finger inserted into the infant's mouth. The intra-uterine movements of the child may become more active, and even convulsive movements may occasionally be noticed. In asphyxiated children either no respiratory efforts at all are noticed after birth, or only imperfect and intermittent ones. The body is motionless and the child appears to be dead except for the continued action of the heart.

Two degrees of asphyxia of intra-uterine origin are observed: a milder form, *asphyxia livida* and a severer form, *asphyxia pallida*. The symptoms, prognosis and treatment of the two are very different.

1. Asphyxia Livida.—In this milder form the skin is dark bluish-red in color, the heart's action is strong although decidedly slow, and the pulse in the umbilical cord is full and strong and the tension high. The conjunctivae are injected and the face turgid. Respiratory efforts are absent or occur only occasionally, and at first very superficially, and are attended by a contortion of the face. Coarse râles may be audible in the lungs. Stimulation of the skin causes an energetic inspiratory effort, and the finger introduced into the mouth for the purpose of cleansing it produces attempts at vomiting or swallowing. A very characteristic symptom of asphyxia livida is that the muscle-tonus is preserved; *i. e.*, although the child is motionless, yet it is not absolutely flaccid when it is lifted.

2. Asphyxia Pallida.—In this variety, which is usually the result of intracranial hemorrhage (Ford[5]), the skin is pale and corpse-like, and the heart's action very weak and usually rapid. The vessels in the cord appear to be empty, and the pulse there is entirely absent or extremely feeble. Generally there are no true respiratory efforts, and any occasional attempts at inspiration which may occur seem to depend solely on the action of the diaphragm, the thorax moving not at all, and no grimace of the face attending them. No râles can be heard; this showing that the efforts at inspiration have been absent or entirely futile. Stimulation of the skin is without result, and the finger in the pharynx produces no reflex movements of its muscles or of the palate. The great characteristic of this grade of asphyxia is complete loss of muscle-tonus. The child is absolutely limp, the jaws fall, the head drops completely in some direction if the child is lifted, and the anus is open.

(*B*) Extra-uterine Asphyxia.—In asphyxia of extra-uterine origin the symptoms vary somewhat, depending upon the cause. The skin is usually dark reddish-blue. The heart's action is strong, and the vessels of the cord are filled with blood. The pulse, however, is not at first slow, and although it becomes so later it finally, as a rule, grows rapid again. This distinguishes the condition from intra-uterine asphyxia. Respiration is wanting or occasional only, and is not attended by râles. This lack of râles shows the absence of fluid from the respiratory tract, an evidence that the condition is extra-uterine in nature. In asphyxia in premature infants respiration may continue irregular and very superficial for days, and is almost entirely diaphragmatic. The children lie for the most part with eyes closed, motionless and somnolent, and make no sound or only occasionally utter a feeble cry. The face is dark-red and somewhat swollen; edema of the extremities and scrotum develops; the temperature is subnormal; there is loss of weight.

Course and Prognosis.—**Asphyxia livida,** when not excessive, will nearly always yield quickly to appropriate treatment. In the course of a few seconds or possibly minutes respirations become more frequent and effective, and are finally succeeded by loud crying. Many infants, however, pass from the milder form into the severer degree The result in **asphyxia pallida** is always more doubtful. The duration is variable. Some infants die almost immediately, while others may continue for hours without any apparent change; or, after improvement begins, may relapse if treatment is not persisted with. Kermauner[6] in 13,913 births found asphyxia in 802, with a mortality of 16.7 per cent in those spontaneously born, and 12.4 per cent in instrumental cases. If recovery ensues intermittent and occasional respirations begin and are perhaps followed by a slight cry, and finally satisfactory breathing is established. The longer the duration of the second stage of labor, the worse is the prognosis. The prognosis is graver, too, in proportion to the weakness of the pulse or of the heart-sounds. The presence of any complication, such as intracranial hemorrhage likewise makes the prognosis unfavorable. Yet even in the severer grades of intra-uterine asphyxia the majority of infants will recover. Even those who have seemed hopeless, and who for hours have appeared to be dead, may still survive. Asphyxia of extra-uterine origin generally runs a rapid course if dependent upon some malformation or some disease of the respiratory apparatus; when the result of premature birth it may continue, as stated, for days.

Regarding the after-effects of the disease upon an infant who has survived, it has been maintained that long-continued severe asphyxia is liable to produce idiocy or paralytic conditions. Although it seems more probable that such disorders are the result of some injury to the brain at birth, of which the respiratory condition was but a symptom, it is conceivable that the congestion accompanying the asphyxia may have produced the breaking of blood-vessels within the cranium, and thus have become the first cause of later nervous or mental disorders. The results of experimental work on animals done by Ford[5] are against this view. Aspiration-pneumonia may develop in an infant after its recovery from asphyxia.

Diagnosis.—It is important to determine the cause of the asphyxia. If due to intracranial hemorrhage with its *compression of the brain* there are produced slowing of the pulse and irregularity of respiration, the asphyxia is usually mild but responds poorly to treatment, and the fontanelle may be bulging.

Intense anemia resulting from tearing of the umbilical cord during birth may simulate asphyxia pallida closely. The history of the case should settle the diagnosis in this respect.

Treatment. (*A*) Asphyxia of Intra-uterine Origin.—The condition should be prevented as far as may be by careful obstetrical care. Whatever the degree of asphyxia present after the birth of the infant the first indication is to free the respiratory passages as far as possible. A finger should be introduced into the mouth and pharynx in order to remove any mucus or fluid present. There should be careful protection against chilling. The infant may be slapped sharply with the flat hand in the attempt to produce a respiratory effort reflexly through cutaneous irritation. It may also be suspended with the head downward for a moment in order to favor discharge of fluid and to bring about a congestive stimulation of the respiratory centers. In well-marked cases of **asphyxia livida,** it is recommended that the cord be tied and ½ fl. oz. (15) or less of blood allowed to escape. Slapping the infant with a cold wet towel or plunging into cool water and then immediately into a hot bath, and similar procedures, are methods long in vogue

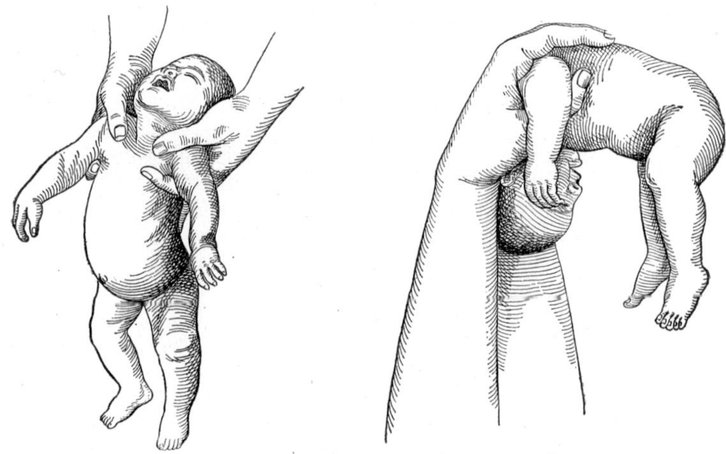

Fig. 28.—Schultze's method of artificial respiration. (*a*) Inspiration; (*b*) expiration. (*B. C. Hirst, Obstetrics, 8th Ed.* 816.)

for starting efforts at respiration by cutaneous stimulation. Henderson[1] objects to these procedures on the ground that they are liable to be exhausting, and because they are based upon the erroneous theory that respiration can be stimulated in this way; while the stimulation really requires the presence of carbon dioxide in the blood and its action upon the respiratory centers. It is true that the use of cold and similar methods is liable to be exhausting and to cause dangerous chilling if not employed with discretion; but it is likewise a matter of common clinical experience that in moderately severe cases of asphyxia livida the cutaneous irritation by cold or in other ways is usually followed by at least temporary efforts at breathing. Rhythmical traction of the tongue as recommended by Laborde[7] is also a powerful reflex stimulation for the awakening of respiratory efforts, provided there is any reflex excitability remaining.

In **asphyxia pallida,** or in cases of asphyxia livida which do not quickly respond, cutaneous stimulation will do no good and artificial respiration should be begun promptly. Various methods have been employed, among which may be mentioned those of Schultze[8] (Fig. 28), Hall,[9] Silvester,[10] Laborde,[7] Byrd,[11] Dew,[12] Ssokolow,[13] Minkévitch,[14] Rosenthal,[15] Greenwood,[16] and Prochownick.[17] The object is first to secure expiration in order to remove aspirated liquid, and then to favor inspiration by compression of the thoracic wall. To obtain these results the body may be rhythmically swung as recommended by Schultze[8] (Fig. 28), or the lower extremities alternately flexed on the chest and then extended (Dew,[12] Byrd,[11] Ssokolow,[13] Fig. 29), or modifications of these procedures employed. Among other methods is mouth to mouth insufflation, which has long been used and which has the advantage that it supplies the infant with an air-mixture containing carbon dioxide (oxygen 16 per cent, carbon dioxide 4.38 per cent; Mathieu and Holman[18]). A clean towel or several layers of gauze are placed over the infant's mouth, and only the first part of the air from the operator blown in. The infant's nostrils should not be compressed

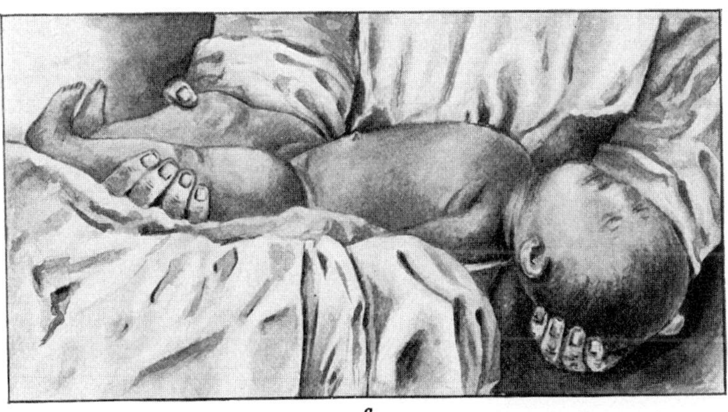

a

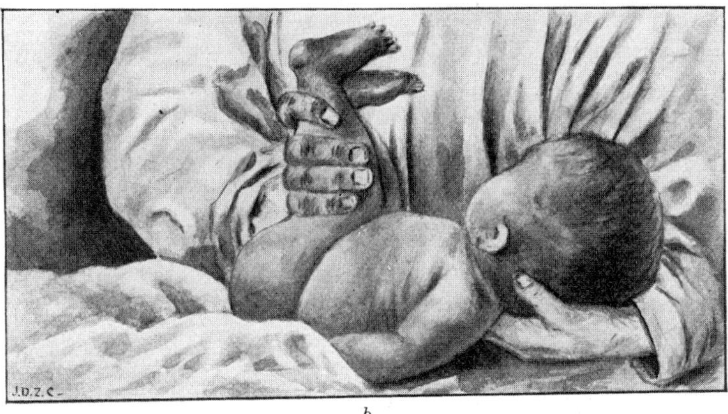

b

Fig. 29.—Method for inducing artificial respiration in the newborn. (*a*) Inspiration; (*b*) expiration. (*After Ssokolow, Monatsschr. f. Kinderheilk., Orig.* 1911, **10,** 459.)

and the blowing should be gentle to avoid danger of rupturing the pulmonary alveoli. In place of this method a soft rubber catheter, fitted with a saliva-trap, may be passed into the trachea and the operator's breath blown gently into this about several times a minute. The chief objection to this method is the difficulty of passing the tube through the larynx instead of by mistake into the esophagus. Henderson[1] recommends especially inflation with oxygen containing 5 to 6 per cent of carbon dioxide, using a special apparatus for administering this and giving it for two to three seconds every three to four minutes, and when respiration is established stopping the inflation but continuing the inhalation until recovery is complete. A respirator devised by Shaw and Drinker[19] has been used with success by

Murphy and Coyne;[20] Murphy, Bowman and Wilson,[21] and others. Flagg[22] also discusses the subject of mechanical appliances for the treatment of asphyxia.

Some method of direct insufflation is particularly indicated when great debility or low temperature of the infant interferes with such vigorous procedures as that of Schultze.

(*B*) Asphyxia of Extra-uterine Origin.—When dependent upon anomalies or upon intra-uterine disease but little can be accomplished by treatment. When associated with prematurity there is usually no need to remove aspirated fluid, since efforts at intra-uterine respiration have not taken place. Cutaneous stimulation may be tried and, if not successful, artificial respiration employed. Other methods than that of Schultze are, however, usually to be selected, on account of the lack of elasticity of the chest walls and the danger of chilling of the body. Inhalation of oxygen may be used when there is cyanosis. The great danger of relapse in this form of asphyxia should be borne in mind, and repeated warm baths may be serviceable.

For the treatment of asphyxia of any kind small doses of alcohol and of cardiac stimulants may be useful. Oberbeck[23] used alpha-lobelin in doses of $\frac{1}{20}$ grain (0.0032) hypodermatically and Wilson[24] injected the drug into the umbilical vein.

References

1. J.A.M.A., 1928, **90,** 583; 1931, **96,** 495. 2. Medicine, 1921, **2,** 534. 3. Am. J. Dis. Child., 1931, **42,** 1372. 4. Monatschr. f. Geburtsh. u. Gynäk., 1850, **6,** 112. 5. Bull. Johns Hopkins Hosp., 1928, **42,** 70. 6. Wien. klin. Wchnschr., 1926, **39,** 1070. 7. Les tractions rhythmées de la langue, 1897. 8. Der Scheintod d. Neugeborenen, 1871. 9. Lancet, 1856, **2,** 124. 19. Brit. M. J., 1858, 576. 11. Baltimore M. J., 1870, **1,** 646. 12. Koplik, Dis. of Inf. and Child., 1910, 196. 13. Monatschr. f. Kinderh., 1911, **10,** 457. 14. Semaine méd., 1902, **22,** 372. 15. Therap. Monatsh., 1893, **7,** 555. 16. Lancet, 1921, **1,** 964. 17. Zentralb. f. Gynäk., 1894, **18,** 225. 18. J.A.M.A., 1929, **92,** 1917. 19. J. Clin. Investigation, 1930, **8,** 33. 20. J.A.M.A., 1930, **95,** 335. 21. Am. J. Dis. Child., 1931, **42,** 1075. 22. J.A.M.A., 1928, **91,** 788. 23. M. J. and Rec., 1925, **122,** 40. 24. Am. J. Obst. and Gynec., 1928, **16,** 329.

CHAPTER IX

SUDDEN ARRESTS OF RESPIRATION IN THE NEW-BORN

To this condition attention was called by Still[1] and later by Kirkwood and Myers.[2] We have encountered 1 very typical case in an infant of six weeks, which ended fatally. It develops usually in infants but a few days old, but sometimes of several weeks. The **cause** is obscure. There is no history of difficult labor, and no association of previously existing asphyxia or cyanosis, nor is there any necessary evidence of general feebleness or malnutrition. The disease would appear to depend upon some affection of the respiratory center. No **lesions** have been found, except in the case of Kirkwood and Myers, in which hemorrhages of microscopic size were discovered just above the level of the olivary body. The thymus gland apparently cannot be implicated in such cases.

The **symptoms** consist of repeated attacks of sudden failure of respiration. Without warning or previous atelectasis, and while the infant is lying quietly, there is a sudden cessation of breathing, followed by pallor or a leaden color of the skin. Breathing returns after artificial respiration is employed, and in a short time the infant seems again perfectly normal;

but in a few hours a second attack develops and is relieved as before. This process continues for a day or two, or possibly even for a week or more, with several attacks each day; and finally, as a rule, the infant dies in an attack. This occurred in 4 of Still's 5 cases, and in that of Kirkwood and Myers, as well as in our own.

Treatment is difficult since the attack comes on without any warning. Consequently constant watching is the only thing possible, in order that artificial respiration and the administration of oxygen with 7 per cent carbon dioxide may be begun immediately.

References

1. Lancet, 1923, **1,** 431. 2. Lancet, 1923, **2,** 65.

CHAPTER X

PULMONARY ATELECTASIS IN THE NEW-BORN

Etiology.—The name denotes a persistence of, or a return to, the unexpanded fetal condition of the lungs. It is peculiarly a disease of the new-born, although under certain circumstances it may develop in older subjects (see p. 746). In Cruickshank's[1] report of 800 necropsies on infants in the first month of life, 67.5 per cent died from asphyxia and atelectasis, or the pneumonia consequent upon them. In some cases the infants are born asphyxiated, respiration is absent or incomplete, and the lungs never expand properly even under the influence of artificial respiration (Fig. 30). (See p. 227.) In other instances, especially in premature children or those who are weakly from other reasons, respiration is established for a time and there is at first no evidence of asphyxia. Soon, however, the poorly distended lungs become gradually more and more collapsed, owing to the weakness of the child and the yielding character of the thorax.

Pathologic Anatomy.—The lungs may be found completely or partly atelectatic. Emphysema may be present in portions, and pneumonia is frequently combined with the other lesions.

Symptoms.—In children who are asphyxiated at birth, and either show little or no tendency to recovery or relapse promptly, the symptoms of atelectasis are those already described under Asphyxia. In those in whom the atelectasis develops later, the pulse will be found weak and slow and the respiration rapid, irregular, shallow, and attended by evident retraction of the intercostal spaces and of the lower portion of the thorax at the insertion of the diaphragm. The infant is somnolent and lies generally with eyes closed, crying but little and never loudly, and making feeble, if any, efforts to suck. The temperature is persistently or only at times subnormal. The physical examination of the lungs generally gives a somewhat impaired percussion-note over the lower posterior portion of the chest. Sometimes, however, no distinct alteration of note can be discovered if numerous inflated areas of pulmonary tissue are present. The respiratory murmur is feeble, with fine râles at times, but as a rule no bronchial breathing is discovered.

This condition may continue for weeks. Recovery may take place after several relapses, or death may occur suddenly, often with convulsions and without there having been any very positive sign which indicated the actual state of the lungs.

Prognosis.—When the disease is present at birth and is accompanied by asphyxia livida, and where no congenital malformations or other pathologic conditions are present the prognosis is generally favorable. When atelectasis occurs in premature infants the result is more uncertain on account of the constant danger of relapse.

Diagnosis.—The disease is to be distinguished principally from the hypostatic pneumonia which is liable to develop in weakly infants. The

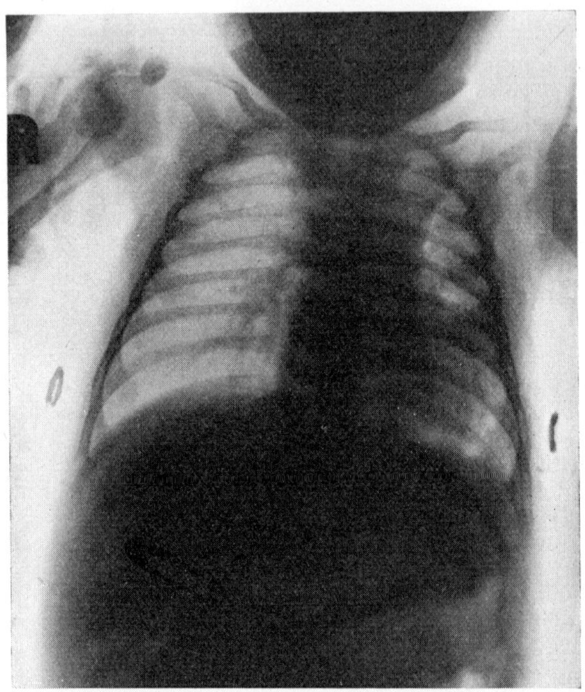

Fig. 30.—Female infant aged three months. Children's Hospital of Cincinnati. Necropsy-diagnosis atelectasis of lower left lobe congenital in origin.

absence of fever and of bronchial respiration constitute the chief diagnostic evidences against pneumonia. The roentgen-ray picture is often a valuable aid.

Treatment.—Although varying with the nature of the causes and symptoms, treatment is practically identical with that recommended for asphyxia, including the administration of oxygen with 5 to 7 per cent carbon dioxide. Henderson[2] recommends this as a prophylactic measure also, employing a suitable inhaler and mask, and giving the inhalations every ten minutes three times a day during the first few days of life. It must never be forgotten that atelectatic infants must have an abundance of fresh warmed air and must not be allowed to lie too long in one position. They should be roused from their somnolent condition at frequent intervals and carried about cautiously, and in general treated like premature infants (p. 213).

References

1. The Causes of Neonatal Death; Med. Res. Counc. Spec. Rep. Ser. 1930, No. 145, 12. 2. J.A.M.A. 1931, **96,** 495.

CHAPTER XI

CONGENITAL ASTHENIA

In this category belong the infants born with a low weight, and with a power of resistance to deleterious influences and a capacity of thriving under ordinary circumstances much below normal. The condition is different from that of premature birth, although often associated with it. Premature birth is doubtless the most frequent cause, but not every case of prematurity exhibits debility, while, on the other hand, infants born at full term may be suffering from asthenia. Such cases of congenital asthenia may be the result of prenatal influences such as prolonged illness of the mother, and particularly such conditions as syphilis, tuberculosis, alcoholism, and the like. In some of these the baby, although born at term, is physically immature, the maternal condition having interfered with intra-uterine development. In other cases the fact that the infant is one of multiple births accounts for the asthenia. The condition is much the same whatever the cause, and the symptoms and treatment are fully considered in the chapter on Premature Birth. There is often a difference, however, in the prognosis. If a prematurely born infant with asthenia dependent upon no maternal disease can be maintained alive until its organs reach the power of functionating properly, the prognosis is good; whereas the infant with constitutional debility, perhaps depending upon prenatal influences, may show little increase of energy as time passes.

CHAPTER XII

DISEASES OF THE UMBILICUS

Affections of the navel are among the common pathologic conditions of the new-born. In 2603 births Porak and Durante[1] found some such abnormality in 832 or 32.6 per cent although this was of an important nature in but 333; viz., 12.8 per cent. All the severer forms have become much less frequent since antisepsis has been practised more perfectly. The studies of Laurinsich[2] show that ordinarily the umbilical stump and surrounding area contain few bacteria, and that these are chiefly saprophytes. Even in the cases where pathogenic organisms are found there is not necessarily any inflammation present.

The various umbilical disorders, with the exception of hernia which will be discussed later (p. 621), may be subdivided as follows:

DELAYED HEALING OF THE UMBILICUS

(Excoriation; Blennorrhea; Umbilical Ulceration, etc.)

Under this title are grouped several minor affections of the umbilicus which are clearly allied.

In place of skinning over with epithelium a few days after the fall of the cord, the umbilical wound sometimes projects slightly and becomes irritated by the dressing applied, constituting the so-called **excoriatio umbilici.** If a flat, red surface is visible, resembling mucous membrane, and secreting pus more or less abundantly, **blennorrhea of the navel** is spoken of. Should the process extend in area or in depth a condition of genuine ulceration is produced with a granulating surface, sometimes covered with necrotic tissue and constituting an **ulcus umbilici**. This ulcer may develop a false membrane, and is then entitled **croup** or **diphtheria of the navel**, without the process necessarily being of a truly diphtheritic nature.

Etiology.—An average time for the separation of the cord is the fifth day, and for the healing of the wound the twelfth to the fifteenth day. It is only when the inflammation increases after the cord has separated that the process can be called abnormal. In some cases local irritation by the dressing or lack of cleanliness are the causes of inflammation. In many instances a local infection is present, and this is nearly always the case when ulceration develops. Diphtheritic infection of the stump is not very rare, and cases have been reported by Henkel,[3] Foth,[4] Comby[5] and others.

Symptoms.—No general symptoms attend these different forms of delayed healing of the umbilical wound, and no danger to life exists provided they remain purely local. When there are decided constitutional symptoms accompanying the umbilical lesions described, infection has certainly extended beyond the umbilicus.

Treatment.—As a prophylactic measure the stump of the cord must be kept as dry as possible. Antiseptic and aseptic treatment is necessary from the moment of birth. Daily dressings may be made using a powder of salicylic acid and starch (1:5). Powdered gypsum has also been recommended as have boric acid and iodoform. The dressing should be one which will not exclude the air too greatly, otherwise the desired rapid drying and mummification will be hindered. Treatment should continue even after the cord has separated.

Should there be delay in healing, washing with hydrogen peroxide and painting with a 1 per cent solution of nitrate of silver are often of service. The dry dressing with one of the powders should be renewed once or twice daily. In diphtheria of the stump 500 to 1000 units of antitoxin should be given subcutaneously.

FUNGUS OF THE UMBILICUS

(Granuloma; Sarcomphalos; Umbilical Polypus)

After the separation of the cord an abnormal growth sometimes develops at the navel. This may be hidden by the overlying skin, or may project as a round, red mass of granulation tissue the size of a pea or larger. The surface is moist, discharges sero-purulent fluid, and bleeds slightly when irritated. Unless treated the growth may persist for months. The general health of the infant is unaffected. Fungus is to be distinguished only from a persistent Meckel's diverticulum (p. 636). The tendency to recovery unaided is slight, and the umbilical wound cannot heal while the fungus is present. Treatment consists in the application of astringents, preferably nitrate of silver, followed by a dressing of powdered boric acid. This may be repeated every few days if necessary. If the fungus is of considerable size it may be ligated. When exuberant granulations have disappeared an antiseptic dressing may be applied until the wound becomes covered with epithelium.

OMPHALITIS

(Periomphalitis)

Etiology.—The term is used to designate a phlegmonous inflammation of the navel and especially of the surrounding tissues. It is not of frequent occurrence, Hennig[6] finding but 12 cases among 7000 sick infants. The cause is a pyogenic infection.

Symptoms.—The disease begins usually in the second or third week of life, after separation of the cord and as a sequel to a delayed healing of the umbilical wound, which may exhibit ulceration with secretion of pus. The skin around the navel is swollen, red, hot, shining and projecting, with a disappearance of the normal folds. The subcutaneous tissue is infiltrated and hard, and the slightest pressure causes intense pain. The inflammation may remain comparatively superficial, or may extend in depth, even involving the peritoneum. It may even attack the greater part of the abdominal wall. In some such cases it is very probable that an erysipelatous infection has been added to the omphalitis, or has been present from the beginning. The general condition of the infant is always affected. There are restlessness, loss of appetite, and fever. Pain is a prominent feature, and on this account there is little movement of the abdomen or lower limbs, the thighs are generally held rigidly, respiration is superficial, and loud crying is avoided. The emptying of the bladder and of the bowels is also painful.

Course and Prognosis.—The duration and course of the disease is variable. In the mild cases the exudate is rapidly absorbed. A few pustules or quite small cutaneous abscesses may form in the vicinity and recovery is complete in a few days. The severe cases may last for weeks, the infiltration being slowly absorbed, or an abscess developing and discharging; and the prognosis is always dubious, inasmuch as gangrene, extension to the peritoneum, or involvement of the umbilical vessels may take place. The more rapidly abscess forms the better for the infant.

Diagnosis.—This is usually easy except to distinguish from a primary umbilical erysipelas. This disease, however, generally spreads more rapidly and has a characteristic color.

Treatment.—Prophylaxis is of great importance. If omphalitis has already developed the umbilical wound should be cleansed carefully and then powdered thickly with boric acid, iodoform, salicylic acid and starch (1:5), or other antiseptic powder. If there is much infiltration of the tissues and abdominal pain, the inflamed area may be covered with a warm, wet antiseptic dressing. Any abscesses which form should be incised early. Attention must be given to the nourishment of the infant, forced feeding being used if necessary, and stimulants being required in many cases. The bowels should be emptied by injections, as the infant cannot make any effort to assist at evacuation, and catheterization of the bladder may be necessary.

GANGRENE OF THE NAVEL

Etiology.—Gangrene may be a sequel to severe cases of omphalitis, ulcer, or inflammation of the umbilical vessels. It is now very rare as a purely local affection, since better antiseptic precautions are observed; but is still seen, though infrequently, as a secondary manifestation of a general septic infection. It may exceptionally follow severe general diseases, especially diarrhea of a choleraic nature, even in children over a month old and previously healthy. The existence of great debility, as in cases of premature birth, favors its development. An especially potent factor is lack of cleanliness about the umbilical wound. It formerly occurred at times in epidemic form.

Pathologic Anatomy and Symptoms.—The inflammation already present develops into a greenish or black offensive mass surrounded by a red areola, and the edges of the wound become discolored and break down, causing a more or less rapid loss of substance, either in area or in depth. In the latter case the process may extend to the peritoneum, and even into the intestine, producing perforation and fecal fistula. If the spreading is toward the periphery the greater part of the superficial abdominal wall may be destroyed, involving more or less the muscular layer and even extending to the bladder. Severe hemorrhage may occur if the umbilical vessels are involved. General sepsis may be produced by way of the vessels or of the peritoneum. The constitutional symptoms attending gangrene are always severe. There are great prostration with coldness of the extremities, quick and weak pulse, and little or no fever. Rapid collapse is frequent. Occasionally the process is not so serious, the gangrene may not extend far, and, the reactive inflammation producing pus, the dead tissue is thrown off and the cavity fills with granulations. The diagnosis offers no difficulty.

Course and Prognosis.—The average duration of fatal cases is about five days, and the prognosis is exceedingly bad, the mortality being over 85 per cent (Fürth[7]).

Treatment.—This is similar to that for omphalitis. The early employment of the thermo-cautery may be efficacious.

UMBILICAL ARTERITIS AND PHLEBITIS

Etiology.—Both of these conditions are of comparatively unusual occurrence. The investigations of Runge[8] show that inflammation of the arteries is far more common than that of the vein, the arteries being involved in all of 55 cases and the vein in but 1. The cause of disease of the umbilical vessels is always an infection of the umbilical wound, even although this may not be apparent. It is most likely to occur before the stump of the cord has completely separated, since the granulations which develop later protect to some extent against infection. It may appear as an epidemic in lying-in institutions, although this has become very much less frequent since better methods have prevailed. The infection may be acquired from the lochial discharges of the mother, or be transmitted by the hands of the physician or nurse, infected umbilical dressings, or even apparently by the air of an infected room or the water used for bathing. Any irritation or infection of the umbilical wound predisposes to it, as does the presence of undue moisture in the stump of the cord. Various organisms have been found here and in the umbilical wound in cases of infection of the vessels, among these being varieties of staphylococci, the streptococcus pyogenes, the bacillus coli, the pneumococcus, and the bacillus pyocyaneus.

Pathologic Anatomy.—The process begins as an infection and inflammation of the perivascular tissue which becomes infiltrated and swollen. It next extends to the vessel-walls and a septic thrombus forms in the vessel. The disease remains local in the majority of cases, resulting in suppuration in or about the affected portion of the vessel or between the abdominal wall and the peritoneum, and the final discharge of pus. In a smaller number of cases the process spreads by continuity along the perivascular tissues, the sepsis reaching the general system through the perivascular lymph-channels. The umbilical wound may appear perfectly normal or may exhibit the lesions of ulcer or of omphalitis. Even if the stump of the cord is mummified and still persists, foci of suppuration may be discovered about the periphery of the region of beginning detachment. Some of the lesions of a general septic infection may be present, such as have been described in considering Sepsis in the New-born (p. 210). The liver may be involved directly by continuity from the umbilical vein.

Symptoms and Diagnosis.—The navel may show local irritation or suppuration, but when only the deeper portion of the vessels is involved there is no umbilical disease visible. In some cases the thickened arteries may be felt through the abdominal wall. Abscess may form above the peritoneum and spread in different directions. Septicemia and pyemia may develop with accompanying restlessness, diarrhea, anorexia, fever and prostration. Icterus may occur when the umbilical vein carries the infection to the liver. In the cases with deep seated infection the symptoms are prone to be few, vague, and uncharacteristic, and it may be that death occurs unexpectedly and the diagnosis is only at necropsy, unless there has been distinct evidence of disease of the umbilical wound. In other cases symptoms of widespread pyogenic infection render the diagnosis of the disease of the umbilical vessels probable, but not certain. It may happen that there are few symptoms but that death occurs unexpectedly, and only at necropsy is the deep umbilical infection found.

Complications.—Pneumonia is that oftenest seen, and may be the only one. It occurred in 22 of Runge's 55 cases. All the widespread local pyemic lesions of septic infection may occur as complications, among these empyema, peritonitis, subcutaneous abscess, nephritis, and the like. In 340 necropsies on new-born infants Runge found 36 cases of general sepsis, in 30 of which its origin could be traced to the navel (see p. 216). Erysipelas may sometimes develop as a complication.

Course and Prognosis.—In nearly all instances the duration of the disease is short, ranging from a few days to several weeks. The greater number of deaths in Runge's cases occurred on the eighth day of life. The prognosis is always grave. It is probable that recovery occurs in many instances if the process does not spread beyond the vessels. Should the sepsis become general, death is almost inevitable.

Treatment.—Prophylaxis is the most important. Careful antiseptic treatment of the umbilicus is necessary from the moment of birth, as already described (p. 55). The child should be at once removed from the vicinity of the mother if she has any evidence of sepsis. If the navel is already diseased it should be treated as indicated (p. 237). It may be possible to open the stump in some cases to permit surgical drainage. For treatment of sepsis see the appropriate section (p. 216).

OMPHALORRHAGIA

(Umbilical Hemorrhage)

This is not a distinct disease, but a symptom of different conditions, itself of enough importance to warrant separate consideration. It is customary to recognize 2 forms (*a*) *accidental*, proceeding from the umbilical vessels, and (*b*) *idiopathic* or *spontaneous* coming from the umbilical tissues.

Etiology. (*A*) Accidental Hemorrhage.—Severe hemorrhage from the umbilical vessels may occur before the fall of the cord as a result of imperfect ligation of it. Usually hemorrhage from such cause will not take place except in the first ten or fifteen minutes of life, but in asphyxia it may occur later, since there results a maintenance of the blood-pressure in the umbilical arteries, and the muscle of the arterial walls fails to contract and close the lumen properly. In like manner gangrene of the umbilicus or imperfect mummification allows the vessels to open again and blood to escape. It is possible, too, that a bath too prolonged and too hot may relax the vessels and permit of hemorrhage. Hemorrhage very rarely results from rupture of the cord during birth in the case of healthy infants.

After the separation of the cord a slight oozing from the umbilical vessels is not uncommon but is rarely severe.

(*B*) Idiopathic Hemorrhage.—Bleeding of this variety from the umbilical wound, decidedly more common than from the vessels, is a very dangerous affection, the causes of which are diverse and little understood. Grandidier[9] writing in 1871 collected 220 cases from medical literature. Townsend[10] reported 14 cases in 7225 births. Winckel[11] observed it in only 1 of 5000 births. In Ritter's[12] 190 cases of hemorrhage in the new-born, 132 (69.5 per cent) were from the umbilicus, and in 97 the hemorrhage was limited to this region. The condition would appear perhaps to be more frequent than these statistics indicate, inasmuch as many cases are never reported. It occurs oftenest after the complete separation of the stump of the cord. Males exhibit it oftener than females. (For further discussion of the cause of hemorrhage see p. 219.)

Symptoms.—Severe **accidental hemorrhage** is usually sudden and profuse, and may terminate life quickly unless checked at once. It occurs generally a few minutes after birth, or, in the case of premature infants with evidences of asphyxia, during the first few hours of life, or occasionally later; sometimes even after the cord has fallen. After the separation of the cord the hemorrhage is usually in the form of oozing only.

No general symptoms attend the accidental hemorrhage other than those of anemia, nor is there bleeding from other parts of the body.

Idiopathic hemorrhage usually occurs somewhere between the fifth and the tenth days of life. It is very frequently combined with the occurrence of bleeding in other parts of the body (see p. 220). Beginning slowly it becomes fairly free and saturates the dressing, yet it appears to be capillary in origin. Sometimes it is profuse from the start. A characteristic of the disease is that effort to check the bleeding by local treatment has but a temporary effect, if any. The infants may appear at first perfectly healthy in every other respect, or may have seemed not quite well before the hemorrhage began, or have looked ill and been somnolent or cyanotic or exhibited diarrhea, vomiting or decided icterus; or these symptoms may develop later. In all such cases the umbilical bleeding is probably but a part of some general disease, evidences of which eventually appear. Not infrequently bleeding takes place not only from the navel, but into the subcutaneous tissues about it. As the hemorrhage continues anemia becomes profound and death occurs, sometimes preceded by coma or convulsions.

Prognosis.—The prognosis in accidental hemorrhage is favorable if the bleeding is not too profuse at the beginning and is discovered and checked at once. In idiopathic hemorrhage it is unfavorable. Older statistics give from 25 to 35 per cent of recoveries only, but the prognosis has improved by newer forms of treatment. If a general condition such as sepsis, acute fatty degeneration or syphilis is present the prognosis is influenced by the primary disease. Death may occur in less than twenty-four hours and the average duration of life from the onset in fatal cases is only two to three days.

Treatment.—Prophylactic treatment for **accidental hemorrhage** consists in the proper ligation of the umbilical cord not too close to the body, in gentle handling of it afterward, and in the proper treatment of asphyxia as soon as possible. Should hemorrhage occur a new ligature must be tied at once. If there is no room to apply this, or if there is free hemorrhage after the separation of the cord, it may be necessary to apply a compress or even to push two needles through the skin, above and below the seat of bleeding, and ligate around these. If the bleeding is very slight the application of an astringent powder or the use of compresses moistened with tr. ferri chloridi or liquor ferri subsulphati may suffice. For the anemia which may have developed are to be employed free stimulation, abundant nourishment, the maintaining of the heat of the body, and later, measures to aid the enriching of the blood. If there has been great loss of blood, transfusion should be given. In the case of **idiopathic hemorrhage** the treatment is that described for Hemorrhage in the New-born (p. 219). Styptic applications may be tried locally, such as alum or tannic acid, and especially the use of firm compresses moistened with tincture of the chloride of iron. These may be fastened in place with broad bands of adhesive plaster crossing over the navel and drawn firmly, finishing on the back. It has also been recommended to pour moistened plaster of Paris on the navel and allow it to remain for several days. Acupuncture with the application of a ligature about the needles may be employed in the manner already described.

PROTRUDING MECKEL'S DIVERTICULUM

(See also Diseases of Meckel's Diverticulum, p. 636)

This rare affection at first sight resembles Fungus of the Umbilicus (p. 236). It consists of a prolapse at the navel of the terminal portion of the omphalomesenteric duct, which has failed to close and to disappear early in fetal life. It is generally patulous throughout, forming a fistulous tract from the umbilicus to the small intestine. In appearance it is usually a reddish tumor of glistening surface, moist with mucous secretion. Microscopical examination shows that it is of the same structure as the intestinal wall and that the surface is composed of mucous membrane. It is generally of the size of a pea or bean, although sometimes much larger, and shows a central opening through which a small amount of fecal matter may be discharged from time to time. This condition may last for years, or the duct may close spontaneously. In some cases the fistula is much larger, and the posterior wall of the intestine, and finally even quite a large portion of the bowel may project through it in the form of two intussusceptions each with its central opening. The treatment of the protruding diverticulum, if small, consists in the application of a ligature. The larger protrusions are more difficult of cure, and more extensive operative procedures are necessary.

References

1. Arch. de méd. d. enf., 1905, **8**, 465. 2. Pediatria, 1924, **32**, 1022. 3. Deutsche med. Wchnschr., 1919, **45**, 1411. 4. Deutsche med. Wchnschr., 1921, **47**, 1261. 5. Arch. de méd. d. enf., 1921, **24**, 437. 6. Gerhardt's Handbk. d. Kinderk., **2**, 131. 7. Wien. Klinik., 1884, **10**, 331. 8. Krankh. d. ersten Lebenst., 1893, 88; 136. 9. Die freiwilligen Nabelblutungen d. Neugeb., 1871. Ref. Runge, Die Kranhk. d. ersten Lebenst., 1906, 224. 10. Boston M. and S. J., 1891, **125**, 218. 11. Lehrb. d. Geburtsh., 1893, 854. 12. Oester. Jahrb. f. Pädiat., 1871, **1**, 190.

CHAPTER XIII

MASTITIS

The activity of the mammary glands so frequently present in the new-born, producing enlargement with secretion of fluid, may pass into an actual inflammatory condition, and is then known as mastitis.

Etiology.—The condition is not an uncommon one, and either sex may be attacked. As a rule it occurs only in a breast in which secretion has been free and has continued for some time. Infection is facilitated by lack of cleanliness or by undue manipulation of the breast.

Symptoms.—Mastitis begins usually in the second or third week of life, but may occur later in infancy. The breast, generally only one, shows local inflammation and enlargement. Suppuration may take place and a circumscribed abscess form. Less frequently there are multiple abscesses. The general symptoms of infection may attend the suppurative process. Occasionally the inflammation spreads beyond the gland to the surrounding connective tissue, and in rare instances this perimastitis may involve much of the anterior and lateral walls of the thorax.

Prognosis.—The prognosis of mastitis of the new-born is nearly always good. Even in the cases where abscess forms recovery follows unless suppuration is very extensive. Yet permanent injury may easily remain, the secreting power of the gland in later life in females being destroyed or impaired, or the nipple being retracted or otherwise distorted.

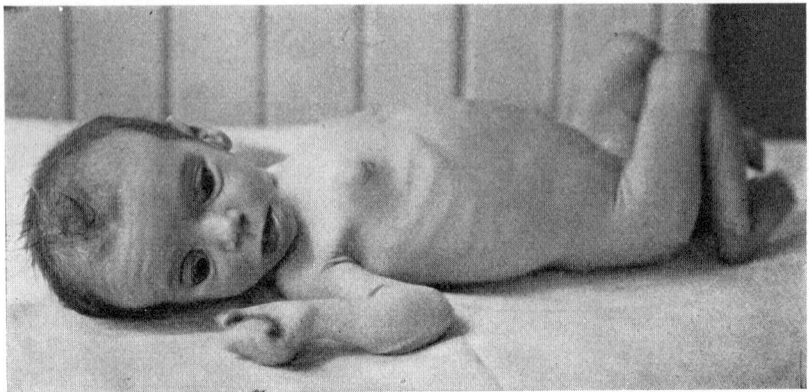

Fig. 31.—Mastitis. Male infant, aged twenty-five days.

Treatment.—The disease should be prevented by careful prophylactic measures. All pressure or rubbing of the breast of the new-born is to be avoided, and cleanliness is to be enforced. If the gland is more swollen than usually occurs, and inflammation is feared, a wad of aseptic absorbent cotton may be laid over it to protect from pressure and to prevent infection. If mastitis actually begins, hot, wet applications may be employed. Any abscess forming should be opened promptly and freely, and the infant given tonic treatment.

CHAPTER XIV

OPHTHALMIA NEONATORUM

The affection in a severe form is a very uncommon one at the present time. Formerly it often prevailed epidemically, particularly in lying-in institutions, where from 5 to 20 per cent of the children born might have the infection.

Etiology.—Much the most common etiologic agent is the gonococcus (55 per cent of 233 cases, Waldeck[1]), the disease generally being acquired from the mother's vaginal discharges at the time of birth. Rarely it arises from other sources after birth. Other germs, such as the colon bacillus, pneumococcus, staphylococcus, meningococcus and the like, may be responsible for the disease.

Symptoms.—Except in rare instances, both eyes are affected and usually simultaneously. The infection becomes evident generally by the end of the third day or is often apparent shortly after birth. In all but mild cases, and in all of the gonorrheal type, there is a very marked purulent conjunctivitis, usually with involvement of the cornea and sometimes with such complications as perforation of the cornea and panophthalmitis. There may be secondary gonorrheal infection of the nose or mouth, and occasionally gonorrheal arthritis develops.

Prognosis.—In the mild nongonorrheal cases the inflammation usually disappears in a few days, but in the severe gonorrheal infections the prognosis is grave as regards the loss of vision, and only prompt and thorough treatment can avail. Various statistics show that about 50 per cent of the inmates of blind-asylums had lost their sight through ophthalmia. In gonorrheal cases in which vision is saved the average duration is three to five weeks, and the severe cases longer.

Diagnosis.—It should always be suspected that conjunctivitis in newborn infants is gonorrheal especially when the inflammation is severe. Bacteriologic examination must always be performed. In diphtheritic conjunctivitis, which occurs but rarely in infants, there is a false membrane and the causative bacillus may be found.

Treatment.—To prevent the development of the milder forms of inflammation, the eyes of the infant should be protected from too bright a light and from mechanical injury. As a prophylactic measure against gonorrheal ophthalmia the treatment of Credé[2] should be carried out, as it will reduce the incidence of gonorrheal ophthalmia to 0.1 or 0.2 per cent. This consists in dropping a 2 per cent solution of silver nitrate into the eyes of every child immediately after birth. This procedure should be a routine one in all institutions, and also in private practice where there is the slightest possibility of a gonorrheal ophthalmia developing. Some of the newer silver compounds, such as argyrol, neosilvol and the like, in about 15 to 25 per cent solution may be substituted for the silver nitrate but are perhaps less certain. When the disease develops in an infant in a maternity or hospital ward, the patient should at once be isolated for protection of other infants and also of attendants, and, unless the technique is without question, the nurse in charge should not come in contact with other children. If only one eye is affected attempt should be made to protect the other. The treatment should be directed by an ophthalmologist whenever possible. There must be frequent cleansing and instillation into the conjunctival sac of boric acid solution, or corrosive sublimate in 1:10,000 strength may be used. Once a day or oftener there should be instilled into the eye 2 or 3 drops of 1 per cent solution of silver nitrate, or a 10 to 25 per cent solution of argyrol or neosilvol. Ice-cold compresses should be used, changing them every two to three minutes during thirty minutes, with intermissions of two or three hours.

References

1. J. Michigan M. Soc., 1922, **21**, 501. 2. Arch. f. Gynäk., 1881, **17**, 50; 1883, **21**, 179; Die Verhütung d. Augenentzündung d. Neugeborenen, 1884.

CHAPTER XV

SCLEREMA AND EDEMA

The literature upon this subject is confusing, and various terms have been employed to describe conditions which were sometimes identical, while in other cases one term has been used for disorders which would seem to be without doubt entirely distinct. Thus we read of sclerosis, sclerema, scleroma, sclerema adiposum, scleroderma neonatorum, necrosis adiposa neonatorum, etc., etc. Although our knowledge of the subject is very far from complete, there would appear to be at least 2 conditions clinically and anatomically quite distinct, with which some of the other disorders mentioned may be allied or be identical. Ylppö[1] and others discuss especially also a third form, that of scleredema.

SCLEREMA NEONATORUM

(Sclerosis; Scleroma; Sclerema adiposum)

This disease in its accepted sense appears to have been first mentioned by Uzenbezius[2] in 1722, and apparently first described accurately by Denman.[3]

Etiology and Pathology.—It is an uncommon affection, observed much more frequently in Europe than in America. Writing in 1897 one of us was able to discover but 5 undoubted cases published in the United States, and to these a 6th was added,[4] and another case reported later.[5] Smith[6] reported another American case and Epstein and Barash[7] 2 cases, with a good review of the theories of etiology. Prematurity, asthenia, and unfavorable hygienic conditions predispose to it and it has occurred oftenest in institutions for foundlings. It may develop after the first month and follow some diarrheal or other exhausting disease.

The pathogenesis is even yet not clearly understood. As early as 1875, L. Somma[8] expressed the view that low temperature had a causative influence. Langer,[9] Knöpfelmacher,[10] Lemez[11] and others contended that the lowering of body-temperature dependent upon inanition produces a hardening of the subcutaneous adipose tissue; this "fetal" fat, due to its low percentage of olein and high percentage of stearin and palmatin, having a higher melting point than in later life. Other investigators, however, could not find any chemical difference in the fat and skin of scleremic and non-scleremic babies respectively; Chen,[12] for example, discovering no difference in melting point, solidifying point, iodine number, saponification value, and acetyl number, and Smith[6] noting a higher content in fatty acid but no difference in oleic acid. Finkelstein and Sommerfeld[13] believe there is a change in tissue-colloids, but that chilling is not causative. It is to be remarked, too, that sclerema is not produced in the great majority of infants suffering from collapse-temperatures, and further that it does not appear in infants in whom there is not a good development of subcutaneous fat. It has never been shown that any type of microörganism is causative. Trauma is held to be a factor by a number of authors, some of whom believe it acts in conjunction with abnormality of the fat. After a careful review of the pathologic anatomy, with personal cases, Harrison and McNee[14] share the views of those who think the process is a primary inflammation of unknown origin. A particular variety, which should probably be considered as an entity, is that due to the application of forceps or prolonged pressure from hard labor. Gelbjerg-Hansen[15] believes that in some of the cases there is a pancreatic fault present, and employs the term *necrosis adiposa neonatorum*, and Fabyan[16] also reports a case of subcutaneous fat necrosis in infancy. It is uncertain, however, whether these cases belong in the category of sclerema, and it is likely, as Gelbjerg-Hansen[15] maintains, that necrosis adiposa neonatorum is to be regarded as an entirely distinct disease.

Pathologic Anatomy.—Incision of the skin is not followed by exudation of blood or serum. The subcutaneous tissue appears remarkably dry, this being one of the chief characteristics. In some of the reported cases little has been found histologically, but usually there are shown increase of the trabeculae of the subcutaneous tissue; fat globules (many of them deprived partly of fat) between the trabeculae; slits or clefts adjoining and surrounding the fat globules; phagocytic cells; occasionally deposition of lime salts and of certain crystals the nature of which is not known but which are supposedly of fatty origin. There is, however, little uniformity in the pathologic findings. Just what the relationship of sclerema and fat necrosis may be seems uncertain, and cases are reported in which necrosis appears to have been entirely absent or to have played a subordinate part.

Symptoms.—The two characteristic symptoms are fall of temperature and a hard swelling of a portion of the skin. Occasionally at birth, but oftener when the greatly debilitated child is a few days or even weeks old, induration of the skin is discovered. This change begins usually in the feet and calves and rapidly spreads perhaps over the whole body. It is generally most decided in the cheeks, buttocks, back and thighs, the parts which have the most fat being chiefly involved. Consequently the penis, scrotum, palms and soles escape. The affected tissues seem to have an almost stony coldness and hardness and will not pit on pressure. The limbs, and sometimes the whole body, are more or less stiff and immovable. The skin cannot be lifted from the subcutaneous tissue. It is pale, flat, waxy, and sometimes in places discolored bluish or yellowish, resembling an old bruise. The temperature of the body is generally very low, sometimes not over 90 F. (32.2 C.) in the axilla, or even less than this. The child has an almost inaudible cry. The respiration and cardiac action are very feeble; the fontanelle is sunken; the infant becomes somnolent and will not take nourishment. Atelectasis is very prone to develop.

Occasionally cases are not so severe, the temperature is not markedly low, there is an absence of discoloration, and the child does not show so great a degree of inanition and debility. We have observed at least 4 cases of this nature which seemed best denominated sclerema, but which were yet clearly not instances of the typical disease as described. To such cases the title scleredema might perhaps better be applied. It is for this type that Marfan and Debray[17] prefer the term "Curable Induration of the Skin." The form due to the *application of forceps* is localized in the region where pressure was applied. It disappears after weeks or months.

Diagnosis.—This is easy in typical cases and rests upon the symptoms as described. The adherence of the skin to tissues beneath and the absence of pitting, distinguish it from any forms of edema. *Scleroderma* is a disease of adults, exceedingly rare in infancy. The hardening is more local, the course is chronic, there are no nutritional disturbances, and the prognosis is better.

Prognosis.—This is extremely unfavorable in typical cases. The great majority die in a few days. Occasionally when the disease is not too extensive, the general condition of the infant better, and treatment commenced early, recovery will slowly take place in the course of some weeks. This was true of the 4 personal cases referred to, but, as stated, it is questionable whether these can rightly be put in the category of sclerema.

Treatment.—This is supportive with the application of local heat. Wolff[18] had good results by submitting the infant to a continued temperature of 104 to 107.6 F. (40 to 42 C.). Bourne[19] reported cure in an infant given daily $\frac{1}{4}$ grain (.016) of thyroid extract.

OEDEMA NEONATORUM

(Scleredema; Acute Edema)

Although edema from various causes may develop in infancy, there is a form oftenest seen in the new-born to which the name Oedema Neonatorum is given. This condition is considered by some writers to be an edematous form of sclerema and the same causative factors are supposed to be operative. It is very probable that more than one disorder is included under this title.

The chief features distinguishing it from sclerema are the swelling of the skin, the presence of pitting, the presence of fluid in the tissues and its escape from the incised skin, and the fact that the skin is not adherent to the parts below it.

Ylppö,[1] von Reuss[20] and others make a special division for scleredema as distinguished from other forms of edema. The skin is very hard, and, although it pits, it is with a doughy resistance. The parts involved are especially the feet, calves, and outer parts of the thighs, but any region may suffer, including usually the genitals, and also at times the palms and soles. The symptoms in general are very similar to those of sclerema and the prognosis in severe cases is unfavorable, although better than in this disease.

There has further been described by Schridde,[21] and the observation confirmed by others (Chiari,[22] Wienskowitz[23]) a special form of widespread edema which is congenital and which has been designated by Chiari[22] *fetal erythroblastosis*, characterized by a universal anasarca; hydrops of the serous cavities; enlargement of the liver and spleen; a very large number of erythroblasts in the blood with a great diminution of other elements; numerous erythroblasts in the liver, spleen, kidneys and other organs; and an abnormal deposit of hemosiderin in the spleen and liver. This form of edema is seen chiefly in premature infants born of mothers with nephritis, which has been the cause probably of a toxic disturbance of the blood-making functions of the child. Still another form is a chronic genital edema occurring in premature new-born infants, or at a slightly later period (p. 847). Edema may occur also as a symptom of erysipelas, acute nephritis in the new-born, or an advanced marantic state.

Treatment.—The treatment of oedema neonatorum depends somewhat upon the cause. In the cases of scleredema it is the same as for sclerema.

References

1. Pfaundler und Schlossman Handb. d. Kinderh., 1923, 3. Aufl., 1, 564. 2. Ephemerides naturae curiosorum, Ref. Underwood, Treat. on Dis. of Childh., 1793, 112. 3. Ref. Underwood, Treat. on Dis. of Childh., 1793, 113. 4. Griffith Med. News, 1897, **71,** 428. 5. Griffith, Arch. Pediat., 1906, **23,** 97. 6. J. Cutan. Dis., 1918, **36,** 436. 7. Am. J. Dis. Child., 1930, **40,** 337. 8. Ref. Epstein and Barash, Am. J. Dis. Child., 1930, **40,** 337. 9. Wien. med. Presse, 1881, **22,** 1375. 10. Jahrb. f. Kinderh., 1897, **45,** 177. 11. Ztschr. f. Kinderh., 1928, **46,** 323. 12. Nat. M. J., China 1930, **16,** 360. 13. Monatschr. f. Kinderh., 1923, **25,** 105. 14. Arch. Dis. Child., 1926, **1,** 63; 123. 15. Arch. f. Dermat. u. Syph., 1920, **152,** 91. 16. Bull. Johns Hopkins Hosp., 1907, **18,** 349. 17. Bull. de la soc. de. pédiat., 1926, **24,** 60. 18. Monatschr. f. Kinderh., Referat., 1914, **14,** 66. 19. Lancet 1922, **1,** 368. 20. Die Krankheit. des Neugeboren., 1914, 367. 21. München. med. Wchnschr., 1910, **57,** 397. 22. Jahrb. f. Kinderh., 1914, **80,** 561. 23. Berl. klin. Wchnschr., 1914, **51,** 1725.

CHAPTER XVI

TRANSITORY FEVER IN THE NEW-BORN

(Inanition-fever; Hunger-fever; Thirst-fever, etc.)

In the early weeks of life febrile elevations readily occur from slight causes. In some statistics their incidence is as low as 4 per cent, although Eröss[1] and Lo Cicero,[2] who took frequent temperature observations at short intervals, would place them at from 45 to 50 per cent or more. The fever usually appears from the second to the fourth day of life and may last a few hours or several days. (See Fig. 32.) It is more common in winter than in summer, with no relation to the temperature or humidity of the nursery (Bakwin and Bakwin[3]). A number of **causes** have been considered. It has been held by Sherman and Lohnes,[4] Grulee and Bonar,[5] and others that the rise in temperature may be attributed to the absorption of protein-products, bacterial and otherwise, from the intestinal tract. Jaschke[6] considers it to be dependent on the absorption of pyogenic substances, and Plantenga[7] upon bacterial action. Others, too, believe that slight digestive disturbances may be responsible, or slight infection such as local putrefactive changes in the umbilical cord (Eröss[1]). No doubt all these factors account for some of the cases. The transitory nature of the fever and the absence of discoverable lesions and of leukocytosis largely eliminate from consideration any serious infections or inflammatory changes. Holt,[8] who noted that it was liable to develop at the time of the greatest initial loss of weight, suggested the term "*inanition-fever*," and Müller[9] and others believe that it is dependent upon desiccation of the tissues. There

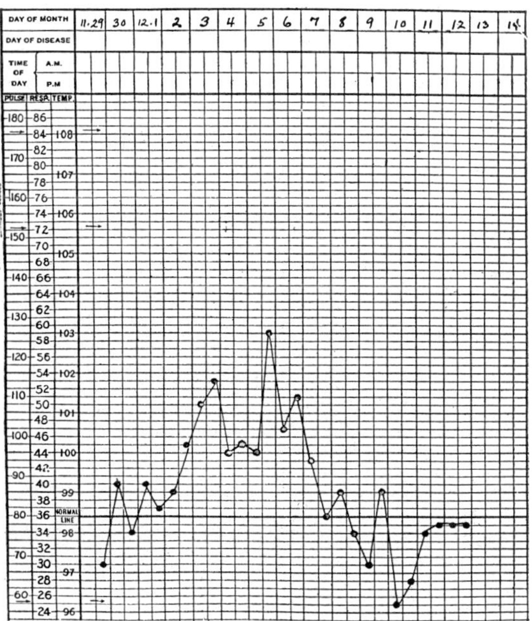

Fig. 32.—Transitory fever in the new-born. Baby M., born Nov. 29. Persistent fever and loss of weight. Weighing before and after each nursing showed an insufficient amount of milk furnished. After supplemental feeding was commenced Dec. 6 the temperature fell and gain in weight began.

is every reason to consider that dehydration is the most likely explanation in the majority of instances. It is well known that loss of water from the tissues or lack of water imbibed can cause febrile rises, and it has been shown by Bakwin[10] that the fever in new-born infants is associated with increase in the concentration of serum-protein; fall in temperature being coincident with an increase in plasma-water. It is seen, too, that those infants who lose most weight are oftenest the ones who have fever, and that the giving of fluids usually causes it to disappear promptly.

The **symptoms** attending transitory fever are more or less characteristic. The appetite is often diminished and the children nurse poorly from the breast or the bottle. In other cases they suck with avidity, as an evidence of hunger and thirst, without obtaining much milk. There is restlessness or, in more severe cases, prostration and little movement of the body. Loss of weight continues while the fever lasts, and is usually greater than in normal infants. The temperature reaches 39 C. (102.2 F.) or often more.

Its duration is two to three days, sometimes with intermissions, and the fall is generally rapid.

The **prognosis** is good in the majority of cases, except that the continued and increasing loss of weight may exert a serious influence upon the insant. The **diagnosis** is on this account very important. A careful examination will usually reveal the causes of fever of any other nature than that now under consideration, and such an examination must, of course, invariably be made. The **treatment** in all cases dependent upon insufficient food or liquid is simple. In addition to the free supply of breast-milk or of water, other measures are entirely symptomatic. Eder and Bakewell,[11] believing that there is an acidosis due to the dehydration, recommend as a prophylactic measure the administration every four hours during the first few days of life 2 oz. (60) of a 5 per cent lactose solution, to which has been added 5 grains (0.3) of sodium citrate. The administration of purgatives has no place in the treatment.

References

1. Jahrb. f. Kinderh., 1891, **32,** 68. 2. Pediatria, 1915, **23,** 768. 3. Am. J. Obst. and Gynec., 1929, **18,** 863. 4. J.A.M.A., 1921, **77,** 1720. 5. Am. J. Dis. Child., 1922, **22,** 44. 6. Ztschr. f. Geburtsh. u. Gynäk., 1916, **78,** 119. 7. Jahrb. f. Kinderh., 1917, **96,** 175. 8. Arch. Pediat., 1895, **12,** 561. 9. Berl. klin. Wchnschr., 1910, **47,** 673. 10. Am. J. Dis. Child., 1922, **24,** 508. 11. Am. J. Dis. Child., 1931, **42,** 1079.

SECTION II

THE INFECTIOUS DISEASES

CHAPTER I

GENERAL

DEFINITION

In the widest sense an "infectious" disease is one due to a specific living organism of some sort which "infects" the human body; while "contagious" indicates merely that a disease may be contracted by one person by contact, directly or indirectly, with another. In the usual narrower sense the term "infectious" denotes a certain general invasion of the organism by specific germs of some sort and with symptoms of a specific nature. The diseases of this class with a comparatively short course are called the "acute infectious diseases"; or, if febrile, the "acute infectious fevers." The others are designated "chronic infectious diseases." Many of the first class are attended by special cutaneous eruptions, and to those the title "acute exanthemata" is often applied. The course of the infectious diseases is often marked by certain stages or periods designated by special terms. That during which the germs are developing in the body without characteristic manifestations is called the *period of incubation*. On this follows the *prodromal stage* or *period of invasion*, during which the *initial symptoms* appear. After this is the stage of the fully developed disease, or *stage of florition*, in the case of the exanthemata called the *period of eruption*. Last comes the *stage of decline*, in the eruptive fevers sometimes designated the *period of desquamation*.

No accurate classification of the infectious disorders is possible at this time of rapidly advancing knowledge. Those which will be discussed here have been separated from other infections as a matter of convenience. At times two or even more acute infectious diseases may affect a patient simultaneously or one shortly after the other. Many of these multiple infections are simply coincidental. We have seen as many as three occur almost simultaneously. In other instances, such as the combination of scarlet fever and diphtheria, it may well be that the lowered local resistance occasioned by one disease predisposes to the other.

METHOD OF DISSEMINATION

The chief source of infection is close contact with or proximity to the patient himself, the disease being communicated to others either before it has been recognized and the individual isolated, or given after quarantine has been removed. It is usually by means of the mucous secretion of the infected person; often through the microscopic drops of mucus which are coughed or sneezed out or carried upon the breath, these reaching the respiratory tract of the previously healthy individual. In numerous instances the disorder has been perhaps so mild that it has not been recognized at all, and the child has remained an undiscovered source of infection. Those who have recovered from an infectious disease but who still harbor its active infectious germs are called "carriers," and the same title is applied to the smaller, but still quite large, class comprising those who have not been ill, but who have been in close contact with patients, and who carry the germs for a considerable time upon their mucous membranes. It is almost solely in this way that the virus is transmitted by a third healthy person, and the danger is probably less than from those who have suffered from the disease. The possibility of the dissemination by air, dust, water, milk, insects, and in other ways will be considered under the headings of the various infectious disorders.

GENERAL RULES FOR THE HYGIENIC CARE AND THE QUARANTINE OF INFECTIOUS DISEASES

The diseases under consideration vary greatly in their relative infectiousness, and in the mode by which the germs are chiefly conveyed. The following rules are those to be applied where rigorous prophylactic measures are to be carried out. Circumstances may well alter either the possibility or the necessity of their application. It has repeatedly been shown in hospital-practice that it is perfectly possible, with proper precaution by the aid of the "box-method," to treat many of the infectious diseases in the general wards without extension taking place (see Koplik,[1] von Pirquet,[2] Richardson,[3] Rundle and Burton,[4] Feer[5] and others on the Box-System and similar methods in hospital practice).

Room.—If the patient is kept at home the room should preferably be in the upper portion of the house. Here the patient is less liable to be disturbed by noises, and here, too, isolation can be better carried out. It should open into another room, which we may call the anteroom. This should be, if possible, a bath-room or a room opening into it. The temperature of the sick-room should be from 65 to 70 F. (18.3 to 21.1 C.). The door entering it from the hallway should be locked. The door from the anteroom into the hallway should be kept closed except at the time of exit or entry.

The sick-room should have all unnecessary articles removed. Only such books and toys may remain as shall afterward be destroyed or sterilized. The room should be kept very clean, all dust being removed by wiping with a 1:1000 bichloride or other antiseptic solution. The bichloride solution must not be used upon metal.

Patient.—The food for the patient and nurse should be brought to the door of the anteroom by an attendant. After the dishes, spoons or other articles have been used, they should be washed, and either boiled or immersed for some time in a 5 per cent solution of carbolic acid. All bed-clothes and body-clothing should be changed frequently and should be put into a 5 per cent solution of carbolic acid or a 1:1000 solution of corrosive sublimate kept in the anteroom. After thorough soaking they should be wrung out, placed in a bucket, and taken by an attendant from the nurse at the door of the anteroom. They may now be washed with the other linen of the house without danger. Old linen or muslin cloths and absorbent cotton or paper napkins may well replace handkerchiefs, since they can be destroyed at once after use. The utmost care should be taken to receive and disinfect or destroy promptly all discharges from the eyes, nose, mouth and, in the case of typhoid fever, the intestine and bladder. When there is free expectoration, paper or other sputum-cups holding a 5 per cent solution of carbolic acid or similar disinfectant may be employed.

Attendants.—The nurse should be dressed in washable material, and should have a cap to cover thoroughly the hair and the neck. She should have her meals in the sick-room or, better, anteroom, and leave it only when about to pass through the house on her way out. Before doing this she should slip off her outer garment, wash her hands and face with soap and water and then with diluted alcohol or some other antiseptic solution, and go directly out without stopping to talk with members of the family. Those of the family who must necessarily enter the room to relieve the nurse should adopt similar precautions. With proper care the confinement of the nurse to the sick-room during the whole of the disease is entirely unnecessary. The physician, too, should on entering the anteroom array himself in a linen or rubber garment. A linen dust-coat is very serviceable for this purpose. He should wear a cap upon his head. Before leaving the anteroom he should remove these articles, and disinfect his hands and face carefully. It is questionable whether the wearing of a face-mask by the nurse gives her any protection, or shields the patient if the nurse is suffering from a respiratory disorder. Whenever possible only immune nurses in perfect health may be employed.

Family.—Other nonimmune children should, when possible, be removed from the house, and should not be allowed to go to school or mingle with others until a time has elapsed equal to the duration of incubation. If obliged to reside in the house they should not associate with other children until the patient is removed from quarantine. In case, however, they have already had the disease, there is no actual reason why they may not safely be with other children if the measures for isolation of the patient are being properly carried out.

Final Disinfection.—When the disease is over the patient may receive a thorough bath with soap and water, followed by an application of an antiseptic solution, such as diluted alcohol or a 1:10,000 bichloride solution. (See p. 194.) He should then be dressed in entirely clean underclothing and removed to another room. The outer clothing in use at the time the disease began, as well as carpets, mattresses, pillows, and the like should be autoclaved, or, if this is not possible, thoroughly exposed to fresh air and sunlight. The woodwork, walls, and furniture should be scrubbed with soap and water and then with a 1:1000 bichloride solution. In such diseases as scarlet fever and diphtheria the walls, if papered, should be scraped and repapered. For all metal work a 5 per cent carbolic acid solution may be used. Fumigation is of practically no value and little employed at present.

References

1. Arch. Pediat., 1911, **28,** 728; 1912, **29,** 5. 2. Ztschr. f. Kinderh., Orig. 1913, **5,** 213. 3. J.A.M.A., 1913, **61,** 1882. 4. Lancet, 1912, **1,** 720. 5. Correspondbl. f. Schweiz. Aerzte, 1919, **49,** 777.

CHAPTER II

SCARLET FEVER

(Scarlatina)

History.—It is probable that scarlet fever was not distinguished from other eruptive fevers until about the middle of the seventeenth century. At this time Sennert[1] gave a good clinical description of an epidemic. Sydenham[2] appears to have been the first to distinguish it clearly from measles, and to apply to it its present name.

Etiology. Predisposing Causes.—Although the disease is far more common in Europe and America than elsewhere, there appears to be little influence that can be attributed directly to *climatic* and *geographical* conditions, except that it is rare in the tropics. The influence of *season* is not very considerable, although the greater number of cases occur usually in the winter and especially in the autumn months. *Sex, hygienic conditions* and the *previous state of health* possess no certain predisposing relationship. Stickler[3] and Kobrack,[4] however, claim that the incidence and severity are less in poorly nourished children than in overfed ones with the exudative diathesis. *Race* is of some importance. Fischer [5] and Kleine and Kroo[6] found scarlatina rare in African natives, and in these the Dick test also was usually negative and the antitoxin content of the blood high. Emerson[7] noted a racial influence in studying various groups in New York; Toyoda, Moriwaki and Futagi[8] observed a difference between Chinese and Japanese; and in Cincinnati we have found negroes less susceptible than whites. The influence of *age* is very great. Although scarlet fever may possibly occur congenitally (Gigon;[9] Liddell and Tangye;[10] Cozzolino[11]), by far the greatest incidence is between the ages of five and ten years, and next between two and five years. The incidence under one year is less than 1 per cent of all cases. Our youngest case was in an infant of three months. However, under six months of age the danger of contracting the disease is so slight that weaning when the mother is suffering from it is hardly necessary. We have seen 3 nursing infants unattacked, although in a scarlet fever ward with their mothers. Lemarquand[12] records 22 similar instances and collected the reports of a number of others.

The *individual susceptibility* varies greatly. Some individuals appear immune although repeatedly exposed, this corresponding closely with the results of the Dick test. (See p. 265.) As previously noted, there seems to be a racial immunity even in localities where scarlet fever had never been endemic. This was illustrated in one of the chief towns in the Faroe Islands, where only 38.3 per cent of exposed unprotected persons contracted scarlatina, whereas 99 per cent contracted measles (Hoff[13]). The spread of scarlatina is much more controllable than is that of measles or chickenpox.

The small number of cases occurring in early infancy is due partly to lack of exposure, but more to the transmission of maternal antitoxin, as shown by the studies of Paunz and Csoma.[14] The skin of the new-born infant is usually not sensitive to scarlatinal toxin even in the absence of antitoxin in the blood (Cooke[15]). The immunity of older persons is probably in part due to repeated exposure to the causative agent which stimulates antitoxin formation, yet without the production of active symptoms. That this is not the entire explanation is shown by the Faroe observations already quoted, in which there was greater immunity in adults, although there had apparently never been exposure to the disease.

Exciting Cause.—It has long been known that streptococci can be obtained from the throat, blood, lymphatic glands and the complicating lesions of scarlet fever patients. Klein[16] as early as 1887, reported the *streptococcus scarlatinae.* (See also serum-treatment, p. 266.) Successful transmission to animals was announced by Landsteiner, Levaditi and Prasek;[17] Bernhardt;[18] Schleissner;[19] and Dochez and Sherman.[20] However, Draper and Hanford;[21] Klimenko;[22] Krumwiede, Nicoll and Pratt;[23] and others could not confirm this. After the development by Dochez, Avery, and Lancefield[24] of a method for differentiation of types of streptococcus haemolyticus, work by Tunnicliff,[25] Gordon,[26] Bliss,[27] Dochez and Sherman,[20] Dick and Dick,[28] Hektoen,[29] Thomson and Thomson,[30] and others seemed to associate a specific type of hemolytic streptococcus with scarlet fever. It should be mentioned that some investigators, such as Kirkbride and Wheeler;[31] Toyoda, Moriwaki, Futagi and Hoshizaki;[32] and Wheeler[33] do not believe that scarlet fever streptococci possess a specificity which distinguishes them from other hemolytic streptococci. However, the experimental production of scarlet fever in man by Dick and Dick[28] and others; the development of an antiserum with curative power by Dochez and Sherman,[20] Blake and coworkers,[34] and Dick and Dick;[35] and the discovery by the last mentioned[36] that scarlet fever toxin produces a cutaneous reaction in those who are susceptible to the disease (p. 265), all argue for a definite causative action of these micro-organisms. Some investigators, as Zlatogoroff[37] and Cantacuzene,[38] favor the view that there is in addition to the streptococcus an associated virus of some sort. Interesting studies by Cooke[39] and by Dochez and Stevens[40] support the idea previously expressed by Meyer[41] and others, that some of the symptoms, such as the rash, may be allergic in nature, Dochez and Stevens[40] maintaining that the scarlet fever streptococcus does not produce a toxin in the true sense, but an "allergin" or "toxallergin." Escherich and Schick,[42] and Zinsser and Grinell[43] also subscribe to the theory that certain of the symptoms and complications, such as arthritis, adenitis and late cardiac lesions, are due to acquired hypersensitiveness to the scarlet fever toxin.

There seems, then, to be no doubt that the hemolytic streptococcus is associated in some way with scarlet fever, and most of the evidence is in favor of etiologic connection of a specific type of it. Certain of the symptoms and sequels, however, can be better explained as allergic manifestations, and this explanation may eventually prove to be the true one.

To be mentioned for completeness only are the diplococcus described by Class[44] and Baginsky and Sommerfeld;[45] the protozoan-like "cyclaster scarlatinalis" of Mallory;[46] the large coccus of Pryer;[47] and the anaerobic diplococcus of di Cristina.[48]

Method of Transmission.—This is usually direct from the sick to the well, or infrequently mediate through fomites. The disease has exceptionally been carried for some distance by the clothing of physicians and nurses, or been transmitted by letters, toys and books, or carried by animals. There are many reports of its spread by contaminated milk. The individual susceptibility to the disease is not as great as with certain other disorders (p. 252). Spread may at times take place by contact with convalescents who have persistent discharges (p. 249), and by means of healthy carriers (Tunnicliff and Crooks[49]). It is also certain that scarlatinal sore-throat may occur without other symptoms of scarlet fever, and that such patients can transmit the disease. The germs do not appear to be carried any distance by air.

Portal of Entry.—This is by way of the nasopharyngeal mucous membrane, but may be through a wound. (See p. 255.)

Period of Maximum Infectivity.—Probably the most active period is that of the height of the eruption, but the latter part of incubation and the beginning of the stage of invasion certainly possess infectious power (see also Prophylaxis, p. 264), and the disease can be transmitted even after the stage of desquamation is over. The duration of the persistence of the infectivity of the virus is uncertain. Formerly it was believed that the tenacity of life was very great, but this is now considered doubtful.

Seat of the Virus.—The secretion from the nose and throat and often from a complicating otitis, empyema, or other source of pus, is undoubtedly infectious. There is doubt regarding the urine and feces, but the desquamation is certainly noninfectious unless contaminated.

Pathologic Anatomy.—There are no definite lesions characteristic of the disease except those of the skin and of the mucous membrane of the mouth and throat. The intense hyperemia present during life disappears after death. There is found, however, a dilatation of the lymphatics and blood-vessels of the *skin*, with a swelling of the cells of the rete, sometimes with extravasations of blood between them. Infiltration of all the layers of the skin by serum and leukocytes takes place, and rapid destruction of the upper cells of the epidermis follows, resulting in desquamation. The *mucous membrane* of the mouth and throat suffers an analogous inflammation with desquamation, particularly well seen on the tongue, and producing, in typical cases, the strawberry appearance. The faucial inflammation may spread to the nose and ears, and thence to the mastoid cells and even the meninges. There is wide-spread involvement of the *lymphatic tissue* throughout the body but especially in the nodes of the neck. The liver and spleen may be enlarged. Endocarditis and pericarditis are not uncommon, and pleuritis and pneumonia may occur. Parenchymatous changes may be found in any of the organs of the body. (See also Complications.)

Symptoms. TYPICAL SCARLET FEVER. **Period of Incubation.**—In general this may be placed at from one day to one week, or exceptionally longer, but in by far the majority of cases from two to four days. As a rule the danger of developing the disease may be considered over after seven days from exposure have elapsed. In cases of surgical scarlet fever, as for instance after tracheotomy or tonsillectomy, the period of incubation is usually very short. Severe cases also appear to have a shorter period of incubation.

Period of Invasion.—The onset is generally of great suddenness. Except in older children there is usually no distinct initial chill, although there may be chilliness and pallor. Convulsions are often among the first symptoms in quite young children. Vomiting, often repeated, occurs at the onset in the great majority of cases. Diarrhea occasionally accompanies it. The temperature rapidly rises to 103 or 104 F. (39.4 or 40 C.) or more, and the face becomes flushed. The pulse is rapid and there is headache and generally sore throat, of which, however, young children often make no complaint. The child looks and feels ill, sleeps badly, and is restless and decidedly prostrated. The lymphatic nodes of the neck begin to enlarge. The eruption is now found in the throat (enanthem), giving a characteristic appearance; the mucous membrane, namely, of the hard and soft palate, the tonsils, and the anterior pillars of the fauces being unusually red, due to the presence here of closely packed, minute, dark-red macules. This condition rapidly spreads to the lining of the cheeks and gums. The macules may be distinctly visible or they may have so fused that only a uniform red flush is perceptible. The tongue is coated with the edges sometimes reddened. The tonsils are swollen and often exhibit whitish spots due to secretion retained in the follicles.

The duration of the invasion is short, from twelve hours or occasionally less up to twenty-four hours. Exceptionally it may reach forty-eight hours. It is of very common occurrence for a child to exhibit the febrile symptoms and vomiting during the night, and to be found with the cutaneous eruption well-developed by morning. In very mild cases there may be no prodromes whatever or none discovered.

Period of Eruption. *The Rash.*—The termination of the period of invasion is marked by the appearance of the rash on the skin. This develops first on the neck and upper portion of the chest; thence spreading rapidly to the rest of the trunk, the arms, and finally the lower extremities. Generally the face is little or not at all involved, the forehead and especially the circle about the mouth standing out prominently and being of a pale-white color in contrast with the rest of the body; the cheeks being flushed, but not the seat of a truly punctate eruption. In exceptional cases, however, there is an extensive development of eruption on the face, but even then the pale oral circle is usually to be found. Viewed superficially the rash seems to be of a uniformly red color, but careful inspection shows it to consist of very minute, closely packed red points situated on a white base. Later the red hue of the punctae grows duskier while the white base takes on a shade of red as well. Though now more confluent the punctate character can still always be discovered. The eruption generally has spread to its full extent in twenty-four hours and often less. Sometimes, however, two or three days are required for this. Its greatest intensity of color may also be reached within twenty-four hours, but is usually not attained for two or three days. Where the integument is softest and finest the eruption is generally especially intense and most confluent. The skin is now hot, dry and somewhat swollen, the swelling being frequently particularly marked on the hands and feet. It often feels slightly rough to the hand rubbed over it. Decided itching is common. Drawing the fingernail over the red skin leaves for a moment a strikingly white line. This, though very suggestive, is not absolutely characteristic.

The rash maintains its intensity for from one to three days and then fades rapidly, following the order of its appearance. The total duration of the eruption is extremely variable. An average may be said to be from three to seven days. A faint underlying yellowish tinge is often discovered when the skin is pressed upon or as the eruption fades.

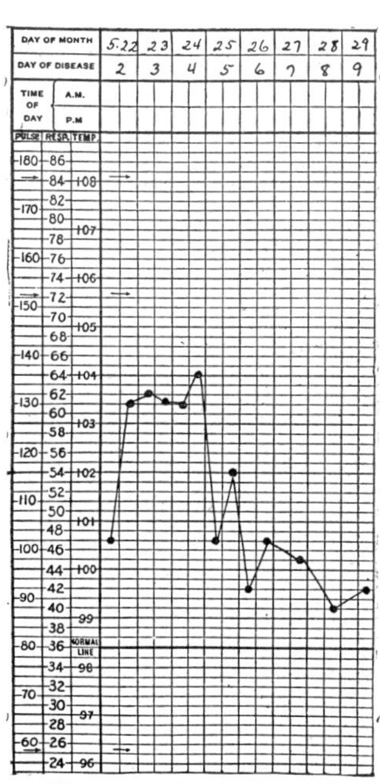

Fig. 33.—Scarlatina. Average case. Andreas L., aged eight and one-half years. May 21, nausea in evening, fever, sore throat; May 22, vomiting, diarrhea, secretion in tonsillar crypts, eruption on body; May 23, sore throat, restlessness; May 24, eruption very abundant; May 25, eruption duskier, tongue entirely denuded; May 27, eruption fading, throat and tongue sore; May 29, sore throat no longer complained of.

Normal Variations of the Eruption.—A number of variations occur in the eruption within the limits of the typical case. The color varies through many shades of red, from a pale rose to that of a boiled lobster, or to a deep red with a slightly brownish or bluish tint. When the eruption is not very extensive it may appear in smaller or larger blotches in some part of the body leaving other parts, especially areas on the extremities, entirely free (*Scarlatina variegata*). Sometimes it is macular in some portions and here strikingly suggests measles. In many cases the skin is unusually rough, due to the presence of much infiltration in the minute red punctae (*Scarlatina papulosa*), while in a large number there is a greater or less development of miliary vesicles (*Scarlatina miliaris*). These vesicles may occur in any part of the body. We[50] have seen them so abundant that the scarlatinal color of the underlying skin was almost totally concealed and the diagnosis made difficult. As a rule, however, they are few in number. Their occurrence does not appear to us to bear any relationship to the intensity of the ordinary scarlatinal rash, the amount of desquamation, or the severity of the case. In rare cases the vesicles may coalesce to a considerable extent, forming small blebs (*Scarlatina pemphigoides*).

In the so-called "*Surgical Scarlet Fever*" the rash develops sometimes first in the neighborhood of a wound, including lesions of the puerperium, and thence spreads over the body; or very soon after the receiving of the wound the rash may appear first on the neck or chest in the ordinary way, and follow the usual sequence in its spread; it being supposed that the infection gained entrance through the wound. In this category belong those cases developing after tonsillectomy, tracheotomy or extraction of abscessed teeth. The symptoms do not differ materially from those of the disease as usually seen. There has been much discussion as to the reality of surgical scarlet fever. There is reason to believe that it does exist, and we have seen it the cause of spread to others. Such patients should, therefore, be kept in scarlet fever wards or under isolation.

Retrocession of the Eruption.—It happens often that the rash soon after its appearance suddenly fades, or, as it is commonly called, has "struck in," the other symptoms persisting or growing worse. This disappearance is often the result of a feeble action of the heart. It is not the cause of unfavorable symptoms, but the accompaniment of them.

Other Symptoms of the Stage of Eruption.—The eruption of the mucous membrane of the *mouth and throat* (enanthem) is reaching its height when that of the skin begins to appear. The intense redness of the mucous membrane persists, and the tonsils, if not already affected, generally exhibit lacunae filled with secretion, while swallowing is painful. The tongue begins to lose its white coating, and by the third to the fifth day of the disease has become entirely denuded, bright-red and with the fungiform papillae swollen and prominent. The result is the "strawberry" or "raspberry" tongue. These titles have often been misapplied to the condition seen during invasion and in many other diseases, where the red papillae, especially on the edges and tip, show prominently through the white coating. In many cases the tongue never becomes denuded throughout. In typical cases the throat improves as the cutaneous rash and the other symptoms abate. By the seventh or eighth day of the disease the tongue appears nearly normal, yet close examination will still show some degree of redness and swelling of the papillae at the edges and tip after other symptoms of the stage of eruption have entirely disappeared. The nose often exhibits a mucopurulent discharge. The lymphatic nodes of the superficies of the body are found swollen, those of the neck, groins and axillae and those below the body of the jaw being most noticeably so, and tenderness on pressure is present. The spleen is often palpable. The *temperature* (Fig. 33) is subject to great variations, and no typical curve exists. As a rule it reaches its height from the second to the third day and continues at 102 to 104 F. (38.9 to 40 C.) with little variation between morning and evening, its elevation being generally in proportion to the severity of the attack. It begins to diminish as the eruption fades, falling by lysis, and reaching normal about the ninth or tenth day. Very often the elevation of temperature lasts a much shorter time than this. The pulse is rapid, often out of proportion to the elevation of temperature. This is generally considered one of the characteristics of the disease. The blood-pressure is sometimes reduced (Rolleston[51]) but its condition possesses little practical significance unless nephritis occurs. The bowels are usually not disturbed, and vomiting is not common during this stage. There are thirst and loss of appetite. Slight delirium may develop during the height of the fever. Either somnolence or restlessness may be present.

The *urine* is high-colored and diminished in amount and, if the temperature is high, may exhibit febrile albuminuria with cylindroids and possibly a few hyaline casts; but blood-cells and granular casts do not occur unless a complicating nephritis develops. The diazo reaction is sometimes positive and urobilin is often found (Rach and Reuss[52]).

The *blood* shows a diminution in the number of red blood-cells and hemoglobin, the percentages returning to normal after several weeks. Leukocytosis develops and may be from 15,000 to 40,000 or more, depending on the severity of complications. In mild and uncomplicated cases the count may return to normal by five to seven days. More characteristic is the polymorphonuclear leukocytosis occurring during the stages of invasion and eruption, which may be from 80 or 90 per cent. The mononuclear cells are diminished. Many studies have shown a diminution of eosinophiles at first, with a rise during defervescence and convalescence which may reach as high as 20 per cent. Iodophilia is reported by Neutra[53] and Magi,[54] and an increase in platelets during convalescence by Schiff and Matyas.[55] Valdimirowa[56] claims that the organic acid content of the blood is increased early in scarlet fever, and Markoma[57] that the chlorine is diminished. In the polymorphonuclear cells of the blood as well as in the internal organs Döhle[58] discovered certain "inclusion bodies" and probably similar bodies were described by Amato.[59] Whatever their nature they are not specific for scarlet fever. While it has often been stated that the Wassermann reaction is positive in scarlet fever, all the later evidence is that when it is strongly so syphilis should be suspected.

Period of Desquamation.—As other symptoms abate and the eruption fades the skin is left dry and rough and desquamation begins, starting in the localities first invaded by the rash. Usually the process may be said

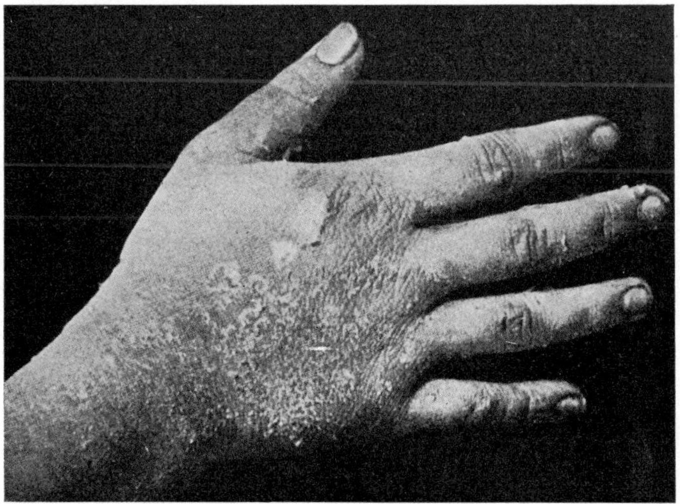

Fig. 34.—Scarlet fever. Well-marked desquamation upon the dorsum of the hands and fingers, showing the lamellar peeling. (*Welch and Schamberg, Acute Contagious Diseases*, 1905, 377.)

to commence at the end of the first week of the disease, but to this there are many exceptions. The scaling is of two forms. The first is a branny desquamation somewhat similar to that seen in measles, and occurs on the head, neck and upper portion of the trunk. Upon the hands and feet the second form is shown as a very characteristic lamellar peeling, the dead skin coming off in larger or smaller strips (Fig. 34) leaving a sharp contrast between the pink new skin exposed and the remaining greyish-white old skin. It begins here often at the tips of the fingers and toes and especially about the roots of the nails. Occasionally the skin is shed from the hands and feet in the form of true casts. The desquamation of the hands and feet is so characteristic that the diagnosis can often be based on this alone. On the rest of the body, and especially well-marked on the lower portion of the trunk, the branny desquamation begins as a small white scale which separates, leaving a pin-hole-like opening to the new skin beneath. The skin surrounding this gradually peels off, enlarging the pin-holes to wider circles which finally fuse.

In some instances the forms may be combined to a large extent throughout the body, except on the hands and feet where only the lamellar form occurs. Very frequently desquamation is absent or difficult to discover. This is especially true if the body has been bathed or oiled often. The scaling continues for from ten days or less up to two or three weeks. It begins last and continues longest on the hands and feet, and here four or even seven or eight weeks may not see it completed. Often it may not have commenced on the hands and feet by the time it is nearly or quite over on the rest of the body. Not infrequently after scaling has apparently ceased it recommences, and this process may be repeated several times. The duration and degree of desquamation usually bear some, but no necessary, relationship to the severity of the case and intensity of the eruption. There is reason to believe that it is even possible for desquamation to occur in regions where there has been no rash whatever; consequently other

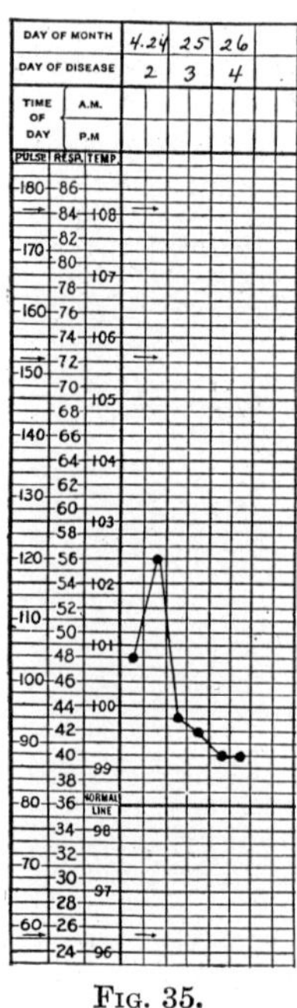

Fig. 35.

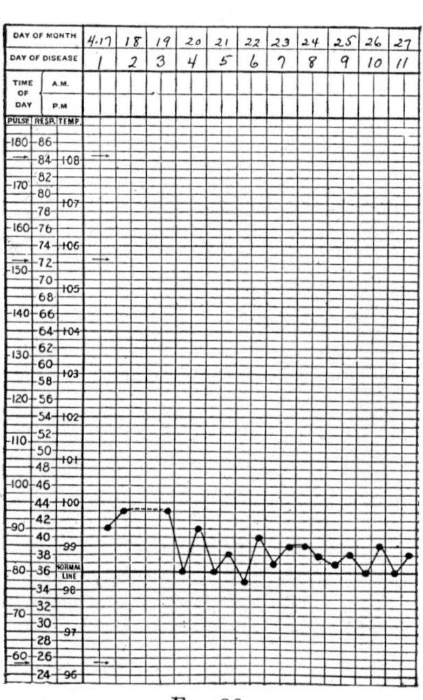

Fig. 36.

Fig. 35.—Scarlatina; abortive form. Weightman F., aged nine years. Apr. 23, vomited; Apr. 24, rash appearing; Apr. 25, rash at height, well developed; Apr. 26, tongue beginning to peel; May 13, desquamation on hands and feet discovered; none found elsewhere.

Fig. 36.—Scarlatina afebrilis. Henry P., aged nine years. Typical rash, slight redness of throat, moderate development of strawberry tongue. Later slight scarlatinal desquamation and albuminuria with casts.

causes than the mere hyperemia of the skin would appear to be active agents in producing it.

Desquamation affects other epithelial structures as well. The nails show the effect of the disorder to a greater or less extent, perhaps in the form of a transverse furrow observed after convalescence, and the hair becomes brittle and falls. The teeth, too, are sometimes affected by the disease and later exhibit erosions. In cases where miliaria has been extensive a fine branny scaling may take place early. This is not to be confounded with the true scarlatinal desquamation which occurs later. During the stage of desquamation all other symptoms are absent in normal cases and the patient feels well.

Atypical Types of Scarlet Fever. (Mild; Severe; Anginose; Malignant; Hemorrhagic).—Different classifications of the varieties of scarlet fever have been made. There are no strict boundaries separating one from another, but a convenient division is the following:

Mild Forms.—The attack may be unusually mild throughout, or some of the symptoms may be absent entirely; (*a*) The whole process may be over in two or three days except perhaps for the desquamation later (Fig. 35) (*Abortive scarlet fever*); (*b*) The eruption may not develop at all (*Scarlatina sine eruptione*); (*c*) Fever may be absent or nearly so (*Scarlatina afebrilis*) (Fig. 36). (*d*) Inflammation of the pharynx may be absent or slight (*Scarlatina sine angina*).

Severe Forms.—(*a*) In the ordinary severe form as most commonly seen all the symptoms of the disease may be present to an unusual degree; (*b*) The severity may depend on the special prominence of one or a few symptoms or complications, the attack being, therefore, "rudimentary" so far as the complete development of the disease is concerned; (*c*) There may occur differences in the development of the eruption. In many severe cases it may be faint, localized, blotchy, and tending constantly to fade; (*d*) There may be long continuence of fever and nervous symptoms without discoverable reason (*Scarlatina typhosa*); (*e*) The anginose symptoms and the cervical adenitis may be unusually severe (*Scarlatina anginosa*); (*f*) Nervous symptoms may be extremely severe, with marked cerebral irritation (*Scarlatina maligna*) (Fig. 37), (*g*) There may be hematuria, purpura, and hemorrhages from other parts of the body (*Scarlatina haemorrhagica*).

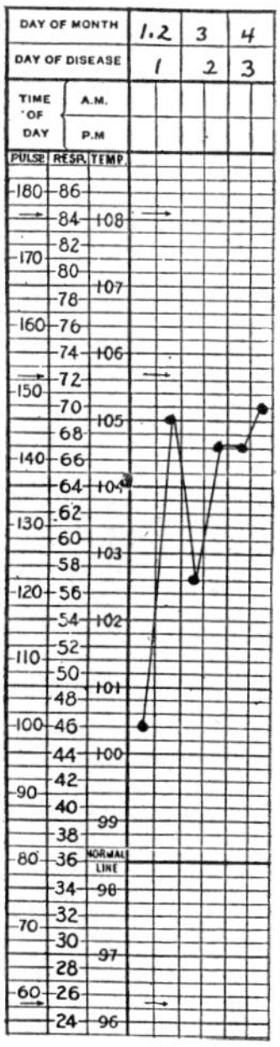

Fig. 37.—Malignant scarlet fever. Domenick S., aged two years. Jan. 2, vomiting, dyspnea and irregular respiration; Jan. 3, red, uncharacteristic eruption, throat red, tonsils enlarged; Jan. 4, wide-spread, abundant petechial eruption combined with the scarlatinal rash, coma, respiration rapid and dyspneic, pulse rapid, tonsillar exudate; Jan. 5, death at 1 A. M.

Complications and Sequels.—It is difficult to state the actual frequency of complications since this varies with epidemics.

Throat and Nose.—It is only when the inflammatory process goes on to the development of a pseudomembrane, perhaps followed by extensive necrotic changes, that the condition can be considered as a complication. This occurs so often that it characterizes one of the variant forms of the disease. Patients previously tonsillectomized have, as a rule, less severe angina and adenitis. Purulent rhinitis may develop.

Ears.—The frequency of otitis media varies, according to our own experience and the figures reported in the literature, from about 2 to 15 per cent or more. It may occur early, or as late as during the second or third week. It is frequently suppurative rather than simply catarrhal, often bilateral, and mastoid disease necessitating operation not uncommonly develops. Younger children are more predisposed to it, as are those with severe angina. Partial or complete deafness is often an unfortunate sequel. Burkhardt-Merian[60] found that of 85 cases of deafness there was a history of scarlet fever in 21 per cent.

Cervical Adenitis.—The lymphatic nodes of the neck are always somewhat enlarged in all cases where sore throat is a prominent symptom. Sometimes they become greatly so, and may advance to the formation of abscess. This takes place oftenest as a sequel in the second week or later. It is attended by fever, but not by any marked septic symptoms, and is relieved by rupture or by incision; but oftenest in our experience the adenitis subsides spontaneously after several days. In severe cases it may go on to cellulitis and sloughing of the tissues of the neck. According to the statistics in the literature cervical adenitis of degree sufficient to be called a complication is found in from 6 to 12 per cent or more of cases. In some epidemics we have seen it as high as 20 per cent.

Arthritis (Fig. 38).—The incidence of this complication varies from about 3 to 20 per cent according to statistics. An average figure according to our own experience would be about 5 per cent. It occurs generally in those past early childhood, and often about the end of the first week; involves especially the hands, fingers and elbows; lasts generally not more than three or four days; and is a mild affection with little or no swelling and redness of joints but, however, with definite pain. The likelihood of its development bears no relation to the severity of the scarlatinal attack. Its nature is that of a synovitis. It rarely terminates in suppuration.

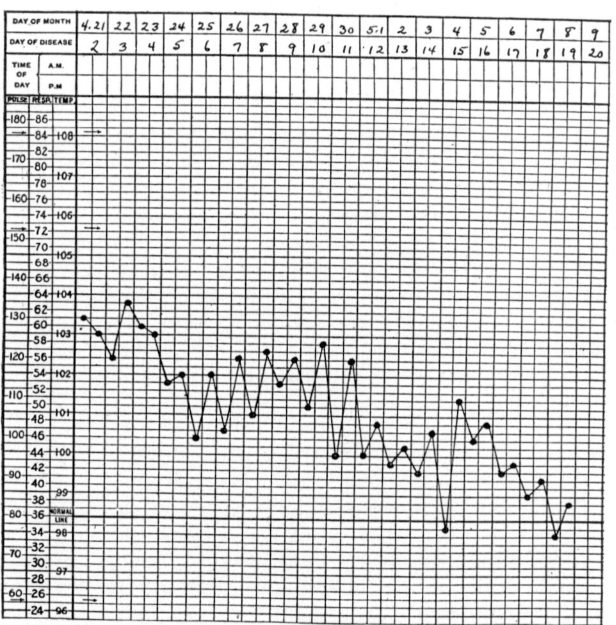

Fig. 38.—Scarlet fever with temperature prolonged by arthritis. Genette F., aged five years. Apr. 20, fever, vomiting; Apr. 21, well-developed eruption; Apr. 22, a few white spots on tonsils; Apr. 23, rash at maximum, tongue peeling; Apr. 24, rash fading; Apr. 26, multiple arthritis, involving fingers, elbows, knees and ankles; May 5, joints improving.

Nephritis.—The incidence and severity of this complication vary greatly in epidemics, figures given in the literature being from 3 to 20 per cent. An average percentage would be 5 or less. In some epidemics under our observation less than 1 per cent of the patients developed nephritis. In the first weeks there may be a febrile albuminuria and cylinduria which cannot properly be called evidences of nephritis; but a severe nephritis may occasionally develop during the height of the disease. This is very common in the malignant cases. The most frequent form, however, is that denominated *postscarlatinal*, occurring in the third or fourth week after the onset. It develops as often after mild as after severe cases, and is of the acute hemorrhagic (glomerular) type. It is usually mild and ends in complete recovery, but it may be severe and uremic symptoms ensue and death follow. In comparatively few instances does chronic nephritis result from it, although some cases relapse and continue for several months. (See Nephritis, p. 817.)

The cause of this late nephritis is not clearly understood. Friedemann and Deicher[61] venture the hypothesis that the antibodies so act on the streptococcus that endotoxins are set free, these causing the nephritis.

Circulatory System.—Functional transitory disturbances of the heart are not uncommon during scarlet fever, but serious lesions directly produced by the disease are less frequent. There is an increase in pulse-rate with the fever, but in the second week a bradycardia sometimes develops. Myocarditis may occur in severe cases and a soft systolic murmur be found, but electrocardiographic studies show that myocardial involvement seldom takes place in cases of average severity. Hypertrophy and dilatation accompanying nephritis are sequels rather than complications. Endocarditis and pericarditis occasionally develop as the result of a complicating nephritis, or more rarely still of a rheumatic synovitis, or as part of septic manifestations. Embolism of the pulmonary or other arteries has been observed. Phlebitis and gangrene have been reported (Hunekens and Siperstein,[62] Silberstein,[63] Fedders,[64] Sutherland[65]). The average frequency of involvement of the heart in scarlet fever is illustrated by Rosenbaum's[66] series of 1770 cases, in which cardiac complications occurred in 106. Twelve of these had had previous endocarditis. In the remaining 94 the following diagnoses were made: myocarditis in 88; endocarditis in 4; pericarditis in 3.

Respiratory System.—The general opinion, with which we are in accord, is that pulmonary complications and sequels are not very frequent. Occasional complications are laryngitis, bronchitis, bronchopneumonia, croupous pneumonia, pleurisy and empyema, and, with a complicating nephritis, edema of the lungs and glottis. Kartascheva[67] in 371 necropsies found ulceration of the larynx, trachea, or large bronchi 46 times.

Gastrointestinal Complications.—These are not, as a rule, troublesome. Catarrhal and ulcerative stomatitis may occur. Vomiting is very common at the beginning of the attack. Diarrhea is a frequent complication. It is generally of a catarrhal nature, but may be inflammatory. Slight icterus is very common.

Nervous System.—Among nervous complications and sequels are especially to be mentioned repeated convulsions. At the onset of the attack these generally have little significance, but later they are suggestive of uremia. Encephalitis sometimes occurs with its various manifestations. Meningitis and thrombosis of the cerebral veins or sinuses may develop as sequels depending upon an otitis. Occasionally a meningitis occurs earlier in the disease and independently of any affection of the ear. Hemiplegia has been known to follow meningeal hemorrhage and encephalitis or be caused by embolism dependent upon an endocarditis. Rolleston[68] collected 75 cases of hemiplegia following scarlet fever; 54 recovered but only 17 completely. Paralysis has also been seen as a result of neuritis or of disease of the spinal cord. Chorea and epilepsy are sequels occasionally reported, and various psychoses are on record. Amaurosis may develop as a result of nephritis.

Cutaneous Complications.—Herpes facialis is one of the most common of these, Rolleston[69] finding it 27 times in 413 cases. Urticaria and erythema may appear after the subsidence of the rash, and eczema as a sequel.

Other infectious diseases may occur in combination with scarlet fever or as sequels to it. One of the most frequent and serious combinations is that of scarlet fever and diphtheria, the latter developing generally in a patient already suffering from the former. It is more prone to appear from the third to the sixth week after the attack of scarlet fever, sometimes earlier or later. Measles and scarlet fever have often occurred together. Many other combinations occur, these being chiefly found in hospitals for contagious diseases due to cross-infection. Tuberculosis may be reactivated.

Among other rarer complications or sequels which have been reported may be mentioned perichondritis of the larynx; esophagitis; necrotic inflammation of the stomach; gastric hemorrhage; optic neuritis; periostitis; peritonitis; noma; furunculosis; vulvovaginitis; myositis; pemphigus; glycosuria; and purpura with leukopenia.

Relapse.—Relapse in our experience is not exceedingly rare. It varies, according to reports in the literature, from 0.2 to 4.2 per cent (McCollum,[70] Sloan,[71] Burton and Balmain,[72] Rolleston,[73] and Lichtenstein[74]). In the cases of Burton and Balmain and of Rolleston, in which the incidence of relapse was 4.16 and 0.2 respectively, antitoxin had been given. In Lichtenstein's second study relapse occurred in 6.2 per cent of serum-treated patients, in 9.3 per cent of those not treated with serum and in 1.5 per cent of those treated with convalescent's serum. Relapse consists in the return of some or all of the symptoms after the disease is apparently over. It is seen oftenest in the fourth week but may occur from the fifteenth to the thirty-fifth day (Lettry[75]), may be milder or more severe than the primary attack, and occurs as frequently in mild as in severe cases.

Recurrence.—Recurrence, while rare, does take place, varying in the experience of those who report on the subject from a small fraction of 1 per cent to 2 per cent (Thomas,[76] Henoch,[77] McCrae,[78] Weissenberg,[79] Gabriel and Zischinsky[80]).

Prognosis.—This varies greatly with epidemics and locality, and the mortality is apparently declining in recent years. From reported statistics the mortality varies from less than 1 per cent to as high as 29 per cent, the higher figures being older European ones. In most cities in the United States recent studies show a mortality of 1 or 2 per cent or even less than 1 per cent. The decline has occurred regardless of antitoxin treatment.

Certain conditions affect the prognosis unfavorably. The mortality in early childhood, especially in infancy, is decidedly higher than later in life. Nephritis and septic complications are unfavorable. The mortality is higher in hospitals, probably because the severer and complicated cases are treated there. Toxic, severe, and malignant cases have a serious prognosis, but death in scarlet fever usually depends upon complications rather than upon toxemia.

Diagnosis.—This is not difficult in typical cases, and rests chiefly on the sudden onset with vomiting, high fever and sore throat, followed by the rapid appearance and characteristic spread of the punctate eruption, and later the peculiar desquamation. In very mild cases, however, as well as in the rapidly malignant ones, the diagnosis is often extremely difficult or even impossible. In the latter the rash may be entirely uncharacteristic or even absent. In the former it may be limited to a small area, poorly developed, or transitory and entirely overlooked; the tongue and throat may not present typical changes, and desquamation may not be discovered. Other cases may present only the affection of the throat without the cutaneous eruption. In some instances no desquamation can be found at any time, especially if inunction has been employed. In negroes the diagnosis is often very difficult, owing to the concealment of the eruption by the dark hue of the skin. In some such cases the redness of the palms and soles is suspicious; in others only the occurrence of nephritis, otitis or other sequel, or of the characteristic desquamation, makes the diagnosis clear. Always it is the clinical picture as a whole rather than any one symptom upon which the diagnosis must be based.

As an aid to the recognition of the scarlatinal eruption Pastia[81] described a uniform linear redness in the transverse fold of the skin at the elbow, more intense than the scarlatinal eruption. It is present at the very beginning of the eruptive stage and lasts after the rash has faded. It appears to be produced by capillary hemorrhages. It is of some diagnostic value and appears to be absent in other eruptive fevers, such as measles. The Rumpel[82]-Leede[83] sign is another supposed evidence of the existence of scarlet fever. It consists in the development of punctate hemorrhages into the skin of the elbow-fold after compression of the upper arm has continued from five to twenty minutes. It is claimed to be especially applicable early in the disease. It can be elicited, however, in other diseases and even in normal children. In the extinction or blanching test of Schultz and Charlton[84] convalescent's serum, normal serum (from persons possessing immunity to scarlet fever), or scarlet fever antitoxin in the amount of 0.5 to 1 cc. is injected intradermally into the area of the rash. If the disease is scarlet fever local pallor should occur, persisting until the rash has disappeared elsewhere. Much study has been made of this test. It would appear that the production of blanching points quite strongly to the existence of scarlet fever, but that the failure to produce it does not exclude the disease. It has been shown further by Toomey[85] that many antitoxins on the market produce little or no blanching, and that even local redness may be produced. Sensitivity to horse-serum confuses the test.

It has been claimed that the Dick test is positive in the early days of scarlet fever and becomes negative about the seventh to the tenth day. To this we[86] have found so many exceptions that we cannot consider it helpful in diagnosis.

Certain diseases are especially to be distinguished from scarlet fever. In *rubella* the absence of general symptoms and of scarlatinal changes in the mouth and throat aid in its recognition. So, too, there may nearly always be found somewhere on the body the characteristic macular eruption of rubella, even when the greater part of the surface is covered by a scarlatiniform rash. Yet differentiation is often extremely difficult (see Rubella, p. 285). *Measles* seldom causes any confusion with scarlet fever. The longer incubation and invasion and the catarrhal symptoms of the former, the buccal eruption, and the slower development of the rash are suggestive.

Diphtheria, if attended by an erythema in the early stages, may not be at first distinguishable from scarlet fever with severe anginose symptoms. The difficulty arises, too, in the cases of scarlet fever in which no rash has been discoverable. The close study of the sequence of symptoms will often be of service. The rash in diphtheria is not very frequent, and is generally confined to the trunk. The discovery of the Klebs-Loeffler bacilli would settle the question, were it not that the two diseases may be combined.

Scarlatiniform erythema is one of the most puzzling conditions so far as diagnosis is concerned. This erythema may be due to sepsis, other infectious diseases, various medicaments, or to acute desquamative dermatitis. It is not infrequent in children with slight disturbance of digestion. Sepsis is the cause in diphtheria, and probably also in the majority of the cases called "surgical scarlet fever." The rash resembles that of scarlet fever in appearance, and may be followed by desquamation. The history of the case, the failure of development of the eruption in the usual sequence and extent, and the absence of the other symptoms of scarlatina aid in the diagnosis. Typhoid fever, grippe and varicella occasionally exhibit an erythema early in the attack. The absence of the scarlatinal symptoms, such as the characteristic throat and tongue, the transitory nature of the rash, and the appearance later of the other manifestations characteristic of these different diseases remove the difficulty in diagnosis. The prodromal erythema of variola is distinguished by its peculiar localization. Various erythemata caused by drugs are at times perplexing. Among these are especially those due to quinine, chloral, salicylic acid compounds, belladonna, antipyrine, and animal sera, especially the diphtheria antitoxin. Local irritants such as mustard-plasters have often been the source of confusion. The occurrence of the atropine eruption has especially been a cause of alarm to parents. In none of these are the other symptoms of scarlet fever present, except that occasionally the eruption may be accompanied by fever and vomiting. Quinine will sometimes produce a scarlatiniform eruption followed by very characteristic scarlatiniform desquamation. Acute desquamative dermatitis (recurrent exfoliating dermatitis) is a peculiar affection which may resemble scarlet fever very closely. Probably many cases supposed to be second and third attacks of scarlet fever are really instances of this cutaneous disease. It is attended by fever, a wide-spread erythematous eruption, and often by desquamation which may even occur in the form of casts of the skin of the hands and feet, as in some cases of scarlet fever. In these respects it cannot be distinguished from scarlet fever. Pharyngeal symptoms are, however, absent. In all these conditions the extinction phenomenon is usually not found. (See p. 263.)

Treatment. (*A*) **Prophylaxis. Quarantine.**—Every case of suspected scarlet fever should be isolated in a hospital or in the home (see p. 250), and kept so until all danger of contagion is over. Six weeks is the usual length of quarantine required, although it can not be insisted that so long is entirely necessary in every case, or long enough in cases with purulent discharges. Desquamation, unless contaminated by secretions, cannot be considered a source of contagion, but all abnormal discharges must be regarded with suspicion. The absence of hemolytic streptococci in 2 or 3 cultures from complicating suppurating processes may be used with reasonable safety as a criterion for removal of quarantine, although this is denied by some authors. On the other hand the presence of undifferentiated hemolytic streptococci in the nose and throat is no proof of contagiousness, since they are so frequently found in normal persons. A number of investigators believe that the specificity of the scarlet fever streptococcus is not sufficiently certain to make this the basis of medical regulations for quarantine. Tunnicliff and Crooks,[49] however, describe a relatively simple method based upon the opsonic index for determining whether streptococci are of the scarlet fever type. Our experience is in accord with Gordon's[87] that convalescents with a continuing rhinitis are more responsible than any other group for the transmission of the disease to others, (p. 253) and that adults, as a rule, are less likely than children to transmit the disease. Children who have been tonsillectomized have a lower incidence of scarlet fever than those not treated. (See p. 540.)

Injection of convalescent's serum as reported by Degwitz[88] and others gives encouraging results, almost always in our experience having prophylactic effect. Five to 10 cc. (.17 to .34 fl. oz.) should be given intramuscularly as soon as possible after exposure, larger doses being somewhat more certain. Its preparation is similar to that for measles (see p. 279), except that it should be secured in from the fourth to the seventh week of convalescence. Normal human serum, or whole blood, given in larger doses than convalescent's serum may also be effective, since even those who have not suffered from a known attack of scarlet fever may yet have antitoxin in the blood. The results with the injection of commercial antitoxins are quite uncertain according to the opinion of most authors. With this we agree, and believe that it should seldom be used, since it may produce a general reaction and is also liable to sensitize the patient to horse-serum. When employed the usual dose is 2.5 cc. (.085 fl. oz.). All of these methods give only passive immunity lasting but a few weeks or less.

There is little doubt of the value of *active immunization* by the injection of increasing doses of scarlet fever toxin as developed by Dick and Dick.[89] Immunity develops after one to four weeks, and practically all persons can be made immune, or at least can be made to give a negative Dick reaction. The usual method is to begin with a subcutaneous injection of the amount of toxin corresponding to 500 skin-test-doses and increase the weekly injections to 80,000 or 100,000 skin-test-doses by the fourth injection. Many persons may be made Dick-negative with smaller and fewer doses, but the ones mentioned above are those recommended by the Dicks. The immunity thus developed lasts usually two or three years or longer and may be checked by Dick-testing, which has shown that only about 10 per cent of persons require a second immunization.

It should be stated, however, that the reactions with this method of prophylactic treatment are often somewhat violent, especially in older persons, and that all the symptoms of scarlet fever, including occasionally even the sore throat, may develop. Even fatal results have followed, possibly through errors in technique. It is probable that the degree of reaction in the Dick test is an indication of the amount of antitoxin in the blood, a markedly positive reaction indicating that little neutralizing antitoxin is present. To patients responding in this way immunizing doses of toxin smaller than usual should be given for fear of producing marked reaction.

The detoxification of toxin by sodium ricinoleate advocated by Larson, Huenekens and Colby[90] is not employed at present, as reactions do not seem to be prevented by its use. There may be mentioned for completeness the preventive vaccination of Gabritschewsky[91] and Wladimiroff,[92] and the mixture of convalescent serum, desquamated scarlet fever skin, and guinea-pig complement employed by di Cristina[93] and other Italian workers.

There is not universal agreement as the reliability of the *Dick test* for immunity. Part of the difficulty no doubt rests upon faulty technique, unreliable preparations, and incorrect interpretation. As described by the Dicks[94] the syringes used must be boiled in distilled water; 0.1 cc. of the diluted toxin is injected intradermally; the reaction read in eighteen to twenty-four hours; and the slightest flush or redness considered as positive if it measures as much as 10 mm. in any diameter. The Dicks also believe that a markedly positive reaction indicates less immunity than a slight one. Many clinicians cannot support the constant reliability of this test. Without denying its value, our own[86] experience leads us to hesitate to place entire dependence on it as a measure of immunity. (For Dick test in early infancy see p. 252.)

(*B*) **Treatment of the Attack.**—The patient should be kept absolutely in bed until desquamation is over, and for at least three weeks even in the mildest cases. The diet should be liquid or soft until the temperature is normal. It is customary not to allow eggs and meat until the end of the third week, although there exists no evidence that feeding these substances increases the incidence of nephritis. Daily warm bed-baths may be given, care being exercised to guard against exposure and chilling. Drafts should be avoided, although some authors claim they are innocuous. The skin should be kept oiled with petrolatum or lanolin, or, if there is itching, a 1 or 2 per cent carbolized oil; or, for young children, a 1 per cent thymol ointment may be employed. Careful examination of the nose and throat should be made daily. Mild antiseptic sprays and gargles may be employed. The urine should be examined frequently. Medication is used only as indicated by the symptoms.

Much has been written regarding serum-treatment. Older anti-streptococcus sera used with more or less success were those of Marmorek,[95] Aronson,[96] and Moser.[97] (See also review by Fedinski.[98]) More recently Dochez and Sherman[20] produced an antiscarlatinal serum by immunization of the horse with streptococci obtained from scarlet fever patients, and Dick and Dick[35] obtained one by injection of the horse with sterile filtrate from broth-cultures (toxin) of scarlet fever streptococci. In the preparation of some commercial sera both these methods are employed. It is impossible to review the literature on this controversial subject. In our own[99] studies, in which careful control was carried out, it was felt that a specific neutralizing effect on the toxin *in vivo* was indicated by the decrease in the duration of the rash, a change in the character and extent of the desquamation, and a reduction in the number of complications. Regarding the last and the effect on mortality there is great difference of opinion. Because of the frequency and severity of serum-reactions the antitoxin should be given only in severe toxic cases, and then early in the course of the disease. There is no doubt that some commercial sera are more potent than others. The usual dose is 15 to 20 cc. (.51 to .68 fl. oz.) given intramuscularly, rarely intravenously. It should not be expected to be entirely efficacious, since recovery from scarlet fever probably depends not upon the development of the antitoxin alone but upon other defensive mechanisms including phagocytosis.

Convalescent's serum has value in treatment as we can attest from our own experience. It should be given intramuscularly in doses of 10 to 60 cc. (0.34 to 2.03 fl. oz.) or larger. So-called "normal serum" or whole blood may be used in still larger doses. (For preparation of convalescent's serum see Measles, p. 279.)

The treatment of certain important symptoms and complications need be mentioned only briefly. *Fever* is better combated by hydrotherapeutic measures than by internal medication. (See Hydrotherapy, p. 190.) These will also benefit *nervous symptoms*, although sedative drugs may be needed and also perhaps lumbar puncture. If *meningitis* develops and is due to the hemolytic streptococcus, antiscarlatinal serum may be given intraspinally. A case so treated by Neal and Jones[100] recovered. For *cardiac weakness* and in *septic cases* with high fever it is possible that digitalis, strychnine, alcohol, or camphor and caffeine hypodermically may be of value. Ordinarily the serum treatment does no good in late septic complications. In *severe angina* local treatment of the throat may be indicated if it does not cause too much disturbance of the patient. Frequently repeated examinations should be made for *otitis media* and paracentesis of the drum and mastoidectomy performed if indicated. *Adenitis* may be treated by the application of an ice-bag, and incision and drainage may be necessary. The treatment of *nephritis* does not differ from that to be described later (p. 825). *Arthritis* may be relieved, or at least the pain of it, by salicylate medication and local applications. The rare purulent form requires surgical intervention. During convalescence anemia, if present, should be treated.

References

1. Med. pract. Wittemberg, 1654, **2,** cap. 12; Ref. Rilliet and Barthez, Mal. des enf., 1891, **3,** 74. 2. Processus Integri; Ref. Williams 20th Cent. Pract. Med. 1898, **14,** 117. 3. Arch. f. Kinderh., 1918, **67,** 15. 4. Ztschr. f. Kinderh., Orig. 1920, **26,** 137. 5. München. med. Wchnschr., 1930, **77,** 1749. 6. Deutsche med. Wchnschr., 1930, **56,** 46. 7. J.A.M.A., 1931, **96,** 2153. 8. J. Infect. Dis., 1930, **46,** 186. 9. Jahrb. f. Kinderh., 1910, **77,** 676. 10. Brit. M. J., 1916, **2,** 389. 11. Pediatria, 1922, **30,** 481. 12. Thèse de Paris, July, 1906. 13. Sundhedskollegiets Aarsberetning, 1876; Ref. von Jürgensen in Nothnagel's Encyclop. Amer. Ed. 228; 382. 14. Klin. Wchnschr., 1928, **7,** 498. 15. Am. J. Dis. Child., 1927, **34,** 969. 16. Proc. Roy. Soc. London, 1887, **42,** 158. 17. Ann. de l'Inst. Pasteur, 1911, **25,** 754. 18. Deutsche med. Wchnschr., 1911, **37,** 791. 19. Jahrb.

f. Kinderh., 1915, **82,** 225. 20. Proc. Soc. Exper. Biol. and Med., 1924, **21,** 184; J.A.M.A. 1924, **82,** 542. 21. J. Exper. Med., 1913, **17,** 517. 22. Jahrb. f. Kinderh., 1913, **77,** 679. 23. Arch. Int. Med., 1914, **13,** 909. 24. J. Exper. Med., 1919, **30,** 179. 25. J.A.M.A., 1920, **74,** 1386. 26. Brit. M. J., 1921, **1,** 632. 27. J. Exper. Med., 1922, **36,** 575. 28. J.A.M.A., 1923, **81,** 1166; 1924, **82,** 301. 29. J. Bacteriol., 1930, **19,** 57. 30. Ann. Pickett-Thomson Research Lab., 1930, 6. 31. J. Immunol., 1927, **13,** 19. 32. Brit. J. Child. Dis., 1930, **27,** 181. 33. J. Prev. Med., 1930, **4,** 1. 34. J.A.M.A., 1924, **82,** 712. 35. J.A.M.A., 1924, **82,** 1246. 36. J.A.M.A., 1924, **82,** 265. 37. Zentralbl. f. Bakteriol., 1928, **106,** 399; 1929, **113,** 97. 38. J.A.M.A., 1930, **95,** 673. 39. Am. J. Dis. Child., 1928, **35,** 991. 40. J. Exper. Med., 1927, **46,** 487; N. Y. State J. Med., 1929, **29,** 22. 41. Deutsche med. Wchnschr., 1923, **49,** 509. 42. Scharlach, 1912; Ref. Swift, Am. Heart J., 1928, **3,** 629. 43. J. Immunol., 1925, **10,** 725. 44. N. Y. Med. Rec., 1899, **56,** 330. 45. Berl. klin. Wchnschr., 1900, **37,** 588. 46. J. Med. Research, 1904, **10,** 483. 47. J. Lab. and Clin. Med., 1922, **7,** 592. 48. Pediatria, 1921, **29,** 1105; 1923, **31,** 1. 49. J.A.M.A., 1929, **92,** 498. 50. Griffith. Jacobi Festschrift, 1900, 182. 51. Brit. J. Child. Dis., 1912, **9,** 44. 52. Jahrb. f. Kinderh., 1910, **72,** 422. 53. Ztschr. f. Heilk., 1906, **27,** 433. 54. Gaz. d. ôsp., 1908, **29,** 433. 55. Monatschr. f. Kinderh.. Orig. 1919, **15,** 259. 56. Ztschr. f. Kinderh., 1930, **50,** 374. 57. Ztschr. f. Kinderh., 1930, **50,** 496. 58. Centralbl. f. Bakt. u. Parasit., 1892, **12,** 909. 59. Sperimentale, 1913, **67,** 455. 60. Volkmann's Samml. klin. Vortr. Chir., No. 54, 1489. 61. Ztschr. f. klin. Med., 1928, **108,** 737. 62. Am. J. Dis. Child., 1923, **26,** 447. 63. Jahrb. f. Kinderh., 1912, **75,** 350. 64. Jahrb. f. Kinderh., 1930, **129,** 270. 65. Brit. J. Child., Dis. 1930, **27,** 102. 66. Arch. Int. Med., 1920, **26,** 424. 67. Pediatria, 1928, **12,** 29. 68. Brit. J. Child. Dis., 1930, **27,** 46. 69. Brit. J. Dermat., 1910, **22,** 309. 70. Boston City Hosp. Rep., 1899. 71. Lancet, 1903, **1,** 436. 72. Lancet, 1928, **1,** 1060. 73. Practitioner, 1930, **125,** 236. 74. Acta pædiat., 1931, **10,** 379; Norsk. Mag. f. Laegavidensk., 1930, **91,** 1133. 75. Thèse de Paris, 1907–8. 76. Ziemssen's Handbk., 1874, B.2, Th.2, 176. 77. Kinderkrankheiten, 1895, 675. 78. Canad. M. A. J., 1911, **1,** 293. 79. Arch. f. Kinderh., 1909, **42,** 17. 80. Jahrb. f. Kinderh., 1930, **127,** 253. 81. Arch. de méd. d. enf., 1911, **14,** 130. 82. München. med. Wchnschr., 1909, **56,** 1404. 83. München. med. Wchnschr., 1911, **58,** 293; 1673. 84. Ztschr. f. Kinderh., Orig. 1918, **17,** 328. 85. Am. J. Dis. Child., 1928, **35,** 607. 86. Eddy and Mitchell, Am. J. Dis. Child., 1930, **40,** 988. 87. J.A.M.A., 1932, **98,** 519. 88. München. med. Wchnschr., 1922, **69,** 955. 89. J.A.M.A., 1924, **82,** 265; 544; 1924, **83,** 84; 1925, **84,** 1481; Am. J. Dis. Child., 1925, **28,** 484; 1929, **38,** 905. 90. J.A.M.A., 1926, **86,** 1000. 91. Russk. Vrach., 1906, 989; Ref. Veldee, J. Med. Cincinnati, 1931, **12,** 91. 92. Arch. f. Kinderh., 1909, **52,** 28. 93. Pediatria, 1916, **24,** 385. 94. Am. J. Dis. Child., 1928, **38,** 905. 95. Ann. de l'Inst. Pasteur, 1896, **10,** 47. 96. Verhandl. Berl. med. Ges., 1902, **33,** 253. 97. Jahrb. f. Kinderh., 1903, **57,** 1. 98. Jahrb. f. Kinderh., 1910, **71,** 189. 99. Veldee, Stevenson and Mitchell, Pub. Health. Rept.. 1931, **46,** 3023. 100. Arch. Pediat., 1927, **44,** 395.

CHAPTER III

MEASLES

(Rubeola. Morbilli)

Measles was differentiated from smallpox by Rhazes[1] about 900 A. D. and from scarlet fever by Sydenham.[2]

Etiology. Predisposing Causes.—*Sex, climate,* and *locality* appear to exert no marked influence on the incidence of the disease, and economic conditions modify it only to a limited extent. *Age* is an important factor. Instances of measles occurring congenitally or within a few days after birth are recorded by Ballantyne,[3] who collected 21 such, and by Mason,[4] Steinschneider,[5] Rocaz,[6] Schulze,[7] Debré, Joannon and Mariani,[8] Musser,[9] and others. We have seen three undoubted instances of this, the mother showing symptoms of the disease in the last week of pregnancy, or, having been exposed, developing it simultaneously with her new-born infant. Herrman's[10] extensive experience is that of others; that infants in the first two months of life whose mothers have had measles are absolutely immune, and that those under five or six months are relatively so. After that time the susceptibility becomes as great as in older children. In Halliday's[11] research the greatest incidence in crowded tenements was in the preschool years, but in better circumstances and in country districts between the ages of five and ten years. That few exposed adults suffer from the disease is because they have already had it. In the epidemic of 1846 in the Faroe Islands, described by Panum,[12] where no one was protected, adults of every age proved as susceptible as children.

The individual susceptibility is greater than in most of the other infectious diseases, and to such a degree that the spread of the infection is little controllable. The Faroe Islands' epidemics demonstrated this especially well (Panum;[12] Hoff[13]). An individual immunity, temporary or permanent, is occasionally met with. A decided *epidemic influence* exists also, measles being more frequent and severe in certain years, and there being no regularity in the return of these epidemic outbreaks. *Season* possesses a slight influence, the disease being more prevalent in winter, and especially in spring, than in summer. This was demonstrated in the study of 530 epidemics by Hirsch.[14] The greater prevalence in the cooler months may depend upon the more intimate indoor association in homes and schools.

Exciting Cause.—As of historical interest may be mentioned the finding of micro-organisms associated with the disease by Canon and Pielicke,[15] Czajkowski,[16] Arsamakov,[17] Lesage,[18] von Niessen,[19] Giarre and Picchi,[20] Zlatogoroff,[21] and Sellards and Bigelow.[22] Caronia[23] and other Italian observers, such as Guardabassi,[24] believe in the causative influence of a small, gram-negative, anaerobic coccus.

More recently Tunnicliff[25] and her co-workers have obtained a gram-positive, filter-passing, anaerobic, green-producing diplococcus from the nose, throat, and blood of patients with the disease. This produced a subcutaneous reaction in nonimmune persons; developed toxin neutralizable by measles convalescent's serum; was agglutinated by such serum; and when injected into horses and goats produced an antitoxin having some protective value. Some investigators have been able to confirm these results. Ferry and Fisher[26] have described a gram-positive, aerobic, green-producing streptococcus (Streptococcus morbilli) which seems to have associations and serologic qualities quite similar to Tunnicliff's diplococcus. There should be mentioned also the so-called "inclusion-bodies" which have been found in the red blood-cells by Doehle,[27] Behla,[28] Rosenberger,[29] and others, and in the skin by Lipschütz.[30] While thought by some to be protozoa, these may be only degenerating cytolysed epithelial cells and leukocytes.

The various experiments upon the transmission of measles to man and other animals are of interest. Inoculation of filter-passing material obtained from the secretions and the blood of patients has apparently been successful with monkeys, rabbits and guinea pigs (Goldberger and Anderson,[31] Hektoen and Eggers,[32] Lucas and Prizer,[33] Nevin and Bittman,[34] Duval and D'Aunoy[35]). Intratracheal injections into such animals of filtered or unfiltered nasopharyngeal washings from cases of measles have produced symptoms somewhat resembling the disease (Blake and Trask,[36] Duval and D'Aunoy,[35] Tunnicliff and Moody,[37] Grund[38]). Whether this condition is actually measles is open to question. (See discussions by Hektoen[39] and Sellards.[40]) It is interesting to mention here that, according to Dormidontov,[41] children have contracted measles when in contact with experimentally infected monkeys. Inoculation experiments with blood from measles-patients, performed accidentally or deliberately upon human beings and claimed to be successful, are those reported by Home,[42] Katona[43] (blood mixed with serum from vesicles), Hektoen,[44] Bauguess,[45] Debré, Joannon and Papp,[46] and Degkwitz.[47] Not all investigators could confirm these results, Sellards,[48] for example, being entirely unsuccessful. Mayr[49] has produced the disease by inoculation with nasal mucus. (See also Preventive Inoculation p. 280.) (For complete review of the bacteriological inoculation studies see Kato.[50])

It may be concluded that there seems to be a close association of green-producing micro-organisms with measles, but that it is probably too early to accept unqualifiedly an etiologic connection; further that there seems to be good evidence that measles has been transmitted experimentally to human beings by the inoculation of apparently sterile material, such as blood and nasal secretions which have been passed through Berkefeld filters. It is possible that the transmission of measles by a filterable virus and its causation by a micro-organism are not necessarily inconsistent, since the germ in some part of its life-cycle may perhaps exist in a filterable form.

Method of Transmission.—In most instances this is by direct contact, only a brief exposure being necessary. Observations reported by Moro,[51] Hoyne,[52] Jasinski and Progulski[53] and others seem to show that the infectious agent may be carried by the air for considerable distances; although the experiments of Grancher[54] and others are opposed to this. The experiences which we have had, in common with others, of the development of measles in a child who has been for months in a hospital ward, or the extension of the disease from one room of a hospital to another with an entirely different nursing staff, certainly argue for the explanation either that the germ is carried by the air or that transmission by fomites or by a third person can at times occur. It is possible that some of these instances are due to the admission to a ward of a child with an abortive form of measles. Wagener,[55] for example, believes that abortive unrecognized attacks may occur in persons who had previously suffered from the disease. Experiences in favor of mediate transmission are on record (Roch,[56] Lanzarini,[57] Rohmer,[58] and others).

The virus enters probably by the respiratory tract or, in rare instances, by inoculation or placental transmission.

Period of Infectiousness.—The etiologic agent probably does not live more than from ten to fourteen days from the onset of the attack. It is likely that the danger of infection exists during the last part of incubation, and certainly so at the onset of invasion and during at least a portion of the period of eruption. The habitat of the virus is the secretions from the nose, mouth and eyes, and the blood; uncontaminated desquamating epidermis probably having no infectious power. The infectiousness lessens rapidly as the catarrhal symptoms disappear. Rooms occupied by patients can be used with safety very soon after the attack is over. In our experience a persistent discharge from a complicating otitis media is not infectious after two or three weeks at the most.

Pathologic Anatomy.—There are few characteristic post-mortem lesions. The principal changes in the skin and the mucous membrane of the eyes and the respiratory and alimentary tract consist of dilatation of the vessels and round-celled infiltration. The buccal eruption, as studied by Hlava[59] and Flamini,[60] consists in interpapillary injection of capillaries, round-celled infiltration, and degenerative changes. The lymphoid tissues throughout the body exhibit decided cellular hyperplasia. Warthin[61] found giant cells in the tonsils and pharyngeal mucosa during the prodromal stage, and Herzberg[62] discovered them in the lymphoid tissue of the appendix. Several authors, as Ford,[63] Greenfield,[64] and Zimmerman and Yannet,[65] have described the lesions which may occur in the nervous system. These consist chiefly of toxic changes; perivascular degeneration of the myelin and white matter; marked glial proliferation; and active phagocytosis of fat. The gray matter is rarely involved. Focal necrosis of the liver has been described (Freeman[66]). Careful histologic studies of fatal cases of measles have been published by Denton.[67]

Symptoms. Ordinary Type. **Period of Incubation.**—As determined by Panum,[12] Lewy[68] and numerous others this lasts fairly uniformly ten to eleven days up to the first appearance of catarrhal symptoms, or fourteen days until the rash develops. Usually there are no symptoms but, as pointed out by Meunier,[69] Heubner,[70] Widowitz,[71] Jakobs,[72] Abercrombie,[73] and Lereboullet and Baize,[74] there may occasionally be early some mild catarrhal manifestations, a brief febrile reaction, and commencing on the

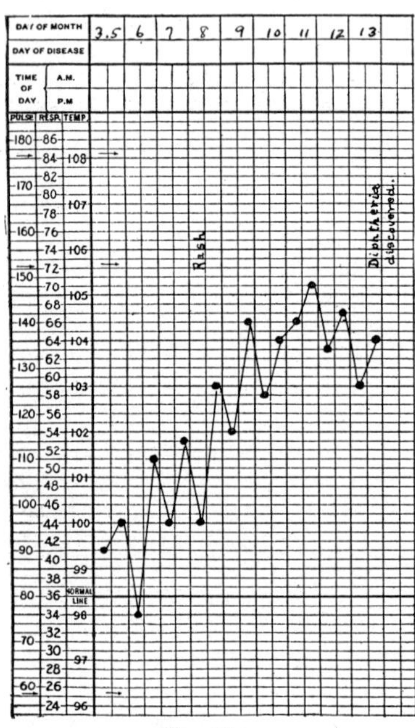

Fig. 40.

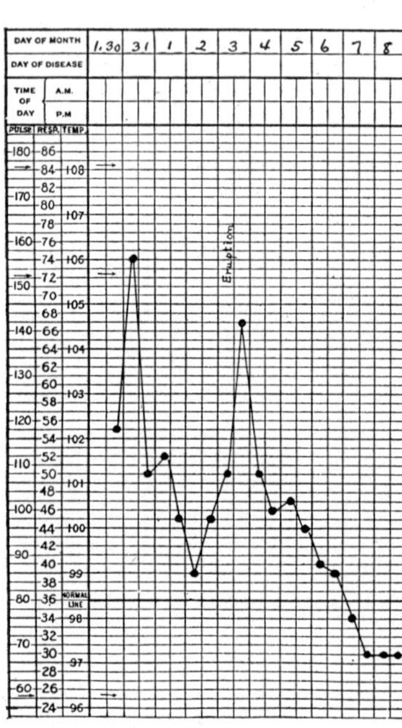

Fig. 41.

Fig. 40.—Measles without pre-eruptive fall of temperature. R. McN., four years old. Mar. 6, vomited; Mar. 8, well-marked catarrhal symptoms, buccal eruption, rash appearing on face and body; Mar. 10, attack severe; Mar. 13, diphtheria discovered.

Fig. 41.—Measles with pre-eruptive intermission in temperature. Lena M. Jan. 30, catarrhal symptoms began; Feb. 2, symptoms very pronounced, fall of temperature to 99; Feb. 3, abundant eruption, general symptoms improved, but temperature elevated; Feb. 8, desquamation.

fourth or fifth day, loss of weight. The blood-changes (p. 273) begin in the incubative period, and sometimes also the buccal eruption. Rolleston[75] maintained that ephemeral eruptions, such as urticaria or erythema, are common in the last part of incubation. There may be a line of congestion on the conjunctival surface of the lower lid, although this is not diagnostic (Stimson[76]).

Period of Invasion.—The onset is usually gradual, with symptoms indistinguishable from those of a severe general cold. Occasionally a convulsion or chilliness ushers in the attack. The child is irritable, tired, and often peculiarly drowsy. Then develop lachrymation, photophobia, redness of the conjunctiva, coryza, sneezing, and often a dry, hard cough. Other common symptoms are headache, sore throat, anorexia, vomiting, diarrhea, and, less frequently, delirium and epistaxis. Congestion of the throat, excoriation of the upper lip, and occasionally a few dry râles are found.

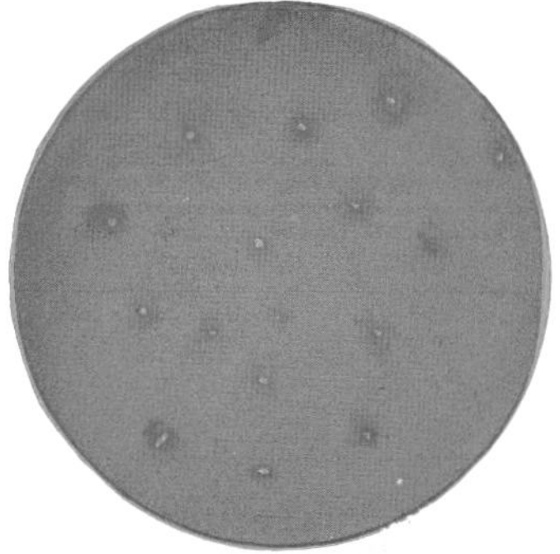

Fig. 1.

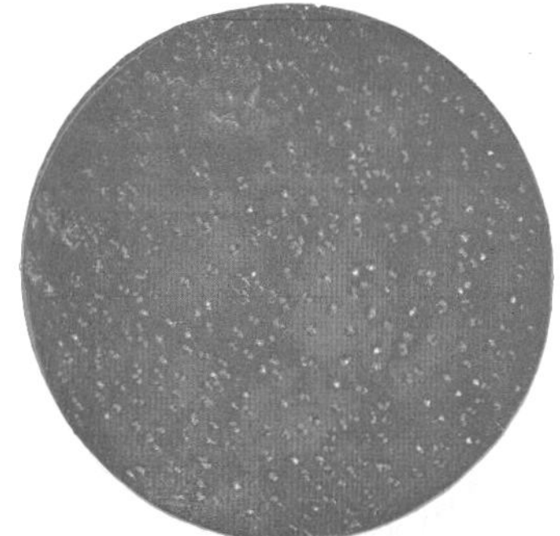

Fig. 2.

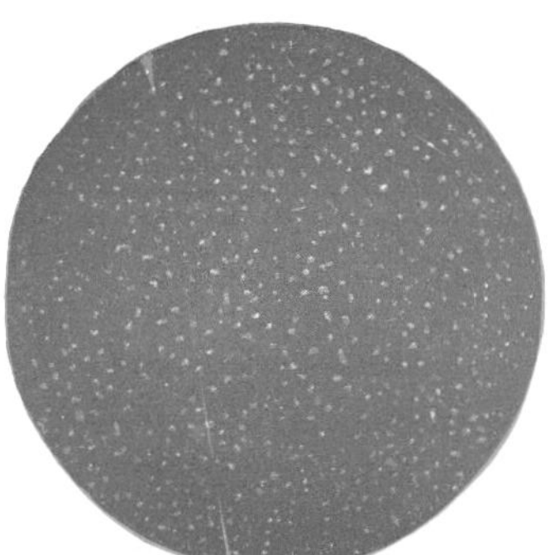

Fig. 3.

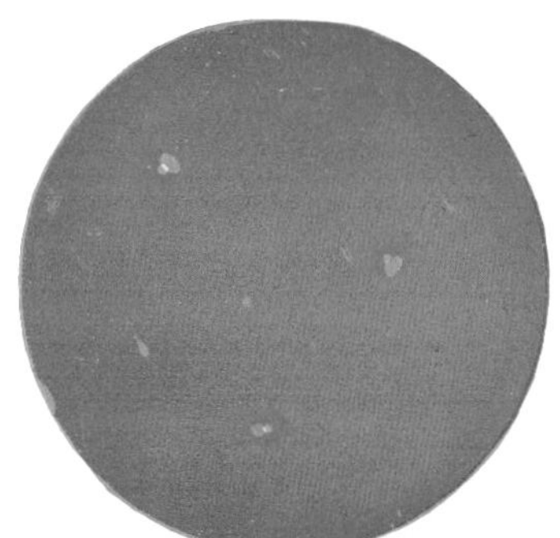

Fig. 4.

Fig. 39.—The pathognomonic sign of measles (Koplik's Spots).

Fig. 1.—The discrete measles-spots on the buccal or labial mucous membrane, showing the isolated rose-red spot, with the minute bluish-white centre, on the normally colored mucous membrane.

Fig. 2.—Shows the partially diffuse eruption on the mucous membrane of the cheeks and lips; patches of pale-pink interspersed among rose-red patches, the latter showing numerous pale bluish-white spots.

Fig. 3.—The appearance of the buccal or labial mucous membrane when the measles-spots completely coalesce and give a diffuse redness, with the myriads of bluish-white specks. The exanthema on the skin is at this time generally fully developed.

Fig. 4.—Aphthous stomatitis apt to be mistaken for measles-spots. Mucous membrane normal in hue. Minute *yellow points* are surrounded by a red area. Always discrete.

(*Medical News*, 1899, 74, 673.)

By the second or third day the characteristic enanthem appears, and consists of small, red macules on the hard and soft palate. It is at its height when the cutaneous rash develops and may persist three or four days more. A condition of another sort, the so-called "buccal eruption" or "Koplik's spots," (Fig. 39) is found upon the lining of the lips and cheeks, oftenest close to the junction of the latter with the upper jaw. It consists of minute bluish-white points each surrounded by a small slightly red areola. It can be seen best in bright daylight. Occasionally it may be found as much as five days before the cutaneous rash develops, but oftener only two or three days before, and quite frequently not until after this is visible. It is almost pathognomonic of measles and is present in from 80 to 90 per cent of the cases. Unless appearing late it disappears by the time the cutaneous eruption is fully developed. Although previously described by Rinecker and Reubold,[77] Monti,[78] Flindt,[79] Filatov,[80] and known to others, its diagnostic importance was not appreciated until this was pointed out by Koplik.[81] Petényi[82] described the occasional appearance a few days before the Koplik's spots of small punctate hemorrhages, 3 to 20 in number, on the buccal mucous membrane.

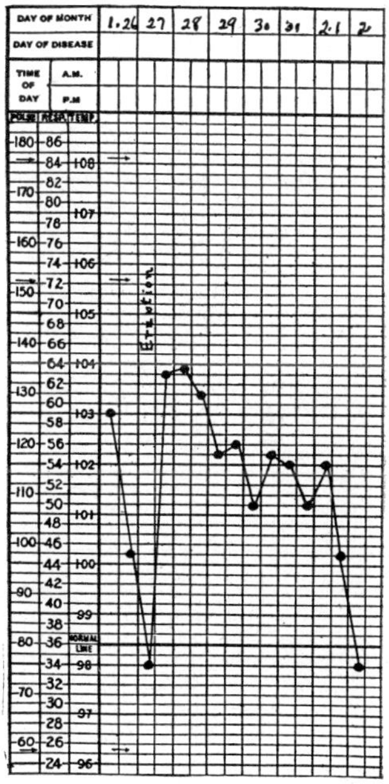

Prodromal cutaneous eruptions are, in our experience, not infrequently observed in this stage, if not seen earlier. They consist of a roughness, reddening, or mottling situated, as it were, *beneath* the surface. In other cases there is a blotchy erythema or an urticaria, or a widely diffused scarlatiniform rash. These usually disappear before the true exanthem of the disease becomes manifest.

Catarrhal symptoms are well marked by the second day of invasion, and increase steadily in severity. The temperature curve is variable. Frequently it increases steadily to 102 to 104 F. (38.9 to 40 C.), with ordinary morning remissions (Fig. 40). In many cases, however, after a sharp initial rise there occurs about the second or third day a decided remission or intermission without amelioration of other symptoms, followed by redevelopment of fever before the eruption appears (Fig. 41). While often considered characteristic, this pre-eruptive fall occurs in only about half of the cases. Occasionally the rash begins to develop before the temperature rises again (Fig. 42). Bologini[83] and Köppen[84] described a slight sensation of crepitation obtained by palpation of the abdomen during the stage of invasion. In typical cases the duration of the invasion is three or four days. (See p. 274.)

Fig. 42.—Measles with pre-eruptive fall of temperature continuing when rash first appeared. Howard M., aged seven years. Jan. 25, catarrhal symptoms and fever; Jan. 26, temperature falling; Jan. 27, abundant eruption on face, spreading to body, temperature still afebrile; Jan. 30, rash almost gone, temperature still elevated; Jan. 31, desquamation.

Period of Eruption. *The Rash.*—This appears by the end of the third or the morning of the fourth day in ordinary cases; sometimes not until the fifth day. It develops first on the forehead, scalp, cheeks, temples, behind the ears, or about the mouth. It then spreads with variable rapidity, but as a rule by its second day is more abundant where first seen, and has also extended over the whole body, possibly excepting the legs, forearms, feet and hands, which may not be involved until its third day. Even the palms and soles finally exhibit it. The *individual spots* are at first of small pin-head size, pale-red, not elevated, round or irregular in shape, and discrete with the surrounding skin healthy. They rapidly enlarge up to the size of a large split pea, becoming distinctly elevated to sight and touch and of a darker red color, commonly with a slightly bluish cast. There exists a decided tendency to grouping, a series of spots becoming confluent by their margins into irregular, short, straight or curved lines—the well-known "crescentic eruption" (Fig. 43). These groupings are separated by small

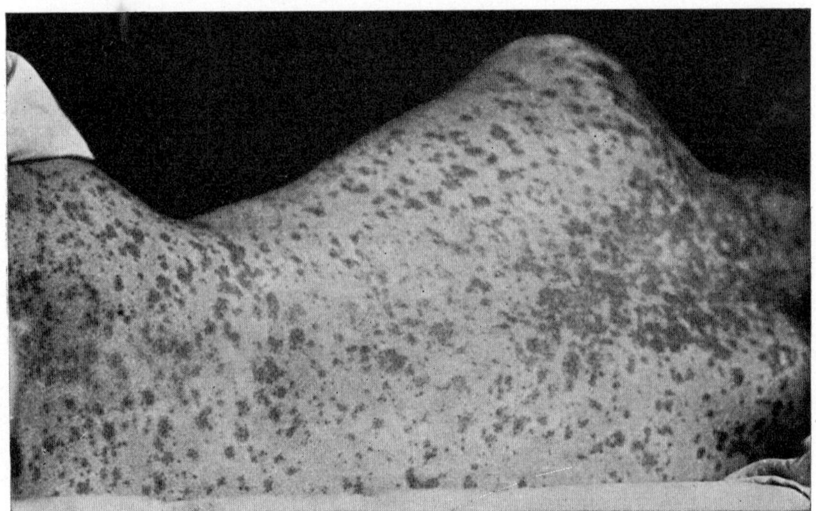

Fig. 43.—Eruption of measles. Boy of twelve years, showing the characteristic grouping exhibited by the eruption.

white channels of healthy skin, the contrast producing the appearance characteristic of this disease. In some portions of the body, especially the face, back, buttocks and the inner surface of the thighs, the rash may become confluent in large areas, principally without intervening channels. Even here, however, the peculiar uneven roughness and lack of uniformity in coloring are quite evident.

The individual spots reach their fullest development in about twenty-four hours, and then begin to fade. Pressure by the finger will at first completely obliterate them for a moment; later a slight discoloration remains. Taken as a whole the rash is at its height on the second or third day and then fades, beginning in the situation where it first appeared. It may consequently be diminishing on the face while not yet at its height on the legs. All traces of it have disappeared by the fourth or fifth day after the first appearance, except a pale-yellowish or brownish pigmentation which very commonly persists for a decidedly longer time.

Other Symptoms of the Eruptive Stage.—The fever generally increases with the rash, reaching its maximum upon the second or third day. Yet there are many exceptions, and the temperature often falls almost by crisis even by the second day of this stage with the rash still at its height. The catarrhal symptoms persist or increase in severity as the rash develops. On the second day of this stage there is present puffiness of the face, which, with the conjunctivitis, coryza, and excoriation of the upper lip, produce a characteristically stupid expression (Fig. 44). Cough is often distressing and numerous râles can be heard in the chest. The tongue is coated and may become dry or even denuded. The inflammation of the fauces continues, but is seldom severe. Thirst, anorexia and diarrhea are common, but vomiting is infrequent. There may be drowsiness or slight delirium. The superficial lymph-nodes throughout the body are swollen and often tender and, as we have found,[85] this is usually so considerable that its well recognized occurrence in rubella cannot be considered a diagnostic symptom of that disease. In our experience enlargement of the spleen during the eruptive stage, with its decrease later, is not so common as Bleyer[86] claims. Friedman[87] could find it in only 12 per cent of his cases. There is often annoying itching of the skin. In the urine may be found albumin, a diazo-

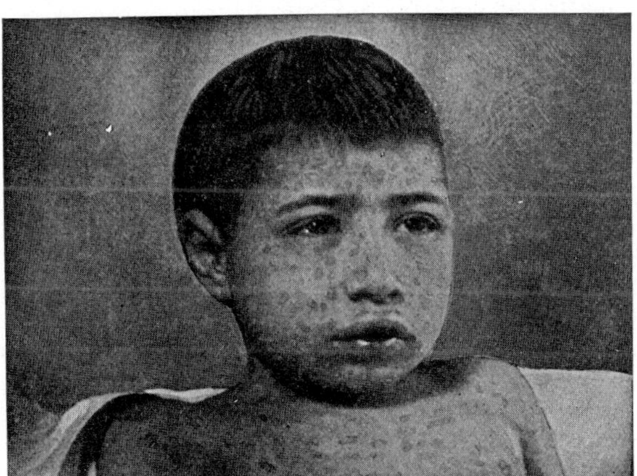

Fig. 44.—Facies in measles. Girl with measles, showing the peculiar heavy and swollen appearance of the face.

reaction, diacetic acid, propeptone, and, according to Rach and Reuss,[88] urobilin. The tuberculin-reaction may be absent during the eruptive stage in persons in whom it was positive previously.[89]

Among the studies of the blood are those by Renaud,[90] Flesch and Schossberger,[91] Hecker,[92] and Lucas.[93] Early in incubation there may be a transient lymphocytosis, but from two to six days before the first symptoms appear a leukopenia and relative diminution of lymphocytes occur. During the invasion the polymorphonuclear cells diminish in number in uncomplicated cases and the lymphocytes increase, and this picture is also characteristic of the early eruptive stage. The eosinophiles are often diminished. A normal blood-picture is attained early in convalescence. Leukocytosis develops if complications are present, and often without these in severe cases. It is stated that during the eruptive stage blood-platelets diminish and bleeding time shortens, Schiff and Mátyas[94] claiming that platelets increase with the fading of the rash.

About the second or third day of the eruptive period the temperature falls by lysis and the catarrhal symptoms improve, although conjunctivitis and cough frequently last for several days. The average duration of fever is about seven days in all. The frequency of pulse and respiration is in proportion to the elevation of temperature. With convalescence the rapidity of the disappearance of symptoms is very striking.

Period of Desquamation.—The eruptive and desquamative stages cannot be sharply demarcated. As a rule the latter begins with the disappearance of the eruption on the seventh or eighth day of the disease, although the actual scaling may not be visible until several days later. The desquamation consists of very fine, branny scales. As a rule it is found first and most markedly on the face, and develops later elsewhere, following the order in which the eruption made its appearance. It continues a few days to a week, or occasionally longer. The amount of it is usually in proportion to the intensity of the eruption, but it is seldom extensive, and often cannot be detected at all. There are no characteristic symptoms, although catarrhal manifestations may sometimes persist.

VARIATIONS FROM THE ORDINARY TYPE.—The duration of *incubation* may exceptionally be as short as five days or as long as three weeks.

The *stage of invasion* may be unusually protracted, extending perhaps six to eight days, Barthez[95] having reported a duration of sixteen days; or it may be abnormally short, lasting only one or two days. We have seen entire local epidemics of measles in institutions characterized by an absence or very slight development of prodromes. In other cases the initial symptoms may be unusually intense; stupor, convulsions, continuously high fever, and severe diarrhea or vomiting being among these. The respiratory symptoms, such as rhinitis or conjunctivitis, may be excessive, and occasionally croup or pneumonia may develop. Violent epistaxis may occur.

The *eruptive stage* is also subject to numerous variations. Thus there is a **mild form** in which the child is scarcely ill at all; **Rubeola afebrilis** (Fig. 45) in which fever is slight or entirely absent; a type in which the eruption strongly resembles rubella; **Rubeola sine eruptione** in which catarrhal symptoms are unattended by a rash; an **abortive form** (Fig. 46) in which, after a well-marked invasion all the symptoms of the eruptive stage disappear with remarkable rapidity; **Rubeola sine catarrho** (Fig. 47) in which the rash is unattended by catarrhal symptoms. While all these forms undoubtedly occur, as shown by their appearance in local epidemics, care should be taken in differential diagnosis that instances of rubella or some disorder of the skin are not mistaken for them. The several **severe forms** of measles are not sharply demarcated. In the **prolonged type** the fever lasts longer than the average time, usually with persistence of catarrhal symptoms, especially bronchitis. In some severe cases all symptoms are intense from the onset or become so soon. In other cases the rash may be poorly developed or late in appearing, or show a tendency to repeated disappearances—the so-called "retrocession of the eruption,"—the child otherwise appearing quite ill. It has been erroneously supposed that this "striking in of the rash" was the cause of the unfavorable symptoms. It is, however, only an evidence of feebleness of the circulation. In some of these cases with retrocession there develops the **typhoid form,** in which there are great prostration, dry tongue, rapid pulse, high fever, low delirium, and perhaps repeated convulsions.

The most severe type is the **malignant form,** in which the symptoms are so intense and the course so rapid that death may take place even before the eruption appears. Such cases sometimes exhibit marked hyperpyrexia. In the **hemorrhagic type,** or "black measles" of the older writers, really a malignant form, bleeding takes place into the areas of the poorly developed eruption, elsewhere into the skin, into the muscles, and from the mucous membrane.

Among **minor variations** from the ordinary type of eruption are *Morbilli papulosi* in which the rash consists of large, deep-red spots, more papular than usual; *Morbilli miliaris* which exhibits minute vesicles upon the usual eruption; the rare *Morbilli bullosi* in which the eruption resembles pemphigus, or lesions of this type are combined with the usual rash (Neff,[96] Morton[97]); *Ecchymotic measles* in which extravasations of blood take place into the rash especially on the extremities. The last form is a very common one, and differs radically from the hemorrhagic measles previously described, in that the grave symptoms which characterize the latter infection are not present. The spots may persist for days or even weeks.

Complications and Sequels.—These occur oftenest and are most serious in early childhood and especially in infancy. Most important and common are those connected with the *respiratory tract.* As complications are severe epistaxis, and severe laryngitis attended by spasm, edema or

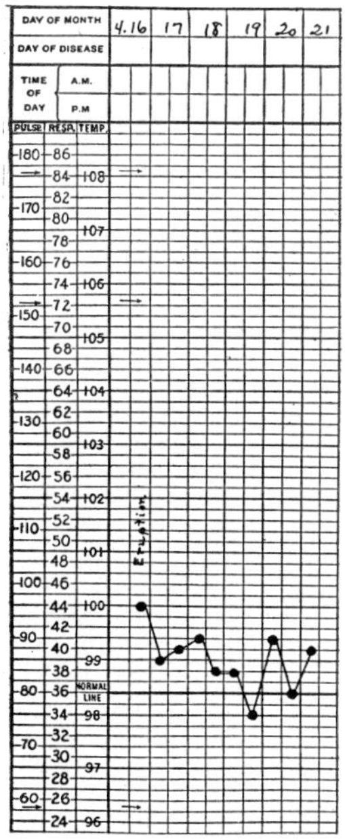

Fig. 45. 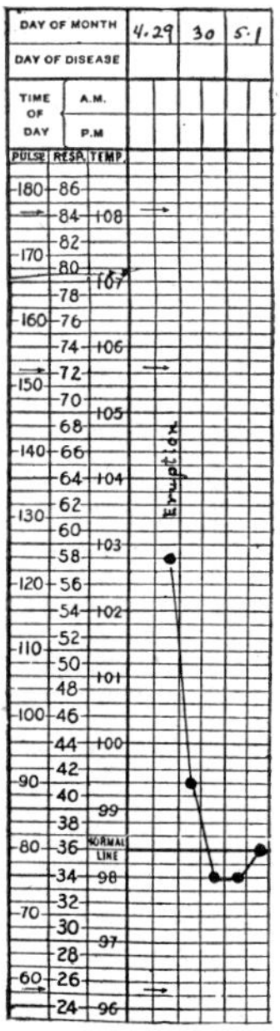 Fig. 46. 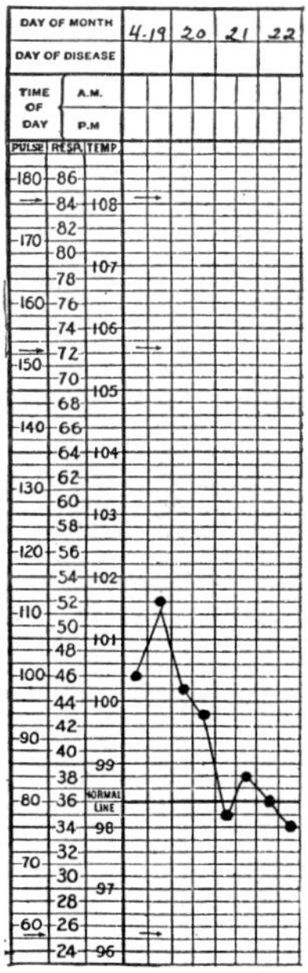 Fig. 47.

Fig. 45.—Rubeola afebrilis. Richard G., aged eight years. Apr. 15, vomited, lachrymation; Apr. 16, vomited again, characteristic rash after a mustard-bath, mild catarrhal symptoms throughout attack, no fever during eruptive period and no indication of it earlier.

Fig. 46.—Abortive measles. Frank A., aged four years. Apr. 29, for three days had coughing, sneezing and drowsiness, typical eruption appeared today on face, catarrhal symptoms continue; Apr. 30, rash spread yesterday, now fading; May 1, rash nearly disappeared.

Fig. 47.—Rubeola sine catarrho. Willie B., aged ten years. Apr. 18, no symptoms noted; Apr. 19, no catarrhal symptoms except a very slight redness of the eyes, eruption developing; Apr. 20, eruption more abundant, no catarrhal symptoms whatever; Apr. 21, rash fading. House-epidemic.

stenosis; as sequels may be chronic nasal discharge and ulcerative laryngitis. Membranous laryngitis may be due to the presence of either a streptococcus or the diphtheria bacillus (see p. 341 and p. 697), and bacteriological examination may be needed to make a positive diagnosis. Tracheitis and bronchitis, while characteristic of the disease, may become sufficiently severe and prolonged to be considered sequels. Kohn and Koiransky[98] have shown by roentgenography that, even in the pre-eruptive stage, abnormal shadows indicating pulmonary infiltration may be present, and persist for as long as six to ten months. Bronchopneumonia, which may be tuberculous in type, is common, especially in infants and young children, and is always serious. It develops oftenest in the eruptive stage. The incidence of pneumonia varies according to the studies of von Jürgensen,[99] Mixsell and Giddings,[100] and Kohn and Koriansky[98] from 6 to about 25 per cent. Croupous pneumonia is of less frequent occurrence. Pleural effusion, or other clinical evidence of pleurisy, is not common, although Kohn and Koriansky[98] frequently found roentgenographic evidence of pleural involvement. Among other uncommon sequels may be mentioned gangrene of the lung and bronchiectasis.

The *gastroenteric tract* furnishes many complications and sequels. Among the former are aphthous and ulcerative stomatitis. Gangrenous stomatitis is rare, yet measles perhaps more than any other disease predisposes to it. (See p. 521.) Membranous pharyngitis, streptococcic or diphtheritic in nature, is not uncommon, as is also severe diarrhea depending upon catarrhal or ulcerative inflammation. Ileocolitis may begin in the prodromal stage of measles and may continue as a sequel, particularly in the summer-time in debilitated young subjects. Appendicitis may occur during the active stage of measles, as we have seen on several occasions. In view of the inflammation of mucous membrane and involvement of lymphoid tissue attending measles it is surprising that this complication is not more frequent. (See Pathologic Anatomy, p. 269.) Instances of appendicitis in measles are reported by Le Lyonnais,[101] Fischer,[102] and others.

Otitis is of frequent occurrence, varying with the epidemic. It may be catarrhal or suppurative. Frequent examinations of the ears are necessary, especially in young infants. In a mild form it is common in the eruptive stage; or it may develop more severely later as a sequel, and may lead to mastoid involvement or meningitis. Of 501 cases of chronic disease of the middle ear reported by Downie,[103] 26.1 per cent owed their origin to measles. Yet chronic otitis occurs much less often than after scarlet fever.

Inflammation of the eyes in the form of conjunctivitis is a regular symptom, but sometimes persists obstinately. Keratitis and iritis may occur as sequels, or even optic neuritis develop (Griscom[104]).

Circulatory affections are uncommon. Endocarditis, pericarditis and myocarditis are rarely seen. Thrombosis of vessels may exceptionally occur (Lutz[105]), and in the extremities this may produce gangrene (Hishon and Rolleston[106]). *Swelling of the thyroid gland* has been reported. *Nephritis* is unusual, but we have seen it occur either with the attack or as a sequel. *Pyelitis* may be initiated, or recurrence of it be brought about. Ulcerative and gangrenous *vulvitis* are rare sequels, to which, however, measles especially predisposes.

Affections of the skin and bones have been recorded as complications, among them gangrene, herpes zoster, herpes labialis, urticaria, erythema, and furunculosis. Generalized cutaneous emphysema, or the rapid development of cutaneous tuberculosis, has also been reported. Arthritis and osteomyelitis may occur. The development of cutaneous hemorrhages has already been mentioned. Purpura hemorrhagica may appear as a rare sequel. It has been made the subject of study by Kelly.[107]

Nervous affections are not common. Boenheim[108] found nervous complications occurring in about 0.4 per cent of 5940 cases of measles. Ford[63] collected 113 such instances and studied 12 others. After the fever has fallen is the usual time of onset. Many of the nervous complications appear to be the result of an *encephalitis* or encephalomyelitis of a toxic nature. (See Pathologic Anatomy, p. 269.) Among others who have reported this complication are Horwitt,[109] Neal and Appelbaum,[110] Musser and Hauser,[111] and Morquio,[112] and we have seen it several times. The dull apathetic condition which may be present for a short time, or even for several weeks, after the disease is over, the convulsions, epilepsy, myoclonia, hemiplegia, asphasia, and the paralyses of various sorts occurring as sequels are probably in most instances the result of this encephalitis. In the acute stages of an accompanying encephalitis there may be little change in the spinal fluid, or only a slight or moderate increase in the cells (which are mostly mononuclear), with a slight protein increase, the sugar being normal or increased in amount.

Some of the paralyses are, however, peripheral in nature rather than cerebral. The subject of paralysis after measles has been reviewed by Allyn,[113] Brückner[114] and others. Acute cerebellar ataxia has been reported following measles (Griffith,[115] Alexander[116]) and bulbar paralysis may occur (Bénard[117]).

Mental retardation after measles has been observed not infrequently, and in 2000 cases of imbecility reported by Beach[118] 11 dated from an attack of measles. Serous meningitis occurs occasionally as a sequel to otitis, or without this; purulent meningitis may appear, or that of a tuberculous nature as a result of a complicating tuberculosis.

Among the *infectious diseases* which may exist in combination with measles, or as sequels or predecessors to it, are diphtheria, scarlet fever and pertussis; and less commonly varicella, erysipelas, influenza, or typhoid fever. Diphtheria seems especially prone to develop during the convalescent stage of measles, and is then often severe (Rolleston,[119] Joannon[120]). Epidemics of pertussis and of measles are particularly liable to occur near each other. The tendency of tuberculosis to be furthered in its development by measles is well known, and not a few of the cases of bronchopneumonia attending the disease are tuberculous in nature, while osseous or glandular tuberculosis may frequently be a sequel.

Relapse.—This is encountered with great rarity, but has been reported by Leach,[121] Goldberger,[122] Macciotta,[123] Hecht,[124] Liebig,[125] van Bogaert, Borreman and Couvreur[126] and others. We have observed it only once, in a case two weeks after the initial attack. Undoubtedly many reported instances were errors in diagnosis. It takes place usually from the second to the fourth week after the onset of the initial attack; consists of the return of all or several of the characteristic symptoms; and is, as a rule, less severe and of shorter duration than the first attack.

Recurrence.—Second attacks of measles are exceptional, many of the so-called "recurrences" being instances of mistaken diagnoses. They have been reported, however, by Maiselis,[127] Berinsohn,[128] de Rudder,[129] Erdheim,[130] and others.

Prognosis.—This is generally good, the mortality averaging about 3 to 6 per cent or less. The incidence of measles is, however, so great that the actual number of deaths from it is large. For example, Comby[131] states that in Paris during nineteen years there were 20,518 fatal cases; and Veeder[132] estimates that between 9000 and 10,000 deaths from measles take place annually in the United States. Godfrey[133] reported that in the period from 1915 to 1924 there were 8036 deaths from measles in New York State. In the Registration Area of the United States in the years 1926, 1927, 1928 there were 18,412 deaths from measles in persons under twenty years of age.[134] Writing in 1926, Bernard[135] stated that the number of deaths was steadily increasing in the United States, so that it exceeded, until the end of the third year of life, the combined number of fatalities from scarlet fever, pertussis and diphtheria. After this age it ranked first of these until the fifth year. His figures show, too, that there was an increasing number of fatal cases in many other countries. The greatest number of fatalities is observed in the second week of the attack.

The mortality varies greatly with *epidemics*, ranging from less than 2 per cent up to 30 per cent or more. *Age* exercises a powerful influence as shown by the studies of Godfrey,[133] Variot,[136] Williams,[137] Henoch,[138] Panum,[12] Kilbourne,[139] Spencer,[140] Halliday,[141] and the United States Census reports.[134] Although in some epidemics the mortality in adults has been high, in general the younger the patient the graver the prognosis, and the number of fatal cases is much diminished after the fifth year. About 75 per cent of all deaths from measles occur in children under three years of age and about 90 per cent or more in children under five years. *Poor hygiene* and *debilitating influences* increase the mortality greatly. *Complications* and *sequels* are far oftener the cause of death than is the toxemia of the disease. Bronchopneumonia, tuberculous or otherwise, probably occasions more deaths than any other complication. Subglottic laryngitis is an occasional cause, as we have witnessed. As previously stated, the combination of measles and diphtheria is a serious one. This is illustrated by the report of Blakely and Burrows[142] on 157 cases of combined measles and diphtheria with 34 per cent mortality. Death after the disease is completely over may be the result of tuberculosis activated by it.

Among *unfavorable symptoms* are high fever, and poorly developed eruption or retrocession of it especially when combined with marked general symptoms. Mortality may be favorably influenced by the administration of convalescent's serum, even when this has been given too late to prevent an attack of the disease. (See p. 279.)

Diagnosis.—This rests principally upon the long prodromal stage with the attending fever and catarrhal symptoms, and the development of the characteristic enanthem and later the exanthem. Before the cutaneous rash develops the enanthem may serve to distinguish measles from a severe cold or grippe. Koplik's spots, while occasionally absent, are probably never present in any other disease, although Michelazzi[143] claims to have found them in pertussis and tonsillitis, and Widowitz[144] and Müller[145] in rubella. According to Wadsworth and Misenheimer[146] the rash is visible under ultraviolet light a few days before it could otherwise be detected. Von Bormann[147] states that if convalescent's serum is injected into the skin before the rash develops it will not occur in that area, but that a rash already present will not be blanched. The leukopenia and other blood changes are of assistance in differential diagnosis, but in some epidemics and in severe cases there may be leukocytosis both in the stage of incubation and later.

Rubella is the disease which most resembles measles, especially in those atypical cases where the rash is morbilliform and the catarrhal symptoms marked. There is diagnostic difficulty, too, in those instances of measles in which the symptoms, including the eruption, are poorly developed. Rubella usually has mild or no prodromes, very slight catarrhal symptoms, rapidly developing eruption with absence of grouping, and an absence of Koplik's spots. As stated elsewhere, the degree of glandular enlargement is not always diagnostic.

Scarlet fever can cause difficulty only in those cases in which it exhibits a blotchy eruption somewhat resembling measles, or in instances of measles where the rash is distinctly confluent. The distribution of the rash of measles on the face and the absence of facial eruption especially about the mouth in scarlet fever are important. There are also the differences in the blood-pictures and in the types of involvement of the throat, mouth and tongue.

Typhoid fever may rarely exhibit a rash suggestive of measles (Fig. 58, p. 307), as may *typhus fever*. Severe and rapidly fatal cases of *cerebrospinal fever* may be confused with malignant measles since both exhibit a sudden and severe onset of cerebral symptoms and a hemorrhagic type of rash. The rash of *variola* may at first suggest measles of the more papular form, but in variola there is an entirely different initial stage of headache, backache, and vomiting, and no catarrhal symptoms. The roseola of *syphilis* may resemble the rash of measles closely, but has no other confusing symptoms. Among *drug eruptions* having a rash which could be confused with measles are those produced by antipyrine, copaiba, luminal, cubebs, and chloral. Serum-rashes are seldom morbilliform in appearance. Urticaria and erythema multiforme may exhibit a morbilliform eruption.

Tunnicliff and Taylor[148] using killed cultures of the green-producing diplococcus previously described (p. 268), obtained positive cutaneous reactions in all persons who had not had measles, and in only 4 per cent of those with a history of it. This test needs further study before it can be employed as a diagnostic procedure.

Treatment. Prophylaxis. Quarantine.—Unfortunately measles is frequently communicated before its existence is suspected, and by the time the diagnosis is made other children have already contracted it. This renders control of infection exceedingly difficult. However, isolation should be established immediately, and every effort made to protect young children and those in a debilitated condition. Quarantine should continue for at least two weeks, although the danger of infection is probably over sooner; and nonimmune children who have been exposed should be kept from contact with susceptible playmates for an equal period in order to permit the usual time of incubation to elapse. Disinfection of the sickroom and destruction of books and toys and the like are not imperative, but thorough cleansing and airing should be carried out. The improbability of the disease being carried by a third person makes immune children practically safe for others. Godfrey[133] points out that in community control it should be remembered that 70 per cent of all the cases and most of the deaths occur in children under three years of age.

Prophylactic Injection of Convalescent's Serum.—Although employed in 1895 by Weisbecker[149] for the actual treatment of measles, convalescent's serum for purposes of immunization appears to have been first used by Cenci[150] in 1907, and several years later by Nicolle and Conseil[151] and Richardson and Connor.[152] Degkwitz,[153] however, stimulated its employment in an extensive way, and since this time a voluminous literature has appeared. It is indicated especially for checking the spread of the disease in institutions, and for the protection of debilitated children or those suffering from other diseases. The immunity conferred is, of course, only passive and temporary, and lasts for two weeks or possibly somewhat longer. The serum is obtained preferably from several donors, free from tuberculosis and syphilis, about seven to fourteen days after defervescence from measles; tested for sterility; and preserved with tricresol. It should be kept in the ice-box and used within a few weeks, but may be active up to three or four months or possibly longer. Dried serum is effective and seems to be active after a number of months (Lichtenstein[154]). Baar[155] secured re-activated serum by injecting adults with the blood of patients in the early stage of measles. Modinos[156] obtained the serum from blister-fluid. Three and a half to 5 cc. (0.12 to 0.17 fl. oz.), or in older children about 10 to 20 cc. (0.34 to 0.67 fl. oz.), are injected intramuscularly before the fourth day after exposure. If given later than this the dose should be doubled. If whole blood, citrated or uncitrated, is used, at least twice the amount needed for serum should be employed. The injection of serum or whole blood from adults who have had measles some years previously, or are presumably immune, seems to afford some protection if administered in double the dose of convalescent's serum. Reitschel,[157] Salomon,[158] Zingher,[159] Karelitz and Levin,[160] and Morales and Mandry[161] have found that this adult's blood possesses some value, but Townsend,[162] Blauner and Goldstein[163] and others have not confirmed this. It is certainly not as efficacious as the serum or blood of convalescents.

Convalescent's serum or blood will afford protection to a large percentage of children. If given as late as the seventh day after exposure, even in larger doses, complete passive immunity usually will not follow, but a modified and mild form of the disease may occur, which quite certainly results in active and, therefore, permanent immunity. In healthy, strong children this modified form with its permanent immunity may be sought deliberately, as recommended by Debré and Ravini[164] and others.

Anderson and Gerard[165] instilled convalescent's serum into the conjunctival sac in order to produce local tissue immunity here and also in the nasal mucous membrane, since the serum would reach the nose through the nasal duct. They claimed good results in developing protection.

Other Forms of Prophylaxis.—It is claimed by Galli,[166] Pontano and Corradi,[167] Mazziotti[168] and others that horse-serum or diphtheria-antitoxin have prophylactic qualities against measles, but our own experience would lead us to doubt this. Tunnicliff and her coworkers[169] and others have been able to obtain some protection by the injection of blood-serum of a goat which had been inoculated with the green-producing streptococcus previously mentioned (p. 268), and Ferry and his coworkers[170] by the employment of antitoxin prepared by injection of horses with the microorganism described by them (p. 268). Halpern,[171] Hoyne and Peacock,[172] and Peterman[173] are apparently favorably impressed with the value of this, but others are sceptical; Park, Williams and Wilson,[174] for example, having had as good results with goat-serum even when the animal had not been immunized, or when it had been injected with other streptococci or diphtheria bacilli. Degkwitz[175] claimed protection by the use of serum from sheep inoculated with Berkefeld filtrates of the nasal secretion and sputum of patients with measles, but later workers could not confirm this. Nobel and Schönberger,[176] Ricciardi,[177] and others reported protective power by the use of a vaccine prepared from Caronia's[23] microörganism.

Preventive Inoculation.—Home;[42] Thomson;[178] Debré, Joannon and Papp;[46] and Petenyi[179] attempted active immunization by the application or, usually, the injection, of small amounts of blood taken from measles patients at the onset of the eruption. (See also p. 268.) Herrman[180] tried with somewhat encouraging results the production of active immunity by inoculating the nasal mucous membrane of infants at the end of the fifth month of life with a specially prepared nasal secretion of patients beginning an attack of measles. The intention was to confer a permanent immunity by the development of a mild form of measles in infants, who, at this age, would have sufficient inherited immunity to prevent a severe attack. Zingher[159] advocated the injection of convalescent's serum about forty-eight hours after the nasal inoculation, made according to Herrman's[180] procedure.

Treatment of the Attack.—(For details of the management of the sickroom, as of quarantine and nursing see p. 250.) Particularly should there be an abundance of fresh air without exposure of the patient, and the air should be moist and the temperature not too low. The eyes should be guarded from undue exposure while there is photophobia, but this should be accomplished by shielding with a screen without making the room dark and shutting off ventilation. The patient should be confined to bed while fever lasts and should be lightly covered. The diet at first should be liquid, avoiding an excess of residue so that diarrhea may not be excited; but precautions must be taken later against debility resulting from insufficient nourishment. A daily bath may be given. The mouth, nose and throat and ears should be examined frequently to discover complications there.

For *fever*, hydrotherapy is best, employing warm tub-baths. Acetylsalicylic acid, phenacetin, amidopyrine (Ronaldson and Collier[181]), or other drugs of this class may be employed in small repeated doses to reduce high fever. *Nervous symptoms*, such as headache, restlessness and the like, or the more serious ones of convulsions and stupor may be treated by hydrotherapy or by bromides or other sedatives, including the coal tar derivatives. In encephalitis Lowenburg and Schaller[182] and McLendon[183] have tried the intraspinous, and also intramuscular and intravenous, injection of convalescent's serum. *Irritation of the eyes* demands protection from the light, douching with boric acid solution, and the application of petrolatum or weak yellow oxide of mercury ointment to the lids. Cold compresses may be necessary. *Inflammation of the throat and nose* may be treated by sprays or drops of alkaline or oily solutions, the latter not being strongly medicated. Of *respiratory complications*, cough may be sufficiently distressing to require sedative remedies. Bronchitis and pneumonia are treated in the usual way. *Itching of the skin* is often helped by petrolatum with 1 per cent thymol, or the application of a powder consisting of camphor 1 dram (3.9); zincum oxidum ½ oz. (15.5); amylum ½ oz. (15.5). Constipation is better relieved by enemata than by purgatives.

During *convalescence* diet should be increased, and, except in the mildest cases, bed-rest continued for at least ten days from the beginning of the invasion. Persistent inflammation of the upper or lower respiratory tract may need appropriate remedies and the patient should be guarded against exposure to cold weather. Any anemia present should be treated. The possibility of tuberculosis as a sequel should always be remembered. Sometimes a change to a warm dry climate is advisable.

The employment of convalescent's serum in the treatment of the disease itself or its complications has been claimed by some to be of benefit. In our own experience we have not seen any noteworthy results; and they are probably not to be expected, especially when complications such as pneumonia are present. We have transfused patients suffering from measles with blood from recent convalescents, doing this when other indications for transfusion existed. Ribadeau-Dumas and Bissaud[184] have also tried this procedure.

References

1. De variolis et morbillis, Haller, 1772. 2. Processus integri; Ref. Williams, 20th Cent. Pract. Med., 1898, **14,** 117. 3. Arch. Pediat., 1893, **10,** 301. 4. Boston M. and S. J., 1908, **159,** 436. 5. Deutsche med. Wchnschr., 1914, **40,** 441. 6. Gaz. hebdom. des sc. méd. de Bordeaux, 1906, **27,** 260. 7. Deutsche med. Wchnschr., 1921, **47,** 271. 8. Nourrisson, 1925, **13,** 249. 9. Med. Clin. N. America, 1927, **11,** 619. 10. Arch. Pediat., 1923, **40,** 678. 11. Med. Res. Coun. Rept. London, 1928. 12. Verhandl. d. physic.-med. Gesellsch. in Würzburg, 1851, **2,** 292; 293; Virchow's Archiv., 1847, **1,** 492. 13. Sundhedskollegiets Aarsberetning, 1876. Ref. von Jürgensen, Nothnagel's Encyclop., Amer. Ed., Measles, 228. 14. Handb. d. histor. geog. Path., 1881, 116. 15. Berl. klin. Wchnschr., 1892, **29,** 377. 16. Centralbl. f. Bakteriol., 1895, **18,** 517. 17. Bolnitch Gaz. Botk., 1898, 40; Ref. Rev. de méd., 1899, **19,** 561. 18. Compt. rend. de la soc. de biol., 1900, **52,** 203. 19. Arch. f. Derm. u. Syph. 1902, **60,** 429. 20. Monatschr. f. Kinderh., 1902, **1,** 577. 21. Centralbl. f. Bakteriol., 1904, **37,** 249. 22. J. Med. Research, 1921, **41,** 241. 23. Pediatria, 1923, **31,** 801. 24. Pediatria, 1927, **35,** 801. 25. J. Infect. Dis., 1922, **31,** 382; 1925, **37,** 193; J.A.M.A., 1926, **87,** 625; J. Infect. Dis., 1927, **41,** 267. 26. J.A.M.A., 1926, **86,** 932; Am. J. Dis. Child., 1929, **37,** 573. 27. Centralbl. f. allg. Path. u. path. Anat., 1892, **3,** 150. 28. Centralbl. f. Bakteriol., 1896, **20,** 561. 29. Am. Med., 1906, **12,** 139. 30. Wien. klin. Wchnschr., 1928, **41,** 365. 31. J.A.M.A., 1911, **57,** 476; 971; 1612. 32. J.A.M.A., 1911, **57,** 1833. 33. J. Med. Research, 1912, **26,** 181. 34. J. Infect. Dis., 1921, **29,** 429. 35. J. Exper. Med., 1922, **35,** 257. 36. J. Exper. Med., 1921, **33,** 385; 413. 37. J. Infect. Dis., 1922, **31,** 382. 38. J. Infect. Dis., 1922, **30,** 86. 39. J.A.M.A., 1919, **72,** 177. 40. Medicine, 1924, **3,** 99. 41. Kazansky Meditsinsky Jurnal, 1931, **27,** 1090; Ref. J.A.M.A., 1932, **98,** 1423. 42. Medical Facts and Experiments, 1759, Pt. 3, 253. 43. Oesterreich. med. Wchnschr., 1842, 697. 44. J. Infect. Dis., 1905, **2,** 238. 45. Am. J. Dis. Child., 1924, **27,** 256. 46. Ann. de méd., 1926, **20,** 343. 47. J. Infect. Dis., 1927, **41,** 304. 48. Bull. Johns Hopkins Hosp., 1919, **30,** 257. 49. Ztschr. d. k. k. Gesellsch. d. Aerzte zu Wien, 1852,

8, 13. 50. Am. J. Dis. Child., 1928, **36,** 526. 51. Monatschr. f. Kinderh., Orig. 1916, **14,** 4. 52. Arch. Pediat., 1920, **37,** 606. 53. Pedj. Polska, 1; 1922. Ref. Groer and Pirquet in Pfaundler und Schlossmann Handb. d. Kinderh., 1923, **2,** 187. 54. Traité des mal. de l'enf., 2 Ed., **1,** 322. 55. Monatschr. f. Kinderh., Orig., 1916, **13,** 477. 56. Arch. de méd. des enf., 1907, **10,** 292. 57. Pediatria, 1907, **15,** 366. 58. Jahrb. f. Kinderh., 1912, **75,** 78. 59. Căsopis lékařů ceských, 1906, 773; Ref. Centralbl. f. inn. Med., 1906, **27,** 923. 60. Riv. di clin. pediat., 1908, **6,** 401. 61. Arch. Path., 1931, **11,** 864. 62. J.A.M.A., 1932, **98,** 139. 63. Bull. Johns Hopkins Hosp., 1928, **43,** 140. 64. Brain, 1929, **52,** 171. 65. Arch. Neurol. and Psychiat., 1930, **24,** 1000. 66. Arch, Pediat., 1900, **17,** 81. 67. Am. J. Med. Sc., 1925, **169,** 531. 68. Ztschr. f. Kinderh., 1920, **26,** 160. 69. Gaz. hebdom., 1898, 1057. 70. Lehrb. d. Kinderh., 1911, **1,** 285. 71. Arch. f. Kinderh., 1923, **72,** 274. 72. Nederl. Tijdschr. v. Geneesk., 1928, **2,** 3914. 73. Brit. J. Child. Dis., 1929, **26,** 15. 74. Arch. d. méd. d. enf., 1931, **34,** 475. 75. Brit. M. J., 1905, Feb. 4, 233. 76. J.A.M.A., 1928, **90,** 660. 77. Virchow's Archiv., 1854, **7,** 76. 78. Jahrb. f. Kinderh., 1873, **6,** 20. 79. Ref. v. Jürgensen, Nothnagel's Encyclop., Amer. Ed., 1902, 286. 80. Dis. of Child., Amer. Transl., 1904, **1,** 97; 1904, **2,** 660. 81. Arch. Pediat., 1896, **13,** 918; Med. News., 1899, **74,** 673. 82. Orvosi hetil, 1929, **73,** 93; Ref. Am. J. Dis. Child., 1929, **38,** 411; Monatschr. f. Kinderh., 1929, **45,** 61. 83. Pediatria, 1895, **3,** 110. 84. Centralbl. f. inn. Med., 1898, **19,** 673. 85. Griffith-Univ. Med. Mag., 1892, **4,** 634. 86. Am. J. Dis. Child., 1926, **31,** 26; 1927, **34,** 176. 87. Am. J. Dis. Child., 1931, **42,** 1114. 88. Ztschr. f. Kinderh., Orig., 1911, **2,** 460. 89. Eddy and Mitchell, Am. J. Dis. Child., 1930, **40,** 771. 90. Thèse de Lausanne, 1900; Ref. v. Jürgensen, Nothnagel's Encyclop. Amer. Ed., Measles, 335. 91. Jahrb. f. Kinderh., 1906, **64,** 724. 92. Ztschr. f. Kinderh., Orig., 1911, **2,** 77. 93. Am. J. Dis. Child.,1914, **7,** 149. 94. Monatschr. f. Kinderh., Orig., 1919, **15,** 254. 95. Barthez and Sanné, Malad. des enf., 1891, **3,** 17. 96. Am. J. Dis. Child., 1920, **19,** 469. 97. Brit. J. Child. Dis., 1921, **18,** 188. 98. Am. J. Dis. Child., 1929, **38,** 258; 1931, **41,** 500. 99. Nothnagel's Encyclop., Amer. Ed., 318. 100. South. M. J., 1923, **14,** 90. 101. Thèse de Paris, 1913–14, No. 109; Ref. Brit. J. Child. Dis., 1914, **11,** 234. 102. Zentralbl. f. Chir., 1928, **55,** 1546. 103. Brit. M. J., 1894, **2,** 1163. 104. Ann. of Ophthalm., 1912, **21,** 42. 105. Berl. klin. Wchnschr., 1913, **50,** 1566. 106. Brit. J. Child. Dis., 1926, **23,** 47; 1928, **25,** 58. 107. Brit. J. Child. Dis., 1922, **19,** 86. 108. Ergeb. d. inn. Med. u. Kinderh., 1925, 28, 598; See Ford, Ref. No. 63. 109. Arch. Pediat., 1924, **41,** 476. 110. J.A.M.A., 1927, **88,** 1552. 111. J.A.M.A., 1928, **90,** 1267. 112. Arch. de méd. d. enf., 1931, **34,** 269. 113. Med. News., 1891, **59,** 617. 114. Jahrb. f. Kinderh., 1902. **56,** 725. 115. Am. J. Dis. Child., 1920, **20,** 84. 116. Edinburgh M. J., 1929, **36,** Nov. 21., Soc. Rep., p. 37. 117. Bull. et mém. soc. méd. d. hôp. de Paris, 1921, **45,** 184. 118. Brit. M. J., 1895, **2,** 707. 119. Brit. J. Child. Dis., 1915, **12,** 21. 120. Prog. méd.. 1927, **42,** 1610. 121. Lancet, 1905, **2,** 1837. 122. Am. J. Dis. Child., 1925, **30,** 55. 123. Il Policlinico, sez. prat., 1925, **32,** 116. 124. Ztschr. f. Kinderh., 1927, **43,** 149, 125. Med. Klinik, 1930, **26,** 968. 126. Presse méd., 1932, **40,** 141. 127. Virchows' Archiv., 1894, **137,** 468. 128. Nederl. Tijdschr. f. Geneesk., 1924, **68,** 1864. 129. Ztschr. f. Kinderh., 1925, **40,** 289. 130. Brit. J. Child. Dis., 1926, **23,** 195. 131. Traité des mal. de l'enf., 2nd. ed., **1,** 347. 132. Arch. Pediat., 1917, **34,** 321. 133. Am. J. Pub. Health, 1926, **16,** 571. 134. Communic. Dis. Control, Rep. of Sec. 2, White House Conf. on Child Health and Protection, 1931. 135. La Rougeole, 1926. 136. Bull. de la soc. de pédiat., 1904, No. 1. 137. 20th Cent. Pract. of Med., **14,** 120. 138. See Williams; Ref. No. 137. 139. Military Surgeon, 1912, **31,** 294. 140. J.A.M.A., 1927, **89.** 1662. 141. Med. Res. Counc. Rep., London, 1928. 142. Boston M. and S. J., 1901, **145,** 89. 143. Gazz. d. osp., 1904, **25,** 35. 144. Wien. klin. Wchnschr., 1899; **12;** 919. 145. München. med. Wchnschr., 1904, **51,** 98. 146. J.A.M.A., 1928, **90,** 1443. 147. Deutsche med. Wchnschr., 1930, **56,** 963. 148. J.A.M.A., 1926, **87,** 846. 149. Ztschr. f. klin. Med., 1896, **30,** 312. 150. Riv. di clin. pediat., 1907, **5,** 1017. 151. Bull. et mém. soc. méd. d. hôp. de Paris, 1918, **42,** 337. 152. J.A.M.A., 1919, **72,** 1046. 153. Ztschr. f. Kinderh., 1920, **25,** 134; 1920, **27,** 171. 154. J.A.M.A., 1931, **96,** 2102. 155. Wien. klin. Wchnschr., 1929, **42,** 949. 156. Bull. et mém. soc. méd. d. hôp. de Paris, 1926, **50,** 406. 157. Ztschr. f. Kinderh., 1921, **29,** 127. 158. Deutsche med. Wchnschr. 1923, **49,** 1151. 159. J.A.M.A., 1924, **82,** 1180. 160. Am. J. Dis. Child., 1927, **33,** 409. 161. Am. J. Dis. Child., 1930, **39,** 1214. 162. Boston M. and S. J., 1926, **194,** 869. 163. Am. J. Dis. Child., 1931, **42,** 803. 164. Bull. et mém. soc. méd. d. hôp. de Paris, 1923, **47,** 226. 165. Compt. rend. soc. de. biol., 1930, **104,** 674. 166. Pediatria, 1922, **30,** 898. 167. Ann. d'ig., 1927, **37,** 515. 168. Riv. di clin. pediat., 1930, **28,** 1049. 169. J. Infect. Dis., 1926, **38,** 48; J.A.M.A., 1926, **87,** 1185; 2139; Boston M. and S. J., 1927, **197,** 272. 170. J.A.M.A., 1928, **91,** 1279. 171. J.A.M.A., 1928, **90,** 1109. 172. Am. J. Dis. Child., 1928, **35,** 1021. 173. Am. J. Dis. Child., 1930, **39,** 294. 174. Am. J. Pub. Health, 1927, **17,** 460. 175. München. med. Wchnschr., 1926, **73,** 191; 248; Klin. Wchnschr., 1926, **5,** 1361; J. Infect. Dis., 1927, **41,** 304. 176. Ztschr. f. Kinderh., 1925, **40,** 197. 177. Pediatria, 1926, **33,** 1333. 178. Glasgow Med. J., 1890, **33,** 420. 179. Orvosi hetil, 1928, **82,** 149. 180. Arch. Pediat., 1915, **32,** 503; 1922, **39,** 607: N. Y.

State J. Med., 1929, **29,** 202. 181. Brit. M. J., 1930, **2,** 994. 182. Arch. Pediat., 1926, **43,** 73. 183. Arch. Pediat., 1926, **43,** 554. 184. Bull. et mém. soc. méd. d. hôp. de Paris, 1918, **42,** 147.

CHAPTER IV

RUBELLA

(German Measles. Rötheln)

THE disease has numerous symptoms. The term "Rubella" was first used by Veale[1] and appears to be the most suited to it. For many years the disease had been confounded with measles and with scarlet fever, but its independence is now fully recognized. The first clear description of its symptoms as we now know them was given by Heim[2] in Germany and by Maton[3] in England.

Etiology. Predisposing Causes.—*Age* is important. The disease occurs oftenest between five and fifteen years, yet adults are frequently attacked. Of 664 cases collected by J. Seitz[4] 45 were in adults. Infants, especially under the age of six months, are relatively immune.

Sex, race, and climate are not etiologic factors. *Epidemic influence* is particularly marked, there being few cases except in epidemic years. Season is not without influence, most epidemics appearing in winter and spring. Concerning the *individual susceptibility,* some regard the disease as only mildly contagious, many persons seeming immune. Our own experience is that it is decidedly contagious, although less so than measles, and that about half of the children exposed will contract it. Older subjects probably possess a greater degree of immunity.

Exciting Cause.—This is undoubtedly a germ, but of unknown nature, although Sindoni and Ritossa[5] describe a gram-positive diplococcus found in the blood. Hess[6] attempted to transmit the disease to apes without success. *Transmission* is probably by way of the secretion from the eyes, mouth, and nose, and possibly by the scales of the epidermis. Indirect infection through a third person, clothing, and the like, is perhaps possible, but certainly very unusual. Transmission by the air probably occurs as with measles, but regarding this there appears to be no data.

The *period of greatest infectiousness* is unknown. The disease is, without doubt, infectious during the stages of eruption, invasion and, it seems likely, the latter part of incubation. Definite knowledge is lacking regarding the infectiousness during desquamation, but it probably ceases as the rash disappears.

Pathologic Anatomy.—There are no lesions characteristic of the disease. The eruption appears to depend upon a capillary hyperemia of the upper layers of the corium with slight inflammatory exudate (Thomas[7]).

Symptoms. ORDINARY COURSE. **Period of Incubation.**—The average would seem to be about two weeks with a range of from one to three weeks, although we[8] have seen it as short as five days. There are no characteristic symptoms other than in some cases slight enlargement of the posterior auricular, occipital, and superficial cervical lymph-nodes.

Period of Invasion.—In the great majority of cases prodromal symptoms are either absent or so insignificant that they are overlooked. When present they consist of mild congestion of the eyes and nose, malaise, enlargement of the superficial cervical nodes, and slight fever; these lasting not more than twelve to twenty-four hours. Stolte[9] noted in many cases a severe night-sweat about forty-eight hours before the rash developed.

Period of Eruption. *Rash.*—Commonly without warning the child is found in the morning covered by the characteristic rash. This appears, as a rule, first upon the face and spreads very rapidly, covering the body within a few hours or a day, and involving sometimes the soles and the palms. It consists of irregularly shaped, pale-rose spots, slightly elevated both to sight and to touch, and varying in size from an ordinary pin-head up to a split pea. The spots are more or less closely placed, but not grouped as in measles. They are for the most part discrete, but often show decided confluence on the face and on regions pressed upon and kept warm in bed. On the trunk the rash is usually paler than elsewhere and of a slightly brownish-red color. Very commonly it passes rapidly like a wave over the body, having almost faded from the face, neck, and trunk by the time the full development is reached on the extremities twelve to twenty-four hours later; the acme on any one part lasting only from a few hours to half a day. This has been considered a characteristic of the disease. Nearly, or fully, as often, however, in our experience, the eruption reaches its greatest development everywhere on the second day, after which it fades with great rapidity. The total duration equals two to four days, although often a much shorter time.

Other Symptoms of the Eruptive Stage.—Appearing with the eruption, or continuing in an accentuated form from the stage of invasion, when this was discoverable, are the trifling respiratory symptoms of the eruptive stage. Often there are no catarrhal symptoms whatever, except moderate involvement of the throat, which is one of the most characteristic and constant manifestations. Even if this is not complained of, on inspection the pharynx exhibits a diffuse redness, and the tonsils are generally swollen. Quite frequently an eruption of yellowish-red or brownish-red spots (enanthem), of pin-head size, is visible over the soft palate, uvula, and the lining of the cheeks. This appears simultaneously with the rash upon the skin and lasts about half a day. Fever is generally slight or absent. It reaches its maximum on the first or second day of the eruptive stage, and either falls suddenly while the rash is still at its height, or diminishes more slowly as this fades. It seldom exceeds 101 to 102 F. (38.3 to 38.9 C.). Not infrequently a subfebrile temperature persists for some days after the rash has disappeared. The tongue is never "strawberry" as in scarlet fever. Enlargement of the peripheral glands throughout the body, and especially of the superficial cervical and posterior auricular glands, is usually present. It is not, however, so diagnostic as was once supposed, since it may occur in measles. Itching and cutaneous edema are sometimes seen, and roughness of the skin (cutis anserina) is common. The stools and urine are unaffected, except perhaps for a slight febrile albuminuria, and that frequently a diazo reaction is found (Nagahara[10]). Vomiting is unusual. The blood has been studied by Hildebrandt and Thomas,[11] Spieler,[12] Kaneko,[13] Hess,[6] and others. The usual finding is a leukopenia with a relative increase of lymphocytes in the eruptive stage. Benzing[14] and Bensa[15] state that the plasma-cells are characteristically increased.

The duration and character of the general symptoms are, as a rule, proportionate to the persistence and intensity of the eruption.

Period of Desquamation.—Spots of a faint brownish or yellowish color are often left for two or three days after the eruption has faded. A very slight, branny desquamation is common but by no means always present. It appears shortly after the disappearance of the eruption and continues one to three days.

VARIATIONS FROM THE ORDINARY FORM.—The symptoms just described are what might be called typical. One of the chief characteristics of rubella, however, is its tendency to variations, many of which occur so frequently that they cannot be called unusual.

The variable length of *incubation* is a normal characteristic. Epistaxis has been recorded as occasionally seen in this period (Squire[16]). The *invasion* is sometimes unusually prolonged. We have known it to last forty-eight hours, and periods as long as six or seven days have exceptionally been reported. The prodromal symptoms may rarely be unusually severe. Among those detailed are decided coryza, vomiting, convulsions, delirium, bleeding from the eyes, ears or nose, edema of the face, dizziness, fainting, severe headache, rigors, croup, and various cutaneous eruptions.

The *eruption* is extremely prone to vary, not only in different epidemics, but in different cases in the same epidemic, and even in different parts of the body in one person. In fact, this multiform appearance is one of the greatest characteristics of the disease. Two types are especially noticeable, and both must be considered as entirely normal forms.

In **Rubella morbilliforme** the spots are fully the size of a split pea and deeper colored than usual, exhibiting the tint of measles and being often characteristically grouped as in that disease.

In **Rubella scarlatiniforme,** on the other hand, the eruption, at first macular and discrete, becomes by the second day widely confluent and is not perceptibly elevated. Careful examination will usually reveal a few macules in the general redness, especially on the brows, wrists and fingers. Nevertheless, in many cases a diagnosis from scarlatina, based upon the eruption, is entirely impossible, especially if the case was not seen at the onset. Filatow[17] believes the scarlatiniform type to be a distinct disease and applies to it the older German title "Rubeola scarlatinosa." In institution-epidemics of rubella, however, we[8] have observed some children with an eruption exactly simulating measles, and others with the most typical rubella scarlatiniforme. All gradations may be found between the two extremes. Sometimes the rash is scarlatiniform in some regions of the body and morbilliform in others.

Other peculiarities of the rash are occasionally seen, such as vesiculation, purpuric development, a marbled appearance, an annular arrangement, a disappearance with reappearance later, a true retrocession with severe general symptoms, or a sensation as of shot beneath the surface. The sequence of its appearance may vary also, the trunk and arms being first involved in some instances, or it may be limited to certain regions or last but a few hours. It is probable also that the disease may rarely occur without eruption.

Considerable variation may be observed in the other symptoms of the eruptive stage. Thus the catarrhal manifestations may be marked, especially in the morbilliform type; sore throat and laryngitis may be severe; the temperature may be high; vomiting may be violent; delirium or convulsions may occur. *Desquamation* may sometimes be unusually abundant and prolonged.

Complications and Sequels.—These occur only rarely. Those oftenest seen are respiratory. Severe *bronchitis* is sometimes witnessed, and *pneumonia* may develop as a complication or sequel. We have seen it follow in 2 instances. *Croup* and *pleurisy* have been reported. *Stomatitis* is an occasional complication. *Intestinal catarrh* is rare, although in an anomalous severe epidemic reported by Cuomo[18] it was witnessed repeatedly.

A secondary *sore throat* occurring rarely as a sequel has been recorded, and *albuminuria* and *nephritis* have been frequent in some entirely anomalous epidemics (Edwards[19]), but ordinarily are most unusual. Wichman[20] had the uncommon experience of seeing *arthritis* in 18 out of 75 cases, and fatal purpura hemorrhagica was reported by Stratford[21] and mengino-encephalitis by Brock.[22] Among other rare complications and sequels recorded, generally in anomalous cases, are thyroid enlargement, conjunctivitis, keratitis, otitis, endocarditis, icterus, urticaria, erysipelas, impetigo, furunculosis, temporary paralysis, serous meningitis, and abscesses in different parts of the body. Other *infectious diseases* may occasionally be associated with rubella.

Relapse and Recurrence.—*Relapse* is very unusual. Isolated cases are recorded in medical literature. It occurred 3 times in 150 cases which one of us[8] has previously reported. It is oftenest seen from one to three weeks after the beginning of the first attack.

Recurrence is rare, one attack fully protecting from another. In 363 cases of rubella Widowitz[23] saw recurrence in but 1 instance.

Prognosis.—This is almost invariably good; certainly so unless the disease has assumed an entirely anomalous form. Certain epidemics have been reported, especially in earlier years, where the mortality reached from 5 to 9 per cent. All such occurrences are, however, very unusual. Death has generally depended upon complications, but occasionally upon the depressing effect of the disease itself.

Diagnosis.—The most important diagnostic signs are the variable duration of incubation, the short or absent prodromes, the slight degree of catarrhal symptoms and of fever, the presence of sore throat and enlarged superficial cervical, occipital and posterior auricular glands, and the characteristic discrete eruption. The combination of the last with insignificant attendant symptoms is very suggestive of the disease. The importance of a correct diagnosis is great, since an error may be sufficient to spread measles or scarlet fever through a house or a school. There is no disease of which it is more true that the diagnosis must be based upon the study of the entire complex of symptoms. In the differential diagnosis from *scarlet fever* the extinction test (p. 263) within its limitations may be of assistance, and the different character of the desquamation is of importance.

Treatment. Prophylaxis.—The contagiousness of rubella and the fact that it is communicated to others even before it is recognized, render prophylaxis exceedingly difficult. It is certainly not communicable for more than eight days from its onset and probably not after two or three days. In view of the difficulties mentioned and the usual mildness of the disease it must be determined by the individual physician and the family, if the diagnosis is certainly established, whether or not isolation in the household is to be attempted. The usual rules regarding association with outside children must, however, be followed.

Treatment of the Attack.—This is purely symptomatic and is, indeed, seldom needed.

References

1. Edinburgh M. J., 1866, 404. 2. Hufeland's Jour. der prac. Arzneykunde, 1812, **34,** St. 3, 60. 3. Med. Trans. Coll. Phys., London., 1815, **5,** 149. 4. Correspondbl. f. Schweiz. Aertze, 1890, **20,** 369. 5. Pediatria, 1925, **33,** 57. 6. Arch. Int. Med., 1914, **13,** 913. 7. Ziemssen's Handb. spec. Path. u. Therap., B. 2, H. 2, 128. 8. Griffith, N. Y. Med. Rec., 1887, **32,** 11; 37. 9. Monatschr. f. Kinderh., 1929, **45,** 206. 10. J. Orient. Med., 1923, **1,** 115. 11. Ztschr. f. klin. Med., 1906, **59,** 444. 12. Wien. med. Wchnschr., 1915, **65,** 919. 13. J. Orient. Med., 1923, **1,** 112. 14. Ztschr. f. Kinderh., Orig., 1920, **16,** 12. 15. Riv. di clin. pediat., 1922, **20,** 513. 16. Quain's Dict. of Med., Am. Ed., 1885, 1382. 17. Arch. f. Kinderh., 1886, **7,** 241. 18. Giorn. internaz. d. sc. med., 1884, **6,** 529. 19. Am. J. M. Sc., 1884, **88,** 448. 20. Hospitalstidende, 1898, **6,** 921. 21. Lancet, 1911, **2,** 156. 22. Lancet, 1929, **2,** 1190. 23. Wien. klin. Wchnschr., 1909, **22,** 1596.

CHAPTER V

THE FOURTH DISEASE, INFECTIOUS ERYTHEMA, AND ROSEOLA INFANTUM

THE FOURTH DISEASE

(Filatow-Dukes Disease)

In 1900 Dukes[1] published the report of three series of cases which, he believed, showed the existence of a fourth eruptive fever in addition to measles, scarlet fever and rubella. He maintained that the affection generally believed to be the scarlatiniform type of rubella was in reality a distinct disorder. This was practically the view advanced by Filatow[2] in 1885, and which had earlier been suggested by Thomas.[3] Zahorsky[4] claims to have observed two small outbreaks. The only reason for maintaining the independence of the affection was that it apparently did not protect from scarlatina. The arguments advanced by Dukes do not seem to us[5] at all convincing, there being no proofs given that the disease was not rubella in two epidemics and mild scarlet fever in the third. This has been practically the position maintained by Williams,[6] Caiger,[7] Pleasants,[8] Poynton,[9] and most of those who have given the matter close attention. As described the rash is scarlatiniform with early and quickly disappearing desquamation, the general symptoms being mild.

ERYTHEMA INFECTIOSUM

The disease appears to have been described by Willan[10] in 1801, who, although he regarded it as measles without catarrhal symptoms, gives a description with a color plate which strongly suggests erythema infectiosum. He emphasizes the fact, too, that it did not protect from measles. It was described also by Tschamer[11] in 1889, who reported on a small epidemic which presented many of the features now recognized as characteristic of the disease. Its independence as a distinct disorder was emphasized by Escherich,[12] and although its position as such is not entirely established, yet it certainly appears in no way to protect against scarlet fever, measles or rubella, nor do these diseases give immunity against it. Reviews on the subject have been published by Escherich,[13] Shaw,[14] Tobler[15] and Stooss.[16] Epidemics have been described by Michalowicz,[17] Heisler,[18] Herrick,[19] Bocchini,[20] and Zappert.[21]

It occurs epidemically especially in spring and summer (Tobler, in winter) and attacks children generally between four and twelve years of age. Adults also contract it, but it is uncommon in infancy. It is only moderately infectious. The nature of the germ is unknown.

Symptoms.—The period of incubation appears to vary from six to fourteen days. Initial symptoms are generally absent or consist only of malaise, discomfort, catarrhal manifestations and sore throat. The rash appears first on the face in the form of a rose-red efflorescence, occupying especially the cheeks, symmetrical in distribution, disappearing momentarily on pressure, and suggesting erysipelas. The skin is swollen and hot and the edges of the affected area are generally slightly raised and sharply defined in an irregular line. The forehead and chin exhibit only discrete small patches of bluish-red color, and the temples, bridge of the nose and the oral circle are uninvolved. On the second day an eruption rather resembling that on the forehead appears on the body, especially the gluteal region, where it is always well-developed, and on the outer surface of the arms and legs, but only to a limited extent on the trunk. It is morbilliform in character, but more macular than papular, with some confluence on the extensor surfaces of the arms, while on the flexor surfaces of the arms and legs it is always less intense. The hands and feet are the last parts to be involved. In many regions on the extremities the rash has a map-like appearance, or is crescentically grouped, or forms annular spots with paler centers, especially while fading. This annular feature is particularly characteristic. On the trunk there are scattered discrete spots, pea-size or larger, sometimes grouped as described; or there may be no eruption whatever.

The rash fades from the face in four or five days, and disappears entirely from the body in six to ten days from its first appearance. No pigmentation or desquamation follows. The mucous membranes exhibit no eruption.

There are practically no symptoms attending the eruption. The blood shows a normal or slightly diminished number of leukocytes for the first few days, but then develops a moderate leukocytosis with some increase of the eosinophiles (Stooss[16]). According to Lawton and Smith[22] there is no leukocytosis, but a tendency to eosinophilia and a relative lymphocytosis.

In the matter of **diagnosis,** the disease is most likely to be confounded with rubella, although it is in reality quite unlike it. In the latter disorder the rash spreads uniformly over the body, is well-developed in the oral circle and on the forehead and exhibits either discrete small macules or a wide-spread confluence over the cutaneous surface. The lymphatic glands are enlarged. None of this is true of infectious erythema. Measles may resemble it, but only superficially in the appearance of the eruption on the extremities; the other symptoms of this disease being lacking. Scarlet fever has but slight resemblance. The general symptoms, the appearance of the throat and the distribution of the rash are characteristic in this disease. The medicamentous and other erythemata have little in common with infectious erythema, and the history, course and distribution of their eruptions aid in distinguishing them.

The **prognosis** is entirely favorable, there are no complications and sequels, and **treatment** is not required.

ROSEOLA INFANTUM

(Exanthema Subitum)

This eruptive fever, the infectiousness of which seems doubtful, has been described by a number of investigators (Levy;[23] Veeder and Hemplemann;[24] Westcott;[25] Greenthal;[26] Park and Michael;[27] Tso;[28] Ruh and Garvin;[29] Conrad;[30] Shima;[31] Glanzmann;[32] Faber and Dickey[33]). The first account of it was given by Zahorsky[34] who named it "Roseola infantum." Veeder and Hemplemann called it "Exanthem subitum," and Westcott, "Pseudorubella." An excellent review is given by Heiman.[35]

Its nature is not certainly determined, but there is reason to believe that it is an independent disorder, since in a few of the reported cases the child had previously had rubella, measles and scarlet fever, or did so later. Infectiousness must be slight, and in none of the published cases has there been more than one case in a family. We have, however, observed two instances in which a second child in a family was attacked five days after the development of the disease in the first patient.

Etiology.—The cause is unknown. The majority of the cases occur in late spring. The *age* ranges from six months to three years, or occasionally up to fourteen years. The first two years of life show the majority of the cases.

Symptoms.—The onset is abrupt with high fever, which continues for three days, generally without other symptoms except malaise. Occasionally the onset is attended by vomiting, and rarely by convulsions.

Sometimes there is diarrhea; but no anorexia, nor catarrhal symptoms other than, very exceptionally, congestion of the throat. Fever continues until the fourth day, or occasionally the third or fifth, and then falls by crisis, and contemporaneously the eruption appears. This is generally seen first on the neck and spreads rapidly to the trunk, upper arms and thighs. The face and the limbs below the elbows and knees are little involved. Its height is reached in a few hours and it has disappeared by the end of forty-eight hours. The rash consists of abundant, pale, rose-red, macular or sometimes elevated scattered spots from 1 to 5 mm. (.04 to .20 in.) in diameter, irregular in outline or less often round, and only occasionally confluent. A crescentic grouping is never present. A whitish areola may surround the lesions. Itching and desquamation are absent. There are no subjective symptoms whatever during this stage, the patient apparently feeling perfectly well. The blood, examined both before and during the eruptive period, according to Veeder and Hemplemann and confirmed by Glanzmann and others, shows a very decided leukopenia, sometimes as low as 3500, with a relatively high lymphocytosis. A decrease in the eosinophiles was noted by Shima.

The **prognosis** is entirely favorable.

Diagnosis.—The chief diagnostic features are the sudden onset, the comparatively long febrile period, the absence of catarrhal or other symptoms, the blood-findings, and the character of the eruption as described.

Treatment other than symptomatic is not required.

References

1. Lancet, 1900, **2,** 89. 2. Arch. f. Kinderh., 1886, **7,** 241. 3. Ziemssen's Cyclop. Pract. Med., Amer. Ed., 1875, 2. 4. Am. J. Dis. Child., 1924, **28,** 261. 5. Griffith, Phila. M. J., 1902, Apr. 12. 6. Brit. M. J., 1901, **2,** 1797. 7. Brit. M. J., 1901, **2,** 590. 8. Phila. M. J., 1902, May 24, 938. 9. Brit. M. J., 1901, **2,** 594. 10. Descript. and Treatm. of Cutan. Dis., 1901, **1,** 234. 11. Jahrb. f. Kinderh., 1889, **29,** 372. 12. Trans. 11th Internat. Med. Cong., 1896. 13. Monatschr. f. Kinderh., 1904, **3,** 285. 14. Am. J. Med. Sc., 1905, **129,** 16. 15. Ergebn. d. inn. Med. u. Kinderh., 1915, **14,** 70. 16. Pfaundler und Schlossmann, Handb. d. Kinderh., 1923, **3,** Aufl. 2B, 235. 17. Przegl. pedj. 4–5; Ref. Jahrb. f. Kinderh., 1910, **71,** 235. 18. München. med. Wchnschr., 1914, **61,** 1684. 19. Am. J. Dis. Child., 1926, **31,** 486. 20. Pediatria, 1928, **36,** 731. 21. Wien. klin. Wchnschr., 1930, **43,** 950. 22. Arch. Int. Med., 1931, **47,** 28. 23. J.A.M.A., 1921, **77,** 1785. 24. J.A.M.A., 1921, **77,** 1787. 25. Am. J. Med. Sc., 1921, **162,** 367. 26. Am. J. Dis. Child., 1922, **23,** 63. 27. Am. J. Dis. Child., 1922, **23,** 521. 28. China M. J., 1922, **36,** 130. 29. Arch. Pediat., 1923, **40,** 151. 30. Virginia M. Monthly, 1923, **49,** 705. 31. J. Orient. Med., 1923, **1,** 61; Ref. J.A.M.A., 1923, **81,** 422. 32. Schweiz. med. Wchnschr., 1924, **54,** 589. 33. Arch. Pediat., 1927, **44,** 491. 34. Pediatrics, 1910, **22,** 60. 35. Arch. Pediat. 1925, **42,** 447.

CHAPTER VI

VARIOLA

(Smallpox)

Smallpox has existed since earliest times in Asia and since at least the seventh century in Europe. The best early description of it was by Rhazes[1] in the first part of the tenth century. It is now seen but seldom in children where the practice of vaccination prevails. Yet in the registration area of the United States[2] for the years 1926, 1927 and 1928, there were 643 deaths from the disease in persons under the age of twenty years.

Etiology. Predisposing Causes.—Race, climate, locality, sex and age exert no influence. The infant may be born with the disease, or having already had it, or may develop it soon after birth as readily as at any later period of life. Vaccination of the mother during pregnancy does not protect the infant (Lieberman[3]). The individual susceptibility is very great, although an immunity, temporary or permanent, is occasionally found to exist in unprotected persons. The affection is prone to occur in epidemics and especially in the winter and spring.

Exciting Cause.—The disease is one of the most contagious known, yet the nature of the virus has never been positively determined. A protozoan-like body was observed by Grünhagen,[4] and this described by Guarnieri[5] as "cytoryctes variolae," and the findings confirmed by Councilman, Magrath and Brinckerhoff,[6] and others; but it is claimed by Proescher[7] and others that these bodies are only protein end-products. Very minute organisms have been found seemingly concerned in the causation of the disease, but it is doubtful whether they are filterable (MacCallum[8]).

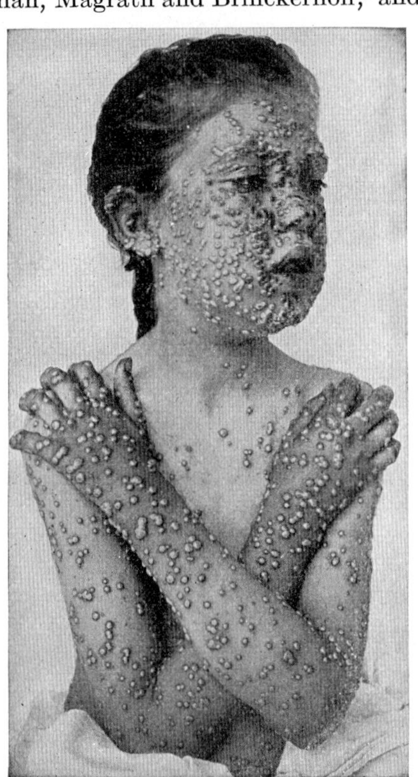

Fig. 48.—Discrete smallpox. Occurring in an unvaccinated girl. Eighth day of eruption. (*Welch and Schamberg, Acute Contagious Diseases*, 1905, *Pl. XV, opp. p.* 177.)

Transmission.—The transmission of the virus by inoculation was long made use of in "variolation." It is communicated also by direct contact, and, as generally believed, to an unusual degree through the surrounding air, from a distance of several hundred yards. This is, however, denied by many. It is readily carried by clothing, insects and the like, or by a third, healthy person. The infection certainly resides in the pustules and the crusts, but apparently not in the mucous secretions unless contaminated by pustular discharge. The blood, however, has been proven to be infectious, and it is also evident that the disease can in some way readily be communicated before the eruption appears. Such a thing as a healthy smallpox carrier does not exist, in the sense in which the term is used for diphtheria and typhoid fever. Danger of infection by the patient ceases by the time the crusts have fallen and the skin has become smooth. The *tenacity of life* of the germ is very great and may continue even for some years. The poison is generally received by way of the respiratory tract and sometimes by the digestive.

Pathologic Anatomy.—Described briefly, the pock begins as a circumscribed hyperemia, with necrosis of the epidermal cells. A reticular framework is produced, with transudation of serum into the lesion. This forms the *papule*, and further transfusion, the *vesicle*. Reticular bands hold down the center and cellular proliferation raises the periphery, and umbilication results, to disappear later under increasing tension. Leukocytes enter the vesicle and produce a *pustule*. If they penetrate deeply into the skin *scarring* results. Analogous changes take place in nearly all the mucous membranes, and sometimes a pseudomembrane is produced. Petechiae may be present on the mucous membranes as well as on the skin.

Hemorrhage may be discovered in the serous membranes, the various organs, the muscles, and the medullary cavity of the bones. Hypostatic pulmonary congestion and bronchopneumonia are common postmortem lesions. In cases which have passed into the suppurative stage, parenchymatous degeneration of the liver, heart, and kidneys is found, and the spleen and lymphatic glands are enlarged.

Symptoms. (*A*) VARIOLA VERA. DISCRETE SMALLPOX (Fig. 48).—In this, the usual form of smallpox, the lesions are everywhere discrete, or confluent on the face and hands only.

Period of Incubation.—This is usually twelve to fourteen days, but may vary from five to twenty or more. As a rule no symptoms are present, but occasionally the last days of this period are marked by malaise, dulness, headache, and loss of appetite.

Period of Invasion.—The onset is generally sudden, with repeated vomiting, prostration, headache, pain in the back, limbs and epigastrium, loss of appetite, coated tongue, thirst, high fever and rapid pulse. Initial convulsions may occur in early life, or a chill in older children. Diarrhea may replace the constipation present in adults. The temperature rises very rapidly to 103 or 104 F. (39.4 or 40 C.) or more. There is restlessness, either sleeplessness or drowsiness, and often delirium.

On the second day the headache, backache, and rapid pulse persist, and occasionally the convulsions, vomiting and abdominal pains also; and the temperature continues unaltered or even rises. Not infrequently, but less often in children, a *prodromal rash* is observed, which is scarlatiniform or morbilliform in type. The scarlatiniform rash is generally limited to the inner surface of the thighs, the lower part of the abdomen, the axillae, the sides of the chest and, according to Tsurumi and Isono,[9] the outer side of the upper arms; but sometimes covers the entire surface and suggests erysipelas. The morbilliform eruption is irregularly distributed, either in limited areas or more widely spread. The prodromal rash may disappear before the characteristic eruption of the disease develops, or may last for a time. Petechiae are sometimes seen in cases destined to be hemorrhagic. The duration of the period of invasion is from two to three days. The general symptoms of the second day continue unabated until the eruption begins to develop.

Period of Eruption. *The Rash.*—On the third or sometimes the fourth day from the onset of the initial symptoms the characteristic eruption begins to show itself. The *individual lesion* consists at first of a red macule which gradually becomes a hard, elevated papule by the second day (the fourth of the disease). It now gives the oft-described sensation as of a shot beneath the skin. On the third day of the eruption a minute vesicle appears in the center and grows slowly to the fifth or sixth day, when it is as large as a good-sized split pea, very firm, of a mother-of-pearl color, circular, slightly flattened on top, often with a central umbilication, and with a narrow red areola. Pricking with a needle allows a small quantity of serum to exude, but the vesicle does not collapse; that is to say, it is multilocular.

By the sixth day of the eruption (the eighth of the disease) suppuration begins and proceeds rapidly, and by the eighth or ninth day is at its height, the vesicle having become a yellow, entirely opaque pustule, of globular form without umbilication, and surrounded by a very distinct areola with much swollen skin about it. The pustule may now rupture, or may remain unruptured and develop a secondary umbilication.

The *regions first attacked* are generally the face and wrists, whence the rash extends to the head, hands, and arms, and in twenty-four hours to the trunk and then to the lower extremities, occupying about three days before it reaches its fullest extent. By this time the entire surface, but especially the face and head, is well covered, the rash having become vesicular in the region first attacked, while still macular or papular elsewhere. The exposed portions of the body show the greatest number of lesions, the trunk being nearly always least involved. In adults the distal portions of the limbs are more affected than the proximal, but this is less well-marked in children. There are more lesions above than below the umbilicus, the flanks are usually clear, and the pit of the axilla is uninvolved. The lesions are separated from each other by skin that is normal except for the swelling, which is especially marked on the face, hands and feet. In some cases the pocks appear everywhere simultaneously; in others first on some other regions than the usual ones. They may number some hundreds in an average case. Those upon the palms and soles consist at first of macules surrounded by an indurated area. They become flattened, deep-seated vesicles, but do not pass through a papular stage.

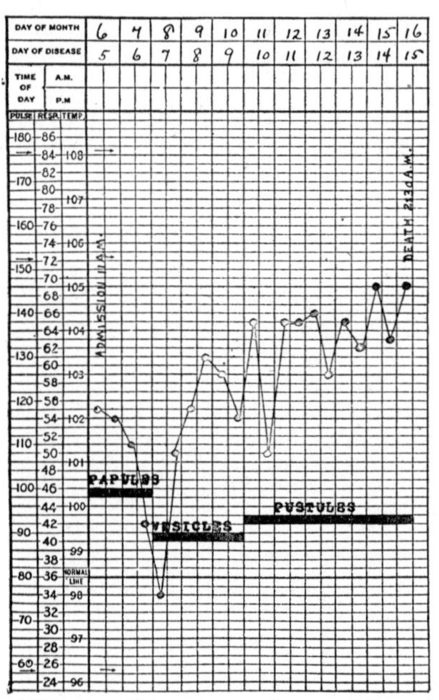

Fig. 49.—Discrete smallpox with typical course. Emily E., aged five years. Never vaccinated. Mar. 2, nausea, headache, aching in legs and back, fever; Mar. 5, amelioration in symptoms, papular rash developing on face; Mar. 7, decided fall of temperature, vesicles appearing; Mar. 10, rise of temperature with pustular stage. From a patient in the Philadelphia Hospital for Contagious Diseases. (*Courtesy of Dr. B. Franklin Royer.*)

Simultaneously with the cutaneous eruption, or a little earlier, lesions may be found on the mucous membrane of the mouth, pharynx, nose, and sometimes the larynx, vagina, rectum and eyes. Their course is similar to that of the cutaneous eruption, except that the vesicles soon rupture and leave ulcerated surfaces.

Symptoms Attending the Eruption.—With the appearance of the cutaneous rash, or shortly after or before it, there is usually a sudden or gradual fall of temperature to normal or nearly so, and the constitutional symptoms improve greatly (Fig. 49). When suppuration begins on the sixth day of the rash, the temperature gradually rises again with morning remissions. This is called the "secondary" or "suppurative" fever. Then follows increase of temperature until about the eleventh or twelfth day of the eruption, when it falls by lysis in favorable cases, the elevation which was reached being generally less than in the stage of invasion. With the onset of the secondary fever the pulse and respiration again become rapid, the heart often weak, and prostration decided. There is severe pain, swelling, tension, and itching of the face, neck and extremities. Every movement or even the pressure of the bed or the bed-clothes may be the cause of great suffering. The eyes may be closed and nasal respiration obstructed; the face so swollen that the patient is unrecognizable. Restlessness, sleeplessness, and delirium are common. The throat is sore and swallowing difficult, thirst excessive, the tongue parched, the breath foul, the teeth and gums covered with sordes, diarrhea may occur, and conjunctivitis and cough are common. The urine often contains albumin and casts. The discharging pus from ruptured lesions produces a very offensive odor.

The blood in smallpox exhibits a diminution of hemoglobin early in the disease. Hoffman[10] in a study of 300 cases found a slight leukopenia in the prodromal stage, but a decided leukocytosis, especially of the mononuclear cells, in the latter part of the eruptive period. There was a moderate eosinophilia during the attack, increasing in the fourth week. Magrath, Brinckerhoff and Bancroft,[11] and others earlier, observed a varying leukocytosis, especially of the mononuclear cells, during the eruptive stage.

Period of Desquamation.—Drying begins about the eleventh or twelfth day of the eruption, generally first in the earliest lesions. By the fourteenth or fifteenth day in average cases the crusts begin to fall. Many, however, are very adherent and do not separate until during the fourth week or later, unless removed forcibly. Following the separation a branny desquamation occurs. On the hands and feet the entire skin may be shed in the form of molds. After desquamation is over there remains a reddish pigmentation, later becoming brownish. The normal color is regained only after weeks or months.

With the beginning of desiccation the swelling and pain in the skin lessen, the areolae about the pustules grow smaller, the temperature begins to fall, and the symptoms in general improve. The itching of the skin is now frequently intense. The hair often falls out temporarily. Feebleness of body and of mind may be present, and disappear slowly only after several weeks. Any scarring left by the disease does not assume the characteristic white appearance for three or four months.

The principal well-defined modifications of the type of the disease are (*B*) *Confluent smallpox*, (*C*) *Hemorrhagic smallpox*, (*D*) *Mild smallpox*, (*E*) *Varioloid*, or *smallpox modified by vaccination*.

(*B*) Confluent Smallpox.—This form is characterized by the tendency of the lesions to fuse, generally with an increase in severity of all the constitutional symptoms. The prodromes are the ordinary ones, but always severe. There is less tendency for the symptoms to subside and the temperature to fall as the eruption develops, this last spreading with great rapidity. In the suppurating stage the entire face may resemble one enormous pustule.

(*C*) Hemorrhagic Smallpox.—This is the malignant form of the disease. The incubation is often very short. The hemorrhagic tendency may develop either in the prodromal or in the eruptive stage. In the former, called **purpura variolosa** or "black smallpox," the symptoms are violent and a purpuric rash appears, at first petechial and later ecchymotic. Much of the surface of the body may exhibit an almost uniform purplish color. Hemorrhage from various mucous membranes may occur. Generally the true eruption of smallpox does not develop; or, if the patient live until the time of the eruptive period, is represented by a few papules only.

In the second variety of hemorrhagic smallpox, called **variola pustulosa haemorrhagica,** the earlier stages of the disease are severe, but the hemorhagic tendency shows itself only as the vesicles or pustules begin to form. Bleeding takes place into the lesions, and in the still severer cases into the surrounding tissues and from the mucous membranes.

(*D*) Mild Smallpox.—Individual cases, or even epidemics, occur in which, although without protection by vaccination, the course of the disease is extremely moderate. The lesions are few in number or entirely absent (**Variola sine eruptione**), and the constitutional symptoms mild or insignificant.

(*E*) Varioloid; Modified Smallpox.—This is the form observed in persons partially protected by vaccination. It is characterized by its mildness more particularly of symptoms after the onset, and the comparatively small number and rudimentary nature of the lesions. The disease, however, does not differ in nature from ordinary smallpox and is as capable of transmitting the unmodified form to unprotected persons. A prodromal rash is frequent, especially of the rubeoloid form. The distribution of the lesions is very variable. Sometimes only about half a dozen may be found, or even exceptionally none at all. They are often confined to the face and hands, but may be more numerous and widespread. Many of the papules never become vesicles, and many of the latter do not suppurate. The entire crop of lesions develops more rapidly than in unmodified smallpox and is present within twelve hours from the first evidence of eruption. With the first appearance of the eruption the initial fever falls rapidly by crisis and is seldom again elevated, and all symptoms promptly disappear (Fig. 50).

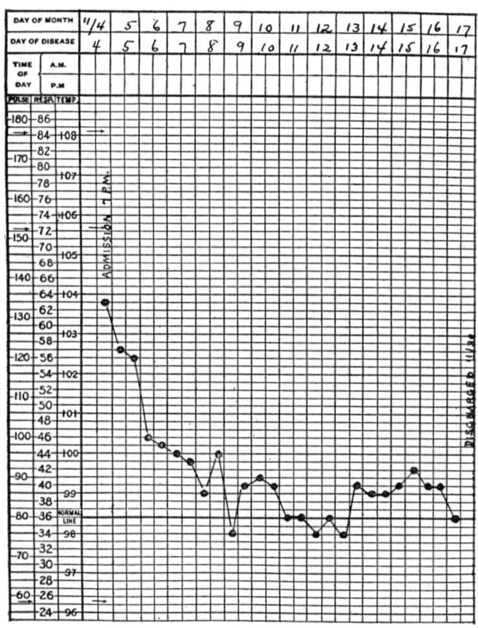

Fig. 50.—Varioloid. Adult. Vaccinated in youth. Nov. 1, headache and backache, high fever, nausea, dizziness; Nov. 3, symptoms continued until this date, when generalized papular eruption developed; Nov. 4, vesicles developed, but nearly all dried in this stage; a few pustules without secondary fever. From a patient in the Philadelphia Hospital for Contagious Diseases. (*Courtesy of Dr. B. Franklin Royer.*)

Complications and Sequels.—Respiratory affections are among the more frequent complications. Laryngitis is common, and in severe attacks involvement of the cartilages may occur, or edema of the glottis cause death. Bronchitis is invariable in severe attacks of smallpox, and bronchopneumonia is common in fatal cases. Lobar pneumonia is uncommon, but pleurisy, especially purulent, is frequent. A pseudodiphtheritic inflammation of the throat is not uncommon. Cardiac complications and nephritis are rare. Otitis is observed occasionally; and conjunctivitis, keratitis, and iritis not infrequently, sometimes followed by more or less permanent impairment of sight. Multiple cutaneous abscesses are a common sequel. Bed-sores or gangrene may develop, and suppurative adenitis is not infrequent. Osteomyelitis may be a sequel, and Chiari[12] and Brown and Brown[13] have described a special necrotic, nonsuppurative form, oftenest occurring in childhood, which frequently destroys the epiphyses. Osteo-arthritis has been reported. Among nervous disorders are neuritis, myelitis, encephalitis and meningitis.

Smallpox may coexist with, follow, or precede other acute infectious diseases, but this appears to be very exceptional. Erysipelas may develop as a sequel during convalescence.

Relapse and Recurrence.—*Relapse; i. e.*, a second attack developing before the poison is out of the system is rarely observed. *Recurrence* of smallpox is sometimes seen, but is very uncommon.

Prognosis.—The character of the epidemic is here one of the important factors, the mortality varying from 70 to 0.01 per cent (Leake[14]). Various other causes influence it. In infancy and early childhood the number of deaths is very large. Statistics of the Hospital for Contagious Diseases of Philadelphia (Welch and Schamberg[15]) gave a mortality of 61.66 per cent in subjects under one year, as compared with a total mortality of 31.79 per cent. The effect of vaccination on mortality is well illustrated by the figures given by Sweitzer and Ikeda[16] in which 107 of the 108 deaths were in unvaccinated persons. A mild initial stage generally presages a mild attack. Severe initial symptoms, however, do not necessarily indicate that the attack as a whole will be severe. Death may occur in any stage of the disease. Among unfavorable symptoms are severe nervous phenomena, abundant eruption on the skin or mucous membranes, marked suppuration, confluence of lesions, hemorrhagic manifestations, intense scarlatiniform prodromal rash, and high fever. The prognosis in modified smallpox is nearly always good, depending upon the degree of protection which vaccination has afforded.

Diagnosis.—The characteristic diagnostic symptoms are the severe pain in the head and back in the initial stage, the sudden drop of temperature about the beginning of the eruptive period, and the well-marked papular stage through which the eruption passes. With great frequency a diagnosis of *grippe* is made at the onset. Early in its development the rash has often been mistaken for *typhoid fever*. At this period, too, it may strongly resemble *measles*, and errors in diagnosis have frequently been made. The absence of the catarrhal symptoms of measles, however, and of the Koplik spots aid in excluding this. The morbilliform prodromal eruption of smallpox may likewise suggest measles. This eruption, however, is not at all elevated as is the rash of measles. The scarlatiniform prodromal rash may lead to the suspicion of *scarlet fever*. Difficulties will necessarily be present in cases in which the vaccination-pocks of *vaccinia* occur in combination with those of smallpox. The *pustular syphiloderm* also may be mistaken for smallpox. The slower onset and course, the appearance of the eruption in successive crops, the history, and the presence of other evidences of syphilis aid in recognizing this affection. *Varicella* occurring in a severe form is the disease causing the greatest diagnostic difficulty. This is especially true in the exceptional cases where the stage of invasion of varicella has been unusually long or well-marked. So, too, mild varioloid may closely simulate ordinary varicella. In varicella, however, there is a rapid development and drying of the vesicles without a papular stage; the occurrence, side by side, of lesions in crops in all stages of development instead of in a single crop; the greatest abundance of the eruption on the trunk instead of on the face and the distal parts; and a lower leukocyte count. These differences make the diagnosis generally clear. Yet in spite of them mistakes are frequently and easily made. Paul[17] developed a method of diagnosis by the inoculation of a rabbit's cornea, while Defries and McKinnon[18] employed the skin of the rabbit.

There are a number of names given to mild smallpox in different countries, among them such titles as Alastrim, Amaas, Kaffirpox, Cuban Itch, Glasspox and Milkpox. Some have considered these to be distinct diseases, but most authorities deny this (Painton,[19] Hoffman,[9] Hill,[20] Leake[14]).

Treatment. Prophylaxis. Quarantine.—Owing to the intense infectiousness any suspected case should be isolated, preferably in a hospital. Everyone exposed should be promptly vaccinated, since by its more rapid development vaccination may modify or even prevent the action of the smallpox infection. The isolation of the patient must continue until every vestige of the disease has disappeared. This takes longest on the thick epidermis of the palms and soles. The time is necessarily very variable, but averages three to six weeks from the onset. The patient, room, and every article which has been exposed should then receive the most thorough cleansing and disinfection. (See p. 249.)

Treatment of the Attack.—This is necessarily purely symptomatic. The patient should be kept scrupulously clean, the bed-clothing light and changed often, the room well-ventilated and moderately cool, the food light but nourishing and administered frequently. Water should be given freely. The aching of the initial stage and the nervous symptoms may require analgesics and sedatives, and the fever may need to be controlled by suitable hydrotherapy.

Many methods have been recommended for the treatment of the cutaneous eruption, particularly as regards the prevention of pitting. Welch and Schamberg[21] believe some good has been accomplished by the employment of tincture of iodine. It may be diluted if necessary. Painting the lesions with a strong solution of potassium permanganate has also been recommended. The tension and itching of the skin may be much relieved by the application of cold, wet dressings changed frequently, or of glycerin and water, or oily substances. The employment of a mask to keep these in place is often serviceable. Except for young children the oily dressings may contain carbolic acid. It is important to keep the crusts always moist with aqueous or oily substances, and frequent warm bathing is useful in favoring their softening and removal, as well as earlier for the relief of the cutaneous discomfort. If irritation, such as by scratching, and secondary infection can be avoided little scarring may result.

The local conditions of the mouth, throat, and nose require astringent and cleansing gargles, washes and sprays. The holding of ice in the mouth, or the employment of cocaine or its derivatives locally, often gives great relief. The eyes must be cleansed several times a day with boric acid or other mild antiseptic solutions. During the suppurative stage the importance of abundant nourishment is very great, and free stimulation is often required. The same methods, with general tonic treatment, are frequently needed during convalescence.

References

1. De variolis et morbillis, Haller, London, 1756. 2. Communic. Dis. Control., Rep. Sec. 2, White House Conf. Child Health and Protection, 1931, 20. 3. Am. J. Obst. and Gynec., 1927, **14**, 217. 4. Arch. f. Dermat. u. Syph., 1881, **4**, 150. 5. Centralbl. f. Bakteriol., 1894, **16**, 299. 6. J. Med. Research, 1903, **9**, 372; 1904, **11**, 12. 7. New York, M. J., 1913, **97**, 741. 8. Medicine, 1926, **5**, 59. 9. J. Infect. Dis., 1921, **29**, 109. 10. J. Trop. Med. and Hyg., 1923, **26**, 217; New York M. J., 1923, **118**, 616. 11. J. Med. Research, 1904, **11**, 247. 12. Beitr. z. path. Anat. u. z. allg. Path., 1893, **13**, 13. 13. J.A.M.A., 1923, **81**, 1414. 14. Pub. Health Rep., 1927, **42**, 221. 15. Acute Contag. Dis., 1905, 275. 16. Arch. Dermat. and Syph., 1927, **15**, 19. 17. Wien. klin. Wchnschr., 1916, **19**, 996. 18. Am. J. Hyg., 1928, **8**, 107. 19. Brit. M. J., 1923, **2**, 1080. 20. Canad. M. A. J., 1924, **14**, 44. 21. Acute Contag. Dis., 1905, 301.

CHAPTER VII

VACCINIA. VACCINATION

Etiology.—The identity of vaccinia or cowpox with smallpox has been disputed, but it seems most probable that it is this disease modified by its occurrence in cattle. The inoculation of the human subject with the vaccine virus is called *vaccination*. Although inoculation with the cowpox virus had been practised previously, the careful testing of the actual protective power and the urging of the procedure upon the medical profession is to be credited to Jenner.[1]

The virus of vaccinia is not definitely known. Various bacteria have been discovered in the lymph, and certain bodies apparently protozoa, and entitled "cytoryctes," have been found in the serum of the vesicle by Guarnieri[2] and others. Paschen[3] claims, however, that these are only end-products, and that the germ is much more minute and still undetermined. This is sustained by Prowazek and Miyaji.[4] Whatever its nature, it must be the same as that of variola.

Vaccination was originally performed with matter taken from a cowpox sore occurring upon a human being. Shortly afterward the virus obtained directly from the cow was employed. Later both bovine and humanized lymph were extensively used, but of recent years only the former. The lymph is usually mixed with glycerin and preserved in glass tubes; the so-called "glycerinated lymph." Glycerin destroys all pyogenic bacteria if thorough ripening has been allowed. Noguchi[5] and others have devised methods for rendering the vaccine sterile.

Age for Vaccination.—The preferable age for vaccination is about three or four months. Later the constitutional effect is liable to be greater. Should smallpox be prevalent vaccination should be done at any age, but otherwise an occasion selected when the infant is in good general condition and free from any irritation of the skin and when the weather is not hot.

Method.—One of the best is the multiple pressure or acupuncture method. The skin, without too much friction, is cleansed with soap and water followed by alcohol, ether or acetone. A small drop of virus is placed on it and then 20 or more punctures or firm pressures made through the drop with a sterilized needle held almost parallel with the skin. The punctures should be confined to an area not over $\frac{1}{8}$ in. (0.3 cm.) in diameter, and should not be deep enough to draw blood. The drop of virus may immediately be wiped off and no dressing need be applied. Later, vaccination-shields should not be worn. The lesion must be kept dry. For protection a piece of sterile gauze may be sewed into the underclothing or loosely applied over the area. If the vesicle or pustule ruptures it may be wiped with alcohol or acetone and dusted freely with powdered boric acid. Bathing should be so conducted during the height of the reaction that water does not touch the lesion. In place of the method by multiple puncture or pressure several shallow scratches may be made with the needle and the vaccine-lymph then applied and gently rubbed in, again taking care, if possible, not to cause bleeding. The *locality* usually selected is the outer surface of the upper arm at about the insertion of the deltoid, or, in girl infants, the outer surface of the leg midway between knee and ankle. A number of writers have advocated the intradermal injection of vaccine, employing about 0.1 cc. of a one to four dilution of it in salt-solution (Toomey and Hauver[6].) This method leaves no scar, but is said by some authors to lead to more complications, and has not been very widely accepted.

Course of Normal Vaccination (Fig. 51).—The development of the vaccine-lesion is practically identical with that of smallpox. (See p. 290.)

The skin shows no characteristic alteration until the third or sometimes the fourth or fifth day. A small, faintly-red macule now appears, changing quickly by infiltration into a papule surrounded by a narrow red areola. By the fifth day of the vaccination a small vesicle develops in the papule, and by the sixth day this covers the vaccinated area and is filled with transparent lymph. The vesicle is multilocular in structure and umbilicated, resembling that of smallpox. From the seventh to the ninth day it reaches its maximum size, is of a pearly-grey color, and ½ in. (1.3 cm.) or less in diameter. The areola about it then extends in width and the lymph becomes cloudy through the production of pus-cells in it. The vesicle is now tense and yellow, the umbilication disappears, the areola grows still more pronounced, and by the ninth day the underlying and surrounding tissues are red and swollen. On the tenth or eleventh day desiccation begins and the swelling and redness diminish rapidly. The pock is now flaccid and depressed, and rapidly dries into a dark crust. This crust is often fully formed by the fifteenth day, although it does not fall off, unless forcibly removed, until about the end of the third week or later, when it leaves a reddish scar which afterward becomes white, depressed, and characteristically pitted (Fig. 52).

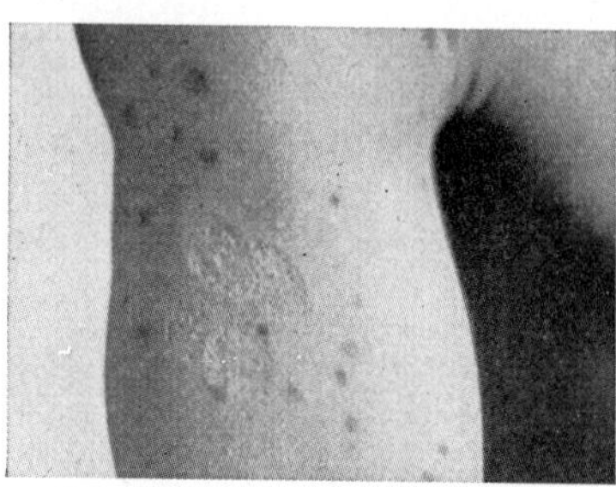

Fig. 52.—Scars of vaccination. Scars from an infantile vaccination, showing pitting and depression beneath surrounding skin. (*Welch and Schamberg, Acute Contagious Diseases*, 1905, *Pl. II.*)

Certain *symptoms* attend the vaccinal eruption, but less often in the early months of life than later. There are itching, tension, and soreness of the lesion, swelling of the lymph-nodes draining the area, and, beginning on the fifth or sixth day and reaching a maximum on the eighth or ninth, the symptoms of infection, including fever and leucocytosis.

Irregularities in the Course of Vaccination.—The lesion may appear later or, less frequently, earlier than usual; fever may be decidedly high; or the local process very severe with secondary vesicles developing. Generally they leave no scars. In rare cases a **spontaneous generalized vaccinia** is witnessed (Fig. 53). In this condition secondary vesicles are found on various parts of the body. They first appear at the time of the maturation of the original pock, or shortly before or after this, and then continue to occur in successive crops, maturing rapidly, the whole process extending occasionally over several weeks, and consequently exhibiting at the same time different stages of development. Fatal cases of generalized vaccinia have been reported by Huddleston,[7] d'Astros,[8] Hegler,[9] and others.

A **vaccinia generalized by autoinoculation** likewise may occur, the child reinoculating itself in various places by scratching or in other ways. The spots are usually very few in number, but they may be found even in the mouth, throat, eyes and nose, Vieu[10] stating that 14 cases are on record of ulceration of the tongue from this cause.

Spurious Vaccination.—Particularly in persons previously successfully vaccinated, but sometimes in primary vaccinations, the so-called *reaction of immunity* may occur, in which the area of greatest redness with slight swelling and itching is reached and has passed within ten to seventy-two hours. In *vaccinoid* the reaction, perhaps with the formation also of a small vesicle, is reached and has ceased by three to seven days. Both of these indicate probable immunity, but revaccination should always be practiced.

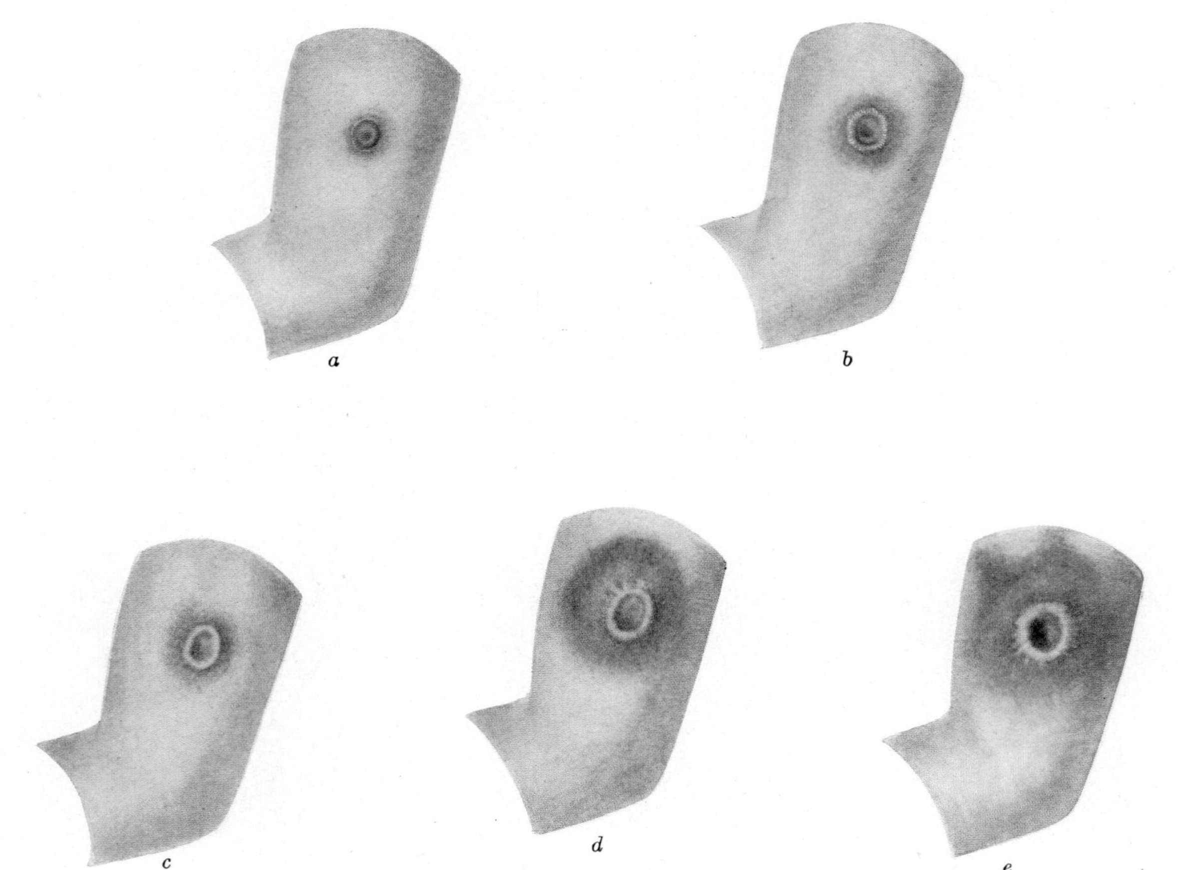
a
b
c
d
e

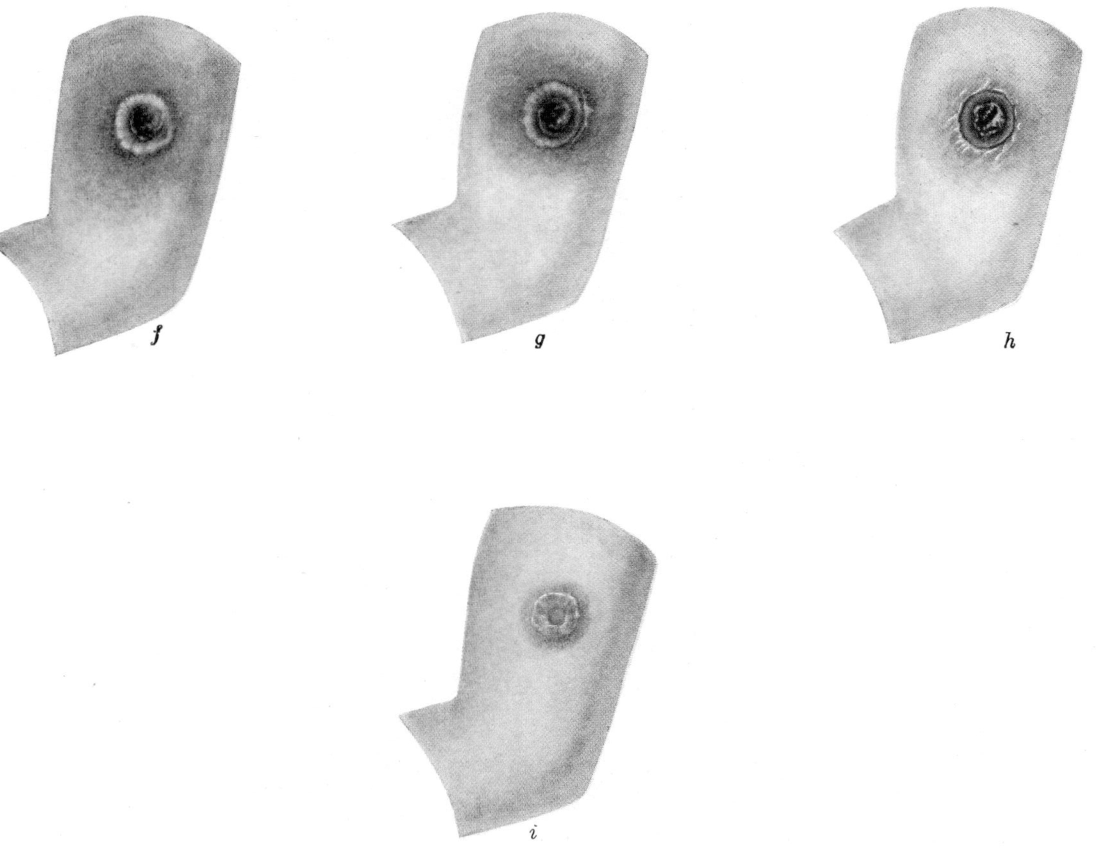

Fig. 51.—Course of normal vaccination. (*a*) fifth day; (*b*) sixth day; (*c*) seventh day; (*d*) eighth day; (*e*) ninth day; (*f*) tenth day; (*g*) eleventh day; (*h*) fifteenth day; (*i*) twenty-fifth day.

Revaccination and Insusceptibility to Vaccination.—As with all infectious diseases certain persons may be temporarily or permanently immune. Repeated vaccinations during infancy may fail to take. In all such cases further attempts should be made at intervals, as there is no certainty that the insusceptibility will be lasting.

Protective Power of Vaccination.—It is unnecessary to quote statistics here, but it may be stated that nothing except the widespread employment of vaccination can account for the great diminution in the number of cases of smallpox. Not only do general statistics throughout the civilized world prove this beyond cavil, but the instances of severe local outbreaks of smallpox in regions where vaccination had been neglected show both the importance of the procedure and that the virulence of smallpox has by no means lessened with the passing years.

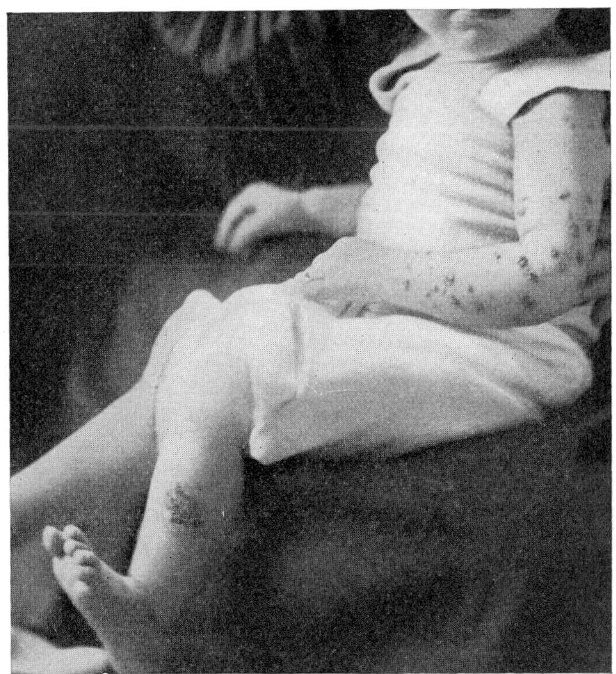

Fig. 53.—Spontaneous generalized vaccinia. Primary vaccination below the knee.

The *duration of the protective power* varies. It is safe to say that revaccination should be performed at the age of five to seven years, again at puberty, and again in early adult life. At times of epidemics everyone who has not had a successful take within a year should be revaccinated. The *degree of protection* afforded depends upon the recency of the vaccination much more than upon the size or number of the scars (Leake[11]).

Complications and Sequels.—Severe local inflammation of the lesion may take place, depending upon trauma or a poor state of health. Secondary infection may lead to ulceration cellulitis or gangrene, and general sepsis has followed this (Brouardel[12]). Eczema, urticaria, erysipelas, and a local or generalized erythema may develop. Among other cutaneous disorders occasionally reported are impetigo, lichen, ecthyma, furunculosis, psoriasis and miliaria;—the etiologic connection of some of these with vaccination being doubtful. Hemorrhagic involvement of the lesion and general purpura have been reported (Schwartz[13]). There is no danger of the transmission of syphilis or tuberculosis with the bovine lymph as now prepared. Tetanus at present is a rare complication, although in 1902 McFarland[14] collected from medical literature 95 cases of this. Some authors hold that vaccination has a deleterious effect on patients with tuberculosis. This need not prevent vaccination if they are exposed.

For a long time nervous symptoms had been mentioned among the occasional complications of vaccination, but apparently encephalitis has become of more frequent occurrence in recent years. In parts of Europe a comparatively large number of such cases have developed, as shown by the numerous reports, as of Bastiaanse,[15] Lucksch,[16] Turnbull,[17] and McIntosh.[18] Bienenstein[19] estimates the incidence of encephalitis in vaccination as 1:1,000,000 in Germany, 1:48,000 in England and 1:4000 in Holland. The cases have not been so frequent in America, but among those reporting them have been Wilson and Ford,[20] Graubarth,[21] Hassin and Geiger,[22] Flexner.[23] We have records of 2 personally observed cases. Myelitis has been reported by Spiller,[24] Perritt and Carrell,[25] Brockbank[26] and others. The pathologic changes consist of degenerative, exudative and proliferative encephalomyelitis involving both the grey and white matter, but particularly the latter, and differing from the lesions in epidemic encephalitis (Flexner). The cause of postvaccinal encephalitis is obscure and it is not clear whether it is due to a peculiar affinity of the vaccine virus for the nervous tissue, a contamination of it, or a sort of activation of, or symbiosis with, some other virus,—the last theory being the least likely. It is much more common in childhood than in infancy. The symptoms, consisting of stupor, convulsions and paralyses of various sorts, manifest themselves from the ninth to the twentieth day after vaccination. The spinal fluid may be normal or show increased pressure, excess of protein and pleocytosis. Of those patients who recover the majority are left without residual nervous lesions.

Mortality.—The mortality from vaccination is a negligible figure if proper precautions are taken. Based upon 32,000,000 vaccinations it was, according to Kübler,[27] 0.000035 per cent. Of the cases of postvaccinal encephalitis about 50 per cent died.

Treatment.—The treatment of the vaccination lesion has already been described. In other respects treatment is symptomatic. In the cases of postvaccinal encephalitis blood-serum from convalescent patients may be given intraspinally.

References

1. An Inquiry into the Causes and Effects of the Variolae vaccinae, etc. London, 1798. 2. Centralbl. f. Bakteriol., 1894, **16,** 299. 3. München. med. Wchnschr., 1906, **53,** 2391. 4. Centralbl. f. Bakt. und Parasitenk., 1914–15, **75,** 144. 5. Arch. Pediat., 1915, **32,** 698. 6. Am. J. Dis. Child., 1928, **35,** 186; J.A.M.A., 1929, **92,** 1005. 7. Med. News, 1901, **79,** 370. 8. Marseille méd., 1912, **49,** 149. 9. Dermatol. Wchnschr., 1914, **58.** Ergänzungsh. 29. 10. Ann. de dermat. et syph., 1930, **1,** 873. 11. Pub. Health Rep., 1927, **42,** 221. 12. 20th Cent. Pract. Med., **13,** 534. 13. Am. J. Dis. Child., 1925, **30,** 856. 14. Proc. Phila. County M. Soc., 1902, **23,** 166. 15. Bull. acad. de méd., 1925, **94,** 815; Nederl. Tijdschr. v. Geneesk., 1926, **70,** 268; 1931, **75,** 586. 16. Schweiz. med. Wchnschr., 1924, **55,** 897; Med. Klinik., 1925, **21,** 1377. 17. Brit. M. J., 1928, **2,** 331. 18. Brit. M. J., 1928, **2,** 334. 19. Ztschr. f. Kinderh., 1930, **49,** 248. 20. Bull. Johns Hopkins Hosp., 1927, **40,** 337. 21. Arch. Pediat., 1929, **46,** 703. 22. Arch. Neurol. and Psychiat., 1930, **23,** 481. 23. J.A.M.A., 1929, **92,** 2190; 1930, **94,** 305. 24. Brain, 1903, **26,** 424. 25. J.A.M.A., 1930, **94,** 793. 26. J.A.M.A., 1931, **97,** 227. 27. Geschichte der Pocken und der Impfung, 1901, 364.

CHAPTER VIII

VARICELLA

(Chickenpox)

Although described much earlier, varicella was first differentiated from variola by Fuller[1] in 1730, and by Heberden[2] in 1767.

Etiology. **Predisposing Causes.**—*Age* is the most important. In the first three months of life there are fewer cases than later, but the disease can occur congenitally. We have seen an infant with the lesions present at birth, and the mother suffering from the disease. In 775 cases admitted to the Cincinnati General Hospital[3] 1.4 per cent occurred in patients under six months of age; 11.7 per cent from six months to two years; 36.5 per cent from two to six years; 24.2 per cent from six to twelve years; 6.8 per cent from twelve to twenty years and 19.4 per cent in patients over twenty years; many of the last group having been sent to the hospital with a diagnosis of variola. Season, climate, and sex exert no particular influence. The individual susceptibility in childhood is great, most of those exposed contracting it, although some seem entirely immune. It is endemic in large cities, and also appears in epidemics.

Exciting Cause.—The cause is unknown. De Korte[4] described an ameba-like body present in the vesicles, Greeley[5] a sporothrix, and Auricchio[6] and MacDonald and MacDonald[7] a micrococcus, and still other germs have been reported. Staphylococci and streptococci may sometimes be found in the vesicular fluid, probably as contaminators. The virus seems to be contained in the fluid from the vesicles. (See p. 305.) Great interest attaches to the relation between this virus and those causing herpes zoster and other forms of herpes, and an extensive bibliography has followed. Many instances have been published in which herpes has developed apparently as a result of exposure to varicella, or the reverse. The two conditions have occurred simultaneously in the same patient. It is also claimed that children inoculated with material from herpes zoster may develop a typical clinical varicella, and further that there is a serologic relationship between the two diseases. Many authors, on the other hand, maintain that these experiences are merely coincidences, and that the two are distinct. It is certainly true that an attack of one of these conditions usually does not protect against the other, as we can testify from our own experience. (For reviews and discussions of this matter consult the publications of Ker,[8] Krauss,[9] Comby,[10] deLange,[11] Bokay,[12] Rivers[13] et al., Cozzolino,[14] and Netter and Urbain.[15])

The *method of transmission* is probably in most instances by direct contact, although the virus can be carried by a third person or by fomites, or be air-borne, and the disease is one of the most readily transmissible known. (For inoculation experiments, see p. 305.) The *period of infectiousness* commences at the beginning of the eruptive stage and probably for about twenty-four hours before this (Gordon and Meader[16]). Its duration is probably not longer than five to eight days after the beginning of the eruption (Thomson,[17] Gordon and Meader[16]).

Pathologic Anatomy.—The only characteristic lesions are the macules and papules, which later develop into superficial vesicles and crusts. The vesicles tend to be unilocular, but are often multilocular. Any other pathologic changes are those incident to irritation or infection, or to the complications.

Symptoms. Ordinary Form.—The *stage of incubation* averages about fourteen days, but is sometimes less and extends occasionally up to three weeks. The *stage of invasion* is usually absent, or there may be slight symptoms of the beginning of infection. At times there is a wide-spread prodromal scarlatiniform or, less often, morbilliform rash seen a few hours before the characteristic eruption. The *individual lesion* is at first a red macule disappearing on pressure, and of the size of a pin-head to that of a split pea or larger. Within a few hours a small vesicle filled with clear fluid develops on the center of the macule; in a few of the lesions preceded by a small papule. Within a day or less the vesicle enlarges to the average size of a split pea, and is round or oval in shape (Fig. 54). A narrow red areola often surrounds it. *Desiccation* now begins at once, the prominent rounded surface flattening a little and the contents becoming turbid. Slight umbilication is common at this stage. After one to two days more

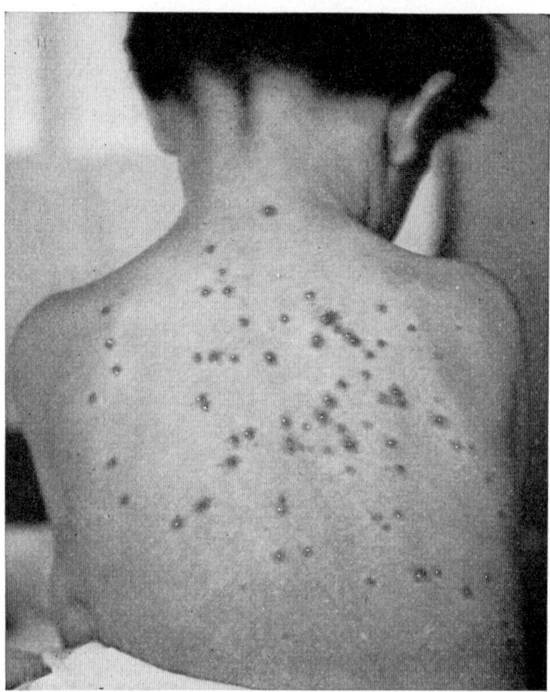

Fig. 54.—Eruption of chickenpox, showing the pearly vesicles. (*From a case in the Children's Hospital of Philadelphia.*)

the areola disappears and a yellowish crust begins to form. This falls off after a period varying from five or six days to two or three weeks, leaving the skin slightly reddened for a time.

This is the course in a typical lesion, but the majority of them never develop further than the macules or papules. Many vesicles, too, never exceed pinhead size and dry rapidly, although some become larger than the average fully developed lesion and dry slowly.

The rash generally appears first on the face and back, less often on the limbs. It spreads rapidly from above downward, and all parts of the body-surface are attacked, including the palms and soles, and mucous membrane of the mouth, throat, nose, genitalia, and sometimes the larynx, trachea and conjunctiva. Upon mucous membranes the vesicle ruptures quickly and resembles aphthous stomatitis.

The number of lesions varies from a dozen up to hundreds, with an average of about 25 to 75. They are generally most numerous on the trunk, especially the back; the forearms, hands, legs, and feet being involved decidedly less. The head is generally little affected, although there are nearly always some lesions on the scalp. They may cluster about a point of irritation; such, for example, as recent skin-tests (Martmer[18]). One of the principal characteristics of the eruption is its appearance in successive crops during the first three or four days, and the presence of lesions in all stages from macules to crusts in the same regions. If secondary infection occurs, decided suppuration may take place and healing be thereby delayed and scarring remain.

Symptoms attending the eruption are slight or absent. In well-developed cases there is moderate fever (Fig. 55), which falls gradually to normal in one or two days, but there may often be no fever whatever. Considerable itching of the skin is frequently present. The *blood* has been studied by Nobécourt and Merklen,[19] Weill and Descos,[20] Mensi,[21] Stroh,[22] Baer,[23] Hoffman,[24] Vitetti[25] and Carrara.[26] In our own[3] studies the leukocyte count was often a few thousand above normal in the first three days of the disease in infants, but in older children there was usually slight, if any, increase in the total number of leukocytes during this period. From the fourth to the ninth day many patients showed a slight leukocytosis, but others no change from normal. No significant change in the differential count was noted. Hoffman and others observed a relative lymphocytosis throughout the attack, and an eosinophilic increase after the first week. Stroh, Baer, and Carrara found a leukopenia at the height of the disease. We have occasionally observed a few myelocytes in the blood and a lymphocytic reaction; the latter being extreme in one unusual case at the Cincinnati General Hospital reported by Goldman.[27]

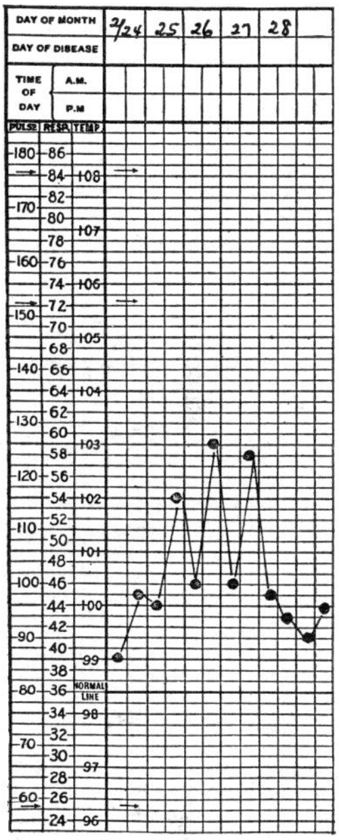

Fig. 55.—Moderately severe varicella with unusually well-developed eruption. Caroline R., aged eight years. Feb. 25, a few vesicles on the body; Feb. 27, child dull; very numerous vesicles, including a large number on the tongue; Feb. 28, improving.

Variations from the Ordinary Course.—There may be unusually severe *prodromes* with vomiting, marked nervous symptoms, and backache. Blood-stained stools have been reported. There are variations in the *eruptive stage*. The prodromal rash may continue into, or first appear during, this period. A **confluent varicella** is very exceptionally observed. **Hemorrhagic varicella** is a rare form characterized by effusion of blood into the vesicles and from the gastroenteric tract. We have seen it occasionally. The subject is reviewed by Storrie[28] and others. **Gangrenous varicella** may develop in debilitated children with septic symptoms and death. In 1 such case which we[29] have observed the bacillus pyocyaneus was recovered from the lesions, in another (Fig. 57) the child was suffering almost simultaneously from rubeola, diphtheria and varicella. Several authors, among them Joe[30] and Zahorsky,[31] have reported diphtheritic infection in the lesions of gangrenous varicella. **Bullous varicella** is a very uncommon variety, the eruption appearing as large bullae reaching an inch or more in diameter. The bullous and gangrenous forms may be combined.

Complications and Sequels.—Nephritis may occur, oftenest at the end of the first or second week. Ochsenius[32] described an instance in which 3 members of the family developed it. Usually recovery follows, but death may occur or the condition become chronic. A varicellous laryngitis may be a severe and fatal complication. We have seen it necessitate intubation. A number of cases of arthritis of a serous or purulent character have been recorded. Among other complications reported are bronchitis, pneumonia, pleurisy, myositis, bursitis, parotitis, ileocolitis, meningitis, osteomyelitis, erysipelas, adenitis, conjunctivitis, corneal ulcer, cellulitis, furunculosis, septicemia, impetigo, otitis, retention of urine the result of swelling of the prepuce, thyroiditis, thrombosis, symmetrical gangrene, appendicitis, subcutaneous emphysema, and bradycardia. Many of these are probably merely coincidental. From some of the suppurative lesions streptococci may be recovered. We have seen fatal purpura occur as a complication, and hemoglobinuria has been reported by Kaiser and Bradford.[33] Varicella may frequently be combined with other infectious diseases.

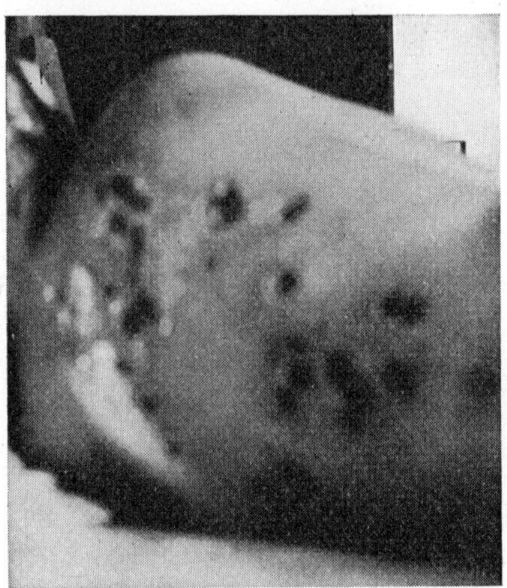

Fig. 56.—Varicella gangrenosa. Boy eight years of age. Lesions shown are those two weeks after onset. Recovery. (*Courtesy Dr. Robert Allen, Glendale, Ohio.*)

Among the most interesting of the complications are those affecting the central nervous system in which there is apparently an encephalitis or encephalomyelitis. Some of the recorded sequels, such as multiple sclerosis, hemiplegia, chorea, transitory blindness, and acute cerebellar ataxia are dependent upon this condition. Among those who have reported nervous complications and sequels are Galli,[34] Krabbe,[35] Winnicott and Gibbs,[36] Tramer[37] and Brain,[38] the last having collected 32 instances, of which 11 were predominantly cerebellar and 8 spinal. We have seen several cases in which the cerebellum seemed more involved, and 2 in which there was an ascending paralysis of the so-called Landry's type. The onset of nervous symptoms is from about the fifth to the twenty-first day. There is a tendency for complete recovery.

Several authors, among them Schiavone,[39] Schwenck[40] and Abraham,[41] believe that chickenpox is one of the diseases which reactivates tuberculosis.

Relapse and Recurrence.—**Relapse** is very rare. It has been observed by Comby,[42] Dawes,[43] P. Freud,[44] and others. **Recurrence** is also extremely uncommon. We have never seen recurrence in a patient who was personally observed in both attacks.

Prognosis.—Fatal cases are occasionally encountered these being almost invariably due to some of the complications or to the severe forms of the disease.

Diagnosis.—*Impetiginous* and *pemphigoid* eruptions may sometimes suggest varicella. The combination of *acne* with varicella may obscure the diagnosis for a time. It may be difficult to distinguish between a combination of varicella and *scarlet fever* on the one hand, and a varicella with a prodromal scarlatiniform erythema on the other. Severe cases of varicella, especially in adults, may strongly suggest *smallpox*, or modified smallpox may resemble varicella. In varicella, however, the prodromes are seldom severe, the eruption selects the trunk rather than the face and distal portion of the extremities, and the lesions are superficial and appear in successive crops, and may involve the deep axilla.

Treatment. **Prophylaxis.**—Isolation should be practised as long as the crusts remain on the body. It is very difficult to combat an epidemic of this disease in an institution, even with a cubicle-system. Inoculation has been attempted with the serum from fresh vesicles by Steiner,[45] Buchmüller,[46] Kling,[47] Rabinoff,[48] Hotzen[49] et al., Nelken,[50] Benini,[51] Finkelstein, Wilfand and Chochol,[52] Petenyi,[53] and others. The reported cases are much at variance, but there seems to be no doubt that in some cases a local reaction, or a slight general eruption, or an eruption like ordinary chickenpox can be so produced and active immunity thereby acquired. Benini injected the vesicle-lymph intracutaneously, and Hess and Unger[54] intravenously. These methods open the possibility of communicating other diseases than varicella. Késmárszky[55] claimed the production of immunity by intracutaneous injection of 0.1 cc. of citrated blood taken from a patient with chickenpox on the second day of the eruption. As shown by Blackfan, Peterson and Conroy[56] temporary immunity can be secured by the injection of convalescent's serum within five or six days after exposure, following the same method employed for measles. In our own experience[57] there seemed to be marked protective value, although others have denied its existence.

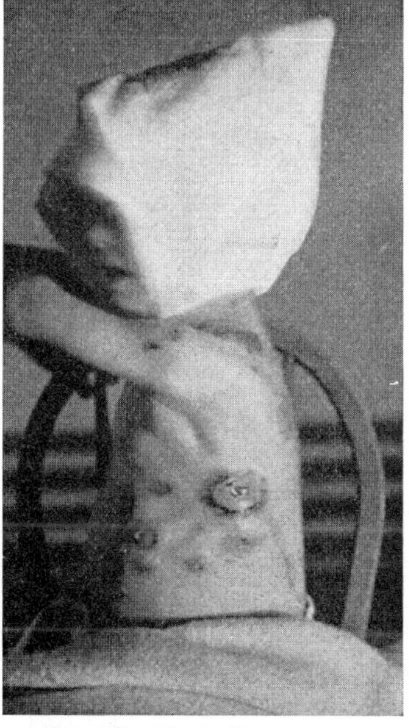

Fig. 57.—Varicella gangrenosa. Occurring in an infant of twenty-two months, a patient in the Children's Hospital of Philadelphia. Diphtheria followed by measles and in a few days by varicella. Large vesicles, some sloughing, developed on whole body, especially the head and back. Death.

Treatment of the Attack.—The treatment is symptomatic. Itching may be allayed by the application of an antipruritic powder, or carbolated or thymolated vaseline (see p. 181), or by the employment of warm baths. Care should be exercised to prevent irritation or scratching of the lesions or the formation of large crusts. *Complications* and *sequels* require appropriate treatment. In gangrenous varicella cultures should be taken of the lesions, and if the diphtheria bacillus is found, antitoxin should be administered.

References

1. Gee, Reynolds Syst. Med., Amer. Ed., 1880, **1,** 124. 2. Med. Trans. Coll. of Phys., London, 1768, **1,** 427. 3. Mitchell and Fletcher, J.A.M.A., 1927, **89,** 279. 4. Practitioner, 1905, **74,** 50. 5. N. Y. Med. Rec., 1914, **86,** 204. 6. Pediatria, 1924, **32,** 1305. 7. Illinois M. J., 1931, **60,** 230. 8. Lancet, 1920, **2,** 347. 9. New York M. J., 1921, **114,** 162. 10. Bull. et mém. soc. méd. d. hôp. de Paris, 1922, **46,** 992. 11. Berl. klin. Wchnschr., 1923, **2,** 879. 12. Jahrb. f. Kinderh., 1924, **105,** 8; 1928, **119,** 127. 13. J. Exper. Med., 1924, **39,** 777; 1924, **40,** 281; 1929, **49,** 899. 14. Pediatria, 1926, **34,** 809. 15. Ann. de l'inst. Pasteur, 1931, **46,** 17. 16. J.A.M.A., 1929, **93,** 2013. 17. Lancet, 1916, **1,** 341. 18. J.A.M.A., 1927, **88,** 1797. 19. J. de phys. et de path. gén., 1901, **3,** 439. 20. J. de phys. et de path. gén., 1902, **4,** 504. 21. Gazz. d. osp., 1912, **33,** 1625. 22. Ztschr. f. Kinderh., Orig., 1920, **26,** 120. 23. Arch. f. Kinderh., 1921, **69,** 198. 24. New York M. J., 1923, **118,** 646. 25. Pediatria, 1928, **36,** 1107. 26. Pediatria, 1930, **38,** 865. 27. Am. J. Dis. Child., 1930, **40,** 282. 28. Brit. J. Child. Dis., 1914, **11,** 62. 29. Griffith, Univ. Med. Mag., 1896, Aug., 837. 30. Brit. J. Child. Dis., 1928, **25,** 111. 31. J.A.M.A., 1930, **94,** 484. 32. Monatschr. f. Kinderh., 1930, **46,** 127. 33. Arch. Pediat., 1929, **46,** 571. 34. Pediatria, 1925, **33,** 681. 35. Brain, 1926, **48,** 535. 36. Brit. J. Child. Dis., 1926, **23,** 107. 37. Med. Klinik, 1930, **26,** 1598. 38. Brit. M. J., 1931, **1,** 81. 39. Semana méd., 1929, **36,** 1495. 40. Ztschr. f. Kinderh., 1930, **49,** 686. 41. Monatschr. f. Kinderh., 1930, **46,** 97. 42. Traité des mal. de l'enf., Grancher, 2nd ed., **1,** 376. 43. Albany Med. Ann., 1903, **24,** 532. 44. Klin. Wchnschr., 1928, **7,** 1739. 45. Wien. med. Wchnschr., 1875, **25,** 304. 46. Mittheil. des Verein der Aerzte in Steiermark, 1866; Ref. Swoboda, Pfaundler und Schlossmann, Handbk. der Kinderh., 1906, 1, b. 724. 47. Berl. klin. Wchnschr., 1915, **52,** 13. 48.

Arch. Pediat., 1915, **32,** 651. 49. Monatschr. f. Kinderh., Orig., 1919, **15,** 576. 50. Monatschr. f. Kinderh., 1926, **32,** 128. 51. Riv. di clin. ped., 1928, **26,** 824. 52. Monatschr. f. Kinderh., 1928, **40,** 489. 53. Orvosi hetil., 1928, **72,** 148; Ref. Am. J. Dis. Child., 1929, **37,** 198. 54. Am. J. Dis. Child., 1918, **16,** 34. 55. Arch. f. Kinderh., 1928, **85,** 1. 56. Ohio State M. J., 1923, **19,** 97. 57. Mitchell and Ravenel, Arch. Pediat., 1925, **43,** 709.

CHAPTER IX

TYPHOID FEVER

Typhoid fever was first clearly distinguished from typhus by Gerhard,[1] in 1836.

Etiology. Predisposing Causes.—The disease is somewhat more prevalent in temperate zones and in autumn and early winter. The influence of *age* is decided and the greatest number of cases are seen in later childhood, youth and early adult life. It is distinctly less frequent up to the age of five years and especially in the first two years of life, but numerous studies have shown that it cannot be called rare (Barthez and Sanné,[2] Schavoir,[3] Montmollin,[4] Crespin and Saracino,[5] Weston and Radbill,[6] and others). We[7,8] have personally seen many cases at this age. Improvement in hygiene has diminished the incidence at all ages in recent years.

Typhoid fever may be found even in the fetus and new-born (*Fetal and Congenital Typhoid Fever*). Cases have been reported by Morse,[9] Vignoli,[10] Gory and Dalsace,[11] and Wing and Troppoli.[12] It may also be acquired shortly after birth, an instance being reported by Gerhardt[13] in an infant of three weeks, and 1 by Weech and Chen[14] beginning about the twenty-sixth day of life. We[15] have observed a case of three months of age.

Apparently there is little if any influence of sex, state of health, or poor hygiene apart from the matter of the transmission of germs. The disease may be endemic, but tends to occur in epidemics dependent upon some factor, such as contaminated water, milk or other food which contains the germs. The *individual susceptibility* is less than in many other diseases; the infrequency in infancy being apparently due to absence of exposure.

Exciting Cause.—This is the *bacillus typhosus* of Eberth, which is found widely disseminated throughout the tissues of the body, and in the blood, bile, sputum, stools and urine.

Transmission.—In the majority of cases transmission of the germs is by the feces or urine. Drinking water and milk (Kober[16]) are the most frequent carriers, as are also flies having access to the infected feces. In the ordinary sense of the term, typhoid fever is but little contagious, and spread of the disease occurs through lack of sufficient care in disinfection. Very rarely it may apparently be contracted through germs transmitted in the milk from a mother suffering with the disease, as in an instance reported by Heiman.[17] In the case of fetal typhoid transmission is by way of the placenta. The *period of greatest infectiousness* appears to be during the second and third weeks of the disease, although the bacilli may be found in the feces earlier than this, and often later until the healing of intestinal ulcers has taken place. The *tenacity of life* of the germ is great, although it may be killed by a temperature of 60 C. (140 F.), by disinfectants, and by sunlight. There may be long persistence of the germ in the intestines, the gall bladder, and the urine.

Pathologic Anatomy. In fetal typhoid fever and in most congenital cases there is absence of intestinal ulceration. In the first two years of life the involvement of intestinal lymph-tissue is more hyperplastic than destructive; and although slight ulceration may occur, yet in some instances there is no intestinal involvement whatever. The mesenteric glands are usually, and the spleen always, enlarged. There are, however, no positive diagnostic lesions at this age. Between the ages of two and six years intestinal ulceration is somewhat more marked, and, toward the end of this period and in later childhood it is more frequent and decided. By the age of puberty the lesions are the same as those in adults. The typhoid bacilli are found in various secretions and excretions, in different organs, the rose spots, and the blood. They may be present in the stools often before the agglutinative reaction can be obtained.

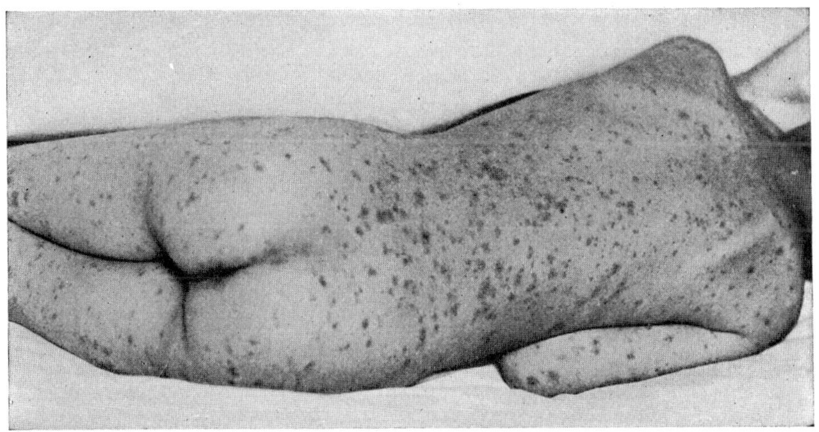

Fig. 58.—Typhoid fever with an unusual degree of development of the eruption. Minnie S., admitted to the Children's Hospital of Philadelphia Feb. 22, aged five years. Illness began five days before. Spots on abdomen observed the day before admission. The day after admission the spots were very numerous, and were seen also on the face. Spleen palpable. Recovery.

Symptoms.—The period of *incubation* is variable, but in general may be placed at one to two weeks. Anorexia, malaise and allied symptoms characterize it. *Invasion* is marked by the development of fever. Its onset may be abrupt and severe, but is oftener slow and insidious, with symptoms little pronounced. In the average case this period continues for about a week before the second, or *eruptive stage,* begins.

Ordinary Course.—Taking the last part of early childhood and the first part of later childhood as furnishing an average type, the principal characteristics distinguishing the disease at this age are: (1) The indefinite and uncharacteristic onset; (2) the short duration and mildness of the attack; (3) the disposition for nervous symptoms to be more pronounced than intestinal ones.

Certain symptoms should be mentioned individually. Of the *gastro-intestinal manifestations,* vomiting is a frequent and sore throat an occasional initial one. Anorexia and thirst are present. The tongue is generally coated and often exhibits the red triangle at the tip and the red edges so frequently described as characteristic. Constipation and diarrhea are about equally common, but this varies with the epidemic. The stools may show the typical pea-soup appearance. Great distention and tenderness of the abdomen is comparatively infrequent. *Enlargement of the spleen* is demonstrable by palpation in 80 to 90 per cent of cases. The typical *roseola* has been stated to be less common in children, but in our experience this is not the case. Morse[18] observed it in 60 per cent of 671 cases, and Henoch[19] found it absent only 19 times in 381 cases. In the average case it is discoverable about the end of the first week. The eruption consists of scattered, round, slightly elevated rose-colored papules which disappear momentarily or on pressure. They come in successive crops, measure about .08 to .16 in. (2 to 4 mm.) in diameter, each lasting about three days. It occurs principally on the trunk, but exceptionally is well marked over the whole body (Fig. 58).

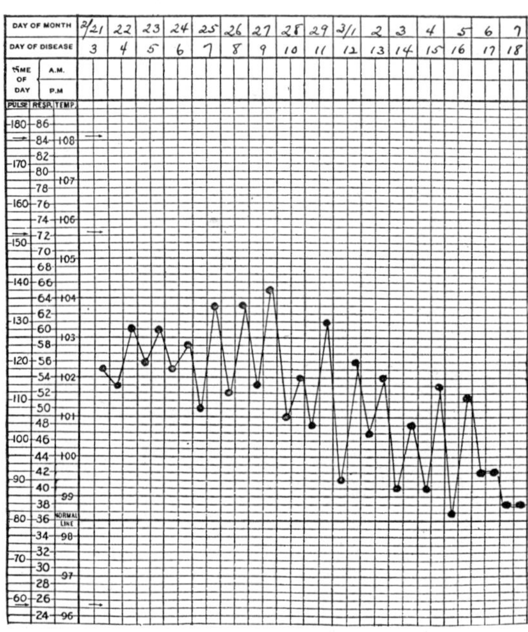

Fig. 59.—Typhoid fever, ordinary form for children. Theresa F., aged seven years. Came home from school with headache on Feb. 19; first seen Feb. 21; had not been in bed. During attack exhibited loss of appetite, enlarged spleen, very little apathy, Widal reaction. Was bright all the time. A few spots first found during a relapse.

The *temperature* often runs a very irregular course, and often a higher one than in adults. In many cases the initial stage is shortened and there is frequently absence of the terminal remittent character (Fig. 59), the final fall being commonly more rapid than in adults, and often almost critical (Fig. 60). The average duration of fever is two to three weeks, but it may be shorter or continue for four weeks or more. There is a tendency to the occurrence of elevations due to insignificant or undiscoverable causes.

The *blood* in typhoid fever shows absence of leukocytosis. The normal leukocyte picture for the different ages must be taken into consideration in this connection (p. 39). Allowing for this, there are usually found a decrease in the polymorphonuclear leukocytes and an increase of the mononuclear cells, with a diminution of eosinophiles. Hemoglobin and erythrocytes are commonly reduced later in the disease. Frequently, but by no means always, any inflammatory complication produces leukocytosis, and this condition, therefore, would not necessarily exclude typhoid fever. The typhoid bacilli may be found in the blood even before the Widal reaction can be obtained. This reaction is usually not discoverable before the beginning of the second week, and it may even not be present until late in the disease or, as we have observed it, not until convalescence; or it may possibly be first found during a relapse. It may continue for months after the disease is over. The *pulse*, as in adults, is not infrequently slower than would be expected from the degree of fever, but dicrotism is not often present, and then generally only, and occasionally, in older children. During convalescence it may be irregular and sometimes very slow. Schlieps[20] claims that the usual irregularities are due to sinus arrhythmia and have no serious import. *Arterial tension* is low.

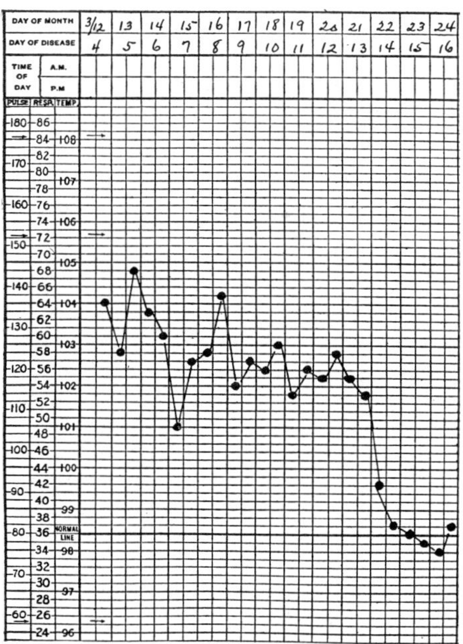

Fig. 60.—Typhoid fever with critical fall. George C., aged seven and a half years. Sudden onset with convulsion. During attack exhibited roseola, splenic enlargement, moderate diarrhea, good general condition. Temperature fell critically on the fourteenth day of the attack.

Cough is common and mild bronchitis is often present. *Epistaxis* is probably less frequent than in adults. *Emaciation* is commonly decided. *Nervous symptoms*, although more marked than gastro-intestinal, as previously stated, are generally less severe than in adults. Moderate initial headache is quite common. In severe cases there may be much pain in the limbs, neck, back or joints. The abdominal reflex is diminished. Some children remain in the best of spirits throughout the attack, but oftener there is a very characteristic decided apathy. Prostration is seldom as great as in adults. Delirium is generally absent or slight, except in severe cases. Convulsions sometimes usher in the attack even in cases which are not later severe. Coma, subsultus and the like are seldom seen at this age.

The *urine* exhibits a decided diazo-reaction. A febrile albuminuria may be present, and also acetone due to the limited diet.

Variations in Type.—Different forms of typhoid fever seen in early life may be classified (*A*) according to the age of the patient, or (*B*) according to the characteristics of the attack in general. These divisions are a matter of convenience only, and the classes naturally overlap to a considerable extent.

(*A*) Based upon *age* the types are as follows:

1. Fetal and Congenital Typhoid Fever.—The distinction between these two varieties is that in the latter the child is born alive. The majority of pregnant women suffering from the disease abort, and the germs may be recovered from the blood and organs of the fetus. The congenital cases are sometimes premature and sometimes born at term. Death nearly always occurs, either in a few minutes or after several days or weeks. The symptoms are usually uncharacteristic. Fever is generally present, and convulsions, icterus, diarrhea, constipation, tympanites, roseola, enlarged spleen, cough, vomiting, intestinal hemorrhage, and purpura have been reported. The mere discovery of a positive Widal reaction cannot be looked upon as diagnostic, since it may be found in apparently healthy children born of typhoid mothers. In an interesting case observed by us the mother died of typhoid fever one week after her infant was born. The infant, while remaining symptomatically well, had a positive Widal reaction at the age of twenty-five days, and three days later a positive stool-culture. The blood-culture on several occasions was negative.

2. Infantile Typhoid Fever.—Here are included cases in which the affection is acquired after birth and during the first two years of life. Especially in the first year there is often absence of characteristic symptoms, the diagnosis being made by blood-culture and later by the Widal reaction and the typhoid roseola. Temperature is generally high and very irregular, and very often a diagnosis of ileocolitis is made. Diarrhea, tympanites, and vomiting are more frequent than later in life. There are often marked prostration, rapid pulse, and restlessness rather than apathy. Bronchitis is common; epistaxis infrequent.

3. Typhoid Fever in Early Childhood.—From the age of two up to six years the attack is usually more benign than at any other period of life. Diarrhea is less common and seldom troublesome; the fever while more characteristic is generally short in its course; nervous symptoms are usually mild; complications not frequent. There are exceptions to this, and the attack may be severe.

4. Typhoid Fever in Later Childhood.—This type, especially after ten years of age, is distinctly more like that seen in adults, and intestinal symptoms and complications are more likely to be witnessed than earlier, owing to the greater tendency to ulceration. The symptoms of the typhoid state are more prone to develop.

(*B*) Based upon *symptoms* as a whole, regardless of age, the following varieties may be mentioned:

1. Abortive Form.—This type is not infrequent. All the characteristic early symptoms may be mild, or present as in the ordinary or severe form, but the course lasts only eight to ten days (Fig. 61).

2. Mild Form.—This is commonly seen in early childhood. There is no diarrhea, anorexia or prostration, and, in fact, practically no subjective symptoms of any severity. Even the temperature may in occasional cases scarcely exceed 100 F. (37.8 C.) (*Afebrile Form*).

3. Nervous Form.—This variety is not uncommon. It may begin abruptly as a pseudomeningitis with repeated convulsions, unconsciousness, restlessness, rigidity of neck, and delirium (*Meningitic typhoid*). These early manifestations tend to cease soon. Sometimes, especially in older children, nervous symptoms may not develop until later. In these cases the spinal fluid is usually normal, except sometimes for increased pressure.

Complications and Sequels.—These are less common in childhood and especially in early childhood and infancy. Those of the *respiratory tract* are perhaps most frequent, and there may be bronchitis, laryngitis, pneumonia and, rarely, ulceration of the larynx with stenosis. We have seen instances of this last condition in which intubation or tracheotomy was required. Some of these cases depend upon perichondritis. Pleurisy, and abscess or gangrene of the lung have been reported, and hypostatic congestion may occur in severe cases. *Circulatory* involvement is rare, but there may be pericarditis and endocarditis, and venous and arterial thrombosis. A hemorrhagic condition, with purpura of the skin and bleeding from the mucous membranes, is uncommon (*Hemorrhagic typhoid*). We have seen epistaxis so severe that it was probably the cause of death. *Disturbances of the digestive system* are important. Vomiting is more common than in adults, and is exceptionally uncontrollable. Parotitis, aphthous or ulcerative stomatitis, pseudomembranous tonsillitis, noma, appendicitis, and fecal impaction are unusual. Intestinal hemorrhage is rare as compared with adult life, and is met with almost only in children of ten years or older (Morse,[18] Costinesco[21]). We[22] have observed it, however, in a number of cases and in one of these in an infant of five months. It has also been witnessed in some of the congenital cases, probably then dependent upon a general hemorrhagic state and septicemia. Intestinal perforation may occur, but is uncommon especially in early childhood. We[22] have observed 9 cases, 1 of them in a girl of four years, and statistics have been published also by Montmollin,[23] Henoch,[19] Morse,[18] Reunert,[24] Schultz,[25] Setbon,[26] Elsberg,[27] Adams,[28] and Jopson and Gittings.[92] It is to be noted that in early life the usual symptoms of perforation, such as fall in temperature, collapse and severe abdominal pain, may entirely fail to develop. Greenwald and Eliasberg[30] report an instance of peritonitis in an infant, which developed without perforation. Typhoidal cholecystitis is probably more frequent than formerly supposed. We have, however, observed it only once. Reid and Montgomery[31] collected 18 cases in children. It may exhibit itself in an acute form with perforation and peritonitis, as in cases reported by Bittner.[32] Slight pain and tenderness over the gall-bladder, disappearing spontaneously, is not infrequent.

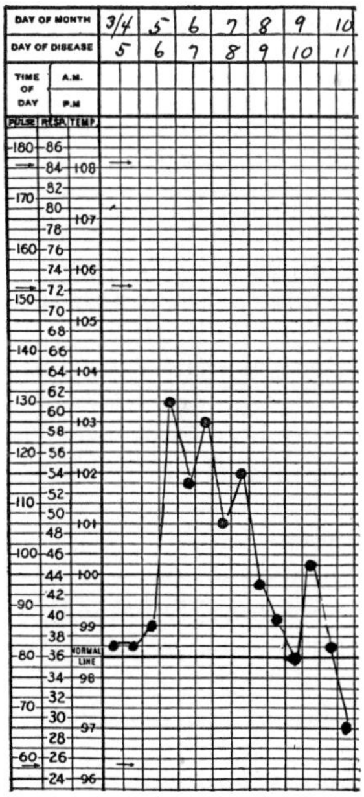

Fig. 61.—Abortive typhoid fever, severe initial symptoms. Annie A., aged seven and a half years. Symptoms of invasion consisted of fever, very frequent vomiting, diarrhea. Then improved, felt perfectly well and was bright, no apathy; vomiting and diarrhea ceased. Enlargement of spleen and roseola (?) present. Widal reaction positive. No fever after tenth day of disease.

Among *nervous complications and sequels* is temporary aphasia, which is witnessed oftener in childhood than later. We have seen it several times. Henoch[19] observed it 20 times in his 381 cases, and Adams[33] reported 4 instances. It sometimes appears to be more the result of apathy, with removal of desire to talk, than of actual inability. Post-typhoidal insanity is unusual, but we have observed it in a number of cases. Chorea is not an infrequent sequel. The majority of cases showing meningeal symptoms are suffering from meningismus or a serous meningitis. Purulent meningitis may occur, due to typhoid or other germs. We have seen only one such instance, but there are reports by Cole,[34] Baumgartner and Olsen,[35] and Weston and Radbill.[36] Hemiplegia has been recorded, and peripheral paralysis resulting from neuritis. As in other infectious fevers, encephalitis may develop. We have seen this with marked mental and physical symptoms, and yet complete recovery followed. *Otitis* is not infrequent. Deafness sometimes appears to depend upon involvement of the auditory nerve or of the labyrinth.

Affections of the *genito-urinary* apparatus may be observed. Among these are cystitis, pyelitis and nephritis; the last usually recovering as convalescence proceeds. Among *suppurative processes* in various regions are furunculosis and subcutaneous abscesses, which are not uncommon, bed-sores, arthritis, and osteomyelitis. Suppuration of the mesenteric glands may suggest intestinal perforation (Rowland[37]). The typhoid spine is observed less often than in adults.

Cutaneous eruptions sometimes are seen as complications, being rubeloid or, less often, scarlatiniform or urticarial. Sudamina are frequent; herpes is rare, but more common than in adults. Other acute *infectious diseases* may complicate typhoid fever, the occurrence of a secondary diphtheria being especially frequent among these.

Relapse and Recurrence.—*Relapse* is perhaps more frequent than in adult life, the age of the child exerting no decided influence. Koplik and Heiman[38] found it in 15 per cent of 160 cases; Adams[33] in 8.7 per cent of 550 cases; and in 75 cases in the first two and one-half years of life observed by us[6] there were 3 relapses. It develops oftenest from the fourteenth to the seventeenth day after the temperature of the first attack has reached normal, and is generally of shorter duration than it. A distinction must be made from *recrudescence,* which lasts but a day or two. Relapse is characterized by return of the usual symptoms, including reappearance of the roseola and enlargement of the spleen. It may occur once or 3 or more times. In 1 case under our personal observation, 3 relapses were witnessed, and David[39] reported 5 relapses in a boy of eleven years. *Recurrence* may be observed once, or, in rare instances, several times, although one attack usually confers lasting immunity.

Prognosis.—In general the mortality in early life may be placed at from 4 to 5 per cent. (Schavoir[40] 1 per cent, Morse[18] 6 per cent.) Of 432 cases in the Children's Hospital of Philadelphia, 23 (5.3 per cent) died.[5] It varies much with age. In infancy the number of fatal cases is large. In our[5] own studies of 278 collected cases under two and one-half years of age, 57 per cent died. This was unusually high, probably because the milder cases were not reported. In the later personal study[8] 75 cases in this age-period had a mortality of only 12 per cent. In early childhood the mortality, when at its lowest, probably does not exceed 2 to 4 per cent. Steadily as puberty is approached the proportion of fatal cases increases.

Among *unfavorable symptoms* are severe diarrhea and vomiting, persistent dryness of mouth, marked abdominal distention, weak and rapid pulse, and stupor, or other severe nervous symptoms. The slow, irregular pulse of convalescence is not unfavorable. Rolleston[41] claimed that the disappearance of the diazo-reaction indicated that temperature was about to fall.

Diagnosis.—In typical cases this rests chiefly upon the course of the temperature, the rose spots, enlarged spleen, absence of leukocytosis, and the Widal reaction. Yet in early life the diagnosis is often difficult, as one or more of the important symptoms may be absent, especially early in the attack. Very important is the obtaining of a positive *agglutinative reaction.* This, however, may be very late in developing, and consequently a negative reaction is of less value. Absence of leukocytosis is a valuable suggestive symptom when combined with fever which continues without definite cause. As the disease progresses the combination of rose spots, agglutinative reaction, enlarged spleen, and low leukocyte count generally makes the diagnosis clear.

Especially in infancy typhoid fever is readily confounded with *ileocolitis.* In this disease, however, the intestinal condition is usually much more severe and a leukocytosis is generally present. *Malaria* of a continued febrile type may closely resemble typhoid fever, but may be recognized by the absence of the Widal reaction and the presence of the plasmodium. Certain cases of *grippe* with prolonged fever and decided prostration may cause perplexity. As these may have enlargement of the spleen and an absence of leukocytosis the diagnosis may have to rest upon the absence of rose spots and the occurrence of the agglutinative reaction. *Acute miliary tuberculosis* is one of the conditions causing much diagnostic difficulty. Like typhoid fever it exhibits fever, splenic enlargement, and absence of leukocytosis or any localizing lesion. The tuberculin reaction cannot be depended upon in this condition. The continuation of the fever beyond the period for typhoid fever, and the failure of rose spots or Widal reaction to appear, and finally, although late, the development of some localization clears up the diagnosis. *Meningitis,* particularly the tuberculous form, presents at first many points of resemblance to typhoid fever, especially of the meningitic type. In this latter condition, however, the nervous symptoms are marked at the onset and generally disappear early, while in all forms of meningitis there is likely to be a leukocytosis. The continued absence of the agglutinative reaction and the result of lumbar puncture will finally distinguish meningitis from typhoid fever. The differentiation from infection by *Brucella abortus* must often be made by the agglutinative reactions, but this condition is rare in infants and children. *Typhus fever,* which is accompanied by leukopenia and a rash, may be differentiated by the positive Felix-Weil reaction and the absence of the Widal reaction.

Treatment. **Prophylaxis.**—There must be careful disinfection of urine, feces, bed-linen, and body-clothing. The attendant's hands should be washed after each handling of the patient. (See p. 250.) Convalescence cannot be considered safe, so far as transmission is concerned, until there have been 3 negative cultures of stools and urine. Urinary antiseptics, such as hexamethylenamine and hexylresorcinol may assist in freeing the urine of the germs. In chronic carriers extirpation of the gall-bladder does not always cause cure of the condition. In 1 case we apparently cured a carrier by duodenal drainage and intravenous injections of mercurochrome.

Prevention of extension in general is accomplished by proper precautions regarding the supply of water and milk, as of other sources of food. Boiling kills the typhoid germ, and so does proper pasteurization.

Immunizing Treatment.—The work originally done by Wright,[42] Pfeiffer and Kolle,[43] and others has shown that injection of vaccine has a definite effect in preventing typhoid fever. It should probably be repeated about once a year in regions where the disease is endemic. Besredka[44] found that many people developed agglutinins for typhoid or paratyphoid fever upon the oral administration of vaccine.

Treatment of the Attack.—This is chiefly symptomatic and an excess of treatment should be avoided. Bond and Barrier[45] claimed good results with mercurochrome given intravenously. There seems to be no value in any attempt to disinfect the intestinal tract. Vaccines and sera have been widely used in treatment since the time of Wright, often with the claim of good results. They have been employed in childhood by Josias,[46] Ortiz, Acũna and Belloc,[47] Kharina-Marinucci,[48] Spolverini[49] and others.

Confinement to bed is imperative, although often not for so long a time as with adults. The diet should be easily digestible and abundant. Boiled sweet milk or some of the acid-milks may form a large part of the caloric intake. Strained vegetables, or carbohydrates in the form of cereals, may also be given. Water should be offered freely and often. When convalescence begins the diet may be increased in quantity and variety.

For *fever* hydrotherapy (see p. 190) may be employed. It is useful not only to reduce temperature but as a quieter of many nervous manifestations. Either sponging or warm tubbing, according to the individual effect produced, can be frequently repeated if the temperature is over 103 F. (39.4 C.). If cyanosis or prolonged weakness of pulse is caused, the water should be warmer, 95 to 100 F. (35 to 37.8 C.), or hydrotherapy abandoned and a careful trial made of antipyretic drugs. These are needed, however, only if the temperature is alarmingly high and the corresponding symptoms severe. For *prostration*, alcoholic stimulants are excellent, and brandy or whiskey given in doses of ½ to 1 fluidram (2 to 4) every three or four hours to a child of two years. If *vomiting* is severe, the milk may be alkalinized, diluted, skimmed or peptonized, or entirely replaced for a time by albumen-water, orange juice, cereals, or broths. *Diarrhea* should not be interfered with unless it is severe, when bismuth in large doses or opium and its derivatives may be administered. For *constipation* only simple enemas or suppositories should be employed. For *tympanites* there should be used turpentine stupes, and a rectal tube, or rectal injections of milk of asafetida. For *nervous symptoms* hydrotherapy is usually the best treatment, but sedatives may be required, and sometimes lumbar puncture is indicated.

Complications and sequels need treatment appropriate for them. In intestinal hemorrhage the foot of the bed should be elevated, an ice-bag applied to the abdomen, and morphine given hypodermically in sufficient dose to quiet intestinal peristalsis. Epinephrine in doses of 5 to 10 minims (0.31 to 0.62) of the 1:1000 solution, given subcutaneously; calcium chloride or lactate (5 to 10 grains (0.324 to 0.648) 4 times daily); or gelatin (10 per cent solution), may be tried. Intestinal perforation demands operative interference at the earliest possible moment. The debility and anemia which often persist after severe cases of typhoid fever require medication with iron, copper, strychnine and other tonics, and often a sojourn at the seashore or in the mountains.

References

1. Am. J. M. Sc., 1836–1837, **19,** 289; 1837–1838, **20,** 289. 2. Mal. des enf., 3rd Ed., 615; **3,** 373. 3. N. Y. Med. Rec., 1895, **48,** 803. 4. Thèse de Neuchatel. 5. Arch. de méd. des enf., 1919, **22,** 183. 6. Arch. Pediat., 1926, **43,** 160. 7. Griffith and Ostheimer, Am. J. M. Sc., 1902, **124,** 868. 8. Griffith, Arch. Pediat., 1912, **29,** 565. 9. Med. News, 1903, **83,** 193. 10. Rev. franc. de gynec. et d'obstet., 1922, **17,** 646. 11. Compt. rend. soc. de biol., 1926, **95,** 1530. 12. J.A.M.A., 1930, **95,** 405. 13. Handbk. d. Kinderkr., **2,** 373. 14. Am. J. Dis. Child., 1929, **38,** 1044. 15. Griffith, Phila. M. J., 1898, **2,** Oct. 15. 16. Am. J. Med. Sc., 1901, **121,** 552. 17. J.A.M.A., 1919, **73,** 913. 18. Boston M. and S. J., 1896, **134,** 205. 19. Lehrb. d. Kinderkrankh., 1895, 773. 20. Jahrb. f. Kinderh., 1911, **74,** 386. 21. Thèse de Paris, 1897, 35. 22. Griffith, Am. J. M. Sc., 1905, **130,** 581. 23. Thèse Neuchatel, 1885. 24. Deutsche med. Wchnschr., 1889, **15,** 1063. 25. Jahrb. f. Hamburgischen Staatskrankenanstalten, 1889, **1,** 7. 26. Thèse de Paris, 1902. 27. Ann. Surg., 1903, **38,** 71. 28. Arch. Pediat., 1904, **21,** 81. 29. Am. J. Med. Sc., 1909, **138,** 625. 30. Am. J. Dis. Child., 1925, **29,** 365. 31. Bull. Johns Hopkins Hosp., 1920, **31,** 7. 32. Prag. med. Wchnschr., 1914, **33,** 279. 33. Trans. Am. Pediat. Soc., 1896. 34. Johns Hopkins Hosp., Rep. 1904, **12,** 299. 35. Arch. Int. Med., 1920, **25,** 537. 36. Arch. Pediat., 1926, **43,** 160. 37. J.A.M.A., 1906, **46,** 507. 38. Arch. Pediat., 1907, **24,** 1. 39. Zentralbl. f. inn. Med., 1912, **33,** 1071. 40. Med. Rec., 1895, **48,** 803. 41. Lancet, 1905, **1,** 290. 42. Lancet, 1901, **2,** 1107. 43. Ztschr. f. Hyg., 1896, **21,** 203. 44. Local Immuniz. Williams and Wilkins, 1927, 137. 45. Arkansas M. Soc. J., 1924, **21,** 71. 46. Ann. de méd. et de chir. inf., 1903, **7,** 438; Acad. de méd., 1906, March 6; Ref. Arch. f. Kinderh., 1908, **47,** 454. 47. Arch. de méd. des enf., 1915, **18,** 575. 48. Pediatria, 1920, **28,** 641. 49. Pediatria, 1921, **29,** 289.

PARATYPHOID FEVER

This disease is produced by the action of the paratyphoid bacillus, either of the varieties "A" and "B" being the agent. The latter is that very much most frequently found. Symptomatically the disorder generally resembles typhoid fever almost exactly, the chief distinction being that the agglutinative reaction with the typhoid bacillus is absent, while it is obtained with the variety of the paratyphoid bacillus which is the causative factor in the case. Sometimes, however, instead of the ordinary typhoidal symptoms, there are those of a dysenteric, choleriform, respiratory, or septic nature; the last especially in very young infants. The affection may occur isolated or in small epidemics, and may affect any age. It appears to be uncommon in the first year of life, but an instance of the A type occurring in an infant of eight months is reported by Eckert[1] and a number of instances by others of infants with Type B. Congenital infection by the B bacillus was observed by Nauwerck and Flinzer,[2] Stolkind and Lorey[3] and others. The lesions appear to be very similar to those of typhoid fever. Decided ulceration of Peyer's patches is uncommon, but this is equally true of typhoid fever in early life. Moreover hemorrhage and perforation have been reported. The diagnosis can be made only by cultural studies of the germs and by the agglutinative reaction. In 117 children with digestive disturbances, not suggesting typhoid fever, Breuning[4] found 11 cases; *i. e.*, 9.5 per cent with paratyphoid bacilli in the stools. As far as experience has yet extended the mortality appears to be decidedly less than that of typhoid fever. The disease as it occurs in infancy and childhood has been exhaustively reviewed by Cannata[5] and later by Marschhausen,[6] Stolkind and Lorey,[3] and Wilde and Wildemann.[7]

Treatment of the disease would be that suitable for typhoid fever. As a prophylactic measure it has been customary to include with typhoid vaccine the paratyphoid bacilli A and B, when inoculations were given.

References

1. Berl. klin. Wchnschr., 1910, **47,** 1102. 2. München. med. Wchnschr., 1908, **55,** 1217. 3. Brit. J. Child. Dis., 1918, **15,** 161. 4. München. med. Wchnschr., 1914, **61,** 1050. 5. Annali di clinica medica, 1911, **2,** 285. 6. Monatschr. f. Kinderh., Orig., 1919, **15,** 615. 7. Arch. f. Kinderh., 1929, **87,** 53.

CHAPTER X

TYPHUS FEVER

Typhus fever has been endemic in Europe, India and China for many centuries, and has occurred in epidemics in the United States. It was first differentiated from typhoid fever by Gerhard[1] in 1836. A variety of it known as Mexican typhus (tabardillo) is endemic in Mexico. The disease described by Brill[2] and termed Brill's disease, is probably identical with Mexican typhus. According to Maxcy[3] a mild form of typhus fever is endemic in the Southeastern States. Clinically Rocky Mountain spotted fever resembles typhus fever, but it is claimed by Ricketts and Walder[4] that the diseases are immunologically distinct.

Etiology.—Yersin and Vassel[5] produced typhus in a human volunteer with blood from a patient; Nicolle, Comte and Conseil[6] transmitted the disease through the body-louse; and Anderson and Goldberger[7] Mexican typhus through the head-louse. Maxcy[3] believes that there is transmission from rodents by the bite of blood-sucking insects, such as fleas and ticks. That Rocky Mountain spotted fever can be transmitted by wood-ticks is shown by the experiments of Ricketts[8] and Maver.[9] The work of Dyer, Rumreich and Badger[10] incriminates the tick as a vector of the Eastern type of typhus fever, and suggests that the rat is a reservoir of endemic typhus and that the rat-flea is a vector.

Certain bacteria believed causative are described by Plotz;[11] and Plotz, Olitsky and Baehr,[12] and other germs have been reported; and there seems to be evidence that organisms of the Rickettsia group are the cause of the disease.

There is apparently no *age* immunity to the disease, and infants and children may be affected.

Symptoms.—The symptomatology of typhus fever and of Rocky Mountain spotted fever may well be considered together. The *incubation period* is probably one to two weeks, and there may be prodromal symptoms lasting several days. The *onset* is abrupt with chills, fever, headache and prostration, and generalized aching. The *fever* rises to 102 to 106 F. (38.9 to 41.1 C.), is characterized by morning remissions, and generally disappears by two weeks or slightly longer. It usually falls by lysis. About the fifth day the *eruption* appears, first on the chest and abdomen and on the inner surface of the upper extremities. It may involve the back and become quite generalized, but the face, palms and soles are invariably spared. It is macular or occasionally papular, and dark-red to purple in color, almost completely fading on pressure. It disappears in a few days, but may last five or six days or longer, and is only occasionally absent. In the disease known as Rocky Mountain spotted fever the eruption is somewhat different, appearing first on the wrist and ankles, then on the back, later becoming generalized, and the palms and soles are often involved. Purpuric staining and petechiae develop, which take several weeks to fade. The *spleen* is enlarged in some of the cases, particularly in the spotted fever group. Nervous symptoms may be marked, and delirium and meningismus develop. There is, as a rule, a normal leukocyte count or leukopenia, but the spotted fever cases may have leukocytosis. The so-called "Felix-Weil reaction" is usually found. This consists in the agglutination of strains of bacillus proteus, particularly that known as X-19.

In infants and small children typhus fever is generally quite mild.

Complications and Sequels are rare in typhus, but in spotted fever marked deafness, visual disturbances and mental confusion have been observed. Bronchopneumonia, thrombosis and suppurative parotitis are reported by Maxcy.

Prognosis.—The mortality is given as 2 to 4 per cent; perhaps higher in the spotted fever group.

Diagnosis.—There may be confusion with typhoid fever, since in both diseases there is leukopenia and an eruption; but the Widal reaction occurs in typhoid and the Felix-Weil reaction in typhus, and the rash is usually more profuse in the latter.

Treatment.—Attempts at immunization by a vaccine of the organism described by Plotz have seemed to have some success. Immunization has also been attempted by inoculation with blood-serum of infected guinea-pigs, material from ticks, or virus obtained from the louse. Passive immunization may perhaps be had by the injection of convalescent's serum. (For discussion see Zinsser.[13])

The symptomatic treatment would be much the same as for typhoid fever (p. 313). In prophylaxis there should be considered the elimination of rodents in view of their probable potentiality for carrying the disease, and of lice and fleas since they are the vectors.

REFERENCES

1. Am. J. M. Sc., 1836–1837, **19,** 289; 1837–1838, **20,** 289. 2. Am. J. M. Sc., 1910, **139,** 484. 3. Pub. Health Rep., 1926, **41,** 1213; 2967. 4. Arch. Int. Med., 1919, **5,** 361.

5. Philippine J. Sc., 1908, **3,** 131. 6. Compt. rend. acad. d. sc., 1909, **149,** 486. 7. Pub. Health Rep., 1912, **27,** 149. 8. Med. Rec., 1909, **76,** 843. 9. J. Infect. Dis., 1911, **8,** 327. 10. J.A.M.A., 1931, **97,** 589. 11. J.A.M.A., 1914, **52,** 1556. 12. J. Infect. Dis., 1915, **17,** 1. 13. Resistance to Infect. Dis., 1931, 4th Ed., 519.

CHAPTER XI

UNDULANT FEVER

(Malta Fever. Brucella Infection)

Etiology.—The micro-örganism responsible for Malta fever was described by Bruce[1] in 1887, and that causing contagious abortion in cattle by Bang[2] in 1897. In 1918 Evans[3] demonstrated the close relationship of these organisms, and it has now become evident that the Brucella melitensis (goat or caprine strain), the Brucella abortus (bovine strain), and the Brucella suis (hog or porcine strain) are quite similar and that all of them may infect man. The designation Brucella is in honor of Bruce. Malta fever acquired from infected goats is common in the Mediterranean countries and is found in parts of the U. S., chiefly Texas, Arizona, and New Mexico. The first human case of melitensis infection in the U. S. was reported by Craig[4] and the first human abortus infection by Keefer.[5] The usual human infection here is with the abortus group. Reviews on the subject are given by Hardy,[6] Hardy et al.,[7] Simpson and Fraizer,[8] Guest,[9] and others.

The *incidence* is greatest in adults, and relatively few cases have been recorded in early life. They do, however, occur, and have been reported in this country by Kampmeier,[10] Kohlbry,[11] King,[12] Simpson,[13] Orr,[14] Hill and Monger,[15] Ey and Van Arsdall,[16] Anderson and Pohl[17] and Coughlin.[18] Infection by the melitensis group of organisms is said to be rare in infants in Europe. While more cases of brucella infection are reported in the male sex in adults, this is a matter of exposure rather than susceptibility. *Individual susceptibility* is not great. *Transmission* is by the ingestion of infected raw milk and, in the case of adults, quite certainly also through the skin of those handling infected meats and animals. In addition to the animals already mentioned, sheep, mules, horses, asses and dogs have been found infected, and guinea-pigs and monkeys may be made so by inoculation.

Pathologic Anatomy.—This has been studied largely in animals, but in only a few human cases. The organisms may be isolated from the blood, urine, intestinal ulcerations and stools, tonsils, complicating lesions, such as of the joints, and the epididymis. In animals they have been found in the genital tract and the mammary glands. Carpenter and Boak[19] isolated them from a human fetus. In human melitensis infection there have been found enlarged liver, congested lungs, ulceration of the intestine, and involvement of the lymph glands.

Symptoms.—The average **incubation period** is probably about two weeks. The **onset** is likely to be insidious, with the usual symptoms of beginning infection, but may be sudden with chills and high fever. These continue, together with malaise, anorexia, headache, backache, constipation, joint pains, abdominal pain, and profuse night sweats. There are marked irritability, restlessness, and insomnia. The fever in abortus infection is much less likely to be undulant in type than in the melitensis or suis infection. In the abortus infection there is a course of irregular fever, reaching 103 to 106 F. (39.4 to 41.1 C.), being highest late in the afternoon or evening. Little is found on physical examination, except enlargement of the spleen in about $\frac{1}{4}$ of the cases, and occasionally enlargement of the liver, a macular eruption, and loss of weight. The febrile period continues for from three to ten or fourteen days, and is followed by a remission of somewhat shorter duration, during which the patient may be subjectively well, except that night sweats may occur. The total duration of the disease is two to four months, but may be shorter or run into many months.

There are many variations. Some cases may be so mild that little general effect is produced and the patient feels surprisingly well (*ambulatory type*); the fever may be *continuous* for six or eight weeks without remission, recovery then coming about gradually; there may rarely be a *malignant* type with severe and fulminating symptoms. In young children there may be nothing characteristic in the symptomatology.

The *blood* almost always shows a definite leukopenia with a relative lymphocytosis, unless complications are present. Beginning in the second week of the disease the patient's blood-serum will usually agglutinate a suspension of the Brucella abortus. A positive agglutination-test with a dilution as high as 1:80 up to 1:100 is considered significant and it may later be positive in much higher titer, such as 1:500 or even to 1:20,000. The titer drops to 1:20 or 1:80 after the disease, one of 1:100 indicating a past infection. There is cross-agglutination between the bovine, caprine, and porcine strains. It is important to emphasize that human cases may occur without a positive agglutination-test, and that a positive test may also be found in those drinking raw infected milk, when clinical disease is not present nor demonstrable in the past history. In some cases the organism may be found in blood-culture, and in culture from the *urine* and *stool*. Growth in such cultures is very slow.

Complications and Sequels.—Very few complications have been reported in children. In older persons a spondylitis has especially been noted and also reported are neuritis, arthritis, endocarditis, bronchitis, epistaxis, orchitis and icterus.

Prognosis.—This is good, the mortality being only about 1 or 2 per cent in abortus cases, or somewhat more in the caprine and porcine ones. High fever and marked nervous symptoms seem to have unfavorable import. Recovery is more rapid in those whose blood shows agglutinating power in high titer (Simpson[13]).

Diagnosis.—The combination of continued fever and leukopenia with indefinite symptoms may confuse undulant fever with typhoid fever, or, when chills and sweats are present, with malaria. *Typhoid fever* may be differentiated by serum-agglutination tests and *malaria* by finding the plasmodium. The agglutination-reaction of undulant fever may be utilized also to distinguish this condition from *tuberculosis*. The arthritic pains of undulant fever, severe as they often are, have caused the diagnosis of *rheumatic fever* to be made, and the spondylitis which occurs not infrequently has been suspected of being tuberculous. In *relapsing* fever the temperature subsides quickly to normal after five to seven days, remains normal for a similar period, then rises again at the beginning of the relapse. Examination of the blood should reveal the spirillum of Obermeyer.

The abdominal pain has led to operations for appendicitis or gall-bladder disease. Many cases of undulant fever have been discovered only by the routine performance of agglutination-tests, and the condition must always be suspected in fever of unknown origin. Cultures from the blood or urine are diagnostic if positive.

Treatment.—The simplest means of *prophylaxis* in children is the boiling or careful pasteurization of milk. The disease is wide-spread in most cattle herds wherever they have been examined. Attempts to immunize the herds by vaccines have not been very successful, and when live vaccines are employed the practice is probably dangerous.

The *treatment of the disease* is symptomatic. During convalescence the anemia and especially the loss of weight need appropriate therapy. Vaccines, autogenous or stock, have been employed quite extensively, sometimes giving the impression of good results. Nonspecific therapy, such as the injection of typhoid vaccines and of milk, has been used. Mercurochrome has been given intravenously by Gage and Gregory[20] and others, and acriflavine by Izar and Mastrojeni[21] in the melitensis infection, and by Hoffman[22] and others in infection by the abortus form. Roger[23] used sulpharsphenamine. In intestinal ulceration with positive stools Leavell, Poston and Amoss[24] found helpful the oral and rectal administration of methyl violet and thionin (25 to 200 mg. each twenty-four hours by mouth) (300 cc. of a 1:100,000 up to 1:25,000 solution by enema).

References

1. Practitioner, 1887, **39,** 161. 2. J. Comparative Path. and Therap., 1897, **10,** 125. 3. J. Infect. Dis., 1918, **22,** 509; 1918, **23,** 354. 4. Intern. Clin., 1906, **4,** 89. 5. Bull. Johns Hopkins Hosp., 1924, **35,** 6. 6. J.A.M.A., 1929, **93,** 891. 7. Nat. Inst. Health Bull., 1930, No. 158. 8. J.A.M.A., 1929, **93,** 1958; Ohio State M. J., 1931, **27,** 21. 9. Ohio State M. J., 1930, **26,** 221. 10. Am. J. M. Sc., 1928, **176,** 177. 11. Minnesota Med., 1929, **12,** 414. 12. New England J. Med., 1929, **201,** 918. 13. Ann. Int. Med., 1930, **4,** 238. 14. Ohio State M. J., 1930, **36,** 1023. 15. J.A.M.A., 1931, **97,** 176. 16. Ohio State M. J., 1931, **27,** 466. 17. Am. J. Dis. Child., 1931, **42,** 1103. 18. Penna. M. J., 1931, **34,** 550. 19. J.A.M.A., 1931, **96,** 1212. 20. J.A.M.A., 1926, **87,** 848. 21. Reforma med., 1927, **43,** 100. 22. J.A.M.A., 1929, **92,** 2169. 23. Marseille méd., 1931, **68,** 694. 24. J.A.M.A., 1930, **95,** 860.

CHAPTER XII

MENINGOCOCCIC MENINGITIS

(Cerebrospinal Fever. Cerebrospinal Meningitis)

Since this disease is so manifestly infectious and often epidemic, it may well be included in the category of Infectious Diseases. While existing at a much earlier period it was first clearly described by Vieusseux[1] in 1805 in Geneva, and shortly afterward in the United States (Danielson and Mann[2]).

Etiology. Predisposing Causes.—The disease is confined to temperate climates, and most epidemics begin in cold weather. More males are affected; race has no influence. Outbreaks are liable to occur under conditions of poor sanitation. Trauma of the head, exposure to heat, and mental and physical over-exertion, seem to predispose. The existence of other diseases and the general state of health are without direct influence.

Age is an important factor, children and adolescents being especially susceptible, although infants in the first year are not exempt. Seventy per cent or more of cases in epidemics occur in patients under ten years of age, and approximately 5 to 15 per cent in the first year. It has been observed even in the new-born (Commandeur and Nordman,[3] Koplik,[4] Miller,[5] Barron,[6] Root,[7] Neal and Jackson[8]). *Individual susceptibility* is slight, it being estimated that in epidemics about 6 in every 10,000 persons contract it. As a rule but a single case occurs in a family; and although we have occasionally seen 2 or more cases in a house, we have never observed the disease develop from hospital contact.

Epidemic influence is very marked. Years may pass with but a few cases in a locality, and then an outbreak occur which may continue for months or years. These epidemics vary greatly in severity and extent, being perhaps limited to one city, or being at other times very wide-spread.

Exciting Cause.—The disease is caused by the *diplococcus intracellularis meningitidis*, or meningococcus, described by Weichselbaum[9] in 1887. There are many different strains of this; Branham, Taft and Carlin[10] having isolated 235 such from the years 1928 to 1930.

The germ was first obtained during life from patients by Heubner,[11] who also produced the disease in animals. It is a gram-negative diplococcus, found in the inflammatory exudate, chiefly within the cells; frequently in the early stages on the nasal, pharyngeal and conjunctival mucous membranes (Goodwin and v. Sholly[12]); and in the blood (Haden,[13] Bloedorn,[14] Herrick[15]). In the last it may sometimes be found before meningeal symptoms, or without their later development. It may be discovered also in the purpuric eruption which accompanies the disease (Babes;[16] Netter, Salamier and Blancher;[17] Sharpe;[18] Brown;[19] McLean and Caffey[20]), or in an accompanying herpetic eruption (Plaut[21]). The *vitality of the germ* seems to be slight, and it is readily killed by low or high temperature.

Mode of Transmission.—Soil and water appear not to be factors; carriage by air is doubtful; spread by domestic animals is possible. Only rarely has conveyance by fomites been proven. As pointed out, transmission from sick to well is the exception, and extension by the schools does not seem to occur.

It is a noteworthy fact, however, as first pointed out by Albrecht and Ghon,[22] that meningococci have repeatedly been discovered on the mucous membranes of healthy persons during epidemics, and especially of those in contact with the patients. Goodwin and v. Sholly[23] obtained them in 10 per cent of contacts; Kutscher[24] in 75 per cent; Glover[25] in from 22 to 38.5 per cent. Norton[26] found that the percentage of carriers varies, being highest during winter and early spring. Between epidemics there are probably very few carriers. The persistence of the germs in the nose and throat after contact or after an attack of the disease is from two to four weeks, but may be for months. Chronic carriers usually have abnormal conditions in the nose and throat. They seldom themselves develop meningitis. While the acquiring of the disease from them seems uncommon, it must be considered that dissemination may occur in this way. It is believed by most authorities that the *mode of entrance* of the germ into the body is directly through the cribriform plate of the ethmoid bone into the meninges. Others think its entrance is by way of the lymph-vessels from the nasopharynx; others that it goes directly into the blood-stream; still others, that the portal of entry is the intestine.

Pathologic Anatomy.—The characteristic lesion is an acute fibrinopurulent inflammation of the piarachnoid of the brain and spinal cord, in the former involving chiefly the base. The choroid plexus is involved, and the ventricles are dilated by cloudy or distinctly purulent fluid. On the cord the exudate is situated chiefly over the posterior portion and especially in the regions below the cervical. The spinal nerve-roots and the sheath of the cranial nerves may be surrounded by it. Meningococci, mostly within the cells, are present in the exudate, as well as in the edematous meningeal tissue which is found between the areas of distinct cellular infiltration. In chronic cases, running a course of a month or more, the exudate has disappeared to a large extent, and its purulent character given place to a condition of a more mucous appearance. The meninges are left edematous and thickened, and the ventricles may be greatly dilated.

The brain-tissue itself is affected to some extent, being congested and softer than normal, and exhibiting cellular infiltration together with meningococci in the superficial layers and especially along the vessels. In chronic cases cocci are scarce and found only with difficulty. The cranial nerves and spinal cord are infiltrated.

Other pathologic changes are those usually associated with infection or due to complications. In chronic cases there are cortical atrophy and sclerosis, and perhaps hydrocephalus.

Symptoms. Ordinary Form.—A general description of the ordinary type follows: The period of *incubation* is not definitely known, but has been variously placed at from one to ten days. The attack may be ushered in by vague *prodromes*, such as malaise, headache and pain in the back, lasting one or two days; but, as a rule, the *onset* is sudden, with fever, headache, prostration, vomiting, pain in the neck, back and limbs, and sometimes chills and convulsions. Stiffness of the neck rapidly develops, and in well-marked cases decided retraction of the head as well. The slightest forcible moving of the head causes a cry of pain. Delirium, great restlessness, and irritability are common. Sensitiveness to light and noise, and cutaneous hyperesthesia are marked. Vomiting, pain, and irregular fever continue, (Fig. 62), more or less opisthotonos develops, and there is often rigidity of the extremities. The face is congested, strabismus or alteration of the pupils appears, sleep is disturbed, and grinding of the teeth or general convulsions may occur repeatedly. There is frequent crying out with pain. Purpura, herpes, or other eruptions of the skin may appear. As intracranial pressure increases the pulse becomes slow and often irregular, the respiration irregular, stupor replaces delirium, and complete coma follows. In infants with open fontanelle the increase in intracranial pressure is readily shown by the tension and bulging in this region.

The *duration* of the disease, even in what may be called average cases, is extremely variable. Roughly speaking it may be placed at from two to four weeks, not including convalescence, but may be much shorter or longer than this. Improvement is characterized by the diminution of the pain and rigidity, permanent lessening of fever, cessation of vomiting, and bettering of the mental state.

Some of the symptoms must be considered more in detail.

Convulsive movements occur in about $\frac{1}{3}$ of the cases in infancy and early childhood; less often in older persons. They may be general and usher in the attack, and then cease; or recur at intervals later, being then either general or local. Sometimes convulsions occur from time to time in the chronic cases after most other symptoms have disappeared. Grinding of the teeth is common and tremor may be observed.

Pain is a very common symptom, beginning early and continuing throughout the acute portion of the attack. It is situated chiefly in the head, but may involve also the back, abdomen and the limbs, especially the lower. It is subject to sudden exacerbations, particularly at night, and is often so distressing that it occasions loud outcries (the "hydrencephalic cry"). It is especially marked on any forcible movement of the body. *General hyperesthesia* is very constant, the patient being greatly disturbed and often crying out on hearing a loud noise, being exposed to bright light, or on the mere touching of the skin.

Muscular rigidity is almost always seen, chiefly in the form of stiffness of the neck and some degree of retraction of the head, and is probably due to irritation of the posterior spinal nerve roots. If the head is lifted forcibly from the pillow the trunk follows it without any bending of the neck taking place. It can, however, be turned from side to side without difficulty. In severe, long-continued cases the occiput may even press against the back beneath the scapulae (Fig. 63). It not infrequently happens, however, that the stiffness of the neck is intermittent. Rigidity with anterior curving of the spine is common, and the children often lie on the side with the arms flexed stiffly and drawn over the chest, the legs flexed, and the thighs drawn to the abdomen—the so-called "gun-hammer"

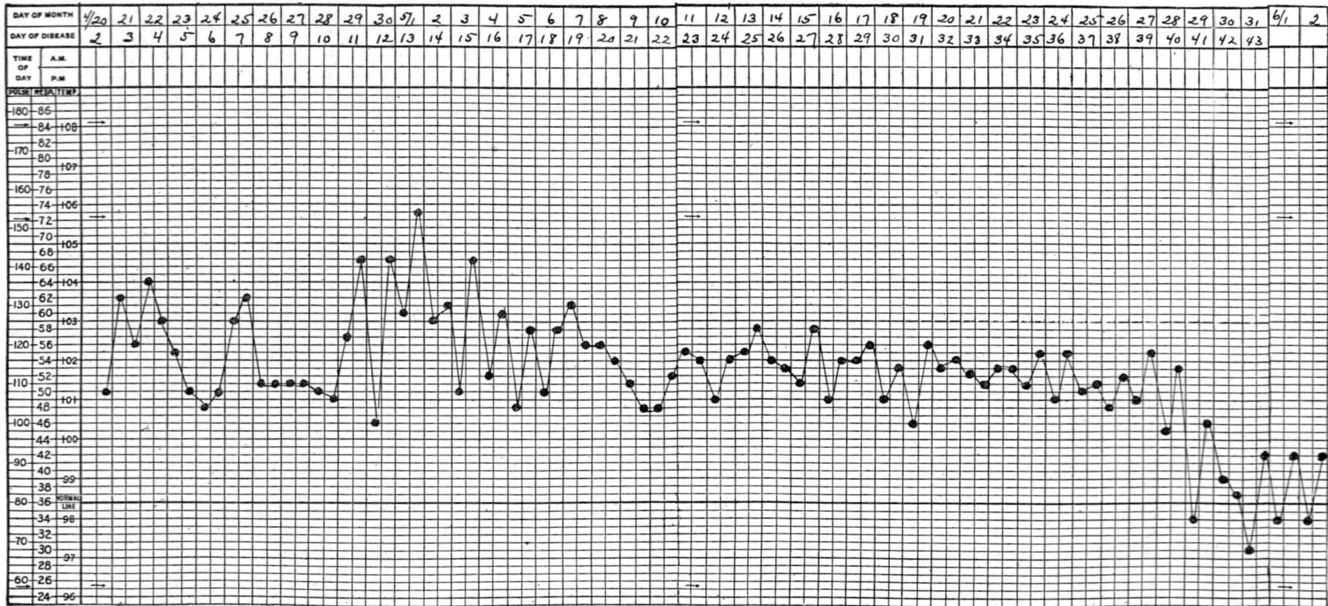

Fig. 62.—Cerebrospinal fever, ordinary form. Louis T. Taken ill suddenly, Apr. 19, with fever, vomiting, pain in head, and stupor. Two other children ill with the disease. Course of the attack characterized by stiffness of neck, irritability, stuporous condition, pain on moving, herpes, Kernig's sign and leukocytosis of 37,800. Very slow improvement began on Apr. 28 in spite of rise of temperature. Decided improvement after May 29. No serum-treatment.

position. In other cases the extremities are rigidly extended. The muscles of the face may be tense and the *risus sardonicus* present (Fig. 64). Trismus may occur and the abdomen is often scaphoid. Brudzinski's sign may early be present, even when rigidity is slight. Kernig's sign is generally observed but may be absent, and the same may be said of the contralateral

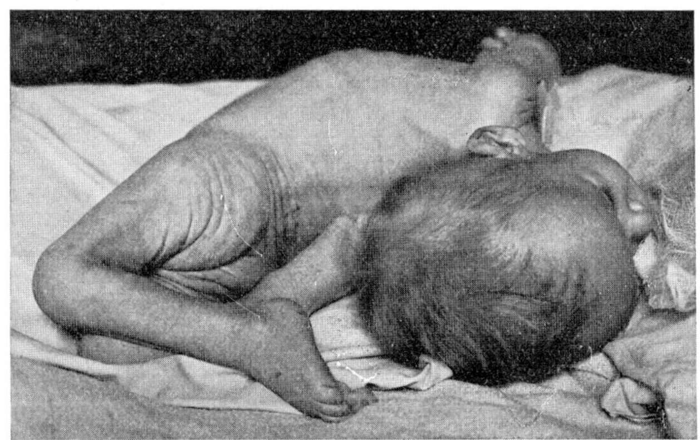

Fig. 63.—Opisthotonos in the subacute stage of cerebrospinal fever. Boy of one year, ill for four or five weeks with irregular temperature, emaciation, leukocytes 33,500, spinal fluid under great pressure and almost clear, 300 cells to the c.mm., 80 per cent polymorphonuclears, meningococci. Death.

reflex, Babinski's sign, and the sign described by Gingold.[27] (For description of these signs, see p. 857.) The *tendon-reflexes* are uncharacteristic, being normal, increased, or absent. The *mental symptoms* are variable. Great restlessness is common early in the attack and may persist. The mind may be clear much of the time, but delirium is frequent and may be intense or even maniacal, the child tossing wildly about the bed or even jumping out of it. In other cases it is merely of the wandering type, and either constant or intermittent; or it may be followed or replaced even at the onset by a more or less apathetic or even stuporous condition. The

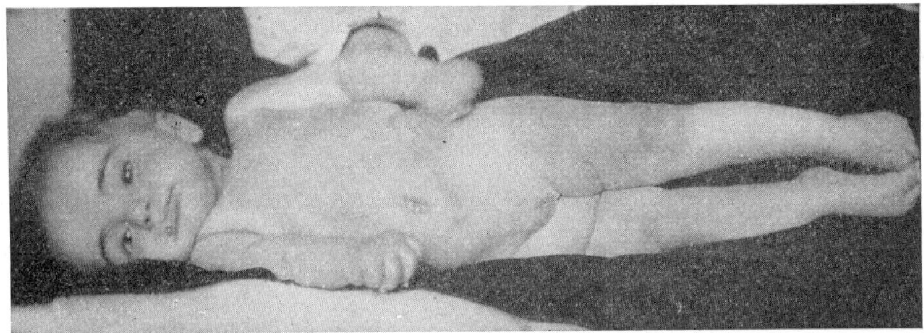

Fig. 64.—Risus sardonicus in cerebrospinal fever. Infant of seven months in the Children's Hospital of Philadelphia. Died after forty-five days of illness. Photograph taken on twenty-first day. Shows the facies as well as the spastic condition of the extremities.

degree of delirium does not appear always to bear any definite relationship to the other symptoms or to the gravity of the attack in general. In severe cases coma is liable finally to supervene, or it can even be one of the earliest symptoms. As in the case of delirium, it may vary greatly from day to day, or coma and delirium may alternate. The expression of the face in the acute condition is that of excitement and irritability, except in the mild cases.

Among *digestive disturbances* vomiting is an early symptom, present in the majority of cases. Generally it subsides as the disease advances. It is cerebral in origin. Anorexia and constipation are usually present.

The *temperature* is irregular and entirely uncharacteristic, and sudden remissions or intermissions as well as sudden rises to 105 F. (40.6 C.) or over are liable to occur. Some patients never exhibit much fever. As a rule there is little connection in acute attacks between the height of the fever and the severity of the disease. Irregularity is especially marked as convalescence advances, or as the disease passes into a chronic state.

The *pulse* bears little relationship to the temperature. It is usually more rapid than normal, especially if there is great general debility. It is subject to sudden changes in rate, and may be slow or irregular if intracranial pressure is increasing. The arterial tension is low.

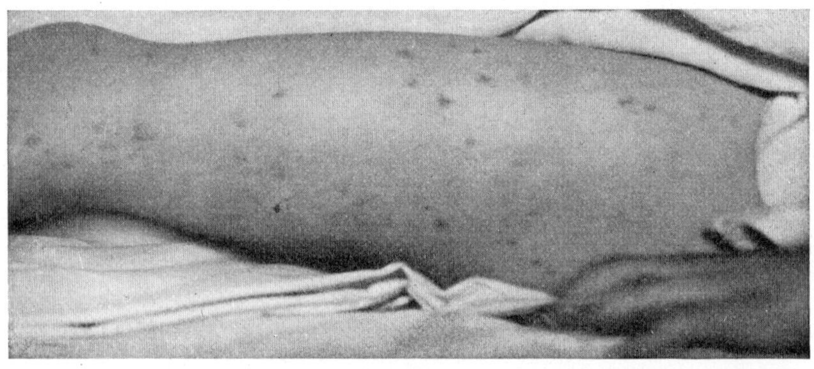

Fig. 65.—Purpuric eruption in cerebrospinal fever. Boy of six and a half years, a patient in the Children's Ward of the University Hospital, Philadelphia. Rash appeared on the fourth day of the disease, abundant on all extremities. Case a severe one; improved temporarily, but terminated fatally.

Respiration is not characteristically affected. Terminally it is often sighing or irregular, or of the Cheyne-Stokes type.

The most frequent of the *cutaneous symptoms* is herpes, which is present in a large proportion of cases. It is usually situated on the face, but sometimes elsewhere. Usually early, it may not develop until later, or it may come out in crops. A petechial or larger purpuric eruption is common, its frequency varying greatly with the epidemic (Fig. 65), but its incidence usually averages about 10 per cent. Its great frequency in earlier epidemics gave rise to the title "Spotted Fever." It may appear early or later, and seems to have little relation to the severity of the attack. In some cases larger cutaneous hemorrhages occur. A well-marked *tache cérébrale* (see p. 858) is a common symptom, as in all forms of meningitis. There may be noted, too, irregular flushing of the trunk where exposed, or of the face. *Emaciation* is decided in long-continued cases.

The *blood* presents an early polymorphonuclear leukocytosis, sometimes reaching 40,000 or more to the cubic millimeter. Meningococci may be found in culture of the blood (p. 320). The *urine* may exhibit a febrile albuminuria and occasionally sugar in small amounts.

The *eyes* may show conjunctivitis. The pupils are variable at first, and later dilate or react slowly. Alternate dilatation and contraction regardless of light or accommodation (hippus) may be present. Strabismus is common; nystagmus may occur. Sometimes the ocular movements are slower than in true nystagmus, and only one eyeball affected; or, if both, the movements may be dissociated (Pieraccini[28]).

The *cerebrospinal fluid* as obtained by lumbar puncture is increased in amount, turbid in acute cases, often quite purulent, and exhibits an increase of globulin. It contains polymorphonuclear leukocytes together with meningococci in varying numbers, free or principally within the cells.

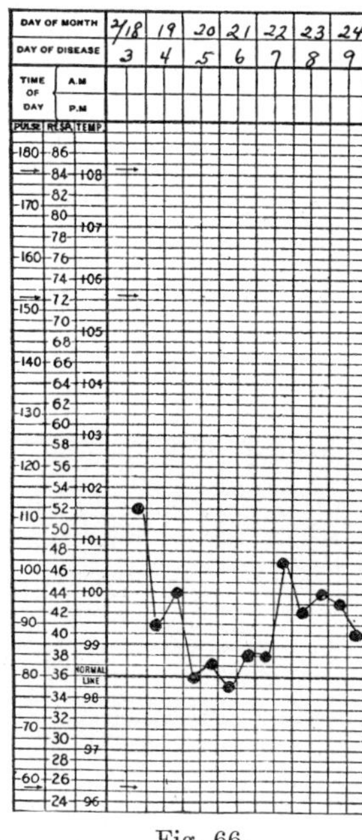

Fig. 66.

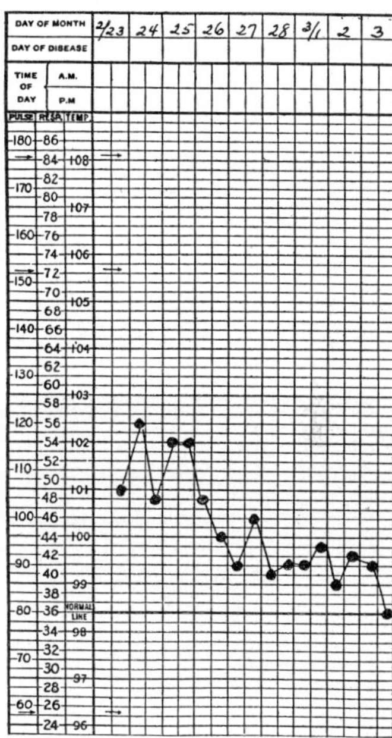

Fig. 67.

Fig. 66.—Cerebrospinal fever, abortive form. Milton L., two years old. Onset with repeated convulsions, prolonged unconsciousness, delirium, fever. Second day showed stuporous condition and fever, the child being apparently very ill. Rapid improvement followed, the mind becoming quite clear by the fourth day, and convalescence being entirely established by the eighth or ninth day. Meningococci found in the spinal fluid.

Fig. 67.—Cerebrospinal fever, mild form. Mary K., aged five years. One of three children of the family ill with the disease. Exact date of onset uncertain, but had been slightly ill for not over a week. Feb. 23, sleeps much of time, mind seems entirely clear, expression placid, apparently no pain, no irritability, no hyperesthesia, abdominal tache marked, neck slightly stiff, head slightly retracted but only if the child lies on her side, no other rigidity, no herpes or petechiae; Feb. 26, improving, much brighter; Feb. 28, greatly better, stiffness of neck gone; Mar. 10, out of bed, entirely well. No serum used. Children's Hospital of Philadelphia.

Sometimes no germs may be found early, but appear subsequently. They frequently disappear early in the attack, and often before the patient has made a complete clinical recovery. In more chronic cases they may persist for months and be found intermittently, or be blocked off in the ventricles or in other locations so that they cannot be recovered by spinal puncture. In such cases, too, the fluid is scanty and may be almost or quite clear and contain few if any cells. The colloidal gold curve is in the meningitic zone (typically 0001123431), *i. e.*, shows complete precipitation only in the last dilutions,—most meningitides giving about the same curve.

Variations from the Ordinary Form.—There may be great variation in the symptoms. Some cases begin with severe manifestations which soon ameliorate, or improvement may begin but be followed by weeks of illness. Other cases start mildly but soon grow severe. Symptoms such as Kernig's and Brudzinski's signs or the Babinski reflex may be constantly or intermittently unilateral (Levinson[29]). The variations are often so decided that a number of special types are described.

1. **Abortive Form.**—The disease begins abruptly and severely, but in two or three days the threatening symptoms disappear and recovery is rapid (Fig. 66).

2. **Mild Form.**—In cases of this sort the symptoms are mild from the onset, or soon become so (Fig. 67).

3. **Severe Form.**—All symptoms are intensified but the course may be short or prolonged.

4. **Malignant or Fulminating Form.**—This is characterized by extremely sudden onset, tendency to collapse, and short course. There may be coma and collapse as the only symptoms; or there may be violent vomiting, intense headache, or repeated convulsions. Wide-spread hemorrhages from the skin and mucous membranes may take place. Death may occur in less than twenty-four hours.

5. **Chronic Form.**—The symptoms at first do not differ from those of the ordinary type but, instead of disappearing, they continue in a modified form. There may be periods when fever and all the symptoms ameliorate,

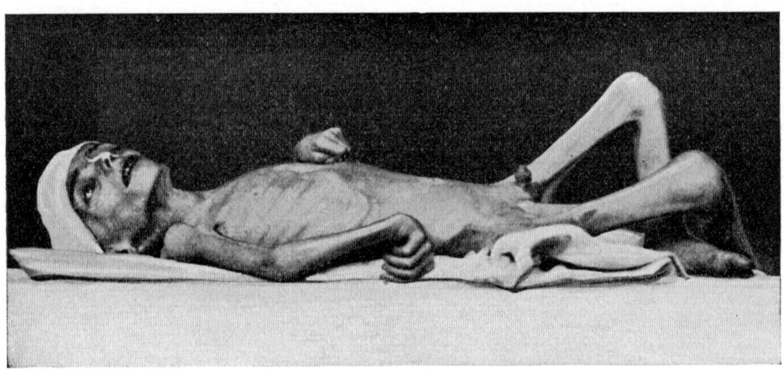

Fig. 68.—Chronic meningitis. Child of four years, a patient in the Children's Hospital of Philadelphia. Duration of disease uncertain. Severely ill six weeks before admission, with persistent wasting and often unconsciousness. Temperature afebrile while in the hospital. Examination of spinal fluid negative. Gradually lost ground and died four months after admission.

and may be absent, or nearly so, for weeks, to be followed by their return, and the disease may be protracted for months. The symptomatology is likely to be variable. Emaciation becomes extreme. We have the records of a case which finally ended fatally after lasting two hundred fifty-one days.

The disease known as *chronic basilar meningitis* which has been described by Gee and Barlow,[30] Still,[31] and others, and which was formerly regarded as a distinct disease, quite certainly is a form of meningococcic meningitis. It may last for several months (Fig. 68).

6. **Intermittent Form.**—In this there are not the longer and irregular periods of freedom from fever characteristic of the chronic form just described, but a temperature curve which strongly suggests malaria. Improvement in symptoms may or may not attend the drops in temperature.

7. **Meningococcemia.**—At times the infection, beginning as a meningococcus-septicemia, may remain as such, but usually after a variable time there is localization in the meninges. In such cases there will be irregular fever and at times the appearance of the macular or petechial eruption, or joint pains, and not infrequently ulcerative endocarditis. We have seen such cases, a number have been reported (Graves, Dulaney and

Michelson[32]), and a review of the earlier literature made by Bloedorn.[14] In one of our cases there was a febrile period during which meningococci, were found in the blood, followed by an afebrile stage of almost three months' duration, and the development then of meningococcic meningitis.

Complications and Sequels.—These are numerous, often serious, and may be the direct cause of death or of permanent disability. The most important are those affecting the nervous system and the special senses. The *eyes* may exhibit optic neuritis or, by extension of the purulent process along the piarachnoid of the nerve, a purulent choroido-iritis. Neuritis of the fifth nerve may be followed by purulent conjunctivitis or keratitis. These conditions may develop early or late in the attack. Complete or partial blindness may result. This occurred in 2 of 44 children reported by McLean and Caffey.[33] The *ears* are often involved in an otitis which, if purulent, may mean the loss of hearing; and there may also be absolute deafness from inflammation of the labyrinth, resulting from extension along the auditory nerve. Moos[34] found 38 deaf mutes in 64 recovered cases of meningococcic meningitis. Deafness occurred in 4 of the 44 cases of McLean and Caffey[33] and in 11 of 144 cases reported by Smithburn[35] et al. In 25 patients of our own followed for a period of from four months to two years persistent deafness was the most frequent sequel, occurring in 4 patients.

Disordered mental states may occur as sequels, among them being aphasia and mental impairment. Of 539 cases of mental defect Looft[36] found 3.7 per cent resulting from cerebrospinal fever. *Headache* is sometimes very persistent. Hydrocephalus is a serious and very frequent sequel. *Paralysis* may involve the eyes or the face; less often the limbs, in the latter case being either hemiplegic or paraplegic in type, and either temporary or permanent. *Inflammation of the nasopharynx* is a frequent complication early in the attack. *Pneumonia* is not uncommon and may in some instances be produced by the meningococcus. *Nephritis* is not frequent. *Arthritis* affecting one or more joints is not uncommon as a complication or sequel. It may be serous or purulent in nature, and the joint-fluid may contain meningococci. Among other complications sometimes seen are pleurisy, pericarditis, pyelitis, parotitis, enteritis, subcutaneous abscesses, urticaria, pemphigus and erythema. Endocarditis, which may be ulcerative in nature, seems especially to accompany the cases of meningococcemia without meningitis.

Cerebrospinal fever may occasionally occur simultaneously with, or as a sequel to, other acute infectious diseases, among these being typhoid fever, scarlet fever, measles, diphtheria and malaria.

Relapse and Recurrence.—In a disease with such a natural tendency to recrudescence it is difficult to determine the frequency of *relapse*. It was observed by Netter[37] from one to three months after apparent recovery in 1.14 per cent of 350 cases. *Recurrence* is certainly rare.

Prognosis.—According to figures from the Registration Area of the United States[38] there was a total of 5955 deaths from this disease in the years 1926 to 1928 inclusive. The variation in the mortality in different epidemics is very marked. More fatal cases occur at the beginning of an epidemic than later. The disease is certainly a serious one, the mortality ranging according to various figures from 20 to 75 per cent or more. As shown by many studies, such as those of Friis[39] and Hirsch,[40] the mortality is especially high in early life. Friis,[39] for example, found it in the first year to be 77.7 per cent; from one to five years 48.7 per cent; from five to ten years 51.6 per cent; from ten to fifteen years 21.4 per cent. In the Federal Census figures just quoted an average of 72 per cent of all deaths were under twenty years of age and 48.5 per cent under ten years of age. A decrease of leukocytosis is said to be a favorable sign, as is, according to Caffey, McLean and Sullivan,[41] an increase in the cerebrospinal sugar.

Death takes place oftenest within the first week, and with those showing improvement in the second week the outlook is brighter; but even then it is impossible to predict the outcome in any given case, either as regards life or persistence of damaging sequels, and the prognosis must always be guarded. The long-continued and chronic forms usually end fatally.

The figures of Friis[39] given above illustrate the mortality before the use of antimeningococcus serum. The effect of serum-treatment on prognosis has been marked. Flexner found that, although the usual mortality had at times reached 70 per cent, in 1294 cases receiving serum it had fallen to 30.9 per cent. The time at which serum is given is of great influence, and in Flexner's[42] series, when it was begun in the first three days, the mortality was but 18.1 per cent. Prior to serum-treatment practically all patients under one year of age died, whereas in Flexner's[42] cases in the first year the mortality was 49.6 per cent. Of 23 infants under three months of age given serum-treatment and reported by Neal and Jackson[8] 11 died. Not only is mortality lessened by serum-treatment, but the attack is shortened and complications and sequels are diminished.

The manner of treatment may have some effect on the mortality. Goldman and Bower[43] found in comparative series that patients treated through cisternal puncture had a 22 per cent better chance of surviving than those treated through lumbar puncture.

Diagnosis.—If the complex of symptoms which has been described is present, the diagnosis is easy, although it must be confirmed by lumbar puncture and the variety and the type of micro-organism found be determined. In mild cases without suggestive symptoms and in malignant cases the diagnosis may be impossible without lumbar puncture. The diagnosis may be especially difficult in young infants in whom vomiting, convulsions and rigidity may be absent, and there may be no symptoms but fever, irritability or drowsiness, and perhaps diarrhea and tenseness of the fontanelle. In such cases it may be only the existence of an epidemic which arouses suspicion. Macewen's sign, in which there is a slightly tympanitic, cracked-pot note elicited by percussion over the region of the lateral ventricles, has been of little value to us unless there is distension of one ventricle only, when the difference between the two sides becomes recognizable.

The character of the spinal fluid is most important diagnostically. There will be discovered numerous purulent cells, and the meningococci which can be found in smears or culture. The infection may, however, be walled off in the ventricles or elsewhere and meningococci not found. Meningococci may also be found in the blood, especially early, and also, as stated, even in the absence of meningitis. They may be recovered from the herpetic or purpuric cutaneous lesions, and from cultures of the nose and throat. (See p. 320.)

Cerebrospinal fever must be differentiated from *other forms of meningeal inflammation*, and this can be done only with certainty by study of the cerebrospinal fluid. In meningismus and serous meningitis the fluid is clear, no organisms are found, and the cell-count is normal or very slightly increased. In tuberculous meningitis, poliomyelitis, and encephalitis the fluid is clear or only slightly opalescent, there is a moderate cellular increase without great predominance of polymorphonuclears, and in the tuberculous variety the causative bacillus may be found. In other forms of purulent meningitis distinction is made only by discovery of the organisms responsible. A test is described by Kafka[44] in which there is ascertained the excretion of sodium fluorescein in the spinal fluid when it is administered by mouth. There is no delay in this in the meningeal irritation of acute infections, tumors, encephalitis, tetany and the like, but this does occur in purulent meningitis of any variety. There seems little necessity for this test in the usual case. *Typhus fever* may occasion confusion because of the purpuric rash, but this is not at first hemorrhagic, as is the case in cerebrospinal fever, and the examination of the spinal fluid will be negative. *Typhoid fever* of the meningitic type may at first cause some perplexity. As a rule, however, the meningitic symptoms soon disappear, and the absence of leukocytosis and the development later of the roseola and the Widal reaction make the case clear, if lumbar puncture has not already done so. Similarly *grippe* may at times resemble cerebrospinal fever closely, but the absence of leukocytosis and the results of lumbar puncture will settle the diagnosis. *Pneumonia* may be ushered in with meningitic symptoms. Both diseases exhibit leukocytosis and herpes. A lumbar puncture should distinguish, except in the instances of combination of the two conditions.

Treatment. **Prophylaxis.**—In view of the lack of exact knowledge of the method of transmission of the disease, preventive treatment is unsatisfactory. Affected persons should probably be isolated, in spite of the lack of evidence of direct communicability. If this is done it should be for fourteen days after the onset, and quarantine continued until no meningococci are found in the nose and throat or in the spinal fluid. Attempt at passive immunization with antimeningococcus serum is unnecessary and probably without effect. There is some evidence that vaccination with killed meningococci may be effective in prophylaxis (Sophian and Black,[45] Black[46]). In epidemics it may seem indicated to search for carriers. The benefit from mild disinfectant nasal sprays in exposed persons is doubtful.

Treatment of the Attack.—Except for serum-treatment, this is largely symptomatic. The patient should be kept very quiet in a darkened room. Strength should be maintained by sufficient nourishment and by alcoholic and other stimulants. Comatose patients should be fed by gavage. Strychnine may better be avoided, since it may increase the excitability. Sedatives should be employed, including morphine, for the relief of the pain. Hydrotherapy is useful in quieting nervousness. There seems to be little value in the application of an ice-bag to the head, and blisters to the back of the neck are useless and only increase the discomfort. In later stages the administration of iodides has been recommended to favor absorption of the meningeal thickening. The removal of spinal fluid by lumbar puncture often gives surprising relief. It should be employed once or twice a day in all cases. If the inflammation has shut off the spinal subarachnoid space, cisternal or ventricular puncture may be necessary.

Serum-treatment.—Kolle and Wassermann,[47] Jochmann,[48] Flexner and Jobling,[49] and others have prepared a serum for use in this disease. That made by Flexner and Jobling is obtained from horses which have been repeatedly inoculated with cultures of the meningococcus. After as much as possible of the cerebrospinal fluid has been drained by lumbar puncture, the serum, slightly warmed, is injected through the needle, which has been left in position. It may be given through a funnel and rubber tube, allowing it to enter by gravity, or a piston-syringe may be used cautiously. Injection should always be made slowly, and the amount should be less than that of the exudate removed. (For performance of lumbar puncture, see p. 151.) The dose should be from 10 to 30 cc. depending on the age and size of the patient. Injections should be made every twenty-four hours, sometimes oftener, during three or four days or more. On the theory that meningococcic infection of the subarachnoid space takes place through the choroid plexus, and that the inflammatory process appears first in the ventricles, some clinicians recommend early intraventricular injections. These do not seem necessary in the average case, especially when they would necessitate trephining, as in the case of patients past infancy. Howell and Cohen[50] found that in certain cases serum introduced subdurally at the outer edge of the fontanelle would reach foci that could not be approached by ventricular or lumbar injections. We[51] favor the approach to the cerebrospinal spaces by cisternal puncture in cases not doing well by lumbar injections, and have performed it many times without in any case seeing harm which could undoubtedly be traced to it. Somewhat smaller amounts of serum should be injected in this way, and very slowly. The procedure is applicable at any age and may effect cure in subarachnoid block in apparently hopeless cases. When there is evidence of blocking of the ventricles, however, puncture and injection of serum into them should be carried out. (See p. 152.) One should always remember that antimeningococcus serum, while possessing slight antitoxic properties, acts chiefly as a bactericidal agent. It must, therefore, be brought into contact with the organisms it is to destroy.

Good results from serum treatment are sometimes immediate and surprising, but oftener there is no immediate effect observable. Even in favorably reacting cases at least five injections of serum should be given, or, better, the treatment continued until no meningococci are found on two successive cultures. Increased cell-count in the fluid and fever may sometimes continue as long as there exists the irritation which the injections may keep up. In this event the injections may be tentatively discontinued, provided meningococci are absent from the fluid and continue to be, and the general symptoms improve. As a rule the injection is without unfavorable results, but occasionally prostration follows, and sometimes the symptoms may become alarming, chiefly in the nature of respiratory failure. In such an event artificial respiration should be employed and atropine given hypodermically. It happens in some cases and in certain epidemics that the serum appears to be without effect. This is often because it does not contain antibodies against the strain of the meningococcus which is operative. Most serum on the market is polyvalent, but that of various manufacturers may continue different strains. For this reason if one serum does not seem to be effective another should be tried. As previously pointed out (p. 320) there are many strains of meningococci. Branham, Taft and Carlin[10] found that of 235 strains isolated by them, 50 per cent were well agglutinated by polyvalent sera from eight manufacturers. The serum used should agglutinate meningococci when it is diluted 1:400 or better 1:1200. While agglutination is a helpful test of the efficiency of a given serum, clinical results will not always be commensurate with it, since it determines only one of the properties of the serum and not the more important bactericidal one. For resistant or so-called "fast" strains, Matsunami, Toyama and Kolmer[52] have tried the addition of 2 to 5 cc. of fresh, sterile human serum to antimeningococcus serum to increase its bactericidal property.

In cases of meningococcemia without meningitis, intravenous injections of serum should be tried. In early severe cases of meningitis intravenous treatment is indicated, but should always be combined with the intraspinal. Certain authors, as Herrick[53] and Haden,[13] have claimed that the mortality can be greatly reduced by combining intravenous with intraspinal treatment. Our own feeling is that serum should be injected intravenously only when there is evidence or strong suspicion that a blood-stream infection is the predominating feature.

In cases of subarachnoid block we have sometimes introduced serum under pressure in the lumbar region and have apparently been able to break up early adhesions. This, however, is a dangerous procedure. Lyon[55] describes a case in which there apparently was an obstruction by exudate in the aqueduct of Sylvius. By a combined ventricular and cisternal puncture and the exertion of pressure (80 mm. of mercury) connection was established, as shown by dye-studies before and after the procedure.

Kolmer[56] recommended in certain cases the injection of 10 cc. of serum into each common carotid artery, following this by drainage of the cisterna and the injection of 10 to 30 cc. of serum there. Neal and her co-workers[57] have published a favorable preliminary report on the use of an antibody-preparation devised by Banzhaf. Convalescent's and normal human serum have also been used. Veillan, Martin and Roux[58] employed successfully in one case intravenous injections of acriflavin. If pericarditis is caused by the meningococcus, the serum should be injected intrapericardially.

After the acute stage of the disease is over little benefit is to be expected from serum-treatment, but it may be tried, using the various routes which have been described. Autogenous vaccine has seemed to have beneficial effect in some cases. For the breaking up of adhesions injections of air have at times been helpful. The treatment of the hydrocephalus which often occurs as a sequel will be discussed in more detail elsewhere. (See p. 949.)

References

1. Hufeland's J. d. pract. Arzneykunde., 1805, **14,** 3 St., 181. 2. Med. and Agric. Reg., Boston, 1806; Ref. Osler, Pract. Med., 1903, 101. 3. Lyon méd., 1907, **108,** 1081. 4. Arch. Pediat., 1916, **33,** 481. 5. Arch. Pediat., 1917, **34,** 824. 6. Am. J. M. Sc., 1918, **156,** 358. 7. Am. J. Dis. Child., 1921, **21,** 500. 8. J.A.M.A., 1927, **88,** 1299. 9. Fortsch. d. Med., 1887, **5,** 573. 10. Pub. Health Rep., 1931, **46,** 897. 11. Jahrb. f. Kinderh., 1896, **43,** 1. 12. Res. Lab., Dept. Health, N. Y. City, 1905, **1,** 177. 13. Arch. Int. Med., 1919, **24,** 514. 14. Am. J. Med. Sc., 1921, **162,** 881. 15. Arch. Int. Med., 1918, **21,** 541; 1919, **23,** 409. 16. Bull. Sect. Sc. Acad. Roum., 1915–16, **10,** 368. Ref. Jahrb. f. Kinderh., 1917, **85,** 151. 17. Brit. J. Child. Dis., 1917, **14,** 264. 18. Arch. Pediat., 1916, **33,** 641. 19. Am. J. Dis. Child., 1924, **27,** 598. 20. Am. J. Dis. Child., 1931, **42,** 1053. 21. Frankfürt. Ztschr. f. Path., 1928, **36,** 18. 22. Wien. klin. Wchnschr., 1901, **14,** 984. 23. J. Infect. Dis., 1906, Supp. vol., 21. 24. Med. Klin., 1907, **3,** 314. 25. J. Hyg., 1918, **17,** 367. 26. Am. J. Pub. Health., 1929, **19,** 1098. 27. Arch. Pediat., 1920, **37,** 19. 28. Riv. crit. di clin. med., 1922, **23,** 181. 29. J.A.M.A., 1928, **90,** 520. 30. St. Bartholomew Hosp. Rep., 1878, **14,** 23. 31. J. Path. and Bact., 1898, **5,** 147. 32. J.A.M.A., 1929, **92,** 1923. 33. J.A.M.A., 1926, **87,** 91. 34. Die Taubstummheit. u. ihre Abhängigkeit von Cerebro-sp. Mening., 1883; Ref. Councilman, Mallory and Wright, Epidem. Cerebro-sp. Mening., 1898. 35. J.A.M.A., 1930, **95,** 776. 36. Nord. Med. Arch., 1901, **2,** No. 4. 37. Bull. de la soc. de méd. d. hôp. de Paris, 1918, **42,** 527. 38. Communic. Dis. Control. Rep. of Sec. 2, White House Conf. Child Health and Protection, 1931. 39. Ugeskrift for Laeger., 1891; Ref. Netter, 20th Cent. Pract. of Med. 14. 40. Die Meningitis cerebrospinalis epidemica, 1866, 33. 41. J.A.M.A., 1927, **88,** 1859. 42. J. Exper. Med., 1913, **17,** 553. 43. Am. J. Med. Sc., 1931, **181,** 414. 44. Ztschr. f. d. ges. Neurol. u. Psychiat., 1912, **13,** 192. 45. J.A.M.A., 1912, **59,** 527. 46. J.A.M.A., 1913, **60,** 1289; 1914, **63,** 2126. 47. Deutsche. med. Wchnschr., 1906, **32,** 609. 48. Deutsche med. Wchnschr., 1906, **32,** 788. 49. J. Exper. Med., 1908, **10,** 141. 50. Am. J. Dis. Child., 1922, **24,** 427. 51. Mitchell and Reilly, Am. J. Med. Sc., 1922, **164,** 66. 52. J. Immunol., 1918, **3,** 157; 177. 53. J.A.M.A., 1918, **71,** 612. 54. J.A.M.A., 1930, **95,** 109. 55. J.A.M.A., 1931, **96,** 1358. 56. J.A.M.A., 1928, **91,** 1427. 57. Bull. et mém. soc. de méd. d. hôp. de Paris, 1929, **53,** 1343.

CHAPTER XIII

ERYSIPELAS

Etiology.—The incidence of erysipelas has diminished very greatly in recent years. Climate and locality have no influence but the disease appears to be more frequent in cold weather. It often occurs in epidemics, especially in unsanitary institutions. Sporadic cases, however, sometimes develop under the best hygienic conditions. *Age* offers no protection, and although more common later, many cases occur in infancy and early childhood and even in the new-born. *Individual susceptibility* exists, some persons being liable to recurrent attacks, and an inherited predisposition being apparently possible. The presence of a *wound* is an important predisposing factor, and infants with umbilical irritation, eczema, lesions of varicella or the like, and those recently circumcised or vaccinated, are especially susceptible. Sometimes the portal of entry is the mucous membranes, with extension later to the skin. Often erysipelas develops without the slightest lesion being discoverable.

Exciting Cause.—This is apparently a streptococcus. Fehleisen,[1] who named this the *streptococcus erysipelatis*, and others have maintained this, and it would appear from the work of Tunnicliff,[2] Birkhaug,[3] and Rivers,[4] that the hemolytic streptococcus found in the disease belongs to a distinct group. (See also Treatment, p. 335.) *Transmission* is by direct contact, fomites, or through a third person. The germ is not diffused by the air to any extent and its vitality is not great.

Pathologic Anatomy.—The skin and often the subcutaneous tissues exhibit all the signs of inflammation, and in some cases suppuration. In the internal organs there may be the parenchymatous changes usually associated with acute infectious diseases; or septic foci, the seat of which depends upon the nature of the complications. Streptococci may be found in the tissues and often in blood-cultures. The infiltration is with round cells, unless suppuration occurs, when polymorphonuclear cells are present.

Symptoms. Incubation.—The period of incubation is generally from one to two or three days.

Symptoms of the Attack.—Initial symptoms may be absent, or consist of chilliness, coldness of the extremities, restlessness, prostration, vomiting, high fever, and occasionally convulsions. Simultaneously, or nearly so, redness, swelling and tenderness of the skin develop in the affected area. The face is the usual starting point (83 per cent of Roger's[5] and 79.8 per cent of Symmers'[6] cases of all ages). The redness exhibits the uniform flush of a dermatitis, unlike that of scarlet fever. Its border is sharply defined, elevated, and either clean-cut or with irregular projections jutting out here and there into the healthy skin. When the process is severe vesicles or bullae form upon the affected skin. Within two or three days the inflammation begins to disappear in the part first involved, and desquamation follows, usually in fine scales, but coarser and in larger pieces if vesicles have been present. In the meantime the border of the infiltrated region has extended more or less rapidly, sometimes a considerable area becoming involved in a few hours, and sometimes the advance being slow.

The manner of the spreading and the degree of swelling depend largely upon the locality. Where the skin is firmly adherent to underlying structures, as at the chin, the patellae and the condyles, the disease often passes around, leaving these areas unaffected. Where the tissue is loose, as at the genitals and the eyelids, the edema is great. When the disease starts at the nose this organ swells rapidly and the rash generally quickly spreads to the cheeks in the well-known butterfly form. It often stops here, but it may involve the eyelids, closing them for days, or may extend over one or both sides of the face and to the ears. The whole scalp may be finally involved. Under such circumstances the head and face seem twice their natural size and the child is entirely unrecognizable (Fig. 69). The inflammation may cease here, or may spread to the body. Developing about a vaccine pustule or other lesion on the arm or leg, it may remain confined to this locality, or may extend rapidly over the whole limb and thence to other parts, but not so often to the head as elsewhere. In some cases the disease appears to start on the mucous membrane of the nose, throat, or mouth and spread to the face, the first symptoms being a severe angina or coryza. In other cases it first attacks the mucous membrane of the vulva and extends to the thighs and other regions, and it has been reported in an adult as a primary lesion in the stomach (Martl and Eisenberg).[7]

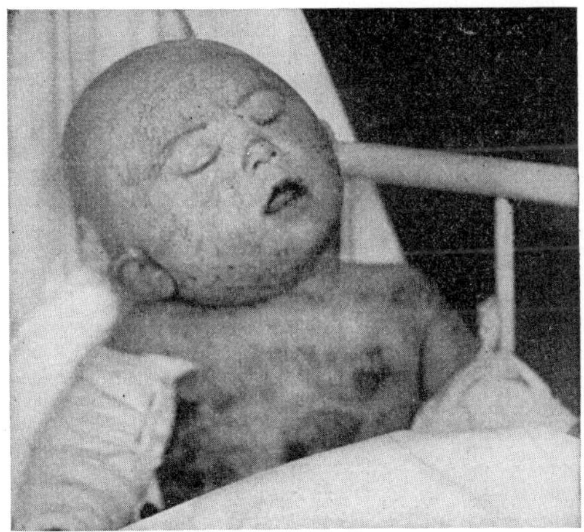

Fig. 69.—Erysipelas with great swelling of the head. Child of fourteen months, in the Children's Hospital of Philadelphia. Disease began in the face, involved the head, closing the eyes, thence spread to the rest of the body. Death nine days after the onset.

The tendency of the rash to spread varies greatly. It may be very slight, the eruption reaching but little beyond the point of original appearance, or it may wander more or less rapidly over the whole body (*erysipelas migrans*), returning and attacking again parts from which it had disappeared but a short time before. This spreading is often with intermissions during which the symptoms ameliorate and the false hope arises that the attack is over.

Symptoms Attending the Eruption.—The temperature as a rule rises very rapidly and remains at 104 F. (40 C.) or more, with but slight morning fall, as long as the spread of the rash is uninterrupted (Fig. 70). In very mild cases fever may be entirely absent or undiscovered. It generally is in proportion to the severity of the cutaneous manifestations. An intermittent extension has an intermittent temperature (Fig. 71); a steady spread, a temperature more continuously elevated. The lymphatic glands in the neighborhood of the dermatitis are nearly always inflamed. The spleen is often enlarged. In severe cases the appetite is poor, the tongue dry, the pulse weak, and respiration sometimes dyspneic. Restlessness, delirium or sopor not infrequently develop. The blood shows a polymorphonuclear leukocytosis most marked in the severe cases. Transient albuminuria is occasionally present. The complex of symptoms varies, being often influenced by the complications.

The *duration* of the disease is extremely variable. As already stated the height of the affection in any one spot is reached in two to three days, and recovery in that region is rapid. An average duration of the entire attack is seven to nine days, but may last less than this or often much longer, and in cases of erysipelas migrans may continue even occasionally for months.

Erysipelas in Early Infancy.—This condition, and especially that denominated *Erysipelas neonatorum*, differs somewhat from the disease as seen later. The regions first attacked are oftenest the umbilicus, vulva, anus, and the lesions of circumcision or vaccination, rather than the head. The onset is more insidious, and the child is restless and fretful, but often

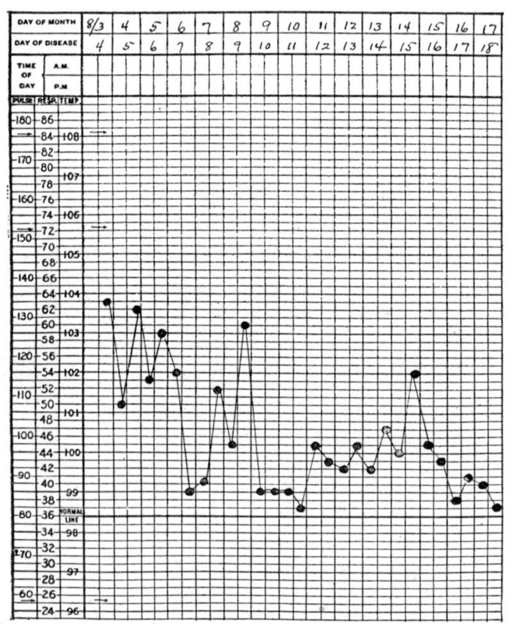

Fig. 70.

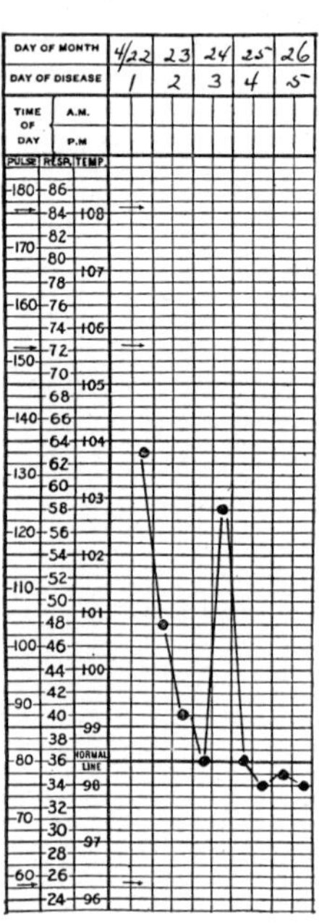

Fig. 71.

Fig. 70.—Erysipelas, average case. Elsie S., aged three and a half years. Aug. 3, fourth day of disease, eruption spreading over left leg; Aug. 5, involving foot; Aug. 6, no extension; Aug. 8, rapid extension to buttock with increase of fever; Aug. 13, fresh extension, involving right leg and trunk; Aug. 14, development of bullae, with increase of fever; Aug. 17, convalescing.

Fig. 71.—Mild erysipelas with recrudescence of fever attending extension of rash. Edith S., aged seven years. Apr. 22, red flush right cheek, extending over nose; Apr. 23, large blebs on right cheek, eye nearly closed; Apr. 24, extension to left cheek with renewed fever; Apr. 26, improving.

without fever for some hours or even days, and sometimes at any time. When fever develops the spleen enlarges, vomiting and diarrhea are likely to occur, and the dermatitis spreads widely. Loss of strength is rapid, septic symptoms appear, the pulse is very rapid and weak, food is refused, collapse supervenes, convulsions may appear, and death may follow within a week or even a day or two from the onset. There is a decided tendency for the disease to assume the wandering type if the infant lives long enough. The eruption differs little from that seen later in life, except that the swelling is liable to be greater and more tense, the redness less intense, the boundary less raised, and desquamation more frequent. The cases which recover generally develop cutaneous abscesses.

Complications and Sequels.—Suppuration in the subcutaneous tissues is not infrequent, and necrosis of portions of the skin has been reported. Bronchitis, pneumonia, peritonitis and empyema may occur. Meningitis is an occasional complication, although many subjects exhibiting its symptoms show no such lesion at necropsy. Less commonly found are edema of the larynx, nephritis, suppuration of joints and lymphatic glands, and endocarditis.

Erysipelas may occur in combination with many other diseased conditions, especially, as indicated, with wounds. It may be a complication of other infectious disorders, as scarlatina, variola, varicella, malaria, typhoid fever, cerebrospinal fever and diphtheria. In the last three it generally develops from a bed-sore or other open wound.

Relapse and Recurrence.—In addition to the frequent recrudescences with pseudocrises so characteristic of the disease, true *relapse* may show itself after several days or even a few weeks, and may be repeated a number of times. *Recurrence* in the sense of a new infection is more common than relapse, occurring in 7 to 8 per cent of cases. In fact, one attack creates absolutely no immunity, but rather seems to predispose to later ones. Perhaps the skin-test with toxin suggested by Birkhaug[8] may prove useful in determining susceptibility. Frequent recurrence is liable to result in permanent thickening of the affected areas, especially the scrotum and the eyelids.

Prognosis.—In the new-born erysipelas is almost always fatal, and at any period of infancy it is serious, especially in the first two or three months of life. Schaffer and Rothman[9] in untreated cases found 80 per cent mortality in the first month; 53 per cent from one to six months; 47.6 per cent from six to twelve months; 14.35 per cent from one to two years. In childhood recovery generally takes place if the disease is uncomplicated and of moderate extent. The prognosis is prone to be worse if the head is attacked, but facial involvement alone responds favorably to treatment. Wandering erysipelas has a graver prognosis than the more limited form. Among unfavorable symptoms are high fever, cerebral symptoms, and a blood-culture positive for streptococci. All complications increase the gravity of the case, and death may follow pneumonia and sometimes peritonitis, meningitis, and involvement of the kidneys. In most studies antitoxin has lowered mortality.

Diagnosis.—The diagnosis rests upon the combination of constitutional symptoms with a dermatitis which is characterized by its sharply defined border and its tendency to extension. The rash of scarlet fever is distinguished by its punctiform character. Deep-seated phlegmonous inflammation lacks the characteristic border, as does also lymphangitis, which follows the course of the lymphatic vessels. Erythema infectiosum (see p. 287), while having a distribution and color upon the face suggesting erysipelas, lacks the sharp outline and the infiltration, and exhibits a morbilliform rash on the trunk and limbs.

Treatment. **Prophylaxis.**—Aseptic precautions should be employed in the care of the umbilical wound or in performing vaccination, circumcision, and the like. Infants and children, especially those with open wounds, should be kept away from patients with erysipelas or any suppurative infections.

Treatment of the Attack.—No drugs are specific, although some clinicians believe that the internal administration of tincture of ferric chloride in large doses gives good results. Quinine and the salicylates have also been employed. Many preparations have been used locally:—ointment or glycerin-solution of resorcin (30 per cent) or ichthyol; powders of iodoform, oxide of zinc, or starch and salicylic acid; solutions of bichloride of mercury (1:2000), boric acid, mercurochrome (2 per cent), lead water and laudanum, and alcohol. Collodion has frequently been painted beyond the margin of the eruption in the hope that the spread of the rash may be prevented by shutting off the lymph-channels, and Hutten[10] employed for this same purpose freezing by ethyl chloride. With a disease which is systemic in nature and with a course so uncertain and erratic, it cannot be definitely proven that any of these methods have certain value. Good results have been reported by Petenyi,[11] Zahorsky,[12] Becker,[13] and Ude and Platou[14] from the local use of ultraviolet rays, employing an artificial source such as a mercury-vapor quartz lamp, and giving usually a strong erythema-dose, but below that which would produce vesiculation. Platou[15] and his coworkers recommend the local application of the roentgen-ray. A form of treatment suggested by Rivers and Tillett[16] from their work on rabbits is the injection of normal or immune (convalescent) serum in the healthy skin at the margins of the eruption, and Musser[17] has reported success in human cases with antierysipelas serum used in the same manner. We have had experience with all of these local treatments and they would seem to be effective in some cases, but should usually be combined in severe ones with serum-treatment or with transfusions.

The antitoxin secured by the injection of animals with the apparently specific type of hemolytic streptococcus and introduced by Birkhaug[3] seems to have definite value. The concentrated form should be injected intramuscularly in doses of from 10 to 20 cc. (0.34 to 0.67 oz.) every twenty-four hours until improvement occurs. Dosage varies more with the severity of the disease than with the age of the patient. Intravenous injection may be followed by severe general reaction. Among those reporting favorable results with the serum are Symmers and Lewis,[18] Symmers,[6] Foote,[19] and Eley.[20] Blake,[21] however, argues that recovery from erysipelas does not depend to any great extent upon the development of antitoxin immunity, and that theoretically antitoxin can be of little use. Convalescent's serum (see p. 279 for preparation), taken a week after recovery, has been employed, and is reported on favorably by Jordan and Dustin,[22] and so-called "normal adult serum" has been used. Transfusion or intramuscular injections of blood often seem of value; Schaffer and Rothman[10] recording a lower mortality as compared with an untreated control group. Gerdes[23] used nonspecific protein therapy (milk injections). For recurrent cases Birkhaug[24] has given a toxin-vaccine preparation. Other treatment is symptomatic.

References

1. Deutsche Ztschr. f. Chir., 1882, **16**, 391. 2. J.A.M.A., 1920, **75**, 1339. 3. Bull. Johns Hopkins Hosp., 1925, **37**, 307; J.A.M.A., 1926, **86**, 1411. 4. J. Exper. Med., 1925, **41**, 179. 5. Arch. gén. de méd., 1901, **188**, 5. 6. J.A.M.A., 1928, **91**, 535. 7. Arch. Path., 1929, **8**, 744. 8. J.A.M.A., 1928, **90**, 1997. 9. Am. J. Dis. Child., 1927, **33**, 116. 10. Beitr. z. klin. Chir., 1925, **133**, 252. 11. Monatschr. f. Kinderh., 1921, **31**, 269. 12. J. Missouri State M.A. 1925, **22**, 61. 13. Strahlentherapie, 1929, **34**, 205. 14. J.A.M.A., 1930, **95**, 1. 15. Arch. Int. Med., 1926, **38**, 573; Am. J. Dis. Child., 1927, **34**, 1030. 16. J. Exper. Med., 1925, **41**, 185. 17. J.A.M.A., 1927, **88**, 1125. 18. J.A.M.A., 1927, **89**, 880. 19. South. M.J., 1930, **23**, 29. 20. Am. J. Dis. Child., 1930, **39**, 529. 21. Trans. Coll. Phys. Phila., 1928, **50**, 3d Ser. 26. 22. J.A.M.A., 1924, **82**, 874. 23. Ugesk. f. Laeger., 1927, **89**, 210. 24. J.A.M.A., 1927, **88**, 885; 1928, **90**, 1997.

CHAPTER XIV

DIPHTHERIA

History.—While diphtheria appears to date from very early times, perhaps the first clear account of it was given by Aretaeus[1] in the first century. It ravaged Europe in the sixteenth and seventeenth centuries, and was described in America by Douglas,[2] in 1736, and very completely by Bard[3] in 1771. It was first called "Diphtheritis" (διφθερα = a membrane or skin) by Bretonneau.[4] The term "diphtheria" should be applied only to the disease caused by the diphtheria bacillus.

Etiology. Predisposing Causes.—The disease is of frequent occurrence in all climates and countries, though perhaps more common in the cooler months of the year. At this season close association in houses is a factor, and perhaps, too, the variation in the antitoxin content of the blood; which studies, such as those of Perkins[5] and his coworkers, show is low in the late winter and spring and rises in the late summer. Humidity has decided influence, probably by increasing the catarrhal affections or, according to Ochsenius,[6] by lowering bodily resistance. This lowering of resistance is brought about also by poor sanitation and impaired health in general, and, for the same reason, other infectious disorders, especially scarlet fever, measles, influenza and pertussis, augment the susceptibility. Tendency to the disease is greater among children in less congested communities, since it is probable that repeated exposure to infection in a dosage insufficient to cause clinical manifestations results in immunity (Zingher[7]).

Age is of importance. The disease is most frequent up to ten years, and particularly from one to five years of age; least so in the first year, and especially in the first six months. In 2600 cases reported by Rolleston[8] there were but 20 in the first year; of 2711 cases Baginsky[9] found only 15 under six months; in 2400 consecutive admissions for diphtheria to the Cincinnati General Hospital reported by Ravenel[10] there were 49 under one year of age. This lesser occurrence in very young infants depends upon a natural immunity at this age, not upon absence of exposure; since new-born infants may become carriers of diphtheria. (The value of the Schick test in young infants will be considered later (p. 347).) Yet new-born infants are occasionally attacked, as shown by the reports of Jacobi,[11] Riesman,[12] Stimson,[13] Becker,[14] Rominger,[15] Brindeau,[16] Comby,[17] and others. The youngest patient we have seen was seven days old. Infection of the fetus with the diphtheria bacillus is also possible (Traugott[18]).

Sex has some influence, most statistics showing that slightly more girls than boys are attacked. There seems to exist sometimes a familial predisposition. Apart from this, the *individual susceptibility* is not great, and the disease may oftener occur in only one child in the family than is true of some other infectious disorders. Diphtheria is *endemic* in large cities, but often becomes *epidemic*.

Exciting Cause.—This is the specific bacillus first recognized by Klebs[19] in 1883 and shown to be the sole cause of the disease by Löffler in 1884. It is straight or slightly curved, rod-shaped, has rounded ends, is about 2 to 3 microns in length, and when prepared with Neisser's stain appears as a brown rod with granules at the poles. It is readily killed by a temperature of 58 C. (136.4 F.) but it is not affected by cold or drying. Normally it is very tenacious of life and may live long on various objects such as toys and the like. It usually disappears from the throat in two to four weeks from the beginning of the disease, but may persist in both the nose and the throat for months in a virulent form, and it sometimes occurs in the discharge from an otitis media or in the urine. At necropsy it may sometimes be found in various organs of the body, as the liver, spleen, lungs, bone-marrow, kidneys, and lymphatic glands; being frequently associated there with streptococci, or less often with staphylococci and pneumococci (Councilman, Mallory and Pearce[21]). Especially in severe cases it may be found in the blood-stream, often with streptococci. Bonhoff,[22] for example, discovered it 13 times in 314 cases, in 10 of which other germs also were present.

Yet the bacilli are not, as a rule, widely distributed, and the disease is *primarily a local one*, the germs growing upon a mucous membrane, whence absorption of the toxin takes place.

Transmission.—Indirect transmission is much the least frequent method of communicating the infection, but it may be acquired through infected milk, domestic animals, books, toys, clothing, and the like. Litterer[23] isolated virulent diphtheria bacilli from fowls, and this can occur without the fowls themselves being ill (Spiegelberg[24]). The belief in extension by means of cats is of long standing. Savage[25] could find in the literature as reviewed by him no certain cases of the disease in cats. Simmons,[26] however, isolated virulent bacilli from cats and found suspicious lesions at necropsy.

In the large majority of cases the germs are communicated directly by unrecognized cases and convalescents, or not infrequently by healthy persons with virulent organisms in the nose and throat. Mild unrecognized nasal diphtheria is a fruitful source of dissemination. Transmission may occur even before symptoms appear, and may take place as long as the bacilli remain virulent.

Carriers.—The remarkable persistence of the germs on the mucous membranes of convalescents or healthy persons, which is frequently seen, accounts for the cases which occur sporadically or without apparent source. Many studies have shown that some persons, especially those who live in cities, carry true virulent diphtheria bacilli on the mucous membrane of the throat, and many others pseudodiphtheritic germs (Mass. Assoc. Boards of Health,[27] Pennington,[28] von Shoolly,[29] Schrammen,[30] Doull et al.,[31] Kliewe and Hofmann,[32] Kollmann[33]). These studies show that the incidence of carriers is from about 1 to 5 per cent, and sometimes much larger, even up to 50 per cent in those who have been recently exposed to the disease. The virulence-test should always be made in doubtful cases, and especially when there has been long persistence of diphtheria bacilli in the throat.

Pathologic Anatomy.—The *primary lesion* is the pseudomembrane, found oftenest upon the faucial and nasopharyngeal tonsillar tissue; very frequently also upon the pharynx, uvula, larynx, trachea and bronchi; and sometimes in the mouth, vulva, vagina, middle ear, conjunctiva, esophagus, stomach and intestine. It occurs occasionally upon wounds, as of circumcision or at the umbilicus in the new-born. The pseudomembrane is usually grayish-white or yellowish-white; sometimes friable and easily removed, often tough and adherent, and separated only with injury to the underlying tissue. In the larynx it is firmly adherent; in the trachea easily detached. In severe cases it soon becomes dark-greenish, blackish, or gangrenous in appearance, with the surrounding tissue deeply congested.

Microscopically the pseudomembrane consists of a necrotic degeneration of the mucous membrane combined with fibrinous exudate from the underlying blood-vessels, which, with the connective tissue, exhibit thickening and hyaline transformation. The diphtheria bacilli do not reach the lowest layers of the exudate.

In some cases the pseudomembrane is represented only by a few small yellowish spots of secretion in the tonsillar crypts (*diphtheritic folliculitis*);

in others there is only a catarrhal condition of the mucous membrane discoverable (*catarrhal diphtheria*). Even in this, however, characteristic necrotic changes can be found in the superficial cells.

The primary lesion is of little importance, except by mechanical obstruction of the larynx. The *secondary lesions* constitute the chief danger. These consist of the widespread cellular degenerative changes caused by the toxin of the diphtheria bacillus, which is produced in the primary lesion and distributed by the blood and the lymph. Other associated microbes in the pseudomembrane probably aid in the process, either by the formation of toxins, or by entering the blood-stream and causing a septicemia. The cervical, bronchial and mesenteric lymph nodes are enlarged, and exhibit congestion, leukocytic infiltration and often hemorrhages. Bronchopneumonic areas are found in over $\frac{1}{2}$ of the necropsies. A serous or serofibrinous pleurisy may occur. Small hemorrhages may be present in the skin, pleura, pericardium and endocardium, and beneath the capsule of the liver and spleen. The cardiac muscle is degenerated in all long-continued severe cases, and Nuzum[34] has reported an increased number of eosinophiles. The spleen and liver are enlarged and soft. The kidneys are large and exhibit changes, but nothing specific for diphtheria (Councilman, Mallory and Pearce[21]), although the interstitial and glomerular types are more common in older children and in long-continued cases. The suprarenal bodies show hemorrhages, or a degeneration and disappearance of the chromaffin substance and of the medullary cells. The brain and spinal cord are little altered, but the cranial and spinal nerves suffer a widespread degeneration.

Symptoms.—These vary greatly with the locality affected, the intensity of the intoxication, and the complications.

ORDINARY TYPE. FAUCIAL DIPHTHERIA. **Incubation.**—The duration of this is difficult to determine, but it is certainly short, varying generally from one to four days.

Invasion.—Although the process is primarily local, the first clinical manifestations are constitutional in nature, and consist in chilliness, slight fever, and anorexia; sometimes vomiting, headache, and cervical adenitis; and occasionally convulsions. There may or may not be complaint of sore throat. Inspection shows only a congestion and perhaps slight swelling of the throat and tonsils.

Symptoms of the Attack.—Within twenty-four hours a small or larger yellowish-white or grayish-white deposit is seen, which resembles ordinary follicular tonsillitis, but which is removable only with difficulty and has somewhat more of a membrane-like character. New membrane forms rapidly after such removal. Sometimes the early appearance of the deposit is more gelatinous.

The pseudomembrane spreads, and, if limited to one tonsil at the outset, extends to the other in from two to five days and then to the uvula, the palatal pillars and the soft palate. Its color becomes a dirty gray, the odor from the mouth is offensive, swelling in the throat increases, and by the end of the first week the fauces, and to some extent the pharynx, may be covered with a thick pseudomembrane sometimes almost closing the throat. The nose is often involved. (See Nasal Diphtheria, p. 340.) Difficulty in swallowing and pain in the throat are variable, and not necessarily related to the extent of the inflammation.

Meanwhile the constitutional symptoms increase in severity. The cervical glands grow larger, generally in proportion to the degree of faucial inflammation. The *fever* exhibits no exact relation to the severity of the symptoms. It is often characteristically low, being around 101 to 102 F. (38.3 to 38.9 C.) (Fig. 72), although sometimes higher. It is generally highest at the beginning of the attack and then falls, although renewed rises may occur as the disease extends to new regions, or as complications develop. The *pulse* is usually weak and much more rapid than might be expected from the elevation of temperature. Blood-pressure is low. The *urine* exhibits albumin and epithelial and hyaline casts in many instances. The excretion of nitrogen is much increased, as the result of destruction of tissue-cells (Howland[35]). Knee-jerks are often absent. The *blood* shows a definite polymorphonuclear leukocytosis, increasing as the disease advances and diminishing during convalescence. Red blood-cells and hemoglobin are reduced in severe cases. The blood-sugar may be

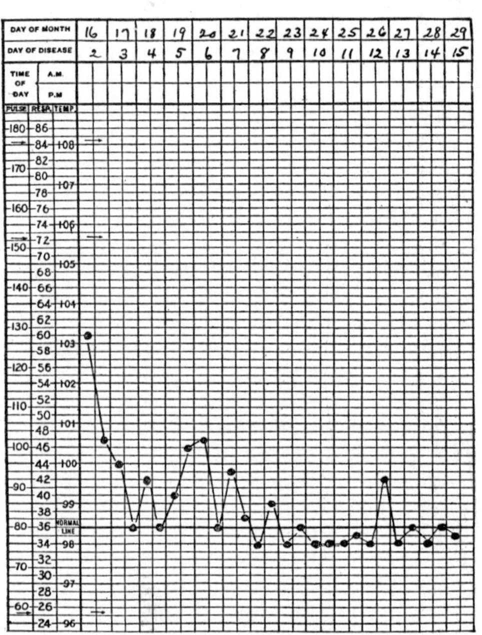

Fig. 72.—Tonsillar and nasal diphtheria. Mary K., aged nine years. Feb. 15, onset with nausea, vomiting, sore throat, and fever; Feb. 16, tonsils and arches covered, nasal discharge; Feb. 18, great improvement; Feb. 21, throat clean. Given 7500 units antitoxin on 16th; 7500 on 17th; 6000 on 18th; 5000 on 19th. Philadelphia Hospital for Contagious Diseases. (*Courtesy of Dr. B. F. Royer.*)

low. (See Prognosis, p. 344.) Blood-calcium is lowered in severe diphtheria (Peola and Inglessi[36]). One of the most marked symptoms is the *prostration*, which is frequently out of proportion to other symptoms. There may early be slight delirium, and later decided apathy, somnolence, or irritability.

At the end of the first week, or frequently not until later, improvement may begin, indicated by the softening and separation of the pseudomembrane and the gradual amelioration of symptoms. The general improvement, and especially the rapidity of disappearance of the pseudomembrane, are greatly influenced by antitoxin-treatment.

Convalescence is usually slow and debility long-continued. Complications occurring at this time will be discussed later (p. 342).

Frequently faucial diphtheria is associated with nasopharyngeal or laryngeal involvement, which modifies the course and duration of the disease.

Nasal Diphtheria.—This may be primary in the nose, and either remain limited here or spread to the nasopharynx, throat, or larynx; or may be secondary to the affection in the fauces or nasopharynx. As a *secondary* affection it is common, and adds to the severity of the case. Respiration through the nose becomes obstructed, and an offensive and irritating discharge causes excoriation and swelling of the nostrils and upper lip. Pseudomembrane may be seen lining the nasal passages, and epistaxis is frequent. Constitutional symptoms are generally severe, and the course prolonged. The disease may extend to the ear.

Primary nasal diphtheria is commonest in infants, very frequently remains for a time undiscovered, and is a fertile source of contagion. When confined to this region either no general symptoms at all are noticed, or there are only slight fever and malaise. These cases may run a somewhat chronic course, the child appearing to have merely a cold in the head; but the irritating nasal discharge is suspicious, especially if it is sanguinolent. *Diphtheria primary in the nasopharynx* is generally severe.

Nasal diphtheria, primary or secondary, is a common form. In 1200 cases of faucial diphtheria Rolleston[37] found involvement of the nose in 41.6 per cent. As a condition limited to the nose he[38] observed it in but 1.5 per cent of 3000 patients.

Laryngeal Diphtheria.—This may more properly be called *laryngotracheal diphtheria.* It is one of the most dangerous forms, causing a large proportion of the deaths. It is almost always secondary to lesions in the nose or the throat, although often appearing primary because these lesions had been slight and overlooked. Laryngeal diphtheria comes on about the fourth or fifth day of the disease; not often after the first week. The first symptoms are hoarseness, a ringing cough, and slightly noisy respiration. If there is no marked pharyngeal involvement there may be little constitutional disturbance, the symptoms being those of laryngeal stenosis. By the second day of the laryngeal attack the voice becomes hoarse or whispering, the cough metallic, and dyspnea severe, both inspiration and expiration being prolonged and labored. There is an anxious expression with restlessness and tossing, and the child often sits upright with his head thrown back, grasping at its throat or at the air with its hands, and drawing its breath only with difficulty and with the aid of all the accessory respiratory muscles. There is moving of the nasal alae and retraction of the epigastrium and of the supraclavicular and suprasternal spaces. Cyanosis becomes marked. Laryngoscopic examination reveals edema of the tissues and the presence of a pseudomembrane.

The symptoms vary, and dyspnea is more marked at some times than others, this change in the picture depending upon the varying degrees of edema present. Occasionally temporary relief is afforded by the coughing up of portions of the pseudomembrane, but the deposit is soon reproduced. Scattered atelectatic areas or massive collapse of the lung may occur with bronchial involvement (Welford[39]). Before antitoxin treatment the majority of cases ended fatally after twenty-four to forty-eight hours, but sometimes not for several days. Death may occur suddenly from suffocation, or more slowly from cardiac failure.

Laryngeal diphtheria appears to be less common than formerly, probably as a result of antitoxin-treatment. In 1962 cases of diphtheria reported by Burrows[40] laryngeal involvement occurred in 17 per cent.

Diphtheria may be classified also according to the character of the symptoms, the severity, and the degree of constitutional infection.

Mild Diphtheria.—Frequently the disease is so mild that it is entirely overlooked, or the diagnosis made only by bacteriological examination. As already stated, primary nasal diphtheria may be of this nature. In other cases there are only the symptoms of a lacunar tonsillitis in which recovery may occur without treatment, or in which after a few days a membrane may develop and the usual course of diphtheria follow, or laryngeal diphtheria occur.

CATARRHAL DIPHTHERIA.—There may be an entire absence of membrane in either nose or throat, the symptoms being simply those of a catarrhal inflammation. Constitutional symptoms may be absent or insignificant, and the diagnosis made only by bacteriological examination. This form, too, may give rise to laryngeal involvement.

SEVERE FAUCIAL AND NASOPHARYNGEAL DIPHTHERIA.—Many of these cases are well called "*septic diphtheria.*" The general symptoms are those of profound sepsis, and, as previously pointed out, streptococci appear to share with the diphtheria bacilli in producing the toxemia. It is in this type that diphtheria bacilli may be found in the blood-stream, with perhaps also other organisms here and in large numbers in the local lesions. The attack may be serious from the onset, or become so only later. The local condition in the fauces and nasopharynx is severe, with great swelling and a wide-spread and sometimes gangrenous pseudomembrane, an abundant offensive mucopurulent nasal discharge, and perhaps hemorrhage from the nose or mouth. All the signs of toxemia are present, such as pallor with cyanosis, cold extremities, and feeble pulse. Petechiae may occur. The prostration is extreme; the temperature variable, and often but little elevated; the cervical glands greatly swollen. The mind may be clear, or there may be delirium or stupor. In cases which recover the pseudomembrane begins to disintegrate about the end of the first week or perhaps later, and the mucous membrane is left denuded or ulcerated. In fatal cases death occurs in about a week from increasing debility or bronchopneumonia, or from uremic convulsions, heart-failure, or the development of laryngeal obstruction.

Malignant Diphtheria is a term applied to the worst type of severe case, in which both local and constitutional symptoms are exaggerated and death occurs in a few days.

UNUSUAL LOCALIZATIONS.—Membrane may appear in unusual regions, either primarily, or secondary to diphtheria of the throat or nose. It may spread to the buccal cavity, lips, or adjacent portions of the face. Occurring on the conjunctiva it is rare. Diphtheria may involve the meninges through extension from the middle ear. The disease may be primary or secondary upon the penis or the scrotum, or upon the vagina or vulva. Any cutaneous wounds, especially that of a tracheotomy or circumcision or unhealed umbilicus, or any eczematous area may be attacked. Occurring primarily on the skin it is uncommon, Billings[41] finding only 27 recorded cases, and adding 2 of his own. Secondary involvement of the trachea and bronchi is common (Fig. 73), but exceptionally the disease may be primary in the bronchi. When these localities are attacked toxin-absorption may not be great, and the condition may be a chronic one. Usually a pseudomembrane forms and there is an irritating and often sanguinolent discharge. In some instances, especially when an open wound is affected, the symptoms may be acute and severe.

Complications and Sequels.—These vary with epidemics and with the time at which antitoxin treatment is given. One of the most frequent complications is *bronchopneumonia*, which is particularly liable to occur in laryngeal involvement, in severe septic cases, and in infancy. It depends not only upon the presence of the diphtheria bacillus, but upon associated germs, as the streptococcus and pneumococcus. It may develop any time during the course of the disease. It is found in over $\frac{1}{2}$ of the fatal cases. Croupous pneumonia is only an accidental complication.

Cardiac failure is one of the most dreaded of complications or sequels. The mechanism of this does not seem to be the same in every instance.

The electrocardiographic studies of Marvin,[42] Nathanson,[43] and Shookhoff and Taran[44] indicated that myocarditis is the important lesion, while those of McCulloch[45] gave evidence of damage both to the intrinsic conducting system and to the heart-muscle. Edmunds and Johnson[46] think that, in addition to myocardial changes, there is a toxic action on the splanchnic nerves, with relaxation of abdominal vessels and a fall in blood-pressure, and a consequent anemia of the medullary centers, this causing a fatal circulatory collapse. Brockington[47] believes that late heart-failure is due to fall in blood-pressure.

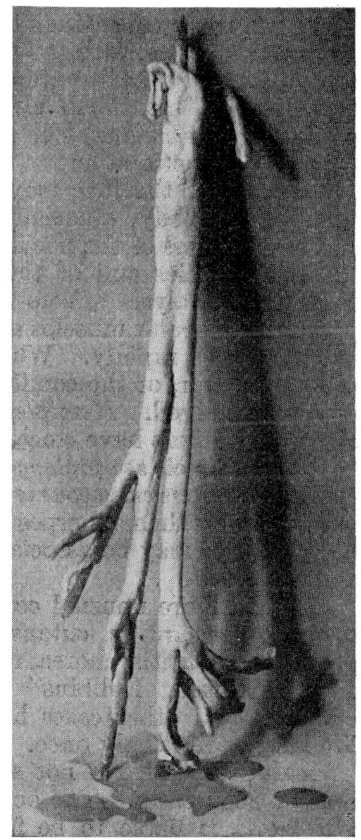

Fig. 73.—Tracheobronchial casts in diphtheria. Boy of five years with laryngeal diphtheria, in the Philadelphia Hospital for Contagious Diseases. Intubation no benefit. Tracheotomy performed and casts removed with forceps through the opening. (*Courtesy of Dr. N. A. Christensen.*)

Heart-failure may occur at any time during the course of the disease, perhaps even on the first day in malignant cases, but is witnessed most frequently as a sequel in the third or fourth week during convalescence, and more commonly after severe attacks of diphtheria. Usually the symptoms come on gradually, lasting three or four days or less, and consist of abdominal pain; vomiting; dyspnea; weak pulse, which is usually rapid and irregular, although sometimes slow; feeble heart-tones, sometimes with gallop-rhythm; enlargement of the liver; and cardiac dilatation. There is pallor and perhaps edema. In other cases heart-failure is abrupt, the child dying suddenly on very slight exertion. Sometimes repeated attacks of failure occur, to be followed finally by recovery or by a fatal ending. Mild disturbances of the heart, as shown by irregular, rapid pulse, faintness and shortness of breath, are very common in diphtheria, White and Smith[48] finding cardiac symptoms in 868 of 946 cases. Bullowa[49] states that the oculo-cardiac reflex, *i. e.*, the slowing of the pulse-rate on ocular pressure, is absent in severe diphtheria, and that this indicates a danger of sudden death.

Nephritis, as evidenced by slight albuminuria with perhaps cylinduria, but without other renal symptoms, is found in probably from $\frac{1}{3}$ to $\frac{2}{3}$ of all cases. It is an indication of the degenerative changes of the renal epithelium. With more decided involvement the urine is somewhat diminished in amount, and there may be leukocytes, epithelial cells and tube casts, usually hyaline; seldom blood. This occurs oftenest in the first or second week. There is generally edema, and recovery as a rule is rapid. In some severe cases a sudden, acute nephritis may develop with complete anuria and symptoms of uremia. Chronic nephritis is an unusual sequel. Occasionally, too, there is found a nephrotic type of renal lesion with edema.

Diphtheritic Paralysis.—This is relatively frequent as a complication or sequel. Rolleston[50] recorded it in 20.7 per cent of 2300 cases. It may occur as a complication; as in the form of early palatal paralysis or as part of the mechanism of heart-failure. As a sequel it is seen especially in the "post-diphtheritic paralysis" affecting various regions of the body. This is observed oftenest after severe attacks in those past the period of infancy, but to this there are many exceptions. The most frequent and usually the first seat is the soft palate, which exhibits paralysis about two or three weeks or more after the onset. The palate is immobile and the speech becomes nasal, and fluids pass into the nose upon attempts at swallowing. With this paralysis is generally associated a loss of the patellar reflex, even when no sign of neuritis is discoverable beyond that of the palate; and, indeed, the patellar reflex may be abolished without any palatal involvement. Early in the attack the paralysis may extend to the pharyngeal and laryngeal muscles, with the result that liquids readily enter the trachea and respiration may be interfered with. Next in frequency and in order of development, but much less common, is paralysis of the ocular muscles, producing strabismus, loss of accomodation, dilatation of the pupils, and ptosis or sometimes other evidence of involvement of the third nerve. The nerves of the face may exceptionally be attacked, or those of other parts of the body, especially the lower extremities. Less often the arms and the muscles of the neck are involved. Paralysis of the abdominal and thoracic muscles and of the diaphragm may occur. In the majority of cases the paralysis affects only the palate and the patellar reflexes, or perhaps the ocular muscles as well, and recovery begins in about two weeks and advances rapidly. When the paralysis is more widespread recovery is much slower, or the condition may end fatally if the respiratory muscles become involved. *Hemiplegia* may occur. Rolleston[51] collected 80 such cases, and others have since been reported.

Other sequels are *prolonged anemia* and *debility*, chronic *rhinitis*, and *otitis media*. Various *cutaneous eruptions* may be seen, among these being a diffuse multiform erythema, herpes and, in malignant cases, purpura. Other *infectious diseases* may be associated, prominent among these being scarlet fever and measles.

Among more unusual complications may be mentioned pleurisy, endocarditis, pericarditis, cutaneous emphysema (the result of necrosis in the pharynx), arthritis, chorea, meningitis, gangrene of the lung, and thrombosis and embolism. Robbins[52] collected 25 cases of gangrene occurring in children, and other cases have been reported by Gunson[53] and Jacobs.[54] We have seen it only once.

Relapse.—This is not so rare; Rolleston[55] finding it in about 1.5 per cent of 2560 cases. The occurrence of measles during convalescence from diphtheria is liable to be followed by redevelopment of the diphtheritic process.

Recurrence.—Recurrence is frequently seen, and some persons even seem predisposed to repeated attacks. As compared with the total number of cases of diphtheria, however, recurrences are not very common, and are prone to be less severe than the first attack. There is a tendency to the acquisition of natural immunity as the person grows older (see p. 346).

Prognosis.—The death-rate from diphtheria has been declining in the United States in recent years. The statistics from the reports of Boards of Health of 78 cities[56] show that the death-rate per 100,000 in 1923 was 13.25 and in 1928, 9.25, and in 1930 in 93 cities[57] the reports give for most of them a death-rate per 100,000 averaging about 5. While the mortality was probably declining even before the introduction of antitoxin, it was certainly also influenced by this. For example, Park[58] shows that the death-rate in New York City had varied from 155 to 280 per 100,000; that in 1895, when free distribution of antitoxin began and it was widely used, the rate dropped more than 33 per cent and that in 1930 it was 2.8 per 100,000.

Yet the prognosis in individual cases is always uncertain, unfavorable symptoms or unexpected complications often developing in cases at first mild. The favorable influence of antitoxin is certainly very great, as is shown, in addition to the figures quoted from Park, by many reports, as those of Burrows,[40] Northrup,[59] Herringham,[60] Zahorsky,[61] Greengard[62] and others. The good effects of antitoxin-treatment have been especially marked in laryngeal cases (Biggs and Guerard;[63] Collective Investigation Committee, American Pediatric Society;[64] McCollum;[65] Siegert[66]), in which antitoxin has not only greatly diminished the necessity for operative treatment, but has also much lowered the mortality of cases requiring intubation. The *promptness* with which antitoxin is given is most important, since it is able to neutralize the toxin only before it has combined with the tissue-cells. In the first report of the American Pediatric Society,[67] the mortality in cases injected on the first day of the disease was 4.9 per cent; this increasing to 38.9 per cent when the first treatment was after the fourth day.

Various factors other than treatment influence the mortality. *Age* is prominent among these, the disease being much more fatal in infancy, largely on account of laryngeal involvement or the development of bronchopneumonia. In 49 cases we have seen in infants under one year of age, 14 died; most of the fatal cases being of the laryngeal type. New-born infants are especially liable to succumb. All studies show that the great majority of deaths are in subjects less than five years old. The *situation of the membrane* and the rapidity of its extension influence the prognosis. Primary nasal diphtheria is generally not dangerous unless it extends to the larynx. In diphtheria of the nasopharynx prognosis is unfavorable. Involvement of the larynx always increases the mortality greatly. In tracheobronchial diphtheria Welford[39] reported a mortality of 95.8 per cent in 24 patients treated with antitoxin and intubation, and Tolle[68] 57.6 per cent in 26 patients treated by antitoxin intravenously and suction of the larynx. The development of *septic symptoms* is unfavorable, as is also evidence of *cardiac weakness*. Very rapid pulse is an unfavorable prognostic indication, and so, too, is bradycardia, especially when combined with low blood-pressure. Yet even cases of heart-block may recover. *Hypoglycemia* (due to the damage of the suprarenals and the tissue-cells) is an indication of the seriousness of the disease (Cartagenova,[69] Lereboullet and Pierrot[70]). *Hemorrhagic conditions* are of very bad import, and the same is true of absence of polymorphonuclear leukocytosis.

Certain complications are serious, among them bronchopneumonia, severe nephritis, marked anemia, and suppurative adenitis. Postdiphtheritic paralysis usually recovers if the heart and respiratory muscles escape. Rolleston[71] and Ronaldson[72] claimed that the more marked the antitoxin reaction the better the prognosis, and that a pronounced serum-rash is a favorable sign. The combination of measles with diphtheria, or the development of one after the other, increases the gravity of the case. Scarlet fever occurring as a complication is unfavorable.

Diagnosis. Clinical.—Even without bacteriological examination the diagnosis of diphtheria is usually easy, except early in the disease or in atypical attacks. It rests, in general, upon the rapid development of pseudomembrane which is removed only with difficulty, and which leaves a bleeding surface beneath; the reforming of the membrane; its tendency to spread beyond the tonsils; constitutional depression out of proportion to local symptoms; decided glandular enlargement in the neck; and the frequent occurrence of paralysis as a sequel. The mode of onset and the temperature-curve are too variable to be of much diagnostic aid.

Mild attacks of diphtheria are most likely to be confounded with *follicular tonsillitis*, especially when the foci of secretion in the latter disease fuse and cover the tonsil. The onset of this condition is generally more sudden, the fever higher, the throat more painful, and there is no spreading beyond the tonsils. Bacteriological examination may be necessary to differentiate. Severe *streptococcic* and *pneumococcic inflammation of the tonsils* can sometimes be distinguished from diphtheria only by bacteriological study.

Primary nasal or nasopharyngeal diphtheria may be unrecognized, but should be suspected when there is irritating and blood-stained discharge. Vincent's infection may occur in the nose and give rise to bloody discharge.

Laryngeal diphtheria must be distinguished from other forms of stenosis. Laryngoscopic examination is helpful. Tolle[68] found that only 61.6 per cent of 344 patients with croup had diphtheritic involvement. In *false croup* there is usually, but not necessarily, relief from obstruction during the day. In *measles* there may be severe stenosis without diphtheritic involvement, but bacteriological examination must be made in these cases. The diphtheria bacillus is the only germ likely to cause an actual pseudomembrane in the larynx, and for this reason laryngoscopic examination is helpful in differential diagnosis. *Thrush, aphthae,* and *ulcerative stomatitis* offer little practical difficulty in diagnosis. *Vincent's angina* is more liable to involve the tongue, cheeks and gums; is necrotic rather than pseudomembranous in nature, and tends to produce a punched-out ulcer. *Foreign bodies* may lodge in the trachea when there is no knowledge of their inhalation and cause stenosis and suffocative attacks, which may simulate diphtheritic croup. The aid of bacteriological examination, roentgen-ray, and laryngoscope should be employed here.

Bacteriological.—In all suspicious cases, cultures should be taken as early as possible. The secretion is obtained by rubbing firmly the affected area, or the posterior portion of the pharynx when the larynx is involved, with a swab of sterilized cotton or a platinum wire loop, and transferring the material to the blood-serum culture-medium. The germs grow sometimes in six hours but better in twelve to twenty-four hours. The culture should not be made immediately after an antiseptic application. It cannot be depended upon in late cases, unless taken from a lower layer of the membrane, since the surface may fail to give a positive culture; nor is a single negative culture sufficient in suspicious cases. Sometimes the diphtheria bacilli can be recognized by immediate staining of smears from the affected areas.

Entire reliance cannot be placed upon the culture alone, and cases which are clinically diphtheritic should be treated as such, even though no specific germs are found. On the other hand, the mere presence of diphtheria bacilli in healthy or even in diseased throats does not constitute diphtheria. A test of the virulence of the germs is sometimes necessary, this being effected by injecting them into guinea-pigs. There may also be found at times the so-called "pseudodiphtheria bacillus," as described by Hofmann-Wellenhof.[73] The xerosis bacillus also possesses a resemblance to that of the diphtheria germ, and there are a number of other types of pseudodiphtheria organisms frequently present. The studies of Guthrie, Marshall and Moss,[74] in which experimental inoculations of human throats were performed, have done much to clear up the differentiation of true disease-producing diphtheria bacilli from the pseudodiphtheria organisms (diphtheroids). An expert bacteriologist can distinguish, even without the aid of the virulence test, many of these diphtheroids from the true Klebs-Löffler bacillus.

Treatment. PROPHYLAXIS. **Natural Immunity.**—It has been recognized for a long time that infants in the early months of life are less susceptible to diphtheria than after this period and during childhood, and that through later childhood there is a slowly increasing return of immunity.

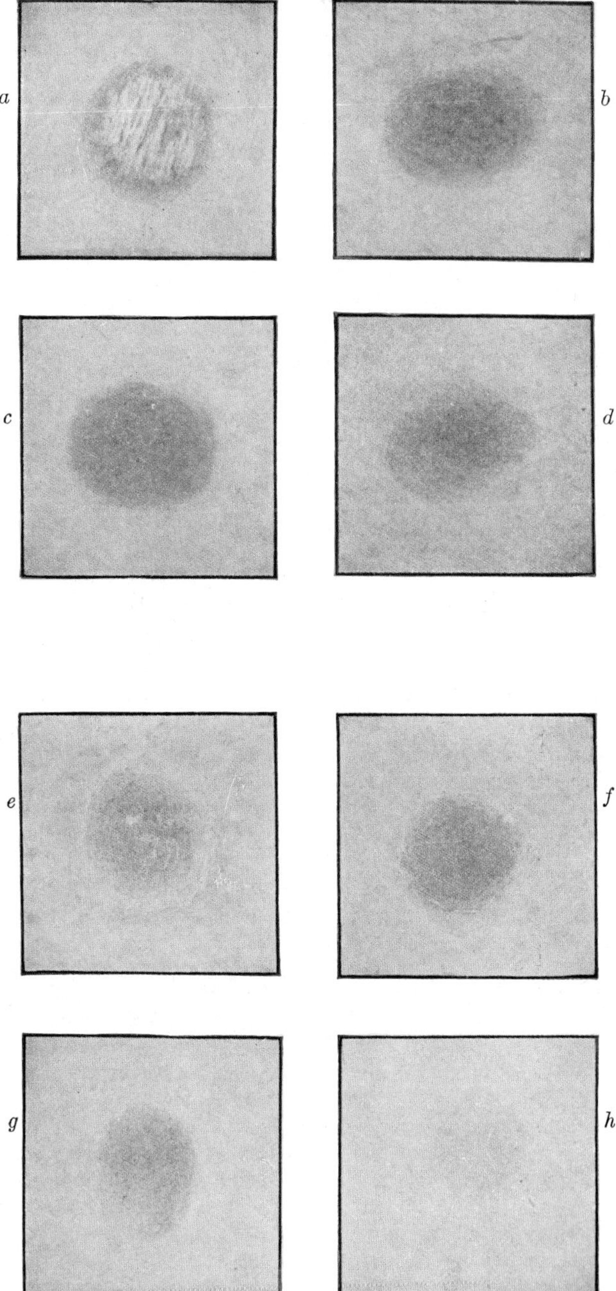

Fig. 74.—The SCHICK reaction in diphtheria. (*a*) to (*d*) Typical positive reactions forty-eight hours after test: (*a*) strongly positive reaction, with vesiculation of the surface layer of the epithelium, which is seen occasionally in individuals who have practically no antitoxin; (*b*) and (*c*) positive reactions; (*d*) a moderately positive reaction; (*e*) fading reaction one week after test; shows redness, scaling and beginning pigmentation; (*f*) after two weeks; (*g*) after three weeks; (*h*) faint pigmentation after four weeks. (*Zingher, Am. J. Dis. Child.* 1916; **11**; 269.)

The investigations of Schick[75] have established these facts on a scientific basis. He found that the intracutaneous injection of $\frac{1}{50}$ of a minimum dose of toxin lethal for a guinea pig, diluted with about 0.1 cc. of salt-solution, will produce in nonimmune persons a local reaction, while in those immune there is no reaction whatever. A positive reaction, demonstrating that the person has no antitoxin in the blood and is, therefore, susceptible, is indicated by a slightly red and edematous spot from 0.5 to 2 cm. (0.2 to 0.8 in.) in diameter, which appears within twenty-four to forty-eight hours (Fig. 74). This disappears within from seven to ten days, leaving a brownish pigmented area with superficial desquamation, the pigmentation persisting for some time. Pseudoreactions appear earlier, are less sharply defined, and disappear within twenty-four hours, leaving no pigmentation. A great many investigators have shown the value of this test. One must remember that it actually indicates only the presence of sufficient antitoxin to neutralize the small amount of toxin injected, and that a negative test consequently does not absolutely guarantee immunity. For example, Flood[6] found that about 45 per cent of a group of children who had a negative Schick test had only $\frac{1}{50}$ of a unit of antitoxin per cc. of blood;—not a large amount. Ordinarily, however, a negative test indicates that an exposed person does not need the passive protection given by antitoxin injection, nor the active immunity produced by injections of toxin-antitoxin or toxoid. We[77] have shown that the test can be used during other acute febrile disorders, since these do not seem to change the reactivity of the skin to diphtheria toxin. It is also interesting that at times a Schick-positive person seems able to carry virulent diphtheria bacilli in the throat without contracting the disease.

There have been several studies which demonstrate rather clearly that the incidence of diphtheria is less in tonsillectomized children. This is certainly because the tonsil tissue offers a favorable site for growth and not because tonsillectomy has any effect in increasing immunity. The latter explanation was the one given by Schick and Topper,[78] who found that 80 per cent of 100 children with positive Schick tests became Schick-negative six months following tonsillectomy. On the other hand, the studies of Geddie,[79] Orosz and Kugler[80] and Dudley[81] do not confirm this view. It does not seem necessary that there must be contact with diphtheria in order that immunity to the disease be secured. For example, in the examination of Eskimos it was found that a large number had negative Schick tests, although they apparently had never been exposed to diphtheria (Bay-Schmith,[82] Heinbecker and Irvine-Jones[83]). (See also p. 337.) Most infants, in cities at least, inherit immunity from their mothers. If the parents are Schick-positive, the new-born infants are also likely to be. Merlini[84] in 34 tests on mothers and their infants under four months of age, found that in all but one the infant reacted positively or negatively in a manner similar to its mother; while 31 infants from five to eight months old differed from their mothers 16 times. If one parent is positive and the other negative, and they belong to different blood-groups, it is probable that the child's reaction will be similar to that of the parent to whose blood-group he belongs (Hirzfeld[85]). Kuttner and Ratner[86] question the reliability of the Schick test in the new-born, and suggest performing it on the mother.

A comparison of statistics from a large number of sources shows that a positive reaction, *i. e.*, an absence of immunity, is present in the new-born in about 7 per cent; in the first year in 34 to 45 per cent; from one to two years in 55 to 60 per cent; from two to five years in about 66 per cent; from six to eight years in 35 to 45 per cent; and from eight to fifteen years in 25 to 30 per cent.

Immunization.—Protection of anyone who has been in contact with a case of diphtheria may be accomplished by the injection of 500 to 1000 units of antitoxin. Passive immunization is afforded in this way, which lasts for about ten days and certainly not longer than four weeks. Protection of this sort is not always necessary. (See also Quarantine, p. 349.)

To produce a more lasting, active immunity, von Behring[87] urged repeated subcutaneous injections of a mixture of toxin and antitoxin, as first suggested for use in children by Theobald Smith[88] in 1909. This preparation contains antitoxin in amounts which over-neutralize the toxin, and after injection there occurs a dissociation of the two and the liberation of toxin, which then stimulates the production of immune bodies. It has also been advised that vaccine of diphtheria bacilli should be combined with toxin-antitoxin in order to bring about bactericidal as well as antitoxin immunity. This possesses little practical value, since antitoxin immunity in diphtheria is the important factor. As shown by many studies, 85 per cent or more of susceptible children will produce sufficient antitoxin, after three hypodermic injections of toxin-antitoxin spaced five days to two weeks apart, to develop a negative Schick test within from three to six months. Very decided, if not absolute, protection against diphtheria will result, which will last, in at least 90 per cent of the children, for more than six years and probably for life. Infants under six months of age should not be injected, both because of the high percentage of natural immunity, and because also of the possibility of severe reaction. After this age, too, when they have lost their inherited immunity, they respond better to active immunizing measures (Blum[89]). Since, as previously mentioned (p. 347), a negative Schick test may occur with a rather small amount of antitoxin in the blood, it would be well to immunize all children aged from six months to two years, and again at the beginning of school-age. In any event the Schick test should be performed from three to six months after the injections have been given, and these repeated if the test is positive. After toxin-antitoxin injection there is probably a so-called "inactive phase" in which there is increased susceptibility to diphtheria. This occurs, too, and perhaps earlier, with toxoid injections (p. 349), and should lead to caution in immunization during epidemics. Patients suffering from other diseases and particularly scarlet fever seem to be difficult to immunize.

The question arises as to the possibility of producing sensitization to horse-serum by injections of toxin-antitoxin. Many have denied that this can occur to the extent of making subsequent administration of horse-serum dangerous. It is pointed out that the probability of acquiring sensitization in the human bears a relation to the quantity of serum injected, and that the amount of horse-serum in toxin-antitoxin is exceedingly small. For example, Zingher[90] observed no instances of anaphylactic shock during a second series of toxin-antitoxin injections. On the other hand, Gordon and Creswell[91] found that 74.1 per cent of persons who had received injections of toxin-antitoxin had a serum-reaction following a subsequent injection containing horse-serum, as opposed to 18 per cent of reactions in those who were being injected for the first time. Cases of sensitization are recorded by Stewart,[92] Gatewood and Baldridge,[93] Lathrop[94] and others; and Waldbott[95] reported the return of asthma in 6 asthmatic children injected with toxin-antitoxin. Our[96] own experience is that the incidence of serum-sickness is decidedly greater in those patients who had previously received toxin-antitoxin mixtures.

Toxin-antitoxin is an unstable product and may become toxic if frozen, probably due to dissociation and to lessening of the antitoxic strength. In some instances of abscess-formation following the injections it was found that the material had been contaminated with staphylococci. Because of the possibility of causing sensitization, and especially for use with allergic patients, attempts have been made to devise preparations free from horse-serum. There can be recommended a sheep-serum toxin-antitoxin which is available on the market. Larson and Eder[97] recommended 2 per cent sodium ricinoleate to detoxify the toxin, but this preparation is little used, since the reactions following it seemed to be marked. Toxoid (anatoxin) is widely employed at the present time. This was recommended by Ramon,[98] and is a serum-free preparation detoxified by the addition of 4 per cent formaldehyde. It is given by subcutaneous injection, the first dose of 0.5 cc. being followed in three weeks by a second dose of 1.0 cc. and a third dose of 1 to 1.5 cc. two weeks later. Often two injections of 1 cc. each are sufficient to produce a negative Schick test. Ramon and Helie[99] claim that within six weeks to two months after toxoid injections 96 to 100 per cent of negative Schick reactions are obtained, with lasting immunity. The concensus of opinion supports this, as also the fact that toxoid is more efficient and quicker in inducing immunity than toxin-antitoxin, although all workers do not obtain so high a percentage of negative tests as that of Ramon and Helie.

Lowenstein[100] recommends the percutaneous administration of toxoid combined with diphtheria bacilli contained in an ointment. Three applications are made, well rubbed into the skin at weekly intervals; the surface not being washed for twenty-four hours afterwards. It is claimed that about 70 per cent of patients became Schick-negative in a few months (Abt and Feingold[101]). Others have obtained smaller percentages; Kagel and Gasul[102] 53.3 per cent in six weeks, and Nobel[103] only 35 per cent in three months. It seems generally considered that immunity is not as well afforded by this ointment as by toxoid given in the ordinary way. Among other immunizing preparations may be mentioned toxin-antitoxin floccules, viz., the precipitate produced when antitoxin, or toxoid, is mixed with toxin. Injection of these floccules has been used with good results by Swyer.[104] Combined immunization against diphtheria and scarlet fever has been attempted by Nureddin[105] who secured 81 per cent negative Schick and Dick tests after six weeks. Zoeller and Ramon[106] used instillation or insufflation of toxoid into the nose and secured immunity.

With toxin-antitoxin, and less so with toxoid, there may be a certain amount of local and general reaction, with fever and body-pains, following the injections. This is less likely to occur in children than in adults. With active tuberculosis present, immunization had better not be attempted.

There seems to be a definite effect of active immunizing procedures on morbidity, and on mortality as well. An extensive community campaign in Detroit was apparently the sole factor in dropping the incidence to $\frac{1}{4}$ that of former years (Geib and Vaughan[107]). Only 2 of 198 persons who died from diphtheria in New York City in 1930 had been actively immunized against diphtheria (Blum[89]), and only 46 of 2391 reported by Challier and Rougier.[108]

Quarantine.—Suspicious cases should be isolated until a bacteriological study has been made. The other children in the family should, if possible, be removed from the house; and not allowed in contact with others until their cultures have been reported. After the diagnosis has been made the same precautions should be followed with other members of the family who continue in close contact with the patient. The Schick test may be used to determine the presence of immunity in those who have been exposed. With these precautions carefully followed the necessity of passive immunization with antitoxin becomes greatly reduced. If, however, exposed children in the family give positive Schick reactions the administration of antitoxin would seem advisable, unless there is some contraindication. Isolation of the patient should continue during convalescence until there have been at least 2 consecutive negative cultures. If cultures cannot be made, quarantine should continue for at least three weeks after all clinical evidence of diphtheria has ceased to exist. In about 80 per cent of cases the bacilli will disappear from the throat in one week, and in 90 per cent in two weeks, after the pseudomembrane has left the throat. Other details of quarantine and disinfection are those appropriate to infectious diseases in general (p. 250).

Management and Treatment of Carriers.—During epidemics in institutions, cultures should be made from the entire personnel, and the Schick test employed to determine the presence or absence of immunity. In those who are not immune and have positive cultures antitoxin had better be given, unless contraindications exist. If, however, the person with a positive culture has no clinical symptoms the culture may be repeated two or three times, and, if it is still positive, a virulence test performed. If this is negative it can be considered that he is not a source of contagion. In nonimmunes with negative cultures these should be repeated two or three times and close observation kept, especially when antitoxin has not been administered. Many measures have been recommended to rid the nose and throat of diphtheria bacilli in the case of carriers. Among them may be mentioned flushing with a 1:10,000 solution of bichloride of mercury or saturated solution of boric acid; local applications of 0.5 to 2.0 per cent mercurochrome (Gray and Meyer[109]); spraying with 2 per cent aqueous solution of gential violet (Saurman[110]); application of iodine and glycerin (Kellogg[111]); application of a solution of nitrate of silver (60 grains: 1 fl. oz.) (4:30) (Hand[112]); spraying with a bouillon-culture of staphylococcus pyogenes aureus (Schiøtz[113]) application of cultures of lactic acid bacilli (Nicholson and Hogan[114]); local treatment with the roentgen-ray (Kahn,[115] Withers, Ransom and Humphry[116]); treatment with the ultraviolet rays (Nagataki[117]). Vaccine treatment with killed diphtheria-bacilli has also been recommended, but the results as reported by Park[58] and Zingher[90] have been disappointing. In many cases of obstinate persistence of virulent bacilli in the throat, often the best means of treatment is the removal of tonsils and adenoids and the correction of any intranasal defects. This, according to the reports of Weaver[118] and others, is often followed by prompt disappearance of the organisms. Personally we have had better success with this treatment than with any other.

TREATMENT OF THE ATTACK. **General and Hygienic.**—The selection and the care of the sick-room have been described. (See p. 250.) Rest in bed, recumbent, is necessary even in a mild attack. The diet should be liquid. Difficulty in swallowing and anorexia may become problems only solved by feeding through a stomach-tube or nasal-tube. Topical applications should not be made if they are exhausting. Very high fever requires hydrotherapy, with due regard to the complete avoidance of exertion and excitement.

Supporting and stimulating treatment may be necessary. Alcohol is, in our opinion, of undoubted benefit if properly used, and may be given in relatively large amounts. In laryngeal stenosis, morphine or its derivatives modify the cough and dyspnea and produce much needed rest. Camphor, caffeine, strychnine and adrenaline are frequently required to combat circulatory disturbances. In partial heart-block, digitalis is contraindicated but it may be employed in complete block. If digitalis cannot be given absolute rest and morphine are the only helpful measures.

Antitoxin-treatment.—This was first brought prominently before the medical profession by von Behring and Wernicke.[119] It consists in the injection of the serum of an animal—usually the horse—which has received repeated injections of diphtheria toxin in increasing doses, and which, as a result, has developed in its blood strong antitoxic properties. The antitoxin neutralizes the toxin already in the patient's blood, checks the growth of the membrane, and prevents the formation of more toxin by inhibiting further development of the bacilli. The strength of the antitoxin is measured by units, each one of which is the amount of the preparation sufficient to neutralize the effect of 100 times the dose of diphtheria toxin that would kill in four days a guinea-pig weighing 250 Gm. (8.82 oz.).

Method of Employment.—Antitoxin is usually supplied in a syringe and with hypodermic needles already sterilized accompanying this. A region is chosen which is not pressed upon in lying, such as the flank or the anterior surface of the thigh. The skin should be cleansed with diluted alcohol or painted with tincture of iodine. The air should be expelled before the needle is thrust under the skin. Intramuscular injection is better than subcutaneous, since in the former there is more rapid absorption and less local pain. Local anesthesia is not necessary. In severe cases, or those seen late, antitoxin should be given intravenously.

Dosage.—In average cases of diphtheria over two years of age, from 5000 to 10,000 units or more should be given. If no improvement follows, this may be repeated within six to twelve hours, and the treatment continued, perhaps in larger doses. Yet if the antitoxin was in sufficient amount in the initial dose, it should remain in the blood and be able to neutralize any further production of toxin; and it is, therefore, questionable whether later doses are needed or have any effect. In severe cases, and especially in laryngeal involvement, 10,000 to 20,000 units or more should be given, often best intravenously. In patients who might be sensitive to horse-serum, or have other evidence of allergic manifestations; in persons who have received previous injections of therapeutic sera; and, perhaps, in all instances if time permits, a preliminary skin-test with the antitoxin or with horse-serum should be made to determine sensitivity. If this is positive, desensitization should be attempted. (See Allergy, p. 484.) In sensitive patients the intravenous route should be used cautiously. If the patient has had antitoxin within six days and without reaction, the danger of reaction from reinjection is slight. Reactions with concentrated serum are less than with unconcentrated, since in the former there is less horse-serum. Serum reaction occurs in 10 per cent or more of antitoxin-treated patients, and oftenest from the fifth to the ninth day. (For symptoms, prevention and treatment of serum-sickness, see Allergy, pp. 485; 488.) Platou[120] recommends the intraperitoneal route for giving antitoxin, as it is thus very rapidly absorbed.

Time of Administration.—The earlier in the disease the antitoxin is administered, the more certain and powerful is its action (see Prognosis, p. 344), and the smaller the amount required to be effective. When given after the third day much less good can be expected, but no case should be considered to have lasted too long to administer the treatment.

Results of Antitoxin Treatment.—Favorable results follow the injection within twelve to twenty-four hours. They consist in a softening and a separation of the pseudomembrane at its edges, diminution of the glandular swelling and of nasal discharge, and an improvement in the general condition. In many cases the throat is clear in three or four days or often earlier. Complications of diphtheria depending on the damage already done by the toxin, or upon septic conditions, are in no way benefited by antitoxin. In the latter conditions and in malignant cases good results have seemed to follow the giving of antistreptococcus serum in addition to the diphtheria-antitoxin (Finkelstein and Konigsberger[121]). As noted under prognosis (p. 345), the good effects of antitoxin are also evident in the reduction of the number of tracheotomies and intubations formerly necessary.

From time to time doubts have been expressed as to the value of antitoxin. It has been claimed that it is not greater than that of simple horse-serum; but this view has not found general acceptance. (For reviews see Calhoun,[122] Ratnoff,[123] and Feer.[124]) Hamburger and Siegl[125] report 20 patients who recovered without antitoxin-treatment, a number of whom had positive Schick tests after recovery. Hentschel[126] reported good results from the use of diphtheria-convalescent's serum, although the pseudomembrane did not disintegrate so readily as with antitoxin.

Local Treatment.—The chief object of this is that of cleansing, but it may also retard the growth of the bacilli, remove them, or check their dissemination. Douching of the nose with warm alkaline antiseptic solutions, normal salt-solution, or a 1 to 2 per cent solution of boric acid may be employed. The injection is preferably given with a fountain syringe or a soft-rubber nasal syringe; the child lying on one side and the fluid, if used in the nose, entering the upper nostril and flowing from the other. Spraying or swabbing of the throat with a diluted peroxide of hydrogen solution is often efficacious. Application of a strong solution of silver nitrate, tincture of chloride of iron and the like is often beneficial, but also often painful. A 1 to 2 per cent solution of mercurochrome is often used. Any local applications which are painful or exhausting to the patient must not be employed. An ice-bag applied externally over the position of the tonsils, and small pieces of ice in the mouth, tend to relieve the pain and difficulty in swallowing.

In laryngeal stenosis a croup tent (p. 188) and inhalations of oxygen are often of great benefit. Local applications of antitoxin seem to be of no value, and this is in accord with the fact that diphtheria bacilli grow without difficulty in antitoxin.

Operative Treatment.—When cyanosis and dyspnea are clearly increasing in laryngeal cases, operative measures are indicated, and they should not be unduly delayed. These consist respectively in tracheotomy and intubation. The latter has largely supplanted the former. Tracheotomy, however, may quickly become necessary after intubation, if no relief is obtained.

The technique of *tracheotomy* need not be described here. Its after-treatment consists principally in keeping the tube clean of mucus and pseudomembrane, and in maintaining the air warm and saturated with moisture.

Intubation.—This was first successfully employed by O'Dwyer.[127] Its technique is difficult to describe and skill in it can be acquired only by practice. For details special publications containing discussions of the subject may be consulted.

A method of performing intubation practically under control of sight is described by Pushkin.[128] Gover and Hardman,[129] Lynah[130] and Tolle[68] recommend that under direct laryngoscopy suction be applied through a metal tube or silk elastic catheter to remove the membrane. One such treatment may be sufficient, or several may be necessary. By this method only about 20 per cent of patients with laryngeal diphtheria require intubation and the mortality is greatly reduced, whereas without this treatment, about 40 per cent of the cases must be intubated (Tolle). If the bronchial tree is involved, intubation and tracheotomy may give little relief. In such cases bronchoscopy with aspiration and removal of the membrane, as recommended by Lynah and others, may be helpful.

Treatment of Complications and Sequels and of the Convalescence.—The exhaustion and *cardiac weakness* following severe cases of diphtheria require especial attention. Rest in bed in the recumbent position must continue so long as there are any evidences of decided weakness of the heart, as shown by rapidity, irregularity, or slowness of the pulse, or weak heart-sounds. Excitement and physical exertion of all sorts must be carefully avoided. Even after mild attacks the patient should be kept in bed for at least a week after the membrane has disappeared, and only cautiously allowed to sit upright, in spite of the fact that the heart may appear to be entirely normal. General tonic treatment is indicated, especially with alcohol, strychnine, and sometimes digitalis. Adrenaline chloride (1:1000) has been given to prevent cardiac failure, the dose being 5 to 10 minim (0.31 to 0.616) according to age. It is further indicated because there may be a low blood-sugar due to damage of the suprarenal glands and depletion of the glycogen store of the liver. Kostyal[131] has advised the use of dextrose and insulin. Pituitrin has also been employed with success.

Other complications or sequels, such as *anemia* and *nephritis,* require appropriate medication.

The treatment of *postdiphtheritic paralysis* depends to some extent upon the part affected. Paralysis of the extremities may be aided by massage and electricity; that of the muscles of deglutition may require gavage. For any form of paralysis the free use of strychnine is to be recommended. When paralysis has developed, relief by antitoxin treatment cannot reasonably be expected, since, as previously stated, the toxin has already combined with and damaged the cells. Antitoxin-treatment unless given early and in large doses does not appear to diminish the number of cases of paralysis, and, according to Kleinschmidt[132] and others, there seems to be no relationship between the development of paralysis and the presence of antitoxin in the blood. Nevertheless, antitoxin-treatment may be tried, since it has been claimed by many, among them Heubner[133] and Labbe,[134] that it does good. In paralysis of the respiratory muscles artificial respiration or the use of respiration chambers may be advised. Marriott[135] reported recovery in a child who was kept alive for five days by artificial respiration in a Gesell-Erlanger apparatus.

References

1. De causis et signis acut. morb. L. 1, Cap. 9.; Ref. Baginsky in Nothnagel's Handbk. d. spec. Path. u. Therap., Diphtheria, 3. 2. Pract. hist. of a new erupt. miliarial fever with angina ulcusculosa, Boston, 1736; Ref. Baginsky Ref. No. 1, 6. 3. Transac. Am. Philosoph. Soc. 1779, **1,** 338. 4. Des inflam. spéc. du tissu muqueux etc. Paris, 1826; Ref. Baginsky Ref. No. 1, 2. 5. Am. J. Hyg., 1929, **10,** 13. 6. Monatschr. f. Kinderh., 1923, **26,** 266. 7. Am. J. Dis. Child., 1923, **25,** 392. 8. Am. J. Dis. Child., 1916, **12,** 47. 9. Nothnagel's Handbk. d. spec. Path. u. Therap., Diphtheria, 52. 10. Am. J. Dis. Child., 1927, **34,** 258. 11. 20th Cent. Pract. Med., **17,** 77, Diphtheria. 12. Phila. M. J., 1898, **1,** 423. 13. New York M. J., 1907, **86,** 1123. 14. Zentralbl. f. Gynäk., 1919, **43,** 996. 15. Ztschr. f. Kinderh., 1920, **28,** 51. 16. Bull. acad. d. méd., Paris, 1921, **86,** 191. 17. Arch. de méd. d. enf., 1921, **24,** 437. 18. Zentralbl. f. Gynäk., 1926, **50,** 3255. 19. Verhandl. d. Cong. f. inn. Med., 1883, **2,** 139. 20. Verhandl. d. Cong. f. inn. Med., 1884, **3,** 156. 21. Bact. and Path. of Diphth., 1901, 16. 22. Ztschr. f. Hyg., 1910, **67,** 349. 23. South. M. J., 1923, **16,** 514. 24. Ztschr. f. Bact., 1915, **75,** 273. 25. J. Hyg., 1920, **18,** 448. 26. Am. J. M. Sc., 1920, **160,** 589. 27. J. Mass. Assoc. Boards of Health, 1902, July. 28. J. Infect. Dis., 1907, **4,** 36. 29. Research Lab. Dept. of Health, N. Y. City, 1905, **1,** 88; J. Infect. Dis., 1907, **4,** 337. 30. Centralbl. f. Bakt. u. Parasit., Orig., 1912–13, **67,** 423. 31. Am. J. Hyg., 1923, **3,** 604; J. Prev. Med., 1928, **2,** 191. 32. Monatschr. f. Kinderh., 1927, **35,** 318. 33. Arch. f. Kinderh., 1929, **86,** 185. 34. J.A.M.A., 1919, **73,** 1925. 35. Arch. Pediat., 1921, **38,** 515. 36. Riv. di clin. pediat., 1930, **28,** 745. 37. Rep. Metrop. Asyl. Board, 1906. 38. Brit. J. Child. Dis., 1917, **14,** 21. 39. Am. J. Dis. Child., 1929, **37,** 944. 40. Am. J. M. Sc., 1901, **121,** 125. 41. Ann. Surg., 1915, **62,** 343. 42. Am. J. Dis. Child., 1925, **29,** 433. 43. Arch. Int. Med., 1928, **42,** 23. 44. Am. J. Dis. Child., 1931, **42,** 811. 45. Am. J. Dis. Child., 1920, **20,** 89. 46. J.A.M.A., 1928, **90,** 441. 47. Lancet, 1931, **1,** 1387. 48. Boston M. and S. J., 1904, **151,** 433. 49. Arch. Pediat., 1923, **40,** 306. 50. Arch. Pediat., 1913, **30,** 335. 51. Clin. J., 1913, **42,** 12. 52. Med. Rec., 1918, **94,** 620. 53. Brit. J. Child. Dis., 1916, **13,** 237. 54. South. M. J., 1923, **16,** 602. 55. Brit. J. Child. Dis., 1907, **4,** 332. 56. J.A.M.A., 1929, **92,** 1759. 57. J.A.M.A., 1931, **96,** 1768. 58. Am. J. Dis. Child., 1931, **42,** 1439. 59. Nothnagel's Encyclop., Am. Ed., Diphtheria, 143. 60. Allbutt and Rolleston's Syst. Med., **1,** 1030. 61. Med. News, 1903, **83,** 1085. 62. Arch. Pediat., 1929, **46,** 441. 63. Med. News, 1896, **69,** 677. 64. Tr. Am. Ped. Soc., 1897, **9,** 32. 65. Proc.

Phila. Co. Med. Soc., 1905, **26,** 80. 66. Jahrb. f. Kinderh., 1900, **52,** 56. 67. Tr. Am. Ped. Soc., 1896, **8,** 21. 68. Am. J. Dis. Child., 1930, **39,** 954. 69. Riv. di clin. pediat., 1927, **25,** 733. 70. Arch. de méd. d. enf., 1928, **31,** 148. 71. Practitioner, 1905, **74,** 660. 72. Brit. J. Child. Dis., 1923, **20,** 129. 73. Wien. med. Wchnschr., 1888, **38,** 60. 74. Bull. Johns Hopkins Hosp., 1921, **32,** 369. 75. München. med. Wchnschr., 1913, **60,** 2608. 76. Am. J. Dis. Child., 1930, **39,** 109. 77. Eddy and Mitchell, Am. J. Dis. Child., 1930, **40,** 985. 78. Am. J. Dis. Child., 1929, **38,** 929. 79. Am. J. Dis. Child., 1930, **40,** 1032. 80. Arch. f. Kinderh., 1931, **94,** 168. 81. Lancet, 1931, **2,** 1398. 82. Klin. Wchnschr., 1929, **8,** 974. 83. J. Immunol., 1928, **15,** 395. 84. Riv. di clin. pediat., 1930, **28,** 789. 85. Ergebn. der Hyg., 1926, **8,** 367. 86. Am. J. Dis. Child., 1923, **25,** 413. 87. Deutsche med. Wchnschr., 1913, **39,** 873. 88. J. Exper. Med., 1909, **11,** 241. 89. J.A.M.A., 1932, **98,** 1627. 90. New York State J. Med., 1923, **23,** 6. 91. J. Prev. Med., 1929, **3,** 21. 92. J.A.M.A., 1926, **86,** 112. 93. J.A.M.A., 1927, **88,** 1068. 94. J.A.M.A., 1927, **89,** 1602. 95. J.A.M.A., 1929, **90,** 290. 96. Veldee, Stevenson and Mitchell, Pub. Health Rep., 1931, **46,** 3023. 97. J.A.M.A., 1926, **86,** 998. 98. Ann. de l'inst., Pasteur, 1928, **42,** 959. 99. Am. J. Dis. Child., 1930, **39,** 685. 100. Wien. klin. Wchnschr., 1929, **42,** 193. 101. Am. J. Dis. Child., 1931, **41,** 8. 102. Am. J. Dis. Child., 1931, **41,** 45. 103. Wien. klin. Wchnschr., 1930, **44,** 75. 104. Lancet, 1931, **1,** 632. 105. Compt. rend. Soc. de biol., 1930, **103,** 1200. 106. Bull. acad. de méd. d. hôp. Paris, 1927, **97,** 849. 107. J.A.M.A., 1931, **97,** 336. 108. J. de méd. de Lyon, 1932, **13,** 1. 109. J. Infect. Dis., 1921, **28,** 323. 110. J.A.M.A., 1924, **83,** 249. 111. Calif. State J. Med., 1915, **13,** 150. 112. Phila. M. J., 1898, **2,** 432. 113. Ugesk. f. Laeger. vidensk, 1909, **71,** No. 49; Ref. J.A.M.A., 1910, **54,** 422. 114. J.A.M.A., 1914, **62,** 510. 115. Am. J. Roentgenol., 1924, **12,** 343. 116. J.A.M.A., 1926, **87,** 1266. 117. J. Pediat., Tokyo, 1931, March 20, No. 370, 425; Ref. Am. J. Dis. Child. 1931, **42,** 1470. 118. J.A.M.A., 1921, **76,** 831. 119. Ztschr. f. Hyg., 1892, **12,** 10. 120. Arch. Pediat., 1923, **40,** 575. 121. Deutsche med. Wchnschr., 1928, **54,** 790. 122. Am. J. Dis. Child., 1921, **21,** 107. 123. Berl. klin. Wchnschr., 1923, **2,** 440. 124. München. med. Wchnschr., 1919, **66,** 343. 125. München. med. Wchnschr., 1929, **76,** 1537. 126. Monatschr. f. Kinderh., 1930, **48,** 50. 127. New York M. J., 1885, **42,** 145. 128. Am. J. Dis. Child., 1930, **40,** 776. 129. Arch. Pediat., 1923, **40,** 170. 130. Laryngoscope, 1916, **26,** 158. 131. J.A.M.A., 1931, **96,** 1329. 132. Jahrb. f. Kinderh., 1917, **85,** 261. 133. München. med. Wchnschr., 1916, **63,** 128. 134. Arch. de méd. des enf., 1921, **24,** 612. 135. J.A.M.A., 1920, **75,** 668.

CHAPTER XV

INFLUENZA

(Grippe)

INFLUENZA, or grippe, has had applied to it a variety of titles. It was described clearly in the twelfth century, and its epidemic, infectious nature recognized since the sixteenth century. This epidemic character is perhaps more marked than in any other affection. It first appeared in the United States in 1627. After an interval of many years the disease reappeared in the great epidemic of 1889, arising in Turkestan and rapidly extending over many parts of the world, including the United States. In 1890 and 1891 there was another outbreak, especially in the United States and England. The malady then became endemic to a limited extent, with exacerbations, until the very severe outbreak of 1918, in which millions of persons in different countries were attacked. Philadelphia suffered especially among the cities of the United States, with about 150,000 cases in the course of two and one-half months, and in this and the succeeding year 1,000,000 cases are said to have been reported in Pennsylvania alone.

The etiologic identity of the early outbreaks with the more recent ones cannot be determined with accuracy, but from a clinical point of view no sharp distinction can be drawn. Similarly there can be no certainty of the relation of sporadic influenza, or grippe, and of the epidemic form until there is more known of the etiologic agent. From a bacteriological standpoint a distinction may be made between those cases seemingly clearly dependent upon the influenza-bacillus (influenza vera), and others, clinically similar, which are apparently due to other germs (influenza nostras). At the present time it seems best, however, to apply the term influenza or grippe to all of them, but excluding from the category cases with the symptoms merely of a severe febrile cold. The subject of grippe in early life has been reviewed by Risel[1] and Moffett.[2] Other excellent reviews are those by Jordan,[3] by Opie, Blake, Small and Rivers[4] on etiology, and by Zinsser.[5]

Etiology. Predisposing Causes.—Climate, race, locality and sex exert no influence. Although it is usually maintained that social conditions are without effect, Sydenstricker[6] found that in epidemics persons of the lower economic level were more frequently attacked. Apparently, while the previous state of health is not a factor, such conditions as bad weather, exposure, insufficient ventilation, and the like increase the susceptibility by predisposing to affections of the respiratory tract.

No period of life is immune. That between five and nine years has a high incidence during epidemics. Even the new-born may suffer from the disease (Strassman,[7] Cannata[8]). It has occurred apparently congenitally, as in a case described by Abt,[9] and as we have seen in new-born infants of mothers suffering from it during the last few weeks of pregnancy. Under such conditions, however, premature labor is often brought about, or miscarriage if the attack is earlier in pregnancy. The *individual susceptibility* is extreme. In some epidemics, such as that of 1918, children were less severely and less frequently attacked than adults.

The relationship of influenza to epidemic encephalitis is discussed elsewhere. (See p. 398.)

Exciting Cause.—There is much evidence to support the etiologic connection of the Pfeiffer[10] bacillus, or influenza bacillus. It is found in the sputum and the nasal secretion. It generally disappears early in the disease or certainly with the return of health, although it may be discovered in the discharges from complicating lesions for months. It is less often present in the blood. At necropsy it may be found in the lungs; Wollstein and Goldbloom,[11] for example, having recovered it in all of 18 infants, although never in pure culture. Suggestive, too, are certain inoculation experiments on monkeys by Blake and Cecil,[12] on rabbits by Walker,[13] and on man by Davis.[14] The fact that many workers have found the influenza bacillus in normal throats or in other respiratory conditions and other diseases, such as measles and pertussis, does not necessarily militate against its causative action in influenza; the situation being somewhat analogous to that of the relation of the pneumococcus to pneumonia in this respect.

Many other organisms have been found in influenza, in the absence of, or in association with, the influenza-bacillus. Among these are the micrococcus catarrhalis, staphylococcus, pneumococcus, and especially the streptococcus (both hemolytic and green-producing strains). Sometimes these are recovered in almost pure culture, and the green-producing streptococcus has been studied particularly by Tunnicliff,[15] Rosenow,[16] Cooper,[17] and Traut and Harrold.[18] While it is hard to deny that these various germs are causative in some epidemics which clinically resemble influenza, it may be that they are secondary invaders, and certainly they may be productive of complications. Olitsky[19] and his coworkers have found a minute, anaerobic, filterable body (Bacterium pneumosintes) which they suggest might be the cause of influenza or, at least, that it prepares the field for secondary invaders.

Gibson and Connor,[20] Nicolle and Lebailly,[21] Long and his coworkers,[22] and others have performed inoculation experiments on animals and man with filtrates of nasal washings, and in some cases apparently obtained positive results.

There is sufficient resemblance between the cases occurring in different epidemics and in certain interepidemic cases to suggest a common cause for all of them. Any difference may be due to variation in virulence of the causative agent, or to different secondary invading organisms. It would seem that most of the evidence favors the influenza bacillus as the initiating agent, although this remains to be proved.

The disease is very contagious, and probably especially so during the first few days. Transmission is generally direct, and the germs are received by the respiratory tract. Indirect transmission is of doubtful occurrence, although it is possible that there may be healthy carriers. Dissemination to any distance by the air is also questionable.

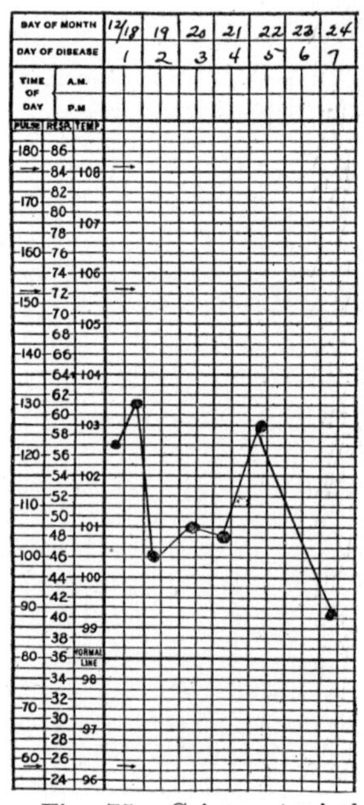

Fig. 75.—Grippe, typical form. Anna S., aged ten months. Cough, running eyes, fever, debility, frequent loose stools, vomited once. Slight preponderance of gastro-intestinal symptoms. Epidemic prevailing.

Pathologic Anatomy.—Apart from a catarrhal condition of the respiratory and alimentary mucous membranes, the lesions are those of the complications. Bronchopneumonia is frequent in many epidemics, and there may be capillary hemorrhages in practically all the viscera. Nasal sinusitis is common. Bakwin[23] described a peculiar degeneration of the rectus abdominis muscle as a frequent finding.

Symptoms.—The clinical manifestations are most varied, differing largely in epidemics.

Typical Form.—The *incubation* lasts from one to three days and is generally without symptoms. The *onset* is sudden with chilliness, fever, and sometimes convulsions. In older children pain in the limbs, trunk, and head may be complained of; in younger ones there is clearly discomfort, the nature of which cannot be determined. The temperature runs an irregular course (Fig. 75) and falls by lysis or crisis in three or four days. The respiration and pulse are accelerated in proportion to the temperature. Vomiting sometimes occurs; diarrhea may develop; anorexia is marked. Prostration, out of proportion to the other symptoms, is a most characteristic symptom. A varying degree of inflammation of the nose and throat, and less of the trachea and bronchi, is present, yet not sufficient to account for the general symptoms. The spleen is not infrequently palpable. Febrile albuminuria is not often found. The leukocyte picture, studied by Bunting[24] and others, shows an early polymorphonuclear leukocytosis, which is followed by a leukopenia with the lymphocytes relatively increased. Leukocytosis develops again if there are secondary infections. In some epidemics and sporadic cases leukopenia is marked and constant, while in others there may be a leukocytosis. The platelets are said to be reduced and the clotting time delayed (Kinsella and Broun[25]). The *duration* of the attack may be only a few days, but debility, anorexia and often neuralgic pain remain for several weeks. The symptoms in early life are generally not as severe as in adults, but to this there are many exceptions.

The ordinary type may be either *mild* or *severe*. In the latter the symptoms and particularly the prostration may be decided, the course prolonged, and convalescence tedious. In this connection it may be noted that certain strains of the influenza bacillus produce toxins lethal for animals, and these may account for some of the toxic symptoms in man (Zinsser[26]).

The different variants from typical influenza depend upon the predominance of symptoms of a certain class. Although there are numerous exceptions, as a rule the nervous and intestinal forms are most frequent in infancy and early childhood and the respiratory in later childhood. In epidemics certain types may predominate, but we have seen different variants in the same household.

Catarrhal or Respiratory Form.—In this form coryza is decided, the pharynx is red, the tonsils swollen with the follicles sometimes engorged; stomatitis may occur; there is annoying cough dependent upon involvement of the larynx, trachea and bronchi; and fever and prostration are present to a degree in no way explained by the local manifestations. The severity of the attack generally diminishes in three or four days, but in severe cases the course is longer and the process readily and rapidly advances to the production of bronchopneumonia, which is much more severe, extensive and fatal than in any other group of cases of this disease. Pulmonary edema and marked cyanosis are prominent features of the toxic cases. There is also a special tendency to the development of otitis and of cervical adenitis. There may be a *laryngeal form* with symptoms of croup. Regan and Regan,[27] Coray,[28] Widowitz,[29] Korsak,[30] and others discuss a severe type of influenzal croup in which intubation may be necessary.

Nervous Form.—In this variety the nervous manifestations predominate, and respiratory symptoms may even be entirely absent. To this class belong a large number of cases in quite early life. In some instances hyperpyrexia, delirium, stupor, or convulsions may occur, so that the case closely resembles meningitis; in others the symptoms of the typhoid state may develop. Still other cases exhibit a continued fever without localizing symptoms, which strongly suggests typhoid fever (Fig. 76). Occasionally there is marked dyspnea of purely toxic origin. Severe cases may sometimes end fatally, although generally in a few days all the alarming symptoms ameliorate, showing that they were toxic and not inflammatory in nature. In other instances actual lesions of the cerebrospinal system develop as complications or sequels. (See p. 358.)

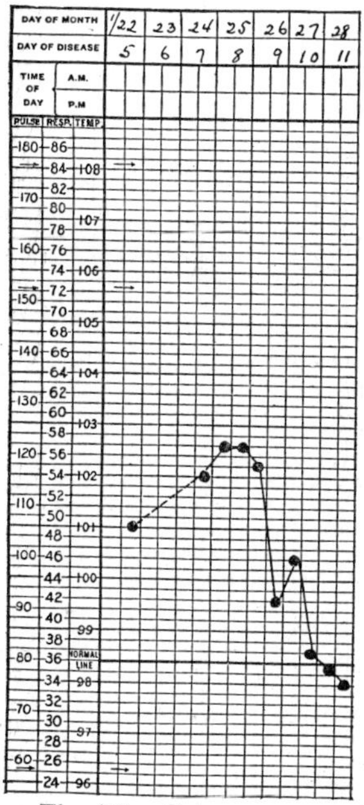

Fig. 76.—Grippe, nervous form. Prolonged febrile type. Louise F., aged sixteen months. Slight cough, apathy, prostration, without any localized symptoms. Fever continued a week or more. Twin sister with same symptoms. Case suggested typhoid fever. Epidemic of grippe prevailing.

Epidemic Pleurodynia.—A peculiar form of acute febrile disturbance, first described by Dabney,[31] and supposed by him to resemble dengue, has since been discussed by Reilly,[32] Payne and Armstrong,[33] Hangar, McCoy and Frantz,[34] Greene[35] and others. It was first called "Devil's grip," and later has received the titles epidemic pleurodynia, diaphragmatic pleurodynia, and epidemic transient diaphragmatic spasm. The cause is entirely unknown, but the disease seems to be associated with influenza, resembling somewhat the nervous form, and it may tentatively be classed as one of the variants of this. It suggests an intercostal neuralgic or a diaphragmatic spasm, is distinctly epidemic in character, occurs chiefly in the late summer months, and cases are acquired by contact. Sex is without influence, and children are attacked as readily as are adults, or even more so. It begins suddenly with severe pain in the lower part of the chest or upper part of the abdomen, which is made worse by deep breathing or movements of the body. With this there are prostration, headache, and fever. The number of leukocytes in the blood is normal or diminished, but there is a relative increase of the polymorphonuclear cells. Physical examination of the chest is entirely negative. At times there is herpes of the face or trunk. Pains elsewhere in the body are usually absent, and there is little, if any, involvement of the nose and throat. The attack may last but a few hours, but is liable to recur, the whole course being from two to three days or sometimes a week.

Gastro-intestinal Form.—The prominent symptoms of this variety, a common one in infancy, are anorexia, nausea, vomiting, abdominal pain, prostration, and diarrhea, the stools often containing mucus and blood. The attack may last only three or four days, but is not infrequently protracted. In other cases the condition is one resembling intestinal toxemia, and there are present the ordinary symptoms of this, with loss of weight, but without diarrhea or vomiting.

Complications and Sequels.—One of the most dangerous and common complications is *pneumonia*, which is usually of the catarrhal variety. It was especially frequent in the epidemic of 1918. It develops during the attack or as a sequel. The symptoms are often more severe than can be accounted for by the physical signs, which are frequently misleading, and the disease is commonly of the wandering type and prolonged, this leading to an incorrect diagnosis of tuberculosis. In other cases it is abortive and lasts but a few days. Leukopenia may be present, in spite of the existence of the pneumonic inflammation. Pleurisy may be an accompaniment and tends to result in empyema. *Sinusitis* and *bronchitis* are practically constant complications of the respiratory type. Influenzal *croup* has already been mentioned as a not uncommon complication.

Otitis, catarrhal, purulent, or often hemorrhagic, is a frequent attendant of the respiratory form, and mastoiditis may follow. *Cervical adenitis* is a striking complication, its incidence and severity varying with the epidemic. *Parotitis* is sometimes observed. *Neuritis* of various forms may constitute a sequel, although not often in children. Anemia, sometimes severe, is a frequent sequel. *Meningitis* depending upon the influenza-bacillus may accompany the attack. Almost invariably, however, influenzal meningitis occurs independently of influenza itself. (See p. 922.) Paralyses, chorea, encephalitis, psychoses, or other *nervous disturbances* exceptionally follow influenza. Cystitis, pyelitis and nephritis are rare. Miller[36] collected 40 cases of acute hemorrhagic *nephritis*, only a few being in children. Among other unusual complications and sequels are peritonitis, ileocolitis, icterus, subcutaneous emphysema, and cardiac dilatation. Bradycardia may be a sequel (Hyman[37]), and heart-block has been reported. *Cutaneous complications* are not rare, especially herpes, urticaria, and a morbilliform, or oftener, scarlatiniform erythema. *Other infectious diseases* may be associated, and the development of tuberculosis as a sequel is not infrequent.

Relapse and Recurrence.—*Relapse*, in the sense of relighting of symptoms before the disease is over, is very common. *Recurrence* is frequent, one attack in no way conferring immunity, or if so, only for a few months.

Prognosis.—While the case-mortality in uncomplicated influenza in interepidemic periods, and in some epidemics, is low (0.5 to 1.0 per cent), the enormous number of persons attacked makes the number of deaths from grippe or its complications large, and the death-rate in communities may increase to 10 or 20 times the normal. It has been estimated that in the epidemic of 1918–19, 6,000,000 persons died of influenza throughout the world. The case-mortality varies, too, in epidemics. Most of the danger is from pneumonia, but gastro-intestinal disorders also increase largely the number of fatalities. The mortality is less in childhood than later in life, except in the first year.

Diagnosis.—This is easy in typical cases during an epidemic; not forgetting, however, the danger at such times of overlooking the possible presence of other diseases simulating grippe. The mildest isolated cases of the respiratory type cannot be distinguished from ordinary catarrh of the respiratory tract; but in all others prostration, out of proportion to other symptoms or to any discoverable cause, is the most important diagnostic indication. Fever, too, not otherwise accounted for is suspicious, as is, in other cases, a rather wide extension of neuralgic pain. Leukopenia, if present, is suggestive of influenza. Cases of the nervous type may resemble meningitis, and lumbar puncture be necessary to make the differential diagnosis. Usually, however, rapid improvement after a few days, and the development of other symptoms, indicate the presence of grippe. In the pleurodynic form there is epidemic incidence and absence of physical signs of pleurisy. Protracted febrile cases may resemble typhoid fever, especially when there is leukopenia, and the Widal reaction or blood-culture may finally be required to settle the diagnosis. The rash of influenza, if present, may resemble that of measles or scarlet fever, but the other symptoms of these diseases, and leukocytosis in the latter, should clear up the confusion. In malaria there is often a more regular temperature-curve and the plasmodium should be found in the blood. In the gastro-enteritis of influenza it is characteristic, except in the prolonged cases, that there is sudden clearing up of the symptoms after a few days. Such complications as pneumonia and cervical adenitis may be difficult to distinguish from these conditions caused by other diseases, except in the presence of epidemics. Dengue may sometimes be observed in children, with symptoms of malaise, vomiting, sometimes convulsions, sometimes morbilliform or scarlatiniform rash, and leukopenia. This disease, however, occurs almost entirely in the tropics and subtropics and in epidemic form.

Treatment. **Prophylaxis.**—Inasmuch as the disease is spread almost entirely by contact, the patient should, if possible, be isolated, especially from infants or delicate children. There seems to be some slight measure of protection for attendants by wearing face-masks and goggles, if these are properly fitted and taken care of. The value of prophylactic vaccines is questionable, whether made from the influenza bacillus, the bacterium pneumosintes, or mixed organisms.

Treatment of the Attack.—There is no specific, and treatment must be symptomatic. Vaccines are without value. Rest in bed is imperative; the diet should be light but nourishing; fever may be treated, if necessary, by febrifuges or hydrotherapy; pain by acetylsalicylic acid or similar drugs; nervous symptoms by sedatives and hydrotherapy.

Complications should receive the treatment appropriate to them. In severe pneumonia with pulmonary edema and cyanosis, in which there is blood-concentration, venesection and fluid-injections may be helpful (Underhill and Ringer[38]).

In convalescence the remaining debility and anemia may require treatment, and often a change of climate is indicated.

References

1. Ergebn. der inn. Med. u. Kinderh., 1912, **8**, 211. 2. Arch. Pediat., 1919, **36**, 578. 3. Epidemic Influenza, 1927. 4. Epidemic Respirat. Dis., 1921. 5. Medicine, 1922,

1, 213. 6. Pub. Health Rep., 1931, **46,** 154. 7. Ztschr. f. Geburtsh. u. Gynäk., 1890, **19,** 39. 8. Pediatria, 1923, **31,** 1137. 9. J.A.M.A., 1919, **72,** 980. 10. Deutsche med. Wchnschr., 1892, **18,** 28; Ztschr. f. Hyg., 1893, **13,** 357. 11. Am. J. Dis. Child., 1919, **17,** 165. 12. J.A.M.A., 1920, **74,** 170. 13. J. Infect. Dis., 1928, **43,** 385. 14. J.A.M.A., 1919, **72,** 1317. 15. J.A.M.A., 1918, **71,** 1733. 16. J.A.M.A., 1919, **72,** 1604. 17. J. Med., 1929, **10,** 175. 18. Arch. Int. Med., 1930, **45,** 412. 19. J.A.M.A., 1920, **74,** 1497; 1921, **76,** 640; 1923, **81,** 744; J. Exper. Med., 1922, **36,** 685; Medicine, 1930, **9,** 387. 20. Brit. M. J., 1918, **2,** 645. 21. Ann. de l'inst. Pasteur, 1919, **33,** 395. 22. J.A.M.A., 1931, **97,** 1122. 23. Am. J. M. Sc., 1921, **159,** 435. 24. Am. J. M. Sc., 1921, **162,** 1. 25. J.A.M.A., 1920, **74,** 1070. 26. Resistance to Inf. Dis., 4th Ed., 1931, 40. 27. Am. J. Dis. Child., 1919, **17,** 377. 28. Correspondbl. f. Schweiz. Aerzte, 1919, **49,** 474. 29. München. med. Wchnschr., 1920, **67,** 1522. 30. Przeglad Lekarski, 1920, **59,** No. 4; Ref. Monats. f. Kinderh., 1921, **21,** 229. 31. Am. J. M. Sc., 1888, **96,** 488. 32. J.A.M.A., 1921, **76,** 1493. 33. J.A.M.A., 1923, **81,** 746. 34. J.A.M.A., 1923, **81,** 826. 35. Arch. Pediat., 1924, **41,** 322. 36. Arch. Pediat., 1902, **19,** 1. 37. Arch. Int. Med., 1927, **40,** 120. 38. J.A.M.A., 1920, **75,** 1531.

CHAPTER XVI

PERTUSSIS

(Whooping-cough)

History.—The first published recognition of pertussis was by Baillou[1] in Paris in 1578. Willis[2] observed it in England in 1658 and described it clearly. After the middle of the eighteenth century it spread widely and is now one of the commonest of the acute infectious disorders over the whole civilized world.

Etiology. Predisposing Causes.—Climate, race and geographical position exert no influence. Pertussis seems to be more frequent in the colder months, probably through more intimate association of children in schools at this time. Epidemics vary, and some statistics, as those of Luttinger[3] and Herrman and Bell,[4] show a greater prevalence during spring and summer. Poor hygienic conditions favor dissemination, and weakly and sickly children contract pertussis apparently more readily than do others. Outbreaks are liable to accompany, or to prevail after, epidemics of measles and influenza.

The influence of *age* is great. Most of the cases occur under six and comparatively few after ten years, as shown by the studies of Szabö,[5] Vladimirov,[6] Baginsky,[7] Luttinger[3] and others. The greater immunity of the first year seen in some infectious diseases does not obtain in pertussis, and even cases of congenital pertussis have been reported by Rilliet and Barthez,[8] Gatti,[9] Cockayne,[10] and Milio, or it may be contracted within a few days after birth (Phillips[12]).

Pertussis is somewhat more prevalent in the *female sex* according to most statistics (Apert and Cambessédès[13]). The *individual susceptibility* is very great and the majority of children exposed contract the disease. Its rarity in adults depends largely upon the fact that so many of them have had it early in life. Unquestionably, however, some children possess a natural immunity. The disease is endemic in larger cities, and epidemic influence is marked.

Exciting Cause.—In 1906 Bordet and Gengou[14] described a very small, ovoid, gram-negative bacillus present in large numbers in the sputum in the early part of the attack. Later investigators confirmed this, and have claimed that agglutination and complement-fixation tests have been specific, and that the disease could be transmitted to apes, monkeys (Klimenko,[15]

Inaba,[16] Sauer and Hambrecht[17]), and puppies (Mallory, Horner and Henderson[18]). The germ is present during the first two weeks in the secretions from the nose and throat in 75 to 90 per cent of cases (Herrman and Bell[4]). While it would seem very probable that the pertussis bacillus is responsible for the disease, this is not entirely accepted. Some workers maintain that agglutination and complement-fixation are not always specific; that the germ can be found in other conditions than pertussis; that it cannot always be discovered in this disease; and that experimental production in animals has failed. The *duration of life* of the germ outside the body is probably brief, and rooms occupied by the patient soon lose their infectiousness.

It should be mentioned that prior to Bordet and Gengou others had described minute bacilli found in the respiratory mucus, among them, Afanassjew,[19] Czaplewski and Hensel,[20] Koplik,[21] Arnheim,[22] and Jochmann and Krause.[23] Pertussis has also been variously described as a pure neurosis of the medulla or the nerves which control cough; a simple bronchial catarrh; a pneumogastric irritation from pressure of enlarged bronchial glands; and a result of sensitization to pollen.

Nature of the Disease.—As will be stated under Pathological Anatomy, there is irritation of the lower, or oftener the upper, respiratory tract, especially in the interarytenoid fossa. As a result of this irritation in the so-called "cough region," a cough is produced by the accumulated mucus. This sets going a series of reflex clonic spasms of the expiratory apparatus, the whoop being due to an inspiratory spasm of the glottis. Many circumstances indubitably indicate, however, that there must exist in addition a general constitutional disorder which determines the peculiar character of the paroxysms, and that this character may depend upon a disturbance of the superior laryngeal nerves and the respiratory centers, brought about by a circulating toxin produced by the germs.

The marked lymphocytosis very commonly present (p. 363) needs explanation. Meunier[24] and others suggest that it may be due to mechanical pressure on the bronchial lymph-nodes produced by the paroxysms. Fukushima[25] believes from experimental investigations that the high lipoid content of the pertussis bacillus stimulates lymphocytosis.

Period of Greatest Infectiousness.—The disease is transmitted early, and probably chiefly, in the catarrhal stage. It is likely that the danger of infection is less in the paroxysmal stage, and disappears entirely before this is over; but to this there are exceptions. Occasionally the infectiousness lasts five weeks or even longer.

Mode of Transmission.—This is by minute droplets of mucus expelled by coughing, which may carry for six feet or more. Exceptionally, if ever, is infection conveyed by a third person, most of such supposed cases having been in reality communicated by someone undergoing an unrecognized attack. On a number of occasions we have seen parents suffering from the disease, in whom the diagnosis had been made only when their children had contracted it from them. (See Recurrence p. 365.) The germs are received through the respiratory tract, except in congenital cases when the infection is blood-borne.

Pathologic Anatomy.—There are no characteristic lesions. During life congestion and swelling of the upper respiratory tract may be observed, especially of the arytenoid region, where there may be ulceration (Meyer-Huni,[26] von Herff,[27] Heinrichsbauer[28]). At necropsy there is very constantly found some degree of pulmonary emphysema, and often various forms of involvement of the bronchi and bronchioles, together with peribronchitis, peribronchiolitis, bronchiolitis fibrinosa, and obliteration and stenotic changes in the bronchi and small bronchioles (Feyrter,[29] Sauer and

Hambrecht[30]). Mallory and Horner[31] observed the Bordet-Gengou bacillus between the cilia of the cells lining the trachea and bronchi. Among other lesions which may sometimes be found, dependent either upon the disease itself or upon complications, are hypertrophy of the tracheal and bronchial lymph-nodes, bronchiectasis, pneumonia, atelectasis, serous meningitis (Reiche[32]), encephalitis (Askin and Zimmermann[33]), degeneration of the nerve-cells of the brain (Husler and Spatz;[34] Ford[35]), dilatation of the heart, and hemorrhages in various organs, especially the brain.

Symptoms.—The attack is divided into four periods which are not sharply differentiated and which vary greatly in length in different cases.

Incubation.—In most cases this lasts seven to fourteen days, sometimes less, rarely longer, and no symptoms are present.

Catarrhal Stage.—The attack begins with symptoms of a tracheobronchitis, some degree of coryza, sneezing and hoarseness, and possibly slight fever, malaise, and irritability. The cough at first is in no way suspicious, but later becomes hard, dry and annoying. Unless there is a coincident bronchitis there will be few if any râles in the chest. The cough gradually becomes more severe, frequent, and paroxysmal in character, and distinctly worse at night. Finally evident whooping develops. The *duration* of the catarrhal stage is variable. Some children begin whooping after two or three days, others only after three or four weeks, or not at all. In general it averages about two weeks, but the younger the child the shorter this period.

Paroxysmal Stage.—The beginning of this third stage is usually dated from the commencement of whooping. A typical paroxysm is very characteristic. Often it comes on without warning, but often, too, the child experiences a slight tickling in the throat or beneath the sternum, an inclination to cough, or a sensation of smothering or of intense anxiety. If previously lying down it sits upright with an anxious expression and perhaps grasps the side of the crib. If moving about it drops its toys and runs to its mother or nurse, or takes hold of some of the furniture of the room. There is a brief moment of holding the breath, a deep inspiration follows, and the attack begins. This consists of a series of short explosive coughs, so rapidly repeated that there is no time for respiration between them. These continue for a few moments and number anywhere from 4 or 5 up to 15 or 20. Meanwhile the face becomes swollen, red, cyanotic, and sometimes quite dark, and the eyes prominent and congested; the tongue protrudes with each expiratory effort; tears flow from the eyes and saliva from the mouth; the veins of the neck are engorged; perspiration breaks out on the face, and the pulse increases in frequency. Finally the cough ceases and the respiration often apparently also, but in a moment a long-drawn, crowing inspiration is heard which is called the "whoop," and depends upon a spasm of the glottis. Immediately after the whoop a second attack generally occurs and after this perhaps a third or fourth or more. The whole paroxysm lasts from a few seconds up to several minutes. In the latter case there may be a momentary period of rest between some of the attacks. Toward the end of the paroxysm very tenacious, ropy mucus is often driven from the mouth by the force of the cough, and this seems to bring relief, and retching or vomiting is liable to follow.

The paroxysms vary from 6 or 8 up to 60 or more in twenty-four hours, not all of them in severe cases being equally marked. They are generally most troublesome at night. They occur without discoverable reason, or are brought on by such slight causes as excitement, crying, swallowing, exercise, sudden change of air, inhalation of the air of close rooms, the use of a tongue-depressor, hearing another child in a paroxysm, and the like. The presence of mucus on some part of the irritated mucous membrane is the commonest immediate cause. Auscultation of the chest during the expiratory efforts reveals no respiratory sound and only the impulse of the cough against the ear. During the whoop only a feeble inspiration is heard or none at all. In bad attacks the urine and feces may be involuntarily expelled and hemorrhage take place from the nose or mouth or beneath the conjunctiva.

More or less fatigue, usually of brief duration, may follow the paroxysm. In severe cases the child may be covered with perspiration after an attack, confused, and quite exhausted. Between the paroxysms a characteristic appearance of the face is often seen, consisting of some degree of swelling and cyanosis, congestion of the eyes, and blueness of the tongue.

The *blood* shows a remarkably high leukocytosis, averaging about 20,000, but often reaching higher figures. This begins early in the catarrhal stage and attains its maximum at the height of the paroxysmal stage, and, in our own experience and that of most clinicians, is a very helpful diagnostic sign which is usually, but by no means always, present. Regarding its incidence there is not entire agreement, and some writers, as Sauer and Hambrecht,[36] think that the leukocytosis is not constant nor decided early enough to be helpful. These authors describe, too, an initial and a terminal leukopenia as quite constant. Leukocytosis reaching 150,000 or over may occur, as reported by Crombie,[37] Seitz,[38] Bourne and Scott,[39] Leitner,[40] Abt,[41] and others. In most of these high counts there was associated bronchopneumonia. In one such case we[42] found a count of 233,600. The important feature of the leukocytosis is that it involves a relative lymphocytosis often of 80 or 90 per cent or more, although in the high total counts the relative percentage was usually less than this. The condition of the blood returns to normal in two or three months. According to Benstz[43] the eosinophiles are diminished. Complications increase the neutrophilic percentage. Regan and Tolstouhov[44] found in the catarrhal stage a diminution of the organic blood-phosphorus and an uncompensated acidosis.

The severity of the paroxysmal stage increases for about two weeks, and then continues for a time unabated. The effect on the patient's general condition depends on the severity of the attack. Usually as the disease advances a few moist râles become audible between the paroxysms. The average *duration* of the paroxysmal stage is about three to six weeks but may be much longer, or may not last for more than a week.

In some cases the paroxysms are so mild or so infrequent that they are disturbing only during the night, if at all. Occasionally no whooping occurs at any time. In infancy and in severe cases whooping may be replaced by dangerous apnea with unconsciousness. In some instances the paroxysm may be accompanied by violent repeated sneezing, or exceptionally this may replace the cough (Szegö,[45] Moncrieff and Lightwood,[46] Reichle[47]). The paroxysmal character of the third stage may disappear for a time if pneumonia develops.

Stage of Decline.—This fourth stage, while not sharply separated from the preceding one, is marked by a lessening in the number and frequency of paroxysms. The cough grows looser and gradually loses its peculiar character, while whooping occurs in only some of the paroxysms. Moist râles are heard in greater numbers in the chest, and the sputum is more purulent. Finally whooping ceases, although more or less cough may continue for an indefinite time. The duration of this stage is very variable, but averages about two to three weeks. It may be indefinitely prolonged by the development of a slight bronchitis, which may cause a return of the severity and an increase in the number of paroxysms, this being particularly true in the winter season.

It not infrequently happens that whooping returns after it has ceased entirely for a time. This cannot properly be called a continuation of the disease, but rather a neurosis without any infectious element. The actual termination of the attack of pertussis may be placed at the time when the whooping and the paroxysmal character of the cough have entirely disappeared for a few days. The total duration of the disease averages about six to eight weeks.

Complications and Sequels.—Of these the *respiratory* are the most frequent. Bronchitis, which is a symptom of the stage of decline, may be regarded as a complication if it is unusually severe or develops early. The most common and one of the most dangerous complications is bronchopneumonia. This is more frequent the younger the child, and occurs especially in feeble or rachitic subjects. It appears oftenest during the height of the paroxysmal stage or later. During it the whooping character of the cough lessens or disappears. The incidence of bronchopneumonia varies statistically from 10 (Rolleston[48]) to 30 (Sée[49]) per cent or more. Atelectasis is of common occurrence in severe cases in infants. Pulmonary emphysema is probably always present, and may remain as a sequel. Among other recorded complications are pneumothorax, pulmonary abscess, croupous pneumonia, pleurisy, and empyema. Of *digestive disorders* may be mentioned vomiting, which may be so severe and frequent after the paroxysms that great emaciation develops. Anorexia, indigestion, diarrhea, ileocolitis, prolapse of the rectum, hernia, ulceration of the fraenulum linguae and stomatitis are often seen.

Nervous complications and sequels are frequent, among the most common being general convulsions, which not rarely end fatally. Some of these are spasmophilic in nature (Powers[50]); others depend upon serous meningitis, encephalitis or intracranial hemorrhage. Hemiplegia, monoplegia, and paraplegia may occur, as also aphasia, blindness, deafness, epilepsy, and various psychoses. When these are temporary they are dependent upon edema and congestion; when permanent upon hemorrhage or perhaps encephalitis. (See Pathologic Anatomy, p. 361.) Among those who have especially studied them are Valentin,[51] Hockenjos[52] and Sears.[53] Myelitis and multiple neuritis are uncommon. Cerebellar abscess and disseminated sclerosis have been reported as sequels. We have seen ataxia of cerebellar nature following pertussis, with the symptoms of nystagmus, a positive Romberg sign, and paresis of the extremities. Complete recovery followed. Strümpell[54] records a case of cerebellar ataxia in which there was also optic neuritis. Spasm of the glottis is a convulsive complication sometimes fatal.

Of *cardiovascular complications* there is frequently seen dilatation of the heart, especially of the right ventricle. In infants Klotz[55] and others have sometimes found a small heart, presumably due to the loss of body-weight. Degenerative changes in the cardiac muscles have been found at necropsy. This is, however, usually only in complicated cases, Ledbetter and White[56] maintaining that generally no damage to the heart occurs, except a temporary mechanical strain. Hemorrhages in various regions are frequent and depend on the intense congestion which the coughing occasions. Epistaxis and subconjunctival hemorrhage are common; hematemesis and hemorrhage from the ears or into the skin unusual. The most dangerous form of hemorrhage is that within the cranium, already mentioned.

Otitis media is not infrequent; albuminuria is often seen during severe attacks; nephritis is an occasional complication or sequel; glycosuria may develop; hematuria and hemoglobinuria have been reported, as also cystitis and pyelitis. Cutaneous emphysema is a rare occurrence.

Other infectious diseases may follow, precede, or accompany pertussis, especially to be mentioned being measles. Tuberculosis in some form, oftenest as bronchial or mesenteric adenitis or tuberculous bronchopneumonia, is a common and dreaded sequel. Nobécourt and Forgeron[57] and others found that a previously positive cutaneous tuberculin reaction is liable to disappear during pertussis. We[58] could not confirm this in our own studies.

Relapse.—As previously pointed out the cough of pertussis has a great tendency to return, but this cannot, strictly speaking, be called a relapse. A true relapse of an infectious nature is certainly uncommon.

Recurrence.—This is very rare, and errors in diagnosis account for many supposed second attacks. LeGendre[59] writing in 1891 found but nine recorded instances of recurrence, and Widowitz[60] observed no second attack in 558 children with the disease. In adult life, however, the immunity may occasionally become exhausted. We have seen quite a few instances in which parents developed a modified second attack, either contracting it from their children or transmitting it to them. From the sputum of some of these cases we have been able to recover pertussis bacilli.

Prognosis.—Pertussis is a serious disease. During one ten-year period approximately 100,000 children died of it in the United States (Johnston[61]), 65,481 died in England and Wales during eight years (Sticker[62]), and Crum[63] estimated that 1 per cent of the total deaths from all causes in 24 countries depended upon it. During the three years 1926, 1927 and 1928 in the Registration Area of the U. S. there were 9128 deaths from pertussis.[64]

The case mortality, too, is considerable, varying from 3 to 15 per cent. In this *age* is a powerful factor, the danger being greater the younger the child. Neurath[65] found a mortality for Vienna, in children under one year of age, of 25.3 per cent and Saget and Van Gelderen[66] for Amsterdam of 42.3 per cent. Studies by Luttinger[3] and Veeder[67] showed the high proportion of the total deaths from the disease which occur in the early years. In the Registration Area of the United States 99.6 per cent of all deaths from pertussis were under twenty years, 67.2 per cent were under one year, 95.9 per cent under five years and 99.1 per cent under ten years.[64] *Sex* probably has some influence, more females dying than males, perhaps because more girls are attacked.

The danger depends more on *complications and sequels* than on the disease itself. Weakly or rachitic infants are especially liable to succumb, and the association with other infectious diseases increases the danger. Obstinate vomiting may induce a marantic stage which is a contributory cause of death. Tuberculosis is a not infrequent fatal sequel. Asphyxia in severe paroxysms may be the immediate cause of a fatal issue in infancy. Complicating convulsions, diarrhea, or pneumonia is a common cause of death. Probably over $\frac{1}{2}$ the fatal cases of pertussis are due to bronchopneumonia.

Diagnosis.—The diagnostic symptoms in typical cases consist in the development of cough, which gradually becomes more and more paroxysmal, and is finally followed by a whoop; the tendency for the cough to be worse during the night; the absence of fever or of evidence of respiratory infection commensurate with the severity of the symptoms; and a lymphocytosis. In order to judge the cough a paroxysm may sometimes be excited by depressing the tongue, or by irritating the nasal or pharyngeal mucous membrane with an applicator or a spray from an atomizer.

Yet early in the attack the diagnosis may be difficult, especially if there is no history of exposure. Vomiting may occur after severe coughing from other causes, and occasionally whooping may also be a symptom of severe bronchitis. In these conditions, however, there will usually be fever and evidence of marked respiratory infection, especially bronchitic râles. In mild cases of pertussis the typical symptoms may be absent; but the prolonged course and its unyielding character are suspicious, especially in the presence of an epidemic. In severe cases in early infancy attacks of apnea, even without a whoop, are strongly suggestive of pertussis. Cough persisting after pertussis might depend upon a beginning pulmonary tuberculosis, and here radioscopy will be of value. A high leukocyte count, especially with a relative increase of lymphocytes, and the absence of fever are helpful diagnostic signs of the presence of pertussis. The concensus of opinion is that the agglutinative and the complement-fixation tests are of little value, and they are seldom employed. A diagnostic test consisting in the intradermal injection of 0.1 cc. of a suspension of killed bacilli has been tried by Modigliani and de Villa,[68] Garzia,[69] and others, but its value has not been proven. Chievitz and Meyer,[70] Lawson and Mueller,[71] Sauer and Hambrecht,[72] and others recommend the "cough-plate" method for early diagnosis. The patient coughs on a Petri dish containing special media, which is held about 4 in. from the mouth. A negative plate does not exclude pertussis, but in a high percentage of cases the specific bacillus may thus be found even before whooping or lymphocytosis develops.

Treatment. PROPHYLAXIS.—Although pertussis is contagious probably for a shorter period, at least six weeks' isolation of the patient should be carried out, or longer if whooping persists. Nonimmune children should, if possible, be sent away from the house, or from the locality where an epidemic is prevailing. Especially to be protected are children less than four years old, or delicate ones of any age. (See Vaccine Treatment, p. 367.)

TREATMENT OF THE ATTACK.—The most that can be expected from any mode of therapy in pertussis is a reduction of the severity. Mild cases may require little if any treatment. The child should be spared medication when there is no real demand for it. The enormous number of remedial measures which have been tried is an indication that none of them have unusual value.

(*A*) **Hygienic Treatment.**—If the weather permits, the patient should be kept in the fresh air as much as possible, and usually confinement to bed is not necessary. In the winter-time airing may best be done in the room with the windows open. Should bronchitis exist there must be fresh air, but cold air is to be allowed cautiously. Fresh air undoubtedly diminishes the number of paroxysms. Clothing should be sufficiently warm but not too heavy. Food should be of high caloric value and easily digestible, and administered in small quantities and frequently when vomiting is troublesome. In such cases so-called "refeeding" may be carried out, according to which food is again given at once, if a child coughs and vomits immediately after a meal. By this method the food is more likely to be retained. Sometimes nutrient enemata are necessary. Sea-air seems to be especially efficacious, and is helpful also during convalescence.

(*B*) **Local Medication.**—This is not as largely employed as formerly. There have been used as insufflations into the larynx or nose powders of quinine, resorcin, salicylic acid and numerous other drugs. As solutions to be sprayed or applied to the larynx, pharynx or nares have been recommended resorcin (1 per cent), cocaine or its derivatives (1 to 2 per cent), hydrogen peroxide, salicylic acid (1:1000), and the like. These insufflations and solutions offer no particular advantage. Inhalations of gaseous or volatile substances may sometimes be helpful, and there may be tried vaporization of such substances as creosote, turpentine, benzine, thymol and eucalyptus. Some have advised anesthetization with chloroform or ether in very severe attacks. Among other treatments have been recommended the fumes of burning sulphur, formaldehyde preparations, ozone, and chlorine gas. Antitussin, an ointment containing diflurphenyl, although a local application, acts systemically with benefit in some instances.

(*C*) **Systemic Medication.**—In the paroxysmal stage sedative treatment is indicated, and during that of decline perhaps either expectorants or drugs to check excessive secretion. Supporting treatment and cardiac stimulation may be needed. The drugs which have been employed during the paroxysmal stage are legion. One of the best is antipyrine, highly recommended by Sonnenberger,[73] which we[74] have used with excellent results in some cases. The dose, according to age, is $\frac{1}{4}$ (0.016) to 2 or 3 grains (0.13 to 0.194) given every three hours. Other sedatives such as bromides, chloral, luminal or its modifications, or even opium and its derivatives may be necessary, particularly at night. Bromoform, recommended by Stepp[75] we have often found serviceable. Gold tribromide in doses of $\frac{1}{30}$ to $\frac{1}{10}$ grain (0.00217 to 0.0065) three times a day is highly praised by Epstein.[76] Belladonna or atropine is often effective and may be combined with the sedatives. Quinine or its derivatives seem to be of value in some instances.

Recommended by various clinicians are such drugs as camphor, hyoscine, cannabis Indica, strontium, asafetida, adrenalin, and thyme or its derivative pertussin. Ephedrine hydrochloride given orally in doses of $\frac{1}{8}$ to $\frac{1}{4}$ grain (0.008 to 0.016) one to three times a day is said by Anderson and Homan[77] and Stewart[78] to give good results. Benzyl benzoate recommended by Macht[79] is little used at present, and we have never seen it produce any noticeable effect. Intramuscular injection of ether first recommended by Audrain[80] and Bedö[81] has been widely employed and claimed to be beneficial, but has not been of much value in our hands. One to 2 cc. (16 to 32 minims) of ether is injected once daily for three or more days. Because of the pain and, not infrequently, the abscesses produced the cure may be worse than the disease. Rectal injections may be given of 20 per cent ether in oil or liquid petrolatum and good results are also claimed for this. Any effects with ether would be of sedative nature and also, it is maintained, by the action on the bronchial mucous membrane of the ether which is excreted through the lungs.

(*D*) **Mechanical and Miscellaneous Treatment.**—Antismallpox vaccination has been claimed to be very effective. It has been employed for a long time, and still is to some extent. We have never been convinced of its effectiveness. A modification proposed by Violi[82] consists in the subcutaneous injection of serum from vaccinated heifers. Treatment with foreign protein, such as the subcutaneous or intramuscular injection of typhoid vaccine or milk, has also been stated to be useful. For control of vomiting and for assistance during the paroxysms an elastic abdominal belt has been recommended highly by Kilmer,[83] Luttinger,[84] and others. The constant galvanic current to the neck and spine, and the use of the pneumatic cabinet has each had its advocates. O'Dwyer[85] obtained relief in severe cases by intubation. Nägeli[86] and Sobel[87] maintain that pulling the lower jaw downward and forward will mitigate the paroxysms. The application of the roentgen-ray to the chest, as advocated by Bowditch and Leonard[88] and others, has been stated to give prompt improvement, perhaps by shrinking the bronchial glands. The concensus of opinion seems to be that there is little value in this treatment. The employment of the ultraviolet ray has also had its advocates.

(*E*) **Vaccine and Serum Therapy.**—Convalescent's serum and whole blood have been used in treatment and to some extent in prophylaxis, and are said to be of service (Sylvestri,[89] Funck and Hellet,[90] Wright[91] and Battley[92]). Jundell[93] used blood from adults with good results. Our own experience with convalescent's serum is not extensive, but also not encouraging.

It is interesting to note that the Council on Pharmacy and Chemistry of the American Medical Association has deleted pertussis vaccine from their publication "New and Nonofficial Remedies." There is a tremendous amount of literature on this subject which it is impossible to quote. Some investigators are convinced of the value of the vaccine both in prophylaxis and treatment; some obtain good results only if it is freshly prepared or given in large doses; others believe that vaccines are entirely inert. In our own opinion there is little if any effect in prophylaxis or in treatment by vaccines, but probably their use should not be discouraged, since they do no harm other than the unpleasant local and general reactions which may follow. For prevention three injections at intervals of two or three days are recommended, giving 25,000,000 to 8,000,000,000 or more of the bacilli; for treatment, five or six injections may be administered at similar intervals. In some vaccines only the pertussis bacillus is present; in others various germs found in the upper respiratory tract are combined with it. Pretet[94] states that the organisms in the vaccine should agglutinate in convalescent's serum when this is diluted 1:5000 or 1:10,000. Kramsztyk[95] used filtrates of pertussis bacillus and other germs found in the pharynx, applied locally by swab or atomizer to the pharyngeal mucous membrane. Morabito[96] combined vaccine with extract of lymphatic glands. Kraus[97] recommended the subcutaneous injection of sterilized sputum from patients with pertussis.

References

1. Geneva Edit., 1762, **1,** 173. 2. Path. cerebri, etc. cap. 12, 1667. 3. Am. J. Dis. Child., 1916, **12,** 290. 4. Arch. Pediat., 1924, **41,** 13. 5. Pest. med.-chir. Presse 1881, **17,** 657. 6. Boln. Gaz. Botk. 1893, No. 12.; Ref. O'Dwyer and Norton, 20th Cent. Pract. Med. **14,** 217. 7. Kinderkrankheiten, 1905, 265. 8. Sanné, Mal. des enf., 1891, **3,** 747. 9. Pediatria, 1914, **22,** 687. 10. Brit. J. Child. Dis., 1913, **10,** 534. 11. Pediatria, 1922, **30,** 297. 12. Am. J. Med. Sc., 1921, **116,** 163. 13. Bull. et mém. de la soc. méd. des hôp., 1920, **44,** 324. 14. Ann. de l'inst. Pasteur, 1906, **20,** 731. 15. Deutsche. med. Wchnschr., 1908, **34,** 2030. 16. Ztschr. f. Kinderh., Orig., 1912, **4,** 252. 17. Am. J. Dis. Child., 1929, **37,** 732. 18. J. Med. Res., 1914, **27,** 291. 19. Petersburg. med. Wchnschr., 1887, **4,** 323. 20. Deutsche med. Wchnschr., 1897, **22,** 586. 21. Brit. M. J., 1897, **2,** 1051. 22. Berl. klin. Wchnschr., 1900, **37,** 702. 23. Ztschr. f. Hyg., 1901, **36,** 193. 24. Arch. de méd. d. enf., 1898, **1,** 193. 25. Orient. J. Dis. Infants, 1928, **3,** 43. 26. Ztschr. f. klin. Med., 1880, **1,** 461. 27. Deutsche. Arch. f. klin. Med., 1886, **39,** 213. 28. Jahrb. f. Kinderh., 1927, **118,** 104. 29. Frankfurt Ztschr. f. Path., 1927, **35,** 213. 30. Arch. Path., 1929, **8,** 944. 31. J. Med. Res., 1912, **27,** 115. 32. Ztschr. f. Kinderh., Orig., 1920, **25,** 28. 33. Am. J. Dis. Child., 1929, **38,** 97. 34. Ztschr. f. Kinderh., 1924, **38,** 428. 35. Am. J. Dis. Child., 1929, **37,** 1046. 36. Am. J. Dis. Child., 1931, **41,** 1327. 37. Edinburgh M. J., 1908, **1,** 222. 38. Am. J. Dis. Child., 1925, **30,** 670. 39. Brit. M. J., 1922, **1,** 387. 40. Jahrb. f. Kinderh., 1928, **121,** 164. 41. M. Clin. N. America, 1931, **14,** 1229. 42. Mitchell and Friedman, Arch. Pediat., 1926, **43,** 617. 43. Nederl. Tijdschr. f. Geneesk., 1916, **60,** 153. 44. J.A.M.A., 1926, **86,** 1116. 45. Arch. f. Kinderh., 1900, **29,** 186. 46. Arch. Dis. Childhood, 1929, **4,** 240. 47. J.A.M.A., 1929, **92,** 443. 48. Brit. J. Child. Dis., 1914, **11,** 38. 49. Arch. gén. de méd., 1854, **2,** 279. 50. Am. J. Dis. Child., 1925, **30,** 652. 51. Thèse de Paris, 1901. 52. Jahrb. f. Kinderh., 1900, **51,** 426. 53. Brit. J. Child. Dis., 1929, **26,** 178. 54. Deutsche Ztschr. f. Nervenheilk., 1915, **53,** 321. 55. Ztschr. f. Kinderh., 1928, **46,** 818. 56. J.A.M.A., 1925, **84,** 1022. 57. Arch. de méd. d. enf., 1922, **35,** 394. 58. Eddy and Mitchell, Am. J. Dis. Child., 1930, **40,** 771. 59. Rév. mens. de mal. de l'enf., 1891, **9,** 496. 60. Wien. klin. Wchnschr., 1909, **22,** 1596. 61. Arch. Pediat., 1895, **12,** 241. 62. Nothnagel's Encyclop. Pract. Med., Amer. Ed., Pertussis, 548. 63. Am. J. Pub. Health, 1915, **5,** 944. 64. Communic. Dis. Control Rep. Sec. 2, White House Conf. on Child Health and Protection, 1931. 65. Pfaundler und Schlossmann, Handbk. f. Kinderh., 1906, **1,** 2; 871. 66. Nederl. Tijdschr. f. Geneesk., 1919, **2,** 1525. 67. Arch. Pediat., 1917, **34,** 321. 68. Pediatria, 1921, **29,** 337. 69. Pediatria, 1923, **31,** 890. 70. Ann. de l'inst. Pasteur, 1916, **30,** 503. 71. J.A.M.A., 1927, **89,** 275. 72. J.A.M.A., 1930, **95,** 263. 73. Deutsche med. Wchnschr., 1887, **13,** 280. 74. Griffith, Therap. Gaz., 1888, Feb., 84. 75. Deutsche med. Wchnschr., 1889, **15,** 639. 76. Arch. Pediat., 1932, **49,** 1. 77. Am. J. Med. Sc., 1927, **174,** 738. 78. Brit. M. J., 1929, **1,** 293. 79.

Bull. Johns Hopkins Hosp., 1920, **31,** 236. 80. Bull. et mém. de soc. méd. d. hôp. de Paris, 1920, **44,** 795. 81. Ztschr. f. Kinderh., 1923, **35,** 325. 82. Gaz. hébdom., 1897, **44,** 904. 83. New York M. J., 1903, **87,** 1101. 84. J.A.M.A., 1922, **78,** 1636. 85. 20th Cent. Pract. Med., **14,** 213. 86. Correspondbl. f. Schweiz. Aerzte., 1889, **19,** 417. 87. Arch. Pediat., 1903, **20,** 418. 88. Boston M. and S. J., 1923, **188,** 312; Am. J. Roentgenol., 1924, **11,** 264; J.A.M.A., 1924, **82,** 1422. 89. Gazz. d. osp., 1901, No. 114; Ref. München. med. Wchnschr., 1901, **48,** 2020. 90. Arch. de méd. des enf., 1925, **28,** 94. 91. Canad. M. A. J., 1927, **17,** 813. 92. Arch. Pediat., 1931, **48,** 675. 93. Acta pædiat., 1927, **7,** 319. 94. Progrès. méd., 1931, 193. 95. Monatschr. f. Kinderh., 1930, **48,** 74. 96. Pediatria, 1929, **37,** 464. 97. Wien. klin. Wchnschr., 1915, **18,** 1405; Deutsche med. Wchnschr., 1916, **42,** 281.

CHAPTER XVII

MUMPS

(Epidemic Parotitis)

The affection was well described by Hippocrates and, although confounded later with other disorders, it was again clearly differentiated toward the end of the eighteenth century.

Etiology. Predisposing Causes. *Age* has a decided predisposing influence, attacks being most frequent at from five to fifteen years, and being not uncommon in young adults. It is infrequent under two years but cases even in the new-born have been reported (Gautier,[1] Demme,[2] White[3]) and it is possible for the infection to be acquired during fetal life (Homans[4]). The youngest case we have seen was in an infant of ten and one-half months.

The influence of *sex* is questionable, although it is claimed that males are oftener attacked than females. Race and climate play no part and the disease is widely spread in all civilized countries. It is most frequent in the colder weather. *Epidemic influence* is very decided, but may be limited to an institution or a portion of a community. Epidemics vary in severity, infectiousness, and tendency to complications, and several years may pass without a case in the community. The *individual susceptibility* is not great except where persons are closely associated.

Exciting Cause.—While the disease is clearly infectious, the nature of the germ is not known with certainty. Different germs have been described by Capitan and Charrin;[5] Ollivier;[6] Bordas;[7] Laveran and Catrin;[8] Mecray and Walsh;[9] Bein and Michaelis;[10] Pick;[11] Haden;[12] Teissier and Esmein;[13] and Kermorgant.[14] These investigators have found such organisms as diplococci and spirochetes associated in various ways, as in the blood, in the parotid secretion or from the parotid by puncture, and in the spinal fluid. Haden claimed to have produced the disease by inoculation of a gram-positive diplococcus into a rabbit's testicle, and Kermorgant by intraperitoneal injection into monkeys, recovering from them a spirochete in symbiosis with a bacterium. Others have had entirely negative results. The experiments in transmission of the disease to monkeys by Gordon[15] and Nicolle and Conseil[16] and to cats by Wollstein[17] would indicate that the virus might be a filterable one.

Transmission and Period of Infectiousness.—Transmission is almost invariably direct and by close proximity, but the germ may possibly be carried by fomites. The period of greatest infectiousness is during the parotid swelling, but numbers of instances prove that transmission can occur some weeks after the swelling is over, as also before it appears. The entrance into the system is usually from the mouth through Steno's duct, but it may be by other routes, as indicated by the occurrence of primary orchitis and congenital cases.

Pathologic Anatomy.—In the few studies made the pathologic process has consisted of catarrhal inflammation of the ducts, an acute interstitial inflammation and a secondary periparotitis, and involvement of the cervical lymph-nodes. Similar changes have been found in the experimental disease in monkeys and cats. Suppuration occurs only with secondary infection. The swelling is usually confined to the parotid glands, but sometimes the submaxillary or, less often, the sublingual are also, or alone, involved. As complications there may occur necrotic changes in the pancreas, orchitis, and meningo-encephalitis.

Symptoms. Incubation.—The average is two to three weeks, but periods as short as three (Demme) and as long as thirty days (Antony[18]) have been reported.

Invasion.—Prodromal symptoms are absent or overlooked, or, if discovered, are slight, consisting of those usual to beginning infection, and continuing for a few hours up to two days.

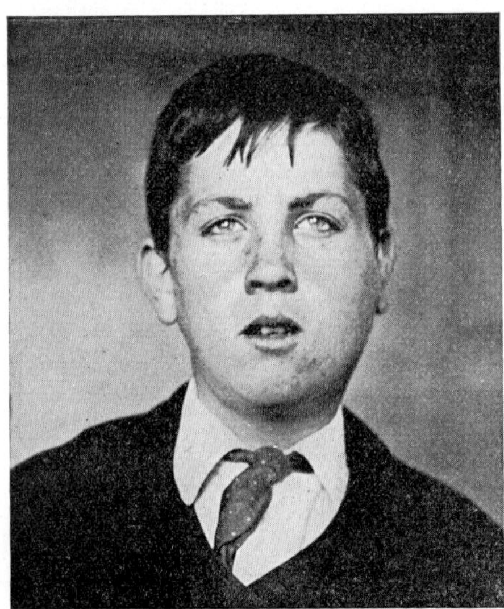

Fig. 77.—Mumps. Swelling of left parotid gland. From a patient in the Children's Hospital of Philadelphia.

Stage of Swelling.—A dull, aching *pain* begins in the region of the ear or the cheek, usually on but one side. This is made worse by pressure, movement of the jaws, or the presence in the mouth of acid or cold substances. It may become quite severe, or be slight in character. Pain in the ear is not uncommon. In the severer cases the mouth can scarcely be opened, chewing is impossible, and speaking and swallowing difficult. A few hours after the first development of pain, *swelling* begins and increases rapidly (Fig. 77). It appears first in the parotid gland, the outline of which can be felt below and in front of the ear. Sometimes only a portion of the gland is attacked at first. As the disease progresses the swelling spreads in every direction and the cervical lymph-nodes and subcutaneous tissue become involved. In well-marked cases it extends well up toward the eye, and from the mastoid process to the anterior portion of the neck. The lobe of the ear seems lifted up and pushed outward. In severe cases there may be edema of the eye-lids or even exophthalmos, or the edema may reach to the clavicle or across the neck. The swelling is hard and moderately tender on pressure, especially over the central portion. The skin covering it is tense and shining, but not reddened. After the maximum is reached, in from two to four days or sometimes longer, diminution in the size of the swelling begins and progresses with variable rapidity.

In the majority of instances, the second parotid is attacked one to two days after the onset of the disease in the first, or the interval may be longer. The degree of swelling in the two glands is frequently different. In some epidemics involvement of both parotids is much less common than in others.

The frequency of involvement of the submaxillary salivary glands varies with epidemics. While nearly always secondary to parotid involvement, it may rarely be primary or even occur alone (Fabre;[19] Wertheimber[20]).

Involvement of the sublingual gland is uncommon. It may exceptionally occur alone or be primary (Fabre,[19] Modigliani[21]).

The degree of *fever* in mumps depends on the severity of the attack. In average cases it may reach 102 F. (38.9 C.), or may be absent in mild attacks. Very frequently, indeed, the child does not feel ill enough to desire to be in bed. The secretion of saliva is often much diminished, or it may be unaffected or occasionally increased. Redness and swelling of the tonsils and throat are not infrequent. Bradycardia is a common symptom according to Teissier[22] and Roux.[23] There may be malaise, deafness and tinnitus, vomiting, diarrhea, or epistaxis. In severe cases there may be headache, delirium, enlargement of the spleen, somnolence, and, rarely, convulsions. The *blood* in mumps shows slight, if any, leukocytosis and sometimes a leukopenia; but always a relative increase in lymphocytes.

The *duration* of the disease in average cases is five to eight days, but in severe cases it may last two to three weeks before the swelling is entirely gone. Constitutional symptoms decline as the swelling diminishes.

Complications and Sequels.—The most important of these involve the *genito-urinary apparatus.* Orchitis is rarely observed in subjects under twelve years of age, although common in adults. It develops oftenest in the second or third week, is generally unilateral, and most frequently on the right side. Sometimes orchitis is primary and occurs alone. The attending symptoms are in part local and in part general. The latter may be severe, consisting of high fever, prostration, and sometimes vomiting, delirium or unconsciousness; but adynamic symptoms with low temperature may be observed. After three or four days the general symptoms disappear, but resolution of the swelling takes somewhat longer. There is not infrequently atrophy of the gland and, if this is bilateral, sterility. Rarely is there loss of secondary sexual characteristics. Uncommonly an analogous inflammation may develop in the uterus, ovaries, female external genitals or the breast. Prostatitis and urethritis are rare complications. Nephritis is an uncommon sequel, is generally of a hemorrhagic nature, and nearly always terminates in complete recovery.

Swelling of the *lachrymal glands* or the *thyroid* or *thymus* is exceptionally seen. Occasionally there is *pancreatitis,* the frequency apparently varying with epidemics. Farmen[24] collected 119 cases. Brahdy and Scheffer[25] reported 13 cases of pancreatitis developing in 263 cases of mumps admitted to the Willard Parker Hospital. Swelling of the cervical lymph-nodes is so common that it can hardly be called a complication, and stomatitis is sometimes seen. Severe *nervous disturbances* occasionally develop. Prominent here is meningitis or meningo-encephalitis. The subject has been reviewed by Feliciano,[26] Acker,[27] and Casparis.[28] The spinal fluid in such cases may be turbid with an excess of cells mostly lymphocytes; the sugar-content may be normal. Meningeal symptoms may occur without actual meningitis, as pointed out by Bonaba,[29] and as we ourselves have observed. Polyneuritis may be a sequel (Rompe[30]). There may be facial paralysis, probably as a result of pressure on the nerve. Paralysis may, however, develop in other parts of the body, depending upon a neuritis or upon meningo-encephalitis. Among other results of the central nervous involvement are aphasia, choreiform states, and severe psychoses, although all these are rare. *Involvement of the ear* has repeatedly occurred with temporary or lasting deafness, generally labyrinthine and usually unilateral (Gallavardin;[31] Boot[32]). The *eye* frequently exhibits conjunctivitis and occasionally keratitis, optic neuritis, iritis, dacrocystitis and ocular paralysis. Woodward[33] collected 23 cases of optic neuritis and neuroretinitis, and others have since been reported. Permanent blindness may result. Polyarthritis has repeatedly been described (Lannois and Lemoine;[34] Sarda[35]). Laryngeal stenosis is an occasional and dangerous complication, dependent upon edema or the pressure of the swelling in the neck.

Suppuration occurs rarely and is a result of secondary infection. Gangrene of the gland is a rare sequel (Demme[2]). Among other rare complications and sequels recorded may be mentioned erythema, purpura, endocarditis, pericarditis, polyneuritis, peritonitis and pneumonia. Mumps may develop in combination with other infectious diseases.

Recurrence and Relapse.—Relapse occurs occasionally in the sense of reawakening of the process in the gland just recovering, or its development in the second parotid some days after the disease is completely over in the first. Second attacks of mumps are only occasionally seen, although some writers think that they are not infrequent. Friedjung[36] saw one patient with 4 separate attacks, and Rommel[37] reports an instance of 5 attacks.

Prognosis.—Mumps causes little danger, especially in childhood, yet complications may exceptionally render an attack severe or even fatal. In the years 1926, 1927 and 1928 in the Registration Area of the United States[38] there were 335 deaths from this disease in patients of all ages.

Diagnosis.—This rests upon the rapid development, the characteristic situation and form of the swelling, and the course of the disease. A useful diagnostic sign is the redness and increased prominence of the opening of Steno's duct in the mucous membrane of the cheek. *Acute cervical adenitis* is a frequent source of error in diagnosis. In it, however, the center of the swollen area appears to be *below the jaw*, while in mumps it is just below the lobe of the ear, and early in the attack the sharp edge of the gland can be outlined. The course of adenitis is much more prolonged and the swelling more tender, with redness of the skin covering it. Mumps primary in the submaxillary gland cannot at first be distinguished from lymphadenitis. The more rapid course and sudden onset of the salivary inflammation, the lesser degree of induration, and the development of cases of parotid disease in the household aid in making a diagnosis. The diagnosis of sublingual involvement should be made only after exclusion of other possible inflammations in the locality. An association with mumps in other salivary glands or attacking other inmates of the house would generally be necessary to make the diagnosis certain. We have seen the swelling due to blockage of the ducts from a salivary calculus diagnosed as mumps. A *secondary parotitis* occurring in the course of other diseases, such as typhoid fever, sepsis, and the like, is slower in development, unilateral, and tends to suppuration. We have more than once seen *diphtheria* supposed to be mumps, the swelling in the lymphatic glands and subcutaneous tissue of the neck being referred by the observer to the parotid gland. Only a careless failure to examine the fauces can account for the error. In *Mikulicz's disease* or in disease due to tumors or to syphilis the enlargement of the glands is chronic and noninflammatory in nature.

Treatment. **Prophylaxis.**—Quarantine to be of any service should continue for three or four weeks or longer from the appearance of symptoms. Hess[39] advised the injection of convalescent's blood, or of that of persons who had had mumps some years earlier. The dose is 2 to 4 cc. given before the seventh day after exposure. Success with this has been reported by Regan,[40] and Barenberg and Ostroff.[41] We have found it of value, but not to the same extent as similar treatment in chicken-pox or measles. In the cases of Barenberg and Ostroff the incidence of mumps was 15 per cent in the treated and 39 per cent in the untreated.

Treatment of the Attack.—This is largely symptomatic. If there is fever, the patient must be confined to bed and given a light diet; especially one that does not require chewing. Sour substances should be avoided lest they increase the pain. Pain may be alleviated by hot fomentations or by a hot-water bag with cotton interposed. The severe nervous symptoms may require treatment with hydrotherapy or sedatives, or perhaps lumbar puncture. It is claimed that the incidence of orchitis can be lowered by injections of convalescent's serum, given early in the disease, but this procedure is hardly necessary in childhood. For involvement of the central nervous system, injections of convalescent's serum may be tried intraspinally, intramuscularly, or intravenously.

References

1. Rév. méd. de la Suisse rom., 1883, **3,** 81. 2. Wien. med. Blätt., 1883, **11,** 1613. 3. Brit. M. J., 1902, **1,** 1537. 4. Am. J. M. Sc., 1855, **29,** 56. 5. Compt. rend. soc. de biol., 1881, **33,** 192; 358. 6. Rév. mens. d. mal. d. l'enf., 1885, **3,** 297. 7. Compt. rend. soc. de biol., 1889, **41,** 644. 8. Compt. rend. soc. de biol., 1893, **45,** 95; 528. 9. Med. Rec., 1896, **50,** 440. 10. Verhandl. 15. Cong. f. inn. Med., 1897, 441. 11. Wien. klin. Rundsch., 1902, **16,** 309. 12. Am. J. M. Sc., 1919, **158,** 698. 13. Compt. rend. soc. de biol., 1906, **60,** 803; 853; 897. 14. Ann. de l'inst. Pasteur, 1925, **39,** 565; Bull. soc. de pédiat. de Paris, 1926, **41,** 18. 15. Rep. Local Gov. Board, London, 1913–14, **43,** 116. 16. Compt. rend. soc. de biol., 1913, **75,** 217. 17. J. Exper. Med., 1916, **23,** 353; 1919, **29,** 377. 18. Semaine méd., 1893, **13,** 99. 19. Gaz. méd. d. Paris, 1887, 7s, **4,** 510. 20. München. med. Wchnschr., 1893, **40,** 656. 21. Pediatria, 1916, **24,** 733. 22. Bull. acad. de méd. Paris, 1912, Jan. 16; Ref. Arch. f. Kinderh., 1913, Suppl., Bd. 41. 23. Thèse de Paris, 1913. 24. Am. J. M. Sc., 1922, **163,** 859. 25. Am. J. M. Sc., 1931, **181,** 255. 26. Thèse de Paris, 1907. 27. Am. J. Dis. Child., 1913, **6,** 399. 28. Am. J. Dis. Child., 1919, **18,** 187. 29. Arch. latino-am. de pediat., 1919, **13,** 130; Ref. Monatschr. f. Kinderh., 1921, **21,** 231. 30. Monatschr. f. Kinderh. Orig., 1918, **15,** 147. 31. Gaz. d. hôp., 1898, **71,** 1329. 32. J.A.M.A., 1908, **51,** 1961. 33. Phys. and Surg., **39,** No. 5; Ref. Centralbl. f. inn. Med., 1908, **29,** 67. 34. Rév. de méd. Paris, 1885, **5,** 192. 35. Montpellier méd. 1888, **10,** 509; 1888, **11,** 15. 36. Wien. med. Wchnschr., 1921, **16,** 637. 37. Pfaundler und Schlossmann's Handbk. d. Kinderh., 1923, **2,** 336. 38. Communic. Dis. Control Rep. Sec. 2, White House Conf. on Child Health and Protect., 1931. 39. Am. J. Obstet., 1915, **72,** 183. 40. J.A.M.A., 1925, **84,** 279. 41. Am. J. Dis. Child., 1931, **42,** 1109.

CHAPTER XVIII

MALARIA

History.—The disease has existed since early times, and different forms of it are well described by Hippocrates. Here will be discussed chiefly the features which are seen in the disease occurring in infants and children.

Etiology. Predisposing Causes.—Malaria is widely distributed, but steadily growing less frequent in temperate climates, although more numerous in some years than in others. More cases are observed in summer and autumn. All *ages* are attacked, and the studies of Koch[1] in Java seem to prove that malaria is very common in infancy in malarial districts. The new-born may exhibit it, cases of fetal infection being on record in which the parasite has been found in the blood shortly after birth. Such instances have been reported by Crandall;[2] Simms and Warwick;[3] Pies;[4] Lemaire, Dumolard and Laffont;[5] Laffont;[6] Bass;[7] Cuadra;[8] Forbes;[9] Trimble;[10] Magid;[11] Alarcon;[12] and Langeron and von Nitsen.[13] The affection is endemic in some regions and rarely seen in others.

Exciting Cause.—Many observations have confirmed the discovery by Laveran[14] in 1880, that the cause of the disease is a parasite of the sporozoa class named the plasmodium malariae. These parasites pass through a definite life-cycle in which they exhibit forms seemingly diverse. In the process they destroy the red blood corpuscles, producing pigment which appears in the leukocytes and in some of the tissues of the body. It was discovered by Golgi[15] that there is more than one variety of parasite, and that each produces a different form of the disease. These are as follows:

1. The parasite of tertian malarial fever (Plasmodium vivax), which has a life-cycle in human blood of about forty-eight hours.

2. The parasite of quartan malarial fever (Plasmodium malariae), which has a life-cycle of seventy-two hours.

3. The parasite of aestivo-autumnal (Tropical) fever (Plasmodium precox), the life-cycle of which is variable, ranging from twenty-four to forty-eight hours. It is in this last form that the well-known crescent-shaped bodies, as well as the flagellated forms, are produced.

Transmission.—Malaria may be transmitted by experimental inoculation with the blood of the patient, as first demonstrated by Gerhardt.[16] Except in this respect the disease is not contagious. It was shown by Manson[17] that it is communicated by the mosquito, and by Ross[18] that the parasite developed in the body of this insect. Grassi and Bignami[19] succeeded in transmitting the disease directly from insect to man. Various species of the genus Anopheles are the only vectors. They acquire the infection only by the sucking of the blood of a malarial patient. In the body of the mosquito the organism then passes through another, viz. a sexual, cycle of development different from that seen in man.

Pathologic Anatomy.—The spleen is always more or less enlarged and very soft, especially in children. It exhibits pigment and broken-down corpuscles. The liver may be hypertrophied and pigmented, and the kidneys enlarged, with pigmentation of the glomeruli. There is sometimes an acute or chronic nephritis, and the gastro-intestinal mucous membrane and even the skin may exhibit pigment.

Symptoms. Period of Incubation.—This is uncertain, and even in experimental malaria it varies from three to twenty-one days.

Typical Form.—The ordinary intermittent form of the disease is seen in adults and later childhood much oftener than at earlier periods. Vague prodromal symptoms are often present, lasting one or more days. There then occurs a typical paroxysm, beginning with such symptoms as malaise, headache, lassitude, general pains, and often vomiting. This is promptly followed by a chill, the *cold stage,* lasting ten minutes to an hour or more. In this, although the patient shivers and looks pinched and blue, and the surface of the body feels cold to the touch, the thermometer shows decided rise in temperature. The second, or *hot stage* follows, with the temperature reaching 104 to 106 F. (40 to 41.1 C.), its maximum being developed during or shortly after the chill. The patient looks and feels hot. The spleen can often be felt. The duration of this stage is from three or four up to twelve hours. This second stage is gradually replaced by the third, or *sweating stage,* with the uncomfortable symptoms disappearing and the temperature rapidly returning to normal. The total duration of the paroxysm averages from six to twelve hours.

The *blood* exhibits, in addition to the parasites, a very decided and rapidly developing anemia in those who have had several paroxysms. There is leukopenia, or at least absence of leukocytosis, and a characteristically relative increase in the number of large mononuclear cells. The leukocytes often contain pigment-granules. Netter[20] found the fragility of the red-cells decreased during the attack. Genoese[21] states that in severe cases in infants the spinal fluid may exhibit during the attack an increase of albumin and sometimes a lymphocytosis. Instead of beginning at almost the same hour on the days of attacks, the paroxysms sometimes "anticipate" slightly (Fig. 78).

In many instances in young children, malaria assumes an irregular, continuous, or remitting type with the various stages of the paroxysm less marked, or not separated at all.

Varieties of the Typical Form.—1. *Tertian Malarial fever* is much the most frequent form in temperate zones. In *Simple Tertian* but one set of germs is present and the paroxysms occur every third, *i. e.*, every other, day, usually at about the same hour (Fig. 78). Should two sets of the tertian organism be present, sporulating on alternate days, *Double Tertian,* or *Quotidian, fever* occurs, the patient having a paroxysm every day (Fig. 79).

2. *Quartan fever* is rare in the Northern United States, and less common in the Southern than are other forms. In it there is a paroxysm every fourth day; *i. e.*, with free intervals of two days. Should two sets of the organism be present, paroxysms occur on two consecutive days, with only

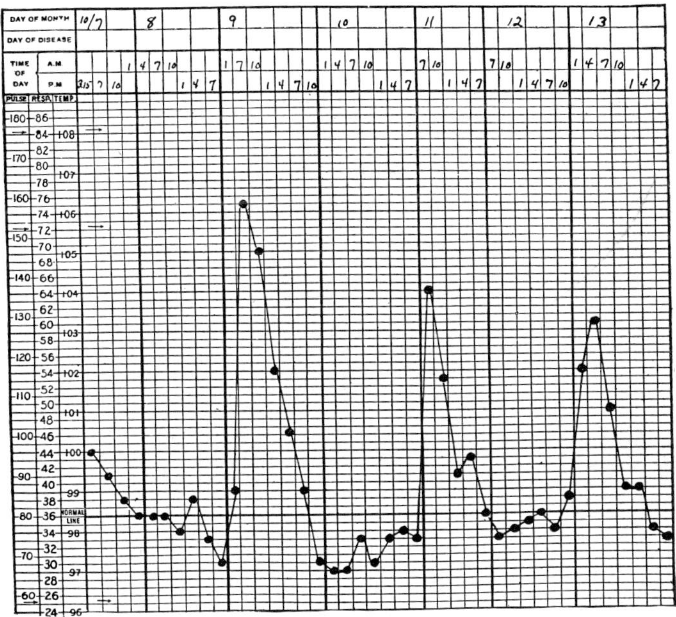

Fig. 78.—Malaria; Simple tertian. John T., aged two years. Oct. 6, fever, thirst, diarrhea; Oct. 7, spleen large, free urination; Oct. 9, plasmodium found in blood; Oct. 13, paroxysm anticipated several hours.

one day free, or if three sets are present, *Quotidian* (*i. e.*, triple quartan) fever is produced.

3. *Aestivo-autumnal fever* (Tropical Fever, Remittent Fever) occurs in both temperate and tropical regions. The severer cases are seen in the Southern United States or farther south. In this variety the attack is usually of the remittent type; *i. e.*, the temperature, although lessening at intervals, does not reach normal; and the paroxysms, if present, are of longer duration. In other cases the individual paroxysms may be little or not at all observed, and in still others the temperature is continuous. Sometimes, although dependent upon the aestivo-autumnal parasite, the attack is distinctly intermittent and either quotidian or tertian in character.

There are *pernicious types* of aestivo-autumnal fever and these may occasionally be produced, too, by the tertian or quartan parasite. In the *algid form,* there is an extreme sensation of coldness and excessive prostration, with the temperature little elevated or often subnormal. Another variety is the *comatose form*, with unconsciousness and high fever. The *hemorrhagic form* of pernicious malaria (Blackwater Fever) is characterized by hemoglobinuria, jaundice, and uncontrollable vomiting. It is very uncommon in childhood.

IRREGULAR FORMS.—It is particularly in infancy and early childhood that variations from definite types of the disease are seen, or that certain symptoms are especially prominent. The typical course is more often absent than present at this time of life. The onset is more abrupt, the whole paroxysm is often shorter, and the division of the attack into stages is frequently absent or little marked. Especially in infants the symptoms may be so irregular and so devoid of periodicity that the disease is fre-

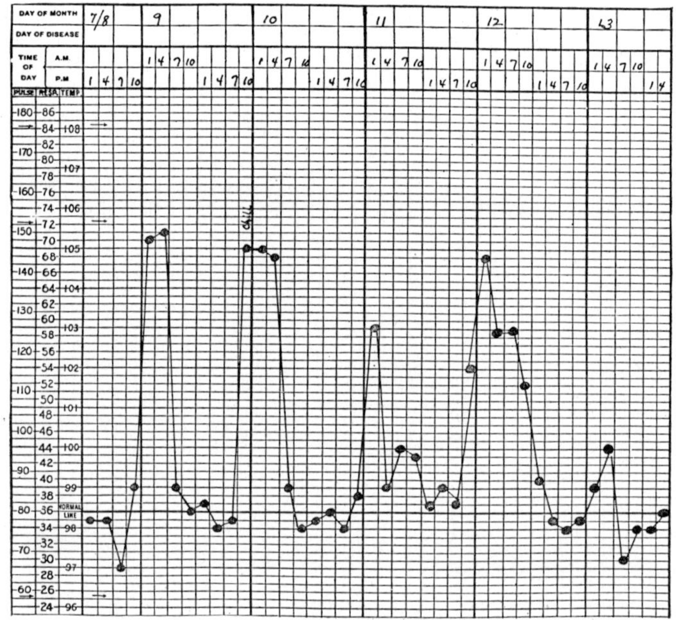

Fig. 79.—Malaria; Double tertian. Lizzie Q., aged eight years. Been having chill every night followed by fever. Vomited once. Examination showed enlarged spleen and parasites in blood. Attacks controlled by 20 grains (1.296) of quinine by mouth and 10 grains (.648) by suppository given on 12th. Previous small doses without effect.

quently overlooked. The chill in early life is usually replaced by mere coldness, pallor, and blueness of the face and extremities; or by yawning and drowsiness, or not infrequently convulsions. Vomiting is a common initial symptom. In the hot stage vomiting may continue and there is coating of the tongue and loss of appetite. Constipation may be present, but diarrhea is very common and sometimes is profuse. The younger the child the more liable is diarrhea to occur. The infant exhibits either drowsiness, or restlessness and crying. The temperature is usually higher in early life and is prone to run a much more irregular course, approaching sometimes, even in tertian fever, a remittent or continuous type (Fig. 80), due, probably, to the presence of a number of sets of the tertian parasite; or fever may be absent in young infants (Mulherin and Mulherin[22]). Nervous symptoms are prominent. Headache and pain in the epigastrium, limbs, or splenic or hepatic region are very frequent, and delirium is not uncommon. Bronchitis is a very common symptom and not infrequently

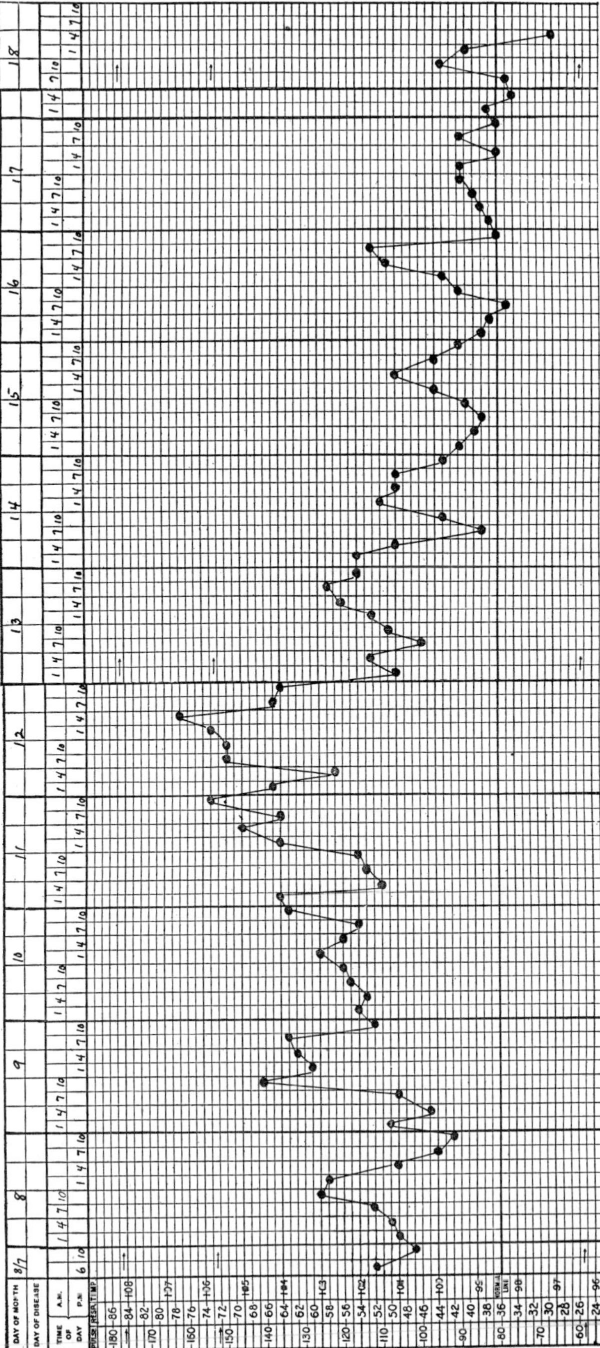

Fig. 80.—Malaria; irregular infantile type. Harriet L., aged nineteen months. Been ill for five days with loss of appetite, malaise, diarrhea and repeated vomiting. Examination showed enlarged spleen and liver and numerous plasmodia in the blood. Given 10 grains (.648) of quinine daily, by suppository, beginning on Aug. 9, without effect; and 10 grains (.648) quinine, taken by mouth, daily, beginning on the 13th.

there may be a degree of pulmonary congestion, especially in infancy, which suggests pneumonia. The sweating stage is absent or little marked in children under two years of age, and when seen is liable to be attended by considerable prostration. According to Mulherin and Mulherin[22] enlargement of the spleen is not discoverable in fully 30 per cent of the cases in young infants. In some cases malaria may be *latent*, the usual symptoms, including fever, being absent, and disease suggested only by such obscure manifestations as a periodical recurring cephalalgia or cardialgia, periodic diarrhea, periodic torticollis, or an obstinate cough which yields only to quinine. The parasite may remain dormant in the system for months, the patient having only at times recurrent attacks.

In patients who have had repeated attacks *malarial cachexia* develops, characterized by large spleen, great anemia, and dropsy of the skin and serous cavities. There may be cough, vague pains, and occasional fever, but nothing characteristic.

Complications and Sequels.—One of the most prominent is bronchitis. Congestion of the lungs often occurs, and exceptionally a pneumonia. Among more or less common complications are obstinate vomiting, severe diarrhea, jaundice, herpes, glycosuria, and vesical irritability. Less common are epistaxis, urticaria, and erythema; and occasionally observed are symmetrical gangrene, endocarditis, torticollis, neuritis, aphasia, hemiplegia or other paralyses, and a hemorrhagic or chronic nephritis. Malaria may occur in combination with, or as a sequel to, other infectious diseases.

Recurrence and Relapse.—The tendency to relapse is one of the great characteristics of malaria. This is due to the fact that the nonsegmented form of the organism may persist in the blood for an indefinite time, but without producing symptoms. On the other hand, infected individuals may finally become immune, and natives of some malarial districts do not readily acquire the disease, apparently because they have developed this immunity through repeated atypical attacks in infancy. It is usually impossible to determine how often a new attack is a *relapse*, due to an infection already present, and how often a *recurrence* through a reinfection from without.

Course and Prognosis.—The duration is uncertain, and unless treated by quinine the disease may continue indefinitely and pass into the chronic stage. In the tertian type particularly it may stop after a week or more, although prone to relapse frequently. Pernicious cases end fatally in a day or two. Malarial cachexia may last for months or years. While the disease is often severe in the tropics and the cause of many deaths, in temperate climates the prognosis is usually good in districts where the malady is sporadic or occurs only exceptionally in epidemic form. This is most true of the intermittent type, particularly if the subject is protected from repeated reinfection. In the Southern United States the aestivo-autumnal form is attended by a rather high mortality in infancy. The prognosis is markedly affected by treatment.

Diagnosis.—The diagnosis is easy in typical cases, but often presents great difficulties in the anomalous and irregular forms, which are especially liable to develop in early life. The most satisfactory diagnostic characteristics are the cure by quinine, if given in sufficient dosage, and the discovery of the parasite in the blood. The search for the parasite is best made a few hours before the paroxysm is expected, since at other times it may not be discoverable. The finding of much pigment free in the blood is suspicious.

Suppurative conditions may simulate malaria closely, and may exhibit an intermittent fever with chills and sweats. These disorders may usually be discovered by careful examination, the fever is only temporarily affected by quinine, and they present a leukocytosis rather than a leukopenia. Malaria may also be closely simulated at times by *tuberculosis* and by *typhoid fever*. It was a habit very common in former years to attribute to malaria various obscure conditions for which no satisfactory explanation could be found. This has been the cause of many fatal errors in diagnosis.

Treatment. Prophylaxis.—This consists in the destruction of the anopheles, the protection from bites of the insects, and the prevention of relapse in those who have had the disease. The avoidance of relapse is to be accomplished by the frequent administration of small doses of quinine at the time of the year when malaria is most likely to occur. Persons obliged to visit malarial regions should take quinine in small doses constantly. It is to be remembered that the anopheles do their biting at night. There should be protection by mosquito netting, and by the application to the skin of ointments containing pennyroyal, menthol, tar, citronella, or other substances disagreeable to the insects. It is interesting that in certain communities where there has been no malaria, but where the anopheles exist, sporadic cases of the disease have been discovered, which could be traced to biting of mosquitos infected by plasmodia acquired from patients with paresis, who had been therapeutically inoculated with the organisms.

Treatment of the Attack.—Quinine is a specific. To subjects old enough it can be given in capsules; for those younger it must be in solution. Either the sulphate (74 per cent quinine), the bisulphate (59 per cent), the hydrochloride (82 per cent) or the dihydrochloride (82 per cent) may be employed. In solutions the last is best on account of its solubility and strength. The taste of these salts may be disguised to a certain extent by the syrups of yerba santa, licorice, cocoa, chocolate, or other pleasant menstruum. The tannate (30 to 35 per cent) is less effective, but in the form of "Quinine chocolates" is often readily taken by children. Quinine ethylcarbamate (aristochin) (96 per cent) is a comparatively tasteless quinine derivative. Quinine should be given in a single large dose two or three hours before the occurrence of the paroxysm, since at this time the parasites are outside the red blood-cells and are more readily killed. If vomiting is produced, smaller doses must be given every two or three hours, beginning three or four hours after the paroxysm is over. In irregular or intermittent forms, and in serious cases, the patient should receive a large dose at once, and then be kept fully under the influence of the drug by small repeated doses.

When not tolerated by the mouth, quinine may be given by bowel in enema or suppository. The dihydrochloride, or the hydrochloride of quinine and urea, may be administered subcutaneously, or, preferably, intramuscularly to avoid danger of abscess. Quinine hydrochloride (10 grains in 100 cc. of solution) can, however, be given intravenously, but there is little evidence that this method possesses any advantage, since the drug does not appear to act directly, but perhaps by the formation of a decomposition-product. When the attack of malaria has been controlled, quinine should be continued in small doses for a few weeks.

Plasmochin (alkyl-amino-6-methoxyquininolinea) is a newer remedy widely used, which has not seemed to be without danger, since it may cause methemoglobinemia. It possesses no marked superiority over quinine.

Dose.—Quinine is borne by children in relatively large amounts. Taking the sulphate as the type, and with due regard to the comparative basic strength of other salts, an infant of one year should receive 6 to 8 grains (0.39 to 0.52) in the course of twenty-four hours, and sometimes much larger doses are needed. In later childhood the dose may be as large as for adults. For parenteral administration the dose is about the same as for oral. For rectal employment it should be two or three times as large.

Treatment of the Paroxysm.—In addition to quinine treatment, warm covers and dry heat in the cold stage, and sponging in the hot stage may be employed.

Treatment of Chronic Malaria.—Quinine should be administered, as well as such tonics as iron, arsenic, and the like to overcome the anemia. Removal from the malarial region is important. The spleen has been extirpated in some cases of chronic malaria, but this does not offer a certain promise of cure. Roentgen-ray treatment of the spleen in chronic malaria causes a diminution of its size, and in some cases a prevention of recurrent attacks. It should not be employed in acute malaria.

References

1. Deutsche med. Wchnschr., 1900, **26,** 88. 2. New York Polyclinic, 1893, **1,** 38. 3. J.A.M.A., 1908, **51,** 916. 4. Monatschr. f. Kinderh., Orig., 1910, **9,** 51. 5. Bull. et mém. soc. méd. d. hôp. de Paris, 1910, **20,** 866. 6. Thèse de Paris, 1910. 7. Arch. Pediat., 1914, **31,** 251. 8. Arch. de méd. d. enf., 1920, **23,** 606. 9. Am. J. Dis. Child., 1923, **25,** 130. 10. China M. J., 1924, **38,** 121. 11. Monatschr. f. Geburtsh. and Gynäk., 1928, **79,** 404. 12. Bull. soc. de pédiat. de Paris, 1928, **26,** 52. 13. Bull. soc. de pédiat. de Paris, 1928, **26,** 98. 14. Bull. acad. de méd. Paris, 1880, **45,** 1346. 15. Gaz. degli osp., 1886, **7,** 419. 16. Ztschr. f. klin. Med., 1884, **7,** 372. 17. Brit. M. J., 1894, **2,** 1306. 18. Brit. M. J., 1897, **2,** 1786. 19. Ref. Mannaberg, Nothnagel's Encyclop., Pract. Med., Am. Ed., Malaria, 117. 20. Rev. méd. de Bogotá, 1919, **27,** 52; Ref. J.A.M.A., 1919, **73,** 72. 21. Il Policlinico, 1919, **26,** 737. 22. J.A.M.A., 1922, **78,** 1873.

CHAPTER XIX

RABIES. RAT-BITE FEVER. TULAREMIA

RABIES

(Hydrophobia, Lyssa)

Etiology.—Rabies is an acute infectious disorder communicated to man by the bite of other infected mammals. Dogs are especially prominent in transmission, because of their great susceptibility to the disorder and their opportunity for attack, particularly on children. It may occur, however, in other domestic animals, such as the cat, horse, and cow, and in many wild animals, as the wolf, skunk, and fox. Possibly it can be transmitted by bats (Lassele[1]). In fact no species of mammal is immune. It is denied that there can be transmission from the infectious saliva brought into contact with unbroken skin or mucous membrane, although such an occurrence is reported by Galtier.[2] It has rarely been conveyed by the bite of a human. Transmission through milk secreted by a rabid cow is improbable (Mugrage[3]).

The specific virus may be found in the saliva and the central nervous system. It is transmitted from the wound of entrance to the central nervous system along the nerve-sheaths, a fact which explains the shorter incubation occurring after bites of the head as compared with bites of the lower extremities. So, too, children, on account of their smaller stature and the shorter distance the virus has to travel, show a more rapid onset of symptoms than do adults. There is also in children the probability of their suffering more numerous bites, with the consequent introduction of larger amounts of virus. Twenty-four per cent of those bitten by rabid dogs develop the disease, according to the estimate of Williams,[4] based on Babes[5] statistics.

The bite of the cat, and especially of the wolf, causes relatively more infections. Part of the low morbidity is explained by the action of clothing in wiping off the virus. Punctured wounds, with the possibility of sealing in of the virus, are more dangerous than lacerations, unless the latter are extensive and offer a larger surface for absorption. Rabies is more frequent in animals in the summer, and the incidence in humans is consequently greater at this time.

Pathologic Anatomy.—In the central nervous system are found minute hemorrhages and areas of softening. The so-called "Rabic tubercles" of Babes,[5] consisting of groups of small round-cells surrounding the blood-vessels and nerve-cells of the spinal cord, have been considered characteristic, but are not always present. The bodies first described by Negri[6] can be found in almost all cases and are pathognomonic. They consist of small, oval or round bodies 10 to 15μ in diameter, with one or more nuclei; are found especially in the hippocampus major, but are often widespread throughout the cellular nervous tissue. It is not certain whether they are forms of micro-organisms or necrosis of nerve-cells. There is often observed the disappearance of the large cells in the cerebrospinal ganglia, and their replacement by small round-cells. Other findings are those of encephalitis and myelitis.

Symptoms.—The *incubation period* is very variable, depending upon the nature of the wound, and may be as short as two weeks, although the average is about six weeks. While it is said that several months or longer may intervene between infection and symptoms, the probability of the development of the disease after three months is slight.

In the *early* stage of the attack, lasting about twenty-four hours, nervous excitability is manifested by irritability and apprehension. General evidences of infection are present, such as slight fever and anorexia, rapid pulse and the like, and the site of the bite may become inflamed and painful or numb. Hoarseness and the characteristic difficulty in swallowing soon appear, and shortly any attempt at drinking, or even external stimuli such as noises or the sight or suggestion of food and water, produce violent laryngeal and pharyngeal spasms. It is from this characteristic that the popular name Hydrophobia is derived. Drooling occurs because of the inability to swallow the saliva. The *second* stage, that of excitement, has now developed, and the nervous symptoms increase in severity and mania may occur, although usually the patient is rational between the spasmodic attacks. Humans seldom injure or attempt to bite attendants. The hoarse sounds made with the contracted larynx have given rise to the false idea that the patient barks. The temperature in this stage may reach 102 or 103 F. (38.9 or 39.4 C.). After two or three days the patient passes into the *third*, or paralytic, stage in which unconsciousness soon appears and death occurs within twenty-four hours from syncope. The mortality is practically 100 per cent.

Diagnosis.—A differential diagnosis should be made from a hysterical condition (*lyssophobia*), in which a neurotic individual, who has been bitten by a dog and dreads the possibility of the development of rabies, presents some of its symptoms. This would be unlikely to occur in a young child. In older children it could be recognized by the lack of severity of the symptoms, as well as the continuance of them beyond a few days, and the final recovery. Tetanus might give rise to confusion if it is of the type in which only the muscles of the head are involved, and laryngeal spasm is associated. Diagnosis of the condition of the attacking animal is of great importance. This should be made by the history of its behavior and by observation of its symptoms, death occurring in the animal in less than five or, at most, ten days. For these reasons it should not be killed, as well as because the Negri bodies in its central nervous system are more likely to be found in the later stages than at the onset of symptoms. Inoculation of rabbits with infected tissue of the central nervous system will produce the disease in them, but only after two or three weeks. Many cities and practically all States make provision for the examination of animals for rabies. The head and neck should be sent packed in ice, or the brain and medulla placed in equal parts of glycerin and water, the mixture having been previously sterilized by boiling.

Treatment.—The most effective *preventive* treatment is the systematic muzzling of all dogs. It is also possible to vaccinate dogs against rabies. This is done by a single injection, or by dividing the dose into six parts. It is not protective against all strains of virus. In the case of children who have been bitten by an animal, the wound should be cauterized as soon as possible with nitric or carbolic acid or formalin, punctured wounds having first been laid open and bleeding encouraged. A diagnosis of the condition of the attacking animal is ascertained in the manner described above, but in suspicious cases the preventive inoculations of Pasteur[7] should be begun without delay. These consist in the daily injections of attenuated virus obtained by drying the spinal cord of infected rabbits, an emulsion of those which have been dried the longest being used in the earlier injections, and about 20 treatments given in all. Several other methods of preparing the vaccine are now recommended, such as killing it by phenol or dialyzing it. The opinion of the International Conference on Rabies[8] was that the virus introduced by Pasteur was preferable to other forms of the vaccine. In cases where the treatment has been started late, or where the wound has been on the face or hands, the first four to six injections are made at intervals of twelve instead of twenty-four hours. Probably the treatment should be given when there is contamination by infected saliva of open wounds, even when there has been no bite. Paralyses, particularly of the ascending Landry's type, may follow the treatment in rare instances. Whether these are due to the vaccine or to the failure of protection is not always clear. Protection afforded by the inoculations is probably of not more than a year's duration. A serum obtained from vaccinated animals and combined with attenuated virus has also been employed as a preventive measure.

The treatment of the attack already developed can be only palliative. The use of the serum from vaccinated animals has been tried in treatment of the attack, but without avail, and we have had no success with injections of serum obtained from persons recently injected with the vaccine. Quiet in a darkened room with avoidance of stimuli of all kinds, the frequent hypodermic injection of morphine in full doses, and inhalations of chloroform during the spasms constitute all that can be done.

RAT-BITE FEVER

This disease is common in Japan, and has been found at times in Europe following lines of marine traffic. Strauch and Bissell,[9] in a review of the subject, state that about 86 instances have been reported in the United States, to which number they add another case; and Reuben and Steffen[10] record 3 more. Dembo[11] and his colleagues report a case in an infant of seven months. Other cases have since been reported.

Etiology.—The bite of an infected rat and also of the cat (Mock and Morrow[12]) transmits the disease. It is probable that the infective agent is a spirochete called the *spirochaeta morsus muris* (Futake[13]). This has been found by different observers in many of the patients, and immune bodies have been demonstrated in the blood of those ill with the disease.

Symptoms.—The period of incubation is about one to three weeks. The onset is sudden, with chills, fever, and inflammatory reaction in the region of the rat-bite. The last may become so marked that necrosis follows. The fever is intermittent, with febrile periods of two to four days and afebrile periods of three to five days. The temperature varies from 101 to 105 F. (38.3 to 40.5 C.). Usually at the time of fever there is a peculiar rash observed, consisting of bluish-red, slightly raised areas varying from $\frac{1}{4}$ to $\frac{3}{4}$ in. (.6 to 1.9 cm.) in diameter, scattered over the neck, trunk, and extremities.

Prognosis.—The disease is usually self-limited after a course of about two months, but some cases are long-continued and result in anemia and malnutrition in much the same way as does malaria. The mortality without treatment is about 10 per cent.

Treatment.—Cauterization of a rat-bite wound is indicated immediately after its occurrence. The treatment is symptomatic unless the infection is severe or long continued, in which event the employment of intravenous injections of arsenical preparations is effective.

TULAREMIA

Tularemia is a disease of squirrels (McCoy and Chapin[14]), rabbits (Wherry and Lamb[15]), and muskrats (Schwartz[16]), and found also in sheep, wood-chucks, cats, sage-hen and certain other birds, ticks and perhaps mosquitos. It is caused by the *Bacterium tularense*, and may be transmitted to man by handling infected rabbits or other animals, or by the bite of a blood-sucking insect, such as the horse-fly. The first human cases in the country appear to have reported by Pearse[17] in Utah, and the disease has appeared in Ohio, West Virginia, District of Columbia, California, Idaho, Wyoming, Colorado, Indiana and North Carolina. It is apparently identical with Ohara's disease in Japan (Francis and Moore[18]). Many cases are probably not recognized, being mistaken for other diseases, as typhoid fever, septicemia, or the like. Clear descriptions of tularemia are given by Francis[19] and Verbrycke.[20]

Symptoms.—A characteristic local lesion appears four or five days after infection at the place bitten; or even without this, as when rubbed into the conjunctiva or when the germs enter through apparently unbroken skin. It consists of a dark or black center, which later becomes necrotic, and is surrounded by an area of very mild inflammation. The neighboring lymphatic glands are decidedly enlarged and not infrequently suppurate. The onset is accompanied by chills and fever, the latter continuing for from one to four weeks and in severe cases rising to 104 or 105 F. (40 or 40.5 C.). The temperature-chart resembles that of typhoid fever, except that there is a rather characteristic fall to normal on the third or fourth day of the disease quickly followed by a rise. There is marked prostration and the usual symptoms attending any febrile state. Local pain in the involved lymphatic glands is often present. Tularemia may occur without a local lesion but with glandular enlargement near the point of entrance, and there is a so-called "typhoid" form without a local lesion of any kind being discovered. The **diagnosis** is suggested by the history of contact with rabbits, and by the characteristic local lesion with glandular enlargement. The white blood-cells number about 12,000 or 14,000 and the blood-serum of the patient will give an agglutinative reaction with the *Bacterium tularense*. The **prognosis** is not grave, as the disease may run a mild course; although in severer cases there is marked prostration and a prolonged convalescence. One fatal instance has been reported (Verbrycke[20]). The **treatment** is symptomatic. Shelton[21] believes that quinine may be useful. Convalescent's serum has been tried in a few instances. Vaccines may be helpful in prognosis and treatment (Foshay[22]).

References

1. J.A.M.A., 1931, **97,** 1976. 2. Compt. rend. soc. de biol., 1890, **42,** 63. 3. J. Lab. and Clin. Med., 1930, **15,** 460. 4. Therap. of Int. Dis., Blumer, Billings, Forchheimer, 1924, **3,** 102. 5. Traité de la rage, 1912. 6. Ztschr. f. Hyg., 1903, **43,** 507. 7. Compt. rend. acad. d. sc., Paris, 1924, **38,** 648. 8. J.A.M.A., 1928, **88,** 1916. 9. Arch. Pediat., 1924, **41,** 315. 10. Arch. Pediat., 1924, **41,** 499. 11. Am. J. Dis. Child., 1925, **29,** 182. 12. Illinois M. J., 1932, **61,** 67. 13. J. Exper. Med., 1916, **23,** 249. 14. J. Infect. Dis., 1912, **10,** 61. 15. J. Infect. Dis., 1914, **15,** 331. 16. J.A.M.A., 1929, **92,** 1180. 17. Northwest Med., 1911, **3,** 81. 18. J.A.M.A., 1926, **86,** 1329. 19. J.A.M.A., 1922. **78,** 1015; 1925, **84,** 1243. 20. J.A.M.A., 1924, **82,** 1577. 21. J.A.M.A., 1925, **84,** 1019, 22. J. Infect. Dis., 1932, **51,** 286.

CHAPTER XX

TETANUS

(Lock Jaw)

Etiology. Predisposing Causes. *Age.*—The great majority of cases in early life occur in the new-born. The influence of age, however, is greatly modified by locality. In some countries Tetanus neonatorum has at times been endemic, and the cause of many deaths. This is shown by the figures of Miron,[1] who stated that of 23,398 infants dying in Roumania in the first month of life, 10,257 were cases of tetanus. It is more frequent in hot climates, but the chief predisposing factor is *absence of cleanliness.* The fact that negro infants in some regions of the Southern States are especially liable to it is due to hygienic carelessness and not to any influence of race. Hines[2] was able to collect from State Boards and U. S. Census Reports a total of 5767 deaths from tetanus in infants under one month of age from the years 1910 to 1927, and a total of 7925 deaths under one year of age from 1906 to 1927. A good review of the literature is given by this author.

The *presence of a wound,* although minute and perhaps undiscovered, is apparently necessary to the development of the disease. Punctured, lacerated and contused wounds, especially of the hands and face, are those particularly dangerous. It may occur several months after an injury has healed if the wound is reopened. It is quite probable that abraded surfaces of the mucous membrane of the intestine offer a portal of entry in some instances. It may follow burns, the wound of ritual circumcision or of vaccination if imperfectly cared for, and rarely suppurating disease of the ears or the eyes. Much the most frequent portal of entry in the new-born is the umbilical wound.

Exciting Cause.—The direct cause has been proved to be the *bacillus tetani,* discovered by Nicolaier[3] in 1884 and isolated by Kitasato[4] in 1889. It is found in garden soil, in the dust of streets, and in the intestinal canal of some herbivora. The bacilli inhabit the superficial portion of a wound, where the virulent poison is produced, and whence rapid absorption of this takes place. The tetanus-toxin exerts a special action on the motor cells in the medulla and on the anterior horns of the spinal cord. The bacilli are spore-formers and therefore tenacious of life, being uninjured by exposure to air or light, and resistant to the temperature of boiling water, or to disinfectants unless their action is prolonged.

Pathologic Anatomy.—There is found congestion of the brain and spinal cord and of their membranes, and often hemorrhage; these changes being probably the result of the convulsive condition rather than of the poison. There are no other characteristic postmortem lesions.

Symptoms. Tetanus Neonatorum.—The **incubation** varies from a few hours to ten or twelve days. Symptoms usually appear toward the end of the first week of life. The **onset** is marked by restlessness and difficulty in nursing, the infant dropping the nipple with a cry of pain. On examination the masseters will be found contracted, and the jaws can be forced open only with difficulty (*trismus*). The eyes are closed, the forehead wrinkled, and the lips pouting. In a few hours the stiffness extends to all the muscles of the body, at times producing arching. Next appears violent increase of the tonic contraction; this coming on in paroxysms which last a few moments, and which are repeated in severe cases perhaps every few minutes, but in milder cases at longer intervals. The paroxysms occur spontaneously or from any slight stimulation. During them the skin of the body and especially of the face becomes red and cyanotic, and the labial commissure is pulled down and outward, producing the *risus sardonicus*. (See Fig. 64 under Cerebrospinal Fever, p. 323.) The whole body is as rigid as a rod of iron, with opisthotonos, retraction of the head, and flexion of the fingers and toes. Respiration is irregular and superficial; swallowing becomes impossible; and the pulse is rapid and weak.

There is variation in the persistence of tonic contraction, especially of the trismus. It may be practically unbroken from the beginning, or complete relaxation may occur for long intervals. Slight clonic movements sometimes accompany the attack. Fever is usually slight or absent, except terminally.

Tetanus in Older Infants and in Childhood.—This differs in no way from that seen in adults. The **incubation** is variable, but usually not over ten days, and the **symptoms** consist of headache, chilliness, fever, stiffness in the neck, and especially difficulty in masticating or in opening the mouth. As the disease progresses the condition is much like that already described for tetanus neonatorum. During the paroxysm the body may assume the position of opisthotonos, but sometimes is straight (orthotonos), or doubled forward (emprosthotonos). The pain is intense. The mind remains clear. In fatal cases the fever is high, the paroxysms frequent, and the duration seldom more than three or four days; sometimes less than twenty-four hours or as long as six days. In cases which recover incubation is longer, the periods of relaxation more prolonged, the paroxysms diminishing in number and severity, and the whole course lasting several weeks. Sometimes only certain regions are attacked, especially the head and neck.

Course and Prognosis.—The *prognosis* of tetanus neonatorum is extremely bad. Hines[2] in an extensive review of English literature could find only 27 cases which recovered. On the other hand, some statistics give a mortality of only 50 per cent. The mortality appears to be inversely proportional to the length of incubation. In tetanus after the new-born period the prognosis is somewhat better. The absence of fever and an incubation of over ten days are the most favorable indications. The average mortality, however, varies from 50 to 80 per cent.

Diagnosis.—Tetanus is closely simulated by *strychnine poisoning*, except that in this condition complete relaxation occurs between the paroxysms and trismus is rare. *Tetany* may sometimes simulate tetanus, but in it the muscles of the limbs are primarily affected, and there is seldom involvement of the neck or jaws. *Meningitis* has been mistaken for tetanus, but there is in this a disordered mental state and the absence of trismus.

Treatment. **Prophylaxis.**—Cleanliness in the care of the umbilical wound is the safeguard against tetanus neonatorum. (See also Antitoxin Treatment.)

General Treatment of the Attack. The first indication is antiseptic treatment and perhaps cauterization of the wound, in order to prevent further production of the poison. The patient should be kept in a darkened room and handled very little, and all other sources of excitation reduced as much as possible. Large doses of such sedatives as chloral, the bromides, phenobarbital, and morphine should be given. Eserine has long been popular. It may be necessary to administer these drugs by bowel or through a nasal tube or by hypodermic injection. Ether or chloroform may be necessary during the paroxysms. Feeding may be accomplished by the rectal or nasal tube if there is inability to swallow.

Magnesium sulphate is a valuable remedy for control of the spasms. It is best given subcutaneously, but may be administered also intraspinally or intravenously. For subcutaneous injection the dose should be 0.6 to 0.8 cc. of a 25 per cent solution per kilogram (4 to 6 minims per pound) of body-weight three to four times a day, or much larger doses may be used. From 10 to 15 cc. (0.34 to 0.51 fl. oz.) or more of a 20 per cent solution may be given by rectum to infants of one year. For intraspinal treatment the dose should be 0.1 cc. of a 25 per cent solution per kilogram. In intravenous injection a 2 per cent solution should be used and not more than 15 cc. per kilogram of body weight should be employed. In case of respiratory paralysis from the magnesium sulphate 5 cc. (81 minims) of a 5 per cent solution of calcium chloride should be administered intramuscularly.

Antitoxin-treatment.—In 1890 von Behring and Kitasato[5] were able to immunize rabbits against, and to cure them of, tetanus by injecting a tetanus-antitoxin, and soon afterward this serum was employed in man. Its prophylactic value is unquestioned, but it must be administered as promptly as possible after the receipt of the wound; 15,000 units, or proportionately less in small children, being injected at once and repeated in ten days. The treatment is advisable whenever the wound is of a suspicious nature, and always when it is punctured or contaminated by dirt, garden soil, or gunpowder. Even if given late it may prolong the incubation period and thus bring about a milder attack. As to the treatment of the disease itself, the results are somewhat uncertain, due probably to the fact that union of the toxin with the cells of the central nervous system occurs very early. In order to reach any of the toxin which is being formed or is still uncombined the attempt should be made to saturate the patient with full doses, and a child of ten years may receive 10,000 units intravenously, followed by an equal amount intraspinally, and shortly afterward a similar dose intramuscularly. The doses vary according to the age and weight of the patient, but under any condition at least half the amount given should be by the intraspinal route.

References

1. II Cong. d. Rüman, Gesellsch. f. d. Fortsch. u. d. Verbreit. d. Wissensch., 1903, Sept. 22; Ref. Schmidt's Jahrb., 1904, B. 281; 206. 2. Am. J. Dis. Child., 1903, **39,** 560. 3. Deutsche. med. Wchnschr., 1884, **10,** 842. 4. Ztschr. f. Hyg., 1889, **7,** 225. 5. Deutsche. med. Wchnschr., 1890, **16,** 1113.

CHAPTER XXI

ACUTE POLIOMYELITIS

(Acute Infantile Paralysis; Meningo-encephalo-myelitis)

History.—The first account of this disease seems to be that of Underwood[1] in 1784, who, however, confessed ignorance of its cause and considered it not a common disorder. It was not until 1840 that a satisfactory description of it was given by Heine.[2] It was designated "Essential paralysis in Children" by Rilliet and Barthez[3] in 1843. Prévost[4] in 1865 and Charcot and Joffroy[5] in 1870 showed the association with lesions of the cells of the anterior horns of the spinal cord. The first study of its epidemic relations was made in Norway and Sweden especially by Medin,[6] and it was called the "Heine-Medin disease" by Wickman.[7] The usual term is "poliomyelitis," although pathologically it should be denominated "meningo-encephalo-myelitis." The term "acute infantile paralysis" really denotes a result of the disorder.

Etiology. **Predisposing Causes.**—*Age* is of great influence. As shown by the studies of Frost,[8] Wickman[9] and others, the majority of cases occur between the ages of one and five years, and especially in the second year. It may be seen even very early in life; Sinkler[10] reporting 1 case at six weeks and 2 at three months, and Gunewardene 1 in an infant of twelve days. In some epidemics the number of cases under one year is about 5 per cent. Practically all statistical reports note a slight preponderance of the disease among males. Everywhere the majority of attacks occur in the warmer *season*, the height of an epidemic in the northern hemisphere being July, August and September and in the southern hemisphere, February, March and April. *Geographical position*, *residence*, and *social position* have no real influence. The action of such factors as other infectious diseases, ill-health, exposure, fatigue and the like seems problematical. There is an impression that the disease is more common in those with light complexion. It occurs in about as many children with tonsils as in those who have had them removed, although rarely tonsillectomy is said to initiate it (Aycock and Luther[12]). The *individual susceptibility* is not great. Flexner and Amoss[13] suggest that there is a protective ability of the healthy mucous membrane to neutralize the virus. The majority of those exposed do not show active symptoms of the disorder, only about 2 per cent being susceptible (Herrman[14]). (See Transmission p. 388.) There have been a number of studies on the question of the development of multiple cases in a family or a household (Committee Report N. Y. Epidemic,[15] Wickman,[7] Everhart and Cole,[16] Robbins[17]). The instances of more than one patient in a family are relatively uncommon (6521 single cases out of 7000 in the New York epidemic of 1916),[15] but considering the total number of cases of the disease multiple household occurrence of the paralyzed and abortive types is not infrequent. This is especially true of certain epidemics (39 per cent in 395 families (Robbins[17]). The *epidemic influence* repeatedly alluded to is of great importance. Formerly a comparatively infrequent disease, in recent years its prevalence has increased enormously. The first local epidemic recorded appears to have been one of 8 or 10 cases in a rural region of Louisiana, reported by Colmer.[18] The first epidemic in Norway is said by Harbitz[19] to have consisted of 14 cases observed by Bull in 1868. A partial list of the reports of other epidemics is as follows: In Vermont in 1894 (Caverly[20]); in Stockholm in 1887 (Medin[6]); in Norway and Sweden in 1905 (Harbitz and Scheel,[21] Wickman[7]); collected list of 35 epidemics up to 1907 (Holt and Bartlett[22]); New York City and vicinity in 1907;[23] in the

United States in 1909 (Lovett and Richardson[24]); in Sweden in 1911 and 1912 (Wernstedt[25]); in Norway in 1911 (Johannessen[26]); in the United States in 1916 (Emerson[27]), and again in 1917 (Lavinder[28]). During the years 1926, 1927 and 1928 there were 4154 deaths from poliomyelitis in the United States Registration Area.[29] A good review of the history and epidemiology is given by McAusland.[30]

Exciting Cause.—That the disease is an infectious one seems to have been first suggested by Strümpell.[31] The investigations fall into two groups, maintaining the presence respectively of a bacterium, and of a filterable virus. Geirsvold[32] early described a diplococcus found in the spinal fluid and the organs. Rosenow, Towne and Wheeler,[33] Rosenow,[34] Nuzum and Herzog,[35] and Mathers[36] found a pleomorphic streptococcus in the central nervous system of patients dying from the disease, and in the throat and spinal fluid during life; have been able with it to reproduce typical symptoms and pathologic changes in monkeys and other animals and to recover the organism from the central nervous system of these animals; and have produced a serum which is claimed to have beneficial effect. (See also Treatment, p. 395.) Olitsky, Rhoads and Long[37] believe, with others, that this streptococcus is not the cause of poliomyelitis. They state that an organism similar to it could be obtained from the brain of a normal monkey and from the air of the laboratory; that injection into rabbits or monkeys produced changes different from those of poliomyelitis; and that there was no difference in the cerebral lesions produced by the streptococcus when inoculated into normal animals and into those which had recovered from poliomyelitis.

Regarding the filterable virus, investigations have been made by Landsteiner and Popper,[38] Flexner and Lewis,[39] Krause and Meinicke,[40] Römer and Joseph,[41] Osgood and Lucas,[42] Pettersson, Kling and Wernstedt,[43] and others. It has been shown that virus can be obtained from the brain, spinal cord, salivary and lymphatic glands, tonsils, nasopharyngeal and oral mucous membranes, blood, and probably the cerebrospinal fluid. This can be transmitted experimentally by inoculation of the monkey's body, including the brain, spinal cord, peritoneum, and subcutaneous tissue. The virus can also be transmitted by introducing it into the stomach and intestine, or by rubbing it upon the nasal mucous membrane. Monkeys are susceptible and can be immunized by injection of this virus. Some investigators have successfully transmitted it to rabbits. Later Flexner and Noguchi[44] discovered very minute globoid bodies in the tissues of the central nervous system, which appeared to have the power of infection.

There is no doubt that a disease resembling poliomyelitis can be transmitted to animals by a filterable virus. Whether this can be harmonized with the studies on the streptococcus remains to be seen. Rosenow and Towne[45] suggest that the globoid bodies of Flexner and Noguchi may be another form of the streptococcus, but Flexner does not agree with this, nor is it clear in his later publications that he is sure of the significance of these globoid bodies. Work by Cooper[47] lends support to the causative action of the streptococcus. It should be stated, however, that many workers believe that the streptococcus is only a contaminating organism or a secondary invader.

Method of Transmission. Infectivity.—It is probable that the virus is acquired from the nasal mucous membrane of an affected individual, enters the human organism of the receptor by way of the nasal mucous membrane, and, according to Flexner and Amoss,[48] reaches the nervous system through the lymph-channels without involvement of the blood. Some students believe that it may enter by way of the intestinal lymphatics (Burrows[49]). The view expressed by Peabody, Draper and Dochez,[50] and by Draper[51] is generally held, according to which poliomyelitis is believed to be a general infectious disease, with a secondary involvement of the nervous system. It is transmitted in some way from sick to well, and probably both directly and indirectly. It is commonly believed that the immunity usually found in adults who have never suffered from poliomyelitis comes about from infection by the virus which resulted in slight or no symptoms. Aycock and Kramer,[52] and Aycock and Luther[53] think that immunity is acquired by exposure to the virus rather continuously in interepidemic periods as well as in epidemics. It may be transmitted by apparently healthy persons acting as carriers, as shown by the fact that the virus can be obtained from their mucous membranes. These carriers may be suffering from the disease in an unrecognized form; they may have been in close contact with patients with the disease; or they may be recent convalescents, or have had the disease some time previously, and have become chronic carriers. It is not certain how often carriers, and especially the chronic ones, are a source of danger. It has also been claimed that the disease may be spread by such agencies as dust (Neustaedter[54]), bed-bugs (Howard and Clark[55]), house-flies (Flexner and Clark[56]), stable flies (Rosenau,[57] Anderson and Frost[58]), and by milk (Aycock[59]), and it is possible that some of these factors are of importance, but further confirmation is needed.

The infectiousness is very probably greatest in the early stages of the disease, but may persist for a considerable time after convalescence. The virus has been found on the nasal mucous membrane of attendants upon patients even seven months after the attack (Osgood and Lucas;[42] Pettersson, Kling and Wernstedt[43]).

Pathologic Anatomy.—This has been studied with especial care in human beings by Wickman[60] and by Harbitz and Scheel,[61] and in monkeys by Landsteiner and Popper[38] and Flexner.[62] There is a disseminated lymphocytic infiltration of the pia and of all parts of the central nervous system, but largely, in most instances, of the gray matter of the cord especially in the anterior horns. Hemorrhages, small or more diffuse, sometimes occur into the gray matter. There rapidly follows degeneration and disappearance of the ganglion-cells of the grey matter, the degree and extent of which vary greatly. The white matter of the cord and the spinal ganglia show similar congestion, edema, and infiltration of the perivascular spaces. The medulla and pons are affected in like manner, but usually to a less degree. The cerebellum and cerebral hemispheres are not so often involved. The anterior horns of the lumbar and cervical enlargements of the cord are the favorite site of the lesions, but the process is, in fact, a diffuse one, involving more or less the entire cord, the meninges of the brain and cord, and portions of the brain itself. The pathologic changes may be much greater in extent than can be anticipated from the clinical picture. In acute cases other organs show such alterations as are seen in any infectious disorder. Hyperplasia of the lymphoid tissue of the intestine, spleen and lymphatic glands is common, and the spleen, lymph-nodes, and thymus may be much enlarged. In cases of long standing the affected portion of the spinal cord is shrunken, and the nervous tissue replaced by sclerotic tissue and neuroglia. From disuse there may be an atrophic condition of the bones in the affected limbs.

Symptoms.—A number of distinct types in addition to the ordinary spinal form will later be described. Many of the statements which follow upon such topics as incubation, method of invasion, and certain of the symptoms apply equally well to all forms of the disease.

1. Spinal Form.—With the exception of the abortive form this is the most frequent variety, consisting of about 90 per cent of the cases in most epidemics.

Incubation.—According to the studies of Aycock and Eton[63] and Aycock and Luther[53] this may vary from six to twenty days. There are no symptoms.

Stage of Invasion.—The onset is usually acute. Analysis of the symptoms at the onset in about 200 cases which we have seen at the Cincinnati General Hospital shows that they appeared in the following order of frequency: Fever, drowsiness, headache, stiffness and pain in the neck, vomiting, restlessness, coryza, photophobia; and, with much less frequency, sore throat, chills, diarrhea, ataxia, hyperesthesia, and sweating. The incidence of these symptoms varies in different epidemics. Respiratory symptoms were most prominent in over ½ of Müller's[64] cases. The tendon-reflexes may in some cases be temporarily increased, but are soon lost. Fever is nearly always present, but is very variable. It is sometimes slight, sometimes continuous, sometimes remittent, sometimes disappearing when the paralysis appears. The symptoms in general of the stage of invasion persist during the first three or four days, seldom lasting more than six or seven days in all. An exception is the initial drowsiness, which disappears soon, and the mind is clear. The pulse is accelerated, often out of proportion to the fever. Retention of urine is not infrequent. Examination of the *blood* may often show moderate leukocytosis. In a series of cases studied by us the leukocyte count ranged from 5800 to 17,900; 50 per cent of the cases having a normal count, or a slight leukopenia for the age of the patient. The total duration of fever from the onset averages about four days, but may range from one to ten days. Pain is a frequent symptom, and this, with hyperesthesia, may continue for weeks. The spinal fluid is clear or slightly opalescent, sometimes forms a fibrin clot, gives a moderate reaction for globulin, and promptly reduces copper solution. The colloidal gold test may show an early transitory reaction in the syphilitic zone (Jeans and Johnston;[65] Regan and Cheney;[66] Regan, Litvak and Regan[67]). (See p. 435.) Pressure is increased in the majority of cases. The microscopical examination of the spinal fluid should be made promptly after it is obtained, since the cells quickly undergo autolysis (Lyon[68]). There is an increase of the cells varying from 20 up to 200 or more. Early in the prodromal stage these may be polymorphonuclear in character, but very shortly the mononuclears become predominant and reach 80 to 90 per cent of the total number before paralysis is manifest. The cellular increase diminishes rapidly as the paralysis appears. There are fewer cells found in the bulbar cases.

The *duration* of the period of invasion varies, the average being about three or four days, but very often prodromal symptoms are absent or overlooked, and the paralysis comes on suddenly while the child is walking or sitting; or the child, apparently previously well at night, is found paralyzed in the morning. In other cases the symptoms may continue for a week before paralysis appears.

Stage of Acute Paralysis.—At the close of the stage of invasion paralysis shows itself; generally at first as a decided weakness of some of the muscles, but increasing in degree and extent during three or four days. Generally there is no increase of the paralysis after acute constitutional symptoms disappear, but exceptionally it develops more slowly. Tendon-reflexes are diminished or lost in the affected muscles. The regions involved vary greatly. Not all the muscles of an affected limb are involved, nor do all the fibers of any muscle participate in the process. When the extremities of both sides of the body are attacked, one side is almost always more severely affected than the other. There may be a combination of different forms of paralysis, such, for example, as involvement of some of the extremities in combination with a facial palsy. The following table is given by Lovett and Richardson[24] based upon 1158 cases:

Table 64.—Regions Paralyzed in Poliomyelitis—America

	Per Cent.
One leg only	27.97
Both legs	23.48
Both legs and arms	11.13
One leg and one arm, same side	9.49
One arm only	7.25
Both arms only	1.98
Face	6.38
Abdomen	5.78
Neck	0.94
Respiration	2.67
Deglutition	0.60

Wickman[69] gives a similar analysis of 868 cases of paralysis as occurring in Sweden.

The *constitutional symptoms* seldom last more than six or seven days in all from the onset, and often a decidedly shorter time. Pain, a frequent symptom, may, however, continue several weeks. There is no anesthesia. The superficial lymph-nodes are enlarged in many cases, and sometimes the spleen also.

Stationary Stage.—This begins with the cessation of constitutional symptoms and of extension of paralysis and lasts from one to six weeks. No change takes place in the paralytic condition except that atrophy rapidly develops. There are no other symptoms, except perhaps a persistence of pain and hyperesthesia. At this time the loss of power seems often very extensive and complete, and it is impossible to predict how complete the paralysis will remain.

Stage of Retrogression.—After the stationary stage improvement begins. The greater part of this will occur in the six months from the onset of the disease; less in the next six months; but some takes place even up to the end of two years or sometimes longer. Meanwhile atrophy becomes more distinct in the muscular tissue which is not undergoing improvement, and by two months from the onset is very decided. The paralysis is flaccid in nature with diminished muscle-tonus and diminution or absence of tendon-reflexes. The affected limb is smaller than normal; there is no anesthesia or analgesia. It is not possible to determine early how much actual destruction of ganglion-cells has taken place. Some cases which at first seem severely paralyzed improve rather rapidly, and in these probably the muscular paralysis has depended chiefly upon pressure of the edema and the cellular infiltration in the cord. The muscle-fibers connected with ganglion-cells which have been destroyed can never regain their power.

Chronic Atrophic Stage.—In the final condition the growth of the affected limb in length and circumference is much interfered with. In addition to muscular atrophy, there is relaxation of ligaments and atrophy of bone. There are coldness and blueness in the paralyzed parts. Contractions begin even during the stage of retrogression, stronger muscles overcoming the weaker paralyzed ones. Talipes and lateral spinal curvature are among common deformities. Muscles most severely affected in the primary paralysis are those which are left with the greatest final paralysis.

Electrical Reactions.—By the beginning of the second week of the attack, both faradic and galvanic contractility are lost in severely paralyzed muscles. Soon, however, there is a reappearance and even an increase in the galvanic response, with the development of the reaction of degeneration. The galvanic contractility soon diminishes, and finally, perhaps after two or three years, all electrical contractility of any sort disappears in the permanently paralyzed muscles. In those which recover the faradic contractility slowly reappears and the galvanic returns to normal. In muscles little affected faradic contractility may never be more than merely diminished.

2. PROGRESSIVE FORM (*Landry's Paralysis Type*).—This uncommon form (4.39 per cent of Wickman's[70] 1025 cases) is characterized by rapid extension of the lesions upward until the medulla is involved. The paralysis begins in the lower extremities, ascending to the arms, involving the muscles of the trunk including those of respiration, and sometimes the diaphragm and even the muscles of deglutition. (See p. 965.) Sometimes the arms are attacked first and the extension is then of the descending type. The course is rapid and usually fatal.

3. THE BULBAR OR PONTINE FORM.—Formerly this condition was termed "Polioencephalitis superior or inferior," according to which nuclei were involved. Lesions may be limited to the nuclei of the cranial nerves, or may be combined with spinal lesions. The facial nucleus is oftenest affected, and the abducent and hypoglossal frequently, but any of the cranial nerve-nuclei may be involved, with the production of the corresponding symptoms, such as paralysis of respiration and of deglutition and disturbance of the heart's action. In some epidemics 5 per cent or more of cases (6.45 per cent in Wickman's series) are of the bulbar type, and McEachern[71] states it may occur in epidemic form.

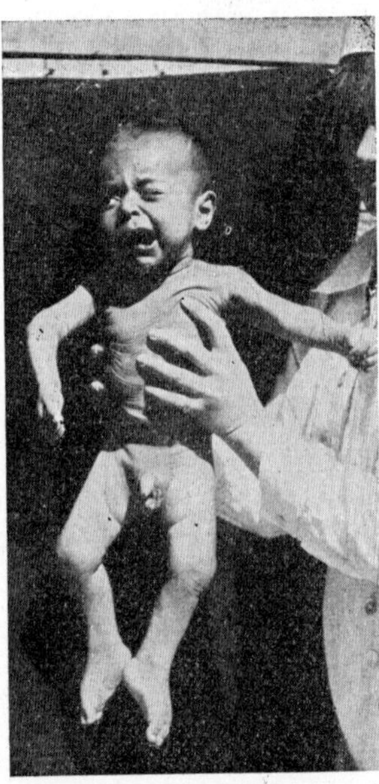

Fig. 81.—Combined lesions in poliomyelitis. Infant of three months in the Children's Hospital of Philadelphia. Facial palsy, flaccid paralysis of the legs, spastic paralysis of the arms.

4. ACUTE ENCEPHALITIC FORM.—Strümpell[31] described this as "acute encephalitis or polioencephalitis of children," and suggested the relationship to poliomyelitis (see p. 953) which is now generally recognized. It is one of the most unusual types. The gray matter of the cortex is involved, but it is possible that certain spastic conditions may be due to involvement of the pyramidal tract high up in the cord and to inflammatory changes in the medulla oblongata, and not to cortical lesions (Rothman[72]). The early symptoms, while variable, suggest those of meningitis. There may be convulsions, somnolence, and paralysis with *increase of tendon-reflexes*. Later spasticity develops; and this may be combined with flaccid paralysis in other regions, due to coincident involvement of the cord (Fig. 81). Fatal cases may occur without development of any paralysis.

5. THE ATAXIC FORM.—Some degree of ataxia is not uncommon. As a chief symptom constituting the form of the disease it is rare (0.43 per cent of Lovett and Richardson's[24] 1158 cases). It involves oftenest the lower extremities, or may be more extensive. It may occur alone or combined with cerebral or spinal symptoms.

6. THE POLYNEURITIC FORM.—This is a rare variety which closely simulates multiple neuritis. There are pain and tenderness in the nerve-trunks and muscles. Pain may be present in the joints as well, and a polyarthritis develop. Paralysis may be extensive, or be slight and transitory or even overlooked. Sensory disturbances are usually absent.

7. THE MENINGITIC FORM.—In this variety, not uncommon in certain epidemics, meningeal symptoms overshadow other manifestations. There may be vomiting, headache, rigidity of neck and back, convulsions, delirium,

and coma variously combined. The diagnosis can be made only if paralysis develops.

8. THE ABORTIVE FORM.—The existence of such cases has been proven by Flexner and Clark[56] and by Anderson and Frost[73] through the discovery of immunizing bodies in the serum of patients with this form of the disease, and by the production of the disease in animals by inoculation with the virus from abortive cases. There is abundant clinical proof that these cases occur, and in them also the spinal fluid exhibits the characteristic changes. There are fever, headache, often vomiting, hyperesthesia, and stiffness of the neck. There may be sore throat, or rhinitis and conjunctivitis. In some instances there is muscular weakness or unsteadiness in gait. After two or three days there is rapid recovery; or there may be very slight transitory paralysis with temporary loss of patellar reflexes. For the abortive cases with evidence of paralysis Müller[64] prefers the term *rudimentary form* in contradistinction to cases without any signs whatever of paralysis, which he calls the *larval form.* Abortive cases are frequent in epidemics and often overlooked. It is probable that in some outbreaks they outnumber cases of any other class.

Relapse.—Occasionally after development of the paralytic symptoms there may be an intermission of six or seven days, after which there is renewed extension of the paralysis and perhaps appearance of other symptoms. In some cases this is probably only a manifestation of the initial lesion; but in others there appears to be a true relapse occurring, it may be, weeks after the primary attack, as in a case reported by Leegaard.[74]

Recurrence.—This is certainly uncommon, but instances have been reported by Lucas and Osgood,[75] Sanz,[76] Francis and Moncreiff,[77] Taylor,[78] Still,[79] and others.

Prognosis.—In European epidemics the mortality has varied from 10 to 17 per cent according to a number of reports (Krause,[80] Wickman,[81] Lindner and Mally,[82] Zappert,[83] Johannessen,[24] Leegaard[84]). Aycock and Eaton[85] reported the mortality from 38 epidemics as averaging 20.8 per cent. The mortality in American epidemics has been somewhat less, except for the epidemic in New York State in 1916, where, according to Nicoll,[86] it reached 25 per cent. During the years 1926, 1927 and 1928 there were 4154 deaths from poliomyelitis in the United States Registration Area.[29] These figures usually do not include the abortive cases, which, of course, give an entirely favorable prognosis. Complications such as bronchopneumonia may be the cause of death. In cases ending fatally death is liable to occur in the first three to five days; after the first two weeks recovery is almost assured so far as life is concerned. The case-mortality is decidedly less in childhood than later (Wickman,[81] Nicoll[87]). In the figures of the United States Registration Area quoted above it was found that 9.7 per cent of the deaths were under one year; 42.1 per cent under five years; 57.1 per cent under ten years; 87.9 per cent under twenty years.

The prognosis, too, varies somewhat with the type of the disease other than the spinal. In the abortive cases it is entirely favorable. In the progressive form there is rarely recovery and death occurs generally in a few days. The bulbar type is dangerous if the nerve-centers controlling respiration and circulation are involved. In the meningitic form the disease is often severe and rapidly fatal.

The likelihood of recovery from the paralytic condition is a matter of prognostic importance. The more promptly improvement begins, the greater the chances of recovery. Not infrequently all traces of paralysis everywhere may disappear, and very great recovery may often take place even in cases of paralysis at first widespread and apparently severe. Lovett and Richardson[24] found that in 16.7 per cent of 150 cases, all evidence of the disease had disappeared within three months. Wickman[88] found that of 530 cases, 44 per cent had no paralysis after one or one and one-half years. The early paralysis of the trunk and neck seen in spinal cases will probably disappear. In the bulbar type, if the patient survives, paralysis generally disappears completely. The polyneuritic cases may or may not recover without paralysis. The ataxia of the ataxic form is never more than a temporary matter. In the spinal cases some evidence of paralysis is very likely to remain throughout life. This varies from complete disability to merely a slight impairment of motion. The muscles of the arms and shoulders seem less prone to undergo improvement than those of the legs. Muscles which have never shown any electrical changes will probably recover completely. Those which have exhibited entire paralysis and complete loss of faradic contractility after the acute stage is over will remain more or less paralyzed. If there is slight return of contraction in the course of a few days longer, partial paralysis will probably follow. If, however, there is continued loss of this for two or three months combined with wasting and loss of power, little improvement can be expected. Nevertheless Lovett[89] found that even as late as three or four years after the attack there was tendency to continued improvement under proper treatment. With this treatment improvement may continue in the lower extremities during three years, and in the upper during four years. It is a matter of controversy whether cases which have been given convalescent's serum are likely to have less paralysis.

Diagnosis.—The most suggestive of the early clinical manifestations are hyperesthesia, sweating, and nervous irritability. If these are combined with other meningeal symptoms or signs of increased intracranial pressure, such as stiffness of the neck, vomiting, somnolence, and a positive Kernig's sign, the diagnosis may be suspected. This would be particularly the case in the presence of an epidemic. Spinal puncture would then be indicated, and the characteristic changes in the fluid found (p. 390) if poliomyelitis is present. It is certain that many very mild and abortive cases can be diagnosed only by examination of the spinal fluid. *Purulent meningitis* of any form may, in the early stages, be differentiated only with certainty by lumbar puncture, the large number of polymorphonuclear cells excluding poliomyelitis. The blood in purulent meningitis exhibits a high leukocytosis. *Tuberculous meningitis* in its early stages is not easily differentiated, particularly since the spinal fluid is very much like that of poliomyelitis. However, the onset is usually more insidious, the paralysis is slower in appearing and is of a spastic type, and the mental condition becomes increasingly stuporous. In the colloidal gold test upon the spinal fluid the reaction in tuberculous meningitis is not in the syphilitic zone; *i. e.*, that of low-dilution, as it is in poliomyelitis.

Acute epidemic encephalitis may readily be confused with poliomyelitis. In the former the characteristic symptoms of lethargy, ophthalmoplegia and asthenia are more likely to be present and continued; while prompt appearance and spread of paralysis of the extremities are in favor of the latter. In poliomyelitis there is likely to be more evidence of meningeal irritation. In encephalitis there may be found in the spinal fluid an increased sugar-content, but in other respects little difference is seen between the fluids of the two diseases. Except in epidemics some cases of the bulbospinal and encephalitic forms of poliomyelitis cannot be differentiated from cases of epidemic encephalitis in which paralysis of the extremities accompanies that of the cranial nerves. In *multiple neuritis* there are, as in poliomyelitis, flaccidity, atrophy, and flail-like freedom of movement at the articulations. There are, however, no cerebral symptoms and no change in the spinal fluid, as would be the case in poliomyelitis of the polyneuritic form. A diminution of the touch-sense indicates the presence of neuritis rather than of poliomyelitis. A *localized neuritis*, as of the arm in obstetrical paralysis, can readily be distinguished by the history of the case. The pseudoparalysis of *infantile scurvy* or *rickets* may easily be confounded with poliomyelitis. In both these conditions there is no diminution of tendon-reflexes, and a careful study of the history and of the symptoms in general should remove all difficulty. Yet we have seen mistakes made in a number of instances. An ordinary *Bell's palsy* should not be mistaken for poliomyelitis, since in the latter there will usually be other paralyses. It is, however, possible to confuse it with some cases of the bulbar type of the disease.

The neutralization test for the diagnosis of poliomyelitis, according to which the blood-serum of the patient is mixed with active virus and injected into the cranial cavity of a monkey, is not a practical one, since antibodies do not form in the patient until the stage of recovery.

Treatment. **Prophylaxis.**—Quarantine of the patient should certainly be enforced, especially during an epidemic, at which time the virulence of the germ appears to be greatly increased. Four weeks would seem ample, unless there is persistent inflammation of the nose and throat. Usually a child who has been exposed may be considered safe if not developing the disease in two weeks. A properly worn mask and goggles may perhaps have some value in preventing the disease in attendants. Any gargles or nasal sprays used for prevention should be of a nonirritating nature. Discharges from the mouth and nose of the patient should be promptly destroyed. Thorough cleanliness and airing of the sick-roon should be carried out after it is vacated. Children should not be taken to localities where the disease is epidemic; or, if already there, they should not associate with those who have recently had the affection, or with those who are ill with any vague symptoms. It is well, too, to prevent their frequenting public places of amusement, and sometimes it is advisable to close schools temporarily. Many experiments have shown that monkeys can be successfully immunized against poliomyelitis by injections of the virus (emulsions of cord and brain). This is not applicable as yet to human beings. Flexner and Stewart[90] and others have recommended injections of 10 to 20 cc. of convalescent's serum for exposed persons. There is no actual proof that this is of value, and the same is true of injections of blood from normal adults (normal adult serum) (Flexner[91]).

Treatment of the Attack.—There is considerable discussion as to the value of lumbar puncture and relief of pressure, and as to the advisability of performing this, but certainly it may be done for diagnostic purposes, and, it seems to us, is indicated therapeutically as long as there is evidence of increased intracranial pressure. It need not be performed after the acute symptoms are over.

Netter[92] in 1910 used injections of blood-serum from subjects who had previously suffered from poliomyelitis. There is controversy as to the value of this procedure. Zingher,[93] Wells,[94] Amoss and Chesney,[95] Aycock and Amoss,[96] Aycock and Luther,[97] Shaw and Thelander,[98] Ayer,[99] MacEachern[100] and his co-workers, and Riley,[101] are among those who report favorable results. To be effective it must be given in the preparalytic stage or certainly very early in the paralysis, and before great damage has been done to the central nervous system. It has been given intramuscularly, intravenously, and intraspinally. The amount injected should be 10 to 20 cc. or more every twenty to twenty-four hours for two or three days. Shaw and Thelander believe that intravenous injection should be given only with homologous (identical type) blood-serum. Normal human serum has also been used and beneficial results claimed. It has been found that the blood of many adults, probably because of the acquiring of immunity through "sub-clinical" infection, has a neutralizing power on the virus (Shaughessy, Harmon and Gordon[102]).

Rosenow[54] reports good results from the injection of a horse-serum which is prepared by repeated injections of the streptococcus previously described. Nuzum and Willy[103] also have recorded benefit from the use of a similar serum prepared from sheep's and rabbit's blood as well as from that of the horse. Rosenow and Nicoll[104] report on 1113 patients who had received this antistreptococcus serum, and claim that, compared with a control group of 278 patients, the mortality and residual paralyses were less. Rosenow's serum is injected intramuscularly in 5 to 10 cc. doses every twelve to twenty-four hours, employing about 60 cc. in all. Neustaedter and Banzhaf,[105] Pettit,[106] and Howitt, Shaw, Thelander and Limper,[107] by injecting horses, goats, or sheep with the virus, have obtained a serum which appears to have some immune properties. These sera have as yet been little used in human cases.

On the other hand there are many clinicians who are not convinced of the value of any serum in this disease. The Harvard Infantile Paralysis Commission (Peabody[108]) could discover no demonstrable value of any such treatment in the preparalytic stage, and observed as many treated as untreated cases developing paralysis, and Lovett[89] in a study based on 5100 cases could not find that either convalescent's serum or any streptococcic serum had proved itself serviceable.

It may be concluded, however, that, until some better method of treatment is found, convalescent's serum should be used whenever available. The Rosenow and other animal sera would seem to require further study before their value can be finally determined.

Complete rest in bed is imperative, and there should be symptomatic treatment of pain, nervous symptoms, fever, and debility. Electricity should not be employed for from three to six weeks or longer after the attack, and not until all pain and hyperesthesia have disappeared. It will then improve the tone and power of the muscles which have been only partially or temporarily injured. The faradic current should be applied to the muscles, and continued for from ten to twenty minutes once or twice a day. If there is no response to the faradic current the galvanic may be tried. Electricity should be employed only in a strength which will produce moderate contractions without pain.

Massage and passive movements may be commenced at the same time as electricity, after all pain and hyperesthesia have disappeared; and it is of especial importance as well that the patient endeavor, no matter how unsuccessfully, to make voluntary active movements. The combination of these various procedures should be persisted with for months or years. Weight-bearing exercises should not be permitted for two or three months, or even much longer, after the acute symptoms are over. Borden,[109] Phillips and Garland,[110] and Bordier[111] believe that roentgen-ray treatment over the spinal segments reduces edema and hastens absorption of the cellular infiltration in the acute stage, and later may stimulate diseased but viable cells of the anterior horn. Meltzer[112] and Taccone[113] recommended intraspinal injections of 0.5 to 2 cc. of a 1:1000 adrenalin solution every few days in the first two to four weeks of the paralysis.

In types of the disease with respiratory paralysis, Durand[114] recommends putting the child chest downward and elevating the foot of the bed, thus permitting the mucus in the bronchial tubes and pharynx to be evacuated. Artificial respiration may also be attempted by means of specially devised respirators, such as the Drinker apparatus, in the hope that recovery will take place if the acute period can be tided over (Drinker and McKhann;[115]

Shambaugh, Harrison and Farrell;[116] Drinker, Shaughnessy and Murphy;[117] Favill and Fentress;[118] Wilson[119]). We have seen this procedure undoubtedly save life.

Mechanical Treatment.—Deformity must be prevented by the employment of mechanical apparatus as early as necessary. Even in the stage of retrogression beginning deformity must be guarded against. The greatest orthopedic skill is required in deciding upon the use of braces and supports, and later upon the advisability of such operations as tendon-transplantation and the like. Under-water gymnastics are helpful in restoring the function of partially paralyzed limbs (Lowman[120]). It should be remembered that atrophy of the bones resulting from disuse may lead to fractures.

References

1. Dis. Child., 1789, 2nd Ed., **2,** 53. 2. Beobachtungen ü. Lähmungszustande der untern Extremitäten, 1840. 3. Malad. d. enf., 1843, **2,** 335. 4. Compt. rend. soc. de biol., 1865, **2,** 215. 5. Arch. de physiol. norm. et pathol., 1870, **3,** 134. 6. Nord. Med. Arkiv., 1896, **6,** No. 1. 7. Beitr. z. Kenntnis der Heine-Medinsch. Krankheit., 1907, 588. 8. Pub. Health Bull., 1911, No. 44, 16. 9. Die acute Poliomyelit., Berlin, 1911, 11. 10. Keating's Cyclop. Dis. of Childr., 1890, **4,** 685. 11. Lancet, 1918, **2,** 847. 12. New England J. Med., 1929, **200,** 164. 13. J. Exper. Med., 1920, **31,** 123. 14. J.A.M.A., 1917, **69,** 163. 15. Med. Rec., 1917, **92,** 477. 16. Atlantic M. J., 1925, **28,** 269. 17. Ohio State M. J., 1928, **24,** 784. 18. Am. J. Med. Sc., 1843, **5,** 248. 19. J.A.M.A., 1912, **59,** 782. 20. Yale M. J., 1894, **1,** 1; J.A.M.A., 1896, **26,** 1. 21. Die acute Poliomyelit. u. verwandte Krankheiten, 1907. 22. Am. J. Med. Sc., 1908, **135,** 647. 23. Rept. on New York Epidemic, Collect. Investig. Committee, 1910, 27. 24. Infant. Paralys. in Massachusetts, 1910, 92. 25. Jahrb. f. Kinderh., 1912, **76,** 605. 26. Jahrb. f. Kinderh., 1912, **76,** 603. 27. Bull. Johns Hopk. Hosp., 1917, **28,** 131. 28. Boston M. and S. J., 1918, **178,** 747. 29. Communic. Dis. Control. Rep. Sec. 2, White House Conf. on Child Health and Protect., 1931. 30. Poliomyelitis, 1927. 31. Jahrb. f. Kinderh., 1885, **22,** 173. 32. Norsk. Mag. f. Laegevidensk., 1905, **66,** 1280. 33. J.A.M.A., 1916, **67,** 1202. 34. J.A.M.A., 1928, **91,** 1594; 1930, **94,** 777. 35. J.A.M.A., 1916, **67,** 1205; 1437. 36. J.A.M.A., 1916, **67,** 1019. 37. J.A.M.A., 1929, **92,** 1725. 38. Ztschr. f. Immunitätsforsch. u. exper. Therap., Orig., 1909, **2,** 377. 39. J.A.M.A., 1909, **53,** 1639; 2095. 40. Deutsche med. Wchnschr., 1909, **35,** 1825. 41. München. med. Wchnschr., 1910, **58,** 568; 945. 42. J.A.M.A., 1911, **56,** 495. 43. Fifteenth Int. Cong. Hyg. and Demography, 1912, **1,** 597. 44. J.A.M.A., 1913, **60,** 362. 45. J. Med. Res., 1917, **36,** 175. 46. J.A.M.A., 1928, **91,** 21. 47. Trans. Am. Ped. Soc., 1931, **43,** 32. 48. J. Exper. Med., 1914, **20,** 249. 49. Arch. Int. Med., 1931, **48,** 33. 50. Clin. Study of Acute Poliomyelit., Rockefeller Inst. Monograph., No. 4; June 24, 1912. 51. Acute Poliomyelitis, 1917. 52. J. Prev. Med., 1930, **4,** 189. 53. J. Prev. Med., 1929, **3,** 103. 54. J.A.M.A., 1912, **59,** 785. 55. J. Exper. Med., 1912, **16,** 850. 56. J.A.M.A., 1911, **56,** 1717. 57. J.A.M.A., 1912, **59,** 1314. 58. U. S. Pub. Health Rep., 1912, **27,** Pt. 2, 1733. 59. J.A.M.A., 1926, **87,** 75. 60. Studien ü. Poliomyelit. acuta. Arbeiten aus dem path., Inst. d. Universit. Helsingfors, 1905, **1,** 109. 61. Path. anatom. Untersuch. ü. akute Poliomyelit. u. verwandt. Krankh., 1902. 62. J.A.M.A., 1910, **55,** 1105. 63. Am. J. Hyg., 1925, **5,** 724. 64. Die spinale Kinderlähmung, 1910. 65. Am. J. Dis. Child., 1917, **13,** 239. 66. Am. J. Dis. Child., 1922, **22,** 107. 67. Am. J. Dis. Child., 1923, **25,** 76. 68. Am. J. Dis. Child., 1928, **36,** 40. 69. Die acute Poliomyelitis, 1911, 44. 70. Die acute Poliomyelitis, 1911, 53. 71. J.A.M.A., 1926, **86,** 90. 72. Am. J. Dis. Child., 1931, **42,** 124. 73. J.A.M.A., 1911, **56,** 663. 74. Norsk. Mag. f. Laegevidensk., 1901, **16,** 377. 75. J.A.M.A., 1913, **60,** 1611. 76. Siglo méd., 1915, **62,** 530; Ref. Brit. J. Child. Dis., 1916, **13,** 56. 77. J. Nerv. and Ment. Dis., 1919, **49,** 273. 78. J. Nerv. and Ment. Dis., 1916, **44,** 207. 79. Arch. Dis. Childh., 1930, **5,** 295. 80. Deutsche med. Wchnschr., 1909, **35,** 1822. 81. Beitr. z. Kenntnis der Heine-Medinschen Krankheit, 1907, 286. 82. Deutsche. Ztschr. f. Nervenh., 1910, **38,** 362. 83. Studien ü. d. Heine-Medinschen Krankheit, 1911, 55. 84. Deutsche. Ztschr. f. Nervenh., 1914–15, **53,** 222. 85. Am. J. Hyg., 1924, **4,** 681. 86. Am. J. Dis. Child., 1917, **14,** 69. 87. Trans. Am. Pediat. Soc., 1917, **29,** 228. 88. Die acute Poliomyelitis, 1911, 78. 89. J.A.M.A., 1921, **77,** 1941; 1922, **78,** 1607. 90. J.A.M.A., 1928, **91,** 383. 91. Science, 1933, **77,** 7. 92. Arch. de méd. d. enf., 1916, **19,** 1. 93. Arch. Pediat., 1916, **33,** 872. 94. J.A.M.A., 1916, **67,** 1211. 95. J. Exper. Med., 1917, **25,** 581. 96. J.A.M.A., 1923, **81,** 474. 97. J.A.M.A., 1928, **91,** 387. 98. J.A.M.A., 1928, **90,** 1923; 1931, **97,** 1620. 99. Am. J. Med. Sc., 1929, **177,** 540. 100. Canad. M. A. J., 1929, **20,** 369. 101. J.A.M.A., 1930, **94,** 550. 102. J. Prev. Med., 1930, **4,** 4637. 103. J.A.M.A., 1917, **69,** 1247. 104. Am. J. Dis. Child., 1927, **33,** 27. 105. J.A.M.A., 1917, **68,** 1531. 106. Compt. rend. soc. de biol., 1918, **81,** 1087; Bull. gén. de therap., 1925, **176,** 389. 107. J.A.M.A.,

1931, **96,** 1280. 108. Boston M. and S. J., 1921, **185,** 174. 109. Arch. Radiol. and Electrother., 1921, **26,** 215. 110. J.A.M.A., 1924, **82,** 1847. 111. Acta psychiat. et neurol., 1927, **2,** 1. 112. Med. Rec., 1916, **90,** 171. 113. Riv. de clin. pediat., 1929, **27,** 883. 114. J.A.M.A., 1929, **93,** 1044. 115. J.A.M.A., 1929, **92,** 1658. 116. J.A.M.A., 1930, **94,** 1371. 117. J.A.M.A., 1930, **94,** 1249. 118. J.A.M.A., 1931, **97, 1464.** 119. New England J. Med., 1932, **206,** 887. 120. J.A.M.A., 1931, **97,** 1074.

CHAPTER XXII

EPIDEMIC ENCEPHALITIS

Terminology.—Among the confusing number of terms used to describe this condition may be mentioned Lethargic encephalitis, Epidemic stupor, Epidemic somnolence, Sweating sickness, Acute infectious ophthalmoplegia, Sleeping sickness, Acute encephalitis, Focal hemorrhagic encephalitis, Postinfluenzal encephalitis, Myoclonic encephalitis, and Nona. To all of these there are objections. The term "Epidemic encephalitis" seems preferable, because the disease usually occurs in epidemic form and its pathologic basis is an inflammation of the brain-substance.

History.—The occurrence of epidemic encephalitis in America was first reported in 1918, and probably was a new disorder here (Tilney and Riley,[1] Bassoe[2]). It was not, however, a new disorder elsewhere. The attention of the medical profession was first aroused by the writings of von Economo[3] describing the epidemic in Austria which began in 1916 and spread widely in different countries. If the difference in terminology is considered, and the symptoms of earlier reported cases studied, it is evident that epidemics of this disorder have visited Europe and Asia for some hundreds of years. The history of encephalitis with comprehensive bibliography may well be consulted in the contributions of Crookshank;[4] Barker, Cross and Irwin;[5] Happ and Mason,[6] and Eckstein.[7]

Relation to Other Diseases.—It is but natural that *poliomyelitis* and encephalitis should be confounded with each other. In both the seat of the pathologic change is in the central nervous system, and epidemic influence and infectious origin are definite, and there are also some symptoms common to both. Nevertheless, the weight of evidence in history, pathology, symptoms, and experiment indicates that each is a distinct entity. In the history of epidemics it can be seen that the two do not occur together; undoubted cases of poliomyelitis are common in the summer and fall, while epidemic encephalitis is a disease of winter. There are differences in pathology and also in symptomatology which will be discussed later. On the other hand, it has been argued that these differences are only those dependent upon the situation attacked by the virus (Burrows,[8] Maggiore and Sindoni[9]) and there are some who maintain that no proof has as yet been offered which clearly separates the diseases in a clinical, epidemiological or pathologic way (Crookshank[10]). Although it has been shown experimentally by Amoss[11] that the blood-serum of recently convalescent cases of epidemic encephalitis was devoid of the power of neutralizing the virus of poliomyelitis, some experiments of Neustaedter, Larkin and Banzhaf[12] appear to prove that this protective power does exist, thus indicating some relationship between the two disorders.

It has been claimed that there is a close relationship between *influenza* and encephalitis, some authors maintaining that the virus causing the two is the same; others only that influenza prepares the ground for encephalitis or, in other words, activates the encephalitic virus. There is no experimental work which establishes any such connection, and in neither epidemic nor sporadic cases of encephalitis can the occasional association be viewed as more than coincidental.

Very interesting is the fact that a virus capable of causing *herpes* in man and a *herpetic keratitis* in animals will produce, when inoculated into such animals as rabbits and monkeys, symptoms identical with encephalitis; and that, furthermore, material from the brains of these animals will in turn produce herpetic keratitis in other animals inoculated (Edel,[13] Doerr and Berger,[14] Lauda,[15] Flexner,[16] Zinsser and Tang,[17] McKinley and Douglass[18]). It has been suggested by Parker[19] that there is only a chance association of the herpetic and encephalitic virus in the material employed. Gundersen[20] from a study of epidemological data thinks that there may be a relation between mumps and epidemic encephalitis.

Some writers claim that certain cases of acute febrile chorea are instances of epidemic encephalitis (Harvier and Levaditi[21]). Certainly there is no reason to classify Sydenham's chorea as epidemic encephalitis, and pathologically they are different (Wilson and Winkelman[22]). Dubini's electric chorea has been regarded as identical with epidemic encephalitis (Cruchet,[23] Litvak[24]). Confusion results from the similarity in symptoms between the choreoid and myoclonic forms of encephalitis and the disease in question. Other diseases thought to possess a near relationship are epidemic hiccup and a disorder entitled Australian X. The latter more resembles poliomyelitis (Flexner[16]).

Etiology. Predisposing Causes. *Age.*—The disease can occur in new-born infants whose mothers were suffering from the malady during pregnancy (Mercier,[25] Klippel and Baruk[26]). It is common in infancy and childhood, as shown by the reports of Heiman,[27] Comby,[28] Moore,[29] Smith,[30] Neal,[31] Hofstadt,[32] Duzár and Baló,[33] Moncrieff,[34] and others. In some epidemics 40 per cent of the patients have been under ten years of age (Neal[31]) and 50 per cent under fifteen years (Smith[30]). Encephalitis is even more common in early life than statistics indicate, many patients having it in a mild and unrecognized form, and in others the true nature of the original illness becoming manifest only after sequels develop. *Sex* has little influence in childhood, although in adults males are more often attacked. *Season* plays a part, and cases are more numerous in the winter and spring months (Wynne[11]). The strong *epidemic influence* has already been alluded to. Sporadic cases are relatively uncommon, and many of them belong in the category of encephalitis following acute infectious diseases. The *geographical distribution* is almost universal, cases being reported from all civilized countries. *Communicability* is slight, and the majority of persons exposed seem to be immune (Smith,[30] Hunt,[35] Happ and Mason,[6] Neal,[31] Ebaugh,[36] Roger[37]). In the experience of these writers instances of home or hospital contagion were absent or very rare. There are, however, reports which illustrate the possibility of direct infection, as those of Claude and Laulerie,[38] Roger and Blanchard,[39] Hofstadt,[32] and others, but mere coincidence may explain some of these. Kling[40] observing an epidemic in a thinly populated section of Lapland found that direct personal contact-transmission can occur, and believes that he has also demonstrated the existence of carriers. The virus appears to be disseminated through the nasopharyngeal secretion, and it may well be that abortive and unrecognized cases occur more frequently than has been supposed, and are sources of infection.

Exciting Cause.—Loewe, Hirshfeld and Strauss,[41] Levaditi and Harvier,[42] McIntosh and Turnbull,[43] Thalhimer,[44] Neal,[45] and others have studied the active cause of encephalitis. The results of the investigations may be summarized as follows: Berkefeld filtrates of brain-material, nasopharyngeal mucous membrane and nasal washings, spinal fluid and blood from cases of epidemic encephalitis have produced in rabbits and monkeys lesions typical of this disease. By means of special cultural methods a minute, filterable organism was discovered in these tissues and secretions, and this same organism later recovered from the brain and nasopharyngeal mucous membrane of animals that had been inoculated with it. The cultures of this recovered organism have again produced the disease when injected into other animals, and the organism has again been isolated. It should be stated that some doubt attaches to certain of these investigations, because such animals as rabbits and monkeys are subject to epizootic encephalitis, and the changes found may be due to this rather than to the experimental inoculations (Lucke,[46] Flexner[16]). It is also claimed that the inoculation of epidemic encephalitic material simply reduces local resistance, so that the virus of the spontaneous epizootic type can act. (See Review in Medical Science.[47])

Micro-organisms other than the type described have been reported by von Wiesner,[48] House,[49] Morse and Crump,[50] Evans and Freeman,[51] and Rosenow and his co-workers.[52] These were mostly green-producing streptococci. Evans[53] has attempted to correlate the studies on the filterable organism with those on the pleomorphic streptococcus, and has obtained the streptococcus by cultivating the virus. The relation between herpetiform viruses and that of encephalitis has already been referred to.

Pathologic Anatomy.—Usually there is little gross or microscopical evidence of pathologic change in the meninges. The brain itself shows gross evidence of edema or congestion, or may appear normal until microscopical studies are made. The essential lesions are (*a*) congestion of vessels and hemorrhagic areas which may be visible macroscopically, but usually are minute and microscopical; (*b*) marked cellular infiltration, consisting of small and large mononuclear and plasma cells which are present in the perivascular and the Virchow-Robin spaces; (*c*) degenerative alterations, such as cloudy swelling, neuronophagia and satellitosis in the nerve-cells, and (*d*) proliferation of the neuroglial cells. While changes may be discovered throughout the brain and even the white matter be involved, it is the gray matter of the mid-brain, the basal ganglia, the pons and the medulla which suffer most frequently and most intensely. The spinal cord, the nerve-roots and the dorsal root-ganglia may be the seat of perivascular lymphocytic infiltration. Numerous spherical homogeneous hyaline bodies are found in the white and gray matter in some cases. Cloudy swelling, congestion, and petechial hemorrhages may be observed in other organs, notably the kidney and the serous lining of the pericardium, pleura and peritoneum.

This description applies to acute cases. In patients dying some time after the active process has ceased there are no characteristic findings that serve to distinguish epidemic encephalitis from any other form.

Symptoms.—The symptomatology is naturally extremely diversified. In epidemics there is a tendency for some one particular type to be prevalent, varying with the epidemic. While there are several ways in which the disease may be classified, it will be discussed here from the point of view of symptoms.

Incubation.—In experimental animals this is as short as five or six days; in human cases the duration is doubtful, Kling[40] giving it as ten days and Roger[37] as one to two months or longer.

Stage of Invasion.—There may be sudden onset with the appearance of the characteristic triad of symptoms; *lethargy*, *asthenia* and *ocular nerve-paralysis;* or these may be preceded for several days by such symptoms as fever, malaise, digestive disturbances, and headache. It is noticeable that the *asthenia* is more marked than the other symptoms warrant. In some cases there may be an interval of several weeks between the onset of general symptoms and the manifestations denoting central nervous lesions. The temperature is usually moderately and irregularly elevated throughout the acute course of the disease (Fig. 82).

In some instances there is little or no febrile reaction, but in fatal cases final hyperpyrexia may occur. Many observers report initial symptoms suggesting infection of the upper respiratory tract. This has furnished one of the arguments for the dependence of encephalitis upon influenza, as also for a primary localization of the virus in the nasopharynx. In many cases, however, respiratory symptoms are absent or very slight.

Disturbances of Consciousness and Mental Symptoms.—The existence of these is very characteristic. They may be so mild as simply to constitute apathy, or so severe that the patient is lethargic or comatose. Like other symptoms the degree of lethargy varies with epidemics, in some of which it is present in all cases and in others in from 30 to 80 per cent. Usually the patient can be roused to answer questions or obey commands, but immediately relapses into the somnolent state. In some instances an exactly opposite condition of marked insomnia is found, either preliminary to or replacing lethargy. Even early, although oftener later, there may be a reversal of the sleep-habit, producing diurnal somnolence and nocturnal wakefulness. Speech is apt to be slow and monotonous, and answers given at a distinct interval after questions. A mask-like facies may accompany the lethargic state, the effect increased by ptosis of the lids and facial paralysis. Any of these symptoms may be present for a few days only, but they usually persist for weeks or even months. A confused mental condition with delirium or excessive talkativeness is sometimes seen instead of, or in addition to, somnolence. Not infrequently there are emotional disturbances during the acute stage, with periods of crying or laughing, delusions, and maniacal states.

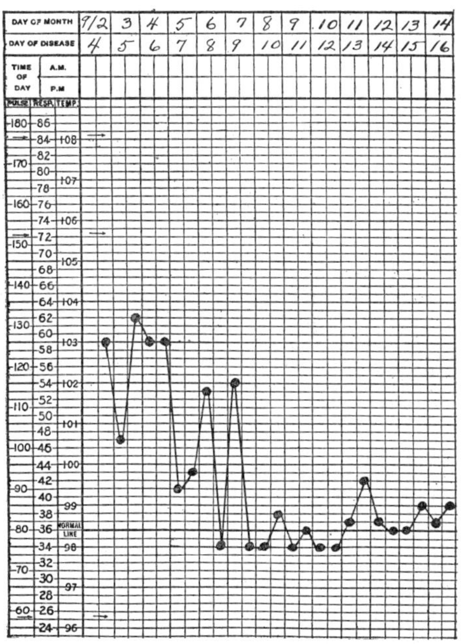

Fig. 82.—Epidemic encephalitis. Moderately mild course; psychic disturbances. Admitted to the Children's Hospital of Phila. on the fourth day of the disease. Unconsciousness, somnolence, restlessness, rigidity of neck, twitching, lateral nystagmus, internal strabismus of right eye. Blood showed 15,900 leukocytes. Spinal fluid 120 cells, chiefly lymphocytes; globulin. Improvement began on tenth day. By eighteenth day mentally bright, but moral sense altered. Residual paralysis of 4th and 6th nerves on right side.

Ocular Disturbances.—These constitute the third of the triad of characteristic symptoms, the cranial nerves involved being usually the 3d and 6th. Transient diplopia is very common (50 to 80 per cent). Ptosis of the upper eyelids is also frequently noted (20 to 95 per cent) and is apt to be continued. The 4th nerve may be involved and assist in causing diplopia by paralysis of the superior oblique muscle of the eyeball. The 2d nerve is affected in some cases, and there may very rarely be optic neuritis. Nystagmus has been observed in some epidemics with considerable frequency, and paralysis of accommodation occasionally. Both early and late in the course there may appear paroxysmal attacks of conjugate deviation of the eyes (Pardee[54]).

Disturbances of Other Cranial Nerves.—There may be involvement of the 5th nerve, causing pain in the head and face; of the 7th nerve, facial paralysis; 8th nerve, tinnitus and deafness; 9th nerve, alteration in taste and dysphagia; 10th nerve, tachycardia; 11th nerve, paralysis of sternomastoid and trapezius muscles; 12th nerve, paralysis of the tongue. (For statistics on frequency of involvement of the cranial nerves consult Smith,[30] Dunn and Heagey,[55] Friesner,[56] Holden,[57] and Howe.[58])

Motor Disturbances.—Some type of motor disorder is frequent (10 to 50 per cent) and this usually occurs with such associated symptoms as lethargy. The paralyses of the cranial nerves have already been noted. In some epidemics as many as 10 or 15 per cent of the cases have shown other paralyses, such as monoplegias, paraplegias or hemiplegias. Generalized spasticity of the muscles may be present, but not so commonly as hypotonia. Catatonia and catalepsy may occur (Musser and Bennett[59]). Frequently seen and of diagnostic importance are *hyperkinetic phenomena.* These consist of quick, jerky movements, which are involuntary and nonrhythmical in character. They may be only fibrillary, or involve an entire muscle or group of muscles; a favorite situation being around the mouth or eyelids. Rhythmic contractions (myoclonia) are of frequent occurrence (Sicard[60]), and are usually bilateral and may be either generalized or limited to the extremities. Reilly[61] described myoclonia of the muscles of the abdomen. This is present in some epidemics but not in others. Fine or coarse tremors of the fingers, bilateral and nonintentional in character, are common (10 to 30 per cent). Tremors of the paralysis agitans type, athetoid or choreiform movements, and ataxia may occur during the acute stage of the disease, but are more commonly sequels. Convulsions are not infrequent at the onset in children. Hiccup is sometimes associated with encephalitis, and at other times occurs as a solitary phenomenon during epidemics of encephalitis, and has been thought to be due to the same virus and to represent diaphragmatic myoclonia.

Disturbances of Sensation.—These are not infrequent. Generalized hyperesthesia and pains may be early and transient symptoms, and may presage the development of hyperkinetic phenomena. Numbness or paresthesia of the trunk, head or extremities is occasionally witnessed. Pain in the head has already been mentioned.

Other Symptoms and Signs.—Other symptoms, the frequency of which varies with epidemics, are profuse and continued sweating; marked salivation; frequently-repeated yawning; alteration in respiratory rate and rhythm with hyperpnea or perhaps with suffocation and cyanosis; and polyneuritis. The superficial reflexes may be unaltered, increased or absent; the part of the central nervous system involved deciding the matter. In the meningeal type the usual signs of rigidity may be found.

Special Types.—It has already been stated that the symptoms vary in their frequency according to epidemics. Usually, even in the special types where there is predominance of one or more symptoms, other symptoms will be found. Thus, in the spinal type, or in the meningeal type, or in the cerebellar type, there will also be periods when perhaps lethargy or ocular paralysis is present. In some instances all the symptoms are so mild that the term *abortive* is justified. These constituted 19 per cent of Howe's cases in children.

Laboratory Findings.—The *blood-examination* shows slight leukocytosis, which may, however, be as high as 20,000 or even 30,000. The polymorphonuclears are relatively increased. The *spinal fluid* is practically always clear, and the number of cells normal or not infrequently increased up to 20 or 30 per cubic millimeter, or occasionally to 100 or 150. Exceptionally cell-counts of 500 or more have been reported. The pressure is slightly increased in about 10 per cent of the cases. The amount of sugar is normal or somewhat increased. This increase is coincident with a hyperglycemia according to Thalhimer and Updegraff.[62] Studies by Halliday[63] indicate that the amount of sugar is normal if the fluid is examined after a twelve hour fast. There is slight increase in albumin and globulin. The colloidal gold test may be positive in the syphilitic zone; *i. e.*, the color changes are most marked in the lower dilutions. Inorganic phosphorus is decreased (Steiner[64]) (the normal being 1.4 to 1.6 mg. per 100 cc.). A characteristic described is a cell-count high in proportion to the amount of globulin (Eskuchen[65]). Pellicle-formation is rare. It should be stated, however, that while the various changes described may be present, it is quite common for the fluid to be perfectly normal. Marked abnormality suggests meningeal involvement.

Complications and Sequels.—Complications such as nephritis and respiratory infections are occasionally seen during the acute course, as in any febrile disease. It is sometimes difficult to determine whether to classify certain end-results as complications or as sequels, since they may begin early and not terminate until after many months, or may even be permanent; or, on the other hand, not commence until some time after the initial symptoms, the patient in the meantime seemingly having become nearly normal. Not infrequently certain conditions, such as myoclonus and mental and behavior disorders, appear to be postencephalitic phenomena, although it is difficult or impossible to elicit a history of acute encephalitis. Some authors have explained the late appearance of sequels and recrudescence of symptoms on the theory that the virus in the nervous tissues is not destroyed, but may resume activity (von Economo;[66] Chiray and Lafourcade[67]). *Sequels* of some kind occur in from 80 to 90 per cent of cases, and about $\frac{1}{3}$ are serious, and either long-continued or permanent.

Postencephalitic phenomena have been statistically studied by a number of writers, among whom should be mentioned Happ and Blackfan,[68] Grossman,[69] Paterson and Spence,[70] Happ and Mason,[6] Leahy and Sands,[71] Comby,[72] Parker,[73] Hohman,[74] Ebaugh,[75] Anderson,[76] Collin and Requin,[77] Kennedy,[78] Kwint,[79] Robb,[80] Stevenson,[81] Howe,[58] and others.

Mental and psychic disturbances are common (50 to 60 per cent of sequels). Among minor manifestations are irritability, emotional instability, inability to focus attention, defective memory, delusions, abnormal drowsiness, and fear and compulsion-neuroses. Disturbances of sleep are frequent (30 to 55 per cent of sequels). There may be marked insomnia, or nocturnal wakefulness and diurnal drowsiness. Wakefulness at night is often associated with hyperkinetic phenomena, or with whistling, singing or constant talking. Drowsiness may be combined with muscular weakness (narcolepsy) (Spiller[82]). Changes in personality and disposition are common (30 to 40 per cent) and are shown by anti-social behavior, such as lying, stealing, incorrigibility, and the like; or the reverse may be demonstrated by amiability in a child previously difficult to manage. More serious mental complications are idiocy, manic depressive insanity or that of the type of dementia praecox, and epileptiform convulsions with mental retardation. Mental and motor sequels are liable to be combined.

Among neuromuscular sequels the so-called "Parkinsonian syndrome" should be mentioned. The occurrence of this in children is variously stated as from 5 to 65 per cent of the sequels. In our experience it has been uncommon, at least in a typically developed form. It is likely to be preceded by a period of excitation and to be slow in developing. Among common motor sequels are tremors, muscular twitchings, choreiform movements, and residual paralyses from involvement of the cranial nerves. Less commonly seen are athetoid movements, blindness and deafness, and such paralyses as monoplegia, paraplegia, hemiplegia and generalized spasticity. A peculiar respiratory syndrome with hyperpnea lasting for a few seconds or a minute and followed by apnea is sometimes seen. Parker[73] reported 7 such cases in children.

Many of the conditions mentioned as sequels may also have been present during the acute course, and this is true of other symptoms as well. Among these are excessive salivation, tics, excessive sweating, yawning, talkativeness, precocious sexual sensations, disturbances of speech, alteration of reflexes, and pupillary changes. Endocrine disorders of the adiposo-genital type have been reported by Hofstadt,[32] Ebaugh[75] and others.

Course and Prognosis.—Mortality in the acute stage is usually high, in most reported series equalling 20 or 30 or even 50 per cent, although it is sometimes only 10 per cent or lower. In young infants the mortality may be very high. After this period the influence of age on mortality seems uncertain. Sudden onset indicates a bad prognosis. It is to be remembered that these figures may give an idea of mortality higher than the actual. They are based mostly upon studies of hospital cases, and as such represent the severe forms of the disease. Many of the milder and all the abortive cases are not included because not recognized.

The *duration* of symptoms in uncomplicated, acute cases varies from two to eight weeks. Of those patients who survive the acute stage some die as the result of complications or sequels, and prognosis must always be guarded. The severity of the attack apparently bears some relationship to the prognosis of functional recovery. A short illness with a few days of lethargy, usually results in complete restoration of health. About $\frac{2}{3}$ of the survivors in ordinary cases will develop sequels, although not all of them will exhibit progressive nervous or mental disorders. Complete recovery occurs in a certain number of cases, the figures varying in the statistical studies from 5 to 30 or even 50 per cent. Improvement in the presence of serious sequels does not begin for several months and may continue for several years. Patients with a well-developed Parkinsonian syndrome hardly ever improve.

Diagnosis.—A typical case of encephalitis with lethargy, asthenia, fever and ophthalmoplegia, especially if occurring at the time of an epidemic, offers no great trouble in diagnosis. From *poliomyelitis* of the encephalitic type a clinical differentiation is often not possible, but in the ordinary type of this disease the predominance of spinal symptoms, the hyperesthesia, the rapid extension of paralysis, and the absence of lethargy help to distinguish it from encephalitis. The cytology of the spinal fluid in the two conditions is so much alike that it is seldom helpful in differential diagnosis. In *tuberculous meningitis* the onset is more gradual, the fever lower at the onset, and the symptoms run a more rapid course with increasing severity and more marked rigidity. The differences in the spinal fluids in the two diseases should settle the diagnosis, except in an early case of tuberculous meningitis before meningeal reaction has become marked. In tuberculous meningitis the increased pressure, definitely increased cell-count, film-formation, and diminished sugar-content are characteristic features. The discovery of tubercle bacilli in the fluid is, of course, at once conclusive. *Syphilis* of the central nervous system has an insidious onset and a chronic course, other evidences of the disease will be found, optic nerve-changes are common, and the Wassermann reaction of the blood and spinal fluid will be positive. *Intracranial tumor* is afebrile in its course and early produces choked disc and, eventually, localizing symptoms. Optic neuritis and choked disc occur with great rarity in epidemic encephalitis, although Holden[57] claims that the 2d nerve is affected in 4 to 5 per cent of cases. *Cerebral abscess* causes septic fever, often localizing symptoms, a high leukocytosis, and possibly a positive blood-culture. A focus of infection may be found, usually in the ear. *Uremia* should be diagnosed by evidences of renal disease and examination of the urine. *Meningitis*, other than tuberculous, will be distinguished by a study of the spinal fluid. *Botulism* exhibits no fever, sensory disturbances, mental impairment, or rigidity; although there may be drowsiness and some paralysis. Toxins of the bacillus botulinus may be discovered in the suspected food. In *poisoning by hypnotic drugs*, there may be a history of ingestion of the drug, often a subnormal temperature, profound coma, and perhaps other evidences characteristic of the action of the drug. In *hysteria* there is not such continuance of tremor, paralyses, lethargy, and the like, nor do ocular paralyses ever occur. *Sydenham's chorea* differs from the choreiform type of encephalitis in its more acute course, in the association with rheumatic manifestations, and in the absence of lethargy or other encephalitic symptoms. In *plumbic encephalitis* there should be a history of exposure to that metal, the lead-line in the gums, the characteristic blood-picture with stippling of the cells, the absence of fever, the deposit of lead seen in the roentgenograms of the epiphyses, and the presence of frequent convulsions. *Encephalitis following acute infections*, such as measles, scarlet fever, pertussis or vaccination, may be suspected by the history of its relation to these conditions. In *Schilder's Disease* there is usually a progressive illness over a period of months, with gradually failing hearing, vision, speech, and mentality, and increasing spastic paralysis.

Loewe and Strauss[83] suggest as a means of diagnosis the intracranial injection into animals of spinal fluid or of Berkefeld filtrates of nasopharyngeal washings, from suspected cases. Sato and Yoshimatsu[84] claim that the myeloid leukocytes present in epidemic encephalitis always give a negative peroxidase reaction, whereas in all other diseases the reaction is positive.

Treatment.—The usual attention given to patients suffering from any infectious fever is indicated. There should be care to keep up fluid intake and nourishment, employing gavage if necessary. In hyperactive conditions intake of food must be sufficient to balance the increased metabolism. Hot packs and warm baths are better than sedative drugs in hyperactive and excitable states. There should be special attention paid to the eyes in cases with ocular paralyses. The bladder should be watched for retention and the skin for irritation. While there is a difference of opinion regarding the advisability of lumbar puncture, it would seem that this should be performed when there is increase in intracranial pressure. The treatment of *sequels* is also mainly symptomatic. In some instances when inversion of the sleeping hours is marked, keeping the patient awake during the day may eventually cause a return to the normal habit. Roentgen-ray treatment of the parotid gland has an inhibitive action in excessive salivation. Scopolamin and tincture of stramonium are said to be helpful in the Parkinsonian syndrome. In hyperkinetic conditions atropine seems to have some effect.

Certain *special forms of treatment* may be mentioned. Helmholz and Rosenow[85] have used a serum obtained by inoculating a horse with the streptococcus previously mentioned. Freeman[86] has employed a vaccine of streptococci obtained from patients with encephalitis. Piticariu[87] gave intravenous injection of the patient's own spinal fluid, and Moore,[88] and Moore and Tucker[89] injected the patient's own blood-serum intraspinally. Convalescent's blood-serum has also been used (Grunewald,[90] Sison[91]), as well as intraspinal injection of convalescent's spinal fluid. Hypertonic salt-solution intravenously may be useful by reducing intraspinal pressure

(Bucks[92]). We have seemingly had excellent results from hypertonic solutions of glucose given intravenously. Strecker and Willey,[93] and Strecker[94] believe that benefit was obtained in the acute stage and in sequels by the use of intravenous injections of a solution of neutral acriflavine. Blood-transfusion has also been employed, and various forms of foreign protein therapy, such as typhoid vaccine, normal horse-serum, diphtheria-antitoxin, sodium nucleinate, and milk, in the hope of influencing persistent sequels. Several investigators have tried the effect of malarial inoculations. It is evident that many of these various forms of therapy need further investigation.

References

1. Neurol. Bull., 1919, **2,** 106. 2. J.A.M.A., 1919, **72,** 971. 3. Wien. klin. Wchnschr., 1917, **30,** 581. 4. Boston M. and S. J., 1920, **182,** 34. 5. Am. J. Med. Sc., 1920, **159,** 348. 6. Johns Hopk. Hosp. Bull., 1921, **32,** 137. 7. Encephalit. im Kindersalt., 1929. 8. Arch. Int. Med., 1920, **26,** 477. 9. Pediatria, 1921, **29,** 682. 10. J.A.M.A., 1923, **80,** 1473. 11. Acute Epidem. Encephalit., Trans. Assoc. for Research in Nerv. and Ment. Dis., 1921. 12. Am. J. Med. Sc., 1922, **163,** 715. 13. Tijdschr. v. Geneesk., 1922, **2,** 263. 14. Schweiz. med. Wchnschr., 1922, **52,** 863. 15. Centralbl. f. Bacteriol., 1924, **91,** 159. 16. J.A.M.A., 1923, **81,** 1688; 1930, **94,** 289. 17. J. Immunol., 1929, **17,** 343. 18. J. Infect. Dis., 1930, **47,** 511. 19. J. Med. Research., 1924, **44,** 289. 20. J. Infect. Dis., 1927, **41,** 257. 21. Bull. et mém. soc. de méd. d. hôp. de Paris., 1920, **44,** 583. 22. Arch. Neurol. and Psychiat., 1923, **9,** 170. 23. Med. Rec., 1920, **98,** 225. 24. La riforma med., 1920, **36,** 322. 25. J.A.M.A., 1921, **77,** 153. 26. Rev. neurol., 1923, **39,** 381. 27. Am. J. Dis. Child., 1919, **18,** 83. 28. Bull. et mém. soc. d. méd. d. hôp. de Paris., 1920, **44,** 161. 29. Northwest Med., 1921, **20,** 176. 30. U. S. Publ. Health Rep., 1921, **36,** 207. 31. J.A.M.A., 1921, **77,** 121. 32. Ztschr. f. Kinderh., 1921, **29,** 190; 272. 33. Jahrb. f. Kinderh., 1922, **99,** 209. 34. Lancet, 1929, **2,** 496. 35. J.A.M.A., 1923, **81,** 1352. 36. Am. J. Dis. Child., 1924, **27,** 230. 37. La médicine, Paris, 1920, **2,** 194. 38. Bull. et mém. soc. de méd. d. hôp. de Paris, 1921, **45,** 36. 39. Bull. et mém. soc. de méd. d. hôp. de Paris, 1921, **45,** 40. 40. Norsk. Mag. f. Laegevidensk., 1922, **83,** 843. 41. J.A.M.A., 1919, **73,** 1056. 42. Ann. de l'inst. Pasteur, 1920, **34,** 911. 43. Brit. J. Exp. Path., 1920, **1,** 89. 44. Arch. Neurol. and Psychiat., 1928, **8,** 286. 45. J.A.M.A., 1928, **91,** 231. 46. Arch. Neurol. and Psychiat., 1923, **10,** 212. 47. Med. Science, 1924, **10,** 355. 48. Wien. klin. Wchnschr., 1917, **30,** 933. 49. J.A.M.A., 1920, **74,** 884. 50. J. Lab. and Clin. Med., 1920, **5,** 275. 51. Pub. Health Rep., 1926, **41,** 1095. 52. J.A.M.A., 1922, **79,** 443; J. Infect. Dis., 1923, **32,** 144. 53 Pub. Health Rep., 1927, **42,** 171. 54. Am. J. Med. Sc., 1928, **175,** 683. 55. Am. J Med. Sc., 1920, **160,** 568. 56. Trans. Assoc. for Research in Nerv. and Ment. Dis., 1921. 57. Acute Epidemic Encephalit., Trans. Assoc. for Research in Nerv. and Ment. Dis., 1921. 58. Bull. Johns. Hopkins Hosp., 1930, **47,** 123. 59. New York M. J., 1923, **118,** 399. 60. La presse méd., 1920, **28,** 213. 61. J.A.M.A., 1920, **74,** 735. 62. Arch. Neurol. & Psychiat., 1922, **8,** 15. 63. Quart. J. Med., 1926, **18,** 300. 64. Jahrb. f. Kinderh., 1929, **124,** 188. 65. Ztschr. f. d. ges. Neurol. u. Psychiat., 1922, **76,** 568. 66. Münch. med. Wchnschr., 1919, **66,** 1311. 67. Bull. et mém. soc. méd. d. hôp. de Paris, 1923, **47,** 406. 68. J.A.M.A., 1920, **76,** 1337. 69. Arch. Neurol. and Psychiat., 1921, **5,** 580. 70. Lancet. 1921, **2,** 491. 71. J.A.M.A., 1921, **76,** 373. 72. Arch. de méd. d. enf., 1921, **24,** 457. 73. Arch. Neurol. and Psychiat., 1922, **8,** 630. 74. Bull. Johns Hopkins Hosp., 1922, **33,** 372. 75. Am. J. Dis. Child., 1922, **25,** 87. 76. Quarter. J. Med., 1923, **16,** 173. 77. Arch. de méd. d. enf., 1923, **26,** 265. 78. Am. J. Dis. Child., 1924, **28,** 158. 79. Ztschr. f. Kinderh., 1926, **40,** 678. 80. Brit. M. J., 1927, **1,** 615. 81. Arch. Dis. Childhood, 1928, **3,** 57. 82. J.A.M.A., 1926, **86,** 673. 83. J.A.M.A., 1920, **74,** 1373. 84. Am. J. Dis. Child., 1925, **29,** 301. 85. J.A.M.A., 1922, **79,** 2068. 86. J.A.M.A., 1927, **89,** 1317. 87. Wien. klin. Wchnschr., 1922, **35,** 441. 88. Calif. State J. Med., 1922, **20,** 387. 89. J. Nerv. and Ment. Dis., 1924, **60,** 347. 90. Deutsche med. Wchnschr., 1920, **46,** 1243. 91. Phillipine Is., Assoc. J., 1924, 306. 92. J. Oklahoma, Med. Assoc., 1922, **15,** 308; Ref. Quart. Cumulat. Index., 1922, 632. 93. Am. J. Psychiat., 1925, **4,** 631. 94. Personal Communication.

CHAPTER XXIII

TUBERCULOSIS

Tuberculosis affects many different parts of the body, the local symptoms usually greatly preponderating over the general ones, and producing clinical pictures essentially different from each other. On this account some of the special forms of tuberculosis will be discussed more in detail in different sections. In the present chapter tuberculosis as a whole will be considered, especially as it affects children.

Etiology. **Frequency.**—As far back as the history of medicine extends tuberculosis has existed as one of the most frequent of diseases. It affects many different varieties of animals, although to unequal degrees; being most prevalent in man, monkeys, cattle and swine; as well as in poultry, although in the last it is a decidedly different disorder. It is rare in sheep, goats, horses, dogs and cats. Guinea-pigs and rabbits are very susceptible if inoculated. The actual frequency of tuberculous infection in man is difficult to determine. Statistical evidence indicates that the disease, or at least the mortality from it, is on the decline in the United States (Shepard[1]). The apparent incidence varies, depending upon whether the study is made by means of physical examination, roentgenogram, tuberculin-reaction, or necropsy. For example, Hetherington, McPhedran, Landis and Opie,[2] observed that the intracutaneous tuberculin-test in school children in Philadelphia was positive in 38 per cent at five years, 71 per cent at ten years, and 81 per cent at fifteen years; but that pulmonary lesions definable by roentgenogram at five years constituted only 5 per cent of all infections, at ten years 11 per cent, and at fifteen years 25 per cent. In 2900 school-children in Christiana, Fröhlich[3] found clinical evidence of the disease in about 5 per cent, but positive tuberculin-tests in about 84 per cent. Vonessen[4] obtained a positive tuberculin test in 57 per cent of 550 children, but discovered manifest lesions in only 2 instances.

Predisposing Causes.—Much discussed in this connection is the influence of *heredity*. The usual view is that children born of tuberculous parents are as free from disposition to the disease as are others; some authors, as Drolet,[5] even claiming that they are more resistant to it. The opposite opinion is expressed by Pearl,[6] whose investigations seemed to indicate that the greatly increased incidence in tuberculous as compared with nontuberculous families cannot be accounted for wholly by contact-exposure. Yet it is fair to conclude that any inherited tendency is of far less importance than the factor of exposure. The effect of association is illustrated by the studies of Armand-Delille and Famin[7] and others, in which it is shown that 50 or more per cent of infants living in contact with tuberculous parents will become infected by the beginning of the 2d year of life. *Race* exerts a certain etiologic influence, but some of the effects attributed to it depend upon other associated conditions. The Indians, Irish, and negroes appear especially predisposed in the United States, the mortality-ratio between whites and negroes varying in the different age-groups between 1:2 and 1:5; and manifest tuberculosis being four times as frequent in the colored from the ages of twelve to eighteen years as in whites (Opie, Landis, McPhedran and Hetherington[8]). The people of primitive races, who have not had tuberculosis as an endemic disease, readily become infected on exposure and develop rapidly advancing forms. *Climate* and *locality* are prominent factors. With some exceptions damp regions predispose, and dry, elevated localities are unfavorable to the occurrence of the malady. The frequency of tuberculosis in children on the continent of Europe would appear from statistics to be much greater than in the United States, and in certain cities the incidence in early life seems to be particularly high. *Unhygienic conditions* are of great importance, the crowding of children in dirty buildings, the lack of fresh air and sunlight, insufficient nourishment, and the like, being prominent predisposing causes. The influence of poor hygiene and improper food became evident in the increase of tuberculosis in Europe during and following the World War (Emerson,[9] Pape[10]). Previously *impaired health* also predisposes, especially derangements of the respiratory mucous membrane, and, to a less extent, those of the alimentary tract, including the tonsils and nasopharynx. Many other disorders exert an influence, particularly measles, pertussis, grippe, and repeated attacks of bronchitis. These various agents may act either by rendering the subject liable to the entrance and development of the germs, or by decreasing the local or general resistance, and thus allowing an infection, already present in the body in a quiescent condition, to assume an active form.

Sex is a factor according to the studies of Opie, Landis, McPhedran, and Hetherington,[8] Gibson and Carroll,[11] Cobbett,[12] and others, girls being more often affected and showing a greater mortality except in the early age-groups.

Age exerts a very positive influence. Congenital tuberculosis is occasionally seen. A number of writers have reviewed the subject, among them Whitman and Green,[13] who estimated that there were on record 113 authenticated cases. Other instances have since been reported. Scheer[14] reports 4 cases and accepts as authentic only 38 of those previously published. Horak[15] admits 114 reported instances of congenital tuberculosis and 519 doubtful ones. Tuberculosis is, however, exceptional in the first three months of life, but increases rapidly in incidence after this period. There exists great variation in the figures obtained by necropsy, depending, among other things, upon the geographical region where the investigations were made. This may be seen in the statistics of Hand[16] from Philadelphia, Feldmann[17] from Hungary, Hamburger[18] from Vienna, Harbitz[19] from Norway, Comby[20] from Paris, and Wollstein and Spence[21] from New York. Other necropsy studies which may be mentioned are those of Cornet[22] and Schlossmann.[23] The usual figure found by these different writers for the first year of life was about 5 per cent; by five years the variation is great, being from 9 to 40 per cent or more; while in the age-period from ten to fifteen years it may be as high as 70 per cent. The figures as given represent, however, only the discovery of tuberculous lesions at necropsy, and they do not always indicate that the death was due to this disease, nor do they reveal the incidence of tuberculosis at different ages in children who do not come to necropsy. In fact, the older the child, the oftener is the tuberculous lesion a latent or healed process.

The question of the frequency of tuberculous infection as shown by the tuberculin-test varies not only with age but also with other factors. The incidence of positive reactions is greater in some localities than others, is greater with the intracutaneous than with the cutaneous method, is greater in groups with poor social status, and is less in childhood in recent years than formerly. Figure 83 given by Smith[29] illustrates some of these differences dependent on locality. Among other studies of importance are those by Lapage[32] for Manchester, McNeil[33] for Edinburgh, Veeder and Johnston[34] for St. Louis, Gittings and Donnelly[35] for Philadelphia, and Dickey and Seitz[36] for San Francisco.

The obtaining of a positive tuberculin-reaction is not a proof that the clinical manifestations which the child may exhibit necessarily depend upon tuberculosis, but only that this infection exists somewhere in the body, perhaps as a small, entirely inactive focus. The test is often positive in children in robust health with no discoverable lesion. Children of the better social class, especially in the younger age-groups, will have fewer positive reactions than indicated in the figures given. The frequency with which tuberculous lesions are found in children dying from other disorders, and the large number of cases in which a positive tuberculin-reaction is obtained in apparently healthy children, support the view of Hamburger,[37] Schlossmann,[38] Wassermann,[39] Köffler[40] and others, that tuberculous infection is liable to be acquired especially in childhood, and, if recovered from, establishes an immunity, but only while the bacilli are lying dormant in the body. This immunity may be overcome by later massive and repeated reinfections (*superinfection*). Adults who have not had the protection of earlier infection are prone, if attacked later, to develop rapidly progressing forms of the disease.

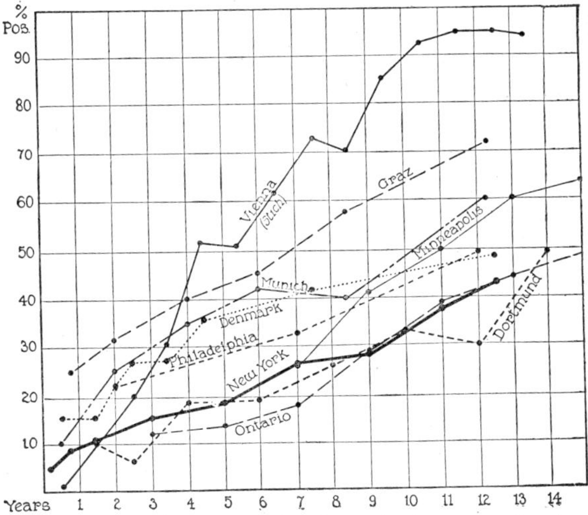

Fig. 83.—Curves marked with names of cities and places showing incidence of positive intracutaneous tests by years. The sources are as follows: Vienna, Hamburger and Monti;[24] Graz, Barchetti;[25] Munich, Barchetti; Denmark, Krogsgaard;[26] Minneapolis, Harrington and Myers;[27] Philadelphia, Opie;[28] New York, Smith;[29] Dortmund, Sander;[30] Ontario, Elliott.[31]

Exciting Cause.—That the disease is an infectious one was believed from early times, but was first clearly proven by Villemin[41] in 1865. That it was dependent upon the tubercle bacillus was first demonstrated by Koch[42] in 1882. Since the studies of Theobald Smith,[43] most authors agree that there appear to be two varieties of the bacillus capable of producing the disease in man: the bovine and the human. The relationship and relative importance of these is still a subject of much discussion. It appears to be proven that the human bacillus can occasionally cause tuberculosis in cattle. In like manner, the bovine germ can certainly produce it in man, but the large majority of cases owe their origin to the human variety. Infection with the bovine bacillus is more common in certain European countries than in the United States; this depending probably upon the condition of the cattle, and still more upon the handling of the milk and the failure to pasteurize it. Statistical studies with somewhat varying conclusions are given by Fraser,[44] Park and Krumwiede,[45] Mitchell,[46] Cobbett,[47] Gordon and Brown,[48] and Rosenau.[49] Tuberculosis of the lungs, meninges, and osseous system in children is nearly always of human origin, but that of the intestine and cervical glands is not infrequently caused by the bovine type. Bovine tuberculosis is more common in children than in adults, causing about 6 per cent of all deaths from tuberculosis, but about 33 per cent in those under five years of age (Cobbett[47]).

The germs are found in tuberculous lesions wherever situated, and in the secretions and excretions from the affected tissues, particularly when the process is active. Outside of the body they are widely diffused and very abundant, the chief source being the sputum, in which they are present in enormous numbers. They are capable of living and remaining virulent for weeks in a dried state in the dust from rooms occupied by consumptive patients, but are killed by a temperature as low as 60 C. (140 F.) if continued for fifteen or twenty minutes. The general opinion is that they are seldom to be found in the blood. It has been claimed by Calmette, Valtis, Négre and Boquet[50] and other workers that the tubercle bacillus may occur in a filterable form, but this has been denied, and remains to be further demonstrated (see Thompson and Frobisher[51]).

Mode of Transmission and Portal of Entry.—The germ enters the body either by the alimentary or, far oftener, the respiratory tract, except in the rare cases of congenital tuberculosis, in which the infection is through the blood, and in the exceptional instances of direct inoculation, as by ritual circumcision or through other lesions in the skin or mucous membrane. The inhaled bacilli tend to go to the alveoli and terminal bronchioles, where they come to rest, because here, in contrast to the remainder of the pulmonary air-passages, there is no ciliated epithelium. Having penetrated cells and tissue-spaces, they then produce tubercles at this point, and are likewise always carried by lymphatic channels to the tracheobronchial lymph-nodes. This primary lesion may be small and difficult to discover, but that it always occurs is maintained by Parrot,[52] Küss,[53] Albrecht,[54] Ghon,[55] and others, and this appears to be the view now commonly adopted. The bacilli may lie dormant in this lesion or in the lymph-nodes an indefinite time. Finally, perhaps, inflammatory changes and softening may occur, and the infection of other organs or of the system at large takes place, extension being by contiguity, bronchial tubes, lymph-vessels or eroded blood-vessels. The younger the patient the less likely are the foci to become dormant.

When the initial infection is by the alimentary tract there is a primary lesion, although small, at the portal of entry, and when this is in the intestine there is secondary involvement of the mesenteric lymph-nodes. The findings of Wood,[56] showing 5.2 per cent of tuberculous infection in 1671 collected cases of extirpated tonsils, point to these structures as one of the portals of entry. Usually in such cases the cervical nodes arrest further extension of the disease. There is no lymphatic connection between cervical and bronchial glands (Beitzke[57]). (See also Tuberculous Adenitis, p. 1059.)

Without reference to the small primary lesion at the portal of entry, but only to the larger ones readily seen, and which would appear to have existed longest, the results of various investigations are contradictory as to the relative frequency of infection of the respiratory and alimentary tracts respectively. Northrup,[58] Holt,[59] Bovaird,[60] Hand,[16] Hamburger,[18] Albrecht[54] and Kudlich[61] found that the oldest lesion was hardly ever discovered in the intestinal tract. On the other hand the studies of Carr,[62] Still,[63] and Leonard[64] show a rather high incidence of primary intestinal tuberculosis. It has been maintained by some that the infrequency of primary lesions found in the alimentary canal is due to the passage of the bacilli directly to the general circulation by way of the thoracic duct, and thence to the lungs and tracheobronchial nodes, instead of producing original lesions in the intestinal wall and in neighboring mesenteric nodes. This would appear to be supported by the experiments of Straus[65] and of Calmette, Guérin and Déléarde,[66] which show that tubercle bacilli injected into the stomach cause general tuberculosis, and that respiratory involvement can be produced in this way without a lesion of the mesenteric lymph-nodes. There does not seem to be satisfactory proof of the truth of this theory, and against it are the investigations of Findlay,[67] Pfeiffer and Friedberger,[68] and others demonstrating the ease with which respiratory tuberculosis can be brought about by inhalation. It would appear to be a justifiable conclusion that all roentgenological and experimental evidence is in favor of the much greater frequency of infection by inhalation.

Directly bearing on this matter is the question of the danger of milk from tuberculous cattle. While it has been shown by Pearson and Ravenel[69] and others that it is possible for tuberculous cattle to excrete bacilli in their milk, even when the udders are not diseased, it is certain that it is not usually the case. Cow's milk can also readily be contaminated by the human bacilli. Proper pasteurization should eliminate such a source of infection.

Pathologic Anatomy. The Histology of Tubercle.—The basis of the pathologic changes of tuberculosis is the miliary tubercle, which is the result of the irritation produced by the rapidly multiplying bacilli. It consists of a gray, translucent body about 0.5 cm. ($\frac{1}{5}$ in.) or less in diameter, surrounded by a reticulum of connective tissue, and is composed of leukocytes at first polymorphonuclear, later chiefly mononuclear, migrating from the neighboring blood-vessels, and of lymphoid and epithelioid cells the result of proliferation of the tissue-cells. Bacilli are present in some of the epithelioid cells. Giant-cells are found in some of the tubercles, their number being inversely proportional to the number of bacilli present. The tubercles may remain scattered and mostly separated from each other, or may be grouped in large masses. As growth progresses degenerative changes take place. Caseation is the most common, the tubercle becoming yellow, containing many bacilli, and finally softening. This is followed by an inflammation of the surrounding tissue and the formation of pus through a mixed infection. Less frequently calcification occurs, seen oftenest in the lymph-nodes. Sometimes, especially if the tubercles remain discrete and miliary, sclerosis takes place, a firm, fibrous structure resulting. Krause[70] terms the tubercle the nodular form of tuberculosis, and the diffuse exudative, inflammatory changes and effusions the non-nodular, the latter being due to allergy (sensitivity) to the protein of the tubercle bacillus. Both of these processes are protective, the nodular successfully walling off the bacilli in 90 per cent of infections and the nonnodular tending to fix them where they lodge.

Regions Oftenest Found Affected by Tuberculosis at Different Periods of Infancy and Childhood.—*Age* is a prominent factor. Taking infancy and childhood as a whole, the statistics compiled by Freeman[71] in 2288 necropsies in tuberculous children reported by different observers show involvement of the lungs in from 71 to 100 per cent; of the bronchial lymph-nodes in from 76 to 99 per cent; of the intestines in from 23 to 55 per cent; and of the mesenteric lymph-nodes in from 16 to 40 per cent. These figures must not be confused with those for the primary or initial lesion already given.

In the *first two years of life* the regions oftenest found diseased are the bronchial lymph-nodes, lungs, and pleura. Involvement of the mesenteric nodes is less frequent than that of the bronchial; that of the cervical nodes not as common as later. Tuberculous meningitis is very common, seen oftenest in combination with other clinical manifestations. Tuberculosis of the peritoneum, the intestine, and the bones is not frequent in infancy. Contrary to the usual experience Merritt[72] found tuberculous ulceration of the intestine in $\frac{1}{3}$ of the necropsies in 75 tuberculous infants under one year of age. At this period of life there is especially to be noted the tendency for tuberculosis to become widespread. (Raczynaki,[73] about 50 per cent of 611 cases up to three years.)

In *early childhood*, from the third to the fifth year inclusive, general tuberculosis and meningitis remain very common, and involvement of the cervical and mesenteric nodes, and of the intestine, peritoneum and bones increases in frequency. Tuberculosis of the lungs is, however, probably the most common form, with that of the pleura and bronchial nodes nearly as often seen as this.

In *later childhood* tuberculous meningitis, although still frequent, is not so often observed as in earlier childhood. Cervical adenitis and involvement of the bones and joints remain common, while tuberculous peritonitis is increasingly often seen.

The kidneys, liver, and spleen may show miliary tubercles on their surface at any age, in cases of general miliary tuberculosis. The larynx is seldom involved. The pancreas, thyroid, thymus, heart, and genito-urinary tract are regions only exceptionally attacked in early life.

Lesions Oftenest Producing Death.—It by no means follows that the parts oftenest affected are those the disease of which occasions the death of the patient. Thus, in infancy, although pulmonary involvement, usually in the form of bronchopneumonia, is the most frequent cause of death, in many pulmonary cases the fatal issue depends actually upon a general miliary tuberculosis, or, oftener, a tuberculous meningitis. Involvement of the bronchial lymph-nodes, although so frequent, rarely produces fatal symptoms. In early and later childhood meningitis, secondary to involvement of the lungs, bones, or lymph-nodes, very often occasions the fatal termination (Shennan[74] 45 per cent of 413 cases). Tuberculous peritonitis is also a not infrequent cause of death in later childhood, while tuberculous pleurisy, although common, is rarely in itself fatal.

Duration of Incubation.—The period elapsing between the time of a known infection of a previously tuberculosis-free child and that when the tuberculin-test responds positively is somewhat variable, but averages for the cutaneous reaction from four to six weeks (Hamburger,[75] Wallgren,[76] Epstein[77]), and somewhat less for the intracutaneous. The determination of the length of clinical incubation is usually difficult and uncertain. It may be a few weeks, or several years, before symptoms of tuberculosis make their appearance.

Clinical Forms of Tuberculosis. (*A*) General Tuberculosis.—This form consists in a wide-spread development of tubercles secondary to some small caseous area. Through the entrance of large numbers of bacilli into the blood the disease is spread more or less diffusely throughout the body, the extent varying with the case. Sometimes the various organs are crowded with tubercles, especially well seen in the lungs; sometimes these are much more scattered and fewer. The symptoms and the rapidity of the course of the disease vary accordingly. The liver is oftener affected in children than in adults. The tubercles are commonly larger in children, and, in the less rapid cases, assume a considerable size through confluence, many of them becoming caseous and breaking down. General tuberculosis may exhibit itself in two forms, (1) the *Typhoid* and (2) the *Marantic*.

1. The Typhoid Form; Acute Miliary Tuberculosis.—This is seen chiefly in infancy and early childhood. The initial symptoms are very vague, consisting of loss of appetite, debility, loss of weight, and other evidences of a general impairment of health. Fever of an irregular and uncharacteristic type soon develops; debility increases; the tongue becomes dry; the pulse and respiration area ccelerated; there are apathy, dulness, sometimes delirium and finally coma. The tympanites and enlarged spleen, with the continued fever and other symptoms, may strongly suggest typhoid fever. In other cases the temperature is almost too irregular for this disease, and often only slightly or, exceptionally, not at all elevated. No cause for the symptoms can be found. Temporary improvement may occur, although the emaciation does not disappear or the strength greatly increase. Finally some localizing symptoms may develop, especially those of pulmonary consolidation or of meningitis; less often of peritonitis. Purpuric spots may occur on the skin and mucous membranes. The course of the disease is rapid, death occurring usually within a few weeks. The differential *diagnosis* from typhoid fever is extremely difficult, especially as a leukopenia may exist in both conditions. Suggestive of tuberculosis is the more irregular fever, the tendency to rapid respiration, the failure of the fever to lessen at the end of three or four weeks, and the persistent absence of the Widal reaction. Finally the development of localizing symptoms, or the suggestion of miliary tuberculosis shown by roentgenograms of the chest, may make the diagnosis of tuberculosis almost certain; but this is usually discovered only a few days before death.

2. The Marantic Form.—Infants not infrequently exhibit a somewhat more chronic form of tuberculosis, closely simulating marasmus (p. 465). The symptoms are entirely uncharacteristic, progressive wasting and anemia being the principal ones. There is at first no fever, or only occasional and irregular elevations, and no respiratory or gastro-intestinal disturbances sufficient to account for the condition. The disease is indistinguishable from other marantic states, except at necropsy. In other instances there develops a few weeks before the end of life more or less constant but moderate fever of irregular type, with slight symptoms and physical signs suggesting bronchopneumonia. Sometimes vomiting or, especially, diarrhea may become troublesome, or the symptoms of meningitis close the scene. Generally, however, death appears to be due to progressive exhaustion. The course of the case is brief, although decidedly more prolonged than in the typhoid form; at longest a few weeks after continued fever or localizing symptoms appear, but often much longer from the first beginning of signs of illness. The *diagnosis* is always difficult and usually impossible, until, perhaps, shortly before death. Even the development of signs of bronchopneumonia is not conclusive, since nontuberculous bronchopneumonia is so frequently a terminal condition in infantile atrophy. The principal diagnostic aid is to be sought in the history. The entire absence of discoverable reason for the continued wasting; the absence of evidences of chronic or repeated intestinal autointoxication; the opportunity for exposure; and the fact that diarrhea, cough, and vomiting have followed emaciation rather than preceded it, are reasons for suspecting tuberculosis. The tuberculin-test may be of value in some cases; in others it is negative on account of the overwhelming nature of the attack.

(*B*) Tuberculosis of Special Regions.—Here are to be included a large number of forms of tuberculosis in which the disease is confined to, or preponderates in, certain regions or organs of the body. Many of the conditions will be simply mentioned briefly here, and fuller description of them given elsewhere.

1. Tuberculosis of the Lungs.—Several varieties of this may be seen:

(*a*) *Acute Miliary Tuberculosis of the Lungs.*—This is the form of the general miliary tuberculosis described, in which the localization from the onset is most prominent in the lungs. It is commonest after the age of infancy. There is a persistent fever of irregular but not hectic type; rapid respiration, which is sometimes dyspneic; prostration; rapid pulse; cough; and sometimes cyanosis. The physical signs in the lungs are often poorly marked and uncharacteristic. Suggestive roentgenographic changes, the so-called "snowflake" appearance, may be found only late in the course of the disease. Still later the evidences of tuberculosis elsewhere may show themselves, the child dying, possibly, from meningitis. The course of the case is usually short. At necropsy the lungs are found filled with miliary tubercles.

(*b*) *Tuberculous Bronchitis.*—This is, strictly speaking, rather an obstinate bronchitis complicating and dependent upon the presence of tuberculous foci somewhere in the lungs. Sometimes it is the first stage of a tuberculous bronchopneumonia. In other instances it is of a chronic nature, and probably depends upon reflex or direct irritation by the tuberculous focus or its

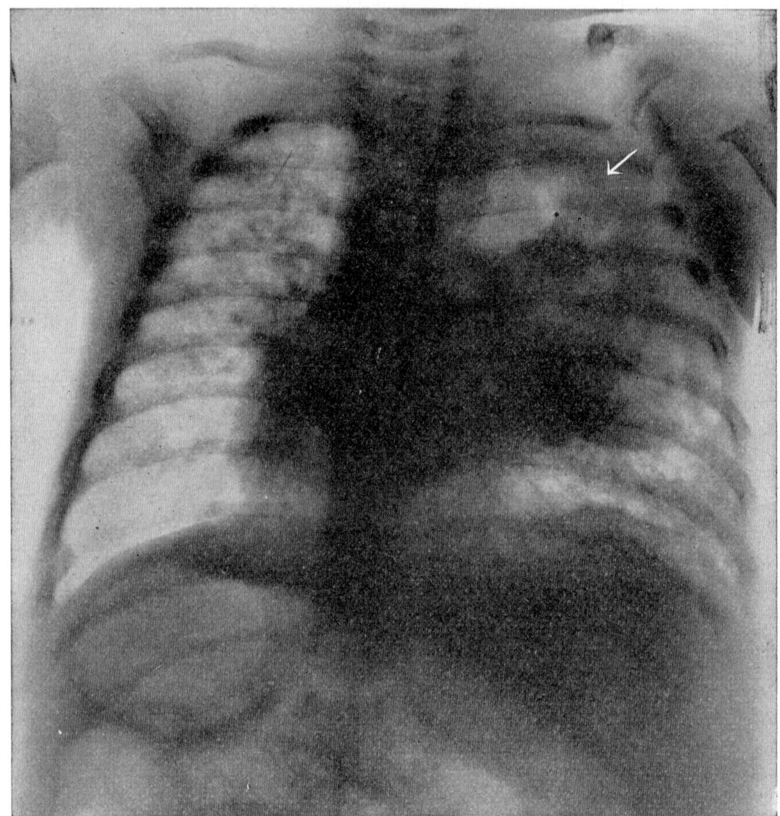

Fig. 84.—Roentgenogram of acute tuberculous bronchopneumonia, with cavity-formation. Mary S.; colored; aged ten months. More or less bronchitis since April. Pneumonia began four days before admission to the Children's Hospital of Philadelphia, June 10. Physical signs of consolidation of upper part of right lobe suggested croupous pneumonia. In hospital five weeks. Roentgenogram July 5th showed consolidation of right lung with cavity at the apex. Necropsy disclosed lesions of tuberculosis. Cavity about 2.5 cm. in diameter with ragged walls; tubercle bacilli in smear from its contents.

secretions. Sometimes the râles are scattered; oftener they are limited to a certain area upon one side. There are no other physical signs. The general symptoms are entirely indefinite and those only of bronchitis, except in the cases which progress unfavorably, when fever finally develops and the condition assumes the characteristics of a chronic bronchopneumonia.

(*c*) *Acute Tuberculous Bronchopneumonia.*—This is one of the most frequent manifestations of tuberculosis in children. It is seen oftenest in infancy and, especially, early childhood; may be primary in the lungs or secondary to tuberculosis in some other part of the body, such as the bones, pleura, peritoneum, and particularly the bronchial lymph-nodes; or may follow some other disease, particularly pertussis, grippe, measles, or even bronchitis or simple bronchopneumonia. The pathologic lesions are the same as those of nontuberculous bronchopneumonia, with the addition of the presence of tubercle bacilli, and the development of tubercles and of the degenerative changes which subsequently take place in these, and which result in the formation of many smaller and larger caseous areas and often finally of cavities (Fig. 84) if life continues a sufficient time; generally small and centrally located, but sometimes of considerable size. We have seen a cavity as large as an average orange, occupying the entire upper right lobe in a child of seven months, and Crespin and Athias[78] report a cavity containing tubercle bacilli in an infant of twenty days. Ghon[79] in 203 necropsies in the first year of life found cavities frequently. Occasionally rupture into the pleural sac takes place. The large, slowly developing, encapsulated cavities characteristic of phthisis in the adult are usually absent in childhood until the age of puberty is approached. With the tuberculous process in the lungs is always associated similar disease of the bronchial lymph-nodes. The clinical picture does not differ materially from that of simple bronchopneumonia. Very frequently, however, the onset is more gradual, the principal early symptoms being cough, loss of weight, debility, increased rapidity of respiration and pulse-rate, and moderate fever of an irregular type. Later dyspnea becomes decided, the cough worse, the temperature higher, and there are cyanosis and increasing weakness. The physical signs are the same as those of simple bronchopneumonia, the lesions usually being scattered to a varying extent throughout both lungs, although most apparent in one. The pseudolobar form is less often seen. When localization occurs it is oftener in the upper lobe and toward the hilus than is the case with simple bronchopneumonia. Yet there is such variation possible in the symptoms and physical signs that the *diagnosis* of the tuberculous nature of the case is often impossible. Suggestive of tuberculosis is the development of bronchopneumonia during convalescence from measles or pertussis, or after a period of wasting and ill-health such as occurs in the general tuberculosis of infants; the discovery of tuberculosis elsewhere in the body; the failure of convalescence to begin at the time which might reasonably be expected in simple bronchopneumonia; and the consequently longer course, continuing perhaps for several weeks. Tubercle bacilli may often be found in the secretion from the lungs. (See p. 421.) The tuberculin-reaction will be positive except in advanced cases. In rare instances hemoptysis may occur. We have seen a profuse hemorrhage fatal in a few minutes in an infant of fourteen months.

(*d*) *Epituberculosis* (*Paratuberculosis, Perifocal Infiltration, Collateral Inflammation, Gelatinous Pneumonia*).—This pulmonary inflammation, to which several names have been given, results from cellular reaction (serum and leukocytes) around the focus which contains the tubercle bacilli. It has been described by Eliasberg and Neuland,[80] Engel,[81] and others. The onset may be acute with fever, or more insidious; the involvement small or including one or more lobes; and the physical signs and roentgenograms much similar to those of a pneumonia, except that there is often a suppression of breath-sounds rather than distinct tubular breathing. Usually the condition is a mild one and the infiltration disappears after a few weeks or months without secondary involvement with tubercle bacilli.

(*e*) *Subacute and Chronic Pulmonary Tuberculosis.*—This may show itself in several forms in children.

(*α*) *Subacute and Chronic Tuberculous Bronchopneumonia* (Figs. 85, 86).—The subacute type of this condition constitutes merely a protracted form of acute tuberculous bronchopneumonia and is directly continuous with it. It may last for some months and terminate fatally, or may, less often, pass into the chronic form. The chronic form may also develop without being preceded by any well-marked acute attack of bronchopneumonia. In some cases there may have been only occurrences of what was supposed to be a bronchitis. Whatever the mode of onset, the recovery is not complete and the child is left with debility and cough. Repeated exacerbations take place at intervals, and gradually decided physical signs of chronic bronchopneumonia develop, if not present previously. Excep-

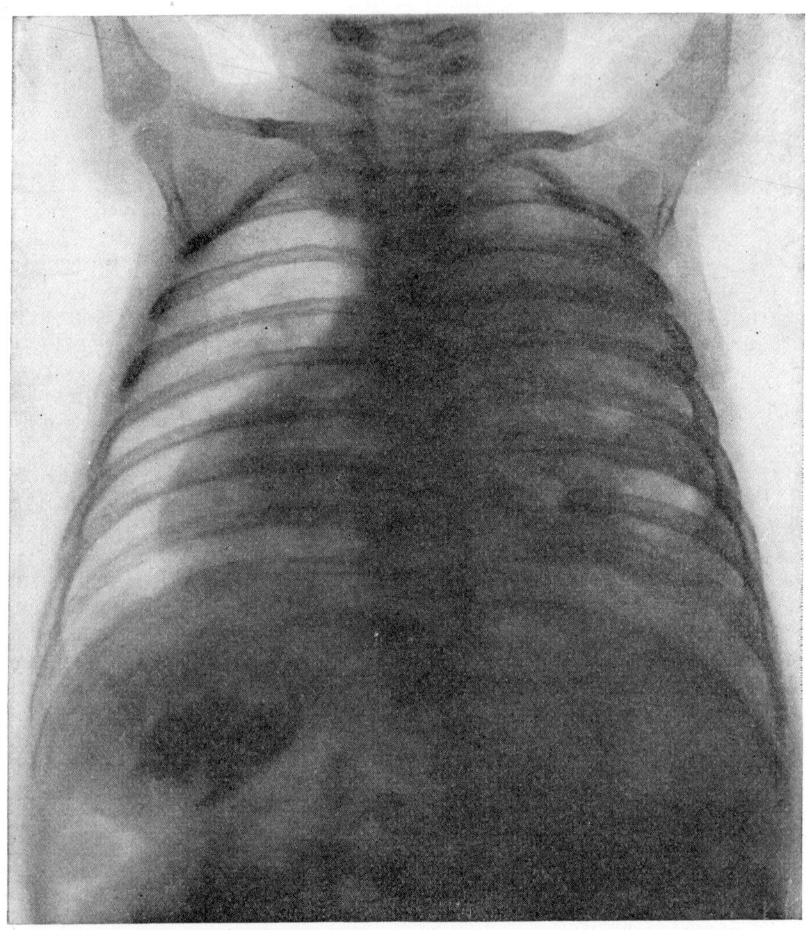

Fig. 85.—Subacute tuberculous bronchopneumonia. Wm. K., age eleven months on admission to the Children's Hospital of Philadelphia. Died at fourteen months. Cough and debility from age of three months. Showed dulness on percussion throughout right lung with crackling râles and feeble breath-sounds, and finally bronchial respiration over upper part with cavernous breathing at the apex. Roentgenogram shows advanced lesions of tuberculous bronchopneumonia in the right lung and to a less extent in the left. Viewed from behind.

tionally the disease may begin insidiously, with wasting, continued fever, and more or less cough. The lesions may not be discoverable, or only unsatisfactorily so by physical examination; but the roentgenogram may show numerous scattered areas (Fig. 86). The disease may continue for months and terminate finally by exhaustion or through the development of some acute tuberculous process.

(β) *Hilus Tuberculosis.*—This is a pulmonary condition arising in connection with tuberculosis of the tracheobronchial nodes, especially those adjacent to the hilus of the lung. It may develop at any period of early life, even infancy. The onset is insidious and the symptoms vague, consisting of malaise, diminished appetite, debility, and possibly evening rise of temperature. There is a positive tuberculin reaction, but an absence of the ordinary physical signs. The involvement of the pulmonary tissue of the hilus cannot be distinguished by physical examination from that of the glands of the hilus which accompanies it. The roentgenogram may show fine lines radiating from the root of the lung (Fig. 87), probably indicating

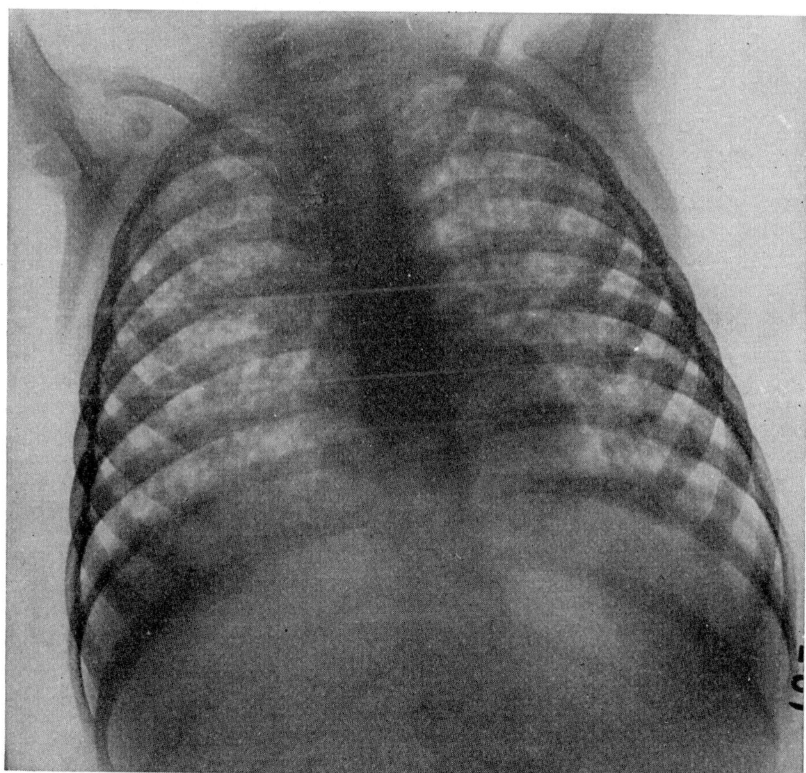

Fig. 86.—Chronic tuberculous bronchopneumonia. George T., age two and one-half years. General poor health in the summer. Ileocolitis in autumn. This followed by impairment of health, troublesome cough, accelerated pulse and respiration and, dating from December, irregular fever. First seen the following April. Under observation had slight cough, emaciation, debility, respiration 30 to 40, irregular fever, positive tuberculin reaction, tuberculide under chin. No tubercle bacilli found. Physical examination of chest revealed only deficient expansion. Died in July. Roentgenogram shows wide-spread infiltration with numerous scattered lesions, larger than those of miliary tuberculosis.

an involvement of the pulmonary parenchyma of the hilus-region. The condition runs the chronic course of tuberculosis of the tracheobronchial nodes.

(γ) *Primary Pulmonary Foci of Ghon.*—The name of Ghon is commonly associated with these lesions, although they were earlier described by others. (See p. 410.) They consist of small, round foci, single or few in number, varying in size, but oftenest about that of a pea. In the large majority of cases the lesion is directly subpleural (90 per cent, Stoloff[82]). Ghon[55] and Schürmann[83] discovered by necropsy, and Stoloff by roentgenographical studies, that the lesion was oftenest in the upper lobes and most frequently on the right side. Around the primary focus, or the tracheobronchial lymph-node, may develop an inflammatory edema and a gelatinous pneumonia, not necessarily specific in nature. In the primary lesion, as also in the tracheobronchial nodes, the infection may lie dormant for an indefinite period, and caseation, calcification, and cicatrization may take place. Especially, however, in youthful subjects, instead of becoming dormant the foci increase in size, remain moderately active, and such symptoms develop

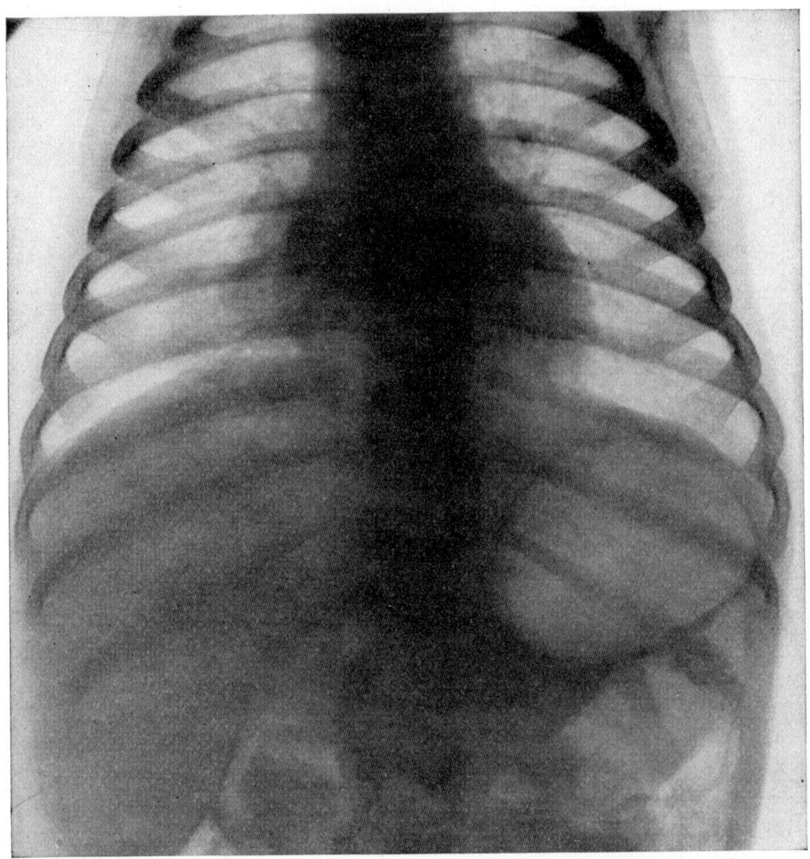

Fig. 87.—Tuberculosis of the bronchial nodes and of the hilus of the lungs. The ray-like shadows indicate the infiltration along the course of the bronchial tubes.

as irregular fever, loss of weight, and chronic cough; with the absence of physical signs, excepting possibly some scattered râles.

(δ) *Phthisis.*—This is the form of the disease so common in adult life. It is rarely found in infancy and early childhood, and even in later childhood it is very much less frequent than after this period. In our experience it occurs much oftener in children of the colored race. Statistics vary considerably, but it is interesting to note that Sawyer[84] in a physical examination of 8000 children under fifteen years of age found only 15 in whom a diagnosis of phthisis could be made with reasonable certainty. Its symptoms, physical signs and treatment are much the same as those of phthisis in adult life, the most important early finding being persistent fine râles at the apices of the lungs. To be noted is the lesser frequency of cough, involvement of the larynx, dyspnea and hemoptysis in children. The disease is to be distinguished chiefly from chronic bronchiectasis, and from those cases of chronic simple bronchopneumonia in which the occurrence of thickening about a large bronchus strongly suggests the presence of a cavity. Abscess of the lung, too, may closely simulate it, but the presence of tubercle bacilli in the sputum, or of the tuberculin-reaction, may settle the diagnosis. The infrequency with which cavity-formation takes place in the cases in children denominated phthisis by many observers raises the question whether many of those included in the statistics should not, strictly speaking, be considered chronic disseminated tuberculous bronchopneumonia, rather than phthisis as it occurs in adult life. No reference is intended here to the rapid production of cavity so frequent in acute tuberculous bronchopneumonia.

2. Tuberculosis of the Lymphatic Nodes.—The involvement of the lymph-nodes is one of the most common forms of tuberculosis in early life, and the frequency of its occurrence is much greater than in adults. That of the internal nodes is often combined with evident tuberculosis of other parts, the symptoms of which give the clinical evidences of tuberculous infection. Included under this heading are general tuberculous adenitis, tuberculosis of the tracheobronchial lymph-nodes, tuberculosis of the mesenteric nodes (tabes mesenterica), and tuberculosis of the cervical nodes. These are described in the section on Tuberculous Adenitis (p. 1058).

3. Tuberculosis of Other Parts of Body.—Tuberculosis may occur in the alimentary tract; in the genito-urinary tract; in the nervous system; in serous membranes, especially the meninges, the peritoneum, and the pleura; in the osseous system; and in the skin. The diseased changes so produced will be discussed under their appropriate headings (see Index).

Prognosis.—It has been frequently stated that tuberculosis is the cause of about $\frac{1}{7}$ of all deaths (11.22 per cent U. S. Census 1900) (Wilbur[85]). In recent years the disease seems to be on the decline (Lee,[86] Kleinschmidt[87]). The causes of this would appear to be the acquiring of immunity by minimal healed infections, the improved living conditions and health of the population in general, improvement in hygienic methods, and better facilities for treatment (Shepard[88]). It is noteworthy, however, that the diminution in the number of deaths from tuberculosis in children has not kept pace with that for later periods of life (Behla,[89] Hoffmann[90]). Further, as already stated (p. 408), such circumstances as the World War, or local conditions of famine, greatly increased for a time the mortality in certain regions.

Prognosis varies with age. In the first year of life the majority of those infected die; in the second year the prognosis is better, and progressively so as the age at which infection takes place advances and the power of resistance increases. Our own experience coincides with a number of published investigations, as those of Langer,[91] Baümler,[92] Söderström,[93] McPhedran,[94] and Myers and Kernkamp,[95] that quite a number of infants may recover, even when infected in the first year of life. Gasul[96] followed for a period of from one to eight years 404 children in whom the diagnosis of tuberculosis had been made from the fourth to the thirtieth month of life. In 221 of these merely a positive tuberculin-reaction was obtained, but in the remainder clinical tuberculosis was diagnosed. The mortality was less than 4 per cent, but highest in those infected during the first six months (17.2 per cent of 29 infants). Some authors, as Klostermann,[97] state that tuberculosis is especially dangerous when contracted during puberty.

There is variation also in prognosis depending on the clinical type of the disease. The primary lesion of Ghon tends to recover without further extension, except in very early life. It is, in fact, by means of this and by tracheobronchial and hilus tuberculosis, which also usually end in recovery, that immunity to later infection may be established. The presence of the foci is, however, always a menace, as dissemination may occur from them. Miliary tuberculosis is almost always rapidly fatal but not invariably so. We have seen two apparently typical cases which recovered. Tuberculous bronchopneumonia is practically always fatal, either in the first attack or in relapses, although in the chronic form it may last for several years. Only isolated instances of recovery from tuberculous meningitis have been reported. (See p. 929.) Favorable termination is frequent in tuberculous peritonitis, tuberculous pleurisy, osseous tuberculosis, and tuberculosis of the cervical nodes. The prognostic indications of the tuberculin-reaction will be referred to later (p. 422).

Diagnosis.—To avoid confusion it should be stated that the terms "incipient" or "minimal" tuberculosis are usually employed to describe a slight lesion, but that the term "early" tuberculosis may be applied to a lesion which is incipient, moderately advanced, or far advanced.

In the diagnosis attention should be given to the history of tuberculosis in the family, especially the opportunity for exposure to infection. There should be investigated also the existence of poor hygienic conditions, and the prior occurrence of such diseases as grippe, pneumonia, bronchitis, pertussis, and measles, because of their predisposing influence in pulmonary tuberculosis. A generally defective state of health may have some diagnostic significance, but malnutrition in itself cannot be regarded as closely related to tuberculosis. For example, Hetherington[98] showed that subnormal weight was not more frequent in children with positive tuberculin-reactions than in others, and that underweight could not be correlated with the graver lesions revealed by roentgenograms. In fact, it is often found that a child with severe tuberculosis of the lungs may be in a good nutritional state, and that his general health has suffered little.

Fever occurs at the time of the initial infection, but may not be discovered. In clinical tuberculosis fever is almost always observed, generally of an irregular type, often slight, and perhaps not constant. It is of diagnostic importance only if other causes for it are entirely excluded. It may be absent in a limited tuberculosis of the hilus and bronchial lymph-nodes. It must always be borne in mind that the oral temperature of many normal children may be almost 100 F. Fluctuation of more than 1.5 degrees in the twenty-four hours has some significance. Ready development of fatigue, and increasing impairment of the general health are common symptoms, but not, of course, specific for tuberculosis. Rapid pulse is usually associated with the fever and present only with it. Cough may be present, but is certainly not a constant troublesome accompaniment of all tuberculous pulmonary lesions. It is generally absent in quiescent lesions as also in involvement of the tracheobronchial lymph-nodes, unless this is extensive. Enlargement of the lymph-nodes discoverable anywhere by any method should receive consideration. Palpable nodular masses within the abdominal cavity are oftenest in early life dependent upon tuberculosis, and ascites at this time is frequently due to this disease. Hemoptysis is rare. Pleurisy should always be regarded with the suspicion that it is tuberculous in nature.

Examination of the blood has possibly some diagnostic value. In many acute forms, including tuberculous pneumonia and miliary tuberculosis, there is often a normal or only slightly increased total leukocyte count. In tuberculous meningitis, however, there may be a decided leukocytosis. A number of observers, among them Cunningham and Tompkins,[99] Becker,[100] Bredeck,[101] Blackfan and Diamond,[102] Hamil,[103] and Reilly,[104] using supravital technique, have found that the monocytes are practically always increased in number and stimulated in phagocytic activity in active tuberculosis, and the lymphocytes decreased; while during healing the number of lymphocytes increase. There is no agreement that the eosinophiles are affected. It has been stated, only to be denied by a number of investigators, that there is a low blood-calcium during the active stage of the disease.

Roentgen-ray examination is of great value in the diagnosis of some forms of tuberculosis in the chest and in the bones and joints. Excellent papers on this subject are those of Pottenger,[105] Bigler,[106] and Opie.[107] Diagnosis can often be made by it of pulmonary lesions before physical signs or symptoms occur. Certain types of lesions cast little or no shadow on the film, and others, which contain calcium, very heavy ones. Small caseated foci are only slightly opaque. Tracheobronchial lymph-nodes, unless calcified or greatly enlarged, may not be seen well in the roentgenogram. Calcification does not prove inactivity in a lesion. When the cervical and the mesenteric lymph-nodes show calcification on the film it is certain that they are tuberculous. Miliary tuberculosis of the lungs generally cannot be demonstrated roentgenographically until it is rather far advanced. Bronchoscopy, with injection of iodized oil and subsequent roentgenographic study, is usually contraindicated in pulmonary tuberculosis, but may be employed occasionally in the differential diagnosis from bronchiectasis or other conditions. Yet it must be admitted that roentgenograms of the lungs in cases of suspected tuberculosis are often misleading, and that the diagnosis from them should be in accord with other physical signs and symptoms.

The value of the complement-fixation test, as first applied in tuberculosis by Widal and Le Sourd,[108] is questioned by a number of authors. The same may be said of the sedimentation test to determine severity and prognosis (Fähraeus[109]) and of the precipitin test. Wilbolz's[110] auto-urine test, in which urine concentrated to $\frac{1}{10}$ of its original volume is injected intracutaneously, is held by most observers to cause a local reaction due to the irritation of urinary salts, rather than to the effect of a specific antigen. Tubercle bacilli should be sought for whenever there is the possibility of their discovery; examining the sputum, spinal fluid, pleural exudate, stools, urine, and discharges from suspected areas. The material should also be injected into guinea-pigs when necessary. Culture of the sputum may help in the differential diagnosis from bronchiectasis, and in certain rare cases of Vincent's infection, or infections of the lungs by mould or yeast. To obtain sputum from young children who do not expectorate, a swab of cotton or gauze may be applied to the throat on a curved metal applicator, and held there during the coughing thus excited. The gastric contents may be withdrawn, centrifuged, examined, and tubercle bacilli found microscopically or by inoculation in cases where the patient has swallowed tuberculous sputum, infected milk, or the discharge from tuberculous tonsils or affected portions of the upper respiratory tract (Meunier;[111] Armand-Delille and Vibert;[112] Poulsen[113]).

The Tuberculin-reaction.—The test may be performed in various ways. (1) When injected *subcutaneously* in doses of 0.1 mg. tuberculin may cause a constitutional reaction with fever. This is not without danger in patients with an active lesion, or even with a latent one, and the method is little employed at present. (2) The *intracutaneous* test (Mantoux[114]) is performed by injecting 0.01 to 0.1 mg. of tuberculin into the superficial layers of the skin. The dose may be increased up to 1.0 mg. if the smaller amounts produce no reaction. Some clinicians increase the dose to as much as 5.0 or even 10.0 mg. The amount to be injected should be contained in 0.1 cc. of solution. A positive reaction is similar to that to be described for the cutaneous test. (3) The *cutaneous* reaction of Pirquet[115] is performed as follows: The skin of the forearm is washed with alcohol or ether, a drop of undiluted old tuberculin* applied and slight scarifications or multiple punctures made through this with a sterilized needle, or scarification done with the special drill-shaped scarifier made for the purpose. A control scarification should be made a couple of inches distant for the purpose of comparison. A positive reaction develops within twenty-four hours, sometimes longer, and consists in a red, slightly indurated maculo-papule 5 mm. (0.2 in.) or more in diameter (Fig. 88). It reaches its height usually upon the second day and fades slowly, often leaving slight scaliness. A papule of smaller size than 5 mm. is not to be considered certainly positive. If the reaction obtained is doubtful or negative, a second trial may be made in a few days or, still better, the intracutaneous test may be used. (4) The *percutaneous* test, devised by Moro,[116] consists in vigorously rubbing into the sound skin for one minute a 50 per cent mixture of tuberculin and lanolin. In twenty-four to forty-eight hours red papules appear, varying in number with the intensity of the reaction. The test is rendered much more accurate if the cutaneous surface-fat is first removed by rubbing with ether. (5) The *ophthalmo-reaction* of Wolff-Eisner[117] and Calmette[118] is obtained by putting into the conjunctival sac one drop of a 0.5 per cent aqueous solution of old tuberculin. The reaction varies from a slight reddening up to a decided conjunctivitis. Owing to the damage to the eye sometimes produced, the test has with reason lost favor.

Our own preference is for the intracutaneous test performed with human tuberculin on one arm and bovine tuberculin on the other, since it gives a greater percentage of positive reactions than the cutaneous, and the dose employed can be made accurate and increased as desired.

Value of the Tuberculin Reaction.—Usually a negative reaction excludes the presence of tuberculosis, especially if it is still so on a second trial with increased dosage, and provided material known to be active is employed. Tuberculin keeps well even when diluted for solutions. In advanced or terminal stages of tuberculosis the test may be negative, and it may be inhibited, too, by such nonspecific conditions as severe inanition, dehydration, or any severe febrile disease such as measles, scarlet fever, grippe, pneumonia, pertussis, typhoid fever, or meningitis (Eddy and Mitchell[119]).

A positive reaction indicates that the patient has tuberculous infection and is sensitive (allergic) to the tuberculin protein, but it is in no sense a proof of the existence of clinical tuberculosis. The reaction once positive almost invariably remains so; but it is possible for such perfect anatomical healing or such complete fibrosis of the infected area to take place that sensitivity ceases, the test then becoming negative. Such instances have been reported by Austrian,[120] Krause,[121] and Myers.[122] Although it is claimed by some investigators, among them Cummins,[123] Lobban[124] and Opie,[107] that the intensity of the reaction or the amount of tuberculin necessary to produce it has prognostic value, this is certainly not our own experience, and we have found with Pinner,[125] that a strong tuberculin reaction cannot be correlated with high immunity or the reverse. It might be mentioned, however, that strong reactions often occur in certain forms of tuberculosis, such as erythema nodosum and phlyctenular conjunctivitis, which are not advanced forms of the disease, and that they are generally stronger in osseous and glandular tuberculosis than in pulmonary forms. We have seen the test markedly positive when careful macroscopical and microscopical study at necropsy failed to disclose the lesion, although it must have been present. Duken[126] reports a similar instance. Obviously a positive reaction in infancy has a more serious import than in later childhood, but any time before puberty it indicates the necessity for careful

* Old tuberculin is prepared by concentrating an old glycerin-broth culture of tubercle bacilli over steam and passing it through a porcelain filter.

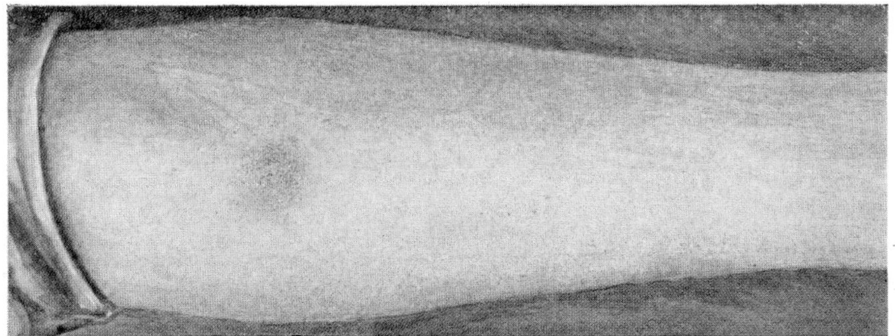

One Plus (+)

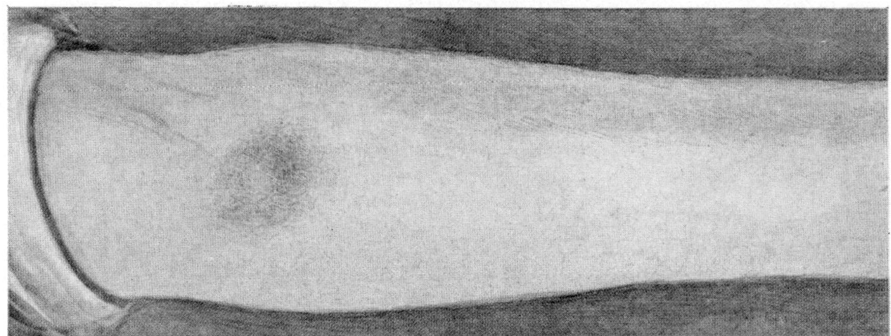

Two Plus (++)

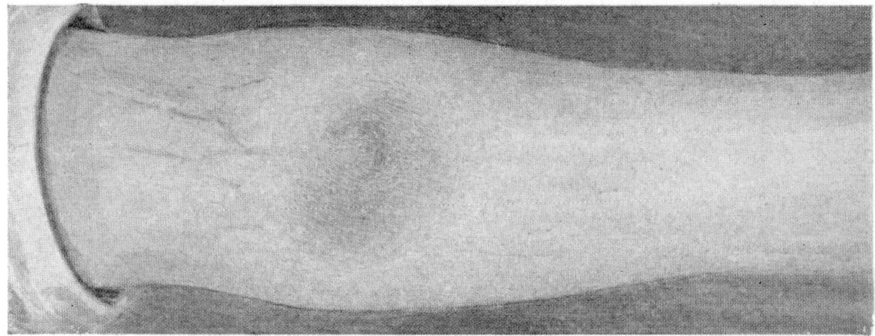

Three Plus (+++)

Fig. 88.—Tuberculin reactions—Mantoux method. (Chadwick and McPhedran, Childhood Type of Tuberculosis; National Tuberculosis Association, 1930.)

study and close observation, and suggests that any symptoms not otherwise explicable may be tuberculous in nature.

Although a small percentage of persons will react only to the human or to the bovine tuberculin respectively, the large majority who react positively will do so to both types. Downing and Higgins[127] believe that in the first stages of the disease the patient will react to but one type, presumably the infecting one, but further work is needed to confirm this.

Treatment. **Prophylaxis.**—The great need is that the infant be guarded against every possible contact with tuberculous subjects including, of course, any member of the family with the disease. Danger of spread from open osseous and glandular tuberculosis is less than from pulmonary forms. If a child must remain in an environment where pulmonary tuberculosis is present, every possible precaution should be employed, such as collection and disinfection of sputum and avoidance of droplet infection. General cleanliness in the care of fingernails, toys, utensils, and the like is important, even though the danger from such sources may be slight. Promiscuous kissing of children should be avoided and, while isolation of an infant is impracticable, the less general its contacts the safer it is. Proper pasteurization of milk should be insisted upon, or only raw milk used from dairies where careful inspection shows the absence of tuberculosis both in the cattle and in the employees. Under general preventive measures are included the maintenance of the best possible health and nutrition, change of climate when indicated and possible, and the avoidance of contact with the acute contagious and respiratory diseases.

Tuberculin seems to have no real value in prevention. B.C.G. (Bacillus Calmette-Guérin) has been widely employed, especially in France and certain other parts of Europe. (See Calmette et al.,[128] Publication League of Nations,[129] Weill-Hallé and Turpin.[130]) In 1930 Calmette[131] stated that over 210,000 children had been so treated, that he believed the procedure to be harmless as well as effective, and that wherever used it resulted in the reduction of infant mortality in general. According to a number of studies, many infants so treated remain clinically free from the disease even after continued exposure to tuberculous parents. B.C.G. is a strain of bovine bacillus attenuated by prolonged culture. Three doses each of 2 cc. of suspension (approximately 400 million bacilli) are given by mouth on the third, fifth and seventh days after birth. Selter,[132] Wallgren,[133] and others give B.C.G. intracutaneously, employing from 0.01 to 1.0 mg. A nodule develops, and often also swelling of the local lymph-nodes, which discharge for several weeks and then heal. With the oral administration a positive tuberculin-reaction may not develop; with the intracutaneous method it usually becomes positive after five to seven weeks. It is a controversial matter whether allergy (sensitiveness to tuberculin) is necessary to the production of immunity, or synonymous with it. Petroff[134] and others believe that there is danger of this attenuated bacillus becoming virulent and causing clinical tuberculosis, and that the use of dead bacilli is preferable. The possibility of securing immunity by injections of killed tubercle bacilli is not admitted by many students of the subject, but some success seems to have accompanied such attempts by Raw[135] and others. Von Ruck and Flack[136] used extractives of tubercle bacilli in preventive vaccination and claimed good results.

In conclusion it must be said, that although some of the various prophylactic measures employing the use of living or of dead tubercle bacilli have seemed encouraging, yet in view of the unfavorable reports which have emanated from various sources, none of the methods can as yet be accepted as definitely beyond the experimental stage.

Treatment of the Attack.—Treatment depending upon localization will be discussed elsewhere in other sections. If there is fever, rest is certainly the most important part of the regime. This may be partial, or complete by constant confinement to bed. The beginning of exercise and its amount are based largely on the return to a normal pulse-rate and normal temperature, and also on the gain in weight and the clinical and roentgenographic evidence of quiescence of the lesion. Fresh air, which may be cold air provided the patient reacts to it properly, is also important. Sanitorium treatment is also helpful, and a climate which is dry and of fairly high altitude is frequently very advantageous. However, when these can not be utilized, much can be done at home by strictly following hygienic measures. The diet should be abundant, but this does not mean that forced feeding with excessive amounts at frequent intervals is advisable. The principles of good nutrition and of proper digestion must not be violated. Sauerbruch, Herrmannsdorfer and Gerson[137] recommend a base-forming diet, low in sodium chloride, protein, and carbohydrate, but rich in fats and vitamins. Others have advocated a diet rich in vitamins, because it would theoretically help in assimilation of calcium. Cod liver oil has been a favorite in this disease for generations, but it should not be given if it interferes with the appetite. Under these conditions a cod liver oil concentrate might be employed. The theory of the so-called "Gerson diet" mentioned above is that it tends to counteract excessive tissue hydration present in tuberculosis and also the demineralization which takes place in the disease. There is no acceptable evidence that the administration of calcium or irradiated ergosterol exerts any favorable influence. Anemia should be treated if present. Cough does not require sedatives unless it is a very troublesome symptom, and the routine use of so-called "cough-syrups" may do more harm than good. The treatment of tuberculosis by injection of gold salts (Sanocrysin), as recommended by Mollgaard,[138] has yet to prove its value and lack of danger.

Heliotherapy has a very definite place in the treatment of tuberculosis, and may be carried out in the home or in any hospital, special equipment and location not being necessary. It is particularly valuable in cutaneous, glandular, osseous, abdominal, and intestinal tuberculosis, but produces also beneficial effect in the pulmonary form if properly employed. In this, however, it should not be used during the acute stages. Heliotherapy has been extensively employed by Rollier[139] in Europe, and apparently first introduced in the United States at Perrysburg, N. Y. (Hyde and Lo Grasso[140]). Certain precautions should be observed, and the patient is first to become accustomed to the open air. Exposure to the sun should stop one-half hour before meals, and should not be begun again within two hours after. If high fever, rapid pulse, or nausea are caused, the treatment should be stopped or curtailed. During the hot part of the day in summer treatment should be suspended. The head and eyes should be protected. The method of gradual exposure is outlined elsewhere (p. 205). Artificial sources of light, while not as effective as sunlight, may also be employed (p. 205). Gerstenberger and Burhans[141] use intensive ultraviolet light-treatment in infants with tuberculosis, apparently with good results. Roentgen-ray treatment of cervical and of tracheobronchial node tuberculosis is helpful in some cases, but only a few clinicians have cared to employ it in pulmonary lesions.

Phrenicotomy, artificial pneumothorax, and oleothorax are measures which cause compression and give rest to the diseased lung. They have their indications in childhood at times; the last two being especially beneficial in the experience of Armand-Delille[142] (with Giroux[143]).

Tuberculin-treatment, which had at one time fallen into disfavor, is advocated by a number of specialists of experience. It is capable of increasing the activity of a lesion, and should be employed only with great care and extremely small initial doses, and only by those especially proficient. It is particularly valuable in ocular tuberculosis. Foreign protein therapy is recommended by some pediatrists (see Czerny[144]).

References

1. J.A.M.A., 1930, **94,** 697. 2. Am. Rev. Tuberc., 1929, **20,** 421. 3. Norsk. mag. f. Laegevidensk., 1914, **75,** 137. 4. Beitr. z. Klin. d. Tuberk., 1922, **49,** 357. 5. Am. Rev. Tuberc., 1924, **10,** 280. 6. Studies in Human Biology, 1924, 273. 7. Bull. acad. de méd., Paris, 1924, **9,** 191. 8. Am. Rev. Tuberc., 1929, **20,** 413. 9. Am. Rev. Tuberc., 1924, **9,** 191. 10. Beitr. z. Klin. d. Tuberk., 1921, **48,** 24. 11. Am. Rev. Tuberc., 1927, **15,** 665. 12. The Causes of Tuberculosis, Cambridge Univ. Press, 1917, 6. 13. Arch. Int. Med., 1922, **29,** 261. 14. Monatschr. f. Kinderh., 1927, **36,** 285. 15. Časop. lek. Česk., 1927, **66,** 411; abst. Am. J. Dis. Child., 1930, **39,** 635. 16. Arch. Pediat., 1903, **20,** 247. 17. Budapesti orvosi ujsáy, 1906; Ref. Jahrb. f. Kinderh., 1906, **64,** 763. 18. Wien. klin. Wchnschr., 1907, **20,** 1069. 19. Norsk. Mag. f. Laegevidensk., 1913, **11,** 1. 20. 17th Internat. Cong. Med., 1913, Sect. 10, 38. 21. Am. J. Dis. Child., 1921, **21,** 48. 22. Nothnagel's Encyclop. Pract. Med., Am. Ed., Tuberc., 307. 23. Beitr. z. Klin. d. Tuberk., 1906, **6,** 229. 24. München. med. Wchnschr., 1909, **56,** 449. 25. Arch. f. Kinderh., 1922, **71,** 180. 26. Acta paediat., 1926, **5,** 103. 27. Am. Rev. Tuberc., 1925, **14,** 454. 28. J.A.M.A., 1926, **87,** 1549. 29. Am. J. Dis. Child., 1929, **38,** 1137. 30. Deutsche med. Wchnschr., 1921, **47,** 532. 31. Tubercle, 1925, **7,** 122. 32. Brit. J. Child. Dis., 1912, **9,** 493. 33. Edinburgh M. J., 1912, **1,** 324. 34. Am. J. Dis. Child., 1915, **9,** 478. 35. Arch. Pediat., 1921, **37,** 78. 36. Am. Rev. Tuberc., 1931, **23,** 13. 37. München. med. Wchnschr., 1908, **55,** 2702. 38. München. med. Wchnschr., 1909, **56,** 398. 39. Ztschr. f. Tuberk., 1921, **35,** 1. 40. Arch. f. Kinderh., 1921, **70,** 95. 41. Gaz. hébdom., 1865, **2,** 795. 42. Berl. klin. Wchnschr., 1882, **19,** 221. 43. J. Exper. Med., 1898, **3,** 451. 44. J. Exper. Med., 1912, **16,** 432. 45. J. Med. Research, 1912–13, **27,** 109. 46. Edinburgh M. J., 1914, **13,** 209. 47. The Causes of Tuberc., Cambridge Univ. Press, 1917, 659. 48. Am. J. Dis. Child., 1923, **25,** 234. 49. Prev. Med. and Hyg., 1927, 166. 50. Compt. rend. acad. de sc., 1925, **181,** 491. 51. Am. Rev. Tuberc., 1928, **18,** 823. 52. Compt. rend. soc. de biol. de Paris., 1876. **3,** 308. 53. De l'hérédité parasitaire de la tuberculose humaine, 1898; Ref. Ghon, Ref. No. 55. 54. Wien. klin. Wchnschr., 1909, **22,** 327. 55. Der primäre Lungenherd bei der Tuberk. der Kinder., Berlin, 1912. 56. J.A.M.A., 1905, **44,** 1425. 57. Beitr. z. Klin. d. Tuberk., 1926, **65,** 291. 58. New York M. J., 1891, **53,** 201. 59. Med. News, 1896, **69,** 656. 60. New York M. J., 1899, **70,** 1. 61. Beitr. z. Klin. d. Tuberk., 1930, **75,** 575. 62. Lancet, 1894, **1,** 1177. 63. Pediatrics, 1899, **8,** 335. 64. Am. J. Dis. Child., 1931, **41,** 513. 65. Arch. méd. exper., 1896, **8,** 689. 66. Compt. rend. acad. d. sc., 1906, **142,** 1136. 67. Brit. M. J., 1902, **2,** 1885. 68. Deutsche med. Wchnschr., 1907, **33,** 1577. 69. Pennsylvania State Dept. Agric. Bull., 1901, No. 75; 65. 70. Am. Rev. Tuberc., 1927, **15,** 137. 71. Med. News, 1905, May 27. 72. Am. J. Dis. Child., 1929, **38,** 526. 73. Jahrb. f. Kinderh., 1901, **54,** 67. 74. Sixth Internat. Congr. Tuberc., 1908, **2,** 4, 367. 75. Pfaundler und Schlossmann's Handbk. d. Kinderh., 1923, **2,** 608. 76. Am. J. Dis. Child., 1928, **36,** 702. 77. Jahrb. f. Kinderh., 1928, **118,** 315. 78. Bull. Soc. de pédiat. de Paris, 1919, Jan.–June, 48. 79. Ztschr. f. Tuberk., 1925, **43,** 3. 80. Jahrb. f. Kinderh., 1921, **94,** 102. 81. Berl. klin. Wchnschr., 1921, **58,** 877. 82. Am. J. Dis. Child., 1927, **33,** 363. 83. Virchow's Arch. f. Path. Anat., 1925, **260,** 664. 84. Brit. J. Child. Dis., 1909, **6,** 205. 85. New York M. J., 1908, **88,** 798. 86. Am. Rev. Tuberc., 1929, **20,** 368. 87. Am. Rev. Tuberc., 1930, **21,** 818. 88. J.A.M.A., 1930, **94,** 697. 89. Berl. klin. Wchnschr., 1913, **50,** 1951. 90. J. Outdoor Life, 1913, **10,** 361. 91. Beitr. z. Klin. d. Tuberk., 1926, **64,** 515. 92. Arch. f. Kinderh., 1928, **84,** 136. 93. Acta paediat., 1928, **7,** Suppl. 2, 167. 94. Am. Rev. Tuberc., 1929, **20,** 533. 95. Am. Rev. Tuberc., 1930, **21,** 423. 96. Am. J. Dis. Child., 1929, **37,** 909. 97. Ztschr. f. Tuberk., 1932, **63,** 167. 98. Tr. Coll. Phys., Phila., 1927, **49,** 129. 99. Am. Rev. Tuberc., 1928, **17,** 204. 100. Ztschr. f. Tuberk., 1928, **51,** 222. 101. Am. Rev. Tuberc., 1929, **20,** 52. 102. Am. J. Dis. Child., 1929, **37,** 233. 103. Am. J. Dis. Child., 1931, **40,** 1023. 104. Am. Rev. Tuberc., 1932, **25,** 178. 105. Am. J. M. Sc., 1928, **175,** 676. 106. Am. J. Dis. Child., 1929, **38,** 978. 107. J.A.M.A., 1930, **95,** 1151. 108. Bull. et mém. soc. méd. d. hôp. de Paris, 1901, **18,** 787. 109. Biochem. Ztschr., 1918, **89,** 355. 110. Cor.-bl. f. Schweiz. Aerzte, 1919, **49,** 793. 111. Presse méd., 1898, **2,** 81. 112. Presse méd., 1927, **35,** 402. 113. Am. J. Dis. Child., 1931, **41,** 783. 114. Compt. rend. acad. de sc., 1908, **147,** 355. 115. Wien. med. Wchnschr., 1907, **57,** 1370. 116. Wien. klin. Wchnschr., 1907, **20,** 933. 117. Berl. klin. Wchnschr., 1907, **44,** 7. 118. Compt. rend. acad. de sc., 1907, **144,** 1324. 119. Eddy and Mitchell, Am. J. Dis. Child., 1930, **40,** 771. 120. Tubercle, 1924, **6,** 29. 121. Am. Rev. Tuberc., 1925, **11,** 303. 122.

J.A.M.A., 1927, **88,** 1457. 123. Brit. M. J., 1929, **1,** 336. 124. Tubercle, 1930, **12,** 19. 125. Am. Rev. Tuberc., 1931, **23,** 175. 126. Ztschr. f. Kinderh., 1927, **43,** 331. 127. Am. J. Dis. Child., 1926, **31,** 178. 128. Presse méd., 1925, **33,** 8251; Bull. de l'acad. de méd., Paris, 1926, **95,** 175. 129. Health, 1928, **3,** 17. 130. Presse méd., 1930, **38,** 1699. 131. J.A.M.A., 1930, **94,** 647. 132. Deutsche med. Wchnschr., 1924, **51,** 1181. 133. J.A.M.A., 1928, **91,** 1876. 134. Am. Rev. Tuberc., 1929, **20,** 275. 135. Brit. M. J., 1924, **2,** 102. 136. Med. Rec., 1921, **99,** 1048. 137. München. med. Wchnschr., 1926, **73,** 47; 108. 138. Chemotherapy of Tuberculosis, 1924; Ref. J.A.M.A., 1925, **84,** 516. 139. Die Heliotherapie der Tuberculose. 140. New York M. J., 1917, **105,** 11. 141. Am. J. Dis. Child., 1926, **32,** 781. 142. Bull. acad. de méd. Paris, 1927, **97,** 600. 143. Bull. soc. de pédiat. de Paris, 1930, **28,** 170 (With Geroux). 144. Jahrb. f. Kinderh., 1926, **114,** 277.

CHAPTER XXIV

SYPHILIS

This disease in early life is represented by two forms: (*A*) Acquired syphilis; (*B*) Hereditary syphilis. The former is far less frequent, and any features which pertain to both forms will be discussed under the Hereditary variety.

(*A*) ACQUIRED SYPHILIS

Etiology.—Infection takes place usually by other paths than the genital tract. The most frequent methods are through kissing by a syphilitic person, nursing from a diseased breast, and contact with infected clothing, drinking cups, nursing bottles, and the like. It is possible, but unlikely, that the disease can be transmitted simply by the milk of a syphilitic wet-nurse without a lesion of the breast. It has been given by a syphilitic operator performing ritual circumcision, and it was communicated by vaccination in the days when human virus was employed. Profeta's law, that an apparently healthy child will not acquire syphilis from contact with its syphilitic mother, indicates only that the infant has acquired immunity because it is, in fact, already syphilitic.

Pathologic Anatomy and Symptoms.—These do not differ materially from those characteristic of adult life, except that the attack is usually milder. Widespread cutaneous eruption is not uncommon, but it is more macular than papular. There is a marked disposition in children to the development of moist condylomata. An initial lesion develops at the point of infection.

(*B*) HEREDITARY SYPHILIS

Frequency.—In older statistics, based solely upon clinical features, the incidence of hereditary syphilis was given usually as 1 per cent or less (Fruhinsholz,[1] Still,[2] Neumann and Oberwarth,[3] Cassel[4]). When cases are included in which the diagnosis rests entirely upon a positive Wassermann reaction, the figures given range from 2 to about 15 per cent. The lower figures are usually those for the white population; the higher ones for the colored. The incidence in the well-to-do groups is less than 2 per cent. The statistics usually do not take into account the numerous instances of still-births, prematurity, and abortions due to this disease. (See studies by Austin,[5] Royster,[6] Jeans and Cooke,[7] Dickey and Sutton,[8] Jenks and Donnelly,[9] McCulloch.[10])

Etiology.—*Exciting Cause.*—The researches of Schaudinn and Hoffmann,[11] confirmed by many others, show that the cause is a spirillum, the *spirochaeta pallida,* or *treponema pallidum,* which is found in the primary lesion and mucous patches in the acquired disease, and in hereditary cases in the various tissues and secretions of the body, especially the liver.

Inheritance.—The father is much most frequently the original source of the disease, but the mother, already syphilitic at the time of conception, may infect the fetus, the father being healthy. Much less often the mother may acquire syphilis at some period during pregnancy, and then transmit it to the fetus (*post-conceptional syphilis*). It is not believed possible that the syphilitic father can communicate it to the fetus without infection of the mother. The true explanation of Colles'[12] law; viz., that the mother of a syphilitic infant will not become infected by contact with it, is that she is immune to reinfection because of already having the disease herself, although without recognized symptoms. Even the fact that such a mother's Wassermann reaction is negative, as it exceptionally is, does not indicate that she is free from syphilis. Transmission of the disease to the fetus is, therefore, always from the mother.

Whether or not the infant of syphilitic parents will be born syphilitic depends on various factors. The nearer to the time of conception the mother acquires syphilis, the greater the danger to her infant. If either parent is suffering from secondary symptoms at the time of conception, transmission is almost certain. If the symptoms are in the tertiary stage, or have been overcome by treatment, the infant may escape. As regards post-conceptional syphilis, the shorter the time between infection and parturition the less liable is the fetus to be syphilitic. If treatment of syphilitic infection of the mother is begun early and is faithfully and thoroughly followed, the infant may escape, as it is usually believed that the fetus is not infected before the fourth or fifth month of pregnancy, or possibly later. Numerous researches show the influence of treatment of the mother during pregnancy, but only those of Bartholomew[13] will be quoted. By comparing 100 treated with 100 untreated women it was found that in the latter group premature births were two times, still-births three times, abortions seven times, and infant-deaths up to ten days of life nine times as frequent as in the treated cases.

There is no acceptable proof that syphilis can be transmitted to the third generation. Among more recent reported cases claimed to be instances of such transmission are those of de Toni,[14] Bondurant,[15] A. Deutsch,[16] and Heck and Eleda.[17] It seems, however, impossible satisfactorily to exclude the fact that the disease might have been acquired in the second generation and was not inherited.

While transmission of the disease by infants with hereditary syphilis is uncommon, it can, nevertheless, occur. Cases are on record in which other children in the family, or nurses in attendance, have contracted it from syphilitic infants.

Pathologic Anatomy.—In cases of early abortion there are often no determinate gross or microscopical changes, but in the fetus approaching full term, or in still-born infants or those dying a few days after birth, the changes are characteristic. The longer the time after birth before symptoms appear, the less liable are the internal organs to be found diseased. In the early alterations there is a diffuse, cellular proliferation arising from the perivascular connective tissue, with involvement of the vessels. Only later is there a tendency to the production of gummata. The most constant and definite pathologic changes are those of the osseous system. In the fetus and in young infants the lesion is usually an osteochondritis, occurring oftenest in the epiphyses. Dactylitis is sometimes observed, especially in early childhood. In later childhood osteochondritis is not often seen, but there is found an osteoperiostitis, particularly of the skull and of the bones of the forearms and legs. Involvement of the joints may also occur in the form of synovitis or chondroarthritis.

Hyperplasia of the spleen is present in the fetus and the new-born. At a later period gummata or interstitial changes may be present. The liver exhibits enlargement and thickening of its capsule. On section it is of a yellowish color, there is increase of interstitial connective tissue, with consequent atrophy of many of the hepatic cells and narrowing of the blood vessels and small biliary passages, and there may be numerous minute gummata. After early childhood the liver less often shows alteration, although gummata of considerable size are sometimes found. The tongue may exhibit condylomata, and these, or chronic inflammation or ulceration, may be present in the pharynx and tonsils. Cellular infiltration and interference with parenchymatous development may occur in the stomach and intestines.

Among lesions frequent or at least not uncommon in infants or even in children are catarrh and ulceration of the nose; the so-called "white hepatization" of the lung; interstitial myocarditis, endocarditis, and gummata of the heart; hydrocephalus; parenchymatous changes in the kidney; and enlargement of superficial lymphatic glands. Less commonly seen are perichondritis or ulceration of the larynx; gummata in the trachea or bronchi, or in the lungs themselves; gummata of the brain and spinal cord; chronic meningitis; interstitial orchitis, or gummata of the testicle. The eyes are oftener involved later, but even in early life there may be iritis, choroiditis, retinitis, and optic neuritis. Keratitis is common among the later lesions. There may be interstitial changes or gummatous infiltration of the pancreas, kidney, thymus, peritoneum, suprarenals, and thyroid gland. Small cystic formations are frequently found in the thymus (p. 1078). Spirochetes may be recovered from all of these tissues.

Symptoms. I. The Early Manifestations of Hereditary Syphilis.—Mothers with recent syphilitic infection, contracted at or near the time of conception, very commonly abort or their infants are still-born at term. Some are born alive with evidences of severe infection, are feeble and atrophic, and are usually capable of living only a few days or weeks. There may be present at birth coryza; pemphigoid eruption of the skin, especially on the soles and palms; enlargement of the liver and spleen; and fissuring and excoriation around the mouth and anus. Still other infants, though feeble and poorly developed, do not at first show the symptoms characteristic of syphilis, but after a short time develop them. The large majority of syphilitic infants, however, appear healthy and well-developed at birth, and symptoms appear only after an interval (*infantile syphilis*). About $\frac{1}{2}$ the cases show symptoms in the first month, especially the latter portion; another $\frac{1}{4}$ or more in the second month; and nearly all the remaining in the third month (Miller[18]). Generally early symptoms do not first appear after the third month.

The earliest symptom in an infant apparently healthy at birth is usually a persistent coryza ("snuffles"). This is soon followed by a hoarse, high-pitched and persistent cry. Shortly cutaneous manifestations appear, frequently accompanied by slight fever; and then, or earlier, evidences of osseous lesions, perhaps with pseudoparalytic conditions. Sometimes severe visceral manifestations are more prominent, although these as a rule manifest themselves, in combination with other symptoms, more in the infant at birth, and are visible evidences of fetal syphilis. The majority of infants who are in good condition at birth, and show no symptoms for some weeks, will present no visceral symptoms of moment. The promptness of the development and the severity of symptoms are in general proportionate to the intensity of the infection. In mild cases the general health and nutrition may remain unaffected. A more detailed description of the symptoms follows:

Cutaneous Symptoms.—The severest symptom of this class, *pemphigus syphiliticus neonatorum*, is oftenest present at birth. It is a bullous eruption with bloody or purulent contents, most frequently found on the palms and soles, but at times widespread. In milder cases of syphilis there is no cutaneous eruption at first, and the earliest evidence of it appears generally about a week after the development of the coryza. The eruption may be circumscribed or diffuse. The *circumscribed* form is oftenest maculo-papular, and occurs as small, slightly elevated, pea-sized or larger macules, associated with papules more or less numerous, situated especially upon the lower extremities, the face, scalp, neck, flexor surfaces of the upper extremities, palms, and soles. Scaling may be present. It is unattended by itching and varies in color from coppery-red to brown or yellowish, according to the age of the lesion. A well-marked annular appearance (Fig. 89) may be

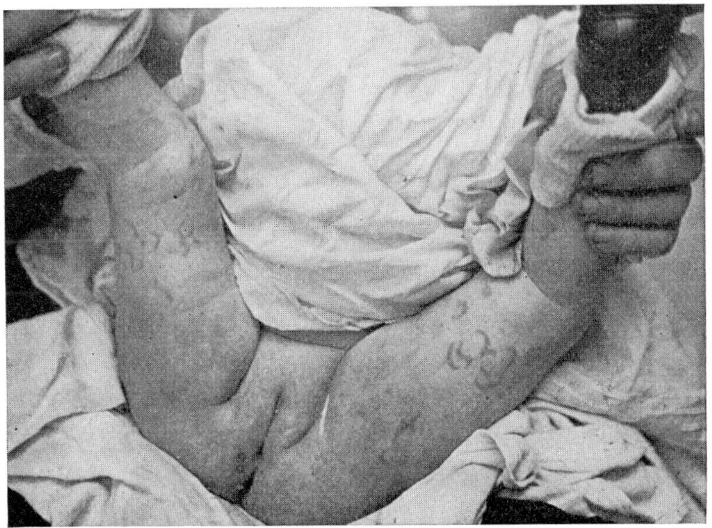

Fig. 89.—Hereditary syphilis, maculo-papular eruption. Unusual degree of annular appearance. (*Courtesy of Dr. J. F. Schamberg.*)

produced in some cases through absorption in the center. In regions with moist surfaces, as the mouth, anal region and genitals, or where the skin is thin and delicate, as behind the ears, between the fingers, or about the navel, there develop flattened elevations,—the "moist condyloma" or mucous patch. The condyloma, however, is not the earliest eruption, being particularly characteristic of the relapses which are so prone to occur. A more papular eruption of a brown-red color is seen oftenest upon the palms and soles and on the forehead. Less often observed, and in severer cases, is a papulo-pustular eruption (Fig. 90), which may terminate in ulcerated or ecthymatous lesions. The roseola of acquired syphilis is rarely, if ever, witnessed in the hereditary form.

The *diffuse* eruption is common and very characteristic, and is not observed in acquired syphilis. It consists of a diffuse infiltration of the skin, situated usually on the palms and soles, face, scalp, genital and anal regions, and the flexor surfaces of the thighs. It presents a somewhat shining surface of a copper-red or brownish-yellow color, and renders the skin distinctly stiffened. Desquamation is slight or extensive (Fig. 91). Fissures in the skin are very characteristic early symptoms. They are often arranged radially, especially at the labial angles and at the anus, are narrow, infiltrated, painful, bleed readily, and may be covered with crusts (Fig. 92). When

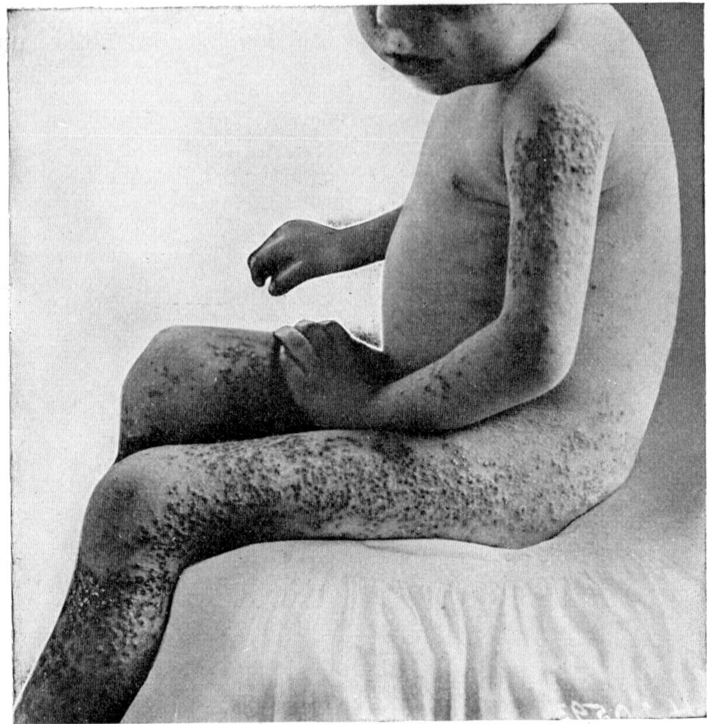

Fig. 90.—Papulo-pustular syphiloderm. (*Courtesy of Dr. M. B. Hartzell.*)

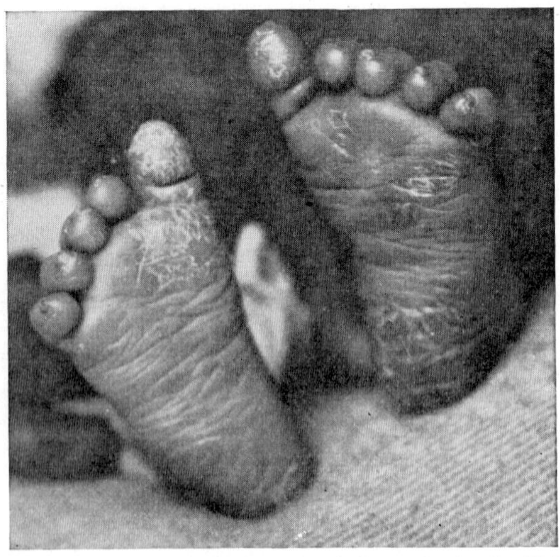

Fig. 91.—Syphilitic scaling of feet. Infant aged six weeks in the Children's Ward of the Hospital of the University of Pennsylvania. Snuffles and cutaneous eruption developed at the age of two weeks.

healed they may leave linear scarring. The nails are often dry, shriveled, exhibit transverse fissures, and may fall off, or a syphilitic paronychia may develop. There may be loss of hair from the scalp (Fig. 93), eyelids, or

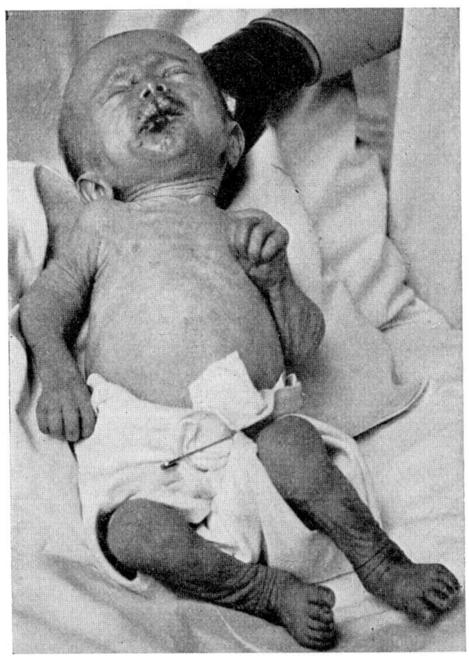

Fig. 92.—Fissures about the mouth in hereditary syphilis. From a female child aged six months in The Children's Ward of the Hospital of the University of Pennsylvania.

eyebrow, or in other cases the growth of hair on the scalp is profuse, producing the so-called "syphilitic wig."

Mucous Membranes.—Lesions of the mucous membranes, other than rhinitis, are usually not encountered until the infant is some months old. Broad condylomata and ulcers may develop upon the mucous membrane of the mouth, tongue, vulva, and elsewhere. "Snuffling" is generally among the first manifestations of the disease and is a very persistent one. It is nearly always present, and frequently at birth, and may be the only symptom. The nasal mucous membrane is swollen and respiration and sucking are difficult. Later there may be mucopurulent discharge, often tinged with blood, and thick crusts block the nostrils. Hoarseness may attend the coryza, being sometimes one of the earliest symptoms. Hemorrhages occasionally occur from the mucous membrane or from cutaneous lesions, or sometimes in the internal organs.

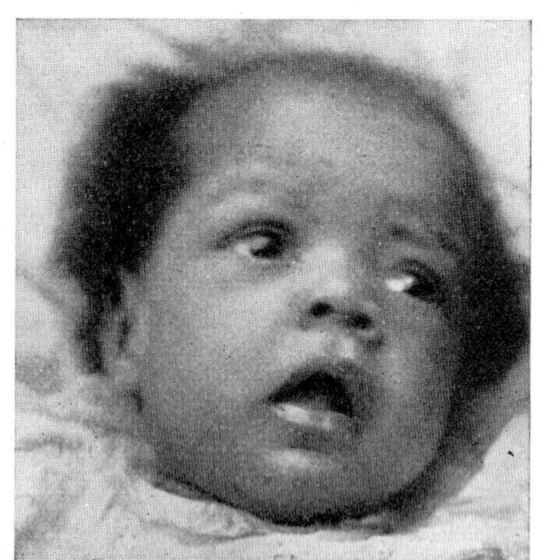

Fig. 93.—Syphilitic alopecia. (*Courtesy of Dr. J. F. Schamberg.*)

Lymphatic-nodes.—These may show moderate enlargement, especially in the axilla, elbow, groins, and neck, appearing as multiple hard bodies without tendency to suppurate. Enlargement of the cubital nodes is suggestive, but not diagnostic of syphilis. In fact the diagnostic importance of enlargement of the lymph-nodes in hereditary syphilis is probably over-estimated.

The Osseous System. (See also p. 1015).—The bones are frequently affected in early life, the most characteristic lesion being an osteochondritis, first described by Wegner.[19] In the exhaustive study by McLean[20] all of his 102 cases had roentgenological evidence of osseous lesions;—osteochondritis in 90.2 per cent, periostitis in 70.6 per cent, osteomyelitis in 46 per cent and osteitis in 6.8 per cent. Sutherland and Mitchell[21] found the frequency of osteochondritis reported by various observers to be from 70 to 93.4 per cent. The disease, which really begins in fetal life, appears first as a tender swelling at the junction of the shaft and epiphysis, oftenest in the extremities, and may advance to complete separation of the epiphysis, with temporary loss of power and pain on passive movement;—the syphilitic pseudoparalysis of Parrot.[22] It is shown in the roentgenogram as a white cap on the diaphysis (dark line in the positive print). Associated with this, or independent of it, may be seen rarefaction of the ends of the bones. The process may involve the joint with secondary suppuration (Fig. 94), or a portion of the shaft of the bone may be attacked. Usually, however, there is a tendency toward disappearance of the osteochondritis after the third month, even without treatment. Dactylitis, in a form described by Hochsinger[23] may develop as an early symptom. (See p. 1015.) The milk-teeth may be decayed or destroyed (Wimberger[24]). Higoumenakis[25] called attention to the frequency of enlargement of the sternal end of the clavicles. Landa and Panow[26] found retardation of ossification of the wrist in 60 per cent of cases. Craniotabes, consisting of thin, softened spots in the skull, is an occasional lesion but not pathognomonic of syphilis. (See p. 1015.) Flattening of the bridge of the nose (saddle-nose) is sometimes an early symptom (Fig. 95). Affections of the eye have been referred to in discussing Pathologic Anatomy (p. 428).

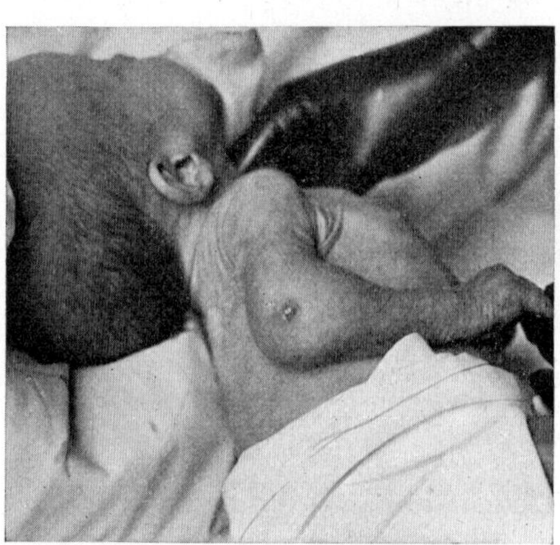

Fig. 94.—Syphilitic epiphysitis with secondary suppuration. Same case as Fig. 92.

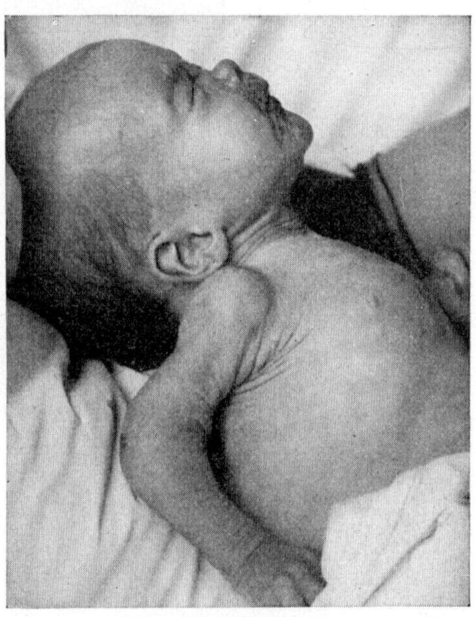

Fig. 95.—Saddle-nose in early syphilis. Same case as Fig. 92.

Visceral Lesions.—These are symptoms more characteristic of syphilis of the fetus and the new-born than of infants past this period. They are well marked in unfavorable cases. The commonest clinical manifestation is enlargement of the liver. Ascites and icterus occasionally result. (See

p. 435.) The spleen also may be much enlarged. Less common are symptoms depending upon lesions of the nervous system. Among them are those of meningitis and the consequent hydrocephalus, cerebral sclerosis, encephalitis, and cerebral and meningeal hemorrhage. Albuminuria may occur, but this does not necessarily depend upon syphilitic nephritis, which is of uncommon occurrence. (See Nephritis, pp. 817; 820.)

General Nutrition.—In severe cases there is rapid emaciation with marked anemia. The skin often exhibits a peculiar *café-au-lait* color, which is either generalized or occurs only in certain localities. The veins of the scalp are sometimes much dilated. In cases which recover the anemia persists after other symptoms disappear. Sometimes the marasmus is the earliest or even the only symptom, and not infrequently fails to yield to antisyphilitic treatment.

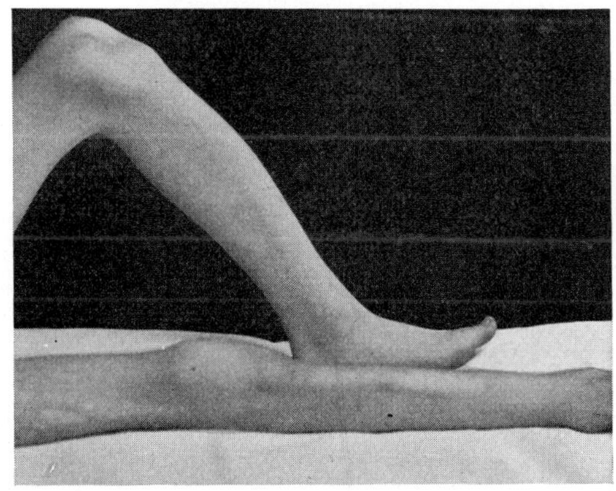

Fig. 96.—Saber tibiae. Boy aged ten years. Children's Hospital, Cincinnati.

The *frequency of occurrence* of the different early symptoms, according to the observations of Still,[27] expressed in percentages is as follows:—Snuffling 70 per cent of cases; cutaneous eruptions 69; splenic enlargement 45, and quite decided in 22; affection of the eyes 15; laryngitis 14; epiphysitis 11; orchitis 8. Hochsinger[28] found enlargement of the liver in 31 per cent of the cases, always attended by splenic enlargement.

II. Later Manifestations of Hereditary Syphilis.—The symptoms just described would be classified as secondary ones in the acquired disease. They appear for the most part in the first and second months of life, and most or all of them disappear after a few weeks of proper treatment. Unless, however, treatment is long continued, there is recurrence of some or all of the original symptoms, but with a special tendency in early childhood to condylomata, which may develop in spite of medication (Hochsinger[24]). In addition to those described new symptoms may appear, which can be classified for the most part as tertiary in type. Prominent among these are gummata in various regions, developing usually after the period of early childhood. In other cases the later symptoms are seen about the time of puberty, or even after this, without any of the earlier secondary symptoms having been observed or recognized (*Syphilis hereditaria tarda*). Some of the later symptoms must be described more in detail:

The **general nutrition** suffers, there being retardation of growth, including bony development, general impairment of vigor, delayed puberty, and anemia.

Osseous changes are present, usually represented by localized gummata or by a hyperplastic osteoperiostitis. The latter chiefly affects the long bones of the extremities and the cranium, (p. 1016 Fig. 248) producing thickening and tenderness, and pain which is most marked at night. Saber tibiae may be produced in this way (Fig. 96). Dactylitis may develop and often goes on to necrosis (p. 1015). Gummata of the bones may occur in various regions and finally break down and form ulcers (Fig. 97). These gummata, or the osteoperiostitis, produce alteration in the shape of the head; the "keel-shaped" cranium, with central frontal deposit, and the "natiform" cranium, with bilateral parietal deposits. Gummata in the nasal septum and hard palate are liable to break down and cause perforations. The saddle-nose developing after early childhood is a result of destructive necrosis in the bone and cartilage (Fig. 98). Painless and often bilateral hydrarthrosis or a hyperplastic synovitis is not uncommon and may result in ankylosis. It involves the knees and less often the ankles, but any joint may be affected. Goff[30] claims that pes cavus, generally bilateral, is a rather constant occurrence. (See also Syphilis of Bones, p. 1015.)

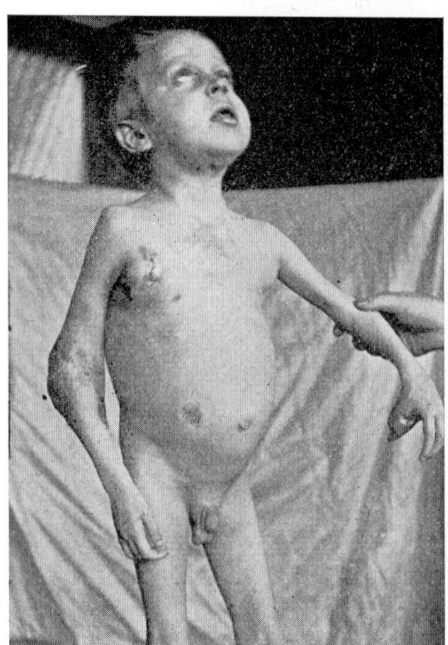

Fig. 97.—Gummata of elbows and chest in hereditary syphilis. (*Courtesy of Dr. H. R. Wharton.*)

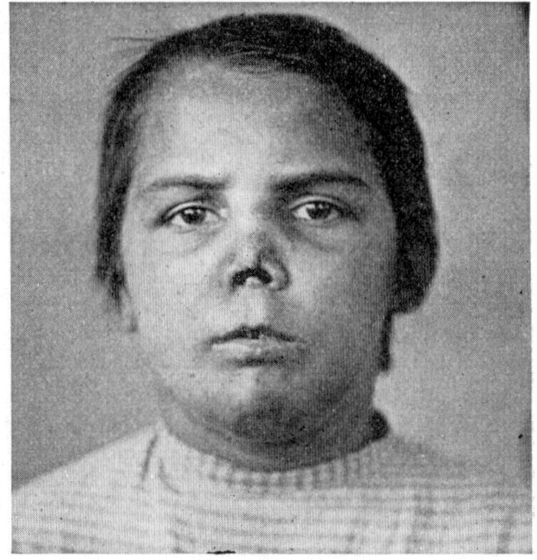

Fig. 98.—Saddle-nose in later hereditary syphilis. (*Courtesy of Dr. Harry Lowenburg.*)

The **skin** may exhibit syphilitic tubercles and gummata in various situations, but less often than in acquired syphilis. These tend to break down and leave ulcers. A papular eruption of the face may develop during relapses. Condylomata, as stated, are particularly liable to appear during relapses, and may, indeed, be the only cutaneous lesion in early childhood, although not so frequent after this period. In general, the longer the time elapsed since infancy, the less pronounced are cutaneous eruptions.

The incisor **teeth** of the second dentition, especially the 2 upper central ones, show characteristic changes, described by Hutchinson[31] (Fig. 99). They are far apart and small, with notching of the cutting surface. In other cases they are tapering and characteristically "peg-shaped." Unerupted Hutchinson's teeth may be demonstrated by the roentgenogram (Stokes and Gardner[32]). The so-called "Fournier's" or "Moon's tooth" is also common, but not entirely pathognomonic. It consists of a six-year-old molar in which the hypoplastic and deformed crown is separated by a circular line of demarcation from the body of the tooth (Stoll[33]). There may be absence of some of the teeth.

Enlargement of the **lymphatic nodes** becomes more common after the first year. The **nervous system** is involved in many ways in the later symptoms of hereditary syphilis. Jeans,[34] Tezner,[35] and others have found evidence of pathologic changes in the spinal fluid in from one-third to one-half of syphilitic infants and children examined. These consist of a positive Wassermann reaction, increased number of cells, positive globulin and albumin reactions, and the characteristic colloidal gold curve, viz. reaction of precipitation in the lower dilution (1:10 to 1:40) (Lange[36]). Chronic meningitis and paralysis of the cranial nerves may develop. Retarded mental development does not appear to be much if any more frequent in syphilitic children than in other groups (p. 905). Juvenile paresis (p. 951) is sometimes seen, and less often, tabes (p. 468). Whether there is a neurotropic strain of the spirochaeta pallida is a controversial matter.

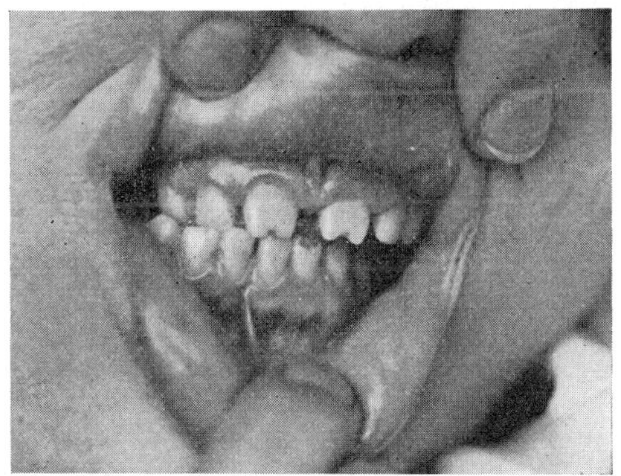

Fig. 99.—Hutchinson's teeth in hereditary syphilis. Boy aged ten years in Children's Hospital, Cincinnati. Wassermann positive.

The **eye**, likewise, exhibits late symptoms, such as keratitis, choroiditis, iritis, and retinitis. Optic atrophy is not very uncommon according to Babonneix.[37] Strabismus may be caused by paralysis of the cranial nerves, and nystagmus has been reported. **Hearing** may be affected by chronic otitis, or by disturbances in the labyrinth resulting in deaf-mutism. Syphilis of the **internal organs** may be among later symptoms, and depend upon interstitial changes or gummata. A clinical picture resembling Banti's disease may be observed (Osler[38]). There may be a disturbance resembling Fröhlich's syndrome. Chronic gastric changes have been reported (Verbrycke[39]); nephrosclerosis is rare (see Nephritis, p. 819); the pancreas and testicles sometimes exhibit lesions. A form of chronic ascites resembling tuberculous peritonitis is occasionally seen. Syphilitic endarteritis may cause areas of gangrene, or, in the larger arteries, produce aneurysm, even in childhood. Clinical evidence of heart-disease is not often found, although pathologically there are frequently changes in the cardiac muscle and the aorta and other vessels (Matusoff and White;[40] McCulloch[10]). Emphysema apparently dependent upon syphilis may occur.

Reviewing the later symptoms as described, some are characteristic of relapses in infancy and early childhood, while others are typically later symptoms and appear oftenest about puberty. Among the former are condylomata, debility, retardation of growth, deformities of the skull, dactylitis, and glandular enlargement. Among the latter are osteoperiostitis, gummata, affections of the teeth, keratitis, labyrinthine deafness, affections of the knee-joints, and retarded mental development and other psychic disorders. The combination of deformed teeth, deafness, and keratitis has been described as "Hutchinson's triad," and is very characteristic among the later manifestations. There is, however, no sharply dividing line between the ages at which the various later symptoms may show themselves.

Prognosis of Syphilis.—The prognosis of **hereditary syphilis** varies with the severity of the infection, the date at which the mother acquired it, and the promptness and thoroughness of treatment. (See p. 427.) In general, the less recent the parental disease, the better the state of infantile nutrition, the greater the delay in appearance of symptoms and the less their intensity, and, especially, the earlier antisyphilitic treatment is commenced after birth, or better, before it, the greater is the chance of the child living. The majority of infants apparently healthy at birth and showing no symptoms for some weeks can be saved by energetic treatment. According to statistics, the mortality varies. The chances of abortion in syphilitic women are about one-third of the conceptions, and about one-third of the infants born at term or near it die within a very short time. The total mortality, including abortions and early deaths, often reaches 70 per cent (Coutts[41], LePileur[42]). Davidsohn[43] gives a mortality of 75 per cent and found that 95 per cent of syphilitic children developed physical signs of the disease before the age of fourteen years. In other series, and especially in better social circumstances, the mortality may be less, varying from about 25 to 40 per cent (Fournier;[44] Hescheles[45]). Orel[46] found that in 100 untreated women, 60 produced living children, and of these only 30 reached the third year. Sullivan observed that while treatment influences clinical symptoms, it was difficult to obtain a negative Wassermann reaction in the patients, and of 60 patients only 20 per cent could be made negative. Morgan[47] had better results and found that if treatment were started early, 80 per cent of the infants could be serologically cured, and if started later about 49 per cent.

Important, too, is the influence of a supply of suitable nourishment, especially breast-milk. The later children of syphilitic parents oftener survive than do the earlier ones. Death is due more often to the general asthenia or to such complications as sepsis and pneumonia than to the lesions of the viscera, unless these are very decided. There is also to be remembered the great tendency to repeated relapses, sometimes occurring in spite of thorough treatment. These, however, constantly diminish in intensity if treatment is continued. There is further a tendency for symptoms of the tertiary type to appear in later childhood, even in cases which have seemed entirely cured earlier. Most of these cases yield to treatment unless there is severe visceral involvement. The nervous manifestations are often entirely resistant to treatment.

The *duration* of the disease is uncertain. Under proper treatment the characteristic cutaneous eruptions generally disappear in three to four weeks, but the rhagades, glandular swelling, and especially the snuffling last longer. The asthenia and anemia may remain after other symptoms have disappeared. Untreated infants lose the cutaneous eruption in a few weeks, but soon relapse. The chance for ultimate recovery depends very greatly upon thorough treatment. Symptoms of the tertiary type yield slowly, but the danger to life is much less.

The prognosis of **acquired syphilis** in infancy is much better than that of the hereditary type, owing to the absence of the severe constitutional impression made by the latter.

Diagnosis.—In syphilitic still-born infants, or in those born prematurely or dying soon after birth, spirochetes may be found in the tissues, there may be syphilitic disease of the placenta, and section of the bones reveals typical changes. Apart from these, the clinical diagnosis in severe cases in the new-born rests upon the enlargement of the spleen and liver, coryza, and osteochondritis. Syphilitic osseous lesions may be demonstrated by the roentgen-ray. In early infancy the most representative symptoms are snuffling, hoarseness, cutaneous eruptions, fissures about the mouth and nose, and malnutrition. Relapses are characterized by return of the symptoms, or the development of condylomata and sometimes of visceral involvement. Among much later diagnostic symptoms of importance are alterations of the teeth, the development of gummata, keratitis, deafness, saddle-nose from destructive lesions, ulcerations of the palate or interior of the nose, saber tibiae, enlargement of the lymphatic glands and of the liver and spleen, and general retarded development.

In mild cases there may be no characteristic symptoms, and the serum-test may be necessary for diagnosis. The known presence of syphilis in the parents, or the occurrence of repeated earlier abortions, is important diagnostically, as is also response to antisyphilitic treatment.

Syphilitic cutaneous lesions are to be differentiated from other eruptions. The circumscribed maculopapular eruption is distinguished principally by its disposition to appear on the face and lower extremities, and the coppery, or raw-ham, tint. The diffuse syphilitic rash may resemble eczema intertrigo, but is scaly, less red, more infiltrated, with diffuse stiffness of the skin, and has the coppery or yellowish-brown tint in place of the intense redness of eczema. The pustular syphilitic lesions have a characteristic dusky-red color unlike the lesions in tuberculosis. Coryza in the early weeks or months of infancy, without fever and resisting local treatment, is suspicious. Scurvy may be differentiated from the osteochondritis of syphilis by therapeutical tests, as well as by other characteristic signs of the two diseases respectively. The syphilitic lesion is nearer the epiphysis, and appears at an early age. Syphilitic involvement of the central nervous system can be distinguished from nonsyphilitic disease by the history, the association with other syphilitic symptoms, and the Wassermann reaction on the blood and spinal fluid.

The Wassermann complement-fixation reaction, as applied by Wassermann, Neisser and Bruck[48] and as modified by others, is diagnostically valuable within its limitations. Many new-born syphilitic infants may have a negative Wassermann reaction for several weeks. On the other hand, a weakly positive reaction in the first month may mean only that reacting substances, but not spirochetes, have been transmitted from mother to fetus. Consequently, if the infant seems entirely healthy and the Wassermann reaction, without treatment, later becomes negative, syphilis cannot be diagnosed. The Wassermann reaction of the mother will usually indicate the presence or absence of syphilis in the offspring. This is, however, not always the case, since a syphilitic woman may have the disease in a latent form, give a negative Wassermann reaction, and yet bear a syphilitic child. Conversely it is possible for a perfectly healthy infant to be born to a distinctly syphilitic mother.

Formerly the complement-fixation test was found positive in other conditions, as scarlet fever, malaria, and the like. Since improvement in the technique the number of these positive results has decreased. In fine, the Wassermann reaction must be looked upon as corroborative evidence, to be considered in conjunction with clinical symptoms. In the presence of symptoms, treatment should be instituted in the face of a negative reaction. The Wassermann reaction may be taken on the cord-blood of the infant at birth, and positive tests may be obtained at times on breast-milk, urine, and other fluids (Klauder and Kolmer;[49] Costellessa;[50] Franken and Rottmann;[51]

Jarcho[52]). What has been said of the Wassermann test applies with practically equal force to the Kahn[53] test (serum diagnosis of syphilis by precipitation). This is widely used, often in conjunction with the complement-fixation test (Caffey and Kreidel;[54] Cookson and Brown;[55] Manace[56]). The Noguchi[57] luetin test is little employed at the present time and its value is doubtful. It consists in the intradermal injection of a suspension of dead spirochaetae pallidae. A local papule appearing in twenty-four to forty-eight hours is an indication of a positive reaction.

Treatment. **Prophylaxis.** The advice originally given by Fournier[58] was to the effect that a syphilitic adult should undergo energetic treatment more or less continuously for from three to four years after the onset of the disease, and for two years there should have been no symptoms. Marriage might by this time take place, although even then without absolute certainty that the disease would not be transmitted. A syphilitic woman should receive treatment during pregnancy, and this commenced at once or as early as possible, for reasons previously stated. Such treatment should be given even in the absence of clinical symptoms, and particularly if the Wassermann reaction is positive. According to Profeta's law (see p. 426) an apparently healthy infant, born of a syphilic mother, may be suckled by her without danger of infection. Naturally if the mother acquires syphilis after the birth of her infant she should not nurse it. Promiscuous kissing of the baby should be avoided. Nurses in attendance should certainly be nonsyphilitic. A wet-nurse must never be employed without examination for syphilis and a Wassermann test being made. In emergency, when breast milk is used from a woman whose Wassermann is unknown, it is better to boil the milk for three minutes.

Treatment of the Disease.—Immediately after birth with infants of parents known to be syphilitic, or in other infants as soon as the diagnosis has been made, treatment should be commenced. With whatever therapy employed, it is important that it be continued for at least a year in infants, and for two years in older children, after the clinical symptoms have disappeared and a consistently negative Wassermann reaction has been obtained. There are four classes of drugs used, (*a*) mercurials, (*b*) arsenicals, (*c*) bismuth, and (*d*) iodides.

(*a*) *Mercury* may be administered by inunction, employing 5 to 10 grains (0.3 to 0.6) of mercurial ointment daily. After preliminary cleansing with soap and warm water this should be gently rubbed into the skin for ten to fifteen minutes, selecting different situations daily. Moll[59] recommends rubbing in the ointment with a shaving brush. Instead of this inunction, if there is extensive cutaneous eruption, a sublimate bath may be given daily. The temperature of the water should be from 100 to 105 F. (37.8 to 40.6 C.), 5 to 15 grains (0.32 to 0.97) of bichloride of mercury added to each five gallons (20 liters), and the infant kept in the bath for from five to fifteen minutes. Mercury may be given internally, either as calomel $\frac{1}{10}$ grain (0.0065), the protiodides $\frac{1}{20}$ to $\frac{1}{10}$ grain (0.0033 to 0.006), mercury with chalk 1 to 2 grains (0.065 to 0.13), or corrosive sublimate $\frac{1}{100}$ to $\frac{1}{50}$ grain (0.0006 to 0.0013) three or four times a day. There are various preparations of mercury which may be used hypodermically, such as the chloride or the salicylate. The usual hypodermic dose of mercuric chloride is $\frac{1}{10}$ to $\frac{1}{8}$ grain (0.006 to 0.008) for small infants, and more for older ones, giving this two or three times a week, or once a week if mercury is being given by mouth also.

(*b*) *Arsenic* in its many forms (salvarsan, neosalvarsan, arsphenamine, neoarsphenamine, silver arsphenamine, sulpharsphenamine, arsenobenzol, sulpharsenol, etc.) is also of value. All of these preparations are for parenteral use, as arsenic has little effect upon syphilis when given by mouth or rectum. An exception is the arsenical preparation stovarsol, which, administered orally in doses of 0.25 Gm. (3.8 grains) twice daily, has been employed with success by Mettel,[60] especially in periostitis. There is much difference of opinion concerning the value of these various forms of arsenic. Arsphenamine and some of the other preparations must be neutralized immediately before use, whereas neoarsphenamine and certain others are already neutralized, and are, therefore, simpler to inject. Sulpharsphenamine may be given intramuscularly, but the other forms of arsenic should be used intravenously or, perhaps, intraperitoneally, as recommended by Rosenberg,[61] and by Grulee, Sanford and Waldo[62] (p. 184). In older children superficial veins may often be found which are suitable for intravenous injection, such as the external jugular or those on the scalp, the arm, or the leg. The longitudinal sinus is a dangerous place to introduce the drug (p. 197).

(c) *Bismuth* has an antispirochetal action. It was first employed extensively for clinical purposes by Fournier and Guénot[63] after experiments by Sazerac and Levaditi.[64] Its preparations are the tartrobismuthate of sodium and potassium in aqueous solution or in olive oil, potassium tartrobismuthate in aqueous solution, bismuth trioxide in olive oil, lipoid-soluble bismuth (biliposol), or bismuth phenylformitate. One preparation is a combination of arsenic and mercury, bismuth arsphenamine sulphonate (Bismarsen), and another a combination of iodides and bismuth, (iodobismitol). Bismuth may be administered by intramuscular injection at intervals of two to four days, 10 to 12 injections constituting a course. Young infants should not receive more than 0.15 grains (0.01) of bismuth at a dose.

(d) *Iodide of potassium* or of *sodium* may be given in doses of 2 to 10 grains (0.13 to 0.65) three times a day to infants, and larger doses to older patients.

Indication for Different Types of Drugs.—*Mercury* has a favorable influence on the symptoms of syphilis, and in young infants seems also to exercise a tonic, in addition to its specific, action and to improve the nutritional state. It should probably always be added to the treatment when arsenic or bismuth is being employed. It rarely produces salivation in early infancy and seldom in childhood. If stomatitis, anemia, or debility is caused by it, the dosage should be diminished or other drugs substituted. *Arsenic* is a recognized adjunct in the treatment of syphilis. Its use is attended by some danger, and death may follow its injection, due either to the toxic action of arsenic or to the death of large numbers of spirochetes in the tissues. It has also been said to have produced an aplastic type of anemia. *Bismuth* is probably inferior to mercury, but is widely employed at present, and is especially valuable when there is intolerance to the other drugs. In some cases bismuth seems to be effective in causing the Wassermann reaction to become negative when mercury and arsenic have failed. The symptoms of over-dose consist of stomatitis, foul breath, polyuria and albuminuria. The *iodides* are of service only for the treatment of the distinctly later manifestations of syphilis, as of later relapses, or of gummata anywhere, or at any time when the viscera or bone is involved. The early relapses with condylomata require the administration of mercury.

There are numerous ways in which these drugs are employed. We are accustomed to the following procedure, the doses mentioned being for infants under one year of age, with 1.5 to 2 times these amounts to be administered to older infants and children:—Twice weekly intramuscular injections are given of sulpharsphenamine in the amount of 0.01 Gm. to each kilogram of body weight, (0.07 grain per pound) the solution being made of 5 per cent strength with distilled water. In place of this neoarsphenamine may be given intravenously in doses of 0.01 Gm. per kilogram (0.07 grain per pound). After this treatment with an arsenical, a bismuth preparation, such as bismuth sodium or potassium tartrate in 1.5 per cent solution, is given intramuscularly in doses of 0.5 cc. (8 minims) once a week for ten doses. After a month the Wassermann reaction is taken and the necessity for further treatment judged by it and the clinical symptoms. Usually at least two courses are employed per year. Mercury may be given continuously, including the time arsenic is being administered, or only during the intervals between the injections.

In so-called "Wassermann-fast" patients, viz., those who persistently give a positive reaction in spite of treatment, some clinicians have employed treatment with foreign protein, using milk, typhoid vaccine, or gonococcus vaccine.

In neurosyphilis, when the medication already outlined does not produce results, the method of Swift and Ellis[65] may be followed. This consists in withdrawing blood from the patient within about one-half hour after the intravenous injection of arsphenamine, allowing it to clot, and putting it in the ice-box for twenty to twenty-four hours, and then injecting from 5 to 15 cc. (0.17 to 0.5 fl. oz.) of the serum intraspinally. Two or three courses of injections at intervals of six weeks may be needed, the result sought being the production of a negative Wassermann reaction, without causing other changes in the spinal fluid. In neurosyphilis an arsenical preparation known as tryparsamide, as first recommended by Lorenz and his co-workers,[66] may be used intramuscularly or intravenously in weekly doses of 0.04 to 0.05 Gm. or less per kilogram of body weight (0.28 to 0.36 grains per pound). It should be used cautiously in disease of the optic nerve.

General Treatment.—This consists in the maintenance of nutrition, especially by the use of breast-milk; the treatment for anemia; and the employment of all hygienic measures, such as fresh air, sunshine and the like.

Local Treatment.—Condylomata and cutaneous ulcers and fissures may be dusted with calomel, covered with mercurial ointment, or painted with a solution of silver nitrate. Ulcers on the mucous membrane should be carefully cleansed, and calomel or silver nitrate applied. Gummatous ulcers may be treated with iodoform or mercurial applications. Coryza is often benefited by a cleansing of the nose, followed by the employment of a diluted yellow oxide of mercury ointment or by the insufflation of calomel well diluted with sugar (1:20).

References

1. Rev. d'hyg. et de méd. inf., 1903, **2,** 1. 2. Pediatrics, 1904, **16,** 577. 3. Arch. f. Kinderh., 1905, **42,** 64. 4. Arch. f. Kinderh., 1909, **50,** 154. 5. Am. J. Dis. Child., 1916, **12,** 355. 6. Am. J. Syph., 1921, **5,** 131. 7. Am. J. Dis. Child., 1921, **22,** 402. 8. California and West Med., 1929, **31,** 242. 9. Am. J. Dis. Child., 1929, **37,** 1198. 10. Am. Heart J., 1930, **6,** 136. 11. Arbeiten aus. d. kais. Gesundheitsamte., 1904–5, **22,** 527. 12. Pract. Observ. on Vener. Dis. and on the Use of Mercury, London, 1837, 304. 13. J.A.M.A., 1924, **83,** 172. 14. Clin. Pediat., 1925, **7,** 289. 15. Arch. Dermat. and Syph., 1927, **15,** 695. 16. M. J. and Rec., 1930, **132,** 78. 17. Dermat. Wchnschr., 1931, **92,** 309. 18. Jahrb. f. Kinderh., 1888, **27,** 362. 19. Virchow's Arch. f. path. Anat., 1870, **50,** 305. 20. Am. J. Dis. Child., 1931, **41,** 130; 353; 607; 887; 1128; 1141. 21. J.A.M.A., 1923, **81,** 1752. 22. Arch. de phys. norm. et path., 1871–2, **4,** 319. 23. Pfaundler und Schlossmann's Handbk. d. Kinderh., 1906, **1,** 2, 916. 24. Ztschr. f. Kinderh., 1927, **43,** 429. 25. Deutsche Ztschr. f. Nervenk., 1930, **114,** 288. 26. Ann. de dermat. et syph., 1930, **1,** 403. 27. Lancet, 1904, **2,** 1402. 28. Pfaundler und Schlossmann's Handbk. d. Kinderh., 1906, **1,** 2, 921. 29. Ergeben. inn. Med. u. Kinderh., 1910, **5,** 84. 30. J.A.M.A., 1926, **86,** 392. 31. Brit. M. J., 1858, **2,** 822. 32. J.A.M.A., 1923, **80,** 28. 33. J.A.M.A., 1921, **77,** 919. 34. Am. J. Dis. Child., 1919, **18,** 173. 35. Monatschr. f. Kinderh., 1923, **35,** 398. 36. Ztschr. f. Chemotherap. u. verwandte Gebiete, 1913, Orig. **1,** 44. 37. Arch. de méd. d. enf., 1927, **30,** 697. 38. Clin. J., 1914, **43,** 462. 39. Am. J. Syph., 1929, **13,** 524. 40. Am. J. Dis. Child., 1927, **34,** 390. 41. Lancet, 1896, **1,** 971. 42. Thèse de Paris, 1851; Ref. Fournier,

L'hérédité syphilitique, 1891, 312. 43. Gesundheits. f. d. Kindersalt, 1926, **1,** 581. 44. L'hérédité syphilitique, 1891, 309. 45. Arch. f. Kinderh., 1926, **76,** 194. 46. Ztschr. f. Kinderh., 1925, **40,** 414. 47. Canad. M. A. J., 1930, **23,** 811. 48. Deutsche med. Wchnschr., 1906, **32,** 745. 49. J.A.M.A., 1921, **76,** 1635. 50. Pediatria, 1923, **31,** 860. 51. Monatschr. f. Geburtsh. u. Gynäk., 1927, **77,** 163. 52. J. Lab. and Clin. Med., 1929, 14, 1097. 53. Arch. Dermat. and Syph., 1922, 5, 570. 54. Am. J. Dis. Child., 1929, **38,** 1206. 55. Brit. M. J., 1930, **1,** 441. 56. Am. J. Dis. Child., 1930, **40,** 63. 57. J. Exper. Med., 1911, **14,** 557. 58. Syphilis et mariage, 1880, 108; 115. 59. Monatschr. f. Kinderh., 1929, **45,** 293. 60. Arch. Pediat., 1931, **48,** 761. 61. J.A.M.A., 1924, **82,** 682. 62. Am. J. Dis. Child., 1928, **35,** 47. 63. Ann. de l'inst. Pasteur, 1922, **36,** 14. 64. Ann. de l'inst. Pasteur, 1922, **36,** 1. 65. New York M. J., 1912, **96,** 53. 66. J.A.M.A., 1923, **80,** 1497.

SECTION III

GENERAL NUTRITIONAL AND MISCELLANEOUS DISEASES

Here may be placed, in addition to nutritional disturbances, a number of disorders the cause and nature of which are not fully understood, or which seem properly to belong in no other category. Among these is Acute Rheumatic Fever, which it seemed better to include here until its etiology is more firmly established.

CHAPTER I

RACHITIS

(Rickets)

Evidences of rickets are found in the skeletons of children of the stone age (Kjerrulk[1]), and the disease existed also in ancient Greece and Rome. It is uncertain whether it was present in ancient Egypt (Findlay[2]). It was first named Rachitis and clearly described by Glisson[3] in 1650. An interesting contribution on the evidences of the disease before that time is that of Foote.[4] Its prevalence varies greatly with locality, but a large proportion of infants brought to hospitals in many of the greater cities of Europe and America exhibit it. It may be estimated that 50 per cent or more of the children of the poor of large cities of the United States suffer from rickets, although the wide-spread application of preventive measures is now diminishing the number of severe cases. (See Geographical Distribution, p. 443.) It is essentially a chronic disorder of nutrition, affecting the bones most strikingly; but general in its nature, and involving as well the ligaments, muscles, mucous membranes, nervous system, and other parts of the body.

Etiology.—Lack of space forbids the mentioning here of any but a few of the investigations on this subject, and only those particularly appropriate to the topics under immediate consideration will be referred to in later sections. Older excellent reviews are given by Howland[5] and by Park,[6] and more recently by Hess[7] in various contributions.

Many influences possess etiologic relationship; all of them intimately associated with three factors: (1) light, (2) proper balance of calcium and phosphorus in the diet, and (3) vitamin D, or the antirachitic substance. The possible mode of action of these will be discussed under Pathogenesis, and their clinical significance under Treatment.

There is little influence of *sex* on the incidence in the human, although in animals (dogs) the female seems to be less severely affected (Stockard[8]). *Diet* is a powerful factor. Clinical evidence of the disease is less frequent in properly breast-fed infants, but milder degrees of it may often be found in them by clinical or roentgenographical study (Eliot[9]). Diets high in carbohydrate especially tend to produce rickets, probably because they are deficient in other respects. Yet the disease may follow overfeeding as well as underfeeding, and great caloric deficiency leads to wasting rather than to the development of rickets. *Race* has an influence, since those with darker skins, as the Italians and negroes, develop rickets readily when they are transported from their native, warmer regions to colder ones. Such *hygienic conditions* as overcrowding, lack of exercise, poverty, and the like increase the incidence of the disease, as does *season,* active manifestations of the disorder being less evident during the summer. *Geographical distribution and climate* are also factors. The disease is especially frequent in northern temperate climates, less common in subtropical countries, and is said to be rare in the tropics and far north, although Brooke[10] noted it not uncommon in the tropics on account of the long wet seasons. Williams[11] found mild rickets frequent in New Orleans, but severe forms uncommon. Torroella[12] found it infrequent in Mexico. It is less common at high altitudes than in low sections of the same country. *Heredity* has probably little, if any, influence, although Siegert,[13] Zimmern,[14] and others have reported cases which seem to support the opposite view. However, Hess and Weinstock[15] point out that races which are particularly predisposed to rickets when they have been transported from warmer to colder climates, have not suffered from the disease in their native environment. The matter of *prenatal influence* will be referred to later. *Age* is an important factor. Rickets is observed especially in the first two years of life, with its height about the end of the first year. It rarely shows itself clinically before the third month and generally not until after the sixth. In roentgenograms it can be found earlier than by clinical examination. In 422 infants younger than six months we[16] found 42 who had roentgenographic evidence of rachitic osseous changes. *Fetal rickets* and *late rickets* are discussed later (p. 452). *Prematurity,* as also *previous diseases* of the infant, may be decided factors. Acute severe digestive disturbance leads to wasting rather than to rickets, but acute disease of other nature may initiate rickets or make it worse if already present. Chronic diseases, as syphilis, tuberculosis, some chronic cutaneous disorders, and prolonged catarrhal states of the gastro-intestinal tract are decided predisposing factors.

Pathogenesis.—Facts ascertained from studies upon rats may be applied in great measure to the problem in infants, although rickets in the two species is not necessarily similar in its production (Mouriquand;[17] Hess and Weinstock[18]).

In some way there occurs a failure of lime-salts to be deposited in the bones, and a cessation in the transformation of osteoid tissue into true bone; and it is evident that ultraviolet light and vitamin D must be operative in regulating mineral metabolism. In the active stage of rickets there is usually a lowered phosphorus-content of the blood and a slightly lowered or normal calcium. There is also an increased excretion of these minerals, more especially of the phosphorus (Schabad;[19] Schloss;[20] Orr, Holt, Wilkins and Boone;[21] Daniels, Stearns and Hutton;[22] Rominger, Meyer and Bomskov[23]). With healing this disturbance of mineral balance returns to normal, being preceded by an increased retention, especially of phosphorus. The calcium of the tissues other than bone is normal in amount (Stöltzner,[24] Brubacher[25]), but the phosphorus is low (Heymann[26]). It would seem that the primary disturbance in rickets is one of phosphorus-metabolism, with faulty deposition of that mineral and of calcium in the bones. It should be stated that Hess[27] and his coworkers have found that rickets can develop when the concentration and the ratio of the calcium and phosphorus of the blood are normal, and that hypophosphatemia is not, therefore, an essential feature. In such cases there must be a local disturbance at the epiphyses causing failure of deposition of minerals. Others, as Shohl and Bennett,[28] have found, too, that the excretion of minerals in rickets is not excessive, and that there is rather a diminished positive balance than an actual negative one.

The question to be considered is the method by which the diverse factors, such as food, sunlight, ultraviolet rays, and vitamin D, act upon the mineral metabolism to cause or to cure rickets. As to the *diet*, that breast-fed infants may develop the milder degrees of the disease may depend upon the lack of richness of the milk in vitamin D (Hess and Weinstock[18]), or upon a poverty of it in calcium and phosphorus (Burhans and Smith;[29] Courtney and Brown[30]). That breast-fed infants do not so often develop rickets as do the bottle-fed, in spite of the normal lower mineral content of human milk, depends in part upon their better retention of phosphorus (Moll[31]); in part upon the less frequent development of gastro-intestinal and other disorders; and in part upon the less alkaline reaction produced by human milk in the intestinal tract. Too great alkalinity of the upper intestinal tract is not favorable to the absorption of calcium and phosphorus, and rickets may thus be produced (Telfer;[32] Jones, James and Smith;[33] Orr, Holt, Wilkins and Boone;[21] Zucker and Matzner;[34] Findlay;[35] Abrahamson and Miller;[36] Grayzel and Miller;[37] Babbott, Johnston, and Haskin[38]). A diminished intake of calcium and phosphorus may lead to rickets, but even more important is a disturbed ratio between them, since it has been shown that an increase of one of these minerals in the diet causes a diminished retention of the other (Salversen, Hastings and McIntosh[39]). This disturbed mineral ratio, as well as the increased alkalinity of the intestinal tract, probably acts by the formation of excessive amounts of insoluble calcium-phosphate. Other elements of the diet besides the mineral content are operative. Thus the low-fat, high-carbonate diets may exert their well-known effect in producing rickets through the lack of retention of minerals which they induce.

That *underfed infants* do not develop rickets has been explained on the basis that the starving body may rectify its abnormal mineral metabolism when the burden of carrying on the metabolism consequent to ingestion of food is removed; and there is also the additional factor that during the lack of growth due to underfeeding minerals are not so much needed for other tissues, and may be utilized by the bones. In *overfeeding* the body's demand for minerals may be so great, on account of rapid growth, that not sufficient is diverted to the formation of bone. There is also probably active the likelihood of disturbing the digestion and other functions by overfeeding, and the consequent interference with normal metabolism. Yet the influence of diet by itself is not always clear, and other factors appear to be involved, since the disease may develop on a diet properly balanced in the amount of minerals and other ingredients, and, on the other hand, can be prevented by ultraviolet radiation or the administration of vitamin D even when an imperfect diet is being given.

The relationship of *sunlight* to rickets is seen in the influence of season, race, climate, altitude, poor hygiene, and, to a certain extent, of age. It is the short ultraviolet rays, under 313 millimicrons in length, that possess antirachitic power, and these can be produced artificially by the mercury-vapor quartz lamp, the carbon-arc lamp, and the tungsten-filament lamp. These rays are effective in prevention and cure; in the latter being demonstrated by clinical improvement, by the return of blood-phosphate and blood-calcium to normal, and by the local healing of the epiphyses as shown in the roentgenogram. The seasonal tide of blood-phosphates, with the ebb in the winter, is related to sunlight; and it has been shown that rickets is uncommon where the minimum seasonal altitude of the sun is not below 35 degrees, and, therefore, ample in ultraviolet radiation (Tisdall and Brown[40]). Exposure to ultraviolet rays decreases intestinal alkalinity and thereby increases mineral absorption (Zucker and Matzner;[34] Tisdall and Price;[41] Grayzel and Miller[37]). The specific action of radiation is probably due to the changes brought about in the ergosterol of the skin (Hess and Smith[42]) (see also p. 445).

Imperfect hygienic conditions favor the development of rickets in part by the insufficient exposure to sunlight, and in part by deficiency in diet. Season is a factor through the favorable influence of the greater amount of sunlight during the summer; and geographical distribution and climate similarly make more tropical regions unfavorable to the development of rickets, because of the greater amount of sunlight and exposure to it, while high altitudes are beneficial because of the more numerous ultraviolet rays. As regards, further, the action of *ultraviolet rays* in preventing rickets in the tropics, the matter is not entirely clear. It has been claimed that pigmented skin, as in the dark races, filters out the ultraviolet rays (Sambon;[43] Hess[44]). Levinsohn,[45] however, claims that some other factor than this must be operative in producing the racial tendency to rickets in dark-skinned races even in temperate climates, since the cholesterol (ergosterol) which must be activated by the light-rays is more superficially placed than the pigment granules. That the rays can penetrate deeper than the epidermis is maintained by Macht, Anderson and Bell,[46] and Lucas,[47] but denied by Hill[48] and others. In any event there still seems some uncertainty about the reason for the racial predisposition of the negroes and Italians in northern temperate localities. Their diet cannot be considered less satisfactory than in the other races of the same social position. It may be that they are less exposed to sunlight, although there is no proof of this, and it is very possible that the darker skinned races need more sunlight to protect them than do those of lighter skin.

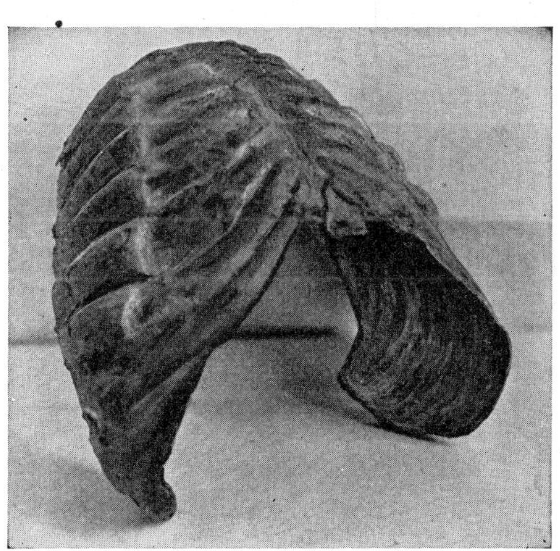

Fig. 100.—Anatomical specimen of rachitic chest. Shows the rachitic rosary produced by enlargement at the costochondral articulations.

The substance *vitamin D* is powerfully antirachitic. It is present in cod liver oil and other fish-oils, and to a less extent in egg-yolk and other substances. (See Vitamins, p. 136.) In its purest form it is found in irradiated ergosterol (viosterol). Hess, Weinstock and Helman;[49] Steenbock and Black;[50] Rosenheim and Webster,[51] and others found that the administration of cholesterol protected against rickets or cured it if present, but only if this substance was irradiated. Later it was discovered (Windhaus,[52] Hess[53]) that it was ergosterol, present with the cholesterol, which was the substance activated by light. Ergosterol is the parent substance, or provitamin, of vitamin D. Cholesterol is probably synthesized in the body and ergosterol formed from it (Schoenheimer[54]). The mechanism of the action of vitamin D is not fully understood, but it has been shown by Grayzel and Miller[37] and others that, as in the case of the ultraviolet rays, it decreased intestinal alkalinity, thus favoring the absorption of calcium and phosphorus. It has also been demonstrated that many fatty and vegetable substances acquire antirachitic properties upon exposure to ultraviolet radiation, or have them increased if present.

Further studies will doubtless reveal more definitely the mechanism by which radiant energy and vitamin D act, or whether there are still other factors operative in the production of rickets. A number of investigators uphold the view that the glands of internal secretion influence the pathogenesis of rickets (Stöltzner;[55] Lehnerdt and Weinberg;[56] Sweet;[57] Jundell;[58] Aschenheim;[59] Vollmer[60]). It has been found that the parathyroids are enlarged in rickets and in calcium deficiency (Pappenheimer and Minor;[61] Higgins and Sheard;[62] Stoltenberg[63]). Numerous other theories as to the etiology and pathogenesis of rickets have been advanced; some of them older views which have been disproven; others more recently advanced and which await further confirmation.

Pathologic Anatomy.—The principal lesions are in the osseous system. The long bones show thickening of the shaft and enlargement at the epiphyseal junctions, especially at the wrists, ankles and costochondral articulations (Fig. 100), in the latter place being particularly marked on the pleural surface. Many of the flat bones are also thickened, the skull exhibiting large bosses, while in other parts of the cranium there are spots of very thin, parchment-like bone (craniotabes). Osseous deformities and fractures occur in many parts of the body. Arrested growth may result as the sequel of the epiphyseal changes. On longitudinal section the epiphyseal junctions are found much wider, thicker, and softer than normal. The medulla of the shaft is red and jelly-like; the cavity broadened and its bony divisions rarefied; the periosteum hyperemic, with friable, spongy, vascular tissue beneath it.

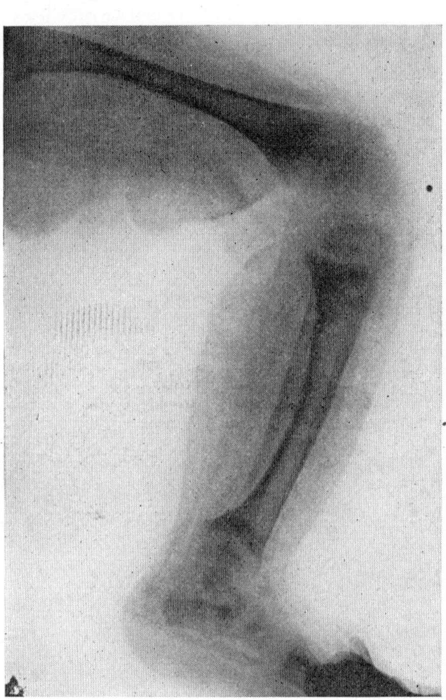

Fig. 101.—Radiograph of left leg in rickets. Moderately advanced stage. Child aged one year. Shows the hazy outline of the epiphysis and of the ends of the diaphysis of the long bones. Children's Hospital of Philadelphia.

Chemically the amount of phosphorus and of calcium in the bone is diminished, but the normal ratio between them is unchanged.

The roentgenographic appearance of the bones is characteristic (Fig. 101). In our[16] own studies on the diagnosis of rickets, we have found most helpful in the early roentgenographic diagnosis a very slight, frayed appearance of the distal ends of the radius and ulna, and sometimes a fine trabeculation of the shafts of these bones. Slight changes may also be found in the metacarpal bones. The presence of lipping of the ends of the bone and the slight spreading have not in themselves seemed to us to be diagnostic.

In brief, the osseous changes in rickets consist in unusual hyperemia; excessive proliferation of cartilage; irregularity in the transformation of cartilage into bone, with disturbance of the normal division into zones; deficient deposit of lime-salts, with consequent over-development of osteoid tissue which fails to change into true bone; thickening of the periosteal layer through undue cellular production, and the formation of masses of osteoid tissue here; absorption of trabeculae in the spongy bone, with consequent increase of the medullary spaces; and hyperemia and widening of the central marrow-cavity.

During recovery from the disease the bony changes disappear through resorption and condensation, and lime-salts are again deposited. The development of very hard, compact, dense, bony tissue (eburnation) may result.

Lesions other than those of the bones may occur. Among these are catarrhal conditions of the lungs with areas of atelectasis and emphysema; enlargement of the spleen, lymphatic glands, and liver; catarrhal inflammation of the gastro-enteric tract; thinness and weakness of the muscles; and dilatation of the ventricles of the brain.

Symptoms.—The constitutional symptoms become manifest about the third month of life and before the more characteristic skeletal changes appear, although the latter can be found microscopically even in the second month. Among the earliest manifestations are head-sweating, restlessness, and rocking of the head on the pillow; these developing gradually and often attracting little attention. In a short time beading of the ribs is noticed in most cases. Other bony enlargements now develop, especially of the

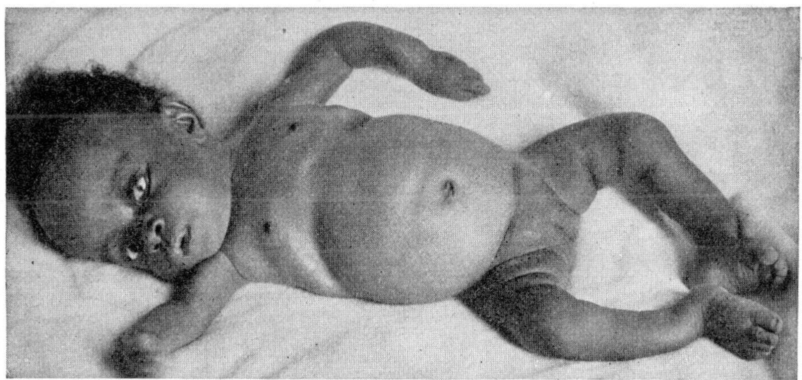

Fig. 102.—Rachitic deformity, showing the curvature of the limbs and the well-marked pot-belly. Patient in the Children's Ward of the University Hospital, Philadelphia.

skull, ribs, wrists, and ankles, while characteristic alterations of the shape of the chest appear and the abdomen becomes pot-bellied. (Figs. 102 and 104.) The general health may remain unaffected at first, but in well-marked cases the child finally grows anemic and suffers readily from respiratory and gastrointestinal catarrhal processes, and sometimes convulsions. The teeth are late in appearing and decay early; the fontanelle fails to close at the proper time; growth of the body is interfered with; and when sitting and walking begin, at a period much later than normal, curvature of the long bones and of the spine is produced. A more detailed description of symptoms follows:

Head.—The head appears, and often is, larger than normal in its horizontal circumference and is usually brachycephalic. The forehead is prominent (Fig. 104), and the occiput and vault flattened. This produces a peculiarly box-like form. The shape, which develops oftenest about the end of the first year, depends largely upon the deposit of rachitic bone, which takes place especially upon the frontal and parietal eminences, along the sutures, and about the fontanelles. The flattening of the occipital region is due to pressure upon the pillow; and should the child while in bed lie very constantly on one parieto-occipital region, great asymmetry of the head may result, one oblique diameter being much shorter than the other, one ear nearer the front, and even one cheek more prominent. The anterior fontanelle is larger than normal, and its time of closing is delayed, this occurring sometimes not until after the second year. A systolic murmur may often be heard above it. In severe cases the posterior fontanelle and the sutures remain open until the end of the first year. In the posterior portion of the skull thin, soft membranous spots are often found in the first

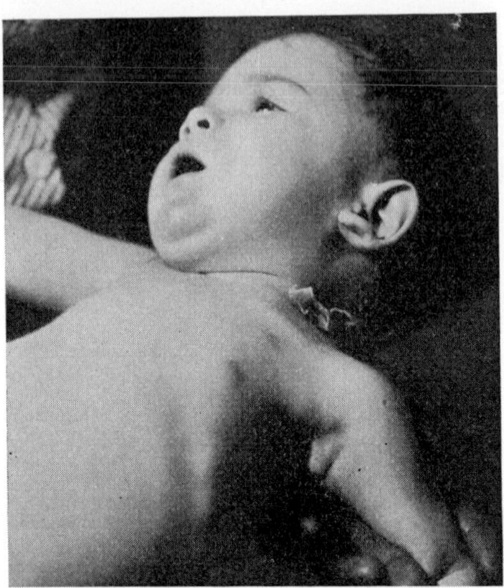

Fig. 103.—Rachitic rosary. Infant, seventeen months of age, Children's Hospital, Cincinnati.

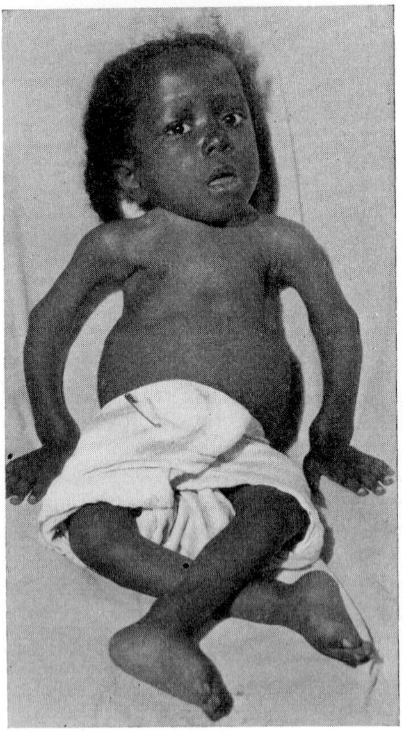

Fig. 104.—Frontal bosses, curvature of arms, deformed chest, pot-belly, enlarged epiphyses. Child three years of age, General Hospital, Cincinnati.

year (*craniotabes*, see p. 999). This condition is not indicative of rickets in the absence of other signs. The veins of the scalp are distended, especially over the temporal regions. The hair is quite commonly worn away from the back of the head by the frequent rocking movements. The face seems small, the upper jaw being narrower than normal and the lower somewhat square. These various deformities usually disappear as recovery takes place, but the relative increase in size may persist in severe cases to some extent throughout life. The temporary teeth usually appear late and out of the normal order, not infrequently none having erupted during the first year. They are generally of good form, although they may decay early. The teeth of the permanent set have often been damaged by the previous rachitic condition, and have a decided tendency to malformation, erosion, and caries.

Thorax.—Beading of the ribs at the costochondral articulations is the most frequent and the earliest osseous symptom. It is quite visible to the eye unless the infant is well covered with fat (Fig. 103). It is very doubtful whether slight enlargement of the costochondral junctions can be considered sufficient evidence in itself to warrant a diagnosis of rickets, but in 600 infants under six months of age we[16] found 18 with a rosary, which, from other findings, could be considered rachitic. In all well-marked cases there is in addition a depression of the cartilages anterior to the epiphyseal enlargements. A flattening or even a concavity of the sides of the thorax in a vertical direction develops, extending backward to the posterior axillary line and downward about as far as the seventh rib (Fig. 104). As a result of this alteration the sternum is unusually prominent, producing a condition suggesting "pigeon-breast," but usually differing somewhat from the typical instances of this seen in certain other conditions, in that the whole sternum is pushed forward in a straight line without any anterior curvature of it. The rachitic thorax also exhibits bulging at the angle of the ribs posteriorly, accompanied by a flattening of the back. These changes produce in well-marked cases a deformity known as the "violin-shaped" chest.

In addition to the vertical lateral depression there is a horizontal one (Harrison's groove) caused by the decided flare of the costal border. This is at about the level of the xiphoid cartilage and corresponds to the insertion of the diaphragm. Occasionally a funnel-shaped depression of the lower part of the sternum occurs. In some cases the clavicles are thickened at the extremities, shorter, and more curved than normal, and may show green-stick fractures.

The thorax as a whole is lengthened in an anteroposterior direction, and is small and narrow, except for the sudden widening of the lower portion (Fig. 104). The deformities are produced by the action of the muscles of respiration, including the diaphragm, upon the very soft bones; and by the pressure of the back against the bed, and of the distended stomach and intestines and the enlarged liver against the costal border.

Spinal Column.—This may be normal, but a certain degree of lateral curvature is common in infants, and may be very persistent. Always seen in marked cases is a long posterior curvature dependent upon the weakness of the ligaments and of the muscles of the trunk. It usually disappears entirely or to a considerable extent when the child is suspended from the arm-pits (Fig. 105).

Pelvis.—In severe cases the pelvis may become permanently deformed, the anteroposterior diameter being shorter and the outlet narrower, with thickening of the crests of the ilia.

Extremities.—Epiphyseal enlargement at the wrist and ankles (Fig. 104) is an early symptom nearly always present, and, less frequently, similar enlargement of the lower end of the humerus and femur and the upper ends of these bones and of the tibia and fibula. The enlargement at the wrists is usually antedated somewhat by the visible rosary. Bending of the shafts of the long bones occurs in the lower extremities, the commonest deformities being knock-knees and bow-legs. (See also p. 996.) The tibia may be bent outward or forward (Fig. 102). The femur is curved only in the severe cases, and generally in a forward and outward direction. Coxa vara is another rachitic deformity. Sometimes a striking distortion results from the child sitting cross-legged, the femora being partly rotated outward and the tibia and fibula of one side fitting into those of the other where pressure one upon the other has been constantly exercised. Bending of the humerus is not common but the bones of the forearm often curve outward (Fig. 104). Green-stick fractures on the concave side of the bone are not infrequent, especially in the forearm and the tibia. Bending is produced largely by the action of position and of muscular pull upon the soft bones, although

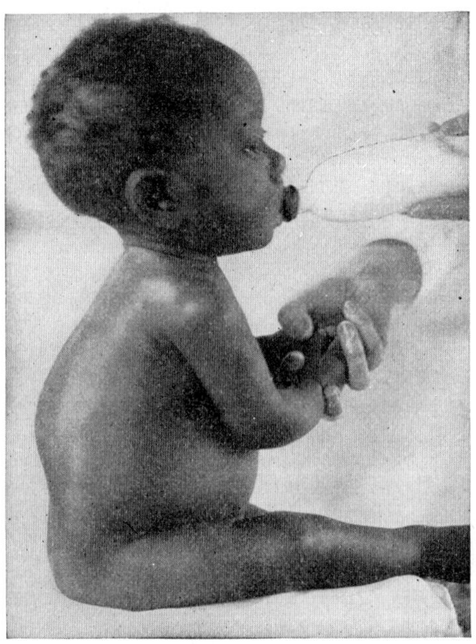

Fig. 105.—Rachitic spinal curvature. Very well marked when child is sitting. *(Courtesy of Dr. H. R. Wharton.)*

partly by asymmetrical growth of the epiphysis. It occurs in the legs even before walking is commenced, but is increased by it. The deformity of the extremities becomes a marked symptom toward the end of the first year.

Growth of the long bones in length is very commonly interfered with, especially in the lower extremities, and in the worst cases permanent dwarfism may be a final result. Occasionally thickening of the fingers occurs. Flat-foot is a common rachitic deformity.

Ligaments.—Relaxation of these aids in producing deformity. It is seen especially in the spine and in the larger joints, aiding in the production of knock-knee, over-extension of the knee-joints, weak ankles, and scoliosis.

Muscles.—These are poorly developed, pale, small, and lack tone. As a result, cases of well-marked rickets are very late in standing and walking, this being occasionally deferred even until early childhood. The lack of muscular power is often, indeed, so great that the diagnosis of paralysis may be made. We have repeatedly seen the mistake occur. The common condition of pot-belly (Figs. 102; 104) depends to a large extent upon weakness of the abdominal muscles, although the weakness of the gastric and intestinal walls, combined with flatulent distention, aids in its production. The abdomen is uniformly distended and tympanitic, but not tender on pressure. Commonly in marked cases there results a diastasis of the external recti of the abdomen, well shown when the child attempts to raise itself from a recumbent position, the intestines then bulging between the layers of muscle.

General Condition.—The skin is usually pale and transparent, with a tendency to enlargement of the veins, especially over the scalp and at the root of the nose. Although the patient is often apparently well-nourished, the tissues are flabby. Severe cases eventually lose in weight and general health, and become anemic with diminished power of resistance.

Digestive System.—Adenoid and tonsillar hypertrophy is common. Rachitic subjects readily develop obstinate catarrhal disturbances of the stomach and intestines, which aid in producing the tympanitic distention and the characteristic pot-belly referred to. Constipation is common, dependent upon the muscular weakness of the abdominal and intestinal walls. Often it alternates with diarrhea. The liver is not infrequently enlarged, but this may be only apparent, due to its displacement.

Respiratory System.—The mucous membranes in rickets are particularly prone to the development of diseased conditions, among them bronchitis and bronchopneumonia. Very characteristic is acceleration of respiration, without fever or other discoverable cause, and often accompanied by moving of the alae nasi and other evidences of dyspnea. The breathing in well-marked cases is largely diaphragmatic, due to the softening and yielding of the framework and the weakness of the muscles of the thorax. The deformities of the chest produce alterations in the physical signs of auscultation and percussion, which may be very misleading in the diagnosis of possible intrathoracic diseases.

Blood.—In the severe cases more or less anemia usually develops. Moderate leukocytosis may be present dependent on complications. During the active stage the inorganic phosphorus of the blood is usually below the normal (4.5 mg. per 100 cc.) but the calcium may be normal (10 to 12 mg. per 100 cc.) or only slightly diminished.

Nervous System.—Prominent among these are restlessness at night, with rocking of the head upon the pillow, and constant tossing off of the bed-clothes. The instability of the nervous system characteristic of rickets would appear to predispose to convulsive conditions of various sorts, as tetany, laryngospasm, and particularly eclampsia. These symptoms are those, however, of spasmophilia, which may be associated with rickets. While this subject will be more fully discussed later (see Spasmophilia, p. 869), it may be stated here that spasmophilic symptoms are present when the blood-calcium is low, and this is not usual in rickets uncomplicated by spasmophilic symptoms. The type of rickets which is associated with spasmophilia is that with slight bony deformity. Pain in the bones, especially evident when the infant is lifted by grasping the chest, is sometimes found. It is probably oftener dependent upon a complicating scorbutus or epiphyseal separation than upon rachitic lesions. In the category of nervous affections may be placed the profuse sweating of the head, which occurs during sleep irrespective of the weather, and which is sometimes sufficient to moisten the pillow. Fever may be present due to complications. In severe cases there may be decided mental backwardness associated with the general weakness.

Lymph-glandular System.—The external lymph-nodes are frequently enlarged. The spleen may be palpable due to its downward displacement, and is enlarged in active and severe rickets.

Fetal Rickets.—Whether this condition exists is much disputed. The diagnosis in some reported cases has rested upon the presence of craniotabes and beading of the ribs in the new-born, which are not in themselves sufficient evidence. Some, too, have been instances of osteogenesis imperfecta or of chondrodystrophy fetalis. (See pp. 1003, 999.) Wieland[64] after careful study did not believe that a single reported case was beyond criticism.

Acute Rickets.—Some cases reported under this term have been instances of scurvy, and others simply instances of severe rickets developing rapidly but differing in no essential feature from ordinary infantile rickets.

Late Rickets.—It is probable that some of the reported cases of late rickets are really instances of osteomalacia, and others belong in the category of renal rickets (p. 821) or celiac rickets (p. 1088). Schmorl,[65] Rendu and Werteimer,[66] and others maintain that true rickets may begin late in childhood, and reports by Hochstetter,[67] Bittorf,[68] Engel,[69] and others indicate that a condition resembling rickets developed after the World War in patients from fifteen to eighteen years of age. Rickets may also persist from infancy into childhood (Bloomberg[70]). In a study of 2 cases of late rickets by Stearns, Oelke and Boyd[71] the content of calcium and phosphorus of the blood and the excretion of these minerals were quite similar to those observed in infantile rickets.

Complications and Sequels.—Respiratory affections, as bronchitis and bronchopneumonia, are common, although Barenberg, Greene and Abramson[72] did not find that mild rickets predisposed to pneumonia. Pulmonary atelectasis is not infrequent in infants with severe deformities of the chest, either in the form of collapse of large areas, or occurring only in the positions corresponding to a marked rachitic rosary. The gravity of all respiratory complications is increased by the yielding character of the chest-walls and the poor expansion of the lungs. A degree of hydrocephalus is a frequent complication in cases with markedly rachitic heads, being the result of the yielding of the cranial bones, which allows fluid to accumulate in the ventricles. Such spasmophilic manifestations as general convulsions, laryngospasm, and tetany are common. Umbilical hernia is frequent, due to distention and thinning of the abdominal wall. Scurvy may be a complication. Bony deformities may remain as sequels, sometimes permanently.

Course and Prognosis.—Rickets is essentially a chronic disease. The active constitutional symptoms usually continue not longer than the termination of the first and seldom more than the end of the second year. Recovery from the bony deformities is much slower. In most cases the enlargement of the epiphyses will finally almost entirely disappear, as will the deformity of the skull. Sometimes, however, the head remains always larger than normal. Even moderate bowing of the legs and other deformities generally disappear spontaneously in a remarkable manner. Recovery is usually complete by the end of the third or fourth year. Bony healing and the disappearance of all symptoms are hastened by active treatment. In well-marked cases of the disease, especially when not well treated, permanent alterations are liable to be present throughout life, in the form of curvature of the bones of the thigh, leg, or forearm, producing bow-legs, knock-knees, and other deformities; distortions of the chest; scoliosis; flat-foot; rachitic pelvis; rachitic coxa vara; and dwarfing from arrested growth of the bones in length. It is also possible for rickets undergoing recovery to exhibit exacerbations, or even to relapse after recovery has apparently taken place; the cause being the renewal of the etiologic factors or the occurrence of some intercurrent disease. That recurrence is not uncommon is indicated by the report of Hess[73] of 31 cases personally observed.

The disease in itself is not dangerous to life, but through its numerous complications or through other intercurrent diseases it is the cause of many deaths. The contraction of the chest and the lack of resiliency in its walls are serious conditions should pneumonia or pertussis be contracted, and severe cases of rickets may die from ordinary bronchitis through the development of atelectasis. The debility and general loss of resisting power predispose to a fatal ending in cases of intestinal disease. Convulsions attending rickets may be the cause of death.

Diagnosis.—Well-developed rickets is not readily confounded with any other disease. Early in its course it is not so easily recognized. The principal early symptoms are the head-sweating and the restlessness at night. Later are evident the enlarged fontanelles, characteristic shape of the head, distended abdomen, alteration in the shape of the chest, rachitic rosary, and the various other deformities described. Roentgenograms, especially as seen in the long bones (see p. 446), are valuable aids in diagnosis. Typical roentgenographic evidence in the epiphyses does not appear as early as does the rachitic rosary, but beading of the ribs is, as stated, not diagnostic without the presence of other symptoms.

Certain other conditions occasion difficulty in diagnosis. *Hydrocephalus* may have a superficial resemblance to the rachitic head. In both the fontanelles are large and the sutures open, but in hydrocephalus the head is of a more globular shape and the sides protrude somewhat beyond the ears, while in rickets the shape is more rectangular, with areas of decided thickening of the bones, especially over the parietal and frontal eminences and about the fontanelles. The tension over the fontanelle is greater in hydrocephalus. *Craniotabes* is not positive diagnostic evidence of rickets, as it may occur in syphilis also, or independently of both of these diseases. *Delayed dentition,* although a symptom of rickets is not diagnostic. *Infantile scurvy* has often been confounded with rickets because the two are so frequently combined; and the names "scurvy-rickets" and "hemorrhagic rickets" have in the past been applied to infantile scurvy. The tenderness of the bones which sometimes seems to be a symptom of rickets is, in most cases, probably due to a certain scorbutic element, which may be quickly alleviated by the administration of orange juice. *Infantile osteomalacia* has been described, but is to be considered identical with rickets in most instances, although probably some of the cases reported belong to the category of osteogenesis imperfecta. A condition of softness of the ribs, flatness of the chest and occiput, and bow-legs has been reported by Hess,[74] in which there are no rachitic osseous changes in the roentgenogram and no response to antirachitic measures.

Osteogenesis imperfecta has often been called "fetal rickets," but is not a rachitic condition. In it there is a remarkable thinness of the flat bones, especially of the skull, with more or less deformity of the long bones. *Osteopsathyrosis,* or *fragilitas ossium,* has likewise often been confounded with rickets. It is true that in severe rickets there is a decided tendency to the occurrence of fractures, yet these are usually of the green-stick variety, due to softness of the bone. In true fragilitas ossium there is nothing of the soft character present, and neither chemically nor microscopically is there anything found resembling rickets. The two conditions are absolutely distinct, as we [75] have pointed out elsewhere.

Infantile myxedema in its early stages bears certain resemblances to rickets. In both there is a delay in dentition and in the closing of the fontanelles, and slowness in learning to walk. In cretinism, however, there is an unusual slowness of growth in length; and the peculiar physiognomy of the disease, with mental impairment and the effect of administration of thyroid extract, soon makes the diagnosis easy. *Paralytic conditions* of various sorts, with wasting of the muscles, sometimes lead to the suspicion of rickets. In all the learning to walk may be long delayed, but in none are the other symptoms of rickets present; while careful study may show the characteristic electrical reactions and other evidences of poliomyelitis, or the spastic condition of a cerebral paralysis. In *syphilis* the pseudoparalysis occurs usually in the early months of life, antedating the weakness of rickets, and the saber-tibia of later syphilitic manifestations is unaccompanied by other conditions suggesting rachitic deformities. The spinal curvature of *Pott's Disease* is short and angular in shape, in contradistinction to the long anteroposterior curve of rickets, and when well-marked does not lessen when the child is lifted by the arms.

Treatment. **Prophylaxis.**—Rickets is to a large degree preventable if proper diet is given and advantage taken of the protection afforded by ergosterol, cod liver oil, and light. Foods too low in mineral and fat should be avoided. It may be mentioned that lactose brings about a more favorable intestinal reaction for the absorption of minerals than do other sugars (Bergeim[76]). Breast-feeding should be employed when possible, since, as stated, while human milk is not rich in the antirachitic factor, severe rickets seldom develops with its use. Breast-milk can be made somewhat more antirachitic by feeding the lactating mother with milk irradiated by ultraviolet light (Scheer and Sandels[77]), or when the mother herself is irradiated (Hess, Weinstock and Sherman;[78] Gerstenberger, Hartman and Smith[79]), but the administration of cod liver oil has no effect (Hess and Weinstock;[15] Gerstenberger, Hartman and Smith;[79] Weech[80]). Cow's milk can be rendered distinctly antirachitic if the fodder is supplemented by irradiated yeast (Steenbock et al.;[81] Hess et al.[82]), and its antirachitic value is increased also by exposure of the cow to sunlight and ultraviolet rays (Steenbock et al.[83]). Fresh and dried milks which have been irradiated are definitely antirachitic (Supplee and Dow;[84] Hess;[53] Nabarro and Hickman;[85] Supplee, Dorcas and Hess[86]), as are also many other food-products such as cereals (Steenbock et al.[87]). *Cod liver oil,* tested for its vitamin D content (see p. 136), may be used, beginning at two months of age or younger with 5 or 10 drops daily, and increasing the amount gradually to 1 dram three times a day at the age of three or four months. Certain extracts made from the nonsaponifiable fraction of cod liver oil are rich in vitamin D. Egg-yolk, while less effective, may be used as a substitute, giving one-half to one uncooked yolk a day, but remembering that it may cause carotinemia. (See p. 1111.) As discussed elsewhere (pp. 136, 445), *irradiated ergosterol* (viosterol) is an effective antirachitic. It should be given in doses of eight to ten drops a day as a prophylactic, and about twice this amount to premature infants.

In regard to the prevention of rickets by prenatal measures, there is some evidence that a mitigating effect can be brought about by treatment of the mother during pregnancy with proper diet, cod liver oil and light (Hess and Weinstock;[88] Greenebaum, Selkirk, Otis and Mitchell;[89] Jundell and Magnusson;[90] Toverud and Toverud;[91] Freund and Schmidt;[92] Macciotta[93]). It must be admitted, however, that the greater influence on rickets is by postnatal measures. In excessive dose—much greater than need ever be employed in practice—it causes hypercalcemia, deposit of calcium in the tissues, and the withdrawal of it from the bones, as shown by Kreitmair and Moll,[94] and others. There is no such danger with the therapeutic doses recommended. *Light* is an efficient preventive of rickets. Heliotherapy is discussed more fully in another place (p. 204). For the prevention of rickets it is not entirely necessary to expose the whole body, and ordinarily one-half hour a day is sufficient. The short ultraviolet rays are filtered out by window-glass; and, to a less extent, by clothing, especially if this is dark in color, as also by moisture and smoke. The ultraviolet content of the sun's rays in January is 20 times less than in July (Luckiesh, Matthew and Pacini[95]), and whenever the sun reaches an altitude of 35 deg. above the horizon marked increase of its antirachitic effect occurs (Tisdall and Brown[40]). The ultraviolet content of skyshine is quite effective, and exposure to it may be carried out when direct sunlight is not available or when the latter is too hot (Tisdall and Brown[96]). A substitute for sunlight is radiation with a mercury-vapor quartz-lamp, as first used by Huldschinsky.[97] (For the technic see Heliotherapy, p. 204.) In our[98] own studies we found that as little as twelve minutes exposure a month to a good lamp would prevent rickets in colored infants. The carbon-arc lamp may also be used, longer exposures being necessary, depending upon the spectrum of the lamp. The tungsten-filament light is antirachitic if employed for a number of hours a day (Gerstenberger and Horesh[99]).

The relative efficiency of cod liver oil, ergosterol, and light has been disputed, some of the differences of opinion being due to the different dosages of the various agents used; to different criteria adopted for proof of prevention and cure; and to the fact that the effect on animals cannot be considered the same as that produced on man. All of these agents are effectively antirachitic if properly employed, and at least one of them should be used routinely for all infants. While they will obviate to a large extent the consequences of a defective diet, they do not do away with the need of proper food or of fresh air and exercise. The special predisposition of *premature infants* to develop rickets is to be noted.

Treatment of the Attack.—All that has been stated in regard to diet, cod liver oil, ergosterol, and radiation applies equally well to the treatment of the developed disease. Cod liver oil should be given in doses of at least 1 teaspoonful (3.9) three times a day, and, in severe cases, viosterol in doses of 15 to 20 drops a day. Contrary to the general opinion cod liver oil can usually be given in hot weather. Probably both these measures should be employed and, in addition, treatment by ultraviolet radiation in the same amount as for prevention. In a few weeks there will often be great improvement or cure, as shown by clinical, roentgenological, and serological observations. When cure is established treatment should be continued to prevent relapse. In late rickets the treatment should be intensive. *Medicinal* therapy other than that mentioned is of little value. There is seldom need to administer calcium, since its intake from milk and other foods is sufficient. In this connection Table 64 may be consulted. Phosphorus in doses of $\frac{1}{300}$ or $\frac{1}{200}$ grain (0.0002 to 0.0003) once a day has been recommended by Kassowitz;[100] Phemister, Miller and Bonar,[101] and, especially when combined with cod liver oil, by Schabad,[102] Compere,[103] and Weese.[104] Hess,[53] however, confirmed the observations made by Monti and others many years ago, that phosphorus by itself had no effect on rickets. The possibility of its toxic action should not be forgotten. Anemia when decided does not respond to antirachitic measures alone (Baumann;[106] Small[107]), and iron, arsenic and copper may be needed. Among preparations used for the treatment of rickets, the value of which has not been established, are thymus gland (Mettenheimer[108]), thyroid gland (Heubner[109] and others), suprarenal gland (Stöltzner[110]), and bone-marrow (Amistani[111]). *Hygienic treatment* is important, particularly life in the open air, massage, and change of climate, when indicated. All other *diseased conditions*, especially digestive disturbances, must be remedied as far as possible.

The development of *deformities* must be carefully guarded against. Rachitic children should be discouraged from walking until the bones have become firm. The wearing of too thick a diaper predisposes to the development of bow-legs. Carrying the infant always on the one arm is very likely to produce scoliosis. Sitting cross-legged may occasion rotation of the femora, indentation of the tibiae, and curvature of the forearms from pressure of the hands against the bed or floor (Fig. 104). Irregular distortion of the head is to be avoided by altering the position in which the child lies. The treatment of deformities already acquired is considered fully in text-books upon orthopedic surgery. Here only may be mentioned the value of massage in strengthening the feeble muscles; the importance of favoring free movement of the limbs by the patient through creeping and any other form of exercise, properly regulated, which does not directly increase deformity; and the correction of deformities by postural treatment and the like, such as lying upon one side with a pillow under it; lying upon the abdomen; the gentle bending of curved extremities by the nurse; etc., according to the nature of the deformity present. Such measures, combined with general treatment, are often completely efficacious without operative or special orthopedic procedures. By the age of three years, however, and often decidedly before this, the ossification of the bones has become too complete to permit of benefit being obtained in this way.

TABLE 64.—CALCIUM-CONTENT AND PHOSPHORUS-CONTENT OF COMMON FOOD-MATERIALS[105]

Animal foods, cereals, etc.	Per cent.		Vegetables.	Per cent.		Fruits.	Per cent.	
	Cal.	Phos.		Cal.	Phos.		Cal.	Phos.
Meats	0.054	1.004	Beans, pea, dried	0.154	0.270	Apples	0.008	0.011
Fish	0.128	1.222	Beans, string, fresh	0.053	0.040	Apricots	0.015	0.025
Eggs	0.071	0.160	Beets	0.014	0.041	Bananas	0.006	0.027
Butter	0.016	0.014	Cabbage	0.041	0.035	Blackberries	0.056	0.036
Butterine	0.016	0.014	Carrots	0.055	0.041	Blueberries	0.032	0.020
Buttermilk	0.123	0.095	Celery	0.067	0.044	Grapes	0.010	0.028
Milk, whole	0.123	0.095	Greens; turnip-tops	0.363	0.043	Oranges	0.031	0.021
Cream	0.105	0.081	Lettuce	0.032	0.032	Peaches	0.011	0.021
Barley, pearl	0.018	0.201	Potatoes	0.011	0.063	Pears	0.013	0.018
Cornmeal	0.006	0.200	Rhubarb	0.043	0.045	Prunes	0.045	0.089
Hominy	0.010	0.309	Spinach	0.046	0.045	Raisins	0.030	0.105
Oatmeal	0.056	0.425	Tomatoes	0.014	0.020	Raspberries	0.051	0.041
Rice	0.009	0.086				Strawberries	0.041	0.030
Wheat flour	0.020	0.094						
Crackers and macaroni	0.020	0.094						
Graham flour	0.026	0.290						
Bread	0.015	0.071						
Maple-syrup	0.088	0.044						
Honey	0.004	0.028						

REFERENCES

1. Hygiea, 1923, **84,** 530. 2. Glasgow M. J., 1919, **91,** 147. 3. Tractatus de rachitide, etc., London, 1650; Ref. Gerhardt's Handb. d. Kinderkr., **3,** 1, 43. 4. Am. J. Dis. Child., 1927, **34,** 443. 5. Medicine, 1923, **2,** 349. 6. Physiol. Rev., 1923, **3,** 106. 7. Rickets, Osteomalacia and Tetany, 1929; Am. J. Dis. Child., 1931, **41,** 1081; 1309; J.A.M.A., 1930, **94,** 1885; 1931, **97,** 370; J. Biol. Chem., 1930, **87,** 37; 1931, **91,** 733; Science 1928, **67,** 333. 8. Am. J. Dis. Child., 1928, **36,** 310. 9. J.A.M.A., 1925, **85,** 656. 10. Arch. Int. Med., 1928, **2,** 281. 11. Am. J. Dis. Child., 1928, **35,** 590. 12. Arch. de méd. d. enf., 1929, **32,** 262. 13. Jahrb. f. Kinderh., 1904, **59,** 237. 14. Nouv. iconog. de la Saltpetrière, 1901, **14,** 299. 15. J.A.M.A., 1924, **83,** 1558. 16. Greenebaum, Selkirk, Mitchell and Bier, Ohio State M. J., 1929, **25,** 34. 17. Paris méd., 1923, **13,** 406. 18. Am. J. Dis. Child., 1927, **34,** 805. 19. Arch. f. Kinderh., 1910, **53,** 380; **54,** 83. 20. Monatschr. f. Kinderh., Orig., 1914, **13,** 271. 21. Am. J. Dis. Child., 1924, **28,** 574. 22. Am. J. Dis. Child., 1929, **37,** 296. 23. Ztschr. f. d. ges. exper. Med., 1930, **73,** 343. 24. Jahrb. f. Kinderh., 1899, **50,** 268. 25. Ztschr. f. Biol., 1890, **27,** 517. 26. Ztschr. f. Kinderh., 1928, **46,** 575. 27. Proc. Soc. Exper. Biol. and Med., 1929, **27,** 140; J. Biol. Chem., 1930, **77,** 37; J.A.M.A., 1930, **94,** 1885. 28. J. Biol. Chem., 1928, **76,** 633. 29. Am. J. Dis. Child., 1923, **26,** 303. 30. Arch. Dis. Childhood, 1930, **5,** 28. 31. Jahrb. f. Kinderh., 1909, **69,** 450. 32. Quart. J. Med., 1922, **16,** 63. 33. Proc. Soc. Exper. Biol. and Med., 1923, **21,** 199. 34. Proc. Soc. Exper. Biol. and Med., 1923, **21,** 186. 35. J.A.M.A., 1924, **83,** 1473. 36. Proc. Soc. Exper. Biol. and Med., 1926, **20,** 1350. 37. Proc. Soc. Exper. Biol. and Med., 1927, **24,** 668. 38. Am. J. Dis. Child., 1923, **26,** 486. 39. J. Biol. Chem., 1924, **60,** 311. 40. Am. J. Dis. Child., 1931, **42,** 1144. 41. Bull. Johns Hopkins Hosp., 1927, **41,** 432. 42. Am. J. Dis. Child., 1931, **41,** 775. 43. J. Trop. Med., 1907, **10,** 67. 44. Lancet, 1922, **2,** 367. 45. Am. J. Dis. Child., 1927, **34,**

955. 46. J.A.M.A., 1928, **90**, 161. 47. Biochem. J., 1931, **25**, 57. 48. J.A.M.A., 1928, **90**, 1310. 49. J. Biol. Chem., 1925, **63**, 305. 50. J. Biol. Chem., 1925, **64**, 263. 51. Lancet, 1925, **1**, 1025. 52. Klin. Wchnschr., 1927, **6**, 666. 53. J.A.M.A., 1927, **89**, 337. 54. Science, 1931, **74**, 579. 55. München. med. Wchnschr., 1921, **68**, 1481. 56. München. med. Wchnschr., 1921, **68**, 1482. 57. Brit. M. J., 1921, **2**, 1067. 58. Hygiea, 1921, **83**, 733. 59. Deutsche med. Wchnschr., 1923, **49**, 85. 60. Jahrb. f. Kinderh., 1922, **99**, 133. 61. J. Med. Research, 1921, **42**, 391. 62. Am. J. Physiol., 1928, **85**, 299. 63. Norsk. Mag. f. Laegevidensk., 1929, **90**, 729. 64. Jahrb. f. Kinderh., 1908, **67**, 675; 1916, **84**, 360; Ergebn. d. inn. Med. u. Kinderh., 1910, **6**, 64. 65. Deutsch. Arch. f. klin. Med., 1905, **85**, 170. 66. Rev. d'orthop., 1921, **28**, 215. 67. München. med. Wchnschr., 1919, **66**, 776. 68. Berl. klin. Wchnschr., 1919, **56**, 652. 69. Berl. klin. Wchnschr., 1920, **57**, 35. 70. Am. J. Dis. Child., 1927, **34**, 624. 71. Am. J. Dis. Child., 1931, **42**, 88. 72. J.A.M.A., 1929, **92**, 440. 73. Am. J. Dis. Child., 1926, **31**, 380. 74. Am. J. Dis. Child., 1931, **41**, 1081; 1309. 75. Griffith, Am. J. M. Sc., 1897, **113**, 426. 76. J. Biol. Chem., 1926, **70**, 35. 77. München. med. Wchnschr., 1930, 77, 1543. 78. J.A.M.A., 1927, **88**, 24. 79. California and West. Med., 1927, **27**, 40. 80. Bull. Johns Hopkins Hosp., 1927, **40**, 224. 81. J. Biol. Chem., 1930, **88**, 197. 82. J.A.M.A., 1931, **97**, 370. 83. J. Biol. Chem., 1930, **87**, 103. 84. J. Biol. Chem., 1927, **73**, 617. 85. Lancet, 1930, **1**, 127. 86. J. Biol. Chem., 1932, **94**, 749. 87. J.A.M.A., 1929, **93**, 1868. 88. J.A.M.A., 1924, **83**, 1558; Am. J. Dis. Child., 1928, **36**, 966. 89. J.A.M.A., 1926, **87**, 1973. 90. Acta paediat., 1929, **9**, 81. 91. Norsk. Mag. f. Laegevidensk., 1929, **90**, 1245; 1930, **91**, 53. 92. Monatschr. f. Kinderh., 1929, **43**, 424. 93. Clin. Pediat., 1930, **12**, 923. 94. München. med. Wchnschr., 1928, **75**, 637. 95. Light and Health, 1926; Ref. Sheard, J.A.M.A., 1927, **88**, 1315. 96. Am. J. Dis. Child., 1927, **34**, 737. 97. Deutsche med. Wchnschr., 1919, **45**, 712. 98. Selkirk, Greenebaum and Mitchell, J.A.M.A., 1928, **91**, 2057. 99. J.A.M.A., 1931, **97**, 766. 100. Wien. med. Blät. 1883, **6**, 1492. 101. J.A.M.A., 1921, **76**, 850. 102. Ztschr. f. klin. Med., 1909, **68**, 94; 1910, **69**, 435. 103. Am. J. Dis. Child., 1930, **40**, 941. 104. Arch. f. exper. Path. u. Pharmakol., 1928, **135**, 111. 105. Bull. No. 27, U. S. Dept. Agric. 106. Monatschr. f. Kinderh., 1928, **39**, 193. 107. New England J. Med., 1929, **200**, 484. 108. Jahrb. f. Kinderh., 1898, **46**, 55. 109. Berl. klin. Wchnschr., 1896, **33**, 700. 110. Path. u. Ther. d. Rachitis, 1904. 111. Pediatria, 1903, **2**, 560.

CHAPTER II

SCORBUTUS

(Infantile Scurvy)

This disease as seen in early life does not differ materially from that long known to occur among sailors and others deprived of suitable food. In infancy it was first described by Möller,[1] but considered by him to be "acute rickets." Barlow[2] in 1883 recognized its true nature, and the disease has often been called after his name.

Etiology.—*Age* is an important factor, the majority of cases occurring in the latter half of the first year and nearly all the remainder before the end of the second year. The disease has been observed in infants as young as three weeks of age (Collect. Investig. Committee;[3] Hill[4]) and may occur even in later childhood (Owen,[5] Miller,[6] Tobler,[7] Weill and Dufourt,[8] Chick and Dalyell[9]). Geographical distribution has no real influence, except in so far as in certain localities there may occur an absence of vitamin C in the diet. The same is true of hygienic conditions. War and famine increase the incidence. For example, 168 cases in children were reported from Leningrad by Schäfgan[10] for the years 1922, 1923 and 1924. The active factor is the employment of an *unsuitable diet* over considerable periods. The unsuitability of the diet appears, however, to vary with the infant, and although the disease may develop on a variety of foods, yet it is beyond doubt that the condition is a deficiency disorder depending upon a lack of the antiscorbutic vitamin C. It is known that prolonged heating of milk destroys to a certain extent this vitamin, and that many of the proprietary infant foods are also important etiologic factors. Yet one infant may have a diet of either of these classes and suffer not at all, while another promptly develops the disease. There is usually, too, a period of latency of weeks or months after the infant is deprived of vitamin C before the symptoms of scurvy appear, and this time is very variable. All these matters point strongly to the existence of an *individual predisposition.* An illustration of this is the fact that the disease may occur in one of twins on the same diet (Brachi and Carr,[11] Wallgren[12]). This would appear to indicate not that vitamin C is not a necessity, but that some infants can do with less of it than can others, and that a diet dangerously deficient in vitamin C for one infant may be satisfactory for another. (See also Vitamins, p. 135.)

Pathologic Anatomy.—There is a replacement of the bone-marrow by an embryonic connective tissue, and an arrest in the formation of bone from the osteoblasts, but not the production of osteoid tissue devoid of lime-salts such as occurs in rickets (Schmorl[13]). In the experimental animal there is little diminution in the amount of calcium and phosphorus in the bones (Brouwer,[14] Salter and Aub[15]). There is said to be calcium-retention in the early stage and calcium-excretion during healing (Lust and Klocman,[16] Frank[17]), but Humphreys and Zilva[18] found no disturbance of calcium-metabolism in experimental animals until the final stage, and considered these changes secondary. Separation of the epiphyses may occur in severe cases as a result of slight trauma. The most characteristic lesion consists in the occurrence of hemorrhage beneath the periosteum, oftenest in the bones of the lower extremities. Hemorrhage may take place, too, in various other tissues of the body such as the muscles, skin, serous or mucous membranes, kidneys, and the internal organs, including the brain. The commonest seat of the hemorrhage after that of the periosteum is in the mucous membrane of the gums, especially about the upper incisor teeth. There may be a local edema in the neighborhood of hemorrhages or elsewhere. The cause of the hemorrhage is not clear. Findlay,[19] Hess,[20] Wolbach and Howe,[21] Nowodworski,[22] and others believe it depends upon weakness of the blood-vessel walls, due to degenerative cellular changes. Barlow[2] reported the existence of enlargement of Peyer's patches, and we have seen this at necropsy. There are changes in the formation of the teeth, consisting of a fibrosis (Zilva and Wells;[23] Hess[24]). Degenerative changes may occur in the central nervous system (Hess[25]).

Symptoms.—The first definite manifestation in most cases is *pain in the limbs,* although anemia, anorexia, and irritability may precede this. It is almost always in the lower extremities, either alone or combined with pain elsewhere. It may develop so suddenly that it is attributed by the parents to an accident, but in other cases the onset is slower. Soon the pain becomes constant and the tenderness intense. Even approach to the bedside may cause the infant to scream through fear of being touched. In the majority of cases there is suffering only when the limbs are moved. Usually there is *pseudoparalysis* depending upon the pain, and this may be the first symptom noticed. With the pain in the limbs often appears *affection of the gums,* this sometimes being the first observed symptom. It is present in the large majority of cases and consists, when well developed, of a deep bluish-purple, spongy swelling of the mucous membrane, generally over the upper incisor teeth (Fig. 106). Slight hemorrhage from the gums or from the palate or pharynx takes place readily, and ulceration is not infrequent. As a rule involvement of the gums occurs only in infants whose incisor teeth have erupted, but this is merely because the disease is seen so much oftener in those past the age of the first appearance of teeth. Often at this time *swell-*

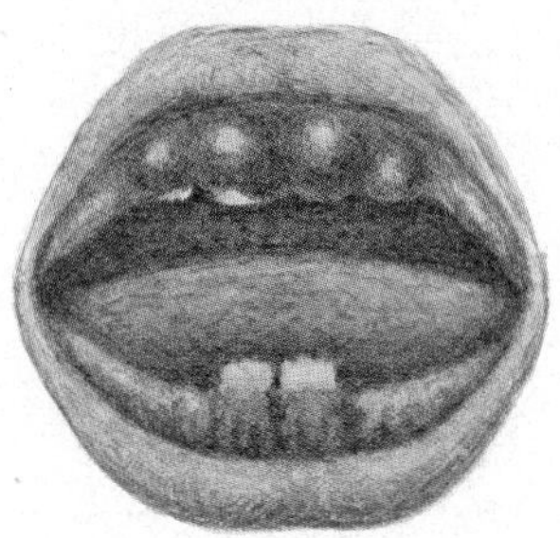

Fig. 106.—Infantile scurvy. Infant of eight months. Well-nourished. Fed upon Horick's malted milk. Fretful, nervous, pain in the legs. Had been suffering for three weeks. Recovered in three days. Illustration shows the swollen, purple gums about the upper incisors, and the purple streaks in the gums of the lower jaw.

ing along the shaft of the long bones can be found, usually near the ankle or the knee but not involving the joint. The swelling may be bilateral, with the skin over it shining and swollen, but not unusually reddened (Fig. 107).

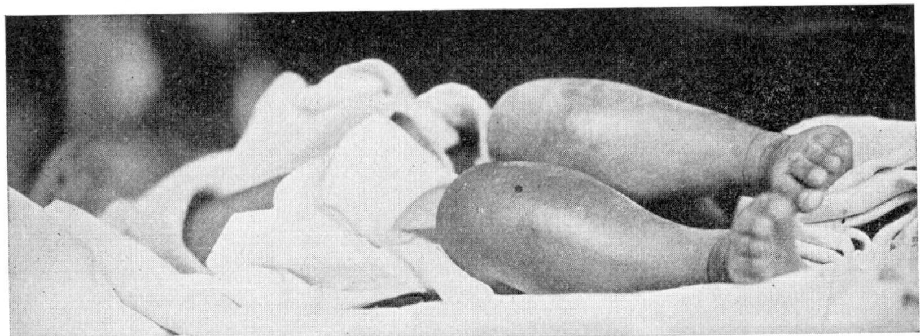

Fig. 107.—Infantile scurvy. Showing swelling of legs. Infant of one and one-half months. Hospital of the University of Pennsylvania. Been fed on a proprietary food. Pain and swelling in both legs about the knees.

It may be slight or extensive, increasing greatly the size of the limb; in severe cases the whole of the affected limb may be edematous. Quite often hemorrhages in the form of ecchymoses or petechiae are seen in various regions of the cutaneous or mucous surfaces. They are often among the earliest evidences of the disease. Orbital hemorrhage producing exophthalmos is not common (Fig. 108). Blood may be vomited or passed by bowel, or there may be hematuria. We[26] have known it to be the only positively characteristic symptom in otherwise doubtful cases.

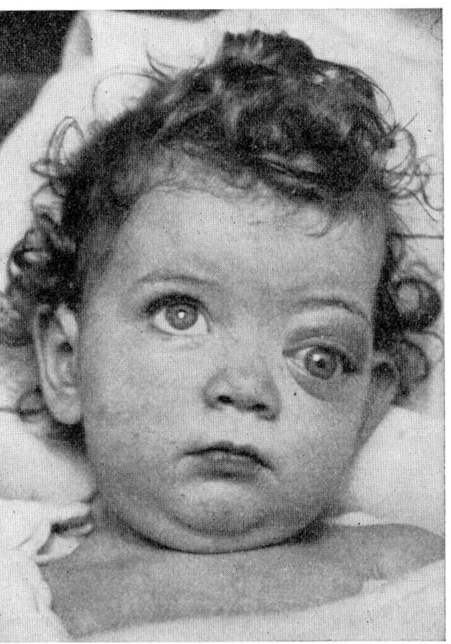

Fig. 108.—Exophthalmos in infantile scurvy. Age fourteen months. Hospital of University of Penna. Severe pain and tenderness in left leg for two months; in right arm for three weeks; left eye-ball bulging outward and downward for ten days. Gums purple.

In the meantime the *general condition* of the child suffers. In severe cases there occur wasting or actual cachexia, mild fever, weak pulse, and anorexia. The blood has been studied by Hess and Fish,[27] Brandt,[28] Bedson,[29] Nowodworski,[22] Carbonara,[30] and others. Anemia, little marked at first, becomes decided as the disease advances, with especial reduction of the hemoglobin and a moderate and inconstant leukocytosis. There may be changes in the size and shape and staining of the red cells; normoblasts may be present; the lymphocytes are often increased; there is diminished viscosity; the coagulation-time is increased; fragility of the red cells is increased; platelets may be normal, decreased, or increased in number; the calcium may be somewhat diminished. Not all observers find the same changes, and they depend in degree upon the stage of the disease. Beading of the ribs is not infrequent, and, according to Hess and Unger,[31] does not always depend upon a complicating rachitis. Certain nervous symptoms, such as paresthesia, anesthesia and the like, occur less commonly than in adult scurvy (Hess[24]).

In some cases the classical symptoms are slow in appearing, but there are such manifestations as failure to gain weight, anorexia, irritability, and perhaps the appearance of punctate hemorrhages in the skin and mucous membrane. To such a condition, apparently due to deficiency of vitamin C, Hess[32] applies the term "subacute or latent scurvy," and Nassau and Singer[33] the title "incipient scurvy." The latter found that in many children these minor symptoms, as described, existed for weeks or months before the ordinary evidences of the disease developed.

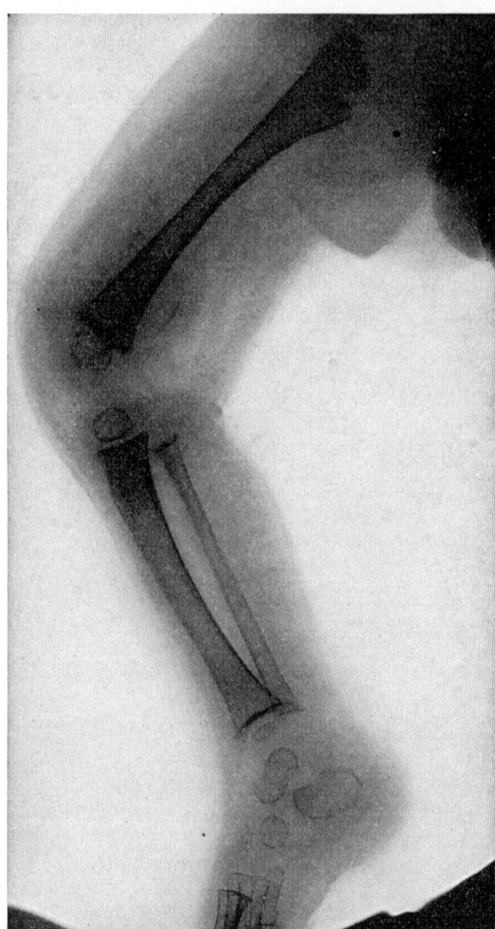

Fig. 109.—Infantile scurvy. White line. Subacute case in an infant admitted to the Children's Hospital of Philadelphia, aged ten months. Knees swollen; tibiae tender on pressure; moves the legs very little; gums swollen and mottled. Note the "white line," (in the negative; naturally black in the print).

Complications.—Rickets may often be associated, since a child suffering from lack of vitamin C is liable to have deficiency in other accessory food factors as well. Yet the two diseases are entirely distinct. In 45 per cent of 340 cases of the American Pediatric Society's Collective Investigation[3] the reporting physicians distinctly stated that rickets was not present, and allowing for possible errors, there would still be enough cases to show the independence of the two disorders. In addition to the hemorrhages already mentioned, bronchopneumonia or severe gastroenteric disturbances are occasionally seen.

Course and Prognosis.—Recovery occurs rapidly in cases correctly treated. Pain ceases in a week or less, and the swelling in the bones and the constitutional symptoms disappear within a few weeks. Subperiosteal hemorrhage, if extensive, may require months to disappear completely. Usually growth is quickly resumed. In unrecognized and untreated cases death is liable to occur after a few months from malnutrition, exhaustion, or some complication or intercurrent disease. When there has been decided involvement of the epiphysis, or displacement of it, shortening of the limb may result.

The **diagnosis** rests upon the symptoms as described. In general it is safe to assume that pain in the limbs or pseudoparalysis developing rapidly in an infant between four months and two years of age is due to scurvy, unless other cause can be found. The type of food which has been taken may be helpful in the diagnosis. The "white line" (black in the positive print) described by Fränkel,[34] which can be seen in roentgenograms at the junction of the epiphyses and diaphyses of the long bones, is a reliable diagnostic sign (Fig. 109). Wimberger[35] described a circular shadow surrounding the centers of ossification in the epiphyses of the long bones, and Pelkan[36] refers to a "ground glass" appearance of the shaft of the bones and a broadening of the epiphyseal line, as well as the circular shadow described by Wimberger; these being apparent before the onset of clinical symptoms. There are also described lateral spurs at the diaphyses. Further careful studies on the roentgenological diagnosis of scurvy are those by Schwartz,[37] Bromer,[38] and McLean and McIntosh.[39] The capillary resistance test (petechiae appearing after application of a tourniquet) may be positive, but is not diagnostic (Dalldorf,[40] Hess[24]).

The diagnosis of *rheumatism* is one oftenest falsely made. This disease is exceedingly rare in infancy; affects the joint and not the bone; there is no involvement of the gums; and the employment of antiscorbutic treatment is inefficacious. The pseudoparalysis of *syphilis* may suggest scurvy. It occurs, however, usually at an earlier age; produces less tenderness; is oftener limited to the arms; is situated at the epiphyses and not in the shaft of the bone; and is associated with other symptoms of syphilis. *Poliomyelitis* causes a true flaccid paralysis with alteration of reflexes, and the exquisite tenderness found in the limbs in scurvy is absent. *Osteomyelitis* invades the joints, if it does not begin there, and is attended by fever and septic symptoms. The frequent presence of *rickets* as a coincident disorder sometimes leads to failure to diagnose scurvy. The painful immobility of the limbs in scurvy may suggest *hip-joint disease* or *disease of the spine*, or the swelling may be mistaken for *malignant growth of the bone.*

Treatment. **Prophylaxis.**—This consists in the administration of a proper diet, containing substances rich in vitamin C. All infants, even breast-fed ones, should receive orange-juice or tomato-juice from the age of about one month. If this is done, a radical change in a diet which is otherwise satisfactory is not so imperative; yet, other things being equal, is certainly advisable. Dried orange-juice is also effective. Smith and King[41] have obtained the active fraction from lemon juice. Even raw milk may not contain a sufficient amount of vitamin C. The giving of pasteurized or boiled milk should not be avoided on account of a diminished content of vitamin C, since its advantages in other respects may outweigh this deficiency, which can be readily supplied by the juices mentioned. Some canned foods are deficient in this factor; others contain it. Treatment of milk by ultra-violet light destroys the antiscorbutic vitamin (Reyher[42]).

Treatment of the Attack.—The administration of 2 or 3 oz. or more of orange-juice or tomato-juice daily will quickly result in cure of the active symptoms. Diarrhea, if present, does not contraindicate the use of these substances, as it may even be controlled by them. Canned tomato juice is equally effective with the freshly cooked. Many other substances contain vitamin C (p. 135), but the two mentioned are the richest in this factor. Fever often develops during the first two or three days of the administration of vitamin C, perhaps due to the rapid absorption of blood from the hemorrhagic areas. We have frequently noted, too, at this time a rapid deposit of calcium in the subperiosteal hemorrhage, as seen in the roentgenogram.

References

1. Königsberger med. Jahrb., 1856–7, **1,** 377; 1862, **3,** 135. 2. Med.-Chir. Tr., 1883, **66,** 159. 3. Tr. Am. Pediat. Soc., 1898, **10,** 5. 4. Arch. Pediat., 1932, **49,** 251. 5. Brit. M. J., 1899, **2,** 1719. 6. Tr. Am. Pediat. Soc., 1924, **36,** 43. 7. Ztschr. f. Kinderh., Orig., 1918, **18,** 63. 8. Arch. de méd. d. enf., 1919, **22,** 561. 9. Ztschr. f. Kinderh.,

Orig., 1920, **26**, 257. 10. Jahrb. f. Kinderh., 1924, **104**, 225. 11. Lancet, 1911, **1**, 662. 12. Acta paediat., 1923, **2**, 37. 13. Beitr. z. path. Anat. u. z. allg. Path., 1901, **30**, 232. 14. Biochem. Ztschr., 1927, **190**, 402. 15. Arch. Path., 1931, **11**, 380. 16. Jahrb. f. Kinderh., 1912, **75**, 663. 17. Jahrb. f. Kinderh., 1920, **91**, 21. 18. Biochem. J., 1931, **25**, 579. 19. J. Path. and Bact., 1921, **24**, 446. 20. J.A.M.A., 1921, **76**, 693. 21. Arch. Path. and Lab. Med., 1926, **1**, 1. 22. Ztschr. f. d. ges. exper. Med., 1927, **58**, 424. 23. Proc. Roy. Soc., London, Ser. B., 1919, **90**, 505. 24. J.A.M.A., 1932, **98**, 1429. 25. J. Infect. Dis., 1918, **23**, 438. 26. Griffith, Phila. M. J., 1901, **7**, 213. 27. Am. J. Dis. Child., 1914, **8**, 386. 28. Arch. f. Kinderh., 1919, **67**, 395. 29. Brit. M. J., 1921, **2**, 1992. 30. Clin. pediat., 1928, **10**, 98; Ref. J.A.M.A., 1928, **90**, 1833. 31. Am. J. Dis. Child., 1920, **19**, 331. 32. J.A.M.A., 1917, **68**, 235. 33. Jahrb. f. Kinderh., 1922, **98**, 44. 34. Fortschr. a. d. Geb. d. Röntgenstrahlen, 1906, **10**, 1. 35. Ztschr. f. Kinderh., 1923, **36**, 279. 36. Am. J. Dis. Child., 1925, **30**, 174. 37. Am. J. Dis. Child., 1927, **34**, 765. 38. Am. J. Roentgenol., 1928, **19**, 112. 39. Am. J. Dis. Child., 1928, **36**, 875. 40. J. Exper. Med., 1931, **53**, 289. 41. J. Biol. Chem., 1931, **94**, 491. 42. Klin. Wchnschr., 1926, **5**, 2341.

CHAPTER III

INFANTILE ATROPHY

(Marasmus, Athrepsia)

THE title "infantile atrophy" was probably first employed by Soranio in the sixteenth century (Albarel[1]), the term "athrepsia" was applied to the disease by Parrot,[2] and the title "decomposition" is used by Finkelstein (p. 552) to cover largely the same condition. Infantile atrophy is a symptom rather than a disease; and when a definite cause is discovered, such as starvation, syphilis, tuberculosis, or a disorder of the gastroenteric tract, it is a *secondary atrophy*. Many cases, however, have no evident cause and should then be termed *primary atrophy*.

Etiology.—The disorder is seen chiefly in infants under one year of age living under bad hygienic conditions and fed artificially. It was formerly the cause of many deaths in asylums for infants, where the term "hospitalism" was often well applied. Gastroenteric affections and parenteral infections frequently precede it. Further causes which seem to be operative are constitutional debility (p. 235) and prematurity (p. 210).

Many theories have been advanced to explain it. Baginsky[3] assumed there was an anatomical basis with destructive change in Lieberkühn's follicles, Bloch[4] that this change was especially in Paneth's cells, and Marfan[5] that the factor was the lack of the specific enzymes of breast-milk acting on infants with feeble digestive power. Bessau and Bossert[6] observed an abnormal proliferation of bacteria in the upper intestinal tract, which would interfere with normal digestion, and Marriott[7] maintains a somewhat similar view, according to which there is insufficient gastric hydrochloric acid to permit of cow's milk, with its high buffer content, reaching an optimum hydrogen-ion concentration in the stomach. Because of this, bacterial growth is not inhibited, rennin action is incomplete, and the chyme is not acid enough to initiate properly the hormone-stimulation of the various enzymes. It has also been maintained that the glands of internal secretion are involved, and diminution of the size of the thymus gland, for instance, has been pointed out by Mettenheimer,[8] and by Stokes, Rührah and Royal.[9] Anderson and Schloss[10] believe that it is not impossible that absorption of foreign protein in the gastro-intestinal tract may play a rôle. Some observers have held that lack of vitamin B is a responsible factor.

In reviewing the theories mentioned it is to be observed that anatomical lesions in the intestinal tract or in the glands of internal secretion, which are other than secondary in nature, have not been found by most observers; that the majority of infants are fed successfully with artificial mixtures the basis of which is cow's milk; and that lack of vitamin B, or allergy to cow's milk, can explain only a small proportion of the cases of atrophy.

The view that primary atrophy is a defect of the physiological processes of the organism, as the result of which the infant cannot utilize the food given, is not well supported by recent evidence. Metabolism studies by Fleming;[11] Fleming and Hutchinson;[12] Parsons;[13] Tisdall, Drake and Brown;[14] Levine, Wilson and Gottschall;[15] Wang, Frank and Kaucher;[16] MacLean and Sullivan;[17] and Wilson, Levine and Kelly[18] have shown that the character of the fundamental metabolism apparently remains normal in infantile atrophy; that the production of heat per kilogram of active protoplasmic tissue appears to be essentially the same as in health; that the actual caloric utilization of food is not disturbed; and that the metabolism and absorption of carbohydrate and fat are normal. That is to say, there is no evidence that there is an abnormal energy-metabolism in the usual case of infantile atrophy.

Certain alterations in the chemical and physical processes of the body are found. Among these are low concentration of protein in the blood;

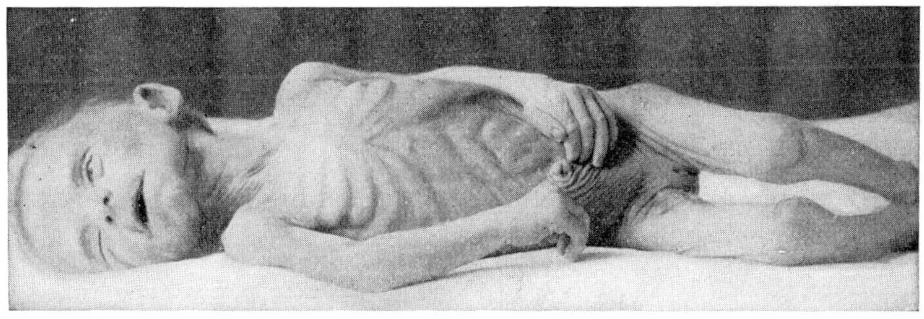

Fig. 110.—Infantile atrophy. Terminal stage. From a patient, aged seven weeks, in the Children's Hospital of Philadelphia. Had been boarded out since birth. Temperature 95 to 98 F. (35 to 36.7 C.). Two to three soft stools daily. Death.

diminution in erythrocytes and hemoglobin; diminution in blood-volume; a low rate of blood-flow; and diminished oxidizing power of the tissues (Marriott,[7] Utheim[19]). There may be a lowering of the alkali reserve but no change in the hydrogen-ion concentration of the blood. All of these alterations are end results rather than primary etiologic factors.

It may be said, then, that infantile atrophy belongs in the category of idiopathic conditions, since there is no evidence that any anatomical or metabolic disturbance has yet been discovered which accounts for the symptoms. It seems to be chiefly the result of chronic inanition, often brought about by underfeeding, defective hygiene, and apparently in some cases by repeated parenteral infections.

Pathologic Anatomy.—Any lesions found must be regarded only as secondary, or as the result of complications. This applies to fatty changes in the liver, bronchopneumonia, atelectasis, atrophy of mucous membrane of the intestine, and involution of the glands of internal secretion. The lymphatic glands are sometimes enlarged. The pathologic picture is that of starvation.

Symptoms.—The essential symptom is progressive loss of weight. The emaciation finally becomes excessive, the face wrinkling all over with each feeble cry, giving the infant the expression of a withered old man (Fig. 110). The fontanelle is depressed and usually small; the bones of the cranium overlap; the chin and cheek-bones are prominent and the eyes large and sunken; the skin of the body is pale and hangs in loose, wrinkled folds. The arms and legs seem to consist of bones with only a thin layer of skin over them; the hands are like claws and they and the feet cold and cyanosed. The outlines of the collar-bones and the ribs suggest a washing-board. The abdomen is sometimes very prominent; sometimes sunken with the thin skin over it showing dilated veins and revealing the outlines of the intestines beneath. The temperature is usually subnormal (Fig. 111), the respiration superficial, the circulation poor, and more or less anemia is present. Toward the end of life edema may occur especially of the face and extremities but sometimes of the whole surface. (See p. 467.) At this period a gain in weight may give false encouragement. It is, however, a bad symptom, due to the deposit of liquid in the tissues. The appetite is usually diminished, sometimes voracious. The stools are often regular and well-digested, oftener contain mucus and undigested food. Yet no matter how normal the stools, the loss of weight continues. Vomiting occurs easily. Albuminuria is absent. The infant is at first fretful and cries often; later apathetic and lying with little movement. The muscles are usually flabby and relaxed, but in some cases a condition of hypertonia is observed, producing arching of the back, retraction of the head, and flexion of the thighs upon the abdomen. (See p. 872.) The whole aspect is one of the most shocking in the realm of pediatrics. The infant appears to be merely a skeleton with a thin covering of skin.

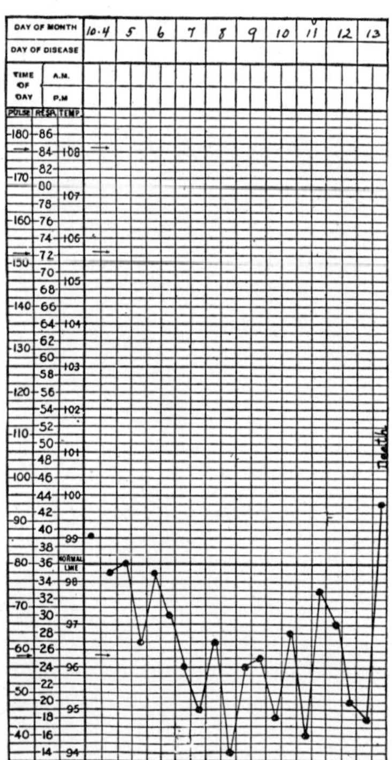

Fig. 111.—Infantile atrophy, with hypothermia and terminal increase of temperature. Infant of three months, University of Pennsylvania Hospital. Emaciation, much crying, no vomiting or diarrhea while in Hospital. Death. Necropsy findings negative.

Complications.—Infantile atrophy is often complicated by the development of furunculosis and other cutaneous abscesses; erythema, chiefly of the nates, scrotum, and back of the thighs; hernia; and thrush. Petechiae, especially on the abdomen, often develop shortly before death. (See p. 252, Fig. 1038.) Bronchopneumonia, atelectasis, and gastrointestinal derangements are frequent. Convulsions may terminate the scene.

Prognosis.—This is always grave, the majority of well-established cases ending fatally from progressive wasting, from complications, or unexpectedly, and sometimes suddenly, from causes not ascertainable. Anything which causes loss of water from the tissues, such as excessive evaporation during hot weather, or vomiting or diarrhea, is especially liable to precipitate the termination. Apart from this, there is a tendency for the disease to grow steadily worse. In some cases there is temporary improvement which is followed by sudden, rapid, renewed loss of weight. Sometimes increase of food is followed by a paradoxical reaction with loss of weight, without discoverable reason, or due to initiation of diarrhea. The longer the condition has lasted and the older the infant the greater the prospect of cure. Recovery may be slow but finally complete, and the child in later years may appear no worse for the illness in infancy.

Diagnosis.—Every effort should be made to determine whether the atrophy is secondary to starvation, tuberculosis, or other cause. The presence of a tuberculin reaction, or the discovery of some localized tuberculous symptoms indicates tuberculosis, but not infrequently the diagnosis of the disease may be evident only at necropsy. Conditions dependent upon starvation from lack of sufficient food (*inanition*), without any complicating gastro-intestinal defect, will improve following a proper diet. Syphilitic atrophy should be diagnosed by the presence of symptoms of this disease and the help obtained from the Wassermann reaction.

Treatment.—In the way of prophylaxis may be mentioned continuance of breast-feeding, careful supervision of artificial feeding, avoidance of parenteral infections, and such general care as the securing of an abundance of fresh air and avoidance of excessive summer-heat. For the developed condition it is often found that breast-milk is helpful, especially when there is no great tendency to diarrhea, and this often seems to be the only measure that will succeed. In artificial feeding the same rules hold good as attend the treatment of indigestion (see p. 571 and p. 601), but all dietetic measures are necessarily experimental as long as the nature of the cause is not understood. Prolonged starvation-treatment, such as might be advisable in acute digestive disorders, must be avoided in this disease. While easily digested food of a low caloric value given frequently and in small amounts may be necessary at first, it is often found that the intake can soon be fairly rapidly increased. In general it may be stated that the acid high-protein foods offer the best chance of success at the beginning, although, in other instances, high-carbohydrate foods act satisfactorily. Fat often is poorly tolerated, but this should not be taken for granted, since, as previously stated, the fat absorption is normal in many cases. The food should contain the essential vitamins, but in few instances is it necessary to administer an excess of these. Orange juice or tomato juice may be given if it agrees, and perhaps in some cases preparations containing especially vitamin B. (See p. 135.) It is necessary in some way to give a food of higher caloric value than the weight would indicate is needed, *i. e.*, the infant must be fed according to what it should weigh rather than what it does; and this is difficult owing to the feebleness of the digestive powers. If fat cannot be digested, as so often happens, the deficit must be supplied in other ways.

The fluid intake must be carefully watched, and more than the average of 2½ to 3 oz. of fluid per pound of body weight (163 to 195 cc. per kilogram) per day may be required. When there is dehydration or acidosis, such as occurs during attacks of diarrhea, the treatment is similar to that for acute gastro-enteric intoxication. (See p. 587.) Of great value are repeated injections of blood. (See p. 199.) An abundance of fresh air and individual attention to the infant's needs are very important. In institutional practice sometimes the best plan of treatment is to send the child home, provided the conditions there are suitable, and that detailed care can be given. There is nothing specific in ultraviolet ray therapy, although, if properly employed, it is certainly not contraindicated. Alcoholic stimulants in moderate doses are serviceable and may increase the appetite. Subnormal body temperature must be combated by suitable means, such as those used for premature infants. (See p. 213.) General massage with oil has been used and may be of value, but not by absorption of the oil, since it has been shown that nutrient substances cannot be absorbed through the skin (Winternitz and Naumann[20]).

Among other treatments which have been advocated are nonspecific protein therapy by injection of animal sera (Freeman,[21] Epstein[22]); the injection of sodium cacodylate (¼ to 1 grain) (0.016 to 0.065) every four days

(Clarke and Dow[23]); the subcutaneous injection of lipoid solutions (Buschmann[24]); and the use of thyroid extract (Nobécourt, Liège and Guérin[25]).

References

1. Ann. de méd. et de chir. inf., 1905, **9,** 1. 2. Prog. méd., 1874, **2,** 637. 3. Brit. M. J., 1899, **1,** 1084. 4. Jahrb. f. Kinderh., 1906, **63,** 421. 5. Nourrisson, 1921, **9,** 193. 6. Jahrb. f. Kinderh., 1919, **89,** 269. 7. Am. J. Dis. Child., 1920, **20,** 461. 8. Jahrb. f. Kinderh., 1898, **46,** 55. 9. Am. J. M. Sc., 1902, **114,** 847. 10. Am. J. Dis. Child., 1923, **26,** 451. 11. Quart. J. Med., 1921, **14,** 171. 12. Quart. J. Med., 1924, **17,** 339. 13. Lancet, 1924, **1,** 687. 14. Am. J. Dis. Child., 1925, **30,** 829. 15. Am. J. Dis. Child., 1928, **35,** 615; 1928, **36,** 470; 740. 16. Am. J. Dis. Child., 1928, **36,** 979. 17. Am. J. Dis. Child., 1929, **37,** 1146. 18. Am. J. Dis. Child., 1930, **39,** 736. 19. Am. J. Dis. Child., 1920, **20,** 366; 1921, **22,** 329. 20. Deutsche med. Wchnschr., 1929, **55,** 1828. 21. Arch. Pediat., 1917, **34,** 425. 22. Monatschr. f. Kinderh., 1923, **25,** 72. 23. Am. J. Dis. Child., 1920, **19,** 260. 24. Monatschr. f. Kinderh., 1926, **34,** 472. 25. Arch. de méd. d. enf., 1930, **33,** 647.

CHAPTER IV

MALNUTRITION

Under this rather vague term may be discussed secondary atrophies in infants, and subnormal nutritional states in older children. The term "Inanition," literally "emptiness," should be employed to express an unusual degree of malnutrition in reality dependent upon starvation.

Etiology.—Malnutrition is extremely common, and depends upon various causes. Based upon a strict application of 7 per cent deficiency in height-weight relationship (see p. 12 and p. 467), Emerson[1] estimated that at least one-third of school-children are malnourished, and at least one-half decidedly underweight. Constitutional debility (p. 235) or prematurity (p. 210) may be the background for subnormal strength, weight, and resistance to disease. Malnutrition is especially common in children of the active nervous type. In the majority of cases, however, the condition is not a constitutional one, but is acquired later. Such chronic diseases as tuberculosis, syphilis, rickets, diabetes, malignant growths, and chronic disorders of the gastro-enteric tract are frequently primary causes. Alteration of the glands of internal secretion may result in undernutrition, and it is possible that such a cause may be operative in certain cases when clear-cut symptoms of the glandular disturbance are not present. Particularly to be mentioned here is a hyperthyroid state. Talbot[2] emphasizes one form in which there exists tuberculosis of the mesenteric lymph-nodes interfering with absorption from the intestinal canal. An acute gastro-intestinal disorder may leave chronic malnutrition in its train. Repeated parenteral infections, with the attendant anorexia, not infrequently lead to malnutrition. Bad hygiene unquestionably predisposes. In many cases, especially in infancy, the fault lies in a failure to offer a sufficient amount of food to the infant. In subjects past the age of infancy probably much the most frequent cause is a combination of faulty food-habits, poor training, either neglect or pampering of the child, and lack of fresh air and exercise.

As in the case of infantile atrophy (p. 463) there seems to be no essential fault in metabolism. The studies of Wang, Hawkes and Hays,[3] Stearns and Moore,[4] and others have shown that children with malnutrition are able to absorb and store nitrogen and to retain calcium and phosphorus normally. Rupp and Schlutz[5] noted gastric motility lessened in malnourished children. Loeber and Weinberger[6] often found gastric hyperacidity, this being somewhat contrary to previous studies, such as those of

Sauer, Minsk and Alexander,[7] and others, who more frequently observed hypoacidity.

Symptoms.—In *infants* the growth of the body in weight, and often in length as well, is much below normal. The strength is poor, the muscles flabby, and sitting and standing are delayed. There may be evidences of such associated conditions as disturbed digestion and rickets, although it is noteworthy that the latter is often absent in the severest cases. An interesting variety of malnutrition is that of **acute inanition,** the direct result of starvation combined with some of the causes mentioned. It sometimes follows a previous moderate malnutrition, sometimes occurs rapidly without this. There are a sudden and dangerous loss of weight, dehydration, sunken fontanelle, hollow eyes, and other symptoms similar to those described under infantile atrophy (p. 463), but distinguished from this condition by the prompt improvement which comes about with treatment, if this has not been too long delayed.

Another interesting form in infants is **malnutrition from excess of starch.** This appears to be common in certain regions where a diet largely of cereal decoctions is employed. It has been designated Mehlnährschaden (Czerny and Keller,[8] Klose[9]) by German writers. It follows too long continuance of an amylaceous diet. The symptoms would seem to depend not so much upon the excess of starch as upon the relative deficiency of protein and fat, and perhaps also in some instances of vitamins; the disease being one of deprivation. Three types may be recognized: First the *hypertonic form* in which there is a rigid condition of the muscles, with opisthotonos and flexion of the extremities. This is the least common variety; and hypertonia may be seen in other nutritional disturbances than those dependent upon a starchy diet. (See p. 872.) Second, an *atrophic form* presenting the appearance of ordinary inanition but often with hypertonia associated. It occurs especially when no salt has been added to the diet. Third, the *hydremic form,* in which salt has been added freely to the food, or has been insufficiently excreted from the body. The retention of water creates the appearance of good nutrition, but gradually edema becomes noticeable and the increase in weight is decided. This form corresponds in some respects to the edema which has been designated hunger-edema, nutritional edema or epidemic dropsy. In some of these cases there is found a low serum-protein which interferes with osmotic pressure, and edema occurs due to excessive filtration of fluid. In all forms the skin is pale and pasty, and infections develop readily, chief among them being suppurative processes of the skin. Xerophthalmia may occur when there is deprivation of vitamin A.

In *older children* the symptoms of malnutrition show themselves in various ways, such as anemia, cold extremities, flabby muscles, nervousness, anorexia, constipation, and insomnia. The child may fatigue easily, especially as evening approaches, but at the same time may be restless and active. Mentality may be above the average, although even such children easily become mentally tired, and school-work becomes difficult. The so-called "fatigue-posture" is found, in which there are flat chest, round shoulders, and prominent abdomen. The body may be thin but the face fat. Slight causes produce outbreaks of indigestion, and there seems to be little resisting power to illness of any sort. It should be remembered that the child should not be considered malnourished on the single criterion that the weight is 7 per cent below the normal for the height. (For discussion of relation of weight to height, see p. 12.) Associated symptoms of malnutrition which point to an endocrine basis, when they cannot be accounted for otherwise, are delayed development of the epiphyses, irregularities in dentition, and delayed puberty.

Course and Prognosis.—This varies with the age and the cause. Infants with congenital asthenia cannot be expected to become hardy with any rapidity. When some existing or previously existing disease is discovered, the prognosis depends upon the nature of this or the possibility of removing it. There is always the danger of a fatal termination from the occurrence of complicating or coincidental disorders. The immediate danger is much greater in young infants than in older children. The prognosis is uncertain in those nutritional disturbances depending upon an excessively starchy diet, although some patients improve rapidly when proper food is given. Acute inanition from insufficient nourishment usually offers a favorable prognosis if it has not advanced too far. However, the patient may have developed an intolerance for food, and the prognosis is then unfavorable. In a child recovering from long-continued malnutrition, Stearns and Moore[4] found that gain in weight began before growth in height, but that once the latter was started it was very rapid.

Treatment.—This depends upon the cause. The first effort must be to discover any dietetic or hygienic error. In *infants* who are breast-fed it is particularly the amount of nourishment received that should be investigated, although sometimes it is found that the composition of the milk is at fault. With weakly infants it may be necessary to express the milk and feed with a dropper. In infants artificially fed who refuse their nourishment, feeding by gavage may be necessary. In young infants with digestive disorder breast-milk may be almost essential for recovery, and when artificial feeding is unavoidable the food must be carefully selected according to the indication of the symptoms. (See chronic gastritis, p. 571; chronic intestinal indigestion, p. 601; infantile atrophy, p. 465.) As soon as digestion permits, the food should be of sufficient strength to supply the caloric needs. It may be found that in some cases high protein food agrees; in others high carbohydrates are well tolerated; and in still others fat may be employed in some of the special mixtures, even though indigestible when given in an ordinary milk formula. Among foods which are sometimes helpful are protein-milk, buttermilk, malt-soup, butter-flour mixture, lactic acid milk with corn syrup, and thick cereal feeding. (See Index.) The diet should always be one which is not deficient in vitamins, and in some cases preparations of vitamin B may be beneficial.

Hygienic treatment, such as fresh air and sunlight, is next in importance to diet. At the same time, the enthusiasm for open-air treatment should not lead to exposure and chilling, especially when there is a tendency to low body-temperature. Since the need for water in the tissues is sometimes pressing, fluid intake must be adequate, and parenteral injections of salt-solution and glucose employed, or transfusion given if necessary. This need is usually not as great as in severe cases of infantile atrophy. (See p. 465.)

In *older children* the causes of malnutrition are so manifold that only careful study may reveal them. All the aids of the history may be needed, combined with the physical examination, and often the roentgenological study of the chest or the gastro-intestinal tract and gastric analysis. In the frequent cases in which no physical underlying cause is discoverable the condition probably depends upon faulty feeding-habits, which are discussed in the section on Anorexia Nervosa (p. 559). Unless there is indigestion, there should be a liberal diet, properly balanced in fat, carbohydrate, and protein. (See Chap. VI.) The correct diet will usually contain sufficient vitamins, but in some cases an additional intake of them may be indicated.

The whole course of the child's daily life must be supervised by the physician and the amount of exercise and rest prescribed, since dietary measures alone are often not sufficient. Perhaps the amount of school-work may need to be diminished, extra hours spent in such studies as music and the like discontinued, and outdoor play encouraged. Any focus of infection, such as diseased tonsils or teeth, which may be thought to be operative should be cared for, but only when distinctly indicated and as part of the general treatment. Massage and gymnastic training are suitable for those children who take too little exercise. It is often difficult to determine whether the fatigue-posture is congenital and the cause of symptoms, or is acquired and the result of the malnutrition. In any event, an attempt should be made to correct it. We have had good results from the employment of the following exercises in which the child must use specific muscles: (1) Stand with heels together and 6 in. (15 cm.) from the wall; inhale, rising on toes; raise arms forward and upward and backward; touch wall with tips of fingers; exhale, slowly lowering the arms to the sides and heels to floor. (2) Lie flat on floor. Toes hooked under chair or dresser; raise body from floor, keeping knees flat and elbows and hands folded across chest. These exercises to be done five and later fifteen times morning and night. When the fatigue-posture is marked and has been long-continued, it may be difficult to correct by exercises alone, and a proper support worn for several months should be used as an adjunct to other measures. Rest, recumbent, in the middle of the day, not insisting upon sleeping in the case of those in later childhood, is sometimes remarkably efficacious, and improvement may be impossible without it. During the rest-hour, or at night, the child may sleep on its back with a small pillow between the shoulders, or on its face with a pillow under the abdomen. A cool morning sponge may have a stimulating effect, provided the after-rubbing brings about a good reaction. Change of environment and particularly a sojourn at the seashore are efficacious.

Drugs occupy a minor position, and they should be used chiefly for symptoms as the need arises. Gastric analysis may demonstrate the need for proper medication. Constipation may temporarily require medication, but is better treated by dietetic and other measures. Cod liver oil is not a specific, but may be given if it does not decrease appetite. When it is suspected that there is an endocrine basis, the stimulating effect on metabolism of thyroid extract may be tried. Topper[10] found that thyroid extract stimulated growth in height even in children who did not have decreased basal metabolism, and its administration in small doses (0.015 to 0.5 Gm.) ($\frac{1}{4}$ to 8 grains) did not increase the metabolic rate. The anemia which is so common a symptom may require treatment directed to it. The treatment of the loss of appetite is discussed under Anorexia Nervosa (p. 559).

References

1. Nutrition and Growth in Children, 1922. 2. Med. Clin. N. Amer., 1927, **10,** 1175. 3. Am. J. Dis. Child., 1928, **35,** 968. 4. Am. J. Dis. Child., 1931, **42,** 774. 5. Am. J. Dis. Child., 1930, **39,** 241. 6. Am. J. Dis. Child., 1931, **42,** 767. 7. J.A.M.A., 1922, **70,** 184. 8. Des Kindes Ernährung, etc., 1906, **2,** 62. 9. Med. Klinik., 1915, **11,** 881. 10. Am. J. Dis. Child., 1931, **41,** 1289.

CHAPTER V

RHEUMATISM

ACUTE RHEUMATIC FEVER

Etiology. Predisposing Causes. *Age.*—Rheumatism of any form is very rare in infancy. We[1] have seen but one instance of articular involvement at this period. Miller[2] writing in 1899, found only 19 recorded cases under one year of age in addition to one of his own, and other instances of articular or cardiac rheumatism under two years of age have occasionally been reported (Smith;[3] Denzer[4]). A few instances of apparently congenital rheumatism have been recorded (Abrahams;[5] Poynton and Paine[6]), and Richdorf and Griffith[7] observed polyarthritis in an infant of six days whose mother was suffering from the disorder. Between six and nine years is the most likely time in early life for the first manifestations to appear. All statistics show that girls are more often attacked than boys, in the ratio of about 3:2. The *individual susceptibility* is not great, not much more than 1 per cent of hospital admissions of children being for disease of this nature (Baginsky;[8] Wachenheim[9]). *Inheritance* seems to be a factor, Kephallinos[10] discovering evidence of it in 50 per cent of his cases, and Poynton, Patterson and Spence[11] in 40 per cent. St. Lawrence[12] found that in 100 families with rheumatic cardiac disease there were two or more instances of it in 29 per cent; an incidence too high to be accidental. Faulkner and White[13] observed that in families in which there had been no previous rheumatic disease the incidence was less than one-half that which existed in families where rheumatism had earlier occurred. Draper, Allen and Spock[14] believe that there is an "age-resistance" character, children of parents who had had rheumatism being liable to suffer their first attack at the same age as it had occurred in the parent. *Epidemics* have been reported in schools or institutions and in family groups. Paul[15] points out that extension in a family is most likely to occur in children from five to ten years of age, and Paul and Salinger[16] show that sudden appearance of both primary and secondary outbursts of rheumatism frequently accompanied the development of recognizable forms of the disease in other members of the family group. Bradley[17] found in two epidemics in schools that there was parallelism with epidemics of hemolytic streptococcic sore throat. This apparent epidemic influence might equally well argue for faulty environmental conditions or for direct infection, but in familial spread it also suggests a hereditary agency. *Climate* is a factor, and rheumatism is more prevalent in the cooler and damper season of the year, and in certain localities where these conditions especially obtain. There seems to be a lesser incidence in rural districts than in urban communities. In hospital statistics rheumatic fever is more common in the northern than in the southern part of the United States (Seegal and Seegal[18]). It is the season of worst weather conditions that apparently predisposes. In England, for example, this is in the late autumn, while in the studies of McCulloch and Jones[19] in St. Louis, and of Sutton[20] and Coburn[21] in New York, the peak of incidence was in the spring. In individual instances, too, coldness or dampness and exposure seem to initiate attacks. Cases are more common in the white *race* than in the colored. In New York City, Sutton[20] found that Italians, Irish, and native-born Americans were more susceptible than Spaniards, Armenians and Jews. Infection of the *upper respiratory tract* in the epidemic form, or in the chronic form in the individual, has some sort of association with rheumatism. Boas and Schwartz[22] also called attention to association of infection of the *lower respiratory tract* with rheumatic manifestations. The relation of *diseased tonsils* and *adenoids* to rheumatism is a matter of dispute and difficult to evaluate. It is discussed at length in the section on Hypertrophy of the Tonsils (p. 540). In this connection it may be said, that while removal of diseased tonsils and adenoids is probably indicated in children of rheumatic families as a precautionary measure, and in patients who have manifested rheumatic disease, there is no assurance that this will prevent the occurrence or recurrence of the condition. There is no evidence that any relation exists between carious teeth and acute rheumatic fever.

Exciting Cause.—Probably Popoff[23] in 1887 was the first to report the presence of micro-organisms in association with acute rheumatic fever. Many observers have since discovered germs in the blood, heart, joints, and tonsils. An important contribution is that of Poynton and Paine[24] who described the "streptococcus rheumaticus." Among others who have found streptococci are Coombs, Miller and Kettle,[25] and Rosenow,[26] who also produced arthritis and carditis in animals by inoculation. Cecil, Nicholls and Stainsby[27] frequently isolated a streptococcus of the viridans type in cases of acute rheumatic fever, and Leichtenstratt[28] found streptococcus viridans in the rheumatic nodules. Small[29] believes in the specificity of a nonhemolytic streptococcus recovered chiefly from the throat of active cases of the disease, which produces a condition in animals resembling rheumatism. With this germ he prepared a vaccine and an antiserum, which are claimed to be beneficial. Birkhaug[30] has isolated from tonsils, blood, feces, urine, and cardiac vegetations a nonmethemoglobin-forming streptococcus.

On the other hand is the fact that in the great majority of cases blood-cultures have given negative results, and that there are decided differences in the varieties of streptococcus which have been claimed to be the active agents.

Some students of the disease, among them Swift and his co-workers,[31] and Zinsser and Yü,[32] favor the theory that allergy to the streptococcus may be the cause of such rheumatic symptoms as joint-pains; the micro-organisms themselves resting latent in such organs as the heart-muscle and spleen. Cecil, Nicholls and Stainsby[27] believe that allergy influences the picture, but that the articular manifestations depend primarily on the localization of bacteria there.

There seems to be no doubt of the association of infection particularly of the upper respiratory tract and acute rheumatic manifestations; and the causative rôle of micro-organisms, such as the streptococcus, while not as yet proven, must be regarded as very possible. Perhaps some of the rheumatic manifestations may be allergic, as claimed. Whatever may be determined finally regarding the relation to infection, there certainly exists a powerful constitutional susceptibility or tissue-predisposition as a background, in which case infection could then act in the nature of a "trigger-mechanism."

For the sake of completeness should be mentioned the claim of some authors that there is an association of acute articular rheumatism with tuberculosis, basing this chiefly upon the results of tuberculin testing, and the theory that the general sensitiveness induced by tuberculosis may allow other infections to act (Reitter[33]).

Pathologic Anatomy.—The articular lesions in acute cases consist of hyperemia with turbidity of the fluid, and slight infiltration of the neighboring connective tissue. In the experience of some observers streptococci are found in and around the joints, but most investigators have failed to discover this. Purulent inflammation occurs only as a complication. Fibrous nodules are sometimes present beneath the skin in various regions in children. These consist of inflammatory connective tissue, fibrin, and cells, the center of the lesion being a thrombosis. Cardiac lesions will be considered elsewhere (p. 780). Here may be mentioned the bodies described by Aschoff[34] in 1904, and known by his name. These are microscopical nodules found attached to the adventitia of the blood-vessels of the myocardium, and are composed of large cells containing numerous nuclei, together with leukocytes and connective tissue fibres. A further consideration of the pathology is contained in the communication by Swift.[31]

Symptoms.—It must be realized that so-called "acute rheumatism" is a chronic disease with a tendency to recurrence, and that between the different manifestations there may be a latent period of from one to two years or more. It shows itself in children in a manner different from that exhibited in adults, and the symptoms in early life are manifold. While acute arthritis is the type, yet there may be no involvement of the joints at all, or this may occur secondarily. In fact, any one of the rheumatic manifestations such as heart-disease, articular involvement, chorea, or subcutaneous nodules may occur initially. In the rheumatic syndrome must be included tonsillitis, since it so often precedes or accompanies other signs of the condition.

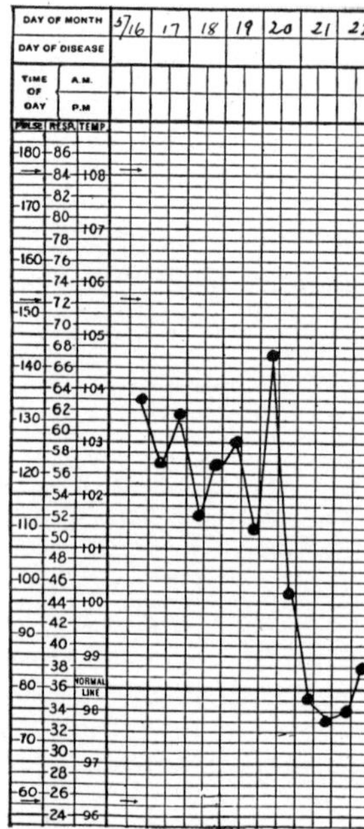

Fig. 112.—Acute articular rheumatism. Alice W., aged six years. After becoming overheated by skating, developed headache, fever, and pain in the knees, ankles and feet. On entrance to the Children's Ward of the University Hospital, Philadelphia, May 16, exhibited pain, redness and swelling of both knees, tongue coated. No cardiac murmur present. Leukocytes 30,200; May 22, swelling and pain nearly gone. A faint systolic murmur audible.

Acute Articular Rheumatism.—Occasionally preceded by malaise or sore throat, the attack generally begins acutely with fever, anorexia, and articular involvement. The intensity of these symptoms varies greatly. In early childhood they are less marked than later, but at any time in early life are usually not so decided as in adults; the redness, swelling and pain of the joints being less evident, sweating absent or slight, and the fever less and soon disappearing (Fig. 112). Generally the lower extremities are first affected, the ankle or knee on one side being most often attacked, with the hip usually next in order of frequency. The disease may remain limited to a single joint, but as a rule the corresponding joints of the other leg are soon involved, and perhaps those of the upper extremities as well. Not infrequently the upper extremity may be attacked alone or primarily. Sometimes the disease appears in the cervical vertebrae; less often in the fingers, toes, or other joints. Quite often one joint improves as another becomes affected, although the inflammation may reappear in the first joint as the course of the disease progresses. As a rule not many joints are involved.

In mild attacks, as observed especially in early life, the patient may not feel ill, fever is insignificant, and the child does not wish to stay in bed unless the lower extremities are affected. Often only lameness is produced without actual inability to walk. The discomfort is frequently so insignificant that it has been given the common title of "growing pains." Sheldon[35] found that in 52 of 277 children with rheumatic heart disease, pain in the limbs for several months was the only preceding evidence of rheumatism. Not all so-called "growing pains," however, have a rheumatic significance. They are found as frequently in children who do not have, and who never develop, any other signs of rheumatism as they are in the rheumatic group (Selkirk and Mitchell;[36] Seham, Shapiro and Hilbert[37]).

Well-marked typical attacks of the adult type are not often seen until toward the end of later childhood. Delirium and other cerebral disturbances are rare at any period of childhood, and abdominal pains simulating appendicitis are less common than in adults. Pleurisy may sometimes be an initial symptom.

The *duration* of acute articular rheumatism is variable, averaging about one to two weeks, but there is a remarkable tendency to relapse. Less commonly than in adults do cases pass into the chronic form.

Cardiac Rheumatism.—As already stated, this is sometimes the first manifestation of the disease, being evidenced by fever and vague general symptoms, and a cardiac murmur then being discovered. Sutton states that from 15 to 20 per cent of children with rheumatic heart disease do not have any previous history of acute articular involvement, growing pains, or chorea. Oftener than otherwise, however, cardiac symptoms are secondary, the manifestations being frequent as a complication of chorea, and occurring after mild as well as severe articular rheumatism, although more common in the latter. It is especially in early life that cardiac involvement is liable to follow. Eventually a large percentage of children with rheumatism develop cardiac lesions (60 to 70 per cent) (Coombs;[38] Kephallinós;[10] Ingerman and Wilson[39]). Coombs[40] stated that he had never seen a child pass through an attack of acute rheumatism without cardiac involvement, and electrocardiographic studies, as those of Cohen and Swift,[41] and Master and Romanoff,[42] show 100 per cent involvement of the myocardium with acute rheumatic manifestations. As discovered clinically, cardiac involvement appears usually at or before the end of the first week of the rheumatic attack. A valvular lesion, generally mitral, persists in probably 50 per cent or more of the cases of articular rheumatism in children, appearing in later attacks oftener than in the first. Pericarditis develops in 10 to 20 per cent of the cases in children. (See pp. 780; 784; 785.)

Chorea.—From 30 to 50 per cent of children with chorea exhibit other rheumatic manifestations. Chorea may develop before or, oftener, after arthritis. The symptoms of the latter may suddenly disappear as the chorea develops. Frequently there is no articular involvement, but endocarditis follows the chorea. It is rare for chorea and acute joint manifestations to occur simultaneously. We do not recall having seen such a situation, and only a few are reported in the literature (Lepehne[43]). It should be observed that not all cases of chorea can be called rheumatic. (See also Chorea, p. 874.)

Subcutaneous Fibrous Nodules (Nodosis rheumatica).—This affection was first described by Meynet[44] in 1875, and in 1881 Barlow and Warner[45] reported 27 cases. It is rare in France; common in England and Germany. Its incidence in the United States has been variously reported and seems to vary with locality. Bronson and Carr[46] found it in 45 per cent of 38 children with rheumatism; Ingerman and Wilson[39] in 11 per cent of 185 cases; Wallace[47] in 12 per cent of 124 cases; Merritt[48] in 11 per cent of 224 cases. It seems to be more frequent in patients with cardiac involvement and apparently increases the gravity of the prognosis. It is oftener seen in children than in adults. The nodules vary in size from that of a pinhead to that of a small nut; are not reddened or tender; are found oftenest upon the back of the head and distributed somewhat symmetrically about the joints, especially the hips, knees, and ankles, along the tendons and the vertebrae, and upon the pinnae of the ear. They vary in number from 1 to 50 or more, develop generally after the arthritis appears, and may last for months (Fig. 113).

Cutaneous Manifestations.—Erythema of various sorts is prone to occur, and sometimes purpura, often associated with the arthritis. *Purpura rheumatica*, so-called, probably has no direct connection with rheumatism. (See p. 1040.)

Tonsillitis.—As stated, inflammation of the tonsils or pharynx may be promptly followed by articular inflammation or cardiac disease, and there is a special tendency to tonsillitis in rheumatic subjects. It is a question whether the tonsillar inflammation is a manifestation of rheumatism, or the source from which it arises. (For discussion, see p. 540.)

Muscular Rheumatism. Rheumatic Myalgia.—It is disputed whether this condition is actually rheumatic in nature. In some cases it certainly seems to be, since we have seen such conditions as acute torticollis either occurring with or quickly followed by arthritis and cardiac involvement.

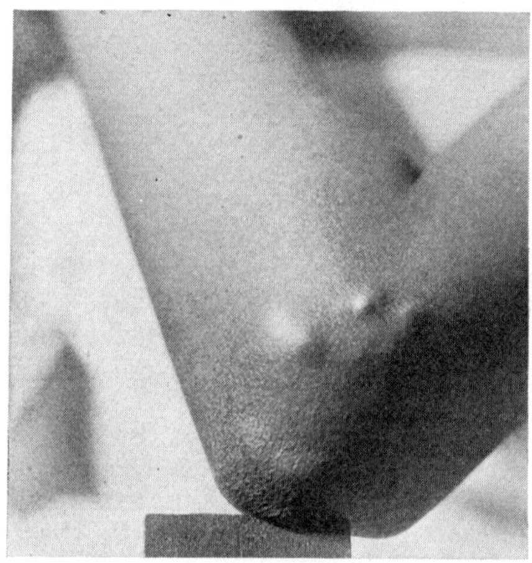

Fig. 113.—Rheumatic nodules at the elbow. Colored girl of ten years of age in Cincinnati General Hospital. Had polyarthritis and endocarditis. Later developed pericarditis. Died three weeks after picture was taken.

(See p. 472.) The "growing pains" already referred to (p. 472) are sometimes myalgic and of a rheumatic nature, but oftener probably located in the joints.

Complications.—Among the disorders which may occasionally complicate rheumatism are nephritis, peritonitis, pleuritis, pneumonia, bronchitis, iritis, trigeminal neuralgia, sciatica, venous thrombosis, epistaxis and mastitis. By some authors many of these complications are regarded as visceral manifestations of rheumatism, which take the place of an acute attack of polyarthritis.

Recurrence and Relapse.—One attack of rheumatism is more liable than otherwise to be followed by later ones, especially in childhood. The severity of the recurrences is in no way dependent upon that of the primary attack. The great tendency to relapse has already been referred to (p. 473). These relapses may occur in spite of the greatest care, or may be brought about by slight exposure, such as leaving the bed too soon after convalescence has seemed established. The disease may appear in the joints previously affected, or in others.

Prognosis.—In childhood the prognosis for recovery from individual attacks is good, and the course of arthritis is shorter and the symptoms milder than in adults. Endocarditis, if slight, is frequently entirely recovered from; if more severe, valvular disease may remain, but even then compensation may be good. (See p. 793.) On the other hand the prognosis of rheumatism in early life is, on the whole, more serious than later on account of the greater tendency for recurrences of arthritis or chorea to take place, and the consequent greater danger that endocarditis will develop in some of them if not in the primary one. The prognosis for ultimate recovery must, therefore, be most guarded. Rheumatic pericarditis is usually a part of a pancarditis and is a serious lesion, and extremely liable to lead to loss of compensation. Subcutaneous nodules are usually associated with serious rheumatic disease and have a consequent unfavorable import. Bronson and Carr,[46] for example, found that in 21 children with rheumatism but without nodules there was only 1 death, whereas in 17 with nodules there were 6 deaths. The large majority of deaths from rheumatism occur before the age of twenty years, and particularly in later childhood near puberty, the disease being at its worst from the sixth to the twelfth year (Poynton, Agassiz and Taylor[49]). The cause of death in early life is nearly always cardiac involvement. Auricular fibrillation is a bad prognostic sign.

Diagnosis.—This is not always easy because of the different guises under which the disease may appear. Acquired valvular disease of the heart is practically always due to rheumatism. The differentiation of an organic from an accidental or functional cardiac murmur may be difficult. Assistance is obtained from the history, such as the past occurrence of growing pains, minor joint-pains or actual arthritis, repeated sore throat, chorea, or torticollis. The electrocardiogram may be of help in detecting minor derangements of the heart. The family history may be of importance. (See also p. 470.)

A number of conditions may be confounded with an attack of acute articular rheumatism. *Osteomyelitis* is less often multiple in localization, exhibits more severe constitutional symptoms, and involves the shaft and epiphysis rather than the joint itself. *Secondary arthritis* after acute infectious diseases is usually monarticular, sometimes polyarticular, and is recognized by the previous history. *Gonorrheal arthritis* is generally monarticular, but more often multiple in early life than later. It is, however, nearly always combined with vulvovaginitis or ophthalmia. *Syphilitic arthritis* is usually localized in both knee-joints, is chronic and with little pain, is generally associated with other signs of syphilis, and a positive Wassermann reaction will be found. *Septic arthritis* is purulent and accompanied by other signs of sepsis. Acute rheumatism of the hip-joint may strongly suggest *appendicitis*. *Scorbutus* and *syphilitic epiphysitis* occur in infancy at a time when rheumatism is extremely rare. *Multiple neuritis* and *sciatica* exhibit no articular involvement. *Poliomyelitis* can be mistaken for rheumatism only early, when there is fever and pain on being moved. *Tuberculous coxitis* can be differentiated by careful examination and by its chronic course and monarticular character. *Retropharyngeal abscess* has been mistaken for rheumatic torticollis.

Cutaneous tests with streptococci for susceptibility have not been sufficiently studied to make them of assured value.

Treatment. **Prophylaxis.**—The effect of therapy both in prophylaxis and in treatment of the disease is extremely difficult to evaluate, because of the natural tendency to self-limitation of certain of the manifestations, and the long latent period between attacks. Certainly all possible foci of infection, such as diseased tonsils, sinuses, and upper respiratory infections in general, should be appropriately treated. It must be emphasized, however, that removal of the tonsils offers no certain promise of prevention of rheumatic manifestations. (See p. 540.) Diseased teeth should receive attention, although they may have no direct causative influence (p. 471). Children with a decided family history of rheumatism, or who have suffered from previous attacks, must be scrupulously guarded against exposure to cold and damp; the hygiene of the mouth, clothing and out-door life carefully regulated; and the general health and resisting power kept in the best condition. A change to a proper climate may be a very great factor in prevention of recurrences. This was especially well shown in the studies of Coburn,[21] in which persons predisposed to rheumatism were greatly benefited by removal from New York to Porto Rico, and where, interestingly enough, hemolytic streptococci seemed to disappear from their throats.

Wilson and Swift,[50] and Swift[31] and his co-workers, have employed intravenous and intramuscular injections of a vaccine of hemolytic streptococci, and believe that some effect was obtained in prevention of recurrences of rheumatism. There is no proof that diet has any influence in preventing the manifestations, although the restriction of carbohydrates has sometimes been recommended.

For the prevention of cardiac involvement during other rheumatic manifestations there is little that can be done except rest. This should be kept up as long as there is fever, even though there is no clinical evidence of heart-disease. In view of what has been previously stated, it is better to consider that there is cardiac involvement, even if only of the myocardium, in every case of acute polyarthritis and chorea. Salicylates have no proven value in preventing cardiac involvement.

Treatment of the Attack.—During the acute febrile stage of articular rheumatism, the diet should be liquid, and the patient kept at rest in an equably heated but well ventilated room. The clothing must be of flannel, and of a type easily changed if wet by sweating. The affected joints may be wrapped in cotton, or warm moist applications used for relief of pain; all motion avoided; and the bed-clothes prevented from pressing on tender regions. The treatment of developing endocarditis will be considered later (p. 790). In the line of medicinal treatment there is no doubt that salicylates control both pain and fever. Whether they are specifics or not is another matter. It is at least interesting to restate the hypothesis that some of the rheumatic manifestations are due to allergy (p. 471), and that salicylates are supposed by some authors to have a beneficial action on this. (See p. 488.) No generally acceptable proof has ever been offered, however, that salicylates exert any specific action in rheumatism. Master and Romanoff[42] in a controlled study could not find that the course of rheumatism was shortened or the cardiac complications prevented. Sodium salicylate may be administered every three hours in doses of 5 to 8 grains (0.3 to 0.52 Gm.) to a child eight or ten years of age, or oil of wintergreen (methyl salicylate), acetylsalicylic acid, phenyl salicylate, or other salicylic acid derivatives may be given. Sodium bicarbonate in at least one-half the dose of the salicylate is an advisable addition. The danger of salicylate poisoning must always be borne in mind, and we have seen it occur when unusually large doses were continued over a period of several days. Oil of wintergreen may be used locally on joints or by inunction in the armpits and other regions. Constitutional effect can be produced in this way. Salicylates may be given by rectum. There is no value in continuing drug-treatment for long after the symptoms have disappeared. If salicylates fail to relieve pain, antipyrine or phenacetin may be employed, or some of the newer preparations such as neocinchophen, novatophan, tolysin, etc., can be tried. Opiates are necessary only in severe cases unrelieved by other remedies.

The antiserum and vaccine, or soluble antigen, of Small[29] is reported on favorably both in treatment and prevention by Riesman and Small.[51]

Some careful students of rheumatic disease, among them Wilson,[52] found no effect produced by this procedure and it is evident that it needs further study.

Every attention should be given to the general health, the administration of a nutritious diet, and the treatment of anemia and the like.

CHRONIC RHEUMATISM

Chronic Arthritis

Etiology.—The etiology of the different varieties of chronic rheumatism is not well understood. Foci of infection in the tonsils, sinuses, joints, and teeth seem to be related to chronic rheumatism, particularly of the atrophic type; or at least their eradication may be helpful in improving the condition. A number of writers stress the intestinal tract as a possible focus of infection. As in acute rheumatism, there is probably in the chronic disease an underlying predisposition to the rheumatic state, inasmuch as the greater number of persons with focal infection show no evidence of rheumatism. There is a metabolic disturbance in the nature of a delay in the removal of dextrose from the blood, a lowered basal metabolism, and a sub-oxidation of the tissues, as shown by the studies of Pemberton,[53] Fletcher,[54] Llewellyn,[55] and others. It is probable that these changes are of a secondary character, or that they occur locally, due to mechanical causes such as vasoconstriction. In atrophic arthritis Rosenow[56] and Paston[57] isolated streptococci from the lymph-nodes, and others, as Cecil, Nicholls and Stainsby,[58] from the blood and joints in a high percentage of patients, whose sera gave, in addition, a strong specific agglutination for these organisms. There are a number of reports showing that some cases of chronic arthritis are associated with dysenteric infection of the intestinal tract. The work of Freiberg[59] suggests that in these there is a local allergic reponse to the dysenteric infection. Other cases of chronic arthritis seem to be etiologically associated with hyperthyroidism, syphilis, and undulant fever. (See these sections.)

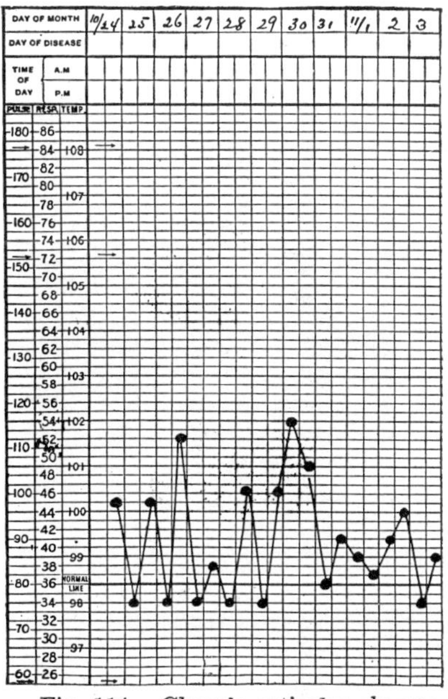

Fig. 114.—Chronic articular rheumatism. Ignatio C., aged seven years. Children's Hospital of Phila., October 25. At twenty months of age in bed three or four months on account of painful swelling of knees and fingers. Then well until last Dec., when hands, elbows, and all joints of the lower limbs gradually became swollen and painful and neck stiff. Been in bed since then. Examination showed poor nutrition; bad teeth; wrists, elbows, ankles, fingers, and toes swollen but not tender; neck stiff; fixation at hips; knees swollen and tender; spleen not enlarged. Leukocytes 12,000. Pirquet-reaction negative. No improvement during brief hospitalization.

Pathologic Anatomy.—In the *atrophic* type there is destruction of cartilage by overgrowth of the synovial membrane and growth of granular tissue from the bone beneath. In the *hypertrophic* type there are fibrillary degeneration of cartilage and overgrowth of the bone at the margin of the joint and elsewhere.

Symptoms.—The simplest and seemingly the best classification of chronic arthritis is that as described under pathologic anatomy. Atrophic arthritis is also variously termed rheumatic arthritis, proliferative arthritis, arthritis deformans and chronic infectious arthritis. Some would classify arthritis deformans as a distinct type, others regard it only as an end-result of the atrophic type, and some make chronic infectious arthritis a separate division. Some cases seem to have no relation to acute articular rheumatism, but, from the beginning, are chronic. Others follow upon a typical attack of acute rheumatism, or are the final result of a series of recurrences or relapses. While chronic rheumatism is comparatively uncommon in early life, we have seen a considerable number of cases, and usually of the atrophic type. The articular involvement may begin in the larger joints, but there is a tendency to primary localization in the hips, small joints of the fingers, jaws, and the neck. The disease spreads

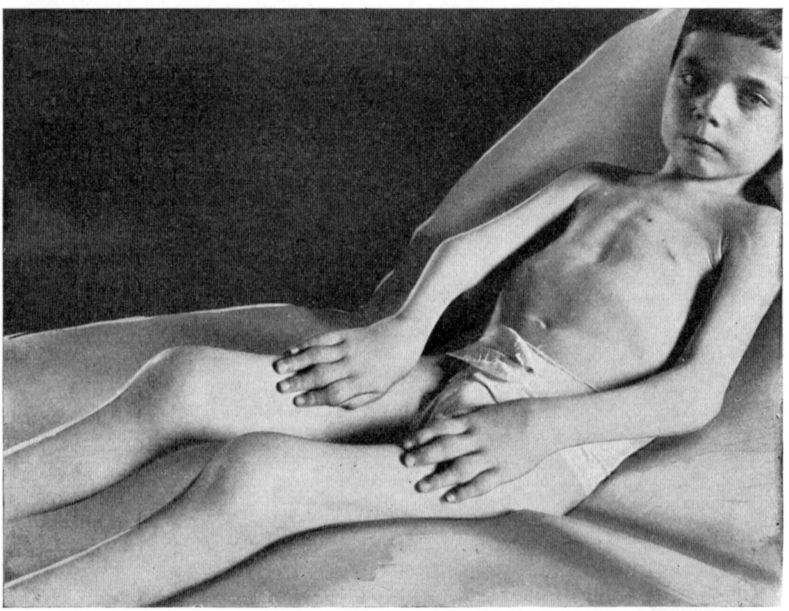

Fig. 115.—Chronic articular rheumatism. Showing enlargement of the elbows, hands and knees. Same case as in Fig. 114.

from joint to joint without disappearing in those first affected, until the majority of the articulations are involved. This is especially true of the cases without initial acute attacks. There are increasing debility and anemia, with cold sweating. Endocarditis is much less common than in acute articular rheumatism. Fever is usually mild or absent (Fig. 114). Periods of improvement occur, but usually without complete disappearance of symptoms. The joints are swollen and distorted and grate when moved, and the neighboring muscles are atrophied. Finally great deformity may develop due to destruction of the cartilages, bony structures, and periarticular tissues (Fig. 115). The hypertrophic form practically never occurs in childhood, but is associated with middle life or later, and is often related to the menopause and hypothyroidism. There is a dry type of slowly-developing arthritis, usually with little swelling and few general symptoms.

A special form of arthritis has been described by Still[60] which is possibly rheumatic, possibly tuberculous, or possibly dependent upon some chronic infection of other nature. It is characterized by progressive involvement of the joints, which become enlarged and stiff, although not very painful, but which do not undergo destructive processes. There is more or less fever, and always enlargement of the spleen and of the lymph-nodes. The liver may become enlarged, and amyloid disease may develop (Carroll and Nelson[61]). The prognosis in some cases of this condition, usually called Still's Disease, is better than in other forms of chronic arthritis.

Diagnosis.—In chronic rheumatism the principal diagnostic problem is to determine the cause, if possible. Search should be made for any foci of infection and for the existence of such diseases as tuberculosis, syphilis, dysentery, undulant fever, or hyperthyroidism, which may be etiologic factors.

Treatment.—In the treatment of subacute and chronic rheumatism the effort must be made, as with diagnosis, to discover the cause. Some cases of chronic arthritis, particularly of the atrophic (chronic infectious) type, may respond to the eradication of foci, provided the disease in the joints has not been too destructive. Autogenous vaccines made from germs obtained from the nose and throat or from foci may be tried. Foreign protein therapy by hypodermic injections of milk, Coley's fluid, peptone and proteoses, or typhoid vaccine has been used by a number of clinicians. There is no doubt that in some cases this is effective if given before there is permanent joint-injury, but it must be only part of the general treatment. Injection of bee-sting toxin has been recommended by Wasserbrenner.[62] Pemberton[53] found benefit following a diet which was restricted in caloric value and in starches and sugars. There is no good clinical or experimental evidence to contraindicate red meat in the diet. Baking the joints is very helpful in some cases, and Röhr[63] recommends roentgen-ray treatment of them. Massage and passive movement must not be used during an exacerbation. The production of passive congestion by the Bier method has been recommended. Rowntree and Adson[64] obtained some relief in arthritis of the lower extremities by bilateral lumbar sympathetic ganglionectomy. Cases depending upon dysentery, hypothyroidism, hyperthyroidism, or undulant fever should be treated accordingly. Benefit has been claimed for the administration of thyroid extract in some cases even without hypothyroidism. Iodides may be of value at times. Several authors have reported good results from the intravenous injection of salts of ortho-iodoxybenzoic acid (amiodoxy P-benzoate), giving 100 cc. of a fresh 1 per cent solution every third day. Others have found it without value. Injections of sulphur have been used by Habler and Weitzenfeld.[65] Attention to general health and the treatment of anemia and the like are important. The patient often becomes depressed and must be kept interested and amused.

References

1. Griffith, Arch. Pediat., 1908, **25**, 265. 2. Arch. Pediat., 1899, **16**, 686. 3. Arch. Pediat., 1922, **39**, 799. 4. J.A.M.A., 1924, **82**, 1243. 5. Med. Rec., 1896, **50**, 547. 6. Researches on Rheumatism, 1914, 389. 7. Am. J. Dis. Child., 1926, **31**, 250. 8. Berl. klin. Wchnschr., 1904, **41**, 1213. 9. Arch. Pediat., 1908, **25**, 669. 10. Wien. klin. Wchnschr., 1906, **19**, 563. 11. Lancet, 1920, **2**, 1086. 12. J.A.M.A., 1922, **79**, 2051. 13. J.A.M.A., 1924, **83**, 425. 14. J.A.M.A., 1929, **92**, 2149. 15. J. Clin. Investig., 1931, **10**, 53. 16. J. Clin. Investig., 1931, **10**, 33. 17. Quart. J. Med., 1932, **1**, 79. 18. J.A.M.A., 1927, **89**, 11. 19. Am. J. Dis. Child., 1929, **37**, 252. 20. Am. Heart J., 1928, **4**, 145. 21. The Factor of Infection in the Rheumatic State, 1931. 22. Am. Heart J., 1927, **2**, 375. 23. Medit. Prebavlena K. Moskowa Sboneskie, 1887; Ref. Dunn, J.A.M.A., 1907, **48**, 494. 24. Lancet, 1900, **2**, 861; 1910, **1**, 1524. 25. Lancet, 1912, **2**, 1209. 26. J.A.M.A., 1913, **60**, 1223. 27. J. Exper. Med., 1929, **50**, 617. 28. Monatschr. f. Kinderh., 1929, **43**, 462. 29. Am. J. M. Sc., 1927, **173**, 101; 1928, **175**, 638; 650. 30. J. Inf. Dis., 1927, **40**, 549; 1928, **42**, 25; 1929, **44**, 363. 31. J.A.M.A., 1929, **92**, 2071; Am. Heart J. 1931, **6**, 625; Am. J. M. Sc., 1931, **181**, 1. 32. Arch. Int. Med., 1928, **42**, 301. 33. Wien. klin. Wchnschr., 1928, **41**, 473. 34. Verhandl. d.

deutsch. path. Gesellsch., 1904, **8,** 46; Brit. M. J., 1906, **2,** 1103. 35. Lancet, 1930, **2,** 394. 36. Am. J. Dis. Child., 1931, **42,** 9. 37. Am. J. Dis. Child., 1931, **42,** 503. 38. Bristol Med. Chir. J., 1907, **25,** 193. 39. J.A.M.A., 1924, **82,** 759. 40. Brit. M. J., 1930, **1,** 227. 41. J. Exper. Med., 1924, **39,** 1. 42. J.A.M.A., 1932, **98,** 1978. 43. Ztschr. f. Kinderh., 1926, **41,** 394. 44. Lyon méd., 1875, **20,** 495. 45. Trans. Internat. Med. Cong., 1881, **4,** 116. 46. Am. J. M. Sc., 1923, **165,** 781. 47. Arch. Pediat., 1924, **41,** 731. 48. Am. J. Dis. Child., 1928, **35,** 823. 49. The Practitioner, 1914, **93,** 445. 50. Am. J. Dis. Child., 1931, **42,** 42. 51. Ann. Int. Med., 1929, **2,** 637. 52. J.A.M.A., 1930, **94,** 842. 53. Am. J. M. Sc., 1914, **147,** 423; 1921, **161,** 517; 1929, **178,** 593; 606. 54. Arch. Int. Med., 1922, **30,** 106; Arthritis and Rheumatoid Conditions, 1929. 55. Lancet, 1925, **1,** 1205. 56. J.A.M.A., 1914, **62,** 1146. 57. J.A.M.A., 1929, **93,** 692. 58. Arch. Int. Med., 1929, **43,** 571; Am. J. M. Sc., 1931, **181,** 12; J.A.M.A., 1931, **79,** 1146. 59. Arch. Surg., 1929, **18,** 645. 60. Med. Chir. Trans., 1897, **80,** 47. 61. Arch. Pediat., 1927, **44,** 187. 62. Wien. klin. Wchnschr., 1928, **41,** 1255. 63. Strahlentherapie, 1931, **42,** 423. 64. J.A.M.A., 1927, **88,** 694. 65. Deutsche med. Wchnschr., 1928, **54,** 566.

CHAPTER VI

CONSTITUTION AND THE DIATHESES

Among the students of constitution should be mentioned Kretschmer,[1] Draper,[2] Pende,[3] and Stockard;[4] and in children especially Masslow,[5] Bakwin and Bakwin,[6] and Lucas and Pryor.[7] (See also p. 14.)

By *constitution* may be designated the aggregate of characters which determine the individual's reaction to environment, and it is usually stated that these attributes are transmitted through the germ-plasm and are little, if any, influenced by environment. This definition is not greatly different from that which may be given for the term *diathesis,* by which is indicated a constitutional tendency to the development of certain sorts of diseases varying with the individual; a tendency which makes the same acting cause vary in the character of the symptoms produced. The influence of constitutional tendencies was strongly emphasized for a number of years, and then for a long time ignored. Recently it has become evident that neither infection nor any other active cause is sufficient by itself to account for the development of certain disorders in certain persons; and that diatheses do, in fact, exist. Without the necessity of employing either of these terms, there is recognized the inheritance of peculiarities of metadolism, of body-structure, and of tissue-predisposition, resulting in such conditions as hemophilia, albinism, blue sclera, hemolytic icterus, cleidocranial dysostosis, and the like, some of which are transmitted according to Mendelian laws, the predisposition residing in the chromosomes.

It is not necessary to discuss the various classifications of constitution, some of them quite detailed. Further statistical and biometrical studies are needed before these can be adapted more definitely to clinical practice and tendencies to disease, and physical and mental characteristics linked to them. There are, however, two main corporeal types, typical examples of which are not often seen; gradations and combinations existing among them. These are the *linear* or tall, thin type, which is apt to be associated with an active, nervous disposition; and the *lateral* or short, round type, associated with a more phlegmatic disposition and greater physical power.

With regard to the *diatheses,* various ones have been described; the definitions differing somewhat with the writer, and the boundary-lines not being sharply marked. There is frequently a combination of certain of them in the same individual. The neuropathic, including spasmophilia, is described elsewhere (p. 869), and here will be considered only the exudative and lymphatic diatheses.

EXUDATIVE DIATHESIS

Etiology.—This title was applied by Czerny[8] to subjects in whom, with other symptoms, there is a tendency to *exudation*, or inflammation, of the skin and mucous membrane. It covers many of the symptoms formerly described as "scrofulous," but is in no way connected etiologically with tuberculosis. It occurs chiefly in the first year of life, but to a lesser extent also after this period. It is to a considerable degree hereditary and familial. A number of authors attribute the condition to dysfunction of the autonomic nervous system. Apart from the constitutional tendency, the symptoms are brought on or increased by an improper diet, such as one containing an excess of food of any sort, particularly one too largely of milk, and, most of all, of fat. It is possible that in some cases the protein may be especially at fault. The question arises whether there is some direct association between the exudative diathesis and allergy. (See Allergy, p. 485.)

Symptoms.—The disease manifests itself in infancy by an unusual disposition to the development of seborrhea of the scalp and face, and later of eczema; the latter often extending over much of the body. Catarrhal inflammation of the upper and lower respiratory tracts is frequent. Some enlargement of the lymph-nodes may be found, but decided and extensive hypertrophy is not a characteristic. The infants are usually too fat, but flabby and anemic, and readily suffer elevations of temperature. In other cases they are thin even before symptoms appear, or become debilitated and lose flesh through the constant irritation and loss of sleep brought about by the itching of an eczema, or without this. The blood, as in allergy, shows an increase of the eosinophilic cells. It is claimed that the retention of chlorides is increased. Herlitz[9] found diminished sugar-tolerance when the cutaneous eruption first began, although later the tolerance became normal. The fat-content of the blood is said to be diminished (Schippers[10]).

After the period of infancy eczema may be replaced by asthma, recurrent bronchitis, obstinate cough, pruritus, lichen, or urticaria. The geographical tongue is a common symptom. Vasomotor disturbances are frequent, such as palpitation, rises of temperature, and the like. It is uncertain whether the phlyctenules which appear on the conjunctiva in children are symptoms of the exudative diatheses, or are always actual tuberculous lesions.

In the category of the exudative diathesis perhaps belong, too, many of the cases of *arthritism* in children, described by Comby,[11] and others. The symptoms of this are variable and multiform. Prominent among them are those just detailed, and in addition attacks of vomiting (recurrent vomiting), arthralgia, headache, neuralgia, vertigo, and various other nervous and vasomotor disturbances.

Course and Prognosis.—The tendency to eczema diminishes greatly after the first year, and in general the exudative manifestations are prone to ameliorate and soon to cease. Generally they are gone by the time puberty is reached. They do not often in themselves constitute an element of danger.

Diagnosis.—This rests upon the symptoms as already outlined. Scrofulo-tuberculosis may, it is true, develop in children with the exudative diathesis, but the eczema and catarrhal condition of the latter have nothing in common with the glandular inflammation, chronic conjunctivitis and keratitis, and severe chronic catarrhal processes of the former; although it is possible that the existence of the exudative condition predisposes to a tuberculous infection producing the symptoms often called scrofula. Status lymphaticus is characterized by decided hypertrophy of the lymphatic tissues throughout the body, including the thymus gland, and by a tendency to sudden death; but not by eczema or catarrhal processes. It is, however, frequently combined with the exudative diathesis.

The diagnosis is aided by the efforts to discover whether any protein can be found to be causative. (See Allergy, p. 486.)

Treatment.—Only the passing of time will cure the constitutional predisposition, and treatment is chiefly dietetic. The fat in the food must be reduced, and, indeed, the total amount of food given usually diminished as well, and care taken to prevent the children from gaining weight rapidly. Starchy addition to the diet should be commenced at once on the appearance of symptoms, and this made to replace milk to a considerable extent.

LYMPHATIC DIATHESIS

(Lymphatism. Status Lymphaticus)

This disorder would appear to be a constitutional condition in which there are present a diminished resistance of the entire organism to morbid influences, and a predisposition to sudden death. Anatomically there is a tendency to general hyperplasia of the lymphoid tissues throughout the body, including the thymus gland. It must be borne in mind, however, that in normal children, and even in the new-born, cervical, axillary, and other glands are discoverable by careful palpation. (See p. 43.) The close association of lymphatism with sudden death and thymic enlargement was emphasized by Paltauf,[12] while Escherich[13] maintained that the condition was a toxemia, the origin of which was the hypertrophied thymus gland. It is possible that lymphatic overgrowth is the direct cause of the symptoms, and that the enlargement of the thymus gland is a concomitant accidental or compensatory process. The theory has been advanced by Heubner[14] and others, and has much in its favor, that the disorder is a constitutional anomaly consequent upon some chemical alteration of the tissues, independent of lymphatic or thymic enlargement, although these are likely to appear among the later symptoms. Personal experience has led us to the belief that the enlargement of the thymus, and perhaps too of the lymphatic glands, is a secondary matter, and can be entirely absent in cases of sudden death, and present in those dying of other causes. The extensive studies of Hammar[15] confirm this view. (See also Sudden Death, p. 174, and Enlargement of the Thymus, p. 1077.)

Etiology.—A distinct family disposition is seen in many instances. We[16] have reported the occurrence of nine sudden deaths from lymphatism in one family of children. The disease is observed especially in infancy and early childhood, but may exist in adult life. Even the new-born and very young infants may exhibit it; and many instances of death have been wrongly attributed to suffocation through overlying, or brought about in other ways. Sex, race and season exert no influence. Rickets, spasmophilia, and the exudative diathesis may be associated with the lymphatic diathesis but have no etiologic connection.

Pathologic Anatomy.—The noteworthy feature often found at necropsy is the hyperplasia of lymphoid tissue. This is seen particularly in the thymus gland, which is frequently abnormally large. In determining the existence of enlargement the great variation in size of the normal thymus gland in different children is to be taken into account, as well as the age of the patient. (See pp. 43, 1074.) In addition to this lesion there is commonly more or less hypertrophy of the lymphoid tissue throughout the body. There is usually moderate enlargement of the spleen, with prominence of the Malpighian bodies. The liver is often fatty and the cardiac muscle may show degeneration. Hypertrophy of the heart has been observed by Riesenfeld[17] and Rieder.[18]

Symptoms.—These are often vague or even unnoticed; often sufficiently well-marked, but varied. The frequent association of the exudative diathesis accounts for the tendency to seborrhea and eczema so often seen. Hypertrophy of the tonsils, the nasopharyngeal lymphatic tissue, and the superficial lymph-nodes is generally discovered. The spleen is often found enlarged, and sometimes hypertrophy of the thymus gland may be discovered through percussion or more often through roentgenography. (See Diseases of the Thymus Gland, p. 1074.) The combination of the neuropathic diathesis or of spasmophilia frequently observed accounts for the occurrence of convulsions, dyspnea, fever from insignificant causes, and larynogospasm; but it is not certain how often this is the case, and how many instances, especially of the last mentioned, depend purely upon lymphatism. The children are usually phlegmatic, flabby, fat, inactive, pale, and of little strength. There is increased susceptibility to disease, and infections of any sort may produce an unusually well-marked reaction.

Of all symptoms, however, the most important is the danger of sudden death. This often appears to be respiratory from asphyxia and cyanosis, but probably in most cases is cardiac, as was pointed out by Pott,[19] the accident occurring without discoverable reason; or following very insignificant trauma, such as a hypodermic injection, an exploratory puncture, the giving of diphtheria-antitoxin, and the like; or being produced by the shock from cold water, the use of a tongue-depressor, the administration of an anesthetic, or the occurrence of some mild acute disease; or often without there having been any previous symptoms whatever. The patient suffers from a sudden, apparently suffocative attack, throws the head back, turns pale, or perhaps bluish, and sometimes dies in an instant; or the child may possibly be found dead in bed without any symptoms having been observed. Sometimes attacks which appear to be laryngospasm, or symptoms suggesting asphyxia from other causes, may be present for several hours; or there may be a series of short attacks of the nature described occurring during some weeks or longer, and the patient at last dies in one of these. We have known such short attacks to be of very great frequency. Thus in one case the mother, a foreigner with little command of English, said of her child that it "died every day."

Prognosis.—For the milder cases the prognosis is on the whole good, the pathologic tendency disappearing as the patient grows older, and particularly as puberty is approached. On the other hand, there is always the possibility of sudden death.

Diagnosis.—This can be made if, with the symptoms described, the distinct evidences of lymphatic hyperplasia are discoverable. A roentgenogram may show hypertrophy of the thymus gland. Discovery by the same means of enlarged tracheobronchial lymph-nodes does not determine whether these are dependent upon tuberculosis or upon the lymphatic diathesis. Similarly the hypertrophy of the tonsillar tissue of the fauces and nasopharynx is not by itself sufficient to warrant a diagnosis of lymphatism, although it is a characteristic of this condition. Often, in fact, lymphatism is entirely unsuspected until sudden death occurs and necropsy shows general hypertrophy of the lymphatic tissue of the body.

Treatment.—The only treatment possible is the careful regulation of the diet and hygiene. Gymnastic exercises and massage may improve the general health. Suitable tonics may be employed to increase the patient's strength and remove anemia. Great care must be taken to avoid the causes which bring about a sudden fatal termination. The use of an anesthetic must be refrained from if it can be avoided, and, indeed, no operation performed which can in any way be omitted. Cool bathing may be dangerous, as may any sudden mental or other physical shock. Even the giving of antitoxin is to be regarded with anxiety, and the objections to it must be carefully weighed before a decision is reached. When the symptoms have clearly pointed to pressure by the thymus gland roentgenological treatment is indicated, but in all other cases it seems doubtful whether apparent improvement can properly be associated with the shrinking of the thymus gland, inasmuch as its enlargement is probably the result and not the cause of lymphatism and its dangerous symptoms

References

1. Körperbau und Charakter, 1922. 2. Human Constitution, 1924. 3. Constitut. Inadequacies, 1928. 4. The Physical Basis of Personality, 1931. 5. Acta paediat., 1927, **7**, 60. 6. Am. J. Dis. Child., 1929, **37**, 461. 7. J.A.M.A., 1931, **97**, 1127. 8. Jahrb. f. Kinderh., 1905, **61**, 199. 9. Acta paediat., 1928, **7**, 1; 286. 10. Nederl. Tijdschr. v. Geneesk., 1920, **2**, 1081. 11. Arch. de méd. d. enf., 1902, **5**, 1; 65. 12. Wien. klin. Wchnschr., 1889, **2**, 877; 1890, **3**, 172. 13. Berl. klin. Wchnschr., 1896, **33**, 645. 14. Lehrb. d. Kinderh., 1911, **2**, 33. 15. Ztschr. f. Kinderh., 1916–17, **15**, 225; Upsala Läkaref. Forhandl., 1922, n. f. **27**, 147. 16. Griffith, New York M. J., 1909, **90**, 444. 17. Jahrb. f. Kinderh., 1917, **86**, 419. 18. Jahrb. f. Kinderh., 1922, **97**, 9. 19. Jahrb. f. Kinderh., 1892, **34**, 118.

CHAPTER VII

ALLERGY

Great confusion exists in the terminology of this subject, and only further study can settle the differences in the opinions expressed. For the present it may be assumed that the word *allergy* (first used by von Pirquet[1] in connection with tuberculin) denotes an altered power of reaction of tissues to certain agents, which in the same dose are harmless to the normal organism. It may be inherited or acquired, antigenic (capable of inciting antibody-formation) in character or not, and in the direction of increased or reduced sensitivity (Wells[2]). The term *atopy* has been used either as synonymous with allergy, or as confined to inherited hypersensitivity in which specific antibodies are found in the blood-stream. The title *anaphylaxis* designates, in a strict sense, the experimental acquisition of hypersensitiveness, brought about by previous injections of proteins (Coca[3]). In all probability allergy and anaphylaxis are identical (Ratner, Jackson and Gruehl;[4] Ratner;[5] Peshkin[6]). Until it is definitely settled whether nonprotein substances can cause antibody-formation, or, in other words, act as antigens, or allergens, the term "*idiosyncrasy*" might be employed for allergic-like reactions against certain drugs, light, and material apparently lipoid in character. What follows is in outline, particularly insofar as the subject bears upon early life, and groups all the manifestations under the one title, allergy.

Etiology.—The mechanism by which allergy is brought about is not fully understood. (For further discussion of this see Wells,[2] and Coca[7].) Allergy may occur from the ingestion of animal and vegetable proteins; from the inhalation of plant-pollens or other products of vegetation, or of emanations from animals; by contact of the intact or broken skin or mucous membrane with plant or animal hairs; and by parenteral injection of blood from other animals. Possibly certain symptoms produced by some animal parasites are allergic in nature. Some effects caused by bacteria are due to their antigenic properties.

Infants who have received only human milk may react to substances never ingested by them. This might be due to inherited tendency but, on the other hand, it has been shown that breast-milk may transmit protein (Shannon;[8] Donnally[9]) ingested by the mother and unaltered. That this can then render infants sensitive by absorption from their intestinal tract has been demonstrated in athreptic infants by Anderson and Schloss[10] and in normal infants by Grulee and Bonar,[11] Walzer,[12] and Coca.[13] It has been shown by Kuttner and Ratner,[14] Ratner, Jackson and Gruehl,[4] and Ratner[5] that the human placenta is permeable to certain proteins and hypersensitiveness could be transmitted in this way.

The average frequency in children of positive response to cutaneous tests with proteins, yet without clinical evidence of allergy, is about 10 to 15 per cent, but in subjects with eczema, hay fever, and asthma this may be as great as 35, 50, or even 70 per cent, the proteins naturally varying with the case.

Symptoms.—In *hypersensitiveness to food-proteins*, and less commonly among these to *cow's milk*, the ingestion of even a small quantity of the substance may result immediately in projectile vomiting; swelling of the mucous membranes with sneezing; erythema, urticaria, and in some instances dyspnea and shock. The symptoms are not often so decided and acute, and it is possible that certain more or less chronic gastro-intestinal disturbances, especially if associated with cutaneous manifestations, may be allergic in nature. *Serum-sickness* may occur in two forms. In the first, which is rare, there develop within a few minutes great dyspnea, cardiac embarrassment with dilatation of the right heart, cyanosis, vomiting, and perhaps convulsions and death. Similar symptoms with death have also followed the injection of pollens. Waldbott[15] reviews 9 fatal cases, 6 due to diphtheria antitoxin, 2 to tetanus antitoxin, and 1 to ragweed-pollen. These serious reactions occur almost invariably after the first injection, rather than after later ones. If serum has been given within six days and no reaction has occurred, there is little danger in repeating the dose. Ratner[16] found that in some instances of reaction to horse-serum the patients were sensitive to horse-dander, and that an anaphylactic relationship existed between this and horse-serum. The second, or usual, type of serum-reaction gives symptoms only after an interval of about a week, this being shortened when there have been several previous injections. There may be only erythema and urticaria, or in addition, or independently, fever, malaise, leukopenia, eosinophilia, albuminuria, pain and swelling of the joints, edema, sneezing, enlargement of the lymph-nodes, and poly-neuritis. In this connection may be mentioned the possibility of producing sensitization by injection even of the small amount of horse-serum present in diphtheria toxin-antitoxin (0.0001 cc. in each dose), or of the occurrence of symptoms from its injection in a subject already allergic. This danger has been denied, but there seems little doubt that it exists. Ordinarily, however, there is a quantitative relationship, and serum-sickness is more liable to occur after large doses than after small ones. According to Park[17] 1 in 20,000 serum-injections is followed by alarming symptoms and 1 in 50,000 by death. *Local necrosis* (the phenomenon of Arthus[18]) may occur at the site of serum-injections, usually only after several previous injections of the same type of serum have been given. After *blood-transfusion* allergic phenonema may rarely follow.

Allergy as related to asthma (p. 710), hay-fever (p. 689), urticaria (p. 1094) and eczema (p. 1103) will be discussed in the respective sections. A large number of other conditions have been attributed to allergy, among them being erythema multiforme, dermatitis venenata, certain cases of cyclic vomiting (Schloss;[19] Le Boutillier[20]), abdominal pain and other intestinal symptoms (Duke;[21] Rowe[22]), headache (Brown[23]) and epilepsy Spangler;[24] Lewin[25]). The connection of these with allergy is problematical, and especially in the case of epilepsy, allergy, if present, would seem to be only an initiating factor. In the category of allergy have also been placed by some the modified local reaction occurring in a successfully vaccinated person, and the local and general symptoms following the injection of tuberculin, as well as infection by the tubercle bacillus.

It is interesting to note that Balyeat[26] is convinced that allergic children are above the physical and mental norm.

Diagnosis.—An inherited tendency to hypersensitiveness may be suspected if the family-history reveals the occurrence of eczema, asthma, hay-fever or urticaria. Contact with, or the inhalation, ingestion, or hypodermic injection of the offending proteins, may be followed by definite allergic manifestations, and the avoidance of these proteins may result in cessation of symptoms. The test with purified protein-substances may be made on the scarified skin or intracutaneously. A large variety of proteins ready for use in testing are procurable. When in paste form a small amount is gently rubbed upon the skin which has been previously slightly scarified. If the powdered form is employed it is necessary first to apply a drop of a decinormal sodium hydrate solution to the point of scarification, after which a small amount of the protein material is mixed with this solution and rubbed in. The amount of paste or powder which can be carried on the end of a small flat wooden toothpick is sufficient, a fresh toothpick being used for each protein to avoid contamination. In scarifying it is better not to draw blood. A small scratch, $\frac{1}{8}$ in. (0.32 cm.) long, may be made with a scalpel, or a Pirquet borer or a Hagedorn needle may be employed. The scarification may be done on the forearm or back, the latter region being preferable in a struggling child. A positive reaction appears in five or ten minutes and persists for about thirty minutes. It consists of an urticarial wheal 5 mm. (0.2 in.) or more in diameter, with irregular raised edges surrounded by a red areola. A smaller wheal, or the occurrence of erythema alone, constitutes a doubtful reaction. Occasionally the reaction is delayed. A control test, in which protein is not employed, should always be made on the sensitive skin near the bend of the elbow.

The intracutaneous test, although more sensitive, is more prone to cause general reactions. Such occurrences, either from intracutaneous tests or from injections for the purpose of desensitization, have been reported by Schloss,[19] Gerstenberger and Davis,[27] Park,[28] Cooke,[29] Waldbott,[15] and Lamson,[30] the last three authors recording instances with a fatal issue. Ophthalmic and nasal tests are sometimes used in the diagnosis of hay-fever.

A negative cutaneous reaction does not necessarily mean that the patient is not sensitive to the particular protein, nor does a positive one indicate that he will develop allergic symptoms when brought into contact with the substance employed in the test. In other words, cutaneous sensitivity is not necessarily synonymous with sensitivity of other parts of the body. It is not always possible or desirable to do many tests in an individual case. The history may suggest the causative substance. Certain manifestations point toward definite groups of proteins. Thus hay-fever is frequently dependent upon pollens; asthma upon pollens, animal emanations or hairs; gastro-intestinal and cutaneous symptoms upon ingested animal or vegetable proteins. To spare unnecessary scarifications in a child the proteins may be mixed, and a group of several tested together; a negative reaction ruling out the group, a positive one necessitating individual tests of the proteins of the group.

Treatment.—The patient should be protected from proteins which offend, whether by contact, ingestion, or in other ways. If this is done, sensitiveness may cease after several months. Other proteins may at times be successfully substituted in the diet. Thus human milk or goat's milk (p. 82) may be given instead of cow's milk. Hill[31] recommends a preparation devoid of cow's milk and consisting of soy bean, olive oil, barley flour and salts ("Sobee"). In mild cases the protein may be altered without changing its variety. For example, milk boiled for an hour or two, or dried or evaporated milk, may sometimes cause no symptoms in infants sensitive to raw milk. A proprietary heat-treated milk denominated Hypo-allergic Milk is available. Heat probably acts by changing the milk-proteins in a way which makes it difficult for them to be absorbed by the intestinal tract, and this fact may be taken advantage of with other proteins. Thus wheat may be tolerated in toast or in some of the prepared cereals when not borne otherwise, or a baked potato may be harmless although one less heated by boiling may not. When cutaneous tests are not performed, or if there is some question of their interpretation, a simple diet may be ordered, and one new food added at a time while symptoms are watched for. Care must be taken, however, that children be not kept too long on a diet restricted in protein or improperly balanced in other ways.

When it is not possible or advisable to eliminate the offending proteins from the diet, the effort may be made to create tolerance for them. In allergy to cow's milk, for example, as little as 0.1 cc. (1.6 minim), or less if this produces symptoms, should be given and this amount slowly augmented, always keeping it below that which causes symptoms. Usually after 5 or 10 cc. (0.17 or 0.3 fl. oz.) can be tolerated the advance may be made rapidly. The same procedure may be followed with such proteins as egg-albumin or beef-juice.

Another method of desensitization is by hypodermic injection, especially practiced with pollens or animal emanations. This is not without danger (p. 485). Dilutions of the protein are made varying from 1:1,000,000 up to 1:10 in a centinormal sodium hydroxide solution. A cutaneous test is first done with these, and 0.1 cc. of that dilution which does not cause a reaction is then injected. After several injections of this dilution are given at three day intervals, increasing 0.1 cc. with each treatment, a stronger one is tested on the skin, and if no reaction occurs the dilution of this strength is injected in increasing amounts, the process being continued until tolerance is established to strong dilutions such as 1:100 or even 1:10.

In patients in whom allergy is known or suspected to be present, or, in fact, in anyone receiving serum, it is well to make a cutaneous test with a drop of the serum, or an intracutaneous test with 1:5 or 1:10 dilution of it. If this proves positive, and even when it is negative in persons with a strong family or personal history of allergy, the so-called "rapid desensitization" originally recommended by Besredka[32] should be carried out. An injection of 0.1 cc. of serum or less is given intramuscularly or subcutaneously, followed in one-half hour by 0.3 cc., in one hour by 0.5 cc., and in two hours by 1.0 cc. In two hours more, if no symptoms have occurred, subsequent injections may be given every three or four hours in gradually increasing doses. Such a procedure does not guarantee absence of reaction. In such cases, too, intravenous injections of serum should be avoided since they are more likely than subcutaneous or intramuscular ones to produce severe reactions. Certain therapeutical goat and sheep sera are available, and may be employed in case of sensitivity to horse-serum. It has also been recommended by Cooke,[29] Insley,[33] and others that a tourniquet or blood-pressure apparatus be applied above the point of injection and the pressure gradually released so as to permit less rapid dissemination of the protein into the tissues. The more acute manifestations of allergy may be relieved by injection of 0.2 to 0.5 cc. (3 to 8 minims) of a 1:1000 solution of adrenaline, repeated every ten minutes if necessary. Hypodermic injections of atropine and pituitrin are also effective in some cases. It is held by Duke;[34] Derick, Hitchcock and Swift;[35] Kinsella[36] and others that salicylates have an ameliorating effect on some of the allergic manifestations. The administration of preparations of calcium and of phosphorus has been found of benefit by Sterling.[37]

References

1. Wien. med. Wchnschr., 1907, **57,** 1370. 2. The Chemic. Aspects of Immunity-1925. 3. J. Immunol., 1920, **5,** 363. 4. J. Immunol., 1927, **15,** 249. 5. Am. J. Dis. Child., 1928, **36,** 277. 6. Am. J. Dis. Child., 1928, **36,** 89. 7. Coca, Walzer and Thommen, Asthma and Hay Fever, Etc., Pt. 1., 1931. 8. Am. J. Dis. Child., 1921, **22,** 223. 9. J. Immunol., 1930, **19,** 15. 10. Am. J. Dis. Child., 1923, **26,** 451. 11. Am. J. Dis. Child., 1921, **21,** 89. 12. J. Immunol., 1926, **11,** 249. 13. J. Immunol., 1930, **19,** 405. 14. Am. J. Dis. Child., 1923, **25,** 413. 15. J.A.M.A., 1932, **98,** 446. 16. J.A.M.A., 1930, **94,** 2046. 17. Am. J. Pub. Health, 1928, **18,** 354. 18. Compt. rend. soc. de biol., 1903, **55,** 817. 19. Am. J. Dis. Child., 1920, **19,** 433. 20. Arch. Pediat., 1922, **39,** 308. 21. Arch. Int. Med., 1921, **28,** 151. 22. J. Lab. and Clin. Med., 1927, **13,** 31; J.A.M.A., 1931, **97,** 1440. 23. Wisconsin M. J., 1920, **19,** 337. 24. Med. J. and Rec., 1925, **122,** 317. 25. J.A.M.A., 1931, **97,** 1624. 26. Am. J. Dis. Child., 1929, **37,** 1193. 27. J.A.M.A., 1921, **76,** 721. 28. Am. J. Dis. Child., 1920, **19,** 46. 29. J. Immunol., 1922, **7,** 119. 30. J.A.M.A., 1929, **93,** 1775. 31. J.A.M.A., 1929, **93,** 985. 32. Comp. rend. soc. de biol., 1908, **65,** 478. 33. J.A.M.A., 1930, **94,** 765. 34. Arch. Otolaryngol., 1928, **8,** 573. 35. J. Clin. Investig., 1928, **5,** 427. 36. J.A.M.A., 1929, **93,** 1534. 37. J. Lab. and Clin. Med., 1928, **13,** 997.

CHAPTER VIII

DISTURBANCES OF ACID-BASE BALANCE OF THE BODY

(Acidosis; Alkalosis)

Under normal conditions the balance between acid and basic substances in the blood and tissue-fluids is maintained with remarkable constancy by means of "buffer" substances, such as hemoglobin, bicarbonate, proteins other than hemoglobin, and phosphate. Base bicarbonate ($BHCO_3$)* and carbonic acid (H_2CO_3) may be considered as a system which normally exists in the ratio of about 60 vol. per cent $BHCO_3$: 3 vol. per cent H_2CO_3, and this constitutes a "first line of defense" against changes in the acid-base balance. When abnormal acids (β-oxybutyric in diabetes, starvation, etc.) or an excess of normal acids (lactic acid in exercise; acid phosphate in renal disease and anhydremia; CO_2 in respiratory diseases or with narcotics, etc.) must be neutralized, the acid carbon dioxide is rapidly excreted through the lungs, and the base, previously bound as bicarbonate, is thus freed, or available, and combines with these acids. This base bound as bicarbonate is spoken of as "alkali reserve of the body," after the designation by Van Slyke and Cullen.[1] The ratio of base-bicarbonate to carbonic acid determines the hydrogen-ion concentration of the blood-plasma, which, if the normal 60:3 relationship is maintained, ranges from about 7.3 to 7.5 pH. (The hydrogen-ion concentration ($H+$) is expressed in terms of pH. It must be remembered that as $H+$ increases, pH decreases and vice versa.) There are other means for maintaining acid-base equilibrium in the body. For example, the base of the blood-phosphate neutralizes acids and excretes them as acid-phosphate through the kidney, provided this is functionally active; a certain amount of the acid is excreted as ammonia-salts; and hemo-

* $BHCO_3$ contains both sodium and potassium bicarbonate.

globin, by virtue of its ability to change its acid strength with changes in its oxygen content, takes care in the respiratory cycle of about 90 per cent of the acid-base shift incidental to the production and elimination of carbon dioxide.

"Acidosis," in its true sense, denotes that the hydrogen-ion concentration has shifted to the acid side (lowered pH), and that the alkali reserve is lowered (lowered $BHCO_3$), *i. e.*, the acidosis is "uncompensated." Often, however, the respiratory mechanism, by elimination of the acid carbon dioxide, keeps the pH within normal limits, and the acidosis is "compensated."

"Alkalosis" by analogy indicates an increase of the alkali reserve, and the terms "compensated" and "uncompensated" denote that the increased alkali reserve is associated with a normal or with a high pH respectively.

Much confusion has been caused by failure to distinguish between the conditions of acidosis and ketosis, and those of acetonuria and ketonuria. "Ketosis" is an acidosis of the body resulting from accumulation of ketone bodies (β-oxybutyric acid and aceto-acetic acid); "ketonuria" or "acetonuria" literally meaning only that the urine contains these substances. Ketonuria may or may not be associated with an acidosis. Accumulation of the ketone acids in the body in certain forms of acidosis leads to an increase of ketones in the urine, but in the acidosis from the retention of other acid substances this elimination of ketone need not occur. On the other hand, ketone bodies are often normally present in the blood and urine of healthy children (Veeder and Johnson;[2] Moore[3]) and are always increased in starvation due to any cause, often then without acidosis. Ketonuria frequently accompanies severe vomiting, and is often present even though the blood-picture may be one of alkalosis. The most common mistake in terminology is the employment of the terms "acidosis" and "alkalosis" in the sense of primary diseases. A disturbed acid-base balance is always the result of some physiological derangement, and if severe and of long duration this disturbance will in turn cause damage to the tissues and organs because of the change in cell-environment.

Because of confusion concerning the terms "acidosis" and "alkalosis" recent investigators are abandoning them, and describing disturbances of the acid-base balance in terms of the primary causes. In the most recent and complete discussion of this subject Peters and Van Slyke[4] divide abnormal acid-base conditions into those due to metabolic disturbances and those due to respiratory causes, and use the terms "carbon dioxide excess and deficit," and "alkali excess and deficit."

PRIMARY ALKALI DEFICIT

(*A*) Metabolic Type.—This is the most frequent of the clinical conditions for which the term "acidosis" has been employed. It is due either to *loss of alkali* or to *retention of acids.* Loss of alkali is most common in severe diarrhea. When loss of water is excessive and dehydration results, the initial alkali deficit, due to loss of base secreted and passed into the intestine, may be aggravated by unusual accumulation of acid, either from faulty metabolism or faulty elimination. Retention of acid, which includes production of organic acids faster than they can be excreted, is common in diabetes, nephritis, starvation, dehydration, and in practically all moribund states. The relation between dehydration and acidosis is most intricate. It is usually stated that acidosis is a result of dehydration, but it is probable that the reverse is often true. The most common symptom of this type of acidosis is hyperpnea (deep, exaggerated breathing), which may or may not be evident when the alkali reserve is diminished to one-half the normal, but which always develops as the acidosis increases beyond that point.

Other symptoms vary. There may be restlessness, headache, nausea, convulsions, or drowsiness. In the final stages coma is usually present, and the hyperpnea increases until shortly before death. The only circulatory symptom is tachycardia. The **diagnosis** depends upon the symptoms described; the association of these with a condition liable to result in acidosis; and an examination of the blood for its carbon dioxide (CO_2) value and perhaps its pH value, both of which may be decreased, the latter in uncompensated acidosis. A knowledge of the "CO_2 content" is preferable to that of the "CO_2 capacity," since the former gives the actual value in the circulating blood, while the latter may vary with the cell-volume and cause confusion in anemia and other conditions. Even in health both CO_2 and pH may vary in the same individual within a small range. The CO_2 content is an index of the alkali reserve; a diminution of it indicating acidosis and an increase alkalosis. In the venous blood taken without stasis the CO_2 content ranges from about 55 to 75 vol. per cent, and the pH from 7.33 to 7.51 (Earle and Cullen[5]). In the way of **treatment** there should be an attempt at prevention by recognition of the causes of acidosis and prompt control of diarrhea, free administration of fluid in illness, careful regulation of diabetes, attempts at elimination and diuresis in nephritis, and the like. When the condition is established its treatment differs with its cause. In *diarrhea* and *enteritis*, restoration of fluid is important, and, since there has been actual loss of base, bicarbonate is useful. There are at present two distinct schools of thought, one holding that restoration of fluid with normal salt solution and glucose is sufficient; the other that bicarbonate also is needed. (See Gastro-enteric Infection p. 590.) Bicarbonate of soda should be given preferably only after a blood-examination has been made to determine the degree of alkali deficit; and sufficient bicarbonate may then be administered to restore it to normal. If the examination is not feasible, coma or impending coma may be used as a criterion, and usually hyperpnea also, although this latter may occasionally be found in alkalosis. Under any condition the administration of bicarbonate should be stopped when the urine becomes alkaline to phenol-red (pH 7). In normal infants from 2 to 3 Gm. (31 to 46 grains) and in older children from 4 to 5 Gm. (62 to 77 grains) will usually render the urine alkaline, but in acidosis perhaps from four to ten times this amount will be required (Howland and Marriott[6]). In urgent cases a 4 to 5 per cent solution of sodium bicarbonate may be given intravenously, employing from 75 to 100 cc. (2.5 to 3.3 fl. oz.) or more of this, and determining the amount and the frequency of administration by examination of the CO_2 content of the blood, or, less safely, by the reaction of the urine. Soda may also be given by hypodermoclysis (p. 184). Palmer and Van Slyke[7] found that 0.026 Gm. of $NaHCO_3$ per kilometer is required to raise the plasma CO_2 content 1 vol. per cent. The usual dose of 0.5 Gm. per kilo raises the CO_2 by about 20 vol. per cent. In any case, not more than half the amount of bicarbonate calculated to restore the plasma $BHCO_3$ to normal should be given without the determination of the resulting level in the plasma. (See also Gastro-enteric Infection, p. 590.) In *diabetic coma* prompt and adequate insulin therapy can restore the body to a normal acid-base balance within twenty-four hours. When insulin is employed most authorities agree that bicarbonate is not needed. Glucose should also be given in 5 per cent solution, using 100 to 200 cc. (3.3 to 6.7 fl. oz.) or more by mouth, hypodermically, or intravenously. (See Diabetes p. 499.) In *retention of acid waste-products* due to damaged kidneys the acid-base balance may be temporarily restored to normal by adequate bicarbonate administration. In severe nephritic conditions convulsions may be quieted and coma relieved. When the condition is an acute one, such a procedure may be life-saving, but in the terminal stage of nephritis the relief is only temporary. It should be remembered that in renal disease the symptoms of acidosis are often indistinguishable from those of uremia, and the diagnosis and treatment must depend on blood-analysis; and also that acidosis may be combined with uremia. (See Nephritis, p. 827.)

(*B*) Respiratory Type.—This form of acidosis occurs when there is an excess of carbon dioxide in the blood, as in asphyxial states or with a poor elimination of the acid in respiratory diseases. There will here be a lowered pH but an increased CO_2 capacity or tension. Its treatment consists in the correction or alleviation of the cause, and the administration of oxygen if dyspnea exists. Other treatment is not necessary.

PRIMARY ALKALI EXCESS

(*A*) Metabolic Type.—This form of alkalosis arises in two ways. (1) Loss of hydrochloric acid from the stomach during severe and persistent vomiting. Loss of gastric secretion may also cause dehydration, and the clinical symptoms of this are often indistinguishable from those of acidosis. (2) Excessive base, usually due to the administration of alkali, as sodium bicarbonate and less often other sodium salts.

In *diabetes*, when a large amount of base has been held in combination with the ketone acids, insulin therapy allows these acids to be metabolized rapidly, and it has been found that under such conditions insulin shock may be accompanied by a primary alkali excess. This serves as an additional warning against the promiscuous employment of alkalis in diabetes.

The **symptoms** in milder cases of alkalosis consist of nausea, vomiting, malaise, numbness, tingling, and headache; but when the condition becomes more severe tetany, convulsions and stupor occur. It may be mentioned here that the tetany of infantile spasmophilia is usually not accompanied by alkalosis (p. 870). Unless tetany supervenes, symptoms of alkalosis may be confused with acidosis. The diagnosis is assisted by laboratory examination. The urine may be alkaline, but is not necessarily so; the CO_2 content of the blood will be increased, and, if the alkalosis is uncompensated, the pH will be increased (lowered hydrogen-ion concentration). The preventive **treatment** consists in removing the cause of vomiting, or care in the administration of alkalis, as the case may be. If the bicarbonate content of the blood is dangerously high, (*i. e.* if the CO_2 content is over 100 vol. per cent), hydrochloric acid or ammonium chloride may be administered by mouth. Hydrochloric acid may also be given by continuous proctoclysis in 0.5 per cent solution, about 100 to 500 cc. (3.3 to 16.9 fl. oz.) of this being used, preferably checked by the CO_2 content of the blood rather than simply by change in reaction of the urine. In the case of extreme urgency this solution of hydrochloric acid has been given intravenously. In alkalosis from vomiting, where chloride (acid) has been lost to a much greater extent than sodium (base), the administration of sodium chloride solution is indicated (Drake et al.[8]).

(*B*) Respiratory Type.—This uncommon form of alkalosis could arise by removal of carbon dioxide from the blood (primary CO_2 deficit) as a result of voluntary hyperpnea (prolonged deep breathing), or hyperpnea resulting from encephalitis, or that due to elevation of temperature. In this type a low carbon dioxide tension of the blood and of the alveolar air may be combined with an increased pH of the blood. The **treatment** consists primarily in removing the cause of the hyperpnea. Other treatment is not indicated unless there is tetany, when inhalations of 10 per cent carbon dioxide with 90 per cent oxygen may be given for periods of five to ten minutes; or, by a closely applied mask, the patient may be forced to rebreathe the expired air and thus increase the carbon dioxide tension. In tetany, too, calcium may be given by mouth, preferably as the chloride or as the gluconate, and the latter may also be administered intramuscularly or intravenously (p. 198). If the hyperpnea is continued, as in encephalitis, the respiratory rate may be lowered by careful administration of morphine or other hypnotics.

References

1. J. Biol. Chem., 1917, **30,** 289; 369; 401; 405. 2. Am. J. Dis. Child., 1916, **11,** 291. 3. Am. J. Dis. Child., 1916, **12,** 244. 4. Quantitative Clinical Chemistry, 1931, **1,** Ch. 18. 5. J. Biol. Chem., 1929, **83,** 539. 6. Am. J. Dis. Child., 1916, **11,** 309. 7. J. Biol. Chem., 1917, **32,** 495. 8. Am. J. Dis. Child., 1930, **40,** 705.

CHAPTER IX

DIABETES MELLITUS

Diabetes mellitus is a disease of metabolism in which carbohydrate is not efficiently utilized by the body, thereby causing a derangement of the normal metabolism of proteins and fats as well as of carbohydrates. It is probable that the sugar absorbed from the intestine is no longer properly changed from an inactive into an active form, so that it can be stored in the liver as glycogen or oxidized in the tissues, but that it circulates in increased quantities in the blood (hyperglycemia) and is excreted in the urine (glycosuria). It therefore becomes lost to the body as a source of energy. As a result the store of glycogen is rapidly exhausted and protein is attacked as a source for glucose. As carbohydrate is necessary for the normal metabolism of fat, incomplete combustion of fat occurs in diabetes, resulting in acidosis and coma.[1]

The foregoing is an exposition of the "nonoxidation" theory. In the "overproduction" theory, which is not so widely accepted, it is presumed that the hyperglycemia and glycosuria are due to overproduction of glucose from protein and fat, and that this is great enough to cause excretion of excess sugar, even in the presence of the ability to oxidize it. (See Soskin.[2])

Only the salient features of diabetes, especially as applied to children, can be discussed here.

Etiology.—Although less frequent in early life than later, many children have diabetes. Statistically about 4 to 6 per cent of cases commence in the first ten years of life, and the age of puberty shows a high incidence (Van Noorden,[3] Dickenson,[4] Joslin[5] and others). Even infants in the first year are attacked, as shown by a number of reported cases. Stern[6] recorded a case in which the disease appeared to be congenital, Cuno[7] one in an infant of three weeks, and Kochmann[8] an instance at four and one-half months. The youngest cases we have seen were in infants of fifteen and sixteen and one-half months respectively. In childhood diabetes is somewhat more frequent in girls than in boys. *Heredity* plays an important part, being a factor in from 10 to 40 per cent of cases according to published statistics. If those cases in which the parents do not show symptoms until after the children have developed the disease are included, the incidence of the hereditary factor is greatly increased (Bunce and Dougherty,[9] Curtis[10]). Pointing also to a hereditary influence is the fact that when one child has diabetes, the others are liable to develop it. Consanguinity, if the taint exists, is a predisposing factor. Gout, nervous disorders, tuberculosis, and syphilis of the parents have also been considered causes by some authors. Excessive consumption of sugar sometimes results in a permanent glycosuria, but probably only in a potential diabetic. Mills,[11] for example, found there was no uniformity between intake of sugar and deaths from diabetes in various countries. Diabetes occasionally follows nervous shock, and not infrequently first appears after acute diseases and infections, tonsillitis being especially prominent in this connection. The pancreatitis which occurs as a complication of mumps may be followed by diabetes. All of these causes, too, probably act usually only in the presence of a potentiality for the development of the disease, although it is possible that some of them exert a direct toxic action on the pancreas where the diabetic taint does not exist. In adults obesity predisposes to diabetes, but this is true to a much less extent in children. It has been remarked by several authors that the potentially diabetic child is physically (including bony development) and mentally precocious (Morrison and Bogan,[12] White[13]). Joslin[14] could not discover that Jewish children were particularly predisposed, although this is known to be the case in Jewish adults and to be associated in them with obesity. Priesel and Wagner[15] believe that the higher incidence in Jews is because of inbreeding. Glycosuria following trauma of the head and intracranial tumors should not be classified with true diabetes mellitus. According to Mills[16] there is a climatic influence in diabetes, the regions possessing the most changeable and stimulating climate being the ones with the greatest incidence of the condition.

Pathologic Anatomy.—There is usually no gross alteration in the pancreas, except perhaps a slight diminution in size. On microscopical examination the organ may be normal, or it may appear that the islands of Langerhans are diminished in number and there may be hydropic degeneration of their cells.

Symptoms.—These do not differ materially from those in the adult except that the onset is frequently more rapid and the course shorter. In some cases nothing is noticed until coma develops. The chief symptoms consist in wasting, great appetite, polyuria and polydipsia. In the beginning, and perhaps during several months, the manifestations may be but little marked and the child does not seem ill. After a variable length of time the symptoms increase in severity unless proper dietetic and insulin treatment is instituted. In untreated cases the teeth decay readily, the skin is dry and harsh, perspiration is diminished, constipation is frequent, there is decided debility, the temperature is subnormal, and wasting is progressive and finally extreme. A yellow discoloration of the skin (xanthosis) may occur when large amounts of vegetables are consumed.

When the disease is not controlled, the total secretion of *urine* may reach three or four times the normal amount, or more. It is pale in color, acid, with a high specific gravity, and the percentage of sugar varies from a small amount up to 5 or even 10 to 12 per cent. The total quantity of sugar excreted in twenty-four hours may reach 6 oz. (170) or over. A small amount of albumin and a few casts are frequently found. As acidosis develops the acetone bodies are found in the urine, although their mere presence is not diagnostic of change in the acid-base balance (p. 489). With the glycosuria there is always elevation of the sugar in the *blood*, so that from the normal 80 to 120 mg. per 100 cc. there may be an increase up to 400 mg. or more. At 180 mg., or even before this, there is usually the appearance of sugar in the urine, and when the blood-sugar reaches 400 mg. coma is imminent. The blood may also exhibit an increase in the cholesterol and other lipoids.

Complications.—Various cutaneous eruptions and infections are not uncommon. Gangrene is rarely seen in early life, and the same is true of cataract, optic neuritis, and retinitis. Nephritis of moderate degree is not infrequent. Tuberculosis may develop and bronchopneumonia is not unusual. Arteriosclerosis from the high lipoid content of the blood seldom occurs until after puberty. One complication of treatment is atrophy of the subcutaneous fat at the site of insulin injection. Such complications as acidosis and coma will be discussed later.

Course and Prognosis.—In cases not treated with insulin the course is rapid, lasting only a year or two before death, the child gradually, in spite of careful regulation of diet, becoming emaciated and developing coma. Some of the acute cases have apparently lasted only a short time, and we have seen the interval from apparent health, without recognized symptoms of any sort, to death in coma equal only a few weeks.

With the newer methods of treatment, including insulin, the prognosis has been greatly modified. The striking effect of insulin in prolonging life is well shown by Joslin,[17] and nutrition can be most satisfactorily maintained. Boyd and Nelson[18] believed that if uncomplicated diabetes was adequately controlled, the growth-response was greater than in non-diabetic children. Further evidence of the good outlook is the fact that treated diabetic children were found to possess a normal basal metabolism (Topper[19]). This optimism is not shared by everyone. For example, Spencer[20] observed that even with the best of care diabetic children showed a rate of gain in weight below the normal. Whether true diabetes once established may be cured is doubtful. Tolerance for carbohydrates may improve from time to time. The severity of the disease may be estimated by the amount of carbohydrate restriction necessary to free the urine of sugar and reduce the blood-sugar to normal limits. The degree of lipoid and cholesterol increase in the blood is of some value in determining prognosis. These are high in severe cases and in acidosis.

In addition to proper dietary control and insulin administration, the prognosis depends on the incidence of infections and the possibility of carrying out a proper hygienic regimen.

Diagnosis.—The diagnosis rests upon the symptoms that have been described and on the discovery of glycosuria and hyperglycemia. The blood-sugar is increased over the normal upper limit of 120 mg. per 100 cc., the blood-fat is usually over the normal of 700 mg. and the cholesterol over the normal of 170 mg.

Diabetes is especially to be distinguished from other conditions in which there is glycosuria. *Transitory glycosuria* following gastro-intestinal and infectious diseases lasts only a few weeks and is not attended by the characteristic symptoms of diabetes. *Alimentary glycosuria* may sometimes occur, but disappears immediately upon diminishing the excessive carbohydrate intake. *Renal glycosuria* presents a normal or subnormal blood-sugar and no other signs of diabetes. The urinary sugar is usually persistent, less than 1 per cent, is unaffected by carbohydrate intake, and the glucose tolerance test shows a normal curve. Very rarely renal glycosuria and diabetes mellitus may be represented in the same patient (Curren and Mills[21]). In *hyperthyroidism* there may be hyperglycemia and glycosuria, but the differential diagnosis should be obvious, remembering, however, that a patient with hyperthyroidism may also be a true diabetic. The so-called "*glycosuria innocens*," in which the blood-sugar is normal and the urinary sugar unaffected by insulin or by carbohydrate intake, is very rare in childhood. A case of this occurring in a child is reported by Rau.[22] It should be remembered, too, that there may be other substances in the urine which will reduce copper solutions, and that consequently other tests, such as fermentation, phenylhydrazin, or the use of the polariscope, must be employed before a positive diagnosis can be given in some cases. In *pentosuria* reduction of copper solutions is slower and more boiling is required, and there are no such symptoms as polyuria and polydipsia. Pentose and lactose are not fermentable. Levulose is fermentable, but is levorotatory.

The differential diagnosis between diabetic coma and insulin shock will be discussed later (p. 501). In a patient seen for the first time during coma differentiation must be made from other conditions, such as *cerebral hemorrhage* or *uremia*. It is only necessary to call attention to this, and to state here that in cerebral hemorrhage there will occasionally be found a glycosuria, but not a hyperglycemia. Not infrequently patients developing acidosis have been operated on because of abdominal pain, tenderness, vomiting, and leukocytosis leading to a diagnosis of appendicitis.

Treatment. **Prophylaxis.**—In the potentially diabetic child there should be avoided obesity, infection, and overeating, especially of carbohydrates. Foci of infection should be removed.

General Discussion.—There is sufficient knowledge about diet and insulin to permit, within certain limitations, of almost mathematical precision in the use of them. In an individual case the carbohydrate-tolerance can be ascertained, and the assistance required of insulin can be calculated in terms of units of this substance. In this chapter we shall endeavor to outline a method which is as simple as is consistent with safety.

Insulin.—Before discussing the details of treatment a brief consideration of insulin is necessary. This substance is an aqueous solution of the active principle, or hormone, of the islands of Langerhans of the pancreas. It was isolated by Banting and Best, working in Macleod's Laboratory at the University of Toronto.[23] The extracts for clinical use were first prepared by Collip,[24] and the effect on human cases of diabetes reported by Banting, Best, Collip, Campbell and Fletcher,[25] since which time an extensive literature has arisen. As prepared for use, the glucose-equivalent of one unit of insulin is about two; *i. e.*, it is standardized so that one unit will enable a diabetic patient to metabolize about 2 Gm. of glucose-forming food. It should be remembered that there is an individual variation in this respect, and also that with each added unit given less and less glucose per unit is burned up.

Insulin should be administered subcutaneously, care being taken that it is not injected too near the skin or intramuscularly. In the extreme of coma it may be employed intravenously. When ingested it becomes inert. When dissolved on the tongue or used by inunction it is absorbed slightly, but in ineffectual amount. It is best injected one-fourth to one-half hour before each meal in severe cases with diacetic acid in the urine; but in milder types twice or perhaps even once a day. After the injection of insulin the blood-sugar begins to fall and the effect lasts from six to twelve hours. Insulin by no means replaces dietary measures, but simply assists them by supplying the deficient pancreatic hormone. In order, then, to regulate the amount of insulin to be given it is necessary to know how much glucose is ingested and how much the patient can metabolize. It must not be administered at all if a diet can be found which will keep the patient's urine sugar-free, and which is so balanced that the fatty acids will be metabolized beyond the ketone-stage, while at the same time the individual is maintained in a normal nutritional state, with allowance for necessary activity. Practically all diabetic children will be benefited by its use, the severity and progressive character of the disease at this age making it difficult to give a diet which will keep them free of urinary sugar and of ketone-bodies, while supplying enough food for growth and development. Boyd,[26] for example, found that only 15 per cent of diabetic children could take an adequate diet without the aid of insulin.

Diet.—The diabetic *diet* should be planned with three definite factors in mind: (*a*) The protein-content, (*b*) the relation between ketogenic and antiketogenic substances, (*c*) the glucose-tolerance of the individual. It may be assumed that in a child at least 1 Gm. of protein will be required per day for each pound of body-weight. Protein-containing foodstuffs are selected which will furnish this amount. It has been shown by Woodyatt[27] and by Shaffer[28] that there is a rather definite quantitative relation between the amount of glucose and the amount of fatty acid which can be metabolized without the acetone bodies remaining and the consequent danger of acidosis. That is to say, ketogenic food-substances must be balanced against antiketogenic food-substances. It may be said that, if the diet contains not more than 2.5 Gm. of fat for each gram of carbohydrate plus each gram of protein, ketosis will not occur. This proportion is based upon the fact that the total fatty acid in the diet should not be more than 1.5 times the total available glucose. The fatty acid (ketogenic) fraction is formed by 90 per cent of the fat and 46 per cent of the protein; and the glucose (antiketogenic) fraction by 10 per cent of the fat, 58 per cent of the protein and 100 per cent of the carbohydrate. This may be expressed by the formula $\frac{K}{A} = \frac{0.46P + 0.90F}{0.58P + 0.10F + C}$. $\frac{K}{A}$ should not be more than 1.5. To put this in a more convenient form, Fat (Gm.) = 2 Carbohydrate (Gm.) + 0.5 Protein (Gm.), indicating that the number of grams of fat in the diet must not exceed a figure obtained by adding twice the number of grams of carbohydrate and one-half the number of grams of protein present in the food.

This means, then, that in continuing the planning of the diet, in which protein has already been supplied in the proportion of 1 Gm. per pound of body-weight, the remainder of the food must be added so that there is 1 Gm. of carbohydrate and not more than 2.5 Gm. of fat per day for each pound of body-weight. A convenient computation devised by W. E. Nelson of Cincinnati, for a child of four to ten years of age is to give 2 Gm. of fat; 2 Gm. of carbohydrate; and 1 Gm. of protein per pound. This gives 30 calories per pound, which is approximately correct for the age. (See Table 66, p. 501.) Children are prone to the development of acidosis, and it is well to keep the fat lower than would be permissible in adults; not much more than 2 Gm. of fat being allowed per pound of body-weight. This is especially important in initial diets until the glucose-burning power of the body is ascertained.

Before proceeding with treatment and the prescribing of the diet, the cases must be divided into three groups:—(*A*) Those uncomplicated cases in which diacetic acid is absent from the urine; (*B*) Those in which diacetic acid is present; (*C*) Those in which there are symptoms of acidosis and threatening coma. Diacetic acid rather than acetone should be the criterion, because the test for the latter is too delicate. The presence of diacetic acid in the urine indicates a real danger, as it shows a positive disturbance of fat-metabolism.

(*A*) Treatment of Uncomplicated Cases (no diacetic acid).—The details may best be illustrated by giving the procedure to be followed in a hypothetical case. Suppose that a diet is to be prescribed for a diabetic child whose weight is 50 lb. Table 65 on page 500, is consulted and the foods for twenty-four hours selected are ordered either by weight or by household-measure as shown in the table on p. 497.

The diet just described has fulfilled certain requirements previously outlined. It has also furnished vitamins and residue. Its digestibility is not as great as that of a nondiabetic diet, because of the high fat-percentage and the overbalance of animal protein. Variety can be obtained by substitution of various vegetables, cereals and fruits, and, as increases are made, the selection can be from foods of different character.

There remains to be ascertained whether such a diet is of sufficient caloric value to maintain the child in a good nutritional state and allow

	P. (Gm.).	F. (Gm.).	C. (Gm.).
Egg (100 Gm. or 2 av. size)	13	12	0
Lean meat (100 Gm. or size of 1 chop)	25	12	0
Butter (30 Gm. or 2 butter-balls)	0	24	0
20 per cent cream (100 cc. or 3½ fl. oz.)	4	20	4
Olive oil (13 Gm. or 1 tbsp.)	0	13	0
Orange (60 Gm. or ¼ av. size)	0	0	5
Oatmeal (100 Gm. or 2 tbsp.)	5	2	20
Macaroni (50 Gm. or 2 tbsp.)	1.5	0.5	8
10 per cent vegetables (100 Gm. or 2 tbsp.)	1	0	6
5 per cent vegetables (100 Gm. or 2 tbsp.)	1	0	3
Soda cracker (6 Gm. or 1 cracker)	0.5	0.5	4
	51.0	84.0	50.0

for activity and growth. If the number of grams of protein and of carbohydrate are each multiplied by four (caloric value of 1 Gm. of protein and carbohydrate) and the number of grams of fat by 9 (caloric value of 1 Gm. of fat), the total caloric value of the diet can be obtained. Thus in the diet above planned the caloric value is 1160. If the patient under consideration is nine years of age, the caloric requirement per pound per day is about 27 (see Table 66, page 501), and the total calories in the diet should be about 1350. On the diet planned, therefore, it is unlikely that there will be sufficient food allowance for activity and growth, although there may be enough for maintenance. This becomes more apparent if the normal weight is considered (see Table 67, page 501). The diabetic patient who has not been under treatment is usually underweight, but has a caloric requirement which should be judged on the basis of normal weight, and the effort should be to bring the weight gradually up to this standard, or slightly above it. Care should be taken not to confuse real gain in weight with that which may occur with the edema attending undernutrition and the administration of sodium bicarbonate, or large amounts of salts in broths and vegetables. If the patient becomes sugar-free in four or five days and continues so on the diet as planned, if diacetic acid is absent from the urine, but the caloric intake remains too low, then the food may be increased every two or three days by adding about 5 Gm. of carbohydrate and twice as much (10 Gm.) fat, the protein remaining about the same. It is not necessary that the carbohydrate and the fat be raised at the same time. In the basic diet it will be noted that the fat is well under the upper limit permitted, and it may be increased before carbohydrate is added, provided it does not supply more than 2.5 Gm. per pound per day, and does not overbalance the ketogenic-forming material,—this latter consideration being determined by the use of the formula $F = 2C + 0.5P$. If glycosuria persists on the initial diet, or on the subsequently increased ones before the caloric intake is sufficient, insulin must be given. It is possible, of course, to diminish the carbohydrate to less than that recommended in the initial diet, *i. e.*, below 1 Gm. per pound, but a child whose tolerance is below that amount should be treated with insulin rather than starved.

There are several methods of regulating the dose of insulin, of which the following is satisfactory: Determine the amount of sugar in a twenty-four hour specimen of urine and give as the day's dose one-half as many units of insulin as there are grams of sugar. If only 5 units are necessary this dose may be administered before the morning meal; up to 30 units may be given, equally divided, before the morning and evening meal; over 30 units should be divided in three equal parts and given before each meal.

Children are especially liable to develop untoward symptoms due to hypoglycemia caused by too much insulin, and if the urine tests indicate that large doses are necessary (over 20 units) it is better to begin with one-half the indicated dose and gradually increase. When the urine has been found free from sugar for three days, the diet may be increased in the manner previously described. If sugar reappears before a diet of proper caloric value has been reached, the insulin dosage must be increased as indicated by the amount of sugar appearing in twenty-four-hour specimens. If the urine is not examined quantitatively for sugar, insulin should be begun in doses as small as 1 or 2 units three times a day, and increased in increments of 1 unit until the qualitative test for urinary sugar is negative. The aim should be to give the smallest efficient dose of insulin. Constant observation of the nutritional state of the patient is necessary, and the urinary sugar should be estimated frequently, in order that an increase or decrease in glucose-tolerance will be met by a corresponding change in insulin-dosage.

(*B*) Treatment of Cases with Diacetic Acid in the Urine.—The appearance of diacetic acid in the urine indicates faulty metabolism of fat and the danger of acidosis and coma. If only a small amount of diacetic acid is found, the diet should be altered in such a way that the fat is decreased and the carbohydrate increased, the dose of insulin being increased approximately 1 unit for each gram of carbohydrate added. For example, if the patient were on a diet such as that prescribed on page 497, most of the fat could be removed by eliminating the butter, cream and olive oil; and the oatmeal, macaroni and vegetables increased or other carbohydrate added as follows:

	P. (Gm.).	F. (Gm.).	C. (Gm.).
Egg (100 Gm. or 2 av. size)	13	12	0
Lean meat (100 Gm. or size of 1 chop)	25	12	0
Orange (250 Gm. or 1 av. size)	1.5	0	20
Oatmeal (200 Gm. or 4 tbsp.)	10	4	40
Macaroni (100 Gm. or 2 tbsp.)	3	1	16
10 per cent vegetables (100 Gm. or 2 tbsp.)	1	0	6
5 per cent vegetables (100 Gm. or 2 tbsp.)	1	0	3
Bread (30 Gm. or 1 slice)	3	0	16
	57.5	29	101

This diet would furnish only 895 calories, but partial starvation is advisable in the face of a possible acidosis. When the diacetic acid has disappeared from the urine, fat and protein are added to the diet in about 5 Gm. amounts daily, the carbohydrate and the insulin being diminished until the patient can be treated in the manner outlined for uncomplicated cases.

(*C*) Treatment of Cases with Acidosis and Threatened Coma.—With large amounts of diacetic acid in the urine, and the onset of such symptoms as restlessness, nausea, vomiting, drowsiness, leukocytosis and slight hyperpnea, the patient should be put to bed, external heat applied, an enema given and the stomach lavaged. Fluid is forced, and the only food allowed is clear broth free from fat; orange-juice; oatmeal gruel; or 5 per cent glucose solution. If nausea and vomiting are present 5 per cent glucose should be given by rectum. It is very desirable that a blood-sugar examination be made and that the CO_2 combining power of the blood-plasma be determined. (See p. 490.) It is possible, but unusual, for coma to occur with normal blood-sugar and in the absence of ketonuria. In such cases there may be reduction of the dextrose in the red blood cells and probably also in the tissues (Foshay[29]). Enough glucose should be given to produce the excretion of a small amount of sugar in the urine. The urine should be examined every few hours for sugar and acetone. From 15 to 30 units of insulin should be administered, the amount depending upon the urgency of symptoms, the age of the patient, the degree of the reaction for diacetic acid in the urine, or the results of blood-analysis; but in any event each unit of insulin should be buffered by the oral administration of 10 cc. ($\frac{1}{3}$ oz.) of orange-juice or 1 Gm. ($\frac{1}{10}$ heaping teaspoonful) of glucose or sugar. Subsequent injections of 10 to 20 units should be given every two to four hours, the amount and frequency being determined by the same considerations as in the case of the original dose. If acidosis has proceeded to the stage of *coma* the same plan should be followed, but the insulin dosage should be greater (30 to 50 units). In advanced cases insulin and glucose should be given intravenously, a 5 per cent solution of the latter being injected at the rate of 10 cc. a minute. If the intravenous route is difficult or impracticable, subcutaneous or intraperitoneal injection may be employed. The amount of glucose used will depend on the symptoms, the age and weight of the patient, and the laboratory examinations; but at least 1 Gm. of it must be employed for each unit of insulin. When this would mean that an excessive amount of fluid must be injected intravenously, part of the glucose-solution may be administered by some other route than the intravenous, or a stronger solution used. In estimating the amount of insulin it should be remembered that coma is much more dangerous than insulin-shock.

The value of soda in acidosis has been questioned. Certainly insulin has rendered it less necessary, but yet it should be used in acidotic states, especially when there is respiratory distress or hyperpnea. In the precomatose stage a teaspoonful of sodium-bicarbonate in 4 or 5 oz. of water may be given every half hour for several doses; if coma is present it may be added in 3 per cent strength to the glucose solution given intravenously. (See p. 490.) An alkaline or neutral reaction of the urine is an indication for the cessation of soda-medication. Methyl red should be used as the indicator, the red color changing to yellow in an alkaline solution.

Hypoglycemia (Hyperinsulinism, Insulin-shock).—If an overdose of insulin has been administered; *i. e.*, more than can be buffered by the available glucose, certain symptoms will arise within from one to five hours. These are not usually observed until the blood-sugar is below 80 mg. per 100 cc. but they may appear at a level of 110 mg. per 100 cc. if a previously high concentration has been too rapidly lowered. Marked shock occurs when the blood-sugar reaches 40 mg. per 100 cc. Early symptoms of hypoglycemia are sudden hunger, weakness, restlessness and nervousness, pallor or flushing, dilated pupils and increased pulse-rate. At this stage the ingestion every ten minutes of such small amounts of carbohydrate as a teaspoonful of corn-syrup or sugar, the juice of an orange or a piece of candy will relieve the symptoms. If a large overdose of insulin has been given there appear the symptoms of sweating, tremor, apprehension, vertigo, diplopia and delirium and, if carbohydrate is not supplied, convulsions, collapse, unconsciousness and death. In advanced states carbohydrate must be administered by stomach-tube, and if improvement is not quickly noted 20 cc. (0.68 fl. oz.) of a 50 per cent solution of glucose should be injected intravenously. If the latter solution is not available, 10 to 15 minims (0.62 to 0.92 cc.) of a 1:1000 solution of adrenaline or of pituitary extract may be injected subcutaneously, but not intravenously. Hypoglycemia should be avoided by the careful balancing of the glucose-intake and insulin-injection. When, for any reason, food is not taken or vomiting and diarrhea occur, the insulin should be discontinued.

Table 65.—Values of Foods as Prepared for Use. (Not Including the Addition of Any Butter, Oil, Lard, Sugar or Flour Which May Have Been Employed)*

	Various ordinary portions.			100 Gm. portions.		
	P (Gm.).	F (Gm.).	C (Gm.).	P (Gm.).	F (Gm.).	C (Gm.).
Foods Highest in Protein						
Dried beef (30 Gm. or 1 oz.)	12	2	0	40	6	0
Lean meat (100 Gm. or size 1 chop)	25	12	0	25	12	0
Chicken, stewed (100 Gm. or 1 slice size 1 chop)	22	5	0	22	5	0
Chicken, roasted (100 Gm. or 1 slice size 1 chop)	20	16	0	20	16	0
Sweetbread (100 Gm. or 4 h. tbsp.)	20	9	0	20	9	0
Cottage cheese (30 Gm. or 2 h. tbsp.)	6	0.5	1	20	1.5	3
Fish boiled (100 Gm. or 4 h. tbsp.) Cod, flounder, whitefish, shad, trout, salmon, haddock.	18	5	0	18	5	0
Egg (50 Gm. or 1 av. size)	6.5	6	0	13	12	0
Egg white (33 Gm. or 1 av. size)	4	0	0	12	0	0
Milk, whole (30 cc. or 1 fl. oz.) sweet or lactic acid	1.2	1.2	1.2	4	4	4
Skimmed milk (30 cc. or 1 fl. oz.) sweet or lactic acid	1.2	0	1.2	4	0	4
Gelatin (30 Gm. or 1 h. tbsp.)	1	0	0	3	0	0
Broth (30 cc. or 1 fl. oz.)	0.75	0	0	2.5	0	0
Foods Highest in Fat						
Olive salad oil or lard (13 Gm. or 1 tbsp.)	0	13	0	0	100	0
Butter (15 Gm. or 1 ball or 1 r. tsp.)	0	12	0	0	85	0
Bacon (30 Gm. or 1 large slice)	3	20	0	10	72	0
Egg yolk (18 Gm. or 1 av. size)	2.5	6	0	13	33	0
Cream, 20 per cent (30 cc. or 1 oz.)	1.2	6	1.2	4	20	4
Cream, gravity or 16 per cent (30 cc. or 1 oz.)	1.2	5	1.2	4	16	4
Baked custard (50 Gm. or 1 h. tbsp.)	3.5	3.5	1	7	7	2
Foods Highest in Carbohydrate						
Sugar (10 Gm. or 1 h. tsp.)	0	0	10	0	0	100
Cereals						
Shredded wheat (30 Gm. or 1 biscuit)	3	0	23	10	0	75
Cornflakes (20 Gm. or 1 h. tbsp.)	1.75	0	15	8.75	0	57
Bread, wheat (30 Gm. or 1 small slice 3 × 3½ × ½ in.)	3	0	16	10	0	53
Gluten bread (40 Gm. or 1 small slice 3 × 3½ × ½ in.)	12	0	12	30	0	30
Rice (100 Gm. or 1 h. tbsp.)	3	0	24	3	0	24
Oatmeal, Ralston's, Pettijohn's (50 Gm. or 1 tbsp.)	2.5	1	10	5	2	20
Macaroni or hominy, boiled (50 Gm. or 1 h. tbsp.)	1.5	0.5	8	3	1	16
Cream of wheat / Farina } (50 Gm. or 1 h. tbsp.)	0.75	0	5.5	1.5	0	11
Saltine cracker	0	0	2			
Butter-thin cracker	0	0.5	2.75			
Soda cracker (3 in. sq.)	0.5	0.5	4.25			
Graham cracker	0.75	0.75	6			
Green and Root Vegetables						
Potato { Baked (40 Gm. or 1 h. tbsp.)	1	0	10	2.5	0	25
Potato { Boiled (50 Gm. or 1 h. tbsp.)	1	0	10	2.0	0	20
Lima beans (49 Gm. or 1 h. tbsp.)	3	0	12	7.5	0	30
Green peas (30 Gm. or 1 h. tbsp.)	2	1	4	6.5	3	13
10 per cent vegetables (50 Gm. or 1 h. tbsp.) String beans, carrots, turnips, beets, squash, onions, pumpkin.	0.5	0	3	1	0	6
5 per cent vegetables (50 Gm. or 1 h. tbsp.)	0.5	0	1.5	1	0	3
Fruits						
Apricot, dried (8 Gm. or 1 av. size)	0	0	5	3	0.5	62
Prune (10 Gm. or 1 small)	0	0	6	1.75	0	60
Plum (35 Gm. or 1 av. size)	0	0	7	0	0	20
15 per cent fruits (25 Gm. or 1 tbsp.) Raspberries, blueberries, cherries, currants.	0	0	3.75	0.75	0	15
Banana (195 Gm. or 1 av. size)	1.5	0.75	28	0.75	0	14
Pear (150 Gm. or 1 av. size)	0.75	0.5	20	0.5	0	13
Pineapple (50 Gm. or ½ slice)	0	0	5	0	0	10
Apple (150 Gm. or 1 av. size)	0.5	0.5	16	0	0	10
Grapefruit (200 Gm. or ½ av. size)	1.5	0.5	20	0.75	0	10
10 per cent fruits (25 Gm. or 1 h. tbsp.) Blackberries, strawberries, gooseberries.	0.5	0	2.5	2	0	10
Orange (125 Gm. or ½ av. size)	0.75	0	10	0.5	0	8
Peach (125 Gm. or 1 av. size)	0.5	0	10	0	0	8
Lemon (65 Gm. or 1 av. size)	0.5	0	3.5	1	0	6

* Amounts less than 0.5 have been omitted as negligible.

Tbsp. = Tablespoonful. H.Tbsp. = Heaping Tablespoonful. Tsp. = Teaspoonful. R.Tsp. = Rounded Teaspoonful. See also Tables 58 and 59, pp. 130–132.

To determine whether insulin shall be given in coma, it may be necessary to distinguish between diabetic coma and insulin shock. For this purpose the following table of contrasts may be found useful:

	Onset.	Vomiting.	Abdominal pain.	W.B.C.	Hyperpnea.	Skin.	Urine.	Blood.
Coma	slow	common	frequent	leuko-cytosis	present	dry	sugar present	hyper-glycemia
Insulin-shock	sudden	seldom	absent	leukopenia	absent	moist	sugar usually absent	hypo-glycemia

Occasionally patients become sensitive to the animal protein contained in insulin.

MISCELLANEOUS.—There is nothing gained by keeping diabetic children in bed, and during exercise more sugar is oxidized. Fatigue and exposure to cold should be avoided. If lack of strength renders rest in bed necessary, massage should be employed.

Infections temporarily, and often permanently, lower glucose-tolerance. During the acute stage of any infection the food-intake in diabetic patients should be diminished one-half or one-third, and after the acute stage the glucose-tolerance must again be ascertained before the full diet is resumed. Tonsillitis seems to be especially prone to cause a decrease in the ability to metabolize carbohydrate. If the tonsils are badly diseased they may be removed, the operation having become a much safer procedure since insulin-treatment has been instituted.

It is hardly necessary to say that the diabetic patient should be under close observation. If it is possible to do so, a blood-sugar analysis should be made every week or two. The urine must be examined frequently for sugar and diacetic acid. Even children can be instructed to perform these latter tests themselves, and the older ones acquire adeptness in cal-

TABLE 66.—AVERAGE CALORIC REQUIREMENTS

Age (yrs.).	Cal. per lb.	Cal. per kilo.
2–4	34	75
6–7	32	70
7–10	27	59
10–14	22	48

TABLE 67.—APPROXIMATE WEIGHT AT DIFFERENT AGES

Age (yrs.).	Av. wt. lb.	Av. wt. kilo.
2	27	12.25
3	32	14.5
4	37	17
5	42	19
6	45	20
7	49	22
8	53	24
9	58	26
10	64	29
11	70	32
12	78	35.5
13	87	40
14	96	43.5

culating diets. Joslin's Diabetic Manual is very helpful in this connection. The patient or the patient's attendant should be instructed in the dangers of diabetes and in the mishaps of treatment, and it is well to have these written down so that they may be referred to in an emergency. A list of instructions would include: (1) The early symptoms of acidosis and the measures to be employed; (2) the early symptoms of hypoglycemia and the treatment to be given; (3) the indication for the cessation of insulin-injections, such as the refusal of food and the presence of vomiting and diarrhea; (4) the danger of infections and the fact that they lower carbohydrate-tolerance and consequently require a diminution in food-intake. Children must be under close surveillance lest they supplement their restricted carbohydrate in a surreptitious manner.

Search is being made for substitutes for insulin, none of which is as yet proven satisfactory. Collip[30] and others discovered that many plants yield an insulin-like substance, glucokinin. Extract of blueberry-leaf contains myrtillin, which reduces the amount of blood-sugar (Allen[31]). Mills[32] found that plant extracts rich in vitamin B favorably influenced diabetes. The oatmeal diet originally suggested by von Noorden[33] probably owed its value to an insulin-like property in the oatmeal. Blotner and Murphy[34] found that an aqueous extract of liver possesses an insulin-like action. Synthalin (an alkaline guanidin derivative) has been used by Frank, Nothmann, and Wagner.[35]

References

1. Rept. of Insulin Committee, Univ. Toronto; J.A.M.A., 1923, **80,** 1847. 2. Biochem. J., 1929, **23,** 1385. 3. Pfaundler und Schlossmann, Handb. d. Kinderh., 1923, **1,** 639. 4. Diabetes, 1875, 66. 5. Treatm. of Diabetes Mellitus, 1923. 6. Arch. f. Kinderh., 1889–90, **11,** 82. 7. Jahrb. f. Kinderh., 1910, **71,** 623. 8. Jahrb. f. Kinderh., 1922, **94,** 20. 9. J.A.M.A., 1929, **92,** 52. 10. J.A.M.A., 1929, **92,** 952. 11. Arch. Int. Med., 1930, **46,** 582. 12. Am. J. M. Sc., 1927, **174,** 313. 13. J.A.M.A., 1930, **95,** 1160. 14. J.A.M.A., 1924, **83,** 1847. 15. Klin. Wchnschr., 1929, **8,** 1398. 16. Arch. Int. Med., 1930, **46,** 569. 17. J.A.M.A., 1931, **97,** 597. 18. Am. J. Dis. Child., 1928, **35,** 753. 19. Am. J. Dis. Child., 1931, **42,** 760. 20. Am. J. Dis. Child., 1928, **36,** 502. 21. J. Lab. and Clin. Med., 1928, **13,** 646. 22. Deutsch. med. Wchnschr., 1929, **55,** 1338. 23. J. Lab. and Clin. Med., 1922, **7,** 251; 464. 24. Canad. M. A. J., 1922, **12,** 142. 25. Canad. M. A. J., 1922, **12,** 141. 26. Canad. M. A. J., 1927, **17,** 1167. 27. Arch. Int. Med., 1921, **28,** 125. 28. J. Biol. Chem., 1921, **47,** 433; 1921, **49,** 143; 1922, **54,** 399. 29. Am. J. Physiol., 1925, **73,** 470; Arch. Int. Med., 1927, **40,** 661. 30. J. Biol. Chem., 1923, **56,** 513. 31. J.A.M.A., 1927, **89,** 1577. 32. Am. J. M. Sc., 1928, **175,** 376; 384. 33. Die Zuckerkrankheit und ihre Behandlung, 1912. 34. J.A.M.A., 1930, **94,** 1811. 35. Klin. Wchnschr., 1926, **5,** 2100.

CHAPTER X

DIABETES INSIPIDUS

This uncommon disease is characterized by a lasting excessive secretion of urine, combined with great thirst. It is to be distinguished from simple polyuria. (See p. 806.) It was first clearly distinguished from diabetes mellitus by Willis.[1]

Etiology.—According to the statistics given by Roberts,[2] Strauss,[3] Stoermer,[4] and Rowntree,[5] the incidence under ten years of *age* varies from 5 to 30 per cent of the cases. Rarely the disease appears to be congenital. In adults more males are affected, but in children the influence of *sex* is inconsiderable. *Heredity* is a powerful predisposing factor. The symptoms of diabetes insipidus may follow trauma of the head, tumors of the brain, especially those involving the pituitary body, meningitis and encephalitis acute infectious disorders, and syphilis. The relation between diabetes insipidus and the pituitary body and its neighboring structures is discussed elsewhere (p. 1088). In those cases in which there are associated a polycystic and fibrous form of osteitis (Heard et al.[6]), defects in the membranous bones and exophthalmos (Denzer[7]), and xanthoma (Griffith,[8] Rowland[9]), the polyuria is probably only an incidental part of the general picture of disturbance of the lipoid metabolism. (See Diseases of Spleen, etc., p. 1052.) In the majority of instances of diabetes insipidus no cause can be discovered, and at necropsy there may be no lesions.

Symptoms.—The most marked early symptoms are polydipsia and polyuria, the onset of these often being sudden. A remarkable amount of fluid may be imbibed, and the daily secretion of urine may reach from 5 to 15 quarts (4.7 to 14 liters), or occasionally as much as 35 to 40 quarts (33 or 38 liters). The urine is pale, with a specific gravity of from 1.001 to 1.005; there is no sugar; albumin is rarely found, and casts practically never. The phenolsulphonephthalein elimination is normal or but slightly diminished. The total solids are usually normal. Sometimes inosite and increase in purine bases have been found. Most patients pass more urine during the night than during the day. The skin is pale and dry, the temperature is sometimes subnormal, there may be anorexia or excessive appetite, the blood exhibits nothing characteristic. The general health may be little affected, but there are often emaciation and lack of bodily and mental development. In the cases due to central nervous lesions other symptoms develop depending upon these.

Course and Prognosis.—In cases symptomatic of central nervous lesions the disorder may last for years. In other cases death ensues from emaciation and debility. Tolerance may sometimes be acquired, but recovery in well-established cases is rare.

Diagnosis.—Study will reveal whether the symptoms are due to brain-tumor or other intracranial lesions. Polyuria following infectious fever or associated with hysterical or other nervous symptoms may last a few weeks, but is easily differentiated. Nephrosclerosis is rare in children; the polyuria attending it is not so great as in diabetes insipidus; and there are albuminuria, casts, and other characteristic symptoms. The possibility of syphilis of the central nervous system should not be forgotten.

Treatment.—Polyuria and polydipsia are results, not causes of the disease, and fluid must not be too much restricted. None of the many drugs tried, such as ergot, antipyrine, arsenic, belladonna, or opium seems to be satisfactory. If the Wassermann reaction is positive, antisyphilitic treatment should be given. Pituitary extract was first used by Francisco.[10] Pituitrin given hypodermically, in doses of 0.1 to 1 cc. (1.6 to 16 minims) of the obstetrical or surgical solution, causes a diminution in the polyuria and thirst. Its effect seldom extends as long as twelve hours, and it can be given several times a day over a long period without apparent injury. Its action appears to be upon the epithelium of the renal tubules, causing them to resorb water at a rate increased over normal. Administered by mouth it is valueless, but some relief follows the application of 0.5 to 1 cc. (8 to 16 minims) of it intranasally by spray or on a cotton tampon (Blumgart[11]). If applied by dropper the patient should be reclining with the head thrown back; the object being to have the solution reach the nasopharynx. Lumbar puncture may afford temporary relief. It should be done with caution if brain-tumor is suspected. Galvanization of the spinal column is claimed to have given good results.

References

1. Pharmaceut. ration., 1675, Sec. 4, Cap. 3; Ref. Senator, in Ziemssen's Handb. d. spec. Path. u. Therap., 1876, **13**, 2, 254. 2. Urinary and Renal Dis., 3rd Amer. Ed.,

1879. 3. Dissert. Tübingen, 1870; Ref. Gerhardt, Nothnagel's spec. Path. u. Therap., **7,** 1. 4. Dissert. Kiel, 1892; Ref. Gerhardt loc. cit. Ref. No. 3. 5. J.A.M.A. 1924, **83,** 642. 6. Am. J. M. Sc., 1926, **171,** 38. 7. Am. J. Dis. Child., 1926, **31,** 480. 8. Arch. Pediat., 1922, **39,** 297; 1923, **40,** 630. 9. Arch. Int. Med., 1928, **42,** 611. 10. Gazz. d. osp., 1913, **34,** 1135. 11. Arch. Int. Med., 1922, **29,** 508; Am. J. M. Sc., 1928, **176,** 769.

CHAPTER XI

PELLAGRA

Pellagra (*pelle-agra,* rough skin) was first recognized as a morbid entity by Casál[1] in Spain in 1735, although it had previously been known under various popular names, among them "Mal de la Rosa." It has been of frequent occurrence in the southern countries of Europe and in Egypt and India, and had been observed in the United States for a good many years, a case having been reported by Babcock[2] occurring as long ago as 1834 and one by Gray[3] in 1864. Since 1906 it has been recognized with increasing frequency in this country, occurring particularly in the Southern States, although nearly every State in the Union has suffered from it.

Etiology.—Pellagra attacks all ages, although apparently more common in young adults. It has been observed even as early as two months of age. Studies especially of children are those of Snyder,[4] Weston,[5] Rice,[6] Knowles[7] and Murphy.[8] In America females are more often affected (3:1), although there is not this marked sex-distinction in early life, or in adults in other countries. Those living in rural districts and in warm climates are more frequently attacked. The active symptoms oftenest appear in the spring and summer months. Unsanitary conditions and debilitated health predispose, and especially long-continued gastro-intestinal disease. While not contagious, several pellagrins may occur in the same family because of the incorrect dietary factor common to all.

Goldberger[9] and his co-workers began the study of pellagra in 1914 and have since then issued numerous publications. These investigations at first pointed to a deficiency in certain amino-acids as the essential etiologic factor, but later it was shown that the deficiency was very probably the so-called "vitamin B-2" (vitamin G, or P-P (Pellagra-preventing) vitamin). (See Vitamins, p. 135.) Mellanby[10] suggests that deficiency of vitamin A may also be associated with lack of vitamin G in the causation.

Other theories concerning the cause of pellagra may be mentioned. It has long been known that it occurred among those who eat corn-meal, and Lombroso[11] especially championed the theory that this caused a food-intoxication, perhaps depending upon a mould which infected the corn. Others have maintained that the disorder was an infectious one transmitted by insects, Sambon[12] believing that the Simulium fly was the vector; Roberts,[13] the mosquito; and Jennings and King,[14] the Stomoxys calcitrans (stable-fly). Harris[15] reported the production of the disorder in monkeys by inoculation with a filterable virus, but others fail to confirm this. Siler, Garrison and MacNeal[16] and others also favored the theory of infection as a cause. Jobling and Arnold[17] isolated a photodynamic organism from the stools of pellagrins, which they believed needed further study. The fact that lesions occur on exposed parts has also led to the thought that photo-sensitizing substances might be in some way responsible. Sabry[18] believes that the disease is due to a poison (dioxyphenylalanine) which occurs in beans, as well as in maize and other cereals, or which may be formed in the body. Bliss[19] suggests that iron deficiency is the underlying factor, and Alessandrini and Scala[20] that the action of silicon in drinking water is the cause. Stewart[21] thought that dysthyroidism was the etiologic factor.

While, then, there is by no means entire agreement as to the exact causation of pellagra, all modern work indicates that the dietary factor is at least important, and that the malady is very possibly a deficiency disease.

Pathologic Anatomy.—The lesions of the skin are at first those of erythema, but finally of atrophy, pigmentation, and sclerosis. Pigmentation may take place in the viscera; the kidney may be sclerotic; the liver and spleen may be smaller than normal; brown atrophy of the cardiac muscle is common; the general musculature atrophies; the fat of the body diminishes; and there is increased fragility of the bones. There may be marked inflammatory changes in the brain, meninges, and spinal cord, chiefly the last.

Symptoms and Course.—The method of onset and the symptoms seen are subject to considerable variation. The latter can be divided into *cutaneous; digestive;* and *nervous.* Any one of these groups may appear

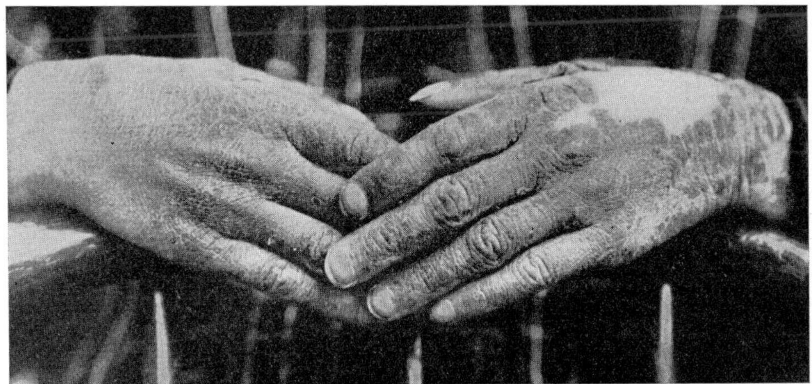

Fig. 116.—Pellagra. Case in a girl of nine years, in the Children's Medical Ward of the Hospital of the University of Pennsylvania, under the care of Dr. M. B. Hartzell. (*Courtesy of Dr. Hartzell and of the J. B. Lippincott Co.*)

first or be most prominent. The **cutaneous** are the characteristic manifestations. These may come on suddenly or very insidiously, the first change being a symmetrically developed erythema on the exposed parts of the body, such as the backs of the hands, the face and the neck; or in other cases, if the patient does not wear shoes, also on the feet and legs up to the knees. It resembles sunburn, and in mild cases, and especially in young children, may easily escape recognition. In typical instances the erythema becomes darker-red and livid, and is followed in about two weeks or more by drying, scaling (*dry type*) and pigmentation of the epidermis (Fig. 116). At the wrists or on the forearms it is sharply demarcated from the healthy skin above it, giving sometimes the appearance of a glove ("pellagrous glove"); or this may be seen on the foot and leg also ("pellagrous boot"), or around the neck ("Casál's necklace"); in fact wherever the covered joins the exposed skin. In some cases vesicles and bullae develop (*wet type*), or there may be suppuration beneath the scaly, crusted epidermis. After a few months in the milder cases recovery occurs and the skin resumes its normal appearance. With, or preceding, the cutaneous symptoms there are **digestive** disturbances, generally most marked in young children. These consist of severe diarrhea, stomatitis, salivation, vomiting, anorexia, and abdominal pain. **Nervous** and **general** symptoms, too, may develop at any period. The child may be little ill, or there may be malaise, wasting, vertigo, depression, insomnia, headache, and cramps in various parts of the body. Occasionally severer nervous symptoms, such as paresthesia and exaggerated reflexes, indicating lesions of the cord, may be early manifestations. There may be a secondary anemia, but no leukocytosis or eosinophilia.

This is, perhaps, the history of the first attack. Entire recovery may take place, or there may be recurrences from year to year as spring comes on. Other regions of the body may become involved, as the entire forearms, the shoulders, and the genital region; and rarely the eruption is universal. In later attacks the skin is often not so vividly red as in the first, but becomes infiltrated, fissured, and atrophic, assuming a parchment-like character, with exacerbations of the erythema in the spring. The nervous symptoms become more marked in later attacks. Mental disturbances are comparatively uncommon in children, except for a degree of dulness or irritability. In the final stage there is profound prostration and great emaciation.

Prognosis.—The mortality in America in the 15,870 cases collected by Lavinder[22] equalled 37 per cent. There is always a tendency to recurrence. There is reason to believe that, although pellagra is more rapidly fatal in infancy, in children from the age of four to ten years the course is mild. The prognosis depends naturally upon the treatment.

Treatment.—It has been reported that infants may develop the disease when nursing from pellagrous mothers. This is probably because breast-milk is deficient in the antipellagrous factor. Soothing applications, such as would be indicated for the treatment of erythema, should be applied locally. Sunshine should be avoided, as this tends to aggravate the eruption. Proper attention should be given to the general health, and tonic measures employed. Anemia should be treated. Bliss[19] is particularly impressed with the effect of medication with iron on the course of the disease. Sabry[18] advises the intravenous use of sodium thiosulphate. The important treatment is dietetic. Corn, maize, and wheat are not so rich in the preventive substance as are the animal products; meat, eggs and milk. Dried yeast, tomatoes, and fresh beef and other animal protein products are particularly recommended. The dietary measures should be used for prophylaxis as well as treatment.

References

1. Hist. Nat. y. Med. de el Princip. de Asturias, 1762. 2. Trans. Nat. Assoc. for the Study of Pellagra, 1912, 18. 3. Am. J. Insanity, 1864, **21,** 223. 4. Am. J. Dis. Child., 1912, **4,** 172. 5. Am. J. Dis. Child., 1914, **7,** 124. 6. Trans. Nat. Assoc. for the Study of Pellagra, 1912, 333. 7. Am. J. M. Sc., 1915, **149,** 859. 8. Arch. Pediat., 1917, **34,** 254. 9. Pub. Health Rep., 1914, **29,** 1683; 1915, **30,** 3117; 1922, **37,** 462; 1923, **38,** 2361; 1924, **39,** 87; 1926, **41,** 297; 1927, **42,** 1299; 2193; J.A.M.A., 1916, **66,** 471; 1922, **78,** 1676; Medicine 1926, **5,** 79. 10. J.A.M.A., 1931, **96,** 325. 11. Trat. profilat. e. clin. della pellagra 1892; German by Kurella 1898. 12. J. Trop. Med. and Hyg., 1910, **13,** 271. 13. Am. J. M. Sc., 1913, **146,** 233. 14. Am. J. M. Sc., 1913, **146,** 411. 15. J.A.M.A., 1913, **60,** 1948. 16. South. M. J., 1918, **11,** 785. 17. J.A.M.A., 1923, **80,** 365. 18. Science, Sup., 1931, **74,** 12. 19. Science, 1930, **72,** 577. 20. Contributo nuovo alla etiologia e patogenesi della pellagra, 1914; Ref. J.A.M.A., 1914, **63,** 868. 21. South. M. J., 1919, **12,** 238. 22. Trans. Nat. Assoc. for the Study of Pellagra, 1912, 27.

CHAPTER XII

ACRODYNIA

(Erythredema; Pink Disease; Dermato-polyneuritis; Swift's Disease)

THE term "acrodynia" is derived from the Greek and denotes "painful extremities." The history of the condition is somewhat obscure, and it is not entirely clear how long the malady has been known. Certainly the erythredema described by Swift[1] in Australia in 1914 is identical with acrodynia as seen in the United States. Bilderback[2] observed instances of the affection in this country as early as 1914, and Byfield[3] in 1915. We have seen a number of typical cases. The title acrodynia was employed by Weston,[4] using the name applied to a disorder seen in France in 1827 and 1829, but which would appear to have been a different disease. Several years later Feer[5] published an extensive contribution upon what he considered to be a hitherto undiscovered neurosis of the vegetative nervous system. Its characteristics, however, appear to be identical with those of the condition earlier described by others and about to be detailed.

Etiology.—Acrodynia, as here described, occurs only in infants and quite young children. The cases are sporadic, but may appear in groups in a way which suggests an epidemic. Sex, season and climate apparently have little influence. Byfield[3] believes that infection of the upper respiratory tract possesses etiologic significance, and that the nature of the disease is a peripheral neuritis mainly involving sensory nerves. Rodda[6] maintains that diseased tonsils are causative. Vipond[7] discovered a gram-positive diplococcus in the lymph-nodes, but in 1 instance only. Helmick[8] suggests that it is an allergic manifestation of some sort. Weston[9] regards it as a deficiency disease with infection superimposed. It has also been suggested that the endocrines are at fault. There is no connection with syphilis. If the disease is a specific infection or due to a dietary deficiency, this yet remains to be shown, and the actual cause is unknown.

Pathologic Anatomy.—This has been little studied. Paterson and Greenfield[10] found the skin normal in 1 case examined. Byfield,[3] Paterson and Greenfield,[10] and Kernohan and Kennedy[11] discovered certain degenerative changes in the peripheral nerves, the nerve roots, the spinal cord, and other parts of the central nervous system. In several reported deaths a complicating acute miliary tuberculosis has been observed.

Symptoms.—The onset lasts two or three weeks or longer, during which the patient is irritable, has anorexia and irregular fever, and frequently rhinitis. There then develops a symmetrical erythema of a decidedly pink color, which is most marked at the ends of the fingers and toes, but extends over the hands as far as the wrists, and the feet as far as the ankles, where it gradually shades off into normal tissue. The cheeks and the tip of the nose are occasionally involved. Pin-head sized papules may develop. The rash is constantly present, although it may fade for a week or two to return later; and at intervals branny desquamation occurs. The skin macerated by perspiration may peel and secondary infection take place. The extremities are cold and clammy and occasionally cyanotic and appear swollen, although edema can seldom be demonstrated. The palms and soles may become pigmented. Elsewhere on the body scattered areas of a vesicular or maculopapular rash may appear.

There is always constant pain in the extremities, which is worse at night. Older children complain of paresthesia, itching, tingling, and burning, and the hands and feet are rubbed in the effort to obtain relief. Occasionally there are motor symptoms of weakness or paralysis. Photophobia is very common, and the child hangs his head or buries it in the pillow. There are great irritability and marked insomnia, perhaps replaced at times by apathy and stupor. Profuse perspiration is always present, and there may be salivation. The most marked gastrointestinal symptom is the anorexia, and there may also be loose, foul stools and occasionally vomiting. In severe cases the teeth may fall out, and ulceration of the gums or even necrosis of the jaw may develop. Occasionally there may be alopecia, sometimes shedding of the finger nails and toe nails, and rarely loss of the digits. The blood may show a secondary anemia, and often a mild polymorphonuclear leukocytosis.

Course and Prognosis.—While the disease usually lasts several months, complete recovery almost invariably follows. Pyelitis is a not infrequent complication.

Diagnosis.—Acrodynia must be distinguished chiefly from pellagra. In the latter the rash on the hands is not so pink in color and there is a sharp line of demarcation where the cutaneous lesions cease (p. 505). Pain and paresthesia are not present. In Raynaud's disease the discoloration is more cyanotic, there is an early stage of coldness and pallor, but none of the constitutional disturbances of acrodynia.

Treatment.—Soothing lotions, such as of boric acid or calamine, may be applied to the extremities, and the child restrained from constantly rubbing them. Atropine may help to check the excessive perspiration. Sedatives are often needed. Arsenic appears sometimes to be helpful. Byfield[3] and Rodda[6] claim good results from removal of foci of infection. The diet should be that suitable for the child's age, and gavage resorted to if anorexia indicates it. McClendon[12] claimed good results in a case in which yeast and viosterol were given. Ordinarily there seems to be little effect from the administration of vitamin B preparations. Raw liver is claimed by Wyllie and Stern[13] to be efficacious. General hygienic measures are important. Local applications of heat or exposure to infra-red light may be helpful, and ultraviolet therapy may be tried. So far, however, there appears to be no specific treatment known.

References

1. Lancet, 1918, **1,** 611. 2. Northwest Med., 1920, **19,** 263; J.A.M.A., 1925, **84,** 495. 3. Am. J. Dis. Child., 1920, **20,** 347. 4. Arch. Pediat., 1920, **37,** 513. 5. Ergebn. d. inn. Med. u. Kinderh., 1923, **24,** 100. 6. Am. J. Dis. Child., 1925, **30,** 224. 7. Arch. Pediat., 1922, **39,** 699. 8. Arch. Pediat., 1927, **44,** 405. 9. South. M. J., 1931, **34,** 378. 10. Quart. J. Med., 1923, **17,** 6. 11. Am. J. Dis. Child., 1928, **36,** 341. 12. J.A.M.A., 1929, **93,** 455. 13. Arch. Dis. Childhood, 1931, **6,** 137.

CHAPTER XIII

POISONING

Poisoning is probably more common than the frequency of diagnosis of it would indicate. The possibility of its occurrence should always be borne in mind in the case of acutely sick children when the cause of their symptoms is not obvious. Poisoning may come about from overdose of drugs used for therapeutical purposes, or from the ingestion by the child, of his own accord, of a wide variety of substances. The carelessness of many parents, and the constant tendency of so many small children to put nearly everything into their mouths, renders the consideration of the subject most desirable. However, only the more important possible sources of poisoning in children can be discussed in this chapter.

Poisoning by Patent Medicines.—It may be difficult to determine the ingredients of various patent medicines, but some idea may be derived from the name, appearance, or odor of them, or the symptoms induced. Even if analysis were always feasible, the results of it might be learned too late to be of service. The publications of the American Medical Association "Nostrums and Quackery" and "Miscellaneous Nostrums" are convenient references.

In an emergency certain general facts may be helpful:

Most patent *liniments* contain such drugs as menthol, capsicum, chloroform, alcohol, and acetone. Many *laxatives* have phenolphthalein or the saline cathartics as their active ingredient; others aloes, calomel and the like; and some strychnine and belladonna. The *headache, cold,* and *grippe cures* usually consist of caffeine, antipyrine, phenacetin, salicylates, bromides, or quinine. The *eczema cures* often have such active ingredients as salicylic acid and carbolic acid. The *digestants* are harmless as a rule, and consist mostly of chalk, charcoal, pepsin and pancreatin. The medicinal constituent of most *worm-syrups* is santonin. Most *tonics* contain gentian and laxatives, and many quinine, strychnine or iron. The numerous *ointments* are quite varied in character, and may consist among other things of carbolic acid, salicylic acid, turpentine and capsicum. There are several so-called "*pneumonia-cures*" and "*salves,*" in which a lard-base is incorporated with such drugs as camphor, turpentine, carbolic acid, quinine, thyme, and eucalyptus. *Asthma-cures* contain the iodides, atropine, and some of them cocaine (noted on package); others have potassium nitrate and stramonium present. The most vicious of all the patent medicines are the so-called "*soothing syrups*" or "*baby's friends.*" In these there are often laxatives such as castor oil, calomel, or some of the saline cathartics, in addition to carminatives. Most important is the fact that many of them contain opium or its derivatives, patent medicine companies having the privilege of using in their nostrums as much as 2 grains (0.13) of opium, $\frac{1}{4}$ grain (0.016) of morphine, 1 grain (0.065) of codeine and $\frac{1}{8}$ grain (0.008) of heroine to the ounce, and there are no restrictions as to the frequency with which purchase may be made.

Insecticides and Rat-poisons.[1]—The composition of these is varied, and may include arsenious oxide, copper hydrate, lead oxide, lead arsenate, tobacco (nicotine), phenol, strychnine, lime, and sulphur. Many of the powders for roaches, water-bugs, ants and the like contain sodium fluoride, white hellebore (veratrum viride), or sodium fluosilicate; in others there is lead, sulphur, lime or phosphorus; and in the liquid preparations phenol, nitrobenzene or mercury. *Fly-poisons* usually consist of some form of arsenic. Some *insect-powders* contain pyrethrum. The *moth-destroyers* are composed of naphthalene, camphor, or cedar-gum. In many insecticides to be used against mosquitoes and bed-bugs there is methyl alcohol or nitrobenzene; and in a few, tartar emetic or tobacco.

Fireworks.—In some of these phosphorus or mercury is present. Several deaths in children are on record from phosphorus-poisoning caused by the ingestion of a variety of fireworks known as "Spit-Devils," "Son-of-a-Guns," or "Devils on the Walk" (Dwyer and Helwig[2]). Another variety, known as "Pharaoh's Serpents" or "Snake-in-the-Grass," contains mercury thiocyanid. We have seen a child of two years of age who ingested three of these, containing about 18 grains (1.15) of mercury in all; but who finally recovered after exhibiting anuria for six days, combined with very palpable enlargement of the kidneys (Friedman[3]).

Food-poisoning.—There are discussed elsewhere the disturbances resulting from indigestion, from allergy, and from the transmission of parasites or bacterial diseases by contaminated food. Certain vegetable and animal foods are in themselves poisonous, among them being some varieties of berries, mushrooms, and fish. There are two common types of mushroom poisoning: (1) that from amanita phalloides, characterized by abdominal pain, diarrhea, vomiting, jaundice, cyanosis, and symptoms of acute nephritis; and (2) from amanita muscaria, characterized by salivation, sweating, constricted pupils and violent gastrointestinal symptoms. In both types there may be convulsions, but particularly in the second, and, in addition, marked mental symptoms such as excitement and hallucinations. Atropine is used in treating the second variety, and in both are employed emetics, gastric lavage, catharsis, application of heat, stimulation, and the administration of large quantities of fluid, perhaps by saline transfusion.

We wish to call attention especially to the form of poisoning induced by the presence in the food of organisms of the paratyphoid-enteritidis or Salmonella group, such as Gärtner's bacillus, B. typhi murium, B. aertrycke, B. suipestifer and B. paratyphosus A and B, and in some instances staphylococci. To such poisoning the term "ptomaine" is often incorrectly applied;—a ptomaine being a toxic protein or lipoid cleavage-product formed by the action of bacteria on animal tissue before its ingestion, or less frequently by certain bacteria in the living intestinal tract. Ptomaine poisoning is rare, but may result from the eating of decomposed meat, or perhaps occasionally of decomposed vegetables. The *symptoms* of food-poisoning are those of violent gastro-enteritis, usually without bloody stools, coming on six to twelve hours after the ingestion of the food. There may be fever, extreme prostration, and evidences of central nervous irritation. The *prognosis* is good, except in very early life. In epidemics of food-poisoning the mortality is variously reported as from 1 to 4 per cent. The *treatment* consists in gastric lavage and the administration of purgatives. Nothing should be done at first to check the diarrhea. Stimulating measures and administration of fluid may be indicated.

Botulism is a special type of food-poisoning due to an anaerobic, spore-bearing organism, the Clostridium botulinum (Bacillus botulinus). This produces a toxin readily destroyed by heat, which has a selective action upon the cells of the anterior horns of the spinal cord and on other nervous tissue. It is probably not formed in the body, but in the food before it is taken, and is found particularly in home-canned vegetables, fruits, and meat; less often in commercially canned substances, as sausage and ripe olives; and rarely in over-ripe fresh fruit. The substances are usually noticeably decomposed. The *symptoms* develop after one to three days or longer, and are chiefly those of involvement of the peripheral nerves, as disturbed vision, dilated or irregular pupils, strabismus, diplopia, or nystagmus. Paralysis of the pharyngeal muscles may occur. There is decided constipation and abdominal distention. No sensory symptoms are present, and the mind generally remains clear. The mortality is high, equalling about 50 per cent. *Treatment* is supportive and stimulative in nature. Atropine should not be given. A serum has been prepared of which 20,000 units should be given intravenously as soon as the diagnosis is suspected, or at the onset of symptoms, since later in the course it has little effect. Ether or luminal is said to have a favorable effect, as also morphine, on the ground that it delays the course of the intoxication and allows a longer time for the antitoxin to exert its influence.

A form of poisoning known as **milk sickness** is produced by drinking milk or eating dairy products derived from cattle with "the trembles," the animals having eaten the white snakeroot or the rayless golden rod. The *symptoms* are continuous vomiting, constipation, subnormal temperature, acetonuria, lipemia, and hypoglycemia. The *treatment* consists in gastric lavage, the administration of alcohol and sodium bicarbonate, and the giving of glucose by enema or parenteral injection.

Poisoning in Other Ways. Dyes.—Some laundry-inks, shoe-dyes, hair-dyes and other dyes contain nitrobenzene or aniline. Poisoning may occur by contact with linen marked with an aniline dye. We have seen this last incident on two occasions in nurseries for the new-born. (See reports on Shoe-Dye Poisoning, by Riviere,[4] Aikman,[5] and Levin,[6] and on Aniline-Dye Poisoning from hospital linen by Zeligs[7] and Weinberg.[8]) (See also p. 512.) There may be a sufficient absorption of phenol or salicylic acid from ointments applied over an open wound or diseased skin to cause general symptoms. Poisoning by the ingestion of lead or arsenic will be mentioned later.

Here may be noted, incidentally, *electric shock.* The symptoms of this are shock and collapse, with respiratory failure. In less severe cases mental confusion may replace unconsciousness. The treatment consists in artificial respiration, which should be continued for a long period before hope is abandoned.

GENERAL SYMPTOMS AND TREATMENT OF POISONING

In addition to the symptoms and treatment already detailed or described later for specific forms of poisoning, certain general therapeutic principles will suggest themselves and the selection of these be indicated by the symptoms present. Among them are gastric lavage and the administration of emetics and purges; demulcent drinks such as milk, white of egg and bland oils in the case of the corrosive poisons; external heat and elevation of the lower part of the body in collapse; stimulants; artificial respiration and administration of oxygen and carbon dioxide; fluid by mouth or parenterally in dehydration. In *poisoning by heavy metals,* such as thallium, zinc, tin, arsenic, lead, mercury, copper and bismuth, the administration of sodium thiosulphate has been recommended as an antidote on the ground that it causes neutralization of these in the stomach and renders more soluble in the tissues any which have already been absorbed. The stomach is washed with 500 cc. (16.9 fl. oz.) of water to which has been added 30 Gm. (463 grains) of sodium thiosulphate, after which a smaller amount is introduced into the stomach and allowed to remain. Intravenously 0.3 to 1.8 Gm. (4.6 to 27.8 grains) of the drug in 20 cc. (0.68 fl. oz.) of distilled water is given every day for four days. Recent reports seem to indicate that this treatment is of comparatively little value.

In the following paragraphs the chief symptoms and treatment of various types of poisoning are given in outline form.

1. Acids.—(Hydrochloric, acetic, sulphuric, nitric, oxalic.) *Symptoms:* Destruction of mucous membrane of mouth; violent gastro-intestinal irritation with pain, nausea and vomiting; bloody diarrhea; prostration; collapse. *Treatment:* Alkalies, as magnesia, chalk, sodium bicarbonate, soap; followed by white of egg and demulcents. Intravenous injections of sodium bicarbonate and of glucose; forcing of fluid. Do not use stomach-tube. In oxalic acid poisoning do not give soda or potash; lime is the best antidote.

2. Alcohol, Methyl.—(Bed-bug poison, boot-leg liquor.) *Symptoms:* Nausea, vomiting, vertigo, delirium, blindness. *Treatment:* Bleeding and intravenous saline injection, emetics, lavage, cathartics, external heat, stimulation or sedatives. Force fluids. No direct antidote.

3. Alkalies.—(Ammonia, spirits of hartshorn, lye, caustic potash, washing soda.) *Symptoms:* Those of gastro-intestinal irritation, as with acids. *Treatment:* Dilute acids, vinegar, lemon-juice, cathartics. Force fluids.

4. Amalgam.—It has been reported that amalgam in fillings for teeth which may contain either copper or mercury may allow sufficient absorption to cause symptoms (Stock[9]).

5. Aniline.—(See Coal Tar.)

6. Antimony.—(Tartar emetic, some of the insecticides.) *Symptoms:* Severe vomiting and diarrhea, collapse, increased flow of saliva. *Treatment:* Tannic acid, strong tea, cathartics, stimulation, external heat.

7. Argyria.—From ingestion of silver salts, or their long continued application to mucous membranes. *Symptoms:* Indelible grayish-blue color to the skin, first noticed on gum margins and finger-nail ends. *Treatment:* Local intradermal injections of 1 per cent solution of potassium ferricyanide in 6 per cent sodium thiosulphate (Stillians and Lawless[10]).

8. Arsenic.—(Fly-poisons, rat-poisons, Paris green, some colored crayons, artificial flowers, wallpaper, and hair tonics.) *Symptoms:* Gastro-intestinal irritation and pain, nausea and vomiting, colic and diarrhea, convulsions. Later, albuminous and scanty urine; and, still later, multiple neuritis and dermatitis, leukopenia and an aplastic type of anemia, alopecia, herpes, pigmentation of the skin. In *subacute* or *chronic* poisoning some of the later symptoms may occur without preceding acute ones. *Treatment:* Ferri hydroxidum cum magnesii oxido (3 oz. (93.)) repeated as necessary, gastric lavage, emetics, castor oil, demulcents, adrenalin, fluids.

9. Atropine.—(Belladonna.) *Symptoms:* Flushing of skin, dilated pupils, dryness of throat, tachycardia, delirium, convulsions. Death from respiratory failure. *Treatment:* Emetics, lavage, cathartics, force fluid, promote respiration; chloroform for convulsions. Use morphine cautiously if at all, because of depressing respiratory action.

10. Barbital.—(Veronal, phenobarbital, luminal, etc.) *Symptoms:* Nausea, muscular weakness, mental confusion and incoördination; later cyanosis, stupor and respiratory failure. In chronic poisoning erythematous rash, poor memory, incoherent speech, ataxic gait, tremors. *Treatment:* Same as for other sedatives (p. 514).

11. Benzine.—(See Hydrocarbons.)

12. Boric Acid.—(As a food preservative; from too free use of boric acid solution on the breast or artificial nipples; mistaken for flour.) *Symptoms:* Anorexia, epigastric pain and colic, vomiting and diarrhea, collapse, cyanosis. *Treatment:* Lavage, purgation, stimulation.

13. Carbolic Acid.—(Some roach and insect poisons, various proprietary antiseptic applications.) *Symptoms:* Gastrointestinal irritation, vomiting and bloody diarrhea, colic, drowsiness, collapse, muscular twitchings, convulsions. Later nephritis with scanty, albuminous, and bloody or smoky urine. *Treatment:* First, white of egg; then lavage with 10 per cent alcohol. Magnesium sulphate. Do not give emetics or oils.

14. Carbon Monoxide.—(Illuminating gas, exhaust of automobile, manholes.) *Symptoms:* Unconsciousness, pinkish flush of skin, brownish-red discoloration of blood due to carbon monoxide hemoglobin. *Treatment:* Artificial respiration; inhalations of oxygen and carbon dioxide; stimulation.

15. Carbon Tetrachloride.—(Anthelmintic.) *Symptoms:* Vomiting, diarrhea, gastrointestinal hemorrhage, tremor, convulsions, collapse, icterus, low blood-calcium. *Treatment:* Calcium chloride intravenously if symptoms are urgent, or otherwise by mouth; parathyroid extract. Before using the carbon tetrachloride build up calcium reserve of body by giving one quart of milk a day, or 3 Gm. (46 grains) of a calcium salt for one week (Lamson, Minot and Robbins[11]).

16. Coal Tar Derivatives.—(Acetanilid, phenacetin, antipyrine, aniline, and certain cold and grippe cures, headache cures, certain hair tonics, and other dyes.) (See also p. 511.) *Symptoms:* Collapse, clammy sweat, vomiting, low blood pressure, somnolence, slow pulse made rapid on exertion, hematuria, death from respiratory failure. Acetanilid and phenacetin and rarely antipyrine may cause cyanosis. This is usually attributed to methemoglobinemia, but Harrop and Waterfield[12] claim that acetanilid and perhaps other aniline substances may produce sulphemoglobinemia, in which cyanosis lasts longer and is darker and more brownish in tint. *Treatment:* Emetics, lavage, external heat and stimulation, large doses of sodium bicarbonate. Oxygen has no effect on the cyanosis, but, with 5 per cent carbon dioxide, it should be used as a respiratory stimulant.

17. Cocaine.—(Asthma cures, nose drops.) *Symptoms:* At first rapid pulse, high blood-pressure, delirium, convulsions, dilated pupils. Later collapse and respiratory failure. *Treatment:* Strong tea, tannic acid, emetics, lavage, cathartics. If collapse; external heat, stimulants. If convulsions; sedatives, especially phenobarbital (Guttman[13]).

18. Copper.—(Certain rat-poisons, blue vitriol or blue stone.) *Symptoms:* Gastro-intestinal irritation, vomiting and diarrhea, the vomitus and stools being greenish or bluish at first; colic; salivation; collapse. Later, if the patient survives, there may be greenish discoloration of skin, gums and teeth; neuritis and nephritis. *Treatment:* Emetics, lavage, demulcent drinks and purgatives, stimulation, external heat, large doses of sodium bicarbonate. The chemical antidote for copper is yellow prussiate of potassium (potassium ferrocyanide), and its ordinary dose is about 5 grains (0.32).

19. Cyanides.—(Certain shoe- and silver-polishes, some insecticides.) *Symptoms:* In large doses death almost instantaneous. In smaller doses; constriction of the throat, mental confusion, irregular gait, dilated pupils, clammy sweat, convulsions, and unconsciousness. *Treatment:* Lavage with 0.3 per cent potassium permanganate, or 30 per cent hydrogen peroxide, or a fresh mixture of ferric sulphide and magnesium oxide; intravenous injections of glucose and insulin; respiratory and cardiac stimulants.

20. Ephedrine.—*Symptoms:* Restlessness, weakness, chills, nausea, tremor, palpitation (Higgins[14]).

21. Fluorides.—(Certain insect-poisons.) *Symptoms:* These develop slowly, usually with gastro-intestinal irritation, vomiting and diarrhea. The action of the fluorides is said to be in precipitating calcium from the tissues. *Treatment:* Emetics, lavage and purgatives. Force fluids.

22. Gasoline.—(See Hydrocarbons.)

23. Hydrocarbons.—(Gasoline, naphtha, benzine and kerosene.) *Symptoms: From inhalation;* burning in throat and chest, vomiting, vertigo, respiratory failure, stupor, convulsions. *From ingestion;* gastro-intestinal irritation, cyanosis, dyspnea, dilatation of pupils, collapse. *Treatment:* Artificial respiration, lavage, stimulation.

24. Jamaica Ginger.—(Certain cheap commercial brands contaminated by triorthocresyl phosphate. These probably no longer procurable.) *Symptoms:* Motor paralysis of extremities. *Treatment:* Of no value after paralysis has developed.

25. Kerosene.—(See Hydrocarbons.)

26. Lead.—(Paint; some rat-poisons and crayons.) *Chronic poisoning* may result from eating paint off cribs or toys, using water from lead containers, the employment of lead nipple-shields, the use of white face-powder by the mother (Fukushima and Matsumoto[15]). *Symptoms:* In *acute cases;* gastro-intestinal irritation, nausea and vomiting, collapse, numbness, paralysis. Later, and in *chronic cases;* multiple neuritis, nephritis, encephalitis, colic, ambliopia, choked disc, blue line in gums, stippling of red blood cells, anemia, increased density of the ends of the bones in the roentgenogram. Diagnosis in chronic cases from examination of blood and "lead lines" in roentgenograms of ends of bones (Vogt[16]). *Treatment:* In *acute cases;* emetics, lavage, magnesium sulphate, demulcents, stimulation, forcing of fluid, relief of intracranial pressure by lumbar puncture and administration of magnesium sulphate. In *chronic cases*, withdrawal of source of lead. Do not employ treatment for removal of lead by administration of acid diet or acid substances (McKhann[17]).

27. Luminal.—(See Barbital.)

28. Mercury.—(Certain rat-poisons, insecticides, fireworks, red crayons, bleaches for the skin, and certain medicinal preparations as calomel, bichloride of mercury, and some patent-medicine laxatives.) *Symptoms:* Gastrointestinal irritation, vomiting and diarrhea, colic, bloody stools, possibly delirium and coma. Later; nephritis and possibly neuritis. *Treatment:* White of egg before lavage; large doses of alkalies by mouth; sodium chloride, 0.7 per cent, intravenously.

29. Methyl Chloride.—(In some electrical refrigerators.) *Symptoms:* Inhalation causes dizziness, nausea, vomiting, mental confusion, anuria, perhaps convulsions and coma. *Treatment:* Alkalies by mouth, oxygen, stimulation. Do not give chloral or chloroform.

30. Naphtha.—(See Hydrocarbons.)

31. Nicotine.—(Tobacco; some insecticides.) *Symptoms:* Depression, clammy perspiration, nausea, vomiting, collapse. *Treatment:* Tannic acid, strong tea, lavage, emetics, cathartics, external heat, stimulation.

32. Opium.—(Paregoric, laudanum, morphine, heroine, codeine, soothing syrups.) *Symptoms:* Contracted pupils, slow pulse and respiration, flushing, and cyanosis. *Treatment:* Tannic acid, strong tea, emetics, lavage with 1:1000 solution of potassium permanganate, stimulation (especially caffeine and strychnine), artificial respiration. Keep patient awake.

33. Phosphorus.—(Certain fireworks and rat- and insect-poisons. Phosphorus in a poisonous form is now rarely used in the manufacture of matches.) *Symptoms:* Usually develop slowly, *i. e.*, after several hours;—Nausea, vomiting (garlic-odor), prostration, intestinal pain. Later; bloody diarrhea, enlargement of liver, jaundice, convulsions, coma, nephritis, sugar in urine, hemorrhage from mucous membranes, increased cholesterol in blood. *Treatment:* Emetics (especially copper sulphate 5 grains (0.32)); lavage with 1:1000 potassium permanganate; hydrogen peroxide or ozonized turpentine ($\frac{1}{2}$ teaspoonful every hour for five doses); cathartics; glucose; stimulation; external heat. Do not give oils. Atkinson,[18] and Dwyer and Helwig[2] recommend 50 to 100 cc. (1.7 to 3.4 fl. oz.) liquid petrolatum to act as a solvent of the phosphorus.

34. Salicylates.—(Headache- and grippe-cures.) *Symptoms:* Flushing of skin, disturbance of vision and hearing, delirium, collapse, slow pulse, clammy sweat, air-hunger, acidosis, pupils at first contracted and later dilated, pulmonary edema. *Treatment:* Emetics, lavage, cathartics, external heat, stimulation, sedatives.

35. Sedatives.—(See also Barbital.) (Bromides, chloral, headache-cures.) *Symptoms:* Drowsiness, coma, subnormal temperature, nausea and vomiting, slow pulse, feeble respiration, diminished reflexes, collapse. *Treatment:* Emetics; lavage; cathartics; stimulation by strychnine, caffeine, pituitary extract; external heat; artificial respiration. In bromide poisoning give intravenous injections of sodium chloride (0.7 per cent solution).

36. Silver.—(*Acute poisoning* from silver nitrate, cosmetics, certain hair dyes.) (See also Argyria for *chronic poisoning.*) *Symptoms:* Immediate vomiting with constriction of throat and pain in stomach, vomitus turns black on exposure to air, bloody stools, vertigo, respiratory failure, paresis, coma. *Treatment:* At first give milk and eggs to form silver albuminate, or sodium chloride or tannic acid to form insoluble silver salts; immediately follow this by gastric lavage.

37. Snake-bite.—2 types of venoms, (1) hemolytic, causing prostration and local extravasation of blood, and (2) neurotoxic, producing paralysis, collapse and respiratory failure. *Treatment:* Venom destroyed by local applications of potassium permanganate, silver nitrate or hypochlorites; ligature above bite and free incision at the bite; small repeated doses of stimulating drugs; "antivenins" specific for each snake. Alcohol is not a specific.

38. Strychnine.—(A few rat-poisons, tincture of nux vomica, some laxative pills.) *Symptoms:* Irritability, nervousness, tetanic convulsions, rapid pulse. *Treatment:* Tannic acid, strong tea, emetics, lavage, chloroform-inhalations, apomorphine, sedatives (bromides, chloral and phenobarbital).

39. Thallium.—(Some rat-poisons, and depilatories.) *Symptoms:* Petechial eruption, stomatitis, abdominal pain, diarrhea, intestinal hemorrhage, eosinophilia, arthritis. In *slow poisoning,* nervous symptoms, gastritis, colitis, testicular atrophy, removal of calcium from bones. *Treatment:* Lavage, emetics, stimulation, purges, administration of calcium. (See also treatment for heavy metal poisoning, lead, etc., pp. 511.)

References

1. Information from Court Proc. and letter from Insecticide and Fungicide Board, U. S. Dept. Agric. 2. J.A.M.A., 1925, **84,** 1254. 3. Cincinnati M. J., 1926, **43,** 193. 4. Ann. de méd et chir. inf., 1911, **15,** 551. 5. Am. J. Dis. Child., 1928, **35,** 1038. 6. J.A.M.A., 1931, **96,** 681. 7. Arch. Pediat, 1929, **46,** 502. 8. Am. J. Obst. & Gynec., 1931, **21,** 104. 9. Med. Klin., 1928, **124,** 1114; 1154. 10. J.A.M.A., 1929, **92,** 20. 11. J.A.M.A., 1928, **90,** 345. 12. J.A.M.A., 1930, **95,** 647. 13. J.A.M.A., 1928, **90,** 753. 14. J.A.M.A., 1929, **92,** 313. 15. Orient. J. Dis. Infants, 1928, **3,** 27. 16. J.A.M.A., 1932, **98,** 125. 17. Arch. Neurol. and Psychiat., 1932, **27,** 294. 18. J. Lab. and Clin. Med., 1921, **7,** 148.

SECTION IV

DISEASES OF THE DIGESTIVE SYSTEM

CHAPTER I

DISEASES OF THE MOUTH, LIPS, JAWS, TONGUE, AND SALIVARY GLANDS

DISEASES AND MALFORMATIONS OF THE JAWS

THE failure of union of the two sides of the upper jaw is described under **cleft palate** (p. 529); and the narrowing caused by adenoids is referred to elsewhere (p. 543). **Prognathism** of the upper jaw is not infrequent. It results in the upper teeth slanting forward beyond the lower. It may be a fault of development, or may sometimes be produced by thumb-sucking (p. 891). Prognathism of the lower jaw is also encountered. Sometimes the lower jaw is abnormally small (**micrognathia**), the teeth failing to come into position below the upper ones when the mouth is closed. When this condition is well-marked in the new-born the tongue may be displaced posteriorly, and difficulty in breathing result. Placing the infant on its face may alleviate this, or splinting of the jaw may be necessary (Eley and Farber[1]). Very occasionally **exostoses** are encountered; or **odontomata** from irregularity in the development of one or more teeth of the second set within the body of the jaws. **Malignant new-growths** connected with the jaw are not of great frequency in early life, the most common being sarcoma. Tumors arising at the junction of the gums with the jaw (*epulis*) are occasionally seen. Generally the growth is a simple granuloma connected with a diseased tooth; but even if sarcomatous, the removal is generally not followed by any return. Maxillary cysts of congenital origin may occur. **Necrosis** of a portion of the jaw may follow alveolar abscess, ulcerative stomatitis, or noma; and in cases of the last-mentioned disorder in which life is not lost great deformity may remain. Osteomyelitis of the jaw is not uncommon in the first two months of life. (For review see Wilensky.[2]) **Ankylosis** of the jaw may result from noma or from traumatism. A **chronic ostitis** may be produced by tuberculosis or syphilis. A rare deformity is **macrostomia** (large mouth).

DISEASES OF THE LIPS

HARELIP.—This common deformity is caused by the failure of the fronto-nasal palate to unite with the lateral process on one side, thus producing a fissure beneath the nostril (single harelip). It is more frequent in white than in negro children. When occurring on both sides double harelip results (p. 529, Fig. 123). The fissure varies in degree from a slight notching to a complete cleft passing into the nostril. In the latter event, particularly if on both sides, cleft palate also is commonly present. Very rarely there is a cleft of the lower lip. The fissure may be great enough to interfere with nursing, with consequent inanition from lack of nourishment. Apart from cleanliness of the mouth the treatment is entirely surgical. Operation should be performed when the infant is in good general condition, and preferably at from two to three months of age, unless difficulty in feeding the child makes earlier interference necessary.

Erosions at the Angles of the Mouth (Faule Ecken, Perlèche).—This condition, long known but first carefully studied by Lemaistre[3] in 1886 and called La Perlèche, (*pour lécher*), is not of very frequent occurrence. It affects especially young children; is favored by debility and uncleanliness; and would even appear to be contagious. A streptococcus has been described by Lemaistre.[3] The lesions consist of small, painful, fissure-like ulcers arranged radially at the labial angle, generally at both sides (Fig. 117). The course is favorable and recovery takes place in from two to four weeks under treatment, leaving no scars in the majority of instances; but without treatment the course may be prolonged and may become chronic. Except

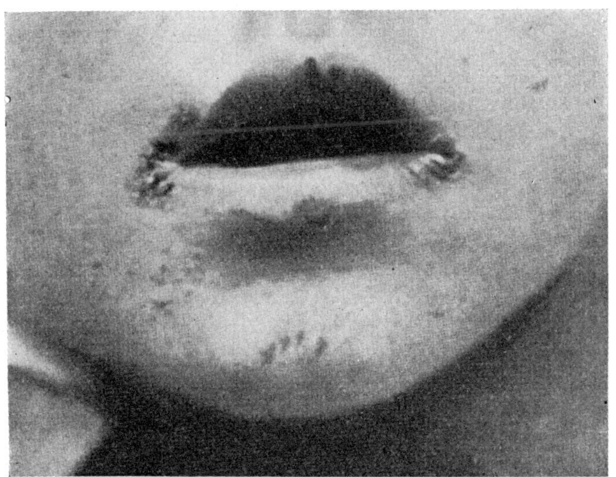

Fig. 117.—Erosions at the angles of the mouth. (*Epstein, Jahrb. f. Kinderheilk.*, 1900, **51**, 317.)

in severe cases there is no lymphatic involvement. The lesions differ from syphilis in that the fissures never extend into the mouth nor deeply into the tissues, and are without induration at the base.

Treatment.—For *prophylaxis* the mouth should be kept clean, and possible infection from other children avoided. For the *developed disease* the fissures should be touched with a 10 per cent solution of nitrate of silver, a crystal of sulphate of copper, burnt alum, or tincture of iodine, and then treated with compound tincture of benzoin, or an ointment of zinc and bismuth or of yellow oxide of mercury applied.

Other affections of the lips, such as syphilitic lesions, herpes, eczema, and the like, are discussed in the sections dealing with these.

ANOMALIES OF DENTITION

Natal Teeth (*Dentitio praecox*).—Exceptionally infants are born with one or more teeth which are nearly always the lower central incisors, and poorly developed. Ballentyne[4] was able to collect but 70 reported cases. There may be a hereditary tendency. We have seen two instances in which the mothers had presented the same anomaly at birth. Unless the tooth is so loosely attached that extraction is necessary, it may be allowed to remain, provided it does not render nursing too painful. Natal teeth may sometimes be supernumerary, and then will be replaced later by the teeth of the first dentition.

Early Dentition.—Dentition may occur as early as the age of three months. This is an occasional characteristic of hereditary syphilis, but is not a proof of the existence of this disease. In some instances it is a familial characteristic. Sometimes a hard white cyst, suggesting an erupting tooth, appears on the alveolar margin in the first few months of life.

Delayed Dentition.—Much more frequent than prematurity of dentition is delay of it. Within normal limits the first teeth may not appear until the age of a year, but a period longer than this is a strong indication of the presence of rickets; less often of cretinism, mongolism, or some other condition.

Irregularities of Dentition.—Disturbed *sequence* in the eruption of the teeth seems to have but little significance, and in our experience has been sometimes both a hereditary and a familial characteristic. It is not infrequently seen in rachitis. The appearance of the upper incisors before the lower has been claimed (Jacobi[5]) to be an attendant upon idiocy with premature ossification of the cranium, but it may occur in normal infants. Irregularities in *shape* and *character* are seen especially in the disposition to caries attending such severe constitutional disturbances as rickets and tuberculosis. Furrowing, erosions, and mottling of the teeth, especially those of the permanent set, may be due to defective formation of the enamel, often dating from stomatitis or some constitutional acute or chronic illness in early childhood, or being hereditary. The peg-shaped or notched permanent incisors in inherited syphilis are also to be noted. (See p. 434.) Other irregularities are sometimes seen, such as that of *size*, some teeth being abnormally small or abnormally large. *Increased rapidity* in the eruption of teeth may follow a febrile condition. The *number* of the teeth is sometimes abnormal, especially in the permanent set, one or more teeth being wanting, or occasionally the number being greater than normal. The abnormality may sometimes be familial. Failure of the temporary teeth to fall out at the proper time is liable to occasion *malposition* of those of the second set. Excessive thumb-sucking sometimes forces the incisors of the lower jaw inward and those of the upper jaw outward (see p. 891), as may also the constant sucking at a rubber "comforter." Lip-sucking, too, may cause depression of the lower incisors. All these faulty habits have, however, surprisingly little effect in producing deformities.

Hereditary Ectodermal Dysplasia.—Here may be mentioned an interesting malformation of the teeth associated with other defects. It has been described by Weech,[6] and Clouston[7] records 119 cases occurring in six generations of one family. Other cases have since been reported. The teeth may be completely absent, or decreased in number, especially in the lower jaw; they decay readily; and the incisors are deformed, in being protruding, aplastic, or misshapen. In addition the skin is thin and often whitish in color and presents a papular eruption. Biopsy may show that the sweat and sebaceous glands are absent. There is no visible perspiration (anhidrosis), and as a result there may be intolerance to external heat. The hair is fine and lanugo-like, and the eyebrows and eyelashes may be absent and the nails atrophic. The mucous membranes are dry and the vermilion border of the lip poorly defined. In some cases there are ocular deformities, such as congenital cataract, and in others deformed ears.

Difficult Dentition.—Unfortunately the custom is wide-spread among the laity, and even to too great an extent in the medical profession, of attributing to "teething," ailments which have no connection with it. Opposed to this view is the modern one that teething is a purely physiologic process and never produces unpleasant symptoms. The truth probably lies somewhere between these extremes, although, with many others, we believe that the rôle played by teething in the production of symptoms is a very small one, and that, as a rule, dentition produces only teeth. The error lies largely in assuming that redness of the gum over a tooth about to appear is an indication of trouble produced by the tooth. As a matter of fact there is scarcely a time in the first two years of life when a tooth is not either pushing through the gum or, more deeply situated, through the alveolar process. If pain and other disturbances are caused by the tooth they should rather occur during the more difficult process—the advance of the tooth through the resistant bony structure—for the thin layer of the gum overlying a tooth which is nearly erupted is comparatively insensitive. Lancing of the gum often relieves a localized catarrhal stomatitis and the accompanying local and nervous symptoms; but it is the stomatitis, not the presence of the tooth, which is causing the disturbance in the majority of cases, and which is relieved by the operation. Nevertheless there are exceptional instances seen in particularly susceptible children when the close approach of a tooth to the gum appears to produce symptoms promptly relieved by lancing. Among these symptoms may be mentioned moderate fever, restlessness, disturbed sleep, fretfulness, loss of appetite, diarrhea, otalgia, salivation, and a constant tendency to put the hands into the mouth. Convulsions may very rarely occur, but we have never seen an instance of this which could unequivocally be attributed to teething. A careful search must be made for all other causes for the symptoms mentioned, and lancing of the gums should be the last, not the first, thought. Gum-lancing, if not followed by a prompt eruption of the tooth, may possibly produce a cicatrix which would increase the supposed difficulty in the eruption.

Alveolar Abscess (*Gum-boil*).—This is a common affection, especially in those whose teeth have been neglected. Pain and swelling result, sometimes with fever. The whole side of the face may be much swollen. The pus usually discharges itself into the mouth, but occasionally externally through the cheek or into the antrum. The treatment should, of course, have been prophylactic, in keeping the teeth clean and free from decay, and in the removal of carious roots. The treatment of the attack consists in the employment of hot applications within the mouth, and the opening of the abscess as soon as possible.

Caries.—This is of extremely common occurrence. Formerly only local causes were sought for, such as lack of care, action of acidophilic bacteria, and the influence of a high carbohydrate diet in favoring the bacterial growth. There have been a number of more recent studies, among them those of Marshall,[8] Howe,[9] Mellanby,[10] McCollum and his coworkers,[11] Grieves,[12] Boyd, Drain and Nelson,[13] Kappes,[14] Bunting,[15] Hanke,[16] and Block;[17] the prevailing opinion being that diets high in mineral and vitamin content aid in the prevention and cure of caries, and that the bacteria are of less importance. Cohen[18] and others think the saliva contains a substance antagonistic to caries. Hess and Abramson[19] can find no connection of vitamin deficiency with caries. Mellanby[10] believes certain cereals have a decalcifying action. Pattison and Proud,[20] Howe,[21] and others think the diet of the mother asserts a prenatal influence on the teeth. Our[22] own observations failed to show any close connection of the maternal diet with dental caries in the child. Nothing, however, yet known militates against the advisability of keeping the mouth and teeth in a clean condition.

The effect of caries is seen locally in the production of such conditions as toothache, foul breath, imperfect mastication, alveolar abscess, gingivitis, and stomatitis. Probably anemia, low-grade fever, and disease in distant parts of the body, such as the joints, the genito-urinary system, the circulatory system, and the like, may result from a persistent gingivitis or from abscess in the jaws the result primarily of caries. Facial tics and habit-spasms seem in some instances to depend upon diseased teeth.

The importance of prevention and treatment of caries is evident. This is accomplished by local cleanliness and the systematic use of the tooth-brush and a simple tooth-paste. Antiseptics have no place, since they can be effective only for a few minutes, if at all. The mouth is normally acid, and its reaction can be changed for only a short period by any substance introduced into it. The diet should contain stale bread, vegetables, and fruits, in order that there may be mechanical cleansing by mastication; and it should be otherwise well-balanced and have a proper mineral and vitamin content. In short, a diet which is correct for the child will also be correct for its teeth. The teeth should be examined by a dentist at regular intervals and caries of both temporary and permanent teeth should receive prompt attention.

PIGMENTATION OF THE MUCOUS MEMBRANE

Pigmentation of the mouth may occur in Addison's disease and possibly in pernicious anemia (Rolleston[23]). It may also be present and very dark, in the absence of disease, in persons of dark complexion or in dark-skinned races. The subject has been reviewed by Weber.[24] Localized upon the tongue it aids in producing the condition known as "black tongue." (See p. 526.)

STOMATITIS

Etiology.—All forms of stomatitis are more frequent in childhood and early infancy than in adult life. An exception to this is pyorrhea, which is very uncommon in infancy and childhood. Traumatism of various sorts, such as rough washing of the mouth or the action of irritating chemical or thermal agents, is active in the production of *catarrhal stomatitis*, as of other forms, and bacterial action and lack of cleanliness are also operative. Diseases of the gastroenteric tract are very commonly attended by catarrhal stomatitis, as are the infectious disorders, especially measles, diphtheria, and scarlet fever. In *aphthous stomatitis* no specific organism has been demonstrated. Gerstenberger[25] believes that the underlying factor is a disturbance of nutrition, perhaps through lack of vitamin B. Ollivier[26] and others claim that the malady is identical with the foot-and-mouth disease of cattle and transmitted from them, but for this view there appears to be lack of evidence. Uncleanliness of the mouth is an important predisposing factor, and disturbances of digestion are not infrequently associated. *Thrush* is an affection known since earliest times, but its nature was not understood until the studies of Berg[27] in 1841 and of Müller[28] in 1842. The causative agent is a mold-fungus of the class of hyphomycetes, variously designated, but oftenest named the "Oidium albicans" (Robin[29]) or the monilia candida (Plaut[30]). Under the microscope can be seen long, fine mycelial threads with numerous gonidia, mingled with epithelial cells, red and white blood-cells, and bacteria. The fungus is subject to considerable pleomorphism in its growth. It may be found in the normal mouth without producing infection, in the stools, and it exists to a certain extent free in the air. It is, therefore, widespread and only awaits favorable conditions for its development. Thrush can be acquired from unclean rubber nipples and even from the human breast, is distinctly infectious, and will spread rapidly in nurseries and hospitals for infants, in spite of careful hygienic precautions. It is seen almost solely at an early age, particularly in the first two or three months of life; but may occur later in marantic or neglected subjects, or even occasionally in vigorous infants in perfect health. *Ulcerative stomatitis* occurs most frequently at from four to eight years of age, seldom before this. Uncleanliness of the mouth, carious teeth, and any debilitating influence predispose to it, and it may accompany measles, diphtheria, scarlet fever, typhoid fever, and other infectious diseases, and may be a symptom of scurvy or be produced by metallic poisoning, especially mercury. It does not seem to develop before the teeth have erupted. It has often appeared in epidemic form in hospital wards. Bernheim and Pospischill[31] found in all but 2 of 20 cases a fusiform bacillus and a spirochete identical with those seen in ulceromembraneous angina (p. 537), but these do not appear to be the etiologic agents in all cases. *Gangrenous stomatitis* is sometimes termed cancrum oris and noma. The last term may also be applied to a condition of the same nature occasionally attacking other parts of the body, as the ear, nose, genitals, or anus. It is fortunately now rare, and even in earlier times was uncommon, Woronichin[32] in 1887 reporting 22 cases among 8286 sick children in hospital-practice, and Ranke[33] in 1888 giving an incidence of 2 in from 4000 to 5000 patients. In a large hospital experience we have seen only a few cases. The disease occurs oftenest between two and five years and occasionally in infancy. According to Heinemann[34] it is twice as frequent in girls as in boys. Local epidemics of noma may occur in institutions (Blumer and MacFarlane,[35] Neuhof[36]), not all the cases, however, being limited to the mouth. Previous bad health is almost a necessity. It develops oftener after typhoid fever, and especially after measles, than under any other conditions, although it may follow pertussis, diphtheria, enteritis, tuberculosis, or other affection producing general debility. It is certainly due to a germ of some sort. Most frequently discovered are the fusospirilliform forms characteristic of ulceromembranous angina (p. 537) although these germs may often be found in the normal mouth, and in this disease may be but secondary invaders. Micro-organisms of other nature have been described by Schimmelbusch,[37] Ranke,[33] Sailer,[38] Durante,[39] and Hellesen.[40] *Herpetic stomatitis* or *simple ulceration of the mouth* may develop as a result of catarrhal stomatitis, from digestive disturbances, or in the course of the infectious diseases, as measles, typhoid fever, and the like. Certain other forms may be classified as *secondary stomatitis*, being secondary manifestations of other diseases. Thus gonorrheal stomatitis may affect the new-born (Rosinski[41]) or older children, in the latter being acquired usually by self-infection from vulvovaginitis. Diphtheritic stomatitis oftenest spreads from the fauces, but we have seen it rarely on the buccal mucous membrane before it could be discovered in the pharynx. A pseudomembranous stomatitis, other than diphtheritic, may follow caustic or thermal irritation, or be produced by the pneumococcus, streptococcus, or staphylococcus. Syphilitis stomatitis often accompanies the hereditary form of the disease, or the primary lesion may occur in the mouth in the acquired form.

Symptoms and Pathologic Anatomy.—In *catarrhal stomatitis* the mucous membrane of the mouth becomes red, hot, and tender, and bleeding may occur; salivation is excessive; taking of food into the mouth is painful; and swelling of the glands beneath the jaw may develop. Fever, if present, is slight. Restlessness, fretfulness and refusal of food are natural symptoms. The constitutional manifestations depend largely upon the condition with which the stomatitis is associated. In *aphthous stomatitis* the lesions consist of patches of irregular shape, varying in size from that of a pin-head to that of a split-pea. They are discrete, or occasionally confluent, and appear first as an elevation of the epithelium with a red margin and a whitish center. In *thrush* the parasite penetrates the lower level of the epithelium, but pus is not produced. The infection may spread to the tonsils and pharynx and rarely to the nasopharynx, middle ear, esophagus, stomach, intestines, larynx, trachea, lungs, and skin. The walls of the blood-vessels and the tissues may be penetrated in some cases (Heller[42]), and general infection and metastasis to distant parts of the body take place (Schmorl,[43] Zenker,[44]

Heubner[45]), or there may be extensive involvement of the skin (Christison[46]). In the mouth small white patches develop of pin-point size and larger, resembling curdled milk. These are situated especially on the dorsum of the tongue, as well as on the lining of the palate, cheeks and lips. They may be few in number but oftener are numerous and coalescent; are raised and covered with epithelium, and when removed usually bleed. Local symptoms are similar to those of catarrhal stomatitis, except that the mouth is rather dry. The lesions of *ulcerative stomatitis* usually begin on the free border of the gums, oftenest of the lower lateral incisors, and upon one side. There is inflammation advancing to ulceration and necrosis, the ulcers being covered by a firmly adherent, yellowish or greenish material. Necrosis spreads rapidly to the cheek and lips and, in severe cases, to the alveolar

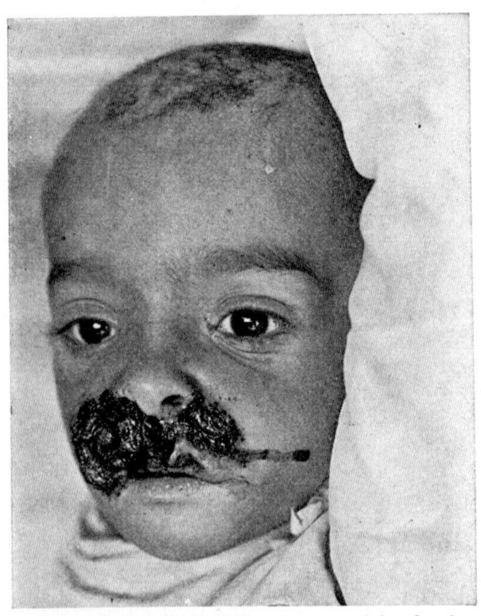

Fig. 118.—Gangrenous stomatitis beginning in the lip. Same case as in Fig. 120. Photograph taken soon after admission to the Children's Hospital of Philadelphia, Oct. 25.

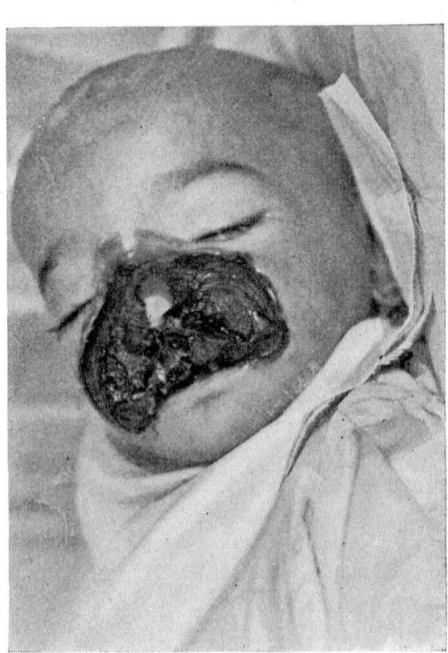

Fig. 119.—Gangrenous stomatitis beginning in the lip. Same case as in Fig. 118. Photograph taken a few days later.

process of the jaws, followed by loss of teeth. The tonsils and palate may be secondarily involved, or the process originate there. The lesions bleed easily and are painful, food is refused, and there are salivation and a very offensive odor of the breath. In severe cases there is enlargement of the submaxillary glands, and decided constitutional symptoms, even of a septic nature. In *gangrenous stomatitis* the process begins probably oftenest on the inner surface of the cheek in the form of a small dark slough, which rapidly increases in diameter and in depth. Meanwhile the substance of the cheek becomes hard and swollen, and the skin red and then blackish, and then perforation occurs. Sometimes the process begins in the substance of the cheek, or rarely on the cutaneous surface. Often, instead of the cheek, the gums or the inner surface of the lip is the primary seat (Fig. 118). In the worst cases both sides of the face rapidly become involved (Figs. 118, 119). In *herpetic stomatitis* the small ulcers are usually single or few in number and exhibit a shallow depression with superficial necrosis. Zahorsky[47] describes a type of herpetic stomatitis under the title of herpangina, which he believes to be a specific infectious disease. This occurs only in summer, and is characterized by the presence of many minute vesicles on the fauces, pillars and soft palate, together with sudden onset with high fever, pain in the neck, back, and extremities, and a short course of two or three days.

Complications and Sequels.—*Ulcerative stomatitis* may have noma developing as a sequel. *Gangrenous stomatitis* is liable to have broncho-pneumonia as a complication; and abscess or gangrene of the lungs occasionally develops. Diarrhea is very common.

Course and Prognosis.—The duration of *catarrhal stomatitis* is a few days to a week, unless prolonged by the continuance of some other disorder. *Aphthous stomatitis,* likewise, usually lasts but a few days, but may in severe cases continue for two or three weeks through the development of fresh crops of the lesions, and the general nutrition may suffer. *Thrush* may last only a day or two under proper treatment, but in debilitated subjects may be obstinate and recurring and add to the danger. Extension to the larynx or esophagus is unfavorable, death having been caused by occlusion of the latter, or fatal hemorrhage from a blood-vessel in this region (Riemschneider[48]). In blood-stream infections a fatal issue may be expected. In the average case of *ulcerative stomatitis* the attack lasts seven to ten days under suitable treatment, but without this it may continue for months. Even with proper care it may become chronic and relapses are prone to occur, or the disease may advance to the gangrenous form. The course of *gangrenous stomatitis* is usually astonishingly rapid, perforation taking place in a few days (Figs. 118 and 119). The issue is fatal in at least 75 per cent of the cases. In the remainder the slough is thrown off after eight or ten days, and exceptionally without perforation having taken place. Extensive deformity is usually left.

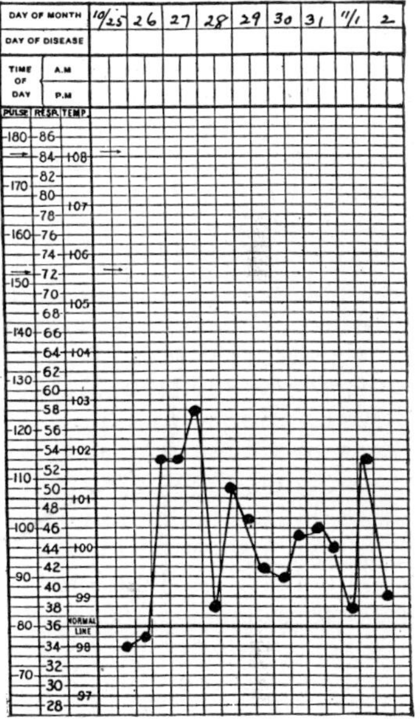

Fig. 120.—Gangrenous stomatitis. Lena P., aged two years, admitted to the Children's Hospital of Philadelphia, Oct. 25, with sloughing in the right half of the upper lip; Oct. 28, gangrene has extended rapidly, and now involves all the region of the mouth (Fig. 119), extending within it and perforating the left cheek; thorough cauterization on this date; Nov. 2, died.

Diagnosis.—The recognition of *catarrhal stomatitis* offers no difficulty. *Aphthous stomatitis* likewise is usually easily diagnosed. When confluent and appearing first or chiefly on the pharynx it might suggest diphtheria, but the presence of scattered aphthous lesions elsewhere in the oral cavity settles the question. The age-incidence of *thrush,* its characteristic curdled milk appearance, and the discovery of the specific mold-fungus should serve to differentiate it from other forms of stomatitis. *Ulcerative stomatitis* might in some cases be confused with aphthae, but the lesions in the former are fewer, deeper, and less discrete, and appear chiefly at the junction of the teeth with the gums, and the odor of the breath is more offensive. In some cases the causative action of scurvy or some other disease, or the influence of mercury, may be discovered. *Gangrenous stomatitis* can scarcely be confounded with any other disease. Well-marked ulcerative stomatitis may cause considerable necrosis and loss of teeth, but the process is very much less severe, does not produce slough, and does not involve the skin. Of the various forms of *secondary stomatitis* the diphtheritic is nearly always associated with diphtheria of the fauces, and the causative germ may be found on culture. The study of smears and culture should also serve to distinguish the various other *pseudomembranous forms* due to pneumococcus, streptococcus, or gonococcus. *Syphilis* of the mouth usually shows itself as mucous plaques or fissures of the labial commissures and should be diagnosed by the associated symptoms and the Wassermann reaction.

Treatment. Prophylaxis.—Both in health and in diseased states care should be taken to keep the mouth clean. Carious teeth should be treated. Traumatism should be avoided. The mouth should be carefully examined when mercury, bismuth, or other heavy metals are being administered. Hygienic and aseptic precautions should be carried out in institutions. Patients with thrush, or ulcerative or gangrenous stomatitis should be isolated. Scurvy and other predisposing diseases should be appropriately treated.

Treatment of the Attack.—Food is best given in a cool form and liquid or soft. In the case of infants, feeding with a spoon may be employed. In bad cases gavage may occasionally be necessary. Pieces of ice may be put frequently into the mouth. The mouth should be kept clean with oft-repeated but very gentle washing with cold water, a solution of potassium permanganate (1:8000), or a saturated solution of boric acid combined with tincture of myrrh (24:1). Painting with silver nitrate (1 to 2 per cent) may be used in *aphthous stomatitis* or the spots touched with burnt alum. The lesions of *thrush* may be cautiously rubbed away with a 5 per cent solution of bicarbonate of soda, and the mouth bathed with a potassium of permanganate solution (1:8000), or with diluted liquor formaldehyde (1 or 2:100). Borax and honey, an old time remedy, should be avoided, but borax in 25 per cent solution in glycerin may be used. Faber and Dickey[49] recommend the application of a 1 per cent solution of gentian violet several times daily, and we have found this is a very satisfactory form of treatment. We have also sometimes found that washing the mouth several times daily with a thick suspension of yeast is helpful. In both *ulcerative* and *gangrenous stomatitis*, especially if the fusiform bacillus and the spirochete can be found, arsenic in some form should be employed, in addition to the constitutional and local treatment described for stomatitis in general. It may be used locally as in Bowman's solution (Liq. pot. arsenitis 12 cc., vin. ipecac 12 cc., glyc. 8 cc.). The arsphenamines or similar preparations may be given intravenously, or sulpharsphenamine intramuscularly in cases not responding to local measures. Sodium perborate made into a paste and applied has been highly recommended by Bloodgood,[50] and chlorate of potash, cautiously given internally and excreted by the saliva, has long been considered a specific in ulcerative stomatitis. In gangrenous stomatitis there is needed in addition prompt and thorough excision and cauterization. General supporting treatment is indicated in all severe cases of stomatitis.

BEDNAR'S APHTHAE

(Pterygoid Ulcer)

This condition, first described by Bednar,[51] is in no way related to aphthous stomatitis. It is seen only in early infancy, and is produced by trauma from too forcible cleansing of the mouth, by pressure of a rubber nipple, or by the mere act of sucking by an infant with catarrhal stomatitis. There develops a superficial ulcer situated on the posterior part of the hard palate in the median line or to one side of it. Sometimes there are two ulcers symmetrically placed. The lesion is shallow, $\frac{1}{4}$ to $\frac{1}{2}$ in. (0.6 to 1.3 cm.) in diameter and covered by a greyish or yellowish-white exudate. It is painful and causes difficulty in sucking, with consequent loss of weight. Catarrhal stomatitis, thrush, or digestive disturbances may occur as complications. The ulcer heals in a few days or weeks with treatment, except in the presence of great debility. Rarely ulceration and necrosis of the bone may develop and the infant die of sepsis. The prophylactic **treatment** consists in the prevention of possible mechanical irritation. A similar caution will generally permit of rapid healing of an ulcer already present. The usual mouth washes may be employed (see catarrhal stomatitis p. 524), and 1 per cent silver nitrate applied occasionally. Cocaine (1 per cent) or one of the newer local anesthetics may be used locally before nursing, if pain is great.

DISEASES OF THE TONGUE

Macroglossia.—This may exist as a rare congenital anomaly of the nature of a diffuse lymphangioma, and reach such size that the tongue cannot be retained in the mouth, and nursing, and, later, speech be interfered with. There may be congenital enlargement of one side of the tongue associated with general hemihypertrophy. We have seen two instances of this. Enlargement not congenital may be seen in cretinism, acromegaly, and to a less degree in mongolism, the process here being due to muscular hypertrophy and interstitial overgrowth. The treatment of congenital macroglossia is surgical. In cretinism the thyroid treatment for this condition is indicated. Very rarely there may be congenital **absence** of a portion of the organ or a split or **bifid** tongue.

Tumors.—These are not frequent, among them being cysts, some of which are dermoids; angiomata; and growths of misplaced thyroid tissue. Surgical treatment is indicated especially when breathing is interfered with. Caution should be observed in removing tumors containing thyroid tissue, lest the gland in the neck be deficient.

Tongue-tie.—By this title is designated a variable degree of shortening of the frenulum, making it impossible to protrude the tongue to the normal extent. Usually it gives no trouble, but uncommonly and in marked cases it may interfere with sucking and later with articulation. Treatment consists in nicking the edge of the frenulum with blunt-pointed scissors, and tearing through the remaining membrane; too deep a cut perhaps causing undue hemorrhage.

Ulceration of the Frenulum.—This is often seen in pertussis and other conditions attended by violent coughing, and results from the forcible impact of the frenulum against the incisor teeth. It occasionally, however, appears without discoverable cause in nursing infants, or in disorders not associated with coughing. It is cured by the application of a 1 per cent solution of silver nitrate.

Sublingual Fibroma (*Sublingual Granuloma; Riga's Disease; Fede's Disease*).—The first account of this affection to attract attention was by Riga.[52] It appears to be not infrequent in Italy for some unknown reason. Cases have also been reported in Poland, Germany, France and elsewhere. A case in a child of American descent was reported by Amberg.[53] It occurs only in the first year of life, especially after the lower incisor teeth have been erupted, and is apparently the result of the irritation produced by sucking. Inflammation results with hyperplasia of the tissues, and a fibrous papilloma is produced. Later a superficial ulcer may form and round-celled infiltration lead to the formation of a granuloma. The lesion is $\frac{1}{4}$ to 1 in. (0.63 to 2.64 cm.) in diameter, somewhat flat, red with a grayish center, and situated transversely at the position of the frenulum. The condition may last weeks or months, but is without danger. It is distinguished from sublingual ulcer by its hypertrophic nature. The lesions may be treated by boric acid and the application of tincture of iodine. In obstinate cases it may be necessary to excise the growth.

Black Tongue (*Nigrities Linguae*).—Brosin[54] in 1888 was able to collect only 40 cases of this uncommon condition. Gottheil[55] reported a case in a child of two years of age. Its cause is unknown. In explanation the action of a mold or germ has been invoked, as has the existence of a hyperplasia of the epithelial layer of the papillae, followed by hardening and change in color. The lesion appears as irregular areas which are smooth, or with elongated papillae (black hairy tongue), situated chiefly near the base of the tongue or running forward in a long black streak. Practically the only subjective symptom is a sense of dryness, and the condition may disappear quickly, but is oftener chronic. Mouth-washes of hyposulphite of soda or hydrogen peroxide may be used, or applications of weak solutions of silver nitrate or salicylic acid. Relapse is very frequent.

Glossitis.—This is uncommon in early life, except as a result of trauma. There may be irritation of the organ by carious teeth or by corrosive or hot fluids, involvement as part of a stomatitis, insect bites or stings, swelling in urticaria or angioneurotic edema, ulceration due to oïdium lactis (Wilkins and Bayne-Jones[56]), or tuberculosis. The entire tongue may become badly swollen, and there is salivation and, rarely, formation of an abscess. The condition usually is not serious. The swelling subsides in a few days, leaving superficial ulceration in the severer cases. The treatment consists in purgation, frequent introduction of ice into the mouth, mildly antiseptic mouth-washes such as indicated for stomatitis(p. 524), and, in bad cases, scarification. The food should be cool, liquid, and given through a nasal tube if necessary.

Tongue-swallowing.—Attention was first called to this condition by Bouchut.[57] It is occasionally seen, especially in infants suffering from nasal obstruction. Inspiration causes a backward displacement of the tongue and its tip until they are pressed against the hard palate, more or less cutting off the entrance of air. Treatment consists in drawing the tongue forward and maintaining it in this position, employing the measures recommended for micrognathia (p. 516). At the same time attempts should be made to open up the nasal passages.

Geographical Tongue.—(Epithelial Desquamation; Wandering Rash; Lichenoid; Ringworm of the Tongue, etc.) The multiplicity of titles indicates the lack of knowledge of the cause of this condition. It is seen in infancy and childhood, and may continue into adult life. It occurs oftenest in subjects with chronic intestinal indigestion or the exudative diathesis. The lesion begins as a small gray patch, the central portion of which soon becomes bright red due to loss of epithelium and filiform papillae. The slightly raised gray border, consisting of epithelial thickening, advances irregularly and rapidly (Fig. 121). Meanwhile the older central portion becomes recoated with epithelium, although the parts just within the border are still bright red. Several patches are often present, some of which may fuse, and new ones may form as the older ones disappear, their outline changing daily. There are no symptoms and the disease is entirely harmless.

DISEASES OF THE SALIVARY GLANDS

Malformations of the salivary glands are unusual, among them being a defective formation and a congenital salivary fistula. **Tumors** are seldom encountered. **Concretions** may rarely be found in any of the salivary ducts, or, less often, in the glands themselves. Neuhof[58] could collect but 7 instances of the disease in children, to which he added three others. A primary purulent **sialo-adenitis** of the submaxillary or sublingual glands is occasionally seen in the first weeks or months of life (Mikulicz and Kümmell[59]). The parotids are not involved. There is swelling of the glands, febrile symptoms develop, and pus is discharged through the ducts. Often

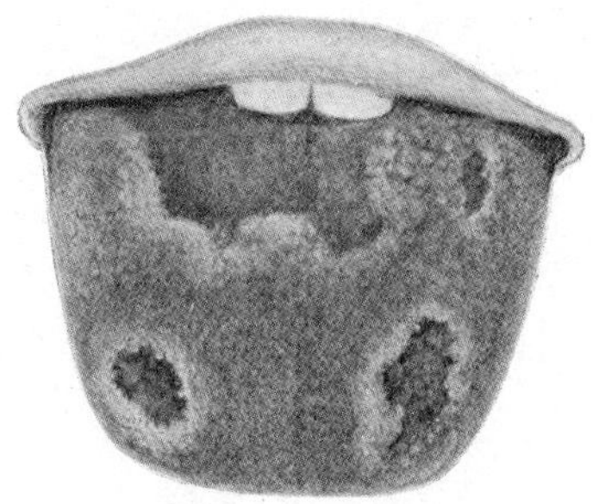

FIG. 121.—Geographical tongue. Showing the denuded areas with elevated thickened margins.

distinct abscess-formation occurs. The prognosis is usually good. **Congenital absence** of the salivary glands may occur. Ramsey[60] reports this in two children in a family, the father of whom presented the same anomaly.

RANULA.—The title designates a cystic formation in the mucous glands or the sublingual salivary glands. It is rarely found in early life, but may even be congenital, and 8 such cases were collected by Leguay.[61] If of considerable size, the tongue is pressed upward and may interfere with sucking.

SECONDARY PAROTITIS.—Secondary parotitis is sometimes seen even in early infancy. Purulent parotitis may occur in the new-born. Plewka[62] has collected 52 such cases from the literature, including one of his own, and Volonte[63] reports a case due to thrush. The subject has been reviewed by Kriss.[64] The secondary form may occur after stomatitis or purulent otitis; or in a worse form, usually advancing to suppuration, it may complicate severe fevers, especially typhoid fever and septic infection (Fig. 122). The germs enter through the duct of Steno, or by way of the blood-vessels

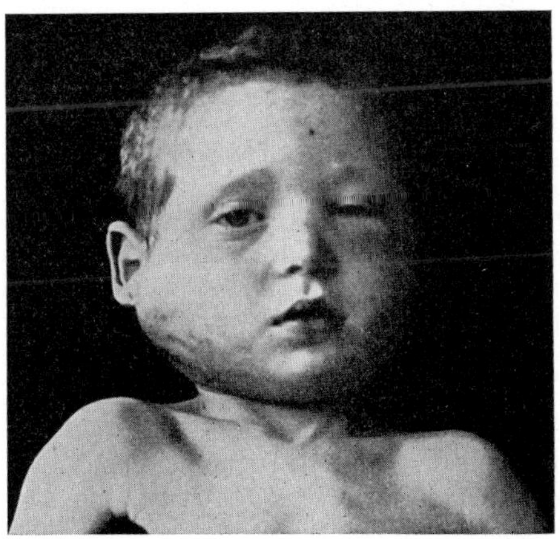

Fig. 122.—Bilateral secondary suppurative parotitis after typhoid fever. Case in a boy of eleven years, in the Children's Ward of the University Hospital, Philadelphia.

in metastatic cases. The process is generally unilateral. The **symptoms** are the usual ones of inflammation, combined with local pain, swelling, and tenderness. After several days resolution begins in favorable cases; but not infrequently there is deep-seated suppuration with increase of swelling and tenderness, discoloration appears, and finally pus is discharged through the overlying skin, or into the mouth either through the duct or the tissues of the face. Necrosis of the jaw or severe hemorrhage may occur; or sometimes death takes place from sepsis. In the line of **treatment** cold compresses should be applied and a purgative given. If resolution does not promptly occur, surgical aid should be sought before fluctuation develops.

MIKULICZ'S SYNDROME.—This condition was first described by Mikulicz.[65] According to Reuben and Douglas[66] there are at least 38 cases reported in children under fourteen years of age. The subject is reviewed by Thursfield,[67] Hochschild,[68] Schaffer and Jacobsen,[69] and Hamburger and Schaffer,[70] and we[71] have published observations upon it. The **etiology** is obscure. It is probably better to reserve the term Mikulicz's disease for cases of unknown origin in which the changes found are those of lymphoma or of chronic inflammation, since swelling of the parotid or lachrymal glands may be caused by tuberculosis, leukemia, or lymphosarcoma. Syphilis is associated in some cases, but whether etiologically is not always certain. We[71] have seen 3 instances of Mikulicz's syndrome, in one of which the specimen obtained by biopsy resembled tuberculosis microscopically, but no bacilli could be found and inoculation experiments were negative. Heerfordt[72] described a case in which there was also present inflammation of the uveal tract. The **symptoms** in typical cases consist only in bilateral painless enlargement of the parotid and lachrymal glands, perhaps with dryness of the mouth and absence of tears. The same symptoms are seen in the pseudo-form, but the characteristic changes in the blood will be present in instances due to leukemia, and there is a greater tendency to enlargement of the lymph nodes and spleen, although there may be some degree of this in the typical form. The course is slow and the **prognosis** good in those cases not associated with other disease. In **treatment** arsenic and iodides may be administered. Roentgen-ray and radium will cause the swelling to disappear and excision is seldom indicated except in the cases due to lymphosarcoma. If syphilis is associated appropriate treatment should be given, and tuberculin treatment has caused improvement in some cases, especially those associated with uveal-tract diseases.

Various other chronic enlargements of the parotid glands have been described, among them a rare familial and hereditary type reported by Hochschild.[68]

Salivation.—Inability to retain the saliva in the mouth is seen in infants of three or four months of age, at which time the secretion is normally fully established. Salivation may depend upon stomatitis, particularly that form caused by the administration of mercury; such reflex causes as nausea or gastralgia; certain nervous affections such, for example, as encephalitis; and upon diabetes, sugar then being excreted by the salivary glands (glycosialorrhea).

References

1. Am. J. Dis. Child., 1930, **39,** 1167. 2. Am. J. Dis. Child., 1932, **43,** 431. 3. Etude sur l'air de la ville de Limoges. De la perlèche, etc., Ref. Epstein, Jahrb. f. Kinderh., 1900, **51,** 317. 4. Edinburgh M. J., 1896, **2,** 1025. 5. Intestinal Diseases of Infancy, 1887, 103. 6. Am. J. Dis. Child., 1929, **37,** 766. 7. Canad. M. A. J., 1929, **21,** 18. 8. Physiol. Rev., 1924, **4,** 564. 9. J.A.M.A., 1922, **79,** 1565. 10. Lancet, 1918, **2,** 767; Physiol. Rev., 1928, **8,** 545; Med. Res. Counc. Rep., 1929, No. 140. 11. Bull. Johns Hopkins Hosp., 1922, **33,** 202. 12. J.A.M.A., 1922, **79,** 1567. 13. J.A.M.A., 1928, **90,** 1867; Am. J. Dis. Child., 1929, **38,** 721. 14. Am. J. Dis. Child., 1928, **36,** 268. 15. Am. J. Dis. Child., 1930, **40,** 536. 16. J. Nutrit., 1931, **3,** 433. 17. Am. J. Dis. Child., 1931, **42,** 263. 18. Am. J. Dis. Child., 1922, **24,** 160. 19. Dental Cosmos, 1931, **73,** 849. 20. Brit. M. J., 1924, **2,** 354. 21. Dental Cosmos, 1928, **70,** 9. 22. Greenbaum, Johnson, Mitchell, Selkirk and Stillwell, J. Am. Dent. A., 1930, **17,** 717. 23. Proc. Roy. Soc. Med. Clin. Sec., 1909–10, **3,** 9. 24. Quart. J. Med., 1919, **12,** 404. 25. Am. J. Dis. Child., 1923, **27,** 309. 26. Rev. mens. d. mal. de l'enf., 1892, **10,** 11. 27. Jour. f. Kinderkr., 1847, **9,** 194. 28. Arch. f. Anat. u. Physiol., 1842, 193. 29. Hist. natur. d. végétaux parasit., Paris, 1853, 488. 30. Kolle und Wassermann, Handb. d. path. Micro-org., 1903, **1,** 575. 31. Jahrb. f. Kinderh., 1898, **46,** 434. 32. Jahrb. f. Kinderh., 1887, **26,** 161. 33. Jahrb. f. Kinderh., 1888, **27,** 309. 34. Ztschr. f. Chir., 1916, **136,** 430. 35. Am. J. M. Sc., 1901, **122,** 527. 36. Am. J. M. Sc., 1910, **139,** 705. 37. Deutsche med. Wchnschr., 1889, **15,** 516. 38. Am. J. M. Sc., 1902, **123,** 59. 39. Pediatria, 1902, **10,** 232. 40. Jahrb. f. Kinderh., 1908, **67,** 294. 41. Deutsche med. Wchnschr., 1891, **17,** 569. 42. 62 Versamml. deutsch. Naturforsch. u. Aerzte, 1889, 342. 43. Centralbl. f. Bact. u. Parasitenk., 1890, **7,** 329. 44. Jahresb. d. Dresdener Gesellsch. f. Natur. u. Heilk., 1861–62, 51. 45. Deutsche med. Wchnschr., 1903, **29,** 581. 46. Am. J. Dis. Child., 1923, **26,** 250. 47. Arch. Pediat., 1924, **41,** 181. 48. Monatschr. f. Kinderh., 1923, **26,** 71. 49. J.A.M.A., 1925, **85,** 900. 50. J.A.M.A., 1927, **88,** 1142. 51. Die Krankheit. d. Neugeb. u. Säugl., 1850, **1,** 105. 52. Movimento med.-chir., 1881, **13,** 22; Ref. Amberg No. 53. 53. Am. J. M. Sc., 1903, **126,** 257. 54. Ueber die schwartze Haarzunge, 1888. 55. Arch. Pediat., 1899, **16,** 255. 56. Am. J. Dis. Child., 1923, **26,** 77. 57. Mal. d. nouveau-nés., 1885, 8th ed., 279. 58. Am. J. Dis. Child., 1924, **26,** 440. 59. Die Krankh. d. Mundes, 1898, 228. 60. Am. J. Dis. Child., 1924, **26,** 440. 61. Thèse de Paris, 1911. 62. Arch. f. Kinderh., 1921, **69,** 279. 63. Rev. méd. del Uruguay, 1923, **26,** 220; Ref. J.A.M.A., 1923, **81,** 787. 64. Ztschr. f. Gynäk., 1931, **55,** 3624. 65. Beitr. z. Chir., Billroth's Festschrift, 1892, 610. 66. Arch.

Pediat., 1930, **47,** 442. 67. Quart. J. Med., 1914, **7,** 237. 68. Jahrb. f. Kinderh., 1920, **92,** 360. 69. Am. J. Dis. Child., 1927, **34,** 327. 70. Am. J. Dis. Child., 1928, **36,** 434. 71. Griffith, Am. J. M. Sc., 1929, **178,** 853. 72. Arch. f. Ophthal., 1909, **70,** 254.

CHAPTER II

DISEASES OF THE PHARYNX AND PALATE

DEFORMITIES AND NEW GROWTHS OF THE PHARYNX AND PALATE

Syphilitic ulceration may take place in the pharynx, oftenest in the palate. **Tuberculosis** of the pharynx, not including the tonsils, is of very

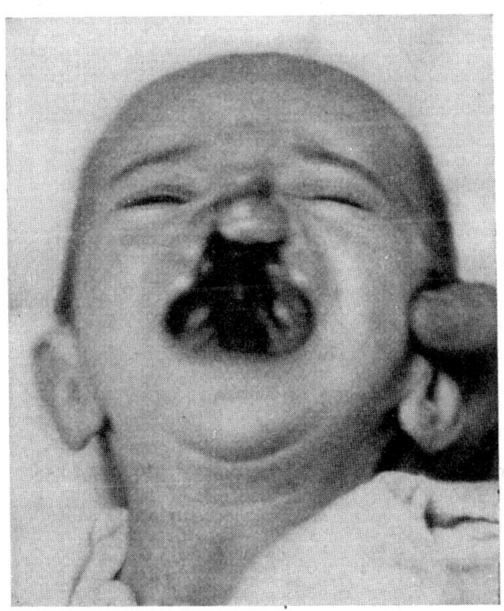

Fig. 123.—Double cleft palate with double harelip. Infant of four months in the Children's Hospital of Philadelphia. Shows double harelip and double cleft palate, with intermaxillary process between the clefts.

infrequent occurrence, and especially so in early life. **Stenosis** may be a congenital deformity, or result from syphilis or trauma. **Morbid growths** are uncommon, those oftenest seen being lymphoma and fibroma. Congential **perforation** of the palate may occasionally be observed. If developing later, it is oftenest the result of hereditary syphilis. **Torus palatinus** is sometimes seen. It consists of an elevated ridge in the midline suture of the hard palate. A **high and narrow arch** to the palate may attend the presence of adenoid growths, or may occur independently of this and be the cause of some of the symptoms usually attributed to the vegetations. It has been supposed sometimes to accompany mental defect, but Case,[1] who carefully examined palates by means of casts, could find no necessary connection between the degree of mental capacity and the height of the palatal arch.

Cleft Palate.—This common condition consists of a congenital fissure of the palate, oftenest of the soft part only, but in bad cases extending through the bony portion and the upper lip. In the worst cases there is a double cleft connecting with a double harelip, and leaving the intermaxillary process completely separated from the jaw on each side (Fig. 123). An opening through the palate interferes with sucking, since the necessary vacuum cannot be formed. As a consequence the nutrition of the infant is severely affected, and special methods of feeding are necessary. A long, large, rubber nipple attached to a glass tube and rubber bulb, as in the Breck Feeder for premature infants, is often of service; or a nipple may be employed to the upper side of which a flap of thin rubber is attached, in order to close the gap in the palate when the infant sucks. In other cases feeding by gavage is necessary. In spite of all care severe cases generally die, not so much from lack of food, as on account of the attending constitutional debility usually present. If the child survives, operation is best deferred until the second year or later.

Paralysis of the Palate and Uvula.—This is seen especially in diphtheria, but may occasionally develop in the course of other infectious diseases, and in certain disorders of the nervous system.

Bifid Uvula.—The uvula may be split into two portions at its tip, or the division may extend throughout the length, producing a double uvula. There are usually no symptoms present.

ACUTE CATARRHAL PHARYNGITIS

(Simple Angina)

There will be described here pharyngitis occurring as a primary affection, including acute catarrhal tonsillitis as a part of the disorder. It is, however, very common as a secondary affection to the acute infectious diseases, especially diphtheria, scarlet fever, grippe, and measles, or accompanying stomatitis, the symptoms being largely the same as in the primary form.

Etiology.—Pharyngitis is exceedingly common at all ages, although less so in early infancy. *Predisposing causes* are exposure to cold, wet, and draughts; overheating and dryness of dwellings; debility; and nasopharyngeal obstruction. The action of hot or caustic substances is an occasional factor. Digestive diseases are not infrequently attended by irritation of the throat. There is, too, a definite predisposition in certain persons or families, in some instances accompanied by a tendency to rheumatic manifestations. The *actual cause* is bacteriological. While no germ seems to be specific, streptococci of various types often predominate in the cultures. The element of contagion is decided.

Symptoms.—Onset is acute, with the simultaneous or later appearance of rhinitis, laryngitis, or tracheitis. This combination is frequently termed *acute upper respiratory infection.* There is a sensation in the throat of roughness, dryness, or even of pain, especially on swallowing; often an annoying cough; and speaking may be painful. In well-marked cases, especially with involvement of the tonsils, there are decided fever, headache, pain in the neck and back, and swelling of the submaxillary lymph-nodes. Infants, of course, make no subjective complaints, but may be quite ill with high fever, vomiting, and perhaps convulsions. Mild cases exhibit merely a slight, bright-redness of the throat; severe ones a deep-red color with swelling. The pharynx, soft palate, uvula, tonsils and pillars may all be involved, or only some of them, and to varying degrees. The mucous membrane is at first dry; later covered with thick, tenacious mucus.

Course and Prognosis.—Recovery may take place in three or four days, but in the frequent cases with rhinitis, laryngitis, or with extension to the trachea and bronchi recovery may be slow. Follicular tonsillitis is frequently associated.

Diagnosis.—Primary pharyngitis must be differentiated from those secondary to some febrile or other disease, especially scarlet fever and diphtheria. In scarlet fever there is a finely punctate enanthem, which usually develops promptly; and there is more fever at the onset, as well as leukocytosis. Diphtheria usually presents an exudate on the throat, and culture of it will reveal the causative bacillus. The pharyngitis of grippe can be distinguished only by the prevalence of other symptoms of the disease in epidemic form.

Treatment.—In **prophylaxis** there should be avoidance of the predisposing factors mentioned, and protection against contagion. Cool morning baths and local cool sponging of the throat may be judiciously tried to increase resistance. For **treatment of the attack** a saline purgative may be administered, a hot general bath or a mustard foot-bath given, and the child then confined to bed and well covered to induce free perspiration. Older children may be given cracked ice, which is allowed to melt as far back in the throat as possible. For fever and pain small doses of salicylates, phenacetin or antipyrine are indicated. Warm solutions of normal saline, bicarbonate of soda, or mild antiseptics or astringents may be employed as gargles or sprays. The throat may be painted with glycerite of tannic acid, or argyrol or other silver preparations. Such antiseptics as mercurochrome or gentian violet are usually unnecessary and may be irritating. Sprays and lozenges containing small amounts of menthol, eucalyptus, and the like often give relief, as do inhalations of water-vapor with benzoin. Cold compresses or small mustard plasters over the tonsillar region are sometimes of value. It may be said that local treatment should be used sparingly, that irritating solutions should never be employed, and, furthermore, that anything which disturbs the patient greatly will do more harm than good.

CHRONIC PHARYNGITIS

This is less often seen in children than in adults, yet is not uncommon. It may follow chronic digestive disorders or repeated attacks of acute pharyngitis, but its more frequent cause is obstruction to respiration through the nose. Disease of the sinuses may also play a rôle. Involvement of the base of the tongue and of the tonsils may occur as complications. The **symptoms** consist of slight discomfort in the throat and efforts to clear it, together with an irritating cough, sometimes moderate and almost continuous, sometimes severe and occurring paroxysmally and only at certain periods, and brought on by the mucus descending toward the larynx. The cough is often falsely assigned to bronchitis. Inspection of the throat shows enlarged, prominent, red or yellowish, distended follicles dotted especially upon the posterior wall of the pharynx, with the surrounding mucous membrane more or less inflamed, or of a pale color and often partly covered by mucopurulent secretion. The vessels may be visibly dilated. There is no fever and no actual pain, unless exacerbations occur. Deafness may develop as a complication, dependent upon accompanying adenoid growths. In advanced cases atrophy of the pharyngeal mucous membrane develops. The course is chronic and the disease yields slowly even under treatment.

Treatment consists in removing any nasal obstruction or affection of the tonsillar tissues; attention to any chronic infection in the nose and to the state of the digestive apparatus; and avoidance of all irritation by exposure and the like. General tonic remedies and change of air are also often necessary. In addition to local treatment to allay irritation there may be needed cauterization of the individual follicles, if not too numerous.

Uvulitis.—This disorder occurs often as one of the symptoms of acute pharyngitis, although sometimes the inflammation may be largely confined to the uvula. Sometimes it seems to be the direct result of trauma. There are swelling and redness of the part, generally with edema and pain on swallowing; and if elongation is present and the uvula comes into contact with the base of the tongue there is a harassing, tickling cough. Applications of glycerite of tannic acid, a weak solution of nitrate of silver, or of epinephrine (1:1000) are of advantage, as is the sucking of ice. In bad cases scarification of the uvula may be required.

Edema of the Uvula.—This is a condition frequently attendant upon uvulitis. Apart from this, edema may occur in nephritis and in allergic and hydremic states. The local treatment is similar to that required for uvulitis. Remedies directed to any more general cause may be needed.

Elongated Uvula.—With acute or chronic pharyngitis, or independently of these and perhaps of congenital origin, some degree of elongation of the uvula may be observed. The only symptoms are an annoying, tickling cough and a desire to clear the throat, worse especially when lying down at night, and produced by the uvula coming into contact with the base of the tongue. The cough may be so severe that vomiting results. Examination of the fauces discloses the uvula touching the tongue if the breath is held or air is expired through the nose. Treatment consists in measures for diminishing the size of the uvula. If the condition is due to inflammation or relaxation, the application of astringent solutions, such as glycerite of tannic acid, or of adrenaline, is often promptly efficacious. Astringent lozenges, as of eucalyptus, are also of service. In obstinate cases, dependent upon a congenital relaxation or upon chronic thickening, amputation of the tip of the uvula may be required, but other treatment should first be given thorough trial.

PSEUDOMEMBRANOUS PHARYNGITIS

(Septic Sore Throat, Pseudodiphtheria)

Etiology.—These titles are but some of those applied to different groups which appear to constitute varieties of one disorder. Pseudomembranous tonsillitis is included in this description. The disease may be primary, or be secondary to some other affection, especially the acute exanthemata, such as measles and, most of all, scarlet fever; although often seen, too, in typhoid fever. It occurs also after tonsillectomy. In many of these secondary cases the disease may closely resemble diphtheria. As a primary affection it may develop without the previous existence of any of the acute infections. Thus in a very severe form, with extension of the necrosis to the nasal mucous membrane and even to the esophagus, it may occasionally be seen in the new-born (Epstein[2]), and in these cases it perhaps complicates Bednar's aphthae (p. 524), or may be consecutive to and associated with thrush. In the form frequently designated *septic sore throat* it has often appeared in epidemics, one of the largest of these having affected over 10,000 persons (Capps and Miller[3]).

The primary cause is undoubtedly microbic. Among the germs found alone or in combination are various forms of streptococci and staphylococci, pneumococci, and influenza bacilli, the hemolytic streptococcus being especially implicated. In some sporadic cases and in epidemics there has been found an encapsulated organism termed the streptococcus epidemicus (Davis and Rosenow,[4] Pilot and Davis[5]). In several epidemics extension has occurred through the milk-supply, and it may perhaps also take place through direct contact.

Symptoms.—The degree of local and constitutional involvement varies greatly. In typical *primary* cases of the *epidemic type* the onset is generally abrupt, with fever, chilliness, pain on swallowing, headache, general pains, sometimes vomiting, and occasionally convulsions. A diffuse, dusky redness with swelling of the pharynx and pillars appears, and in a few hours patches of exudation usually develop on the tonsils and pillars and the neighboring structures, and in some cases the pseudomembrane involves the nose and occasionally the larynx. The process may go on to necrosis and gangrene. In two or three days the cervical lymph-nodes become enlarged and tender, but rarely suppurate. The tonsillar pseudomembrane can, as a rule, be wiped away without difficulty. In milder cases there may be little or no exudate on the throat, or only a lacunar tonsillitis may appear.

In *sporadic* as in many *secondary* cases the disease is usually milder and limited chiefly to the tonsils. Not infrequently, however, especially in secondary cases, the attack is as severe as in typical cases of the epidemic form, with the symptoms intense and even of a septic nature, and the pseudomembrane widespread.

Course and Prognosis.—The prognosis on the whole is favorable. The duration is but three or four days in the milder cases, and recovery is rapid. In the severer forms the course is longer, lasting perhaps one or two weeks, and the result uncertain, the process extending both into the substance of the tonsils and to other regions. In malignant cases death may occur after a few days. Uncommonly, but oftener in the secondary cases, extensive sloughing takes place, all the symptoms of sepsis develop, and the case ends fatally. Occurring in early infancy in debilitated subjects the disease is usually fatal, and in the new-born always so.

Diagnosis.—The affection causing most difficulty in diagnosis is diphtheria. In average cases of pseudomembranous pharyngitis the onset is more sudden and stormy than in diphtheria, and the deposit is oftener limited to the tonsils and is not so closely adherent. There is less swelling of the cervical glands and less prostration of the system, except in some of the severe instances of epidemic septic sore throat. The extension of membrane beyond the tonsils is a strong evidence that the disease is diphtheria. There are, however, so many exceptions to these distinctions that dependence should be placed only upon bacteriologic examination. Secondary cases are usually more easy of recognition, owing to the presence of other diseases, such as measles or scarlet fever; but here, too, a positive diagnosis can be made only by bacteriologic study. A necrotic condition of the tonsils may occur early in acute lymphatic leukemia. In this event there would be little if any fever, and the associated anemia and blood-findings should lead to the diagnosis. In agranulocytic angina, which is rare in childhood, there occurs a leukopenia with decrease of the granular (polymorphonuclear) leukocytes.

Treatment.—Isolation had better be carried out. In cases closely resembling diphtheria, antitoxin should be given without waiting for a culture. In severe cases local treatment as recommended for acute laryngitis (p. 694) or anginose scarlet fever (p. 265) is required. Polyvalent antistreptococcus serum and transfusions may be tried in cases with general symptoms of sepsis, especially if the blood-culture is positive.

RETROPHARYNGEAL ABSCESS

This disorder, although much less common than many other diseases of the pharynx, is seen not infrequently, and retropharyngeal adenitis without symptoms and not advancing to suppuration is probably a comparatively common affection.

Etiology.—Nearly all cases occur in the first three years of life, and especially in the first year. Only when secondary to caries of the vertebrae is it more likely to develop after infancy. Nasopharyngitis commonly precedes the condition, and consequently the abscess is seen oftenest in the winter during the period of catarrhal inflammations. Exceptionally it follows such disorders as scarlet fever, grippe, or measles. Debilitated health is also a factor. The usual germs found in the abscess are streptococci. Waugh[6] claimed that the disease never occurs when the tonsils have been removed, but this is not supported.

Symptoms.—The inflammation is situated in the retropharyngeal lymph-nodes. The first suggestive symptom is difficulty in swallowing, perhaps with regurgitation through the nose and mouth, or vomiting. The difficulty may cause food to be refused. There is a characteristic gurgling or spluttering respiration, as also snoring because of nasal obstruction, but not the stridor of laryngeal disease except in advanced cases. The mouth is kept open and the head thrown back or to one side. The voice is nasal and cough is not uncommon. As a rule more or less fever is present (Fig. 124), and prostration is decided. Direct examination of the pharynx

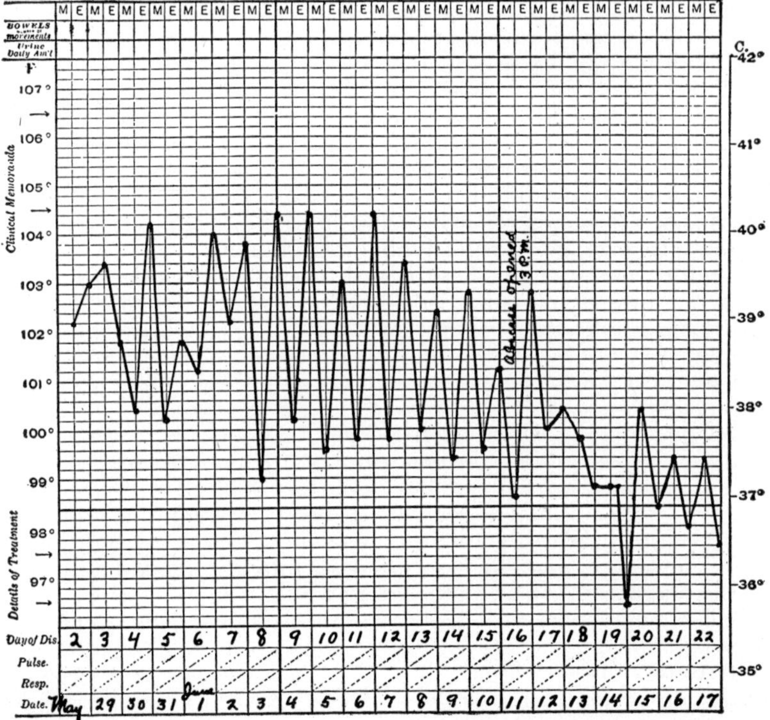

Fig. 124.—Temperature chart from a case of retropharyngeal abscess in a child of twenty months. (*Hand, Annals of Gynaec. and Pediat.*, 1899, **12**, *Jan.*)

reveals, sometimes to the eye and always to the palpating finger, a fluctuating mass projecting forward from the posterior pharyngeal wall, most marked on one side, and sometimes extending so far forward that the uvula is displaced laterally. In most cases the swelling is also visible from without, upon one side of the neck behind and below the angle of the jaw and extending backward and downward. This is dependent either upon the burrowing by pus, or upon involvement of neighboring lymph-nodes.

Early the swelling may be merely indurated and not fluctuating (*retropharyngeal adenitis*). In abscess dependent upon vertebral caries the onset is more insidious, the constitutional symptoms less marked, and there is little fever. In these cases, too, pus may sometimes burrow downward along the spinal column.

Course and Prognosis.—In patients who have had clinical manifestations it is uncommon for retropharyngeal adenitis to disappear without suppuration. The course is rapid and within a week the symptoms are threatening. If there is discovery of an abscess and prompt incision made the prognosis is good. Sometimes in infants the constitutional depression is so severe that death occurs even although the abscess has been opened; or the cavity may constantly refill and gradual failure of strength lead to a fatal issue. The majority of deaths take place in unrecognized cases. Here sudden death may follow from edema of the glottis or pressure upon the larynx; from rupture into the larynx; or from erosion of blood-vessels and fatal hemorrhage. Other causes of death are septic pneumonia or burrowing of pus into the mediastinum or elsewhere. The actual mortality is less than 4 per cent (Bókai[7]). When the abscess depends on cervical caries the course is slower; after operation reaccumulation of pus is prone to occur; and there is greater tendency to burrow, but less danger of asphyxia.

Diagnosis.—The abscess may not always be visible on inspection of the throat but is always palpable. The examination with the palpating finger should be made thoroughly, but quickly in order to avoid interference with respiration. The mass can often be well visualized by a roentgenogram, which reveals a forward displacement of the pharynx, larynx and trachea (Brown and Reineke[8]). Characteristic symptoms are the position of the head, the open mouth, the spluttering respiration, and the difficulty in swallowing. *Laryngeal stenosis* is simulated if the abscess is deeply situated. *Edema of the glottis* has none of the characteristic symptoms, nor is an abscess felt on digital examination. Differentiation should be made between the usual form of abscess and that due to *cervical caries.* In the latter there is the slower course; often previous poor health; the abscess is more medial; there is less likely to be external swelling; and there is greater stiffness of the neck together with other symptoms of involvement of the spine.

Treatment.—The child is held firmly in an upright position with the arms pinioned. A bistoury, wrapped with adhesive plaster except at the tip, is then introduced along the guiding finger, incision made, and the child's head rapidly bent forward and downward to prevent entrance of pus into the pharynx; or the operation may be done with the child's head held in a position lower than the body. A good substitute proceeding is to push blunt-pointed scissors into the abscess, separate the blades, and withdraw the scissors while in this position. This tends to prevent the wound closing too promptly.

References

1. Am. J. Insanity, 1918–19, **75,** 501. 2. Jahrb. f. Kinderh., 1895, **39,** 420. 3. J.A.M.A., 1912, **58,** 1848. 4. J.A.M.A., 1912, **58,** 773. 5. J.A.M.A., 1931, **97,** 1691. 6. Lancet, 1906, **2,** 845. 7. Jahrb. f. Kinderh., 1892, **33,** 360. 8. Am. J. Roentgenol., 1928, **20,** 208.

CHAPTER III

DISEASES OF THE TONSILLAR TISSUE

Tumors of the tonsillar tissue are rare, papilloma, fibroma, and lymphosarcoma being oftenest found. **Tuberculosis of the tonsils and adenoids** of a nature discoverable clinically is very seldom seen. Pathologically, tubercle is present in 5 per cent or less of tonsils examined (White,[1] Weller,[2] MacCready and Crowe,[3] Scarff and Whiteby[4]). In some instances it is found in the adenoids alone. When there is tuberculosis of the cervical lymph-nodes the percentage of tonsillar involvement is much increased.

Acute Catarrhal Tonsillitis is a part of acute catarrhal pharyngitis. (See p. 530.) *Pseudomembranous tonsillitis* has been described in discussing pseudomembranous pharyngitis. (See p. 532.)

ACUTE LACUNAR TONSILLITIS

(Follicular Tonsillitis)

In many cases lacunar tonsillitis shades into the catarrhal form, a few engorged lacunae often appearing in the catarrhal variety and then disappearing quickly. The more typical cases are here described, in which the inflammation is located chiefly in the crypts of the tonsils.

Etiology.—The disease is common at all ages, except in infancy and especially in the first year of life, although it occurs at this period oftener than is usually supposed. Exposure to cold and wet, and digestive disturbances are predisposing causes, and undoubted contagiousness is sometimes seen. In many children there is a remarkable predisposition to repeated attacks. Inflammation of the tonsils must often be considered as part of the rheumatic syndrome. (See p. 474.) In the crypts are found bacteria of various sorts, oftenest streptococci, staphylococci, pneumococci, and influenza bacilli. As a *secondary* affection lacunar tonsillitis is encountered especially in the course of scarlet fever and diphtheria.

Symptoms.—The attack begins with chilliness, malaise, pain in the head and body, anorexia, and fever which often reaches 103 or 104 F. (39.4 or 40 C.). Vomiting and diarrhea may occur, the tongue is coated, the breath heavy, and the cervical lymph-nodes may be swollen. In some cases there is abdominal pain, due, perhaps, to an accompanying inflammation of the mesenteric lymph-nodes (Brennemann[5]). Pain on swallowing and speaking is frequently present, although often less than in catarrhal tonsillitis, and frequently the degree of it is surprisingly slight. Occasionally an erythematous rash is observed. Examination of the throat shows swollen, deep-red tonsils with few or many irregularly shaped, yellowish-white spots of varying size. These are sometimes so closely placed as to suggest a pseudomembrane, but they can usually be removed without bleeding. Usually both tonsils are attacked, but not necessarily equally so or simultaneously.

Course and Prognosis.—The general and local symptoms are usually severe, but the course is of short duration unless relapses occur, or such complications develop as arthritis, endocarditis, or nephritis.

Diagnosis.—When the deposit becomes confluent lacunar tonsillitis may be confounded with *diphtheria,* especially where the latter disease begins as a lacunar inflammation. In lacunar tonsillitis, however, the deposit is an easily removable secretion and not a necrotic destruction of the mucous membrane. Furthermore lacunar tonsillitis usually manifests higher fever at the onset than diphtheria and greater soreness of the throat, and never produces exudate on the pillars or uvula. In some mild cases of diphtheria the exudate may be confined to the lacunae, and in such dependence must be placed on bacteriologic examinations. *Scarlet fever* often exhibits lacunar tonsillitis early in the attack but the other symptoms of that disease should soon develop.

Treatment.—The patient should be isolated and in doubtful cases a culture taken to determine the presence of diphtheria. The local and general treatment is similar to that recommended for acute catarrhal pharyngitis, including cleansing and astringent washes and gargles, and the control of pain and fever. (See p. 531.)

CHRONIC LACUNAR TONSILLITIS

This disorder is sometimes a sequel to repeated attacks of acute inflammation, and is present in many instances of hypertrophy of the tonsils. There is a retention of caseous material in some of the crypts, which may be pressed out, or discharged by coughing; with a resulting fetid odor to the breath. Sometimes the material is retained by adhesions which close the orifice of the crypt. In some cases the tonsils are infected with fungi of various sorts. There are no symptoms except perhaps attacks of coughing and slight pain on swallowing saliva, although not with solid food. Acute exacerbations may occur with fever and increase of pain. Treatment consists in opening and cauterizing the crypts; but removal of the tonsils is indicated.

ULCEROMEMBRANOUS TONSILLITIS

(Plaut-Vincent Angina)

Etiology.—The disease is somewhat contagious, yet predisposition to it must be required since it is found oftenest in debilitated subjects, and the causative organisms, as shown by Pilot and Davis[6] and others, are commonly found within the normal mouth in the tartar on teeth and in the tonsillar crypts. The active cause appears to be a symbiosis of the fusiform bacillus and a spirochete. Both these organisms were referred to by Miller[7] as occurring in the mouth; but their association with this form of tonsillitis was emphasized by Plaut[8] in 1894, and by Vincent[9] in 1898. Vincent[10] claims that he was the first to describe the fusiform bacillus, and that the organisms described by Plaut and Miller are not similar to it. It should be said, also, that although the spirochete and fusiform bacillus may be found in certain cases of bronchitis and of gangrene of the lung, these disorders are not necessarily preceded by the tonsillar infection.

Symptoms.—On one or, less often, both tonsils there develops an exudate covering an ulcer of varying depth. In the *milder* cases the deposit can be readily removed, leaving a bleeding surface beneath. There is little fever or general disturbance. The breath is offensive, and the cervical lymph-nodes enlarge but do not suppurate. In the *severer* cases the ulceration is deeper and the constitutional symptoms more marked.

Course and Prognosis.—In milder cases recovery follows in a few days; in the severer the process may last several weeks, and relapses take place. The disease may prove fatal by spread to other parts of the mouth and pharynx producing a condition similar to, and probably identical with, gangrenous stomatitis (p. 521).

Diagnosis.—From diphtheria the distinction is made by the softness of the exudate and the depth of the ulceration in ulceromembranous tonsillitis, but bacterological examination is often necessary, especially as the two conditions may be combined. We have seen this on a number of occasions. In some cases of ulceromembranous tonsillitis the blood may show a lymphocytosis, and this might lead to a false diagnosis of leukemia. The severe anemia, the hemorrhages, and the fatal issue of the latter disease are distinguishing points. In agranulocytic angina there is necrosis of the tonsillar surface, but the blood reveals a leukopenia characterized especially by a diminished number of polymorphonuclear cells.

Treatment.—This is similar to that recommended for ulcerative stomatitis; namely local cleaning and disinfectant washes; parenteral and local employment of arsenical and other preparations; and supporting measures if needed.

PARENCHYMATOUS TONSILLITIS

(Phlegmonous Tonsillitis, Quinsy, Peritonsillar Abscess)

Etiology.—Quinsy is uncommon in early life and rare in infancy. Graef[11] reports an instance in an infant of six months of age. Even in later childhood it is less frequent than in adults. It is generally a peritonsillar abscess, the process often involving the tonsil as well. Less frequently it develops primarily in the tonsil. Catarrhal or lacunar tonsillitis may act as a predisposing cause, and there exists also a decided family or individual tendency. The exciting cause is infection by some pyogenic organism.

Symptoms.—The attack begins with suddenness and severity, with the symptoms of catarrhal pharyngitis. Rapidly, however, the fever becomes high and the pain in the throat constant and severe, making swallowing, speaking, or opening of the mouth difficult or impossible. The breath is offensive; the tongue badly coated. Inspection at first shows little except a prominence in the tonsillar region upon one side of the throat; but palpation reveals a hard, swollen, and very tender mass. The absence of any positive evidence on inspection is due to the fact that the inflammation is largely at first in the deeper portion of the affected region. As the process advances the whole tonsillar area on one side becomes prominent, with the mucous membrane red and swollen and the mass pushing the edematous uvula to the other side of the throat and often nearly closing the fauces. The other tonsil and the pharynx in general may exhibit a catarrhal inflammation. Finally fluctuation may sometimes be made out, although in other instances this is never discovered.

With these local manifestations there are increasing symptoms of illness; fever continuing high, oppression and difficult respiration being sometimes present, the pulse rapid, and general restlessness and delirium perhaps developing. There may be much pain and tenderness on moving the neck. The patient is able to take almost no food or drink and the general condition is most distressing.

The disease lasts several days or a week, and then an abscess may often be seen to be pointing, generally in the neighborhood of the anterior pillar of the fauces. Pus may be discharged and relief from all symptoms be complete in a few hours. In many cases, however, there is no pus evident and a gradual resolution takes place. Severe hemorrhage has been known to follow the bursting of the abscess, and edema of the glottis also has occurred. The **prognosis** is, however, nearly always good.

Treatment.—Early in the case effort should be made to abort the process by the application of ice-bags externally, combined with the sucking of pieces of ice. Sometimes the application of a hot poultice and the use of hot water as a gargle are more beneficial. Opiates or other analgesic drugs are necessary for the pain. As soon as any region suggesting fluctuation is discovered incision should be made. Even if no pus is found relief may follow the local blood-letting. Complete removal of the tonsils later will prevent further attacks.

HYPERTROPHY OF THE TONSILLAR TISSUE

There is in childhood a special predisposition to hyperplasia of the faucial tonsil and the pharyngeal tonsil (adenoids), and, less frequently in children, the lymphoid tissue at the base of the tongue (lingual tonsil). Often there is also hypertrophy of the follicles visible on the posterior wall of the pharynx. The hyperplasia affects both the lymphatic structure and the connective-tissue, sometimes one or the other predominating.

HYPERTROPHY OF THE FAUCIAL TONSILS

Etiology.—The condition is very frequent in early life. Although sometimes beginning in infancy, the hypertrophy is not generally believed to reach any decided degree until later. In our experience, however, enlargement in the first year is not uncommon. There is often noted a marked family predisposition. The general health appears to exert no causative action, except for the predisposing influence of lymphatism. The repeated occurrence of catarrhal pharyngitis is a factor, although such repeated attacks are often the result rather than the cause of hyperplasia. Tuberculosis has no etiologic connection with ordinary cases of hypertrophy, but the two may be combined.

Pathologic Anatomy.—When not associated with a temporary catarrhal inflammation, as shown by the redness of the mucous membrane, the tonsil is large and pale. When the overgrowth is chiefly in the lymphoid tissue, the tonsil is soft and the lymphoid element projects in the form of nodules. If the fibrous overgrowth is in excess it is hard and firm, broad bands of connective tissue crossing it in different directions. The crypts frequently exhibit yellowish masses, yet without showing signs of inflammation. The hypertrophy is nearly always bilateral, yet one tonsil may be more affected than the other. Frequently tonsillar hypertrophy is overlooked because the organ is deeply situated or submerged behind the pillars, and its actual size is not at first discovered. The overgrowth in these cases is chiefly in depth and width. At the times when an acute inflammation is superimposed, the organ increases much in size and becomes redder.

Symptoms.—Examination shows the presence of enlargement of the tonsils as described. In cases of submerged tonsils palpation with the finger, or causing the patient to gag, reveals the degree of enlargement present. In other instances the tonsils may be so large that they almost touch each other. The general symptoms are not well-marked, many of those attributed to this condition depending in reality upon adenoid overgrowth which so frequently accompanies the hypertrophy of the faucial tonsils. Moderate enlargement of the latter, if occurring alone, produces few symptoms. When, however, the hypertrophy is great there is often a thick tone to the voice as though there were food present in the mouth, and the swallowing of solid food and even the respiration may be mechanically interfered with. As a rule deglutition is not painful. There is a great tendency to repeated, acute tonsillar inflammation, and at this time the symptoms are exaggerated. The lymphatic glands in the neck may become chronically enlarged. Mouth-breathing and snoring occur and deafness may result; but, again, these conditions oftener depend chiefly on the accompanying adenoid hypertrophy. The enlargement of the tonsil may frequently be felt externally. In other cases, without recognizable manifestations other than the chronic tonsillar enlargement observed on inspection, there is a tendency to repeated attacks of fever without discoverable cause, general impairment of health, and other uncharacteristic symptoms. That these are due, in some instances at least, to a mild toxic condition produced by absorption from a chronically inflamed tonsil, seems proven by the disappearance of symptoms after tonsillectomy.

The presence of micro-organisms in the hypertrophied tonsils is important. It has been shown by the studies of Davis,[12] Tongs,[13] Pilot, Pearlman and colleagues,[14] Hambrecht and Nuzum,[15] Pilot and Brams,[16] and others, that the tonsils harbor such organisms as the hemolytic streptococcus in 90 per cent or more of the cases demanding extirpation, while often present also are the pneumococcus, influenza bacillus, fusiform bacillus, streptococcus viridans, and, less frequently, the diphtheria bacillus, diphtheroid bacilli, streptococcus mucosus and others. These organisms are found in greater numbers deep in the crypts than on the surface of the tonsils or on the mucous membranes of the nose, throat and mouth. Removal of the tonsils diminishes the number in the nose and throat. These facts would explain not only the predisposition to local disease of the adjacent mucous membranes which exists with infected tonsils, but also certain cases with rheumatic fever and other forms of acute and chronic arthritis, chorea, endocarditis, nephritis, pyelitis and the like, in which the tonsils seem to act as foci of infection.

Course and Prognosis.—The soft lymphoid tonsils vary in size from time to time, being larger during an acute attack of tonsillitis, and afterward sometimes larger, sometimes smaller than before this. There is a natural disposition for them to become diminished in size as puberty is approached, although increasing connective tissue overgrowth often prevents this, and the fibrous tonsils grow very little smaller with time. The dangers associated with diseased tonsils will be discussed later (see below). The discovery of tubercle bacilli in excised tonsils need not cause undue alarm. MacCready and Crowe,[3] who followed 50 such cases in most instances for from five to ten years, found that the majority did not develop clinical evidence of pulmonary or intestinal tuberculosis.

Treatment.—Local treatment does little if any good. Attention to the general health, plenty of fresh air, the avoidance of repeated respiratory infections, the treatment of anemia, the administration of cod liver oil, and change of residence to a dry climate may all be indicated. Extirpation is, however, the only means of cure. There has been much discussion of the indications for tonsillectomy and the results obtained from it. Among the studies on the subject may be mentioned those of Simpson;[17] St. Lawrence;[18] Ingerman and Wilson;[19] Kaiser;[20] Wilson, Lingg and Croxford;[21] Findlay,[22] McCulloch and Jones;[23] Bradley;[24] Sheldon;[25] Monroe and Volk,[26] and Cunningham.[27] From time to time we[28] have, in association with others, published our observations on this matter. A critical analysis of some of the various published contributions shows that in the evaluation of the results not sufficient attention has been paid to such modifying factors as sex, race, heredity, season, length of time after operation, and particularly the age when this was done. Many of the symptoms and conditions popularly supposed to be associated etiologically with diseased tonsils are those in which the natural course and incidence, regardless of the effect of tonsillectomy, are not known. While all of this evidence cannot be quoted, and much of it is contradictory and more of the nature of supposition than proof, it may be reasonably deduced that tonsillectomy somewhat reduces the incidence and recurrence of rheumatic fever and chorea; may decrease somewhat the occurrence of carditis and seems to inhibit to a certain extent the number of attacks of cardiac decompensation; sometimes lessens for a time the incidence and severity of infections of the upper respiratory tract, although young adults, tonsillectomized as children, may have an increased susceptibility to colds; may increase the number of infections of the lower respiratory tract (bronchitis, pneumonia); lessens the susceptibility to scarlet fever and diphtheria; diminishes the number of sore throats; affords some slight protection against cervical lymphadenitis; may in some instances improve the nutritional state; has no decided influence on the incidence of growing pains. While taken up in more detail elsewhere, it may be mentioned here that the tonsils act as foci of infection in some cases of pyelitis, nephritis, chronic arthritis, and the like. The mere occurrence of a few small lymph-nodes in the neck is no indication for operation, nor is mere hypertrophy of the tonsils without other symptoms. Mouth-breathing, snoring, nasal obstruction, and repeated attacks of otitis media are more closely linked to adenoid than to tonsillar hypertrophy. In general it may be said that great caution must be exercised in the drawing of conclusions and the promising of good results from tonsillectomy.

In spite of the uncertainty of knowledge the physician is confronted with the practical problem of deciding when to recommend the operation. It is manifestly improper for him to advise removal because he can not tell from the simple appearance of the tonsils whether or not they are infected and a source of trouble. A proper decision is in many cases a very difficult one. Consequently, it may, with advantage, be attempted to formulate a *list of indications for the removal of tonsils and adenoids* as follows:—Two or more attacks of sore throat, tonsillitis, or otitis media, one attack of peritonsillar abscess; the occurrence of one of the rheumatic manifestations; a family history of tendency to rheumatic disease including polyarthritis, chorea, and endocarditis; one or more attacks of cervical adenitis, or decided chronic enlargement of the cervical glands; mouth-breathing and nasal obstruction not otherwise accounted for; tonsils of such a size that they are mechanically obstructive. For malnutrition, excessive fatigue, headache, or unexplained fever the tonsils should be removed only after careful study to determine the existence of any other removable cause. Our own experience forces us to the conclusion that little is to be expected from tonsillar enucleation in repeated colds, although the operation should be performed if other indications exist. Under certain conditions, such as in pyelitis, nephritis, and chronic arthritis, when there is reason to believe that absorption from the tonsils is taking place they should be removed.

It is by no means understood just what useful purpose the organs fulfil, and it is a safe dictum that no operation should be performed on any region of the body unless positive indication for it exists. The fact that it is estimated that about $\frac{1}{3}$ of all the operations in the cities of the United States are for the removal of tonsils and adenoids (Collins and Sydenstricker[29]) leads inevitably to the conclusion that they could not all have been necessary or helpful. It is true that tonsillectomy and adenoidectomy—the two procedures usually being performed at the same operation—are usually not dangerous, but such conditions as hemorrhage, pneumonia, pulmonary abscess, pyemia, and septic inflammation of different parts of the body may follow. We have several times seen scarlet fever develop within twenty-four to forty-eight hours after the operation, perhaps due to the release of scarlet fever streptococci which had been retained in the tonsillar tissue. One should not expect results from the operation when the symptoms have in reality been dependent upon infected sinuses, deviated septum, nasal polyps, or other nasopharyngeal disease.

If, however, it is decided that the tonsils should be removed this should certainly be done as thoroughly as possible. Frequently small pieces of tonsillar tissue are found remaining after operation. This was true, for example, in 73 per cent of 403 patients examined by Rhoads and Dick.[30] This tissue, especially if it becomes fibrotic, may be as great a potential source of danger as the tonsils themselves. Particularly in children removal of the tonsils may result in hypertrophy of the other lymphoid tissue in the nasopharynx, such as the adenoids if not extirpated at the same time, or the tissue on the posterior pharyngeal wall. It is to be considered whether this tissue may not act as a focus of infection and at times be more dangerous than the tonsils themselves.

Removal of the tonsils by electric coagulation and desiccation is seldom applicable in children, because of the number of treatments and the attendant pain and sore throat. Treatment by roentgen-ray and radium, which causes shrinkage of the tonsils, is indicated only when tonsillectomy should not be performed, as in hemophilia, lymphatism, nephritis, or cardiovascular disease, although in the last the operation is often well borne. It is our belief that a period of two weeks should elapse between any acute inflammation in the throat and the time of operation. Some clinicians recommend the removal of tonsils during the acute stages of cardiac decompensation or during the active manifestations of arthritis or chorea. We believe that

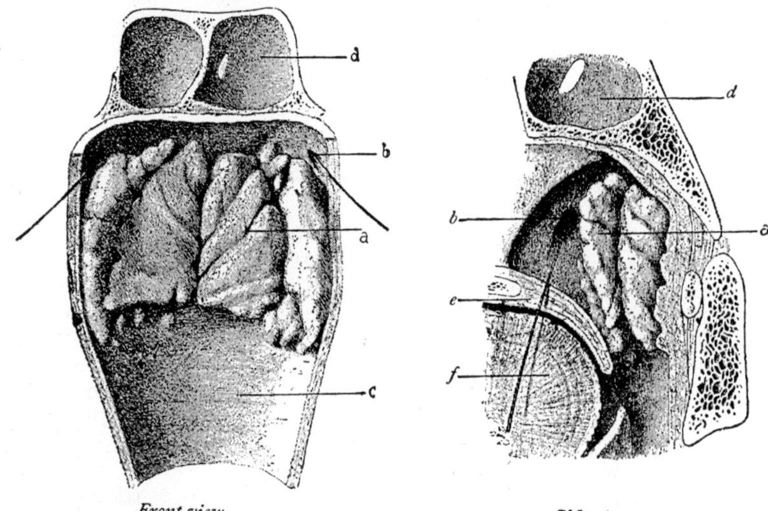

Fig. 125.—Adenoids in situ. *a*, The vegetations; *b*, Eustachian orifice; *c*, the pharynx; *d*, sphenoidal sinus; *e*, velum of the palate; *f*, base of the tongue and epiglottis. (*Lennox Browne, The Throat and Nose and Their Diseases*, 1899, 422; *after Castex and Lacour.*)

there is danger in this, and no advantage. It has also been advocated (Levinger[31]) that tonsillectomy be performed during or shortly after the acute stage of peritonsillar abscess. Mention should be made of the dirty-gray pseudomembrane which often follows tonsillectomy. This may readily cause alarm from its resemblance to diphtheria. Yet if diphtheria should follow tonsillectomy the diagnosis is difficult, as we have observed on a few occasions. Zingher[32] has called attention to this condition. To avoid the uncertainty a culture of the nose and throat should be made before operation. In case of doubt after operation the culturing should be repeated, and antitoxin given if necessary. If the history of the patient is at all suggestive of a hemorrhagic tendency, the bleeding-time and coagulation-time should be determined before operation.

HYPERTROPHY OF THE PHARYNGEAL TONSIL

(Adenoid Vegetations)

Etiology.—This is an extremely common condition in early life, to which attention was first directed by Meyer.[33] Any factor producing nasopharyngeal inflammation is an important cause, and, in general, the disease is subject to the same predisposing and hereditary influences as is hypertrophy of the faucial tonsils (p. 539).

Pathologic Anatomy.—The soft "adenoid" structure which is normally widespread in the nasopharynx, especially on the posterior wall and the roof, undergoes hypertrophy and forms masses of varying size (Fig. 125), reaching even that of a walnut, and attached to the underlying tissue by a broad base. These may more or less completely fill the vault of the pharynx and cut off the passage of air through the choanae. In young subjects they consist of soft, spongy, lymphoid tissue, but after a time this grows denser, fibrous and less vascular, resembling more the connective-tissue hypertrophy of chronically enlarged faucial tonsils. If the tonsils are hypertrophied, the adenoid vegetations usually are so likewise.

Symptoms.—The manifold symptoms may be divided into those chiefly *local* and direct, and those more *general* in nature. Of the former, *mouth-breathing* is one of the most characteristic (Fig. 126). The degree and persistence of this varies with that of the obstruction. In some infants and children it is observed only during sleep, especially if on the back, at which time snoring is liable to occur. In others the obstruction is sufficient to make the sleep very restless, the child trying ineffectually to find some position in which respiration may be easier. In cases of decided adenoid hypertrophy the mouth hangs open during the day as well; the lips are dry; the expression dull or stupid; the color of the face sometimes pale. Alteration in the *shape of the nose* is common. The nostrils are small and narrow, and the lack of use of these for the normal purpose of breathing gives the nose a "pinched" appearance (Fig. 127). Sometimes, however, the upper portion of it seems unduly broad. *Nasopharyngeal catarrh* is an attendant symptom either more or less constantly present, or occurring in repeated attacks from very slight exposure. The voice is altered, developing a nasal, muffled character; the breath offensive; and the taste and smell impaired. A harrassing *cough* is often present, especially at night, the result of the irritation of the larynx by the inspired air, which has not been properly warmed and moistened by passing through the nose in the normal manner. The cough may depend upon bronchitis, to which the affected children are greatly predisposed. *Deafness* is a very common symptom, at first temporary and developing with the catarrh; later more or less permanent unless treatment of the adenoids is promptly undertaken. It is the result of the blocking of the entrance of the Eustachian tubes, and of the catarrhal processes in them or in the middle ear.

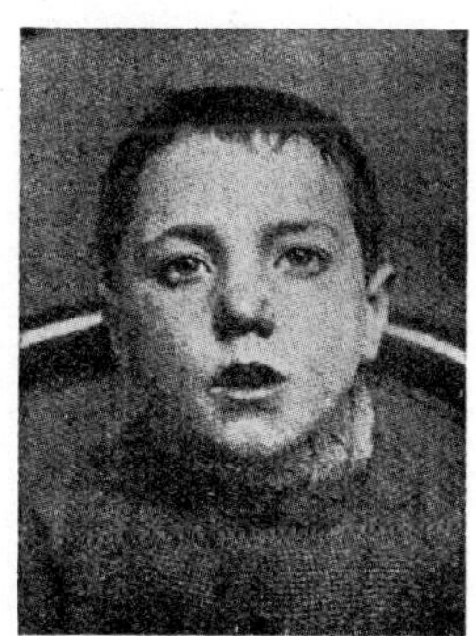

Fig. 126.—Adenoid face. (*Thomson, Clinical Examination of Sick Children*, 1925, 11, *Fig*. 12.)

Permanent *bony deformities* of the structure of the skull may be the result of the pressure of the adenoid tumors or the efforts at respiration. There may be a high and narrow arching of the palate; irregularity in the position of the teeth of the upper jaw, which assumes a somewhat V-shaped form and tends to project forward too greatly; exophthalmos; and a keel-shaped chest with lateral depression of the lower portion of the thorax. This last occurs in patients who have developed adenoid hypertrophy early, and is the result of the unusual efforts at respiration required to obtain a sufficient amount of air in the lungs. It is best seen in rachitic subjects or in those with non-rachitic softening of the ribs (Hess[34]). A number of more or less indirect or general results are evident. There is often a decided *retardation of mental development*, sometimes the result to a certain extent of the impairment of hearing. The stupid expression, dependent in part upon this mental state and in part upon the direct mechanical action of the adenoids in keeping the mouth hanging open and in producing deafness, may, however, give only a mistaken idea that the patient is imbecile. The *growth of the body* is also often interfered with, anemia is common, and the general health suffers. Among other conditions sometimes associated with adenoid hypertrophy and relieved by its removal, are stammering and stuttering, laryngospasm, spasmodic croup, bronchial asthma, hoarseness, headache, night-terrors, enuresis, chorea, scoliosis, cervical adenitis, grinding of the teeth, and convulsive attacks, although the causal relationship of some of these to adenoid

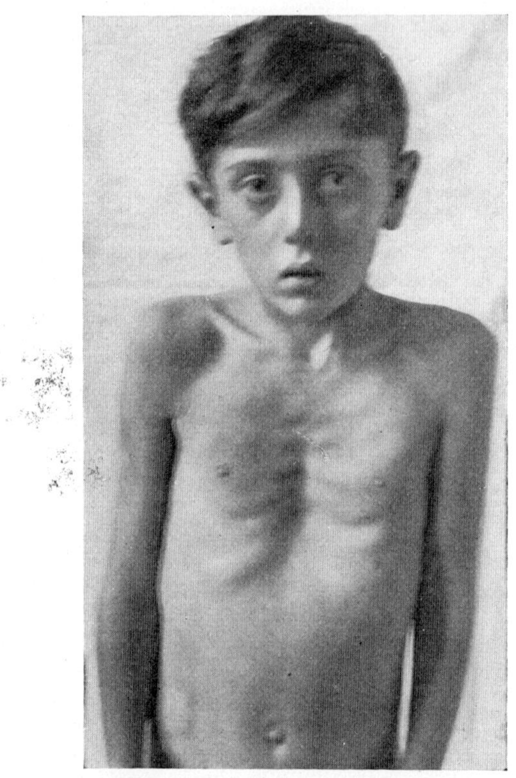

Fig. 127.—Deformity from adenoid growths. Child of seven years and nine months. Shows the narrow nasal bridge and small nostrils, as well as a marked degree of funnel-chest from persistent respiratory tugging.

hypertrophy and infection is by no means clear. Some are more closely related to tonsillar disease.

Course and Prognosis.—Adenoid growths are disposed to increase gradually in size and the symptoms consequently to grow worse, reaching their height about the beginning of later childhood, and continuing until puberty unless relieved by treatment. At puberty there is a tendency for the growths to become smaller and for symptoms to disappear, unless the tissue has become of a fibrous nature. So, too, the condition is always better in summer-time and in a dryer climate, due to the diminution of the catarrhal involvement of the mucous membrane and the shrinking of the growths. Owing to this disposition to grow worse, there is a likelihood of serious deformities and affection of the health developing, particularly when symptoms have appeared during infancy Infection of various sorts, especially by tuberculosis and diphtheria, is liable to occur by way of the adenoids, and the presence of these vegetations makes many diseases affecting the throat run a more serious course. The results from operative treatment are sometimes remarkably prompt and complete; oftener somewhat slower in manifesting themselves; sometimes disappointing if the adenoids have been allowed to remain too long and if bony deformities or nervous symptoms have developed.

Diagnosis.—The existence of hypertrophied faucial tonsils indicates that adenoids are probably also present. The diagnosis can be confirmed by digital or rhinoscopic examination of the vault of the pharynx. Even before this has been made, the diagnosis is rendered very probable by the mouth-breathing, snoring, expression of the face, and frequently recurring nasal catarrh.

Treatment.—The best treatment is early and thorough removal when there are symptoms such as mouth-breathing, affection of speech, otitis, deafness, nasal or other bony deformity, retarded mental or physical development, and persistent or recurring catarrh. If other conditions such as asthma, cervical adenitis, enuresis, night-terrors, headache and the like seem to be dependent upon adenoid hypertrophy, adenoidectomy may constitute part of the treatment. When the growths are small and there is little obstruction improvement may occur with change in climate or measures suitable for the catarrhal condition, and it may be permissible to temporize, especially if the patient is an infant. However, the age for operation is the time when serious symptoms are threatening. The necessity for operation must be determined in the individual case, and it should be surrounded by the same precautions as tonsillectomy, since the same dangers exist. It is customary to remove any adenoid growth present when tonsillectomy is performed, although there may be occasions, particularly in young infants, when adenoidectomy should be recommended alone.

References

1. Am. J. M. Sc., 1907, **134,** 228. 2. Arch. Int. Med., 1921, **27,** 631. 3. Am. J. Dis. Child., 1924, **27,** 113. 4. J. Laryngol. and Otol., 1928, **43,** 328. 5. Am. J. Dis. Child., 1921, **22,** 493. 6. Arch. Int. Med., 1924, **34,** 313. 7. Deutsche med. Wchnschr., 1884, **10,** 395. 8. Deutsche med. Wchnschr., 1894, **20,** 920. 9. Bull. soc. d. hôp., 1898, **15,** 244. 10. J.A.M.A., 1928, **91,** 978. 11. New York M. J., 1923, **117,** 267. 12. J. Infect. Dis., 1912, **10,** 148. 13. J.A.M.A., 1919, **73,** 1050. 14. J. Infect. Dis., 1921, **29,** 47; 51; 55; 59; 62. 15. Arch. Int. Med., 1922, **29,** 635. 16. J. Infect. Dis., 1923, **33,** 134. 17. J.A.M.A., 1916, **66,** 1016. 18. J.A.M.A., 1920, **75,** 1035. 19. J.A.M.A., 1924, **83,** 759. 20. J.A.M.A., 1924, **83,** 33; 1927, **89,** 2239; 1930, **95,** 837; Am. J. Dis. Child., 1929, **37,** 559; 1931, **41,** 568. 21. Am. Heart J., 1928, **4,** 197. 22. Arch. Dis. Childhood, 1929, **4,** 363. 23. Am. J. Dis. Child., 1929, **37,** 252. 24. Arch. Dis. Childhood, 1930, **5,** 335. 25. Lancet, 1930, **2,** 394. 26. Am. J. Pub. Health, 1930, **20,** 495. 27. Arch. Int. Med., 1931, **47,** 513. 28. Gittings and Mitchell, Atlantic M. J., 1924, **27,** 823; Mitchell. Atlantic M. J., 1927, **30,** 481; Mitchell and Renner, Ohio State M. J., 1928, **24,** 365; Selkirk and Mitchell, Am. J. Dis. Child., 1931, **42,** 9. 29. Pub. Health Rep., 1927, No. 175. 30. J.A.M.A., 1928, **97,** 1149. 31. München med. Wchnschr., 1930, **77,** 1666. 32. Am, J. Dis. Child., 1926, **31,** 72. 33. Trans. Med.-Chir. Soc., 1870, **53,** 191; Arch. f. Ohrenh., 1873, **1,** 241; **2,** 241. 34. Am. J. Dis. Child., 1931, **41,** 1309.

CHAPTER IV

DISEASES OF THE ESOPHAGUS

MALFORMATIONS OF THE ESOPHAGUS

THESE are occasionally seen in early life, and most of them are congenital. We[1] have earlier reviewed the subject to some extent, and statistically the diseases have been studied by Cautley[2] and by Plass.[3] Other cases have since been reported. Some of these malformations are incompatible with life and the infant dies a few days after birth; others may be continued indefinitely. Certain of them may be mentioned.

1. Branchial fistulae and cysts are the result of a failure of complete closure of the branchial cleft, which opens in fetal life through the neck into the upper part of the esophagus or the lower portion of the pharynx. This results in a small, external fistula, usually unilateral, and oftenest just above the sternoclavicular articulation, sometimes high in the neck at the inner edge of the sternocleidomastoid muscle. The fistula ends blindly, or may communicate with the alimentary tract. Treatment is usually unsatisfactory and better avoided except in cases with a continual mucous discharge, or where the external opening of the fistula has become clogged and a disfiguring cyst-like mass results. Cysts of a similar appearance, due to other causes, occur in this locality. To all such growths the title *Hygroma* is often applied (Fig. 128).

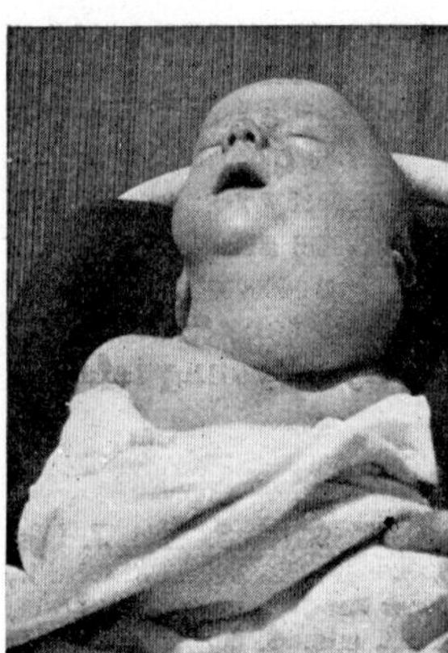

Fig. 128.—Hygroma cysticum. Patient aged seven months, in the Children's Hospital of Philadelphia. Tumor was noticed at birth, grew steadily larger, and finally interfered with respiration and deglutition.

2. Diverticula of the esophagus are occasionally seen, and are probably never really congenital. They occur most frequently as the result of traction exerted by adhesions of the esophagus to the trachea or to a bronchial gland. Their situation is oftenest at the level of the bifurcation of the trachea. The food taken, especially if solid, experiences difficulty in passing into the stomach, and often is regurgitated after a shorter or longer interval, without nausea and without evidence of action of the gastric secretion. In some cases swelling upon one side of the neck is present when the diverticulum is distended by food. The sound when passed may catch in a pocket somewhere in the course of the esophagus, or may at other times pass into the stomach. A roentgenogram taken after the administration of an opaque substance serves to confirm the diagnosis.

3. Congenital absence of the esophagus is very rare. There were found by us but 7 reported cases.

4. Congenital stenosis is uncommon. It is due either to a fold of mucous membrane or to narrowing of the entire wall of the tube. It is attended by the symptoms of stenosis seen in the acquired form. (See p. 548.)

5. Dilatation of the esophagus as a congenital lesion is limited to the portion just above the diaphragm. An acquired secondary diffuse dilatation of the entire length of the esophagus may result. Acquired dilatation is liable also to be a sequence to stenosis of any nature, but is oftenest seen in corrosive esophagitis with stricture. (See p. 548.)

6. A partial or complete **doubling of the esophagus** has been observed in 2 or 3 instances.

7. Sometimes a **tracheo-esophageal fistula** exists without other lesions. This is very rare.

8. Finally there may be a congenital **obliteration of the lumen** of the esophagus in a portion of its extent. Unattended by fistula this is very uncommon. We[1] found but 17 published cases. The most common congenital malformation of the esophagus is a combination of obliteration through more or less of its extent with tracheobronchial fistula (Fig. 129). Of this Plass[3] collected 136 published reports and Hirsch[4] 103. In some cases the defect seems to have been caused by external pressure, as from an aberrant ductus arteriosus (Jacobi and Rascoff[5]). The upper portion of the esophagus is somewhat dilated and ends blindly. The chief symptom of obliteration is the complete inability to swallow food; it being promptly regurgitated through the mouth and nose, producing severe suffocative attacks. Attempts to pass a sound encounter the obstruction, and it can be visualized in the roentgenogram after the swallowing of an opaque substance. Only if there is communication of the esophagus with the trachea or bronchi will there be gas in the stomach. The fistula may be shown, too, by the injection of lipiodol into the trachea (Reid[6]).

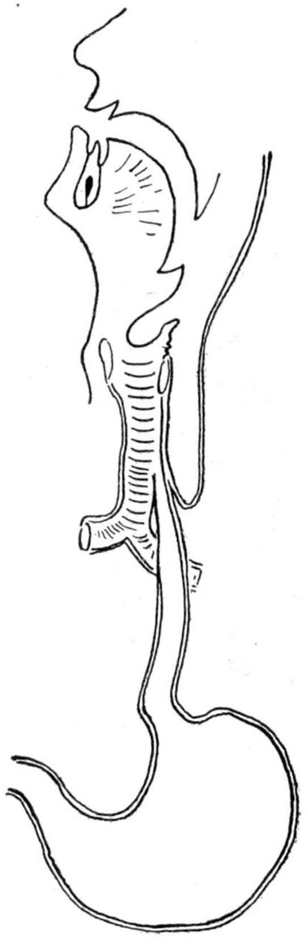

Fig. 129.—Diagram illustrating tracheo-esophageal fistula.[1] (*Griffith and Lavenson, Trans. Amer. Pediat. Soc.*, 1908, **20**, 86.)

SPASM OF THE ESOPHAGUS

(Esophagismus)

This occasionally occurs in children, and we[7] have encountered one very typical instance. A neurotic or psychopathic element exists. The obstruction to swallowing may be constant, or develop only at intervals under increased nervous excitement. In some cases liquids can be taken readily, although solids give trouble; while in others there is difficulty with both. Sometimes hot liquids can be swallowed better than cold. The diagnosis is to be made especially from organic stricture by the fact that an esophageal bougie passes without interference, at least under anesthesia. The prognosis is good so far as life is concerned, but the duration of the disorder is often long. Treatment should be directed especially to the nervous system. Over-anxiety should not be shown by the parents; a skillful nurse is of great aid; and the patient does better if removed from home. General tonic and hygienic measures, change of air, and the like are serviceable. It may be well to pass a bougie daily.

CATARRHAL AND FOLLICULAR ESOPHAGITIS

Acute catarrhal esophagitis may occur under a variety of conditions, and may be seen even in the new-born. It may develop in the acute infectious diseases or pneumonia; attend catarrhal inflammation of other parts of the digestive tract; or follow lacerations produced by the swallowing of foreign bodies or the injury done by the ingestion of hot liquids. The mucous membrane is injected and swollen and the subcutaneous connective tissue edematous. Superficial erosions may occur. The lesions generally last but a few days, and the prognosis is favorable. Symptoms are absent or are uncharacteristic, and consist of mild pain on swallowing. **Chronic catarrhal esophagitis** is of unusual occurrence in early life. It may follow an acute catarrhal process, or be the result of venous congestion in chronic pulmonary or cardiac disease. **Follicular esophagitis** is probably more uncommon than the catarrhal variety. It has been found in typhoid fever and in chronic gastrointestinal and respiratory disorders. The lesions consist in enlargement of the mucous follicles, sometimes attended by superficial erosion of them. **A secondary esophagitis** of a different nature from the lesions described may occur in the course of various diseases, but is rare. Thus diphtheritic or other pseudomembranous inflammation has been found in the esophagus; thrush may extend into it and even obstruct its lumen; pustules of variola have been discovered there; and ulceration may result from perforation of a caseous lymphatic gland. As with the other forms of esophagitis mentioned, the recognition is usually impossible during life. **Papilloma** of the esophagus is a very rare condition described by Johnson.[8]

CORROSIVE ESOPHAGITIS; STRICTURE OF THE ESOPHAGUS

Corrosive inflammation is the variety of esophagitis oftenest seen in children. The most frequent **cause** is swallowing of caustic solutions such as strong acids or alkalies, given to the children by mistake, or carelessly allowed to be within their reach. The **lesions** vary from a superficial necrosis of the epithelium to a destruction of the entire thickness of the mucous membrane. In the severer cases a slough results which, if the patient survives, is at last replaced by cicatricial connective tissue, resulting finally in stenosis. In the worst cases even perforating ulceration of the esophageal wall occurs.

Symptoms.—The early symptoms are immediate pain and burning from the mouth downward, with vomiting of bloody mucus; painful or impossible deglutition; and great thirst. Total collapse may occur at once, and death take place in a few hours or days; or somnolence and fever may mark the severity of the toxic action. If the early danger is passed, there remains for some days the evidence of severe local inflammation, with great pain especially on swallowing. The mucous membrane of the mouth is in places denuded of epithelium. Vomiting of pieces of necrosed membrane may occur. Death may result later from perforation into the peritoneal or the pleural cavity, or improvement gradually occurs, although erosion of the blood-vessels or perforation of an ulcer may unexpectedly take place later. After some weeks or months the symptoms of **stricture of the esophagus** begin, if the corrosive action has been more than merely superficial. There is then an increasing difficulty in swallowing solid food, which often is regurgitated after the attempt is made. Finally, in severe cases, even liquid food is ejected, and examination with the sound shows a more or less complete stricture of the tube. This may be annular or cylindrical in form and its position varies. In the majority of cases in children it is situated in the upper third of the esophagus.

Although the great majority of cases of stricture are dependent upon corrosive esophagitis, there are exceptions of various sorts. Congenital atresia or stricture of the esophagus has already been referred to (p. 546). There may further be mentioned stricture from the lacerations produced by foreign bodies, or by the ulceration of diphtheria, syphilis, or variola, and a spasmodic stenosis occurs in hysteria or rabies. Narrowing by compression from without may take place in cases of retroesophageal abscess, inflammatory enlargement of the thyroid gland, and caseous tracheobronchial glands.

After the development of cicatricial stricture a dilatation of the esophagus, either cylindrical or sacculated, generally forms above it, and food may lie for some time in this before being regurgitated. If the stricture is decided, rapid loss of weight and of general health will occur. There is, however, frequently a variability in the completeness of the obstruction, and children may be able to swallow fairly well at certain times and not at all at others. This probably depends upon a varying increase and decrease in the swelling of the mucous membrane.

Prognosis.—The prognosis of corrosive esophagitis is always serious and uncertain. A large number perish from the primary lesion, and of those who survive a considerable part die of stricture. About 80 per cent of the cases due to lye develop stricture. Cases where the lesions of the mouth and pharynx soon heal probably also have an involvement of the esophagus which is likewise mild, and the prognosis is consequently better.

Treatment.—The first indications for treatment, if the child is seen early enough, are the exhibition of antidotes to the corrosive poison and the washing out of the stomach (p. 200). After this the administration of ice and of demulcent solutions internally is indicated, such as those of flaxseed or gum-arabic, oil, and the like, with morphine hypodermically to relieve the suffering. Any food given must be liquid and perhaps best administered by rectum. In cases in which stricture has developed, the treatment is purely surgical and consists in the systematic and careful use of bougies of a progressively increasing size, beginning with small instruments when necessary. This procedure should not be commenced until at least three or four weeks have elapsed, and all acute symptoms have subsided. If no bougie can be passed, gastrostomy becomes necessary, followed by an attempt to dilate the stricture through the cardia. The use of bougies must be continued for months in order to prevent recurrence of the stricture. In the way of foods recommended are beef-juice, orange juice, milk, cream, eggs, olive oil, sugar, and finely divided or powdered vegetables. Carbohydrate foods, as cereal, rice, and potato, may be predigested (Guerinot[9]). In cases in which food must be given entirely through the gastrostomy opening, even a well-balanced and sufficient diet may fail to support adequately. Jackson[10] found that marked improvement followed having the patient spit the fluid food mixed with the saliva into a funnel attached to the gastrostomy tube. We can confirm this as a valuable procedure.

FOREIGN BODIES IN THE ESOPHAGUS

The lodging of foreign bodies in the esophagus is of not infrequent occurrence. Careful examination with the sound will reveal the body and its position, and the use of the roentgenogram is of great aid in confirming the diagnosis. The place of lodgment is oftenest either at the upper opening, or lower where the left bronchus crosses the tube. Sometimes esophagotomy is necessary. In recent years great advance has been made in the discovery and removal of foreign bodies through the employment of the esophagoscope. Should the object pass into the stomach amylaceous food, such as potato and cereals, should be given freely, in order to render the feces consistent and thus coat the foreign body and protect the bowel from injury.

RETRO-ESOPHAGEAL ABSCESS

(Peri-esophageal Abscess)

This rare condition is sometimes seen in infancy and childhood. But one instance has come to our[11] observation, and a study of the literature up to 1898 revealed 12 others reported in detail.

Etiology.—The causes are similar to those producing retropharyngeal abscess, except that spinal caries appears here to be the most frequent etiologic factor. Among other causes are pleuritis and pericarditis; ulceration resulting from a foreign body in the esophagus, or from a tracheotomy tube or intubation tube; diphtheria of the pharynx; and suppurating lymphatic glands. The abscess forms behind and around the esophagus and often displaces it readily to one side, while it exercises compression upon the more firmly seated trachea or on other parts.

Symptoms.—These are very uncharacteristic and misleading. Dyspnea is nearly always present. Cough, too, is generally observed; sometimes only slight, sometimes spasmodic or brassy and suggesting stenosis. Dysphagia might be expected but seldom occurs, doubtless due to the fact that the esophagus is readily displaced by pressure. Swelling in the neck may result if the abscess is situated behind the upper part of the esophagus.

Prognosis.—This is nearly always unfavorable. Death may result from the pressure of the abscess upon the pneumogastric nerve, or on the trachea with consequent asphyxia; or rupture into the trachea, bronchi or lung may occur and a purulent bronchitis or bronchopneumonia follow. Should the abscess rupture into the esophagus the pus is likely to enter the larynx and produce asphyxia.

Diagnosis.—This generally cannot be more than conjectural, since other pathologic conditions may produce very similar symptoms. If caries of the vertebra is known to exist, retro-esophageal abscess may be suspected if the dyspnea and other symptoms as described develop. If the abscess has a very high situation it may perhaps be reached by the finger thrust deeply downward through the pharynx, or a lateral swelling in the neck may be visible. If there is a history of the swallowing of a foreign body, the roentgenogram may reveal the presence of an abscess.

Treatment.—If the abscess is situated high enough to be discoverable by the finger it may be opened. Otherwise nothing directly in the way of treatment can be done. Tracheotomy may be performed if there is urgent dyspnea, because, with the uncertain diagnosis, some other disorder may be the cause of the respiratory stenosis.

References

1. Griffith and Lavenson, Trans. Am. Pediat. Soc., 1908, **20**, 86; Arch. Pediat., 1909, **26**, 161. 2. Brit. J. Child. Dis., 1917, **14**, 1. 3. Johns Hopkins Hosp. Rep., 1919, **18**, 259. 4. J.A.M.A., 1921, **76**, 1491. 5. Am. J. Dis. Child., 1931, **42**, 1148. 6. J. Pediat., 1932, **1**, 87. 7. Griffith, New York M.J., 1914, **99**, 1113. 8. Am. J. Dis. Child., 1928, **7**, 536. 9. J.A.M.A., 1929, **93**, 375. 10. Arch. Pediat., 1923, **40**, 324. 11. Griffith, Univ. Med. Mag., 1898, **10**, 198.

CHAPTER V

DISEASES OF THE STOMACH AND INTESTINES

In the absence of complete knowledge of the physiology of digestion and of the pathologic lesions found in the digestive tract, any classification of the diseases of the stomach and intestines can be only provisional. That based either upon the lesions alone or upon etiology alone is no more practically useful than is that scientific which rests solely upon symptoms; since the same lesions may be productive of different symptoms, and, on the other hand, identical symptoms may be the result of quite diverse pathologic causes. There are diseases, too, which appear to depend entirely, or in great part, upon functional disturbances rather than upon actual lesions, and it is often difficult or impossible to determine from clinical manifestations how far the disordered condition is due to one or the other factor. The etiologic rôle of micro-organisms and their toxins is also important, the bacteria being either those foreign to the alimentary canal, or those which are natural inhabitants of it, and are without harmful influence under ordinary circumstances. This rôle is, however, uncertain; sometimes the affection being probably chiefly a disturbance of function through the poisonous toxins or other altered chemical conditions; sometimes a distinct pathologic infection produced by the germs; although just which action predominates cannot well be determined. Again it is evident that the diseases of the stomach and of the intestines respectively cannot be always sharply separated from each other, since so often the symptoms of both may appear simultaneously or consecutively, or sometimes those of the one region predominating and sometimes of the other. We have, therefore, adopted a classification based chiefly upon clinical manifestations as connected with the different regions of the gastrointestinal tract; modified by the known pathologic anatomy, and by what we may believe is certainly known of the respective actions of the food-ingredients and of the bacteria. In the study of the subject attention should be given to the anatomy and physiology of the gastro-intestinal tract as discussed earlier (pp. 22; 25; 29).

THE FINKELSTEIN CLASSIFICATION

The theories of Finkelstein regarding nutritional diseases associated with disordered digestion or metabolism, an elaboration and modification of the views of Czerny and Keller[1], have attracted so much attention that a review of them is necessary. The classification is given at length in the article by Finkelstein and Meyer[2] in Feer's work on Pediatrics, and previously in many journal-publications. (See also reviews by J. Hess,[3] Meara,[4] and others; and especially by Snow.[5]) Finkelstein regards the digestive and nutritional disorders as disturbances of metabolism, the result of the toxic action of substances derived from the different normal elements of the food, rather than as dependent upon bacterial activity. The healthy breast-fed baby has a normal tolerance for food; but the artificially-fed infant, especially if weakly, has to deal with food-ingredients not natural to it, and a degree of intolerance for some of these is readily established. The casein of the milk is, according to his view, the ingredient most readily borne; the whey is a source of much trouble. The sugar and the fat readily produce intolerance, but chiefly when given in combination with or contained in the whey. Abnormal fermentation of the food in the digestive tract occurs, for instance, during hot weather from a diminution of the power of digestion rather than from unusual contamination by bacteria.

The development of intolerance may be shown by various digestive symptoms, such as vomiting, diarrhea, and the like, as well as others of deranged metabolism producing nervous manifestations, albuminuria, fever, etc.

Finkelstein divides the disturbances into: (1) Disturbance of balance; (2) Dyspepsia; (3) Decomposition, and (4) Intoxication.

1. Disturbance of Balance.—This is the mildest modification of the food-intolerance. The most common injurious element of the food is the fat, because the increased alkaline secretion of the intestines combines with the fatty acids and produces soap-stools. The chief symptoms are unsatisfactory gain in weight in spite of the administration of food the caloric value of which is sufficient. The most effective treatment is a diminution of the fat and an increase of the carbohydrate element of the diet.

2. Dyspepsia.—This is also a mild form of the disturbance. Its commonest cause is an inability to assimilate carbohydrates, with a consequent fermentation of these in the intestine, and resulting increase of peristalsis, with diarrhea. This fermentation prevents the proper absorption of the fat, which then appears in the stools. Increase in the amount of food produces loss of weight (paradoxical reaction). The symptoms consist in the failure to gain weight, diarrhea, anorexia, vomiting, tympanites and colic. The stools are thin, green, frothy, and contain mucus and white lumps composed of fat and bacteria. Treatment is best carried out by giving human milk. In the absence of this the carbohydrates should be reduced after a brief period of fasting. Often the employment of some other sugar than that of milk is successful; cane-sugar and, still better, dextrin-maltose preparations being less liable to ferment. The fat also should be reduced. Buttermilk is often of service. He regards "protein-milk" as one of the best of foods for the condition (p. 108). Too long a continuance of underfeeding must be avoided.

3. Decomposition.—By this term is indicated a loss of the constituents of the body; a decomposition. It is one of the severe forms of nutritional disorder, the equivalent of the condition ordinarily described as infantile atrophy or marasmus. It depends upon a decided loss of digestive power. There is a great intolerance for fat and carbohydrate. The symptoms and treatment are similar to those described under the heading of infantile atrophy (p. 462).

4. Alimentary Intoxication.—This is a threatening condition of food-intolerance developing as a later stage after that of dyspepsia or of decomposition. The disorder is probably associated with an acidosis. The cause is the administration of food much above the tolerance of the child, and the consequent severe disturbance of metabolism. Food rich in whey or carbohydrate is especially prone to produce the condition; but excess of fat is toxic also. The symptoms and treatment are much like those described under gastro-enteric intoxication (p. 583).

Later Finkelstein and Meyer[6] modified this classification to some extent, among other changes substituting the title "dystrophy" for "disturbance of balance." The division then consists of (*A*) *Nontoxic nutritional disturbance* and (*B*) *Toxic nutritional disturbance*. In the first group are (1) *Dystrophies* with or without diarrhea, and (2) *Decomposition*. In the second group are (1) *Acute dyspepsia* and (2) *Intoxication*. In spite of these changes the discussion of the underlying principles and the symptomatology has been but little altered.

Those who have long followed the increasing purification of the milk-supply, as connected with the lessening morbidity and mortality of infants during hot weather, find it difficult to admit that bacteria play as small a part in the production of summer diarrhea as Finkelstein's claims assign to them. There are, also, sufficient grounds based on experimental work to render it probable that in many cases a change in the character of the food does good by militating against the growth of certain harmful species of bacteria in the intestinal canal, whether or not these possess any distinct infectious power. The influence of dehydration in producing the symptoms of intoxication is likewise to be considered.

VOMITING

Vomiting, although not a disease itself, is so common a symptom that some of its causes and varieties may be reviewed. (See also p. 116.) There is a vomiting center in the medulla. Impulses pass from this during vomiting to the stomach by way of the vagus, to the diaphragm by the phrenic nerve, and to the abdominal wall by the spinal cord and spinal nerves. There follow closure of the pylorus, relaxation of the cardiac end of the stomach, and contraction of the diaphragm and abdominal muscles, and vomiting results.

1. One of the most troublesome forms seen in infancy is due to **overloading of the stomach.** This may occur in a child in other respects healthy. At first it is a mere regurgitation of the excess of food taken; is harmless in itself; and is unattended by evidences of nausea, such as sudden cessation of crying, pallor about the mouth, and the like. If the overloading is persisted in a chronic dyspeptic condition develops.

2. What may be called **nervous vomiting** or **habit-vomiting** is an exceedingly intractible and common form seen in many infants, the reflex arc-pathway apparently being more readily stimulated than normally. In such cases the slightest excitement may produce vomiting; such as crying, sudden movement of the infant by the mother or nurse, or sometimes the mere psychic stimulation connected with taking food, laughing, or even smiling. It is on account of the mental influence that vomiting may be absent during the sleeping hours, but occur after every feeding during the daytime. Doubtless a more or less dyspeptic state is present in most of these cases. A very similar condition is often seen in older children, in which vomiting becomes a habit, and anger or other emotion may readily produce it. Such children vomit when any medicine is given which has an unpleasant taste, or even with any medicine whatever, or if food is urged of which they are not fond. Many of them seem to have the power of vomiting at will. In other instances the vomiting is dependent upon a neurotic or hysterical condition. Some cases of this nature vomit especially in the morning before or after breakfast, the occurrence being connected with the excitement or overwork of school-life. In some of these cases there may be hypoglycemia (p. 556). Still another cause of nervous vomiting depends upon a disturbance of the equilibrium of the body, as in swinging, sea-travel, or railroad-journeys, in these conditions the impulses being carried from the semilunar canals of the internal ear to the vomiting center.

3. Organic nervous diseases are frequently attended by vomiting dependent upon actual pathologic changes outside the stomach, increased intracranial pressure directly stimulating the vomiting center in the medulla. This is especially true of meningitis and of intracranial tumors and abscess and of certain cases of intracranial birth-injury and hydrocephalus. The vomiting is often the earliest symptom noticed, and is sometimes very persistent and often violent and projectile in character. Other evidences of intracranial disease soon develop.

4. Vomiting is nearly always present in **acute gastric dyspepsia** due to the ingestion of indigestible food. It may come on immediately after eating, especially in infancy, but usually occurs after some hours, the contents of the stomach then showing evidence of disordered digestion. It is preceded by nausea, faintness, loss of appetite, and sometimes fever, and may continue after the first emptying of the stomach; mucus and finally bile appearing in the vomited matter. An analogous condition is the frequent vomiting observed in certain cases where there is an abnormality of the gastric secretion, such as hyperchlorhydria.

5. Chronic gastritis is attended by the frequent vomiting of food which has remained too long in the stomach and has undergone decomposition; or the vomitus may be merely an acid, watery liquid.

6. Acute infectious diseases are very commonly ushered in by vomiting. This is especially characteristic of scarlet fever and pneumonia, but is also true of malaria, typhoid fever, poliomyelitis and other infectious disorders. It probably is caused by the direct action of the poison of the disease on the vomiting center. Zahorsky[7] reports an epidemic type of vomiting occurring in the winter months only ("*hyperemesis hiemis*"). The onset is sudden with marked and continued vomiting, prostration, mild diarrhea, and slight fever. Recovery follows in a few days.

7. Toxic vomiting is seen, for instance, in recurrent or cyclic vomiting, being dependent upon some poison in the blood. Uremia may act in a similar manner. Poisonous substances or certain medicaments introduced into the stomach may cause vomiting by direct irritation of the organ, by their influence upon the nerve-centers, or, as in the case of contaminated milk, by the actual absorption of poisonous material produced by the changes which have taken place in the food. Apomorphine, digitalis, tartar emetic, and the like act directly on the vomiting center. The vomiting which often occurs in the later course of diphtheria, typhoid fever, and other infectious diseases, is probably toxic or septic in nature.

8. Vomiting after cough is seen especially in pertussis, but may occur after severe coughing from any cause.

9. Obstructive vomiting is observed in several conditions. One of the most frequent causes is intestinal obstruction, especially intussusception. Congenital obstruction of the duodenum or pylorus is a cause of obstinate vomiting in early infancy. A form of temporary obstruction producing vomiting is a frequent variety depending upon imperfect handling of the infant. Smith and Lewald[8] have shown by roentgenographic examination that all breast-fed and bottle-fed infants swallow air when nursing. If the infant is not held erect after feeding to permit of regurgitation of this, a large air-bubble may collect at the pyloric end of the stomach interfering with the exit of food, and the contents of the stomach may be pushed toward the cardiac orifice and vomited.

10. Appendicitis is commonly productive of vomiting combined with severe abdominal pain early in the attack. Later it may recur from the development of septic poisoning.

11. General **peritonitis** from any source is nearly always attended by vomiting. It is due either to sepsis or to paralysis of peristalsis, which consequently produces practically an intestinal obstruction. Probably of the same nature is the vomiting sometimes occurring in idiopathic dilatation of the colon and in gastroptosis.

12. Passive congestion of the stomach, such as occurs in severe forms of heart-disease, is often attended by vomiting with evidences of chronic indigestion.

13. Reflex vomiting may depend upon many causes, as the presence of worms in the intestinal canal, the putting by the infant of its fingers into its mouth and throat, and the like.

In every case of vomiting the important and often difficult matter is to determine the cause. Treatment is then that indicated for this.

RECURRENT VOMITING

(Cyclic Vomiting)

While a condition of this nature had been reported earlier, the first important description of it appears to have been by Gruère.[9] The title "recurrent" is to be preferred, since "cyclic" implies a regularity which is not characteristic of the disease.

Etiology and Pathogenesis.—The first attack usually develops in early childhood; occasionally in infancy. Sex exercises no important influence. A highly developed nervous organization seems to predispose, but the condition is by no means confined to such children. History of the family may reveal a tendency to migraine or other nervous disorders. As factors initiating attacks may be fatigue, emotional excitement, exposure to cold, or the onset of an acute infection; or the attack may begin without these. Diet has some influence, since alteration of it is effectual in preventing attacks in some cases, although without result in others. So, too, the occurrence of slight premonitory digestive symptoms in some cases suggests an etiologic relationship.

There have been various theories concerning pathogenesis. One no longer held is that the affection is a manifestation of the uric-acid diathesis or "arthritism." Marfan[10] and others have designated it "acetonemic vomiting," on the ground that acetone is so constantly present in the urine. Marfan admits, however, that this may be the result rather than the cause, or may be due simply to starvation. Usually the acetonuria appears after the onset of an attack, although it occasionally precedes it. The presence of acetone-bodies in the urine does not in itself indicate acidosis. (See p. 489.) It has been reported, too, that recurrent vomiting may occur and yet alkalosis develop (Kast, Myers and Schmitz[11]), and this might be expected in some cases from the loss of hydrochloric acid occasioned by vomiting. Yet in many instances there is an acidosis, or at least a lowered CO_2 combining power of the plasma is found. An observation of Ross and Josephs,[12] later repeated by Josephs,[13] showed that there may be a lowered blood-sugar at the height of the attack. Not all of these cases, however, were typical of recurrent vomiting, but the hypoglycemia has been found by others, and we have observed it; and Shaw and Moriarty[14] reported that lowered blood-sugar produced by fasting may be followed by violent vomiting, promptly relieved by the administration of sugar. Salomonsen,[15] however, could not by starvation initiate characteristic attacks in patients with the disease.

Other observations on the disease should be mentioned, although they but confirm the uncertainty as to the cause and nature. Sedgwick[16] and Mellanby[17] reported a urinary excretion of creatinine at the time of the attack, but Rose[18] and Folin and Denis[19] have shown that creatinine is normally excreted by children. Underhill and Steele[20] attributed etiologic significance to adenoids, and Byfield[21] to diseased tonsils. The occasional presence of icterus has suggested that the liver is at fault (Richardière[22]) and the hypoglycemia would also indicate this. Comby[23] thought some cases depended upon chronic appendicitis; Snow[24] that some were caused by intermittent hyperchlorhydria; Talbot and Brown,[25] Kerley,[26] and Sherman and Koenig[27] that one of the factors involved was poor body-mechanics with gastroenteroptosis.

It would seem reasonable to conclude that recurrent vomiting is a distinct clinical entity, and that the same basic cause exists for every case. It must be stated, however, that many of the metabolic disturbances described, such as hypoglycemia, acidosis, acetonuria, and similar conditions, might well be secondary results. Fright, infections, and the like appear to act only as trigger-mechanisms in a predisposed individual. Even the fact that degenerative changes are sometimes found in the kidney, liver, and other organs may indicate only that these are secondary to the metabolic disturbances, rather than primary causes. The toxic changes found in the liver might lead to hypoglycemia and vomiting, and perhaps some of the fatal cases differed in their etiology from typical recurrent vomiting. It is possible that the explanation of recurrent vomiting lies in the fact that the metabolism of fat and carbohydrate in these cases is sufficient under ordinary circumstances, but breaks down under the strain caused by excessive fat-intake or because of lowered resistance due to the factors mentioned.

Symptoms.—The attack may commence suddenly or may be preceded for twelve or more hours by coated tongue, constipation, malaise, irritability, abdominal discomfort, and loss of appetite. Vomiting then begins, at first of the food ingested; later merely serous, mucous, or finally bilious; or sometimes brownish or blood-stained. The vomiting is often forceful, with much retching, and occurs whenever anything whatever is swallowed, or even without this with varying frequency; sometimes in severe cases as often as every half hour. There is little or no elevation of temperature, unless the attack is one which has been coincident with an acute infection; often abdominal pain; and occasionally tenderness, obstinate constipation, urgent thirst, scaphoid abdomen or sometimes tympanites; and in some cases headache. The pulse is sometimes rapid and weak, sometimes slow or intermittent. As the attack continues the coated tongue becomes dry and brown; the prostation extreme; there is an anxious expression of face; the eyes are sunken; there is an odor of acetone on the breath; the urine is scanty and sometimes contains albumin. Acetone and β-oxybutyric acid are found in it later, and in some cases even at the outset. Because of the dehydration the blood may show retention of nonprotein nitrogen. Convulsions may occur. Ross and Josephs[12] have suggested that these may be due to hypoglycemia, but some are apparently uremic in nature. A rather characteristic feature is that the vomiting ceases as suddenly as it began.

Course and Prognosis.—The attack lasts two to four days or longer, but in spite of the extreme prostration frequently present, recovery generally takes place and is prompt. A number of fatal cases are, however, on record. We[28] have seen 2 typical cases terminating fatally with evidences of nephritis. In another case, with final recovery, gangrene of the leg followed a marantic thrombosis. There is always recurrence of attacks at intervals usually of a number of months, and this may continue throughout several years, although as puberty is approached they ordinarily cease. In some instances, as in those reported by Rachford[29] and others, and as we have several times seen, the vomiting has been replaced by migraine in later life.

Diagnosis.—This often presents many difficulties unless there is a history of previous attacks of a similar nature. It is important to make a most careful examination of the body, including the urine, to eliminate the presence of other causative conditions. It is important, also, to remember that vomiting is a symptom of many infectious and toxic states and of poisons, in some of which there may be damage to the liver and a hypoglycemia. The obstinate constipation may suggest *intestinal obstruction,* and we have seen instances in which the differential diagnosis was most difficult. There is seldom, however, severe abdominal pain in recurrent vomiting, and in the case of intussusception there are characteristic distinguishing symptoms. Nevertheless cases showing typical symptoms of recurrent vomiting have been found at necropsy to depend upon obstruction of some sort. *Appendicitis* usually has less severe vomiting and is attended by localized tenderness and more pain, together with fever. At least until there is marked dehydration there is little leukocytosis in recurrent vomiting. Acute *indigestion* has often the history and the evidence of indiscretion in diet and the vomiting is of shorter duration. *Acute febrile diseases* having an onset with vomiting are generally soon distinguished by the development of other symptoms. *Tuberculous meningitis* or other serious disorder of the brain has, it is true, vomiting of a suggestive forceful character, but its other symptoms eventually remove doubt. *Nephritis* may produce uremic attacks with severe vomiting. Other symptoms and the careful examination of the urine will settle the question.

There is a type of vomiting which often occurs in epidemic form and which bears some resemblance to the recurrent variety. The onset is sudden with vomiting as a marked feature, and the ketone bodies appear in the urine in large amount. The clinical distinction of the epidemic type lies in the cessation of the vomiting within six to twenty-four hours, the presence of diarrhea, the higher elevation of the temperature, the occurrence of similar cases in the community, and the absence of subsequent attacks. We do not believe that there is any reason to classify these cases with recurrent vomiting, the latter probably being toxic or metabolic in nature, and epidemic vomiting being an infection with acetonuria as a secondary result of this and of the starvation.

Treatment.—In cases where premonitory symptoms show themselves the attack may occasionally be aborted by stopping all food except carbohydrate, and by procuring a very free evacuation of the bowels by purgatives, such as Rochelle salts, citrate of magnesia, or calomel, but never to the point of increasing the tendency to dehydration. If the attack has already commenced no food or drug of any sort should be given by the mouth, except possibly small amounts of a carbohydrate if these can be retained. The child should be kept as quiet as possible in bed. To relieve the distressing thirst, small pieces of ice may be placed in the mouth, but this should be limited as much as possible, since the irritability of the stomach is very liable to be increased in this way. The nature of the metabolic fault, whether this be causative or merely secondary, suggests the administration of glucose as a corrective measure. This may be introduced in 5 per cent solution by proctoclysis, hypodermoclysis or intravenously, in amounts varying from 100 to 400 cc. (3.38 to 13.53 fl. oz.), depending on the age and weight of the child and the severity of the symptoms. It may also be taken orally if it can be retained. It may be followed by excellent results, especially if given intravenously. The fluid so administered also aids in combating the dehydrated state present, for which saline solution is likewise indicated, since this helps to replace the chloride lost by vomiting. It has also been recommended to give one unit of insulin for every 3 Gm. of glucose injected. This helps in the more rapid utilization of glucose, and in the proportion advised probably will not add to any hypoglycemia already present. In desperate cases blood-transfusion should be performed. If the case is prolonged, rectal feeding may be tried. The oral administration of cocaine hydrochloride seems to be helpful in some instances in quieting the vomiting. An eighth of a grain (0.008) may be given every two or three hours to a child of five years of age. The only other treatment which offers much hope of checking the vomiting is the hypodermic administration of morphine in full but divided doses. The relief is sometimes remarkably prompt and lasting. Bromides and chloral may be tried by the bowel, but are usually unavailing. Bicarbonate of soda is widely used during the attack, but is of little value. Its employment should be restricted to those cases in which acidosis has been demonstrated by laboratory test. As the attack subsides the resumption of the ordinary diet can usually be made rapidly.

Effort should be made in the intervals to prevent the recurrence of attacks. Repeated and continued administration of bicarbonate of soda has been advised, but appears of little value; acidosis being a secondary and not a primary factor. If the tonsils are diseased they should be removed. Faulty posture and gastroenteroptosis should be treated by appropriate measures. (See p. 469.) Care should be taken that the bowels are open daily, and at intervals of a week or two a freely acting purgative should be administered. Excitement and undue fatigue should be avoided. The diet should be digestible and simple. Reducing the amount of fat and increasing that of the carbohydrate within safe limits should certainly be tried, on the assumption that the disease may be associated with faulty metabolism of the fats. We have seen attacks cease to recur following this altered diet.

GASTRALGIA

Gastralgia, like vomiting, is a symptom of various conditions. In the broader sense of pain in the epigastrium, not necessarily arising in the stomach, it is common and may be the result of acute gastric indigestion, spinal caries with pain conducted along the nerves of the abdominal wall, malaria, renal colic, appendicitis, pneumonia, gastric ulcer, diaphragmatic pleurisy and other causes. In some children of delicate constitution or highly neurotic organization there may occur a true nervous gastralgia, apparently of a neuralgic nature, due to many diverse agencies, such as exposure, fatigue, and emotional disturbances. This is more common in childhood than in infancy. In the milder cases the pain is slight and of short duration; in the more severe it may be continuous and so intense that prostration and faintness are present and perforation may be suspected. In infancy symptoms may develop which are apparently those of intestinal colic, but which are relieved by the eructation by the patient of gas from the stomach, thus indicating the true nature of the affection.

A careful study of the various possibilities should be made in order to reach a correct diagnosis of the form of gastralgia present. In the way of **treatment,** the cause must be sought for and removed if possible. In those cases in which the pain appears neuralgic, or due to an accumulation of gas in the stomach, treatment during the attack consists in confinement to bed; abstinence from food; hot applications to the abdomen, such as hot water bags, stupes, or mustard-plasters; the administration of a carminative such as ginger or oil of cloves, best combined with spirits of chloroform or with milk of asafetida or compound spirits of ether; and if necessary the giving of an opiate. Between the attacks efforts must be made to improve the general health and to correct any faults of diet. The best results are sometimes obtained by the administration of quinine or arsenic.

ANOREXIA

This is a symptom common to a great number of diseased states. It accompanies acute febrile disturbances and acute gastric indigestion. Anorexia of a chronic nature is present in ptosis of the gastrointestinal tract, overfeeding and too frequent feeding, there being no opportunity to grow hungry; chronic intestinal indigestion; and anemia. Apparent anorexia may be exhibited by children with disorders of the mouth or throat, because of the pain produced by eating. In some cases alteration in the gastric secretion has been observed, but this is variable, Sauer, Minsk and Alexander,[30] and Rohrböck[31] finding delayed emptying-time and a hypochlorhydria in children with poor appetite, and Berman,[32] Kerley and Lorenze,[33] and Loeber and Weinberger[34] often hyperacidity. There is a group of cases in which anorexia is persistent and causes much parental anxiety. It is, namely, of frequent occurrence for an infant, who has previously nursed well, to refuse entirely or partly one or more bottles a day, and to continue this for weeks, although apparently in good health. In some of these cases it can be discovered by careful study of the caloric intake that more food is offered than needed, or that other fault in the diet exists. In some there is no cause discoverable unless it be the constipation often present.

Anorexia of the sort just described is even more common in older children who are usually of the tall, thin, active, nervous type, often with an increased metabolic rate. The meal-time becomes a struggle on the part of the parents to persuade the child to eat. The causes already mentioned should be sought for. It may be found that the child eats between meals, and then often food of an unsuitable nature. In certain cases there is lack of fresh air and exercise; in others constipation seems to be a cause, or perhaps more often a result. It can occasionally be shown by roentgenograms that the stomach is smaller than normal. Sometimes the child is from birth constitutionally a light eater, and then may either remain in normal health and nutrition in spite of an appetite less than normal or, on the other hand, may become anemic and thin.

Treatment.—A careful search must always be made for any organic cause of anorexia, including, if necessary, gastric analysis. The diet must be studied to determine whether it is calorically correct and properly balanced. Constipation must be overcome and anemia treated if these are present. Exercise out-of-doors may be prescribed, but fatigue avoided, especially near the meal-time, since over-exertion definitely depresses gastric and intestinal secretions. Cool morning bathing, massage, and change of climate may all be efficacious. Meals should not be too frequent and no food allowed between them. For a child with a small stomach small frequent meals may, however, be necessary. If a child refuses one meal it is usually better to offer nothing until the next meal is due. Foods of a concentrated nature should be prescribed, and not liquids of little nutritive value. Usually the best procedure is to reduce the amount of milk or temporarily to stop it entirely, or sometimes to allow skimmed milk, but to diminish decidedly for a time the amount of fat allotted in any form. Lucas and Pryor[35] found it helpful to substitute a quart of fruit juice for the milk. Nearly all pediatrists agree that quantities of milk exceeding 32, or even perhaps 24 oz. a day have a depressing effect on appetite. In case of acute temporary anorexia from any cause, the taking of food should not be urged.

Medication is of secondary consideration. Sometimes an alkaline bitter tonic, as a combination of nux vomica, gentian and bicarbonate of soda, may give results; in other cases a mineral acid, as dilute hydrochloric, is better, the choice being made when possible on the basis of gastric analysis. Often of benefit is a bitter alcoholic tonic or suitable doses of sherry, port, or whiskey. The constipation and the anemia may both need medicinal treatment. Liver, beefsteak, and kidney may not only help anemia but also seem to stimulate the appetite. Perhaps vitamin B preparations may be helpful in certain cases. If cod liver oil is administered it should be not before meals.

Anorexia Nervosa.—This form is of purely nervous origin and in some instances is a hysterical manifestation. The simplest form is that developing from emotional excitement, as anxiety, grief, or pleasurable anticipation. It is the more chronic cases which are most difficult to treat. In this category may be placed some of the instances already referred to of persistently poor appetite in children. Repugnance to food may even result in vomiting what is taken, if the eating of more is urged. An element of hysteria is distinctly shown in some instances. Thus a child who has a reputation for having no appetite subconsciously feels obliged to live up to it. Consequently the anxious urging of food by the parents, and the remarks made in the child's presence regarding the anorexia, tend to fix in his mind the unwillingness to eat. Imitation, too, plays an important rôle, and if other members of the family eat little or openly express dislike for certain foods, the child may do the same. In older children this hysterical anorexia may be a serious menace to health (Forchheimer[36]), and even in infancy may, more commonly than supposed, reach a threatening degree. In an instance previously reported by us[37] an infant twenty-one months of age refused all nourishment but breast-milk, which had become insufficient. After a month of effort gavage was employed and was required for a period of six months. In this case anorexia apparently depended upon fear of anything taken from a spoon or glass, dating from an attack of illness at nine months of age, when medicine was administered in this way.

Treatment.—In the treatment of anorexia nervosa there should be followed the plan of study and the measures already outlined (see above). All anxious discussion of the diet in the presence of the patient must be abandoned, and little notice taken of the anorexia, except that the child should be sent from the table after a reasonable length of time, rather than be permitted to play with its food. No food should be allowed between meals. Change of scene may be of benefit, and sometimes temporary separation of the child from the family is almost essential. Eventually, however, complete cooperation must be obtained in the home. Gavage may be necessary for a time.

STENOSIS OF THE PYLORUS

(Hypertrophic Pyloric Stenosis; Pylorospasm)

An instance of this condition, perhaps the earliest reported, was by Hezekiah Beardsley,[38] although its nature was not recognized at the time. Possibly a still earlier case is that described by Armstrong[39] in 1777 and reported clinically as "watery gripes," although the necropsy revealed pyloric stenosis. A case in infancy was published by Williamson[40] in 1841, and another by Siemon-Dawosky[41] in 1842. No further notice was taken of the subject until the contribution of Hirschsprung[42] in 1888. Ibrahim[43] in 1910 stated that up to the period of writing 598 instances of stenosis had been recorded. So many instances have since then been observed, that the publication of them has ceased and the disease may well be regarded as a fairly common one. An interesting note on the earlier history was published by Foote.[44]

Pathogenesis.—There appear to be certainly two factors in producing stenosis, and consequently two classes of cases, not however, sharply distinguishable: (1) **pylorospasm,** dependent upon a spasm of the muscular layer of the pylorus; (2) congenital hypertrophy of all the tissues, but especially the muscular fibers, viz. **hypertrophic stenosis of the pylorus.** The first element predominates in some cases, the second in others. Perhaps there is a third factor, viz. a swelling of the mucous membrane of the pylorus. In the majority of instances it is probable that a certain degree of hypertrophic stenosis is present, but that the stomach is at first able to overcome this; and that finally a large element of spasm develops in addition and closes the pylorus, while at the same time the expelling power of the stomach diminishes. In other cases spasm is the sole or principal cause, as shown by the numerous instances of recovery without operation, and by the fact that typical symptoms have existed, yet at operation or necropsy no pyloric narrowing has been disclosed. On the other hand the findings at operation or necropsy demonstrate in most instances the reality of organic changes. Hypertrophy of pyloric tissues has also been found in persons dying from other causes, who have exhibited no obstructive symptoms during life.

Thomson[45] believed the spasm to be primary, the result of irritation produced by swallowing liquor amnii, and that hypertrophy follows this. Heubner[46] also views it as primary, as does Haas.[47] The latter and White[48] consider the spasm due to overaction of the vagus. In fact, a number of investigators attribute it to an imbalance of the vegetative nervous system or to a hypertonia. Aldrich[49] and others believe there is an imbalance due to insufficiency of the suprarenals, while Pirie[50] and Gray and Reynolds[51] maintain there exists a hyperadrenalism; a view disproven by Shipley and Blackfan.[52] Cohen and Breitbart[53] suggest the influence of allergy sensitizing the fetus in utero; and Moore, Brodie, Dennis and Hope[54] attribute the spasm to deficiency of vitamin B in the mother. A relationship to spasmophilia has been suggested, as also to enlargement of the thymus, but an etiological connection is not clear.

On the other hand it would appear that more observers regard hypertrophy as being the primary condition, and spasm secondary to and produced by it, and this would seem to be a very acceptable explanation. That the two are interdependent is supported by the fact that tumor may persist without symptoms when spasm has been relieved, and by the experiments of Tumpeer and Bernstein,[55] in which pyloric tumors produced in dogs by the injection of paraffin, failed to cause any symptoms of pyloric stenosis.

Etiology.—Many more boys are affected than girls, and more first-born than later children. We have a number of times seen a familial influence in that more than one infant of the same parents have been attacked. This is referred to by others, among them Caulfield,[56] and Bratusch-Marrain.[57] Cases have been encountered in both of twins. Most cases develop in breast-fed infants, this being probably only an accidental occurrence, since at the early age of onset most infants are being breast-fed. It is rare in negro infants. We have seen only 3 cases in members of this race, in all of them spasm being apparently largely responsible for the quite typical symptoms.

Pathologic Anatomy.—The pylorus is found elongated, thickened, with the stiffness of cartilage, and with the mucous membrane projecting into the duodenum. Incision shows great thickening of the walls, and the lumen occluded by this and by the swelling of the longitudinal folds of the mucous membrane (Fig. 130). The appearance is much the same whether

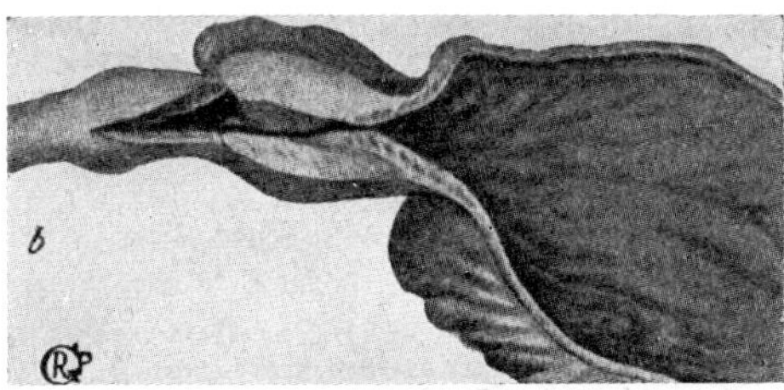

Fig. 130.—Hypertrophic pyloric stenosis in a six weeks old infant. Longitudinal section, showing hypertrophy of circular fibers and extremely narrow lumen. (*Pisek and LeWald, Arch. of Pediat.*, 1912, **29**, 911.)

due to spasm or to hypertrophy. If the organic change is the predominant one there is found evident hypertrophy of the muscular layer, especially of the circular fibers. This has been shown especially well by wax models of the pylorus (Sauer[58]). The stomach may be contracted, but is usually dilated, and the esophagus may share in the dilatation, and both its walls and those of the stomach may exhibit hypertrophy.

Symptoms.—Probably in all cases there is a combination of spasm and stenosis, and although they are sometimes described separately, there is clinically no sharp distinction between the two conditions. Evidences of the disease may occasionally appear in the first few days of life in cases depending on decided hypertrophy (4 per cent in the first week. Holt[59]). In the majority of cases the symptoms chiefly appear in the first three weeks of life, spasm probably being an important factor. A few have been reported (Scott,[60] Rosenheim[61]) which did not begin until two years or later. Perhaps the majority of these were due to spasm, or not identical with congenital stenosis, but others have been proven hypertrophic. Vomiting is at first uncharacteristic and only occasional. Steadily it grows projectile in character and becomes more frequent, taking place after each ingestion of food, either promptly or after a delay of some hours, all or only a portion of the food being lost. If there is *dilatation* of the stomach with retention, there may be the expulsion of more food than was taken at the last feeding, and this may occur perhaps only once or twice a day. By stomach-tube or by roentgenogram food may still be found in the stomach four to ten hours after its ingestion, and several hours pass before any at all enters the intestine, this showing the loss of gastric motor power. The gastric contents contain more or less altered food, often mucus, and sometimes streaks of blood, the last from the trauma produced by the tube. An increase of hydrochloric acid may or may not be present. There is no evident nausea. *Constipation* is a striking feature, its degree depending on the degree and constancy of the stenosis. There may be no fecal matter for days. *Loss of weight* is usually rapid and may proceed to extreme emaciation, although in some cases nutrition is surprisingly well maintained. *Gastric peristaltic waves*, visible through the thin abdominal wall, constitute a characteristic symptom, present in nearly all cases. They are seen especially after food has been taken, or just before vomiting, but may occur at any time, even during sleep, and may be brought into evidence by stimulation through deep palpation or friction of the abdominal wall. They start on the left

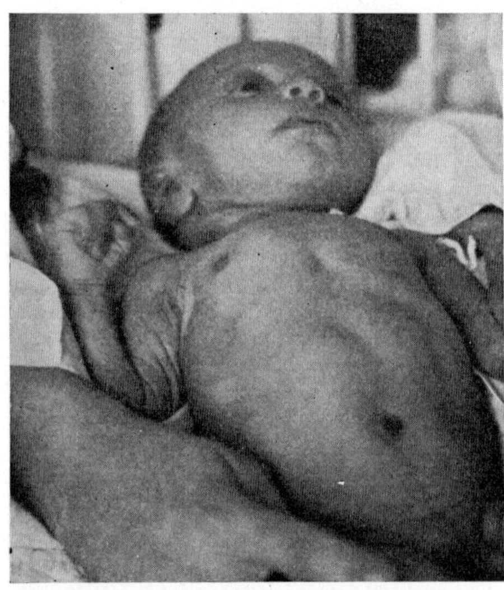

Fig. 131.—Well-marked gastric peristalsis in pyloric stenosis. Ansell G.; aged two months on entering Children's Hospital of Philadelphia, Nov. 3. Constipation, projectile vomiting, steady loss of weight and very marked gastric peristalsis. No tumor felt. Fredet-Rammstedt operation done Nov. 4. Recovery.

side at the costal margin, and pass toward the pylorus, one or two being visible at a time, and suggesting the rolling of two large balls under the abdominal wall (Fig. 131). In the examination it is best to have the light coming from the left and not too bright, the observer situated to the right of the infant with his eyes on the level with the abdomen. *Pain* sometimes seems to follow the ingestion of food, but is not produced by the peristaltic waves. A movable *pyloric tumor* may be felt in many cases slightly to the right of the middle line, under the edge of the liver, or often lower and toward the umbilicus. It is about the size of a small nut and oftenest found when the stomach is empty or the patient under light anesthesia. Some clinicians claim to feel it more readily when the stomach is full. *Fever* develops only with dehydration or complications. The *urine* may be concentrated from lack of sufficient fluid intake. An *alkalosis* may occur from the loss of chloride due to vomiting (Maizels, McArthur and Payne[62]).

Course and Prognosis.—The chances for recovery without operation are better in those cases in which the symptoms develop late, the recovery indicating that spasm was the chief element in producing symptoms. The mortality from the older type of operation, which was usually a gastroenterostomy but sometimes divulsion or pyloroplasty, was often as high as 50 per cent (Ibrahim[43]). With the newer methods (see p. 564) it is less (Richter[63] 13.6 per cent; Strauss[64] 4.6 per cent; Sauer[65] 12 per cent; Tisdall, Poole and Brown[66] 13.2 per cent; Rammstedt[67] 22.5 per cent). In cases treated medically Ibrahim found a mortality of 36.5, Sauer 8.9, Monrad[68] 4.4 per cent after certain hopeless cases were excluded; and Rammstedt 16 per cent. All statistics are to a certain extent misleading, since it is the more serious type of case which is operated on, and the operative mortality depends upon the condition of the patient at the time, which is often bad on account of the delay.

Heidenhain and Gruber[69] attribute certain gastric disturbances in adults to the occurrence of pyloric stenosis in infancy. Ackman[70] related the instance of a man of seventy-two years who had digestive difficulties since infancy, and at whose necropsy pyloric stenosis was found; and Crohn[71] a somewhat similar case in a woman of forty-five. Our experience has been the usual one, well demonstrated by the follow-up studies of Monrad,[68] that once the infant has recovered from the stenosis, whether by surgical or medical treatment, the prognosis is good for future health and for the continuance of gastric function and motility. This last has, too, been demonstrated roentgenologically by Veeder, Clopton and Mills.[72] Heubner,[73] Bendix,[74] and others have claimed that there is a tendency for the patients to develop neuropathic disturbances in childhood or later, but Reiche[75] and Liefmann[76] deny this. If such a predisposition exists it would seem to be a part of the underlying nervous imbalance which several writers assume to be present. Months may pass in those treated medically before the pyloric tumor and the gastric peristalsis disappear, although the vomiting ceases much earlier.

Diagnosis.—The chief characteristic symptoms are the early development; the obstinate, forcible, expulsive vomiting without sufficient digestive disturbance to account for it; the gastric peristalsis; constipation; and, if discovered, the pyloric tumor. Very rarely congenital atresia of the pylorus exists and cannot be distinguished from stenosis except by the completeness of the symptoms and their immediate development. Stricture of the duodenum gives rise to projectile vomiting beginning shortly after birth, but if the constriction is below the ampulla of Vater, the vomitus contains bile. Confusion may arise when the pyloric end of the stomach is constricted from without, as by congenital adhesions or through pressure by the cecum (Toporski[77]); or there may be an hour-glass stomach as in a case reported by Variot,[78] and as we have seen in one instance. All these conditions are rare, and some of them may be diagnosed by roentgenograms. Hoffa[79] in a number of cases found visible gastric peristalsis without any reason to suspect stenosis. It is possible that in these cases peristalsis was really colonic rather than gastric, since the two may readily be confused. In stenosis of the esophagus the food is usually regurgitated almost immediately and unchanged in character, and there is no gastric peristalsis. Greatly delayed emptying of the stomach may be demonstrated by roentgenography after the addition of barium to the food. (See p. 153.) This procedure is not, however, absolutely conclusive and is often unnecessary since the delay can be determined equally well and more conveniently with the stomach tube.

The distinction between cases with a large element of spasm and those with great organic hypertrophy is made chiefly by the more marked symptoms of obstruction in the latter, the earlier beginning, and the less rapid response to medical treatment. These differences, however, while applying to the classes in general, are too varying and uncertain to be of much diagnostic service in the individual case.

Treatment.—In most cases a trial of medical treatment should be made. This consists in efforts to stop the vomiting, the prescribing of the proper food, and the combating of dehydration. The stomach may be lavaged once or twice a day with salt solution or 1 per cent bicarbonate of soda solution, if this does not prove too exhausting. Atropine is of great value, particularly in those cases with a large element of spasm. It has been recommended by many clinicians, and large doses employed, especially by Haas.[47] It should be in *fresh* solution five large drops (approximately 5 minims) (0.31) of which contain $\frac{1}{1000}$ of a grain (0.000065) of atropine. Beginning with $\frac{1}{1000}$ grain three to five times a day, the dosage should be increased rapidly until flushing of the skin and dilatation of the pupils appear and the dosage then slightly decreased. Tolerance soon develops and the amount must then be increased, and usually remarkably large doses may be reached. Fever may sometimes be produced by it. When the frequency of vomiting makes retention doubtful the drug should be given in smaller doses hypodermically. Knöpfelmacher,[80] Bókay,[81] and others have had good results with papaverine hydrochloride. Eckstein[82] used sedatives such as adalin, narkophin and noktal.

Breast-feeding should not be discontinued, although it may be necessary to supplement it. In artificially fed infants human milk should be obtained when digestive disturbance is a complicating factor. The best substitute food is that of a thick nature, as recommended by Birk,[83] Sauer,[84] Moll,[85] Porter,[86] and others. This is more difficult to vomit. A gruel containing 5 to 10 per cent of rice-flour, farina, arrowroot, or other amylaceous substance may be employed, cooked in a double boiler for at least an hour, and made at first with one part of skimmed milk, and later whole milk, and three parts of water; the proportion of the water being rapidly diminished. The amount of food given at any one time should be small, and the intervals short or long as trial shows to be the best; three hour intervals often being satisfactory. Feedings may be given after lavage, and immediate refeeding practised after vomiting. In some cases the mixture need be only sufficiently thick to flow through a large hole in a nipple, in others so thick that it must be fed far back in the mouth with a spoon or wooden tongue-depressor. When dehydration is present small rectal injections of normal salt solution should be given several times daily, or normal salt solution subcutaneously or intraperitoneally, or 5 per cent glucose subcutaneously. Transfusion is often indicated. These measures, too, are helpful before and after operation, except that intraperitoneal injections should not be given under these circumstances. We have seen no improvement following roentgen-ray exposure of the thymus gland as some authors have advocated.

After a fair trial of the methods mentioned without avail the question of operative interference arises. It need not be employed too soon, but it must certainly not be delayed until the infant has become too weak. We do not subscribe to the dictum that every infant should be operated upon as soon as the diagnosis is made. Every case must be a rule to itself. Usually, medical treatment may be tried for at most one or two weeks in infants in good condition, but if there is not prompt improvement or the infant is in poor condition operation should be done at once. The Fredet[87]-Rammstedt[88] operation of simple splitting of the hypertrophied musculature has given such good results that it is now the one almost universally employed. Modifications have been proposed by Strauss,[64] Downes,[89] and others. The older operations of gastro-enterostomy, divulsion, and pyloroplasty have been largely abandoned. Foramitti[90] has successfully incised the anterior gastric wall and introduced a dilator into the pylorus.

The feeding of water, or a solution of glucose or other sugar may be started a few hours after operation, and by six or eight hours diluted breast-milk, whey, boiled skimmed milk, or thick gruels may be used. At first only a few drams at a time should be allowed, given from a bottle or a dropper, but by forty-eight hours at least an ounce may be taken every three or four hours. In about a week nursing at the breast may be resumed cautiously. In the meantime dehydration must be prevented or combated by hypodermoclysis, and, if the malnutrition is severe, by small repeated transfusions. Vomiting is liable to continue for a few days. A semi-recumbent position of the infant in bed tends to prevent this, and, if not successful, lavage may be used. The vomiting generally soon ceases permanently.

CARDIOSPASM

Attention has been called to this condition by Freund,[91] Göppert,[92] Beck[93] and others. It may occur in new-born infants, or in those older (Birnberg,[94] Segar and Stoeffler[95]). Moersch[96] records 34 patients whose symptoms began under fourteen years of age. It is not as uncommon as has been supposed, and we have seen several cases. The principal **symptom** is the prompt vomiting after the first swallowing of food. This is attended by very characteristic actions, viz. regurgitation and repeated reswallowings; distinguished, however, from rumination in that there is no difficulty at all attending deglutition in the latter disease. The passage of a sound encounters resistance at the cardiac orifice of the stomach, and the obstruction to the passage of barium at this point can be determined by the roentgenogram. The entrance of food through a small catheter passed directly into the stomach is not followed by vomiting. In the few cases as yet reported the prognosis appears good. In the line of **treatment** a sound may be passed systematically, or a hydrostatic dilator used. Atropine may be employed in the same manner as for spasm of the pylorus (p. 564).

DILATATION OF THE STOMACH

Moderate dilatation of the stomach is frequent especially in infants. A degree of it sufficient to produce symptoms and demand special treatment is not common.

Etiology.—Dilatation of a *chronic* nature may follow a mechanical obstruction such as stenosis of the pylorus, but the most frequent cause is atony of the muscular walls dependent upon constitutional conditions, notably rickets, infantile atrophy, or decided malnutrition combined with constant overfeeding. This results in indigestion; decomposition and formation of gas, and the accumulation of this and distention of the stomach. It is encountered oftenest at the end of the first or in the second year. A condition of gastromegaly and chronic duodenal ileus is described by Miller and Gage.[97] There may be observed an *acute* dilatation of the stomach, and of the intestine as well, occurring sometimes in the course of respiratory disease or after abdominal operations; and very rarely a sudden and even fatal acute dilatation may develop in infants without any discoverable cause. The disease in this form has been reviewed by Lucas.[98]

Pathologic Anatomy.—The earliest changes are simple relaxation of the gastric walls, but this is followed in the chronic cases by atrophy of all the layers. The shape of the stomach becomes much altered, the greater curvature extending downward much farther than normal and the dilatation being most marked near the cardia. The gastric capacity is greatly increased. Gastroptosis may also be present, and generally, except in cases of pyloric stenosis, an accompanying dilatation and ptosis of the intestine.

Symptoms.—These are principally those of chronic gastric indigestion, (see p. 572) except that when vomiting occurs the amount ingested is often surprisingly large. On physical examination the gastric region is found distended and tympanitic, and sometimes the stomach can be clearly outlined by percussion. A succussion-sound may be elicited. There is delay in the emptying-time of the stomach.

Prognosis.—The outlook is unfavorable when the disease is due to pyloric stenosis, unless relieved by the treatment for this. When dependent upon other causes the prognosis is usually good, if dilatation is not excessive and the underlying factor such as rickets or indigestion removed, although recovery may be tedious. The development of gastric dilatation may constitute a dangerous complication of other diseases, especially pneumonia.

Diagnosis.—To distinguish between a distended colon and a dilated stomach the latter may be filled with water a few hours after a meal and the lower limit of percussion-dulness now sought for. If this nearly reaches the transverse umbilical line the organ is dilated. Roentgenographic examination may also be made.

Treatment.—Correction of the diet is essential. The food should be nutritious and unirritating; suitable to the age and the digestive power of the patient. It must be given frequently and only in small quantities, the amount of fluid especially being reduced in older children. When the appetite is inordinate, not sufficient food should be allowed to satisfy it. As the stomach grows smaller the excessive hunger will disappear. In general those articles of diet are to be avoided which tend to produce an accumulation of gas in the stomach. Systematic lavage daily is of value in cases where dilatation is decided. Every care must be taken to improve the general health by tonic and hygienic measures. Massage is of service, and the administration of strychnine is of value. In cases of acute dilatation the stomach-tube should be passed at once and a hypodermic injection of eserine given.

GASTRIC HEMORRHAGE

Etiology.—This is a symptom already referred to under melaena neonatorum (p. 220) and hemorrhagic disease of the new-born (p. 219). It may also occur in some forms of purpura; scurvy; hemophilia; certain diseases of the blood; cirrhosis of the liver; septicemia and various toxemias; icterus; rupture of the stomach; injury by a foreign body; and from varicose veins in Banti's disease (Wallgren,[99] Smith and Howard[100]).

Symptoms.—These consist solely in the vomiting of blood originating in the stomach. Hemorrhage at first supposed to arise there may come from the nose, mouth, lungs, or the fissured nipple of the mother, the blood having been swallowed and then vomited. Blood from the lungs is bright-red in color, coughed up rather than vomited, and frothy if expectorated directly without previous swallowing. If hemorrhage from the stomach is free, the blood may be bright-red; if it has taken place slowly or if it has been lying for some time in the stomach, it is dark-brown or black in color. The **prognosis** depends on the cause, and is often serious.

Treatment.—While this is of the cause, it is also symptomatic. The patient should be at absolute rest, an ice-bag placed over the epigastrium and small pieces of ice swallowed. Food is prohibited. An opiate hypodermically is of benefit by quieting peristalsis. Adrenalin may be given by mouth in small quantities of water, and gelatin internally is sometimes helpful. Fibrogen has been recommended for hypodermic administration. Whole blood may be given intramuscularly, and, if large amounts of blood have been lost, intravenously.

GASTRIC ULCER

Etiology.—This is an unusual condition in early life. Of reports and collected cases in childhood may be mentioned those of Stowell,[101] Jacobi,[102]

Lockwood,[103] Lee and Wells,[104] Proctor,[105] Sturtevant and Shapiro,[106] Butka,[107] and Loeber.[108] Butka reports a case of perforated ulcer in an infant of six days of age, and Lee and Wells one in which the perforation probably took place before birth. The primary round peptic ulcer is rare, occurring usually only in later childhood, and oftener in girls than in boys. Other causes for ulceration are melena, sepsis, acute and chronic gastritis, corrosive poisoning, and, very rarely, tuberculosis. The peptic ulcer is usually single, the others multiple.

Symptoms.—Sometimes the first indication of an ulcer is its perforation. In other cases there is vomiting of blood and its passage by bowel. There may be pain and tenderness in the epigastrium, or they are referred elsewhere and appendicitis or other intra-abdominal disease is suspected. Often the symptoms are atypical, simulating gastritis, or the lesion may be discovered only at necropsy. The **prognosis** varies with the cause and type and is often serious. The **treatment,** following that indicated for adults, consists in the employment of an unirritating diet, rest, alkalies, and sometimes belladonna. If hemorrhage occurs the treatment already described for this should be employed (p. 566). If it is uncontrollable or if perforation takes place operation is demanded.

RUMINATION

(Merycismus)

This affection is more common than supposed. In our experience close observation of infants believed to be vomiters has disclosed that not a few of them were ruminating. It appears to be analogous to rumination normally occurring in some mammals. Ylppö[109] considers it a nervous condition, its production perhaps aided by dilatation of the stomach and swallowing of air. It is more common in infants than in older children. The disease has also been studied by Aschenheim,[110] Bruning,[111] Schippers,[112] Grulee,[113] Riehn[114] and others.

The **symptoms** consist in a series of repeated regurgitations of small amounts of food taken, occurring some time after its ingestion. Each regurgitation lasts about fifteen to thirty seconds, and the whole attack continues for an hour or two. It may be observed after all or only some of the feedings. Some of the regurgitated food may be swallowed promptly, some may be lost from the mouth, and some may be held in the mouth or pharynx for a time. The return of food from the stomach is often preceded by peculiar chewing movements, with the tongue pushed forward within the oral cavity. Sometimes the procedure is started by the infant putting the fingers into the mouth. Both breast-fed and artificially fed infants are affected, and the nature of the food seems to possess little influence, although some infants will retain solid food, such as thick cereal, and ruminate liquids. Food is usually eagerly taken. The **prognosis** depends on the severity of the condition. Emaciation may be extreme, and in the more persistent types Grulee states that the mortality may be as high as 25 to 50 per cent. Other experiences have not been so unfavorable, Riehn, for instance, losing but 2 out of 17 cases. The **diagnosis** is usually made clear by the nature of the act, and the disorder is not likely to be confused with cardiospasm, pylorospasm or stricture of the esophagus, although it should be remembered that at times rumination is associated with these conditions. In **treatment** the effect of thickening the food with cereals may be tried. If the mouth is held firmly shut after feeding, regurgitation cannot occur. A bandage or cap fitted to the head, to which are attached tapes that can be tied tightly under the chin, may be found effective. This should be applied immediately after feeding and kept on for about two hours, and the procedure persisted in for several days until the habit is controlled. Jenny[115] succeeded in an obstinate case by Siegert's method of closing the cardia after each feeding by a rubber bag inflated through a stomach-tube. Ylppö has had good results by placing the infant upon the abdomen, and restraining the hands from being put into the mouth. The effect is probably partly due to the diversion of the infant's mind which the unaccustomed position produces, since anything which distracts the infant's attention may stop the ruminating for a time. The administration of the bromides appeared to be of service in a case reported by Lust.[116]

FOREIGN BODIES IN THE STOMACH

Foreign bodies may find their way into the stomach of infants and, less frequently, of older children. They may then be vomited, or may pass into the intestine and be voided. The **symptoms** are indefinite. There may be choking at the time of swallowing, possibly pain in the throat, or slight hemorrhage if the body is not smooth. When once in the stomach there are usually no symptoms whatever, although sometimes irritation may be set up by rough and sharp objects, and occasionally obstruction, inflammation, abscess, or perforation may result. Roentgenograms or the fluoroscope will establish the diagnosis except for nonopaque objects. While often passed from the stomach promptly, we have seen foreign bodies remain a week or two before entering the duodenum. In regard to **treatment,** two or three weeks may be allowed to elapse before removal is attempted if there are no symptoms, and especially if the fluoroscope shows the object to be movable. Almost all foreign bodies will eventually pass the pylorus, even if of larger size than its diameter. Once in the intestine, progress to the rectum is almost always uneventful, taking forty-eight hours to a week or more. Aid may be needed to effect passage of the object through the anus. Purgatives and emetics should not be given, but such substances as potato, bread, and cereals may possibly coat the object, and protect the mucous membrane. If interference is indicated, removal with a gastroscope may be accomplished under the fluoroscope. If this fails operation may be necessary.

The **hair-ball** is a special form of foreign body which occurs in children in the habit of chewing hair from the head, fur, wool from blankets, cotton, and the like. When the amount swallowed is not large it may be passed into the intestine and promptly voided; but in some cases it is retained in the stomach and, by continuance of the habit and accumulation, reach such a size that it forms a tumor recognizable by palpation and giving a soft, crackling sensation to the fingers. A rather characteristic roentgenogram may be secured. The symptoms are indefinite and consist at the most of indigestion and gastric distress. Small amounts of the material may occasionally be found in the stool.

MALFORMATIONS, MALPOSITIONS AND NEOPLASMS OF THE STOMACH

Malformations, with the exception of pyloric stenosis, are of great rarity. **Malpositions** are occasionally seen. The stomach may occupy the right side of the abdomen in cases of transposition of the viscera, or may be found partially within the thoracic cavity in diaphragmatic hernia or eventration of the diaphragm. Through the presence of adhesions it may retain the more vertical prenatal position. It may remain of very small size, with thickened walls; a case with a capacity at necropsy of 4 cc. being reported by Piana.[117] It may exhibit complete closure at either orifice, or may be partially divided into two portions by a constricting wall (*hour-glass stomach*). **Morbid growths,** too, are very uncommon in early life. Even tuberculosis and syphilis of the stomach are rare. Osler and McCrae[118] collected 6 reported cases of cancer under the age of ten years. Sarcoma and lymphadenoma are even less often seen. Other instances of morbid growths have since been reported. **Rupture** may take place from injury or from obstruction situated lower in the intestinal canal (Seegar and Schulz[119]).

ACUTE GASTRIC INDIGESTION

This must be distinguished pathologically from acute gastritis, in which there is more than a functional disturbance. Among the **etiologic factors** is the ingestion of unsuitable or too large a quantity of food. In breast-fed infants the condition of the mother, as, for instance, after emotional excitement, sometimes produces milk which causes indigestion. Nervous influences, as fatigue, excitement, and unusually hot weather are operative on the child. Acute gastric indigestion is also often a part of the symptomatology of severe febrile disturbances and infections, there being then a lowering of gastric secretion and motility. **Symptoms** come about from the disturbed function, the food lying too long in the stomach and undergoing abnormal changes. Nausea and pain are complained of by older children, and in those younger these are shown by pallor of the entire face or around the region of the mouth, and by perspiration of the forehead. Vomiting then occurs and gives temporary relief. The vomitus in infancy is sour and there are often curdy masses present; in older children it is sour and may contain undigested food taken several hours previously. A single act of vomiting may empty the stomach, but oftener it is repeated several times. There are often fever, coated tongue, offensive breath, thirst, prostration, perhaps headache, constipation or diarrhea; less commonly convulsions, somnolence, or even coma. Between attacks of vomiting there may be hunger or complete anorexia. The **prognosis** is good, the acute symptoms disappearing in a few hours or a day or two. Death, however, may take place in weakly subjects, or the disease may be followed by more serious digestive disturbances. The **diagnosis** from *acute gastritis* is usually impossible at the beginning. In this disease the course is generally longer and more severe, and the vomitus contains more mucus and may be blood-streaked. Sometimes the question is settled only at necropsy. When vomiting accompanies the onset of *acute febrile diseases*, as pneumonia, grippe, or meningitis, the other symptoms of these disorders will soon develop. In **treatment** the first indication is to empty the stomach and bowels by the administration of a purge. Castor oil is excellent, unless there is too active nausea and vomiting. Calomel in divided doses is often of service. No food should be given, but there is no objection to small pieces of ice or to water, since, if vomited, this washes out the stomach. Lavage and emetics are effective but usually not needed. If vomiting continues repeated doses of bismuth subcarbonate and soda bicarbonate (5 grains (0.32)) may be given, or to infants teaspoonful doses of equal parts of lime-water and cinnamon-water. The application of a hot-water bag or a mustard-plaster to the epigastrium is useful. Return to food should be made cautiously in nursing infants with diluted or skimmed breast-milk; in artificially fed infants with albumen-water, barley-water, or boiled skimmed milk. In older children, because of the hypochlorhydria usually present, foods of low buffer value such as cereals and vegetables are often better tolerated than milk, eggs, and meats. If there are repeated attacks of acute indigestion the diet should be carefully studied to determine the fault.

ACUTE GASTRITIS

This differs from acute gastric indigestion in the presence of distinct organic alterations. It is of much less frequent occurrence and, when present, is usually combined with lesions of other parts of the gastro-enteric tract. Many cases supposed to be gastritis exhibit at necropsy none of its lesions.

Etiology.—The disease can be divided into: (*a*) the *acute catarrhal*, (*b*) the *corrosive*, and (*c*) the *pseudomembranous* forms. The causes in the catarrhal variety are much the same as in acute gastric indigestion, and the disease is more common in infancy than later. In addition to the disturbance of function there is inflammation added, probably dependent upon an infection. The hemorrhagic erosions (*ulcerative gastritis*) sometimes found, may occasionally be produced likewise by sepsis of the new-born, or accompany thrush or intestinal ulceration. In corrosive gastritis the cause is the introduction of an irritant poison. Pseudomembranous gastritis is rare, although much oftener seen in children than in adults. It is usually dependent upon the germ of diphtheria, less frequently on some other germ; and may occur in smallpox, scarlet fever and other infectious diseases, or in sepsis in the new-born.

Pathologic Anatomy.—(*a*) In *catarrhal gastritis* the mucous membrane is swollen, injected, and covered with an abundant, thick layer of mucus, often with a brownish stain from slight hemorrhage. Microscopical examination shows round-celled infiltration of the mucosa and sometimes of the submucosa. There may be localized disintegration of the superficial epithelium, or, rarely, the production of erosions. (*b*) In *corrosive gastritis* when death has occurred promptly, there are found only the evidences of destruction of the gastric walls. If the destructive action has been less intense and life has continued longer the lesions of acute gastritis are present. (*c*) *Pseudomembranous gastritis* exhibits a greyish-green membrane on a part or all of the lining of the stomach, consisting of desquamated epithelium, bacteria, granular matter, and fibrin, and there is an extensive round-celled infiltration of the mucosa and even of the layers beneath.

Symptoms. (*a*) **Catarrhal Gastritis.**—The symptoms at first cannot be distinguished from those of acute gastric indigestion (p. 569), but the vomiting, instead of disappearing, continues even when no food is taken; the ejected matter containing mucus, sometimes blood-streaked. Abdominal discomfort or pain persists, the tongue remains coated, and the breath is heavy. Fever continues, although lower, with great thirst and loss of appetite. Constipation usually gives place to diarrhea, and there is more complete prostration than occurs with mere indigestion. The only evidence of the occurrence of erosion is a greater tendency to bleeding. In older children the pain and vomiting are decided features, but the prostration and fever are generally less. (*b*) **Corrosive Gastritis.**—The symptoms are acute and severe, with accompanying evidence of lesions of the mouth, pharynx, and esophagus. Vomiting occurs immediately, the vomited matter being blood-stained. If death does not quickly result, there develop the symptoms of acute catarrhal gastritis and enteritis in a severe form. (*c*) **Pseudomembranous Gastritis.**—This condition has no characteristics by which it can be distinguished during life. The symptoms may be those of acute catarrhal gastritis or there may be few evidences of disorder of the stomach.

Course and Prognosis.—The symptoms of *catarrhal gastritis* are most severe at the onset. Their duration is a few days to a week, but they may be followed by intestinal symptoms. Recovery usually results. In infancy an initial convulsion or the prostration may cause death. Unless properly treated there is great danger, too, of relapse, or of the occurrence of repeated attacks with a final development of a chronic gastritis. In *corrosive gastritis* the prognosis is grave. Collapse is liable to result promptly and death to follow in a few hours after the ingestion of the poison; or life may be prolonged for a time, but death occur in two to three days from prostration. Older children may survive and later show evidences of chronic gastritis or of lesions elsewhere in the gastro-enteric tract. The prognosis of *pseudomembranous* gastritis is very unfavorable.

Diagnosis.—Milder cases of *catarrhal gastritis* cannot be differentiated with certainty from gastric indigestion, except by the persistence of symptoms. The subacute cases strongly resemble typhoid fever, but are to be distinguished in most instances by the more irregular temperature, which has a tendency to diminish after the onset instead of increasing. The more severe instances suggest the onset of pneumonia, meningitis, or scarlet fever, but can be recognized by the failure in a short time of any of the characteristic symptoms of these to develop. *Corrosive gastritis* is marked by the extremely sudden and severe onset, collapse, the evidences of corrosion about the mouth, and the history of the ingestion of an irritant substance.

Treatment.—The treatment of *catarrhal gastritis* does not differ from that of acute gastric indigestion (see p. 569). The return to food should be even more cautiously attempted than in the milder disease. The treatment of *corrosive gastritis* consists in the immediate administration of the proper antidote if the case is seen early enough. (See Poisoning, p. 508.) After this follows the administration of ice; ice-water; cold demulcent fluids, such as albumen-water and solution of gum arabic; oils; and the like. Prostration is to be overcome by cardiac stimulants hypodermically, or whiskey given by the rectum, and pain and repeated vomiting by the hypodermic use of morphine.

CHRONIC GASTRITIS—CHRONIC GASTRIC INDIGESTION

Gastric indigestion frequently repeated or long-continued will finally produce distinct lesions. Consequently no sharp clinical distinction can be made between the functional and the organic chronic disease. There is usually present also a combination, or even a predominance, of intestinal disturbance (*Gastro-enteritis*) (p. 583).

Etiology.—This disease, more common in infants than in older children, is the result of a single severe attack, or of a series of recurrences, of acute gastric indigestion, or of acute gastritis from which complete recovery had not been made; or it may develop without any previous acute condition. In infancy it may depend upon a food constantly too rich in some ingredient, especially fat, or a diet of other substances than milk entirely unsuitable for the age. Predisposing factors are rickets, tuberculosis, syphilis, or other chronic diseased condition affecting the general nutrition. In older children the continued giving of food of an improper character is probably the most frequent cause; but other factors are hurried eating with imperfect mastication; eating at irregular times, especially between meals; and imperfect hygiene of any sort, including lack of exercise and sleep, over-fatigue, and undue stimulation of the emotions. Chronic gastritis may follow also an acute infectious disorder, or may attend a chronic debilitating disease. There occurs, too, an inherited predisposition, and the presence of a neurotic temperament is often an important factor.

Pathologic Anatomy.—The stomach is somewhat dilated and the mucous membrane is covered with a tenacious layer of mucus; exhibits prominent rugae; is thickened and is greyish in color; or may exhibit hyperemia in spots combined with punctiform hemorrhages. Small hemorrhagic or other erosions may be seen in severe cases, and occasionally more distinct ulcerations. Microscopically there is a round-celled infiltration of the mucosa, with compression and partial destruction of the gastric tubules. The blood-vessels of the mucous and submucous layers are congested, and there may be thickening of the entire wall of the stomach in severe, long-continued cases.

Symptoms.—The symptoms in infancy are somewhat similar to those of acute gastric indigestion, although less severe; but not infrequently the onset is insidious, marked by loss of appetite, coated tongue, occasional nausea and vomiting, and failure of health. Eventually the vomiting becomes the most striking symptom. This may occur promptly after each taking of nourishment, or less often only at longer intervals, the food then being vomited in small amounts and this repeated until the stomach is empty. Often the vomited matter consists only of a very acid, watery liquid, while the solid portion of the food is retained. In long-continued cases with actual inflammation the vomiting of mucus is a prominent feature. The breath has an offensive, sour odor, and eructation of gas of the same character is common. The bowels are usually constipated; sometimes diarrheal. The stomach is often greatly distended by gas, resulting in pain and tenderness, restlessness, fretfulness, disturbed sleep, and difficulty in taking food even though the child be hungry. The appetite may be very large, but is usually much diminished. Examination reveals the distended tympanitic gastric region, and sometimes a constant gastric dilatation. (See p. 565.) The employment of the stomach-tube shows the presence of decomposed food with mucus and many bacteria hours after the organ ought to have been empty. There is nearly always undue acidity, chiefly from the fermentative changes, the hydrochloric acid being generally below normal.

The symptoms described may be nearly continuous, or there may be temporary improvement in which the appetite returns and vomiting is less, to be followed by recrudescences with evidences of acute gastritis. Meantime the health gradually deteriorates, anemia develops, and there is failure to gain or even loss of weight.

In **older children** the symptoms are much the same, except that vomiting is not so frequent, the so-called "stomach cough" is a prominent feature, and frequently headache, debility, disturbed sleep, and similar constitutional symptoms are more pronounced than those evidently gastric in nature. Constipation is the rule.

Course and Prognosis.—The disease in *infancy* is a serious one, particularly if it has been of long duration. Recovery, however, usually takes place under treatment, especially if this is instituted early. Unfavorable factors are bottle-feeding as opposed to breast-feeding, hot weather, and poor hygienic surroundings. The younger the infant the less chance it has. The course is always tedious and relapses are very prone to occur, and there is a predisposition to diarrheal disorders, rachitis, and infantile atrophy. In *older children* the prognosis is more favorable, but the course is liable to be long-continued, and the tendency to relapse may last for years.

Diagnosis.—This is usually easy, if the history of the case is known. In infants the onset of tuberculous *meningitis* is sometimes marked only by vomiting, and confusion may arise until its characteristic symptoms develop. *Stenosis of the pylorus* may readily simulate a chronic gastritis. This is particularly the case when the obstruction has not been absolute, the disease has continued some time, and gastric dilatation has developed. The active gastric peristalsis and the usual prompt and violent projectile vomiting after taking food characterize stenosis, especially early in the case. The combination of emaciation and cough may suggest *tuberculosis* in older children.

Treatment. Infants.—Treatment must vary with the individual case. *Prophylaxis* is much easier than cure, and, on the first warning of danger, as through the repeated development of gastric disturbance, most careful search must be made for the cause, which is oftenest a dietetic one; and this removed before the condition becomes established. Overfeeding is more common than underfeeding, either too great a total amount of food being given, or one too rich in some particular. In many cases the diet is one entirely unsuited to the infant in question, however fitting it may have proved for others. The effort so often made to feed children by a fixed rule is a fertile source of chronic digestive disorder.

With the *disease already established* the whole past dietetic history must be reviewed. Perhaps most frequently the fault will be an excess of or an intolerance for fat. In such cases benefit may often be obtained by giving a fat-poor mixture, using skimmed milk as a basis. In other cases, although much less frequently, the protein occasions difficulty. In this event, peptonizing may be of service, or the administration of casein-free milk in the form of whey. Whey is, indeed, an invaluable remedy in many instances, but is too weak a food for long continuance. Often a diet with high protein-percentage and diminished fat-percentage is serviceable, as obtained by the use of some of the numerous "protein-milks," or "casein-milks" (p. 108). Buttermilk or other lactic acid fat-poor milk is a valuable remedy in such instances, being a food in which the fat is low and the protein in high percentage, already coagulated and broken up into a fine flocculent state. The addition of a cereal and sugar, as commonly advised (p. 105), increases its caloric value. In some instances certain sugars agree better than others, only trial demonstrating which to select. Many cases show entire intolerance for milk for a time, and in these the food may temporarily be albumen-water or a cereal decoction such as barley-water. As this is not sufficient to sustain life indefinitely, a plan often useful is to fortify it after a time by the addition of whey made from skimmed milk, and later by peptonized skimmed milk in small amounts gradually increased. In other cases a cereal decoction may be partially dextrinized, and to this milk be finally added in increasing amounts. Malt-soup (p. 113) is often useful in such instances. In still other cases the fault is an excess of starchy food, and the chief dietetic treatment consists in the decided reduction of the amount given.

It is usually of benefit in beginning treatment to make a radical change from the food which had been given. Whatever diet may be selected, the first effort must be to bring about a cessation of the vomiting, but without striving for a gain of weight. Merely to stop the loss is all that is required for a while. After a time, however, a gradual return to a stronger diet is imperative. The effort should be made to return to a milk-modification containing fat as soon as this can be done with safety.

Some infants do better on small amounts of more concentrated nourishment; others on larger quantities more diluted. As a rule the interval should be long, but only trial will show whether feeding frequently at short intervals and in small amounts may not be better. In some cases food given by gavage will be retained when that taken in the ordinary way is not. In such instances it should usually be in larger amount, sometimes with advantage peptonized, and administered perhaps but three times daily. At times the anorexia is so great that gavage must be used to sustain life. In the line of diet there is often nothing so good for young infants with chronic gastritis as the employment of a wet-nurse.

In addition to the correction of diet, lavage is a most useful remedial measure to rid the stomach of mucus. This should be performed two or three hours after a feeding, once or sometimes twice daily; later less frequently, using a normal salt-solution or a 1 per cent solution of bicarbonate of soda. Sometimes it is of benefit to give food by gavage while the tube is still in position after gastric washing; in other cases better results are obtained by giving no nourishment for two hours after the washing has been performed. Mere feebleness is not a contra-indication to lavage; but in any infant in whom it produces severe nausea, vomiting, prostration, or cyanosis, it should be employed with great caution or abandoned.

The administration of drugs plays a secondary part in the treatment of chronic gastritis. Bismuth is sometimes useful in controlling the vomiting, and occasionally it may well be combined with minute doses of calomel, or with benzoate or bicarbonate of soda. In other instances a mixture of soda, bismuth and spearmint-water is of value in neutralizing acidity and dislodging accumulated gas. Tincture of nux vomica may be administered with soda in cases where there is great loss of appetite. Occasionally dilute hydrochloric acid with pepsin is of service, particularly where examination of the gastric contents shows diminution of the gastric secretion. Tincture of ginger or other aromatic may relieve pain, by causing displacement of gas. Constipation must be overcome by laxatives, especially citrate or milk of magnesia. Among other measures are the maintenance of the body-temperature, if below normal; the exposure to abundant fresh air out of doors or in a sun-parlor; massage; bodily rest; careful handling after feeding, and the avoidance of all excitement.

Older Children.—Prophylaxis here also is important. In the treatment of the disease itself, not only is the diet to be carefully regulated, but late hours, undue mental excitement or strain, bodily fatigue, too long school-hours, lack of fresh air and exercise, and other possible etiologic factors must necessarily be corrected in order to obtain benefit, since so much of the chronic indigestion is of functional origin. Change of climate is often of great benefit. Rest recumbent for an hour daily is of service and, in addition, rest for fifteen minutes before and after each meal. No food should be allowed between meals, and the diet should be plain and digestible, all highly seasoned dishes, fried foods, pastry, puddings, cakes, and sweetmeats being avoided. As a rule, but a limited amount of carbohydrate should be allowed. The diet should consist largely of lean meats; milk not too rich, or preferably buttermilk or other fermented milk; small amounts of toast or zwieback; and later green vegetables carefully tried in small amounts. The increase of carbohydrate vegetables should be made slowly and cautiously until recovery is well advanced. In other cases, because of the diminished gastric acid, low-buffer foods such as cereals and vegetables are better tolerated than meats, milk and eggs. Thorough mastication is important. In severe cases a diet purely of milk, modified in some way and often with the fat largely removed, may be required for a time, while in others milk may need to be withdrawn entirely. Medicinal treatment is similar in many respects to that for infants, and the tonic remedies recommended for anorexia (p. 559) may also often be given with advantage. Constant care for the general hygiene and the diet is required often for years, in order to avoid the great tendency to relapse.

References

1. Des Kindes Ernährung, Ernährungstörungen und Ernährungstherapie, 1906, 2. 2. Feer, Lehrbuch der Kinderh., 1914, 223. 3. Am. J. Dis. Child., 1911, **2**, 422. 4. Arch. Pediat., 1910, **27**, 579. 5. Arch. Pediat., 1909, **26**, 801; Am. J. Dis. Child., 1914, **8**, 163. 6. Feer, Lehrbuch f. Kinderh., 1922, 230. 7. Arch. Pediat., 1929, **46**, 391. 8. Am. J. Dis. Child., 1915, **9**, 261. 9. Précis. d. travaux de la soc. méd. de Dijon, 1838–1841; Ref. Northrup in Grancher and Comby, Traite d. mal. de l'enfance, 1904, **2**, 191. 10. Arch. de méd. d. enf., 1921, **24**, 73. 11. J.A.M.A., 1924, **82**, 1858. 12. Am. J. Dis. Child., 1924, **28**, 447. 13. Am. J. Dis. Child., 1926, **31**, 651; 1929, **38**, 746. 14. Am. J. Dis. Child., 1924, 28, 553. 15. Acta paediat., 1929, **9**, suppl. 1, 1. 16. Am. J. Dis. Child., 1912, **3**, 209. 17. Lancet, 1911, **2**, 8. 18. J. Biol. Chem., 1911, **10**, 265. 19. J. Biol. Chem., 1912, **11**, 253. 20. Am. J. Dis. Child., 1914, **8**, 127. 21. Arch. Pediat., 1921, **38**, 505. 22. Ann. de méd. et de chir. inf., 1905, **9**, 150. 23. Arch. de méd. d. enf., 1905, **8**, 741. 24. Am. J. M. Sc., 1904, 128, 966. 25. Am. J. Dis. Child., 1920, **20**, 168. 26. Arch. Pediat., 1922, **39**, 512. 27. Arch. Pediat., 1924, **41**, 595. 28. Griffith, Tr. Ass. Am. Phys., 1900, **15**, 16; Am. J. M. Sc., 1900, **120**, 553. 29. Arch.

Pediat., 1808, **15**, 607. 30. J.A.M.A., 1922, **79**, 184. 31. Jahrb. f. Kinderh., 1925, **109**, 7. 32. New York M. J., 1921, **114**, 226. 33. J.A.M.A., 1922, **79**, 1814. 34. Am. J. Dis. Child., 1931, **42**, 767. 35. Am. J. Dis. Child., 1931, **41**, 249. 36. Arch. Pediat., 1907, **24**, 801. 37. Griffith, Arch. Pediat., 1908, **25**, 321. 38. Cases and Observations by the Med. Soc. of New Haven County in the State of Connecticut, 1788; republ. by Osler, Arch. Pediat., 1903, **20**, 355. 39. An Acct. of the Dis. Most Incident to Children, 1877, 42. 40. London and Edinburgh Month. J. of Med. Sc., 1841, 23. 41. Caspar's Wchnschr. f. die gesam. Heilk., 1842, 105. 42. Inaug. Dissert. Freiburg, 1879. 43. München. med. Wchnschr., 1910, **57**, 1154. 44. Am. J. Dis. Child., 1919, **15**, 351; 1927, **33**, 294. 45. Scott. M. and S. J., 1897, **1**, 511. 46. Arch. f. Kinderh. 1907, **45**, 96. 47. Arch. Pediat., 1919, **36**, 385; J.A.M.A., 1922, **79**, 1314. 48. Am. J. Dis. Child., 1923, **26**, 91. 49. J.A.M.A., 1930, **94**, 1119. 50. Lancet, 1919, **2**, 513. 51. Brit. M. J., 1921, **2**, 891. 52. Bull. Johns Hopkins Hosp., 1922, **33**, 159. 53. Am. J. Dis. Child., 1929, **38**, 741. 54. Arch. Pediat., 1929, **46**, 416. 55. Am. J. Dis. Child., 1922, **24**, 306. 56. Am. J. Dis. Child., 1926, **32**, 706. 57. Arch. f. Kinderh., 1928, **85**, 93. 58. Am. J. Dis. Child., 1924, **27**, 608. 59. J.A.M.A., 1917, **68**, 1517. 60. J.A.M.A., 1918, **70**, 1913. 61. Berl. klin. Wchnschr., 1899, **36**, 703. 62. Lancet, 1930, **1**, 286. 63. J.A.M.A., 1914, **62**, 353. 64. J.A.M.A., 1918, **71**, 807. 65. Arch. Pediat., 1924, **41**, 145. 66. Am. J. Dis. Child., 1927, **34**, 180. 67. Deutsche med. Wchnschr., 1930, **56**, 348. 68. Monatschr. f. Kinderh., 1927, **37**, 473. 69. Deutsche Ztschr. f. Chir., 1923, **179**, 330. 70. Canad. M. A. J., 1929, **41**, 423. 71. J.A.M.A., 1928, **90**, 197. 72. Am. J. Dis. Child., 1922, **24**, 405. 73. Therap. d. Gegenwart., 1906, N. F. **8**, 433. 74. Med. Klinik., 1909, **5**, 1813. 75. Ztschr. f. Kinderh., Orig., 1919, **21**, 67. 76. Monatschr. f. Kinderh., Orig., 1914, **12**, 714. 77. Jahrb. f. Kinderh., 1910, **72**, 285. 78. Bull. et mém. soc. méd. d. hôp., 1921, **45**, 1454. 79. Monatschr. f. Kinderh., Orig., 1912, **10**, 523. 80. München. med. Wchnschr., 1914, **61**, 284. 81. Jahrb. f. Kinderh., 1921, **94**, 233. 82. Arch. f. Kinderh., 1928, **84**, 314. 83. Dis. of Inf. Trans. by Schultz, 1916, 242. 84. Arch. Pediat., 1918, **35**, 385. 85. Ztschr. f. Kinderh., Orig., 1919, **22**, 147. 86. Arch. Pediat., 1919, **36**, 385. 87. Rev. de chir., 1908, **37**, 208. 88. Med. Klinik., 1912, **8**, 1702. 89. J.A.M.A., 1920, **75**, 228. 90. Jahrb. f. Kinderh., 1929, **124**, 127. 91. Monatschr. f. Kinderh., 1903, **2**, 15. 92. Therap. Monatshefte, 1908, **22**, 390. 93. Monatschr. f. Kinderh., Orig., 1911, **9**, 555. 94. Am. J. Dis. Child., 1929, **38**, 1183. 95. Am. J. Dis. Child., 1930, **39**, 354. 96. Am. J. Dis. Child., 1929, **38**, 294. 97. Arch. Dis. Childh., 1930, **5**, 83. 98. Arch. Pediat., 1909, **26**, 454. 99. Acta paediat., 1927, **6**, Suppl. 1. 100. Am. J. Dis. Child., 1927, **34**, 585. 101. Med. Rec., 1905, **68**, 52. 102. New York M. J., 1909, **90**, 837. 103. Surg. Gynec. and Obst., 1914, **19**, 462. 104. Ann. Surg., 1923, **78**, 36. 105. Surg., Gynec. and Obst., 1925, **41**, 63. 106. Arch. Int. Med., 1926, **38**, 41. 107. J.A.M.A., 1927, **89**, 198. 108. Arch. Pediat., 1929, **46**, 578. 109. Therap. Halbsmonatsh., 1920, **34**, 76. 110. Ztschr. f. Kinderh., Orig., 1913, **8**, 161. 111. Arch. f. Kinderh., 1913, **60**, 116. 112. Nederl. Tijdschr. v. Geneesk., 1914, **1**, 785. 113. Am. J. Dis. Child., 1917, **14**, 210. 114. Monatschr. f. Kinderh., 1921, **22**, 257. 115. Klin. Wchnschr., 1924, **3**, 1915. 116. Monatschr. f. Kinderh., Orig., 1911–12, **10**, 316. 117. Clin. Pediat., 1930, **12**, 431. 118. New York M. J., 1900, **71**, 581. 119. Am. J. Dis. Child., 1930, **40**, 334.

CHAPTER VI

DISEASES OF THE STOMACH AND INTESTINES (*Continued*)

TYMPANITES

Distention of the stomach and intestine with gas may attend diverse conditions, and may become the symptom demanding urgent treatment. It is prominent in chronic intestinal indigestion, acute peritonitis, and sometimes in appendicitis, and is frequently present in typhoid fever and tuberculous peritonitis. In pneumonia it is sometimes excessive and a serious symptom, rachitis is constantly accompanied by it, and in congenital dilatation of the colon the degree of distention is characteristic and remarkable.

The **treatment** is that of the cause, but must often primarily be symptomatic. For this purpose may be employed such measures as turpentine stupes; intestinal douching; the use of the rectal tube, which may be allowed to remain in place for some hours; the administration of carminatives and of asafedita; and in urgent cases the hypodermic injection of eserine, which, because of its depressing action, should be combined with strychnine. We have found pituitrin less effective than eserine, and some clinicians believe it to be contra-indicated. Opium, although it relieves the pain, should be given cautiously, since it tends to increase distention by diminishing peristalsis.

INTESTINAL COLIC

(Enteralgia)

This important symptom consists, in the narrower sense, in the occurrence of intestinal pain in *paroxysms*, depending sometimes on distention, oftener upon a spasmodic contraction of the muscular wall of the intestine perhaps due to a vagotonia. The paroxysmal nature distinguishes it from the more persistent pain accompanying inflammatory conditions or certain nervous disorders, which is to be included under the broader title of *enteralgia*.

Etiology.—Among the causes a common one is swallowing of air by the infant. Any form of intestinal indigestion results in an accumulation of gas. This is observed in the first three or four months of life with especial frequency, and in breast-fed as well as bottle-fed infants, even when the breast-milk seems to be normal and well-digested. Starch if given in great excess is a fertile source of pain in the bottle-fed, although any element of the diet may at times produce it. In older children colic may attend indigestion from the eating of unripe fruit or other unsuitable substances. Many cases of colic appear to have a reflex nervous origin, such, for example, as chilling of the body-surface. Certain poisons, as lead or arsenic, produce intestinal pain, as do frequently also purgative drugs. Peritonitis, enteritis, appendicitis, intussusception, and any condition causing tympanites may cause enteralgia.

Symptoms.—In enteralgia the chief symptom is abdominal pain and in true colic this is paroxysmal. Frequently, especially in the breast-fed, the infant is healthy and thriving except for the colic. The attack begins more or less suddenly; the cry is very loud and unceasing; the face is congested and often somewhat cyanotic, or with pallor about the mouth; the abdomen is distended and tense; the legs are now drawn up upon the abdomen, now momentarily extended; the feet are often cold; the hands are clenched and the arms flexed and drawn to the body. The paroxysm continues a variable time, sometimes several hours with complete or partial intermissions lasting for a few moments only. Finally with the expulsion of gas or feces the symptoms disappear completely and the infant falls asleep. If the colic has been prolonged prostration may follow. In many instances the symptoms are not nearly so severe and the baby is merely fretful and wakeful until relieved. In others with highly sensitive nervous systems convulsions may develop, these occurring usually only in spasmophilic infants.

The frequency of colic varies greatly. In many infants it is only occasional, but in others in the first few months of life it seems oftener present than absent, and is especially liable to occur in the night-time; with the result that the parents, as well as the infant, obtain almost no sleep. It is a noteworthy fact that whereas every one in attendance seems exhausted on the next day, the infant often appears none the worse for its experience.

Diagnosis.—Often the diagnosis is difficult if dependence must be placed entirely on a description given by the mother or nurse. Colic is especially to be distinguished from *hunger*. The cry of colic is generally sharper, more violent, and more paroxysmal; that of hunger more persistent and often more fretful. Frequently the infant with colic refuses food; in other cases it will take it well if the pain is not too severe, and may be temporarily relieved by it. Soon, however, the cry returns in full force, thus excluding the diagnosis of hunger. Continued failure of the infant to gain sufficient weight renders the diagnosis of hunger probable. *Earache* causes persistent screaming, and there is tenderness about the ear. The pain of *peritonitis* and *appendicitis* is to be distinguished from colic by the more continuous character and by other attendant symptoms, especially the tenderness on pressure. In colic gentle pressure is often a source of relief. The pain of intestinal colic is often difficult to differentiate from that of *gastralgia,* which, indeed, it may attend, or with which it may alternate. Older children refer the pain of gastralgia to the epigastrium. In infancy relief of pain by expulsion of gas from the rectum indicates that the disturbance was in the large intestine. Obviously in the differential diagnosis there should be ruled out all organic obstructions and inflammations, lead poisoning, intestinal parasites, and the like.

Treatment.—Among *preventive measures* are the holding of the infant erect after feeding to permit the eructation of swallowed air, and careful regulation of the diet. In nursing infants with colic who are otherwise thriving, breast-feeding should be continued, perhaps lengthening the intervals and shortening the time of nursings; especially since colic lessens greatly after the first four months of life. It is here particularly that one must be sure that it is really colic and not hunger which is at fault. Then, too, in many cases the type and quantity of food has little causative effect, the colic in these being of nervous origin, dependent rather on intestinal spasm than on indigestion. In fact a change from breast-feeding to bottle-feeding seldom is of benefit, and weaning may be more dangerous than is the colic. Sometimes it is helpful to supplement breast-feedings by thick cereal feedings, or to give these to bottle-fed infants. In the case of colicy infants who have been receiving an excess of starch, this must be reduced or omitted, and a high protein diet may be tried. Chilling of the body-surface should be avoided. A stool should be had daily, and it may be well to see that this is secured just before the colic is inclined to be at its worst, probably during the night; using an enema or suppository if necessary. A carminative such as sodamint, cinnamon-water, spearmint-water, peppermint-water, fennel-water, or tincture of ginger is often useful, given before feeding.

During the paroxysm a hot-water bag, mustard-plaster, turpentine-stupe, or spice-plaster may be placed on the abdomen. Rubbing the abdomen with the warm hand is often of service. A fairly large enema is one of the best measures, and the carminatives mentioned are also useful. Emulsum asafoetidae, 10 minims, (0.62) or spir. aether. comp. in about half this dose are among other drugs which may be employed. Small doses of chloral and the bromides, likewise, seem effective in relaxing the muscular spasm. In the worst cases it may be necessary to give a narcotic. Atropine acts almost specifically in those cases in which the infants are of the so-called "hypertonic" type with vagotonia.

UMBILICAL COLIC

This is a disorder first given this title apparently by Wertheimber, according to Knöpfelmacher and Bien.[1] It has also been discussed by Friedjung,[2] Moro,[3] Finkelstein,[4] Stern,[5] Timmer,[6] Hutchison[7] and others. We have encountered it not infrequently. It appears to be entirely of nervous origin, and in some cases may be regarded as a hysterical manifestation. Finkelstein considered it an enterospasm in a neuropathic individual. It is observed oftenest in female children from five to twelve years of age.

The **symptoms** consist in sudden attacks of abdominal pain in the region of the umbilicus. These come on without discoverable cause at any time of the day, or sometimes following moderate excitement; or in other cases are connected with a meal, and yet beginning so promptly, and while still at the table, that indigestion can hardly be considered, and it seems rather the nervous anticipation by the patient of the occurrence of pain which is at fault. The pain may be moderate, but in typical cases is severe and accompanied by drawing up of the thighs, pressure of the arms against the abdomen, crying and sometimes pallor. Vomiting is uncommon. Tenesmus may accompany the pain, but is evidently reflexly produced. The attacks may last only a few moments, or may, with intermissions, continue several hours. They may occur every day or with irregular periods of freedom. The whole condition may last for months or years.

The **diagnosis** is of the utmost importance, especially that from a chronic appendicitis. This disease, however, has usually been preceded at some time by an acute attack. Pain in the umbilical and right hypochondriac region is suggestive of umbilical colic, yet not necessarily so, since the pain of appendicitis may be situated here. Acute appendicitis exhibits fever, leukocytosis, vomiting and general symptoms which do not appear in umbilical colic. Umbilical colic may further be simulated by duodenal ulcer, inflammation of the stomach or intestines, tuberculous disease of the mesenteric or retroperitoneal glands, abdominal purpura, and the like. Careful study will usually exclude these. A case was reported by Landis and Gittings[8] which resembled umbilical colic, but which, on account of other attending symptoms, was ascribed by them to hyperactivity of the sympathetic nervous system (sympathicotonia).

The **treatment** is by suggestion. The most effective is change of surroundings, especially familial, since the discussion of symptoms which is constantly taking place in the presence of the child seems to perpetuate the symptoms. Of drugs, probably the best is atropine in sufficiently large dose. If the case is judged to be one of sympathicotonia, pilocarpine should be given.

THE FECES IN DIGESTIVE DISEASES

(See also pp. 26–29)

When there is gastro-intestinal disturbance it is important to examine all the stools evacuated in twenty-four hours, as otherwise wrong conclusions may be drawn. In older children the character of the abnormal stools varies with the food taken; meat-fiber, vegetable material, milk, and the like showing themselves in different degrees. Mucus may be in large amount in some forms of chronic intestinal indigestion and in colitis. The following description applies especially to the stools of infants:

The normal stool of the breast-fed infant is mustard-yellow in color, smooth, with no evidences of undigested food, and slightly acid. (See Fig. 8, p. 28.) In healthy artificially fed children the normal shade of color is often somewhat lighter, depending upon the amount of fat in the food; a high percentage of this producing a paler stool. At the most there may be small, scattered white masses of undigested fat. In older infants the yellow is somewhat deeper and the stools more salve-like in consistency.

Mucous Stools.—In cases where food has been withdrawn for a day or two, the stools consist of the thin mucoid secretion of the intestine stained a brownish tint (*starvation-stools*). After a purgative, especially castor oil, a large amount of mucus is passed in infancy, often wrongly supposed to have been present before the oil was administered. Mucus occurs readily, too, in many disturbances of the digestive tract in early life, and may indicate only a functional disturbance of the large intestine, or, if persistent, an inflammation. Undigested starch somewhat resembles mucus in appear-

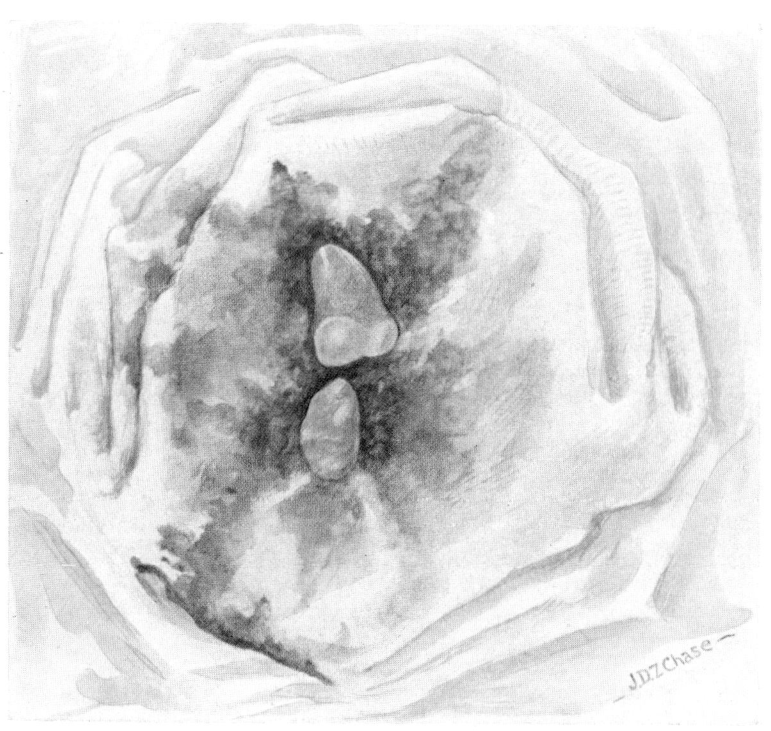

Fig. 132.—A hard protein-curd, broken into two portions.

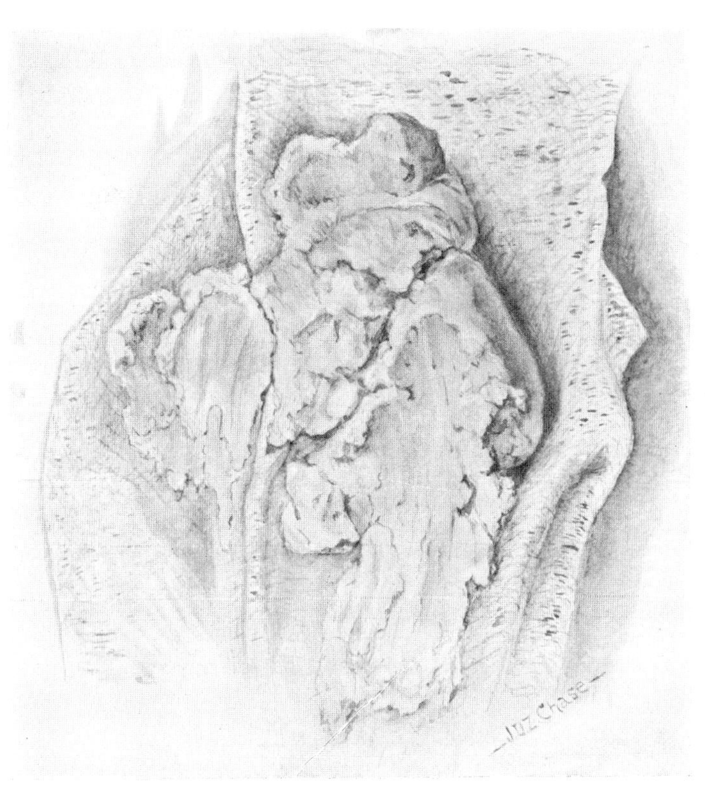

Fig. 133.—The soap-stool. Shows the white, salve-like character.

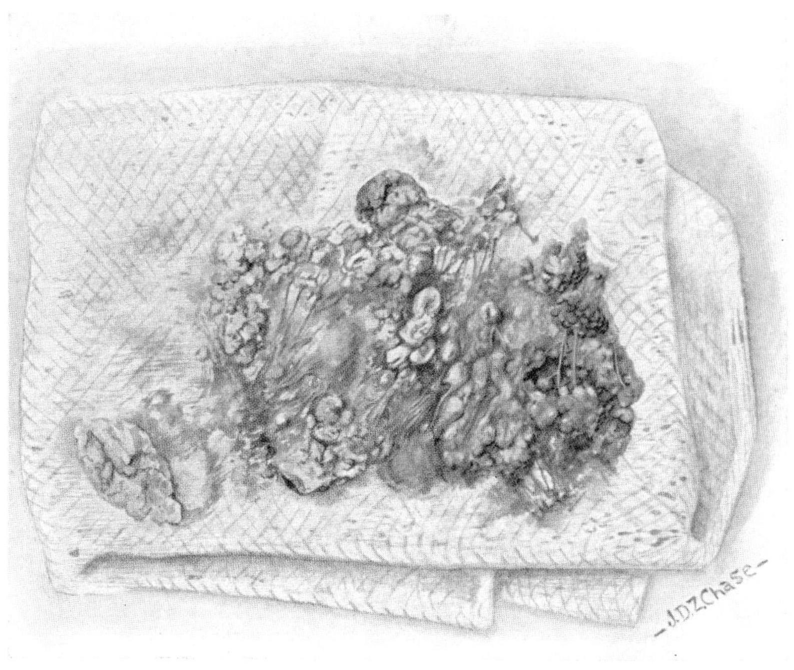

Fig. 134.—The curdy stool. Shows the white, fatty masses, with mucus of a pale-brownish tint.

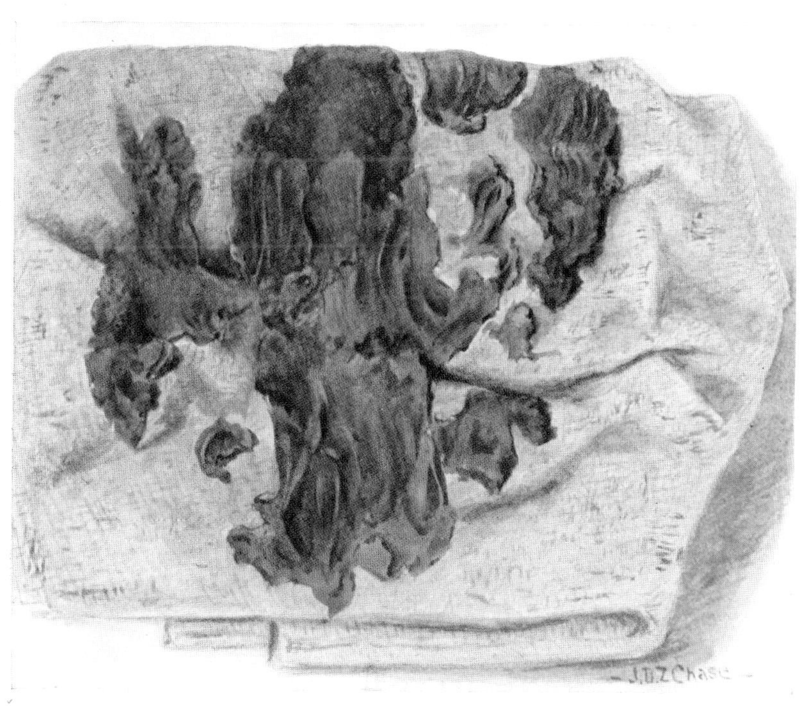

Fig. 135.—The carbohydrate-stool. Smooth, soft, homogeneous, brown mass. Infant fed on malt-soup.

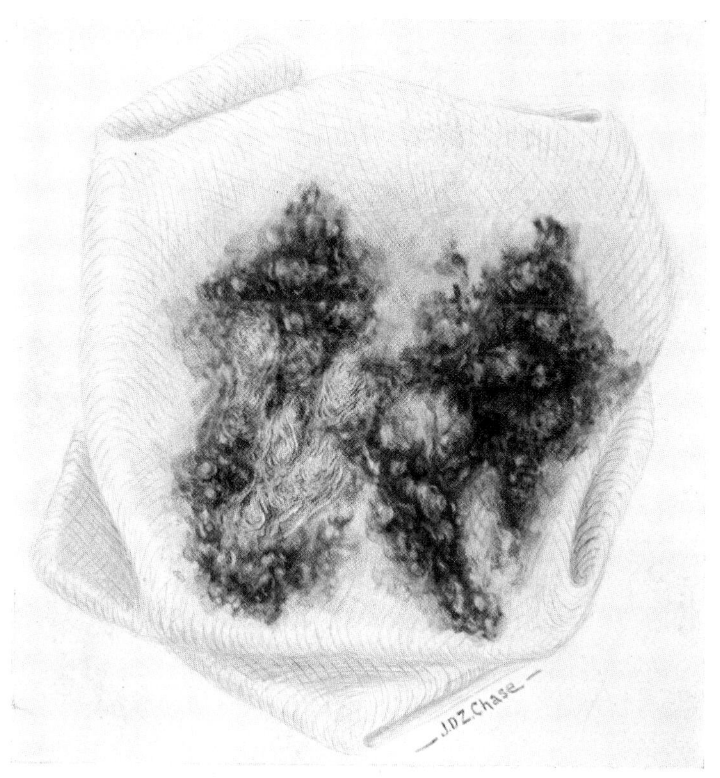

Fig. 136.—The spinach-green stool. With a few lumps of fat-curds and large amount of mucus, a portion of it blood-stained.

ance, but can be distinguished by the iodine reaction. Stools composed almost entirely of blood-stained mucus occur in dysenteric conditions and in intussusception.

PROTEIN-STOOLS.—These are seen especially in infants where the protein of the food is of high percentage and undigested. The odor of putrefaction is discoverable at times, combined with an alkaline reaction. The color is brownish-yellow or sometimes dirty-green, and mucus is always present. Sometimes tough, yellowish protein-curds are found when unboiled milk has been given (Fig. 132).

FAT STOOLS.—The *soap-stool* depends upon a large excess of fatty acids, combined with calcium or magnesium to form a soap. It is white or grey, shiny, fairly firm, homogeneous, crumbly or salve-like, of acid reaction, and has a rancid or sour odor (Fig. 133). It is commonly combined with more or less protein, and, if this is in large amount, the odor is cheesy and offensive from its decomposition, and the reaction may be alkaline. The *fatty stool* is bright-yellow, soft, looks greasy, and will produce a grease-spot if placed upon paper. It contains a large amount of neutral fat and fatty acids. The stools are thin, and may be frequent enough to constitute a fatty diarrhea. The *curdy stool* exhibits numerous large or small curds and is of an acid reaction. The curds are generally soft, white, and composed of fat. They are to be distinguished from the yellow curds consisting of protein material and already referred to. The stool as a whole, apart from the white lumps, is of a green or yellowish color and often diarrheal, and mucus is always present (Fig. 134). The occurrence of curdy stools, as also of soap-stools, is a matter of little clinical consequence unless symptoms of indigestion are present. The term *steatorrhea* is sometimes used to include all conditions, as pancreatic disease, obstruction to the entrance of bile into the intestinal tract, celiac disease, or obstruction to the lacteals, in which there is excess of fat in the stools. Cases of congenital steatorrhea have been reported by Garrod and Hurtley[9] and by Miller and Perkins.[10]

CARBOHYDRATE STOOLS.—Often the stool of this nature is of a normal consistence, homogeneous, smooth, and of a brown or yellowish-brown tint and acid reaction (Fig. 135). If starch has been administered in excess it may be found with the iodine test. In other cases there may be a decomposition of the carbohydrate in the intestine, producing, thin, frothy, acid stools, light yellow or often green in color. The odor is then sometimes that of acetic acid.

GREEN STOOLS.—These are of very common occurrence. The stool may be of a faint pea-green color when passed, or may become so shortly afterward. This probably depends upon unaltered biliverdin, and evacuations of this nature are not to be considered pathologic. In other cases the color is of a deep spinach-green, seen chiefly in the mucus passed in the stool (Fig. 136). In some cases this probably is the result of bacterial action. These green stools frequently have present the white curdy masses already described. Green, watery stools often occur in acute intestinal indigestion, both in breast-fed and artificially fed infants. They may depend upon an excess of either fat or of sugar.

BROWNISH STOOLS.—As stated, these are quite characteristic of many cases where food containing a high percentage of protein or of carbohydrate (Fig. 135) is given. Children fed on whey develop brownish stools, and the starvation-stools referred to (p. 578) have a similar tint.

BLOOD IN THE STOOLS.—This is not necessarily a serious matter. Any moderate congestion of the mucous membrane of the large intestine may develop streaks of blood upon the mucus passed (Fig. 136). Blood-streaks may depend, too, upon hemorrhoids or fissure of the anus, or upon the passage of a large constipated movement. Proctitis of any sort may cause it, especially the gonorrheal type. Combined with a considerable amount of mucus, blood is also seen in intussusception and in ileocolitis. If in large amount and coming from higher in the alimentary canal, the result of ulceration, purpura, or hemorrhage from other causes, the stools are colored a reddish-black. The condition is to be distinguished from the black stools following the administration of bismuth or iron. Occult blood in the stools of new-born infants who have no other evidences of hemorrhage is not uncommon (Bonar[11]).

Intestinal Sand.—Occasionally minute sand-like bodies are found in the stools, and these may be in considerable quantity. They may be visible when the passages are of a diarrheal nature, or discoverable only after washing and straining them from the fecal matter. In some instances the sand consists of the woody cells from the banana; in others it is of a crystalline nature, probably produced in the process of digestion. It is uncertain whether any symptoms are attendant upon its presence.

Micro-chemical Examination of the Stools.—Starch is detected by the application to the feces on a glass-slip of a little diluted Lugol's solution, which colors the granules blue. Sudan-3 stains neutral fat-droplets red, and carbolfuchsin colors fatty acids a brilliant red. The bacteriology of the stools is discussed elsewhere (p. 26). Zahorsky[12] believes that a large number of polymorphonuclear cells indicates an infectious process in the intestinal tract.

DIARRHEAL DISORDERS

While only a symptom, diarrhea is such an important one that its various causes and characteristics should be reviewed. Reference has already been made to the large part it plays in general mortality in early life (p. 173).

Etiology.—*Age* is a powerful factor, the great majority of serious cases being seen in the first two years of life; and although diarrhea is of frequent occurrence in childhood its consequences are less severe. *Season* is of importance, the incidence and mortality seeming often proportionate to the heat of the weather. For example, Wilkins[13] observed that of 628 infants in Baltimore kept under observation from June to November, 27 per cent developed simple diarrhea and 7.5 per cent ileocolitis. *Poor hygiene* and *debilitated health* are factors, and, as stated elsewhere (p. 172), *diet* has especial significance, the likelihood of death being much greater among artificially fed infants. Diarrhea is often an important, or a secondary, symptom of other *diseases*, especially the acute infections. It is frequently difficult to evaluate the factors involved, and to distinguish between diarrhea due to functional disturbance and that dependent on, or associated with, organic involvement of the gastro-enteric tract. The part played by bacteria may also be uncertain. The following classification may be employed as a matter of convenience; although the distinctions cannot be sharply drawn.

1. Diarrhea Due to Locally Acting Mechanical or Chemical Causes.—Among purely *mechanical* causes is the presence in the bowel of a large mass of undigested or of indigestible food, as unripe fruits, green corn, celery-stalks, fig-seeds, etc., which produce increased secretion and peristalsis by mechanical irritation. Some of them may act as *chemical* causes also, as may in infancy some of the food-elements of the milk, especially the fat. Too large doses of purgatives, likewise, start diarrhea chemically.

2. Toxic Diarrhea.—This depends upon the local influence of toxins produced endogenously by bacteria, or upon their action upon the intestinal contents. These toxins may also be absorbed and have a general constitutional effect.

3. Nervous Diarrhea.—Examples of this often encountered are cases due to chilling of the body, high external temperature, emotional excitement, fatigue, and the reflex action immediately following the ingestion of food.

4. Diarrhea of Acute Intestinal Indigestion.—This very frequent type may be the result of some of the causes already noted, and, like the other forms mentioned, is largely dependent upon a functional disturbance.

5. Metabolic Diarrhea.—This comes about through the efforts of the system to eliminate various endogenous poisons and toxins in the circulation, as those produced in uremia, acidosis, and the like.

6. Inflammatory Diarrhea.—Here the condition is the direct result of organic intestinal changes, and the irritation and disturbance of function which these occasion. It is usually caused by bacterial action, and is denominated *infectious;* this in contradistinction to *fermentative*, in which the bacteria apparently responsible act, not on the intestinal wall, but on the intestinal contents. Chemical irritation could also cause organic inflammatory diarrhea, and tuberculous enteritis may be placed in this category.

Symptoms and Treatment.—Diarrhea exhibits symptoms and requires treatment of a nature in accordance with the cause. That from local mechanical or chemical causes is attended by gastric disturbance, abdominal pain, and often fever. Unloading of the bowel by a freely acting purgative is required, as is the temporary withdrawal of food. When there has been decided irritation or much pain, opiates may be needed later. Diarrhea of nervous origin has few symptoms except the looseness of the bowels. It demands the removal of the cause in order to prevent recurrence of the attacks, and for the attack itself opium may be given promptly. On the other hand, in diarrheas of an eliminative nature no opium should be administered early, unless the condition is so severe that exhaustion is feared. Nature's efforts at elimination must not be interfered with. Cases of diarrhea of any sort, if at all severe, should be treated by rest in bed, since exercise tends to prolong the attack. Inasmuch as a large loss of the salts of the body occurs in severe diarrhea, hypodermoclysis or intraperitoneal injection of normal salt-solution is often of great value in supplying the needed sodium chloride and favoring the retention of liquid in the tissues. Certain forms of diarrheal disorders must receive separate consideration.

ACUTE INTESTINAL INDIGESTION

Here may be included those milder cases of digestive disorder dependent upon functional disturbance, in which the local symptoms generally predominate. The distinction between this and the gastro-enteric intoxication to be next described is one chiefly of degree, with intermediate forms. Acute intestinal indigestion is also quite commonly associated, especially in infancy, with acute gastric indigestion (p. 569), and it corresponds in many respects to the Dyspepsia of Finkelstein's classification (p. 551).

Etiology.—Among the principal causes in *infancy* are over-loading of the gastro-intestinal canal with too large an amount of food; the use of a diet unsuited to the patient; nervous or other conditions affecting the milk of the mother; and influences involving the digestive power of the infant, such as undue excitement, acute diseases, rachitis, and the like. The effect of hot summer-weather is especially noteworthy, and particularly so in artificially fed infants, not only through the alteration of the intestinal contents produced by bacterial growth, but through the direct prostrating effect of the high air-temperature upon the child's digestive powers. In *older children* are seen such causes as the ingestion of unripe fruits or indigestible vegetables; fatigue; acute illnesses; chilling of the skin; very hot weather; and similar causes temporarily inhibiting the digestive functions. Sometimes one article of food, as fish, shell-fish, and certain vegetables or fruits, always produces diarrhea in a certain child, perhaps through an allergic influence (p. 484). Bacteria appear to play a very minor rôle, so far as any direct effect upon the intestinal mucous membrane is concerned; although doubtless their action in altering the character of the food taken is of importance.

Pathologic Anatomy.—There are no lesions other than congestion of the mucous membrane and an increase of intestinal secretions.

Symptoms.—These are usually associated with gastric symptoms, and the attack is ushered in by vomiting of short duration. This is attended or followed by fever, which disappears usually within twenty-four to forty-eight hours, or sometimes longer (Fig. 137). There are intestinal pain, anorexia, restlessness, often abdominal distension, prostration, occasionally slight jaundice, and soon diarrhea. In *infancy* the stools may be green from unchanged biliverdin, have a sour or fetid odor, vary in number from a few larger to 15 or more smaller ones, are usually acid, may contain mucus but no blood, are watery and loose and sometimes frothy. In *older children* the stools may contain undigested food, often the particular article which caused the attack; later they are watery, of a yellowish or brownish color, and have an offensive odor.

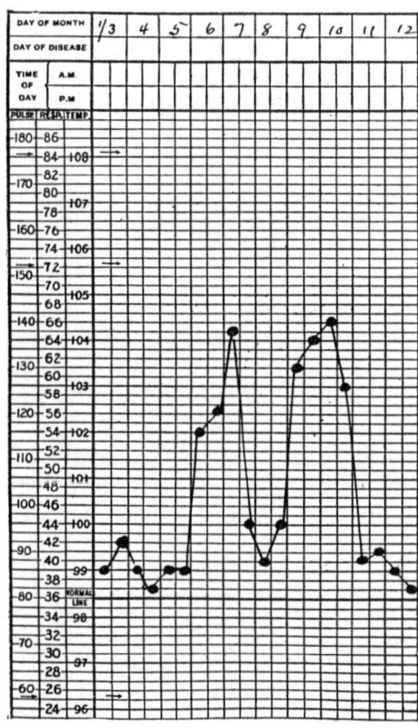

Fig. 137.—Acute gastro-enteric indigestion following change of food. Leonard F., aged ten months. Suffered from vomiting for some weeks. Admitted to Children's Ward of the Hospital of the University of Pennsylvania on Jan. 2, suffering from rickets; Jan. 6, had been doing well, but ceased to gain, change of diet on this date caused vomiting, liquid greenish movements and fever; Jan. 11, fever ceased; condition of stools had improved.

Course and Prognosis.—Under proper treatment the attack is usually over in a few days. When the disease affects infants during hot weather it may pass into gastro-enteric intoxication or ileocolitis. There is, too, a tendency for repeated attacks to occur.

Treatment.—The primary indications are to stop the food and to empty the bowels. In infancy thin barley-water or plain boiled water, perhaps slightly sweetened, should be given for twenty-four hours or more. Then stronger barley-decoctions, or albumen-water or well-skimmed broths may be allowed for another day or two; return to milk being made very gradually, using at first diluted and skimmed milk mixtures. In older children it is often advisable to remove milk from the diet for a few days, allowing only thin cereals, albumen-water, or broths thickened with barley and rice and perhaps well-cooked vegetables. Enemata may be employed if there is much abdominal distension or pain, but purges are required to empty the small intestine as well as the colon. Castor oil and calomel, the latter followed by a saline purge, are the best drugs if the stomach will tolerate them, or the citrate or milk of magnesia may be given alone. If diarrhea persists astringents, as bismuth, must be employed. (For further details see Treatment of Gastro-enteric Intoxication p. 587.)

ACUTE GASTRO-ENTERIC INTOXICATION AND INFECTION

(Summer-Diarrhea; Milk-poisoning, Infective Diarrhea; Acute Gastro-enteritis; Cholera Infantum; Food-intoxication; Alimentary Toxicosis or Intoxication)

This serious and common affection of early life, especially frequent in infancy, has been described under various names. There are no sharp etiologic or pathologic lines of distinction from acute intestinal indigestion (p. 581); the two disorders shading into each other. Clinically the distinction rests upon the greater severity of the local symptoms, and especially on the constitutional involvement.

Etiology.—The *predisposing causes* have been mentioned in discussing Diarrheal Disorders in general (p. 580) and also Acute Intestinal Indigestion (p. 581). Among them are defective hygiene; malnutrition or debilitated health from some acute or chronic illness, as rickets; artificial feeding; excessively hot weather; and increased humidity. These factors act in various ways;—illness, whether digestive or general, by decreasing digestive power; heat by favoring growth of bacteria in the food and also by affecting the gastro-intestinal secretions (Demuth, Edelstein and Putzig;[14] Arnold[15]). Aside from the possibility of bottle-feeding introducing the bacteria or producing digestive disturbance, the nature of its causative action is uncertain. A number of observations by Gerstley, Wang, and others[16] indicate that the indigestibility of cow's milk is not primarily responsible, but rather the effect of milk upon the general body-metabolism and nutrition of the body.

The *direct cause* is not the same in all instances. In some cases it would appear to be a toxin, this being produced either by the action of bacteria on the food before its ingestion; or by the action on it within the alimentary canal of bacteria normal to the tract, which, however, have increased in number and in virulence; or finally, to changes brought about on the food in the canal by bacteria foreign to it which have entered from without. In other cases the bacteria are parasitic and actually attack and invade the intestinal mucous membrane. In another group, as emphasized by Renaud,[17] Floyd,[18] Marriott,[19] Jeans and Floyd,[20] Alden,[21] and others, parenteral infection, often arising in the middle ear, nasal sinuses and mastoid, is responsible. While there is no doubt that this is true, it has been overstressed as we[22] have elsewhere indicated, and in some instances the otitis is undoubtedly secondary to, rather than primary and causative of, the enteritis. A further possibility of bacterial injury, as pointed out by Bessau and Bossert,[23] Moro[24] and others, has been summarized and elaborated by Davison,[25] who suggests the following sequence of events: (*a*) a primary undetermined and varying cause such as fever, overfeeding, etc. and (*b*), as a result of this, reduction in the activity of the duodenal enzymes. There is (*c*) consequent accumulation of undigested material in the duodenum followed (*d*) by invasion from the large intestine of bacilli of the colon-group and (*e*) resulting fermentation and formation of irritating end-products.

Without question micro-organisms such as the dysentery bacillus and the gas bacillus can infect the intestinal tract and cause gastro-enteritis. These produce ileocolitis and will be considered later (p. 590). Other germs which have been viewed as direct causative agents in intestinal intoxication are the streptococcus group, including the streptococcus gastro-enteriditis (Booker[26]); the colon group (Escherich[27]); the bacillus pyocyaneus; bacillus proteus vulgaris; bacillus mucosus capsulatus; and Morgan's bacillus. Organisms of the typhoid group have been isolated in some epidemics, but it is better to consider these as specific in type. Green-producing streptococci seemed quite certainly the pathogenic agents in two epidemics we have seen, and which were studied by Cooper. It is certain that no one germ is specific, and it is often difficult to evaluate what etiological relationship bacteria hold to diarrheal diseases. No one complex of symptoms is brought about by a single species of micro-organisms, and, conversely, one species is capable of producing different clinical manifestations. Furthermore, many of the micro-organisms which have been claimed to be causative may be found in the stools of normal infants (Ford, Blackfan and Batchelor;[28] Davison and Rosenthal[29]).

Pathologic Anatomy.—The changes are chiefly degenerative rather than inflammatory, and may affect the entire gastro-enteric tract. The stomach and small and large intestine are usually distended; the mucous membrane slightly thickened, anemic or congested in patches, and perhaps exhibiting slight hemorrhages. The solitary follicles and Peyer's patches are prominent and congested. Microscopically there is found degeneration of the cells of the mucosa, and in severer cases desquamation of epithelium in places, and perhaps round-celled infiltration. Bacteria may penetrate the intestinal wall where the epithelium has been lost. It is noteworthy how slight are the changes in the intestinal tract, especially macroscopically, as compared with the severity of the symptoms. Other organs such as the liver, kidneys and mesenteric glands may exhibit degenerative toxic changes.

Classification.—The disease may affect either the stomach or the intestines, or diverse symptoms connected with other parts of the body may assume especial importance. In general, however, cases may be divided into three classes, not sharply separated, and being only different clinical manifestations of the same disorder: (1) The ordinary type; (2) alimentary intoxication; (3) choleriform diarrhea.

1. THE ORDINARY TYPE.—The **symptoms** vary as the stomach or the intestine bears the brunt of the attack. In *infancy* they manifest themselves gradually after some evidences of indigestion, or quite suddenly with fever of 101 to 103 F. (38.3 C. to 39.4 C.) or sometimes higher, combined with colic and frequently vomiting. The nervous symptoms are early in developing and may consist only of restlessness; but not infrequently there is great prostration with unconsciousness or convulsions. There is loss of appetite; but sometimes great thirst causes liquid nourishment to be taken readily. The severity and persistence of vomiting vary greatly. The vomited matter is at first the food taken, and later even any water swallowed, or may consist of mucus or bile. Generally vomiting stops soon or becomes a minor symptom. Diarrhea develops, as a rule, within twenty-four hours. The movements are at first chiefly fecal, often with white curdy masses, and usually strongly acid in reaction; later liquid, of a greenish or pale-yellow color and of an offensive odor, and containing but small amounts of fecal matter. A large quantity of gas is often passed by the rectum. The stools vary from two or three to fifteen or twenty in twenty-four hours. They are often preceded by pain and expelled with force and straining, and with some mucus. The development of diarrhea is frequently attended by a diminution or subsidence of fever and an improvement in the nervous symptoms; but if the case continues and if the stools are large, wasting of the body rapidly takes place, the pulse is accelerated and weak, and the prostration is unchanged or grows worse. The urine is usually scanty and often contains albumin, and, in severe cases, casts.

In *older children* the onset is oftenest abrupt; vomiting may occur, but is less frequent than in infancy; and abdominal pain is a more prominent symptom. The nervous symptoms likewise are generally less marked and the temperature is not high. The stools are very offensive, liquid, and usually of a brownish color.

Course and Prognosis of the Ordinary Type.—In the more favorable cases, properly treated, the course is a week or two. Not infrequently, however, the fever lessens but does not disappear, the abnormal stools persist, and the attack assumes the subacute form, with difficulty distinguishable from the later stages of ileocolitis undergoing recovery; while sometimes the condition passes into an actual ileocolitis. In other severe cases the patient may never recover from the initial toxic stage, and death may occur in two or three days. In other instances the fever is moderate at first, but rises to hyperpyrexia just before a fatal termination. In general it may be said that the severity of the attack is not necessarily in proportion to the frequency of the stools. There is always danger that at any time mild instances of the disease may suddenly assume a very severe form and the patient fail rapidly, or that a patient apparently out of danger may experience a mild or severe relapse. The prognosis is, on the whole, favorable in older children, but in infants always uncertain. It is affected adversely by poor hygienic circumstances, previous ill-health, and especially the existence of hot weather. Breast-fed infants develop the disease less often and have a vastly better prognosis.

2. Alimentary Intoxication.—This corresponds to the fourth form of Finkelstein's classification (p. 551), although this might equally well apply to choleriform diarrhea. In older terminology the condition was designated "acute milk poisoning." The **cause** appears to be related to the food, since in favorable cases symptoms cease when the food is withdrawn. The degree of vomiting and especially of diarrhea may be slight, and by no means accounts for the severity of the condition. Furthermore symptoms develop so suddenly that dehydration could play but a minor rôle, and it might be suggested that they were due to a poison formed in the food before its ingestion. This hypothesis is, however, not necessary, since the same explanations may obtain as applies to the production of them in choleriform diarrhea. (See below.) In addition to prostration and collapse the **symptoms** are largely those of a nervous nature or dependent perhaps on acidosis, and consist of restlessness, delirium, hyperpnea, coma, or convulsions. Fever may or may not be present.

Course and Prognosis of Alimentary Intoxication.—In mild cases, seen early and promptly treated, recovery may follow; but in the severe cases the prognosis is unfavorable and death may take place in two or three days.

3. Choleriform Diarrhea.—This is not a common disease. In infants it is designated *cholera infantum;* in older children *cholera nostras,* the latter described by older writers under the title "cholera morbus." The symptom-complex to be detailed has many similarities to that of the acute alimentary intoxication as just described. Distinguishing characters, however, are the persistent uncontrollable vomiting, the profuse unyielding diarrhea, and the excessive dehydration upon which many of the later clinical manifestations depend.

Symptoms.—As a rule the attack is preceded by acute gastro-enteric intoxication of the ordinary type, after which the choleriform symptoms set in with great suddenness. The vomiting continues, and the diarrhea likewise. The vomitus becomes merely a greenish liquid. The stools are watery, of a greenish color, and finally almost colorless and odorless; very frequent and generally large; sometimes smaller and passed every few minutes. Extreme prostration, loss of weight, sinking and filminess of the eyes with ptosis of the lids, shriveling of the face, depression of the fontanelle, and pallor and wrinkling of the skin develop with an astonishing rapidity; all indicating the effects of dehydration. This is shown especially well in the skin, which, being the largest storage place for water with the exception of the muscles, readily loses it upon the general demand for fluid. The whole aspect of the face is completely changed in a few hours. The temperature is usually elevated and hyperpyrexia is common in fatal cases.

The pulse is weak and rapid; the respiration often irregular or the deep and sighing breathing of hyperpnea; the urine is nearly or quite suppressed, and may be albuminous and contain sugar; thirst is very great; the abdomen is shrunken; the tongue coated, or red and dry; and the lips of a bright-red hue. Often the body becomes cold and cyanotic as in the algid stage of Asiatic cholera, although the rectal temperature at the time may show an elevation of 106 F. (41.1 C.) or over. In other cases the rectal temperature is finally subnormal. Nervous symptoms are marked. At first there is usually irritability and restlessness; later there may be a state of apathy or stupor, or coma and convulsions may develop. Leukocytosis is present. In the *cholera nostras* of older children there develop very suddenly severe, almost constant vomiting, abdominal pain, and repeated diarrhea. The stools are nearly colorless, and may be extremely offensive. The temperature is elevated; the cerebral symptoms less marked than in infants, but the same wasting develops.

The symptoms which have just been described are those which may be seen to some degree in any severe diarrheal condition, and it is of practical importance from the viewpoint of treatment to understand the method of their production. Studies by Howland and Marriott,[30] Chapin and Pease,[31] Schloss and Stetson,[32] Schloss,[33] Marriott,[34] Schwartz and Kohn,[35] Mitchell and Jonas,[36] Darrow and Buckman,[37] Schiff, Bayer and Fukujama,[38] Hamilton, Kajdi and Meeker,[39] and others have shown that, when toxic symptoms are present in these dehydrated infants, or in experimental exsiccosis, there is a retention of the nonprotein nitrogen constituents of the blood, a diminution of plasma-volume, and an acidosis. It is believed that these conditions are due to the same cause, viz.: functional failure of the kidney dependent upon lack of water (oliguria), and as a result of this, in spite of the fact that there may be few renal lesions, the patient is practically in a state of uremia. The cause of this type of acidosis is discussed elsewhere (p. 489). In some cases there may be an alkalosis instead of an acidosis. It has been suggested that some of the symptoms may be caused by toxic bodies similar to histamin in nature, produced in the intestinal tract and absorbed. Although work along this line has been done by Mellanby,[40] Schloss,[41] Kohn,[42] Boyd,[43] and Röthler,[44] no positive proof in support of this hypothesis has as yet been given. Dodd, Minot and Casparis[45] have found a guanidine-like substance in the blood in a few cases and suggest that this might be the toxic substance.

Course and Prognosis of Choleriform Diarrhea.—The prognosis in cholera infantum is serious and probably the majority of patients die. The disease may last not over two to three days. In some instances the diarrhea and vomiting continue until death occurs in collapse. In others there may be an abatement or even a cessation of the gastro-enteric symptoms, but nervous manifestations with prostration may persist, and death may take place from convulsions or in coma. This is the condition described as "pseudomeningitis" or "hydrencephaloid." In the case of older children the prognosis is likewise serious but not to so great a degree.

Complications and Sequels of Acute Gastro-enteric Intoxication. In the ordinary type of the disease, if at all long-continued, complications may arise. Bronchopneumonia and otitis are common; furunculosis and multiple abscesses may develop. Urticaria and erythema are oftener seen in older children; forms of stomatitis are sometimes met with; and renal involvement is not infrequent. Sclerema is a complication reported in cholera infantum, but must be rare in this country. Ileocolitis is a not uncommon sequel.

Diagnosis.—*Acute intestinal indigestion* generally exhibits a lower temperature, a shorter course, and much less serious involvement of the nervous system. Often *ileocolitis* cannot be readily differentiated, especially as it is so frequently a sequel to gastro-enteric infection. It generally exhibits a greater amount of mucus in the stools, which are more numerous and smaller, may contain blood, and are passed with pain and frequent straining efforts; while the temperature continues elevated instead of falling in a few days. Only the course of the case can distinguish the symptomatic gastro-enteric manifestations which so frequently usher in various *acute febrile diseases*, and sometimes in the intestinal form of grippe the diagnosis may be difficult throughout. The differentiation from typhoid fever in infancy is at times uncertain. In most cases of acute gastro-intestinal intoxication, however, the course is shorter and the fever falls in a few days, and, in addition, the Widal reaction will be an aid. The nervous symptoms of the severer cases of gastro-enteric intoxication sometimes suggest *meningitis* at the outset. Usually the prompt development of diarrhea, uncommon in meningitis, makes the diagnosis plain. In older children *acute poisoning* by arsenic or similarly acting drugs could produce symptoms suggesting choleriform diarrhea.

Treatment of Acute Gastro-enteric Infection. **Prophylaxis.**—This is of extreme importance. Weaning must be discouraged, especially in summer-time, unless it has been proven beyond doubt that artificial food is necessary. The mother's nipples and the infant's mouth must be kept clean. (See pp. 53–65.) In the case of bottle-fed infants every precaution must be taken to preserve an aseptic condition of the bottles and nipples and of the food employed. (See pp. 101–103.) Great care must be taken, too, in starting an infant on artificial food to employ a weak mixture at first, and to increase the strength gradually. During periods of unusually torrid weather a temporary decided reduction of the strength and of the amount of the food is an excellent prophylactic measure. Abundant fluid must be given. The problem of the supply of proper food to bottle-fed infants among the poor in cities and the instruction of the mothers is a vital one. It is advisable to pasteurize or boil the milk during hot weather, since it is such a good culture-medium for bacteria. In the case of older children care must be taken that no indigestible food, such as unripe fruit, is allowed.

The sustaining of the digestive power of the patient by prompt removal from the city during hot weather is a matter of much importance. The infants of the poor should be sent for the day into the parks, to the seashore, or on the river if these are accessible. The infant should be bathed once a day or oftener. The clothes must be carefully adapted to the state of the weather. Chilling of the surface undoubtedly predisposes, but even to a greater extent does the use of too warm clothing in summer-time. Constant supervision of the children of the poor by district physicians and visiting nurses is of great value in the prevention or early recognition of digestive disorders.

Treatment of the Attack. *Diet.*—Dietetic treatment is by far the most important. On the first evidence of digestive disturbance food must be withheld. Water must be offered freely, since what may appear to be appetite for food is often only thirst. Infants at the breast are best given only water, thin barley-water, or strained broth for twenty-four hours, or even longer if severe symptoms persist. After this period nursing may be cautiously resumed, curtailing the duration of each nursing and perhaps alternating with thin barley-water or strained broth for twenty-four hours, or even longer if severe symptoms persist. Breast-milk is not an ideal food in diarrhea, since it is too high in carbohydrate and too low in protein. We have found it beneficial to augment breast-milk with casein-flour (0.5—1 to 20). In the case of bottle-fed infants the same methods should be followed, except that the return to a milk-food should be delayed longer. While albumen-water and broths may be ordered and are widely used and recommended for this stage, it often seems better to employ starchy foods, such as toast or dried bread, barley-water and other cereal decoctions. The chief consideration is an easily digested food of low caloric value, and when one kind of nourishment is refused some other may be tried. After several days, when symptoms have abated, return to milk may be tried, using diluted and boiled skimmed-milk, buttermilk or other acid-milks, or casein-milk. It is only in the case of infants already marantic that somewhat prolonged starvation may do harm. In any mixture fat and sugar must not be too high, although whey may agree in spite of its high sugar-content and radical difference in composition from the milks just mentioned. For older infants and for children the early avoidance of milk is advisable also, giving broths and gruels for a number of days. If the condition persists the dietetic methods advised for chronic gastric and intestinal indigestion may be employed (pp. 574–610). Recommended more particularly for older infants and children suffering from ileocolitis, but also applicable here, are the fruit-diets which will be discussed in more detail later. (See Ileocolitis, p. 594.) After recovery the tendency to relapse, especially in hot weather, makes it imperative to return to the ordinary diet cautiously; or, indeed, the diet may need curtailing until the cooler season.

Treatment based upon the nature of the bacteria present has been discussed elsewhere[46] and may be epitomized as follows: Two groups of bacteria occupy the intestinal tract, the acid-forming and the protein-splitting, and either may be causative or, at least, in excess. If the first is operative, the stools are highly acid, frequent, often green, and scald the buttocks. In such cases, after the preliminary starving, a high-protein food should be given, such as protein-milk, buttermilk, skimmed acidophilus milk, or boiled, skimmed milk. Both fat and carbohydrate should be avoided or kept low. If the protein-splitting (putrefactive) group of bacteria is predominant, the stools are brown, alkaline and offensive. In such cases the food should be high in carbohydrate, and the protein should be kept low; using, for instance, weak milk-mixtures with the addition of starch or lactose. This is from the theoretical side an entirely reasonable view, and based on these facts the selection of food should be simple; but experience shows that the chief factor in the treatment is the preliminary starvation, when this is not contraindicated, with a subsequent careful, gradual return to full diet; and that even when the stools are highly acid cereals may often be given successfully and acid-milks later if needed.

Hygiene.—The measures suggested for prophylaxis apply here as well. The child should be kept at rest in bed or in its coach, but not necessarily confined to the house except during the excessive heat of mid-day. Fresh air is needed, with light clothing if the weather is hot; chilling by cool draughts, however, being avoided. Against the action of hot weather, or if there is fever, repeated warm tub baths are often of service.

Medicinal and Local Treatment.—This is entirely symptomatic. If the case is seen early, a purgative should be administered. Castor oil is excellent, but only if vomiting has ceased. Calomel with soda is a serviceable remedy, giving $\frac{1}{10}$ grain (0.0065) of the former, with 1 grain (0.065) of the latter, hourly or half-hourly, to a child of six months until from five to ten doses have been taken. Milk of magnesia also is a valuable preparation, alone or following the calomel. For older children the solution of citrate of magnesia, 2 to 4 oz. (59 to 118) is useful. Irrigation of the colon with a normal salt-solution is also advisable in nearly every case in order to empty this part of the intestine promptly. Later it may be done once or twice a day but not continued too long, since it may cause moderate intestinal irritation. Cool irrigation, too, is often a useful means of reducing fever, if this is unduly high. When vomiting is persistent, lavage with a 1 per cent solution of bicarbonate of soda is of service. In place of this there may be given at least ½ dram (2) each of liquor calcis and aqua cinnamomi. In some cases of vomiting bismuth with bicarbonate of soda is of value. Should diarrhea persist to a moderate degree, not too great haste can be permitted in efforts to check it, especially if fever or nervous symptoms continue; since these may be a sign that there are irritating substances still present. Under such circumstances the administration of castor oil, magnesia, Rochelle salts, or other purgative once or twice daily for a few days is often of value.

After the general symptoms have disappeared a continuance of diarrhea may call for direct treatment. Bismuth subcarbonate or subgallate is now useful, 5 or 10 grains (0.32 or 0.65) being given every two hours to a child of a year or less. Kaolin or charcoal may be administered in doses of 15 grains (0.97) or more every two or three hours. These act mechanically by carrying with them large numbers of bacteria as they pass through the intestinal tract, and probably by their adsorptive properties also take up toxic bodies. Astringent remedies such as tannalbin, tannigen and similar preparations, or the older ones containing tannic acid, are to be reserved for cases which pass into a subacute stage, the result of the development of ileocolitis as a sequel. Opium is an invaluable remedy in some instances but a dangerous one in others. It must not be exhibited in the early stages when vomiting and nervous symptoms are present, or where there is reason to believe that the locking up of the bowels would be harmful. Later it is of great service when food and liquid are hurried on and out of the intestine, with consequent prostration and emaciation. Opium in proper dosage acts by increasing the tone of the gut. As a result distention, which is a stimulant to peristalsis, is decreased (Plant and Miller[47]). The dose to be employed varies with the case and the effects produced. (See p. 179.) Colic and distention may often be relieved by the application of spice-poultices or of stupes, or by the employment of a rectal tube or a small enema.

As measures to sustain strength are alcoholic stimulation; the administration of digitalis, caffeine, and camphor; and hot mustard-packs or baths when collapse threatens. Most helpful are small repeated injections or transfusions of blood, which should be employed before the patient is *in extremis*. When dehydration exists, and before it has reached any threatening degree, it must be combated vigorously by fluid administration. Fluids given by mouth may not be retained, but moderate vomiting should not discourage their trial in this manner. Clinically, fluid so introduced often appears to do more good than by parenteral administration, perhaps because it is better retained by the body-tissues and less liable to be lost by diuresis. Proctoclysis is an unsatisfactory method of administration, since diarrhea causes its expulsion; but large amounts of salt-solution may be given subcutaneously, intraperitoneally, or even intravenously in urgent cases. Continuous intravenous administration by a drip method has also been recommended. (For description of methods see Div. I, Chap. X.) Glucose may be employed in 5 per cent solution intravenously or by hypodermoclysis, and also orally or rectally. It seems hardly necessary to use insulin with it as is sometimes recommended. Choremis[48] claims that the isotonic glucose gives the most satisfactory results. The advisability of giving large amounts of sodium chloride has been questioned by Hartmann,[49] Hartmann and Elman,[50] and Schoenthal,[51] who state that the oliguria so often present may lead to an acidosis because of retained chloride. So-called "buffered" solutions are recommended by Hartmann and also by Cunningham and Darrow.[52] We agree with Schloss,[53] and Hoag and Marples[54] that normal salt-solution produces no harmful effects provided that the secretion of urine is established, as it usually is when large amounts of fluid are administered. Furthermore the newer solutions possess no great advantage over those of glucose.

The treatment of *acidosis* and its prevention is largely that by free administration of fluid. When acidosis has been determined by accurate laboratory study sodium bicarbonate may be administered in proper dosage. (See Acidosis, p. 490.) It must never be continued when the urine becomes alkaline, and it may do harm by the production of alkalosis.

Calcium gluconate injected intramuscularly has been recommended by Dodd, Minot and Casparis[45] in those cases in which there is increased guanidine in the blood.

ACUTE ILEOCOLITIS

(Enterocolitis; Follicular Enteritis; Dysentery; Inflammatory Diarrhea; Infectious Diarrhea)

The term "ileocolitis" properly designates a group of cases in all of which the element of inflammation is predominatingly present. There is, however, no sharp boundary line between this disease and acute gastro-enteric intoxication.

Etiology.—Numerous *predisposing factors* are of importance. Thus it is more common in children under two years of age; acute gastro-enteric intoxication has ileocolitis frequently following it; it develops readily in atrophic children the subject of chronic intestinal indigestion; it may be a sequel to acute febrile diseases, as measles, typhoid fever, pneumonia, and diphtheria; it is more frequent in hot weather; and unsatisfactory hygiene of any sort increases its incidence. Perhaps oftenest, however, it occurs as an acute primary disorder not preceded by any digestive or other disturbance. Epidemic influence is positive, especially in tropical countries, although it is more often seen sporadically. Its contagiousness is uncertain.

Ileocolitis is an infectious disease and the *exciting cause* is an organism of some sort. In tropical dysentery this may be the amoeba coli, so named by Lösch,[55] and this parasite may occasionally be encountered in children in the temperate zone. According to Kessel and Mason[56] it is the entamoeba histolytica which is the variety usually active, entamoeba coli and entamoeba nana being less prone to produce symptoms. The dysentery bacillus likewise may be causative and some writers would apply the term "dysentery" only to those cases in which this organism is found. It was first described by Shiga[57] in 1898, and shortly afterward, in 1900, Flexner[58] reported another strain. Since then a number of other strains have been isolated. Duval and Bassett[59] observed the Flexner strain in ileocolitis as well as in other diarrheal conditions in children. In the United States the Flexner type is more commonly causative than the Shiga, but either may occur alone or in combination with other types, such as that of Hiss and Russell.[60] The Sonne[61] type has been found in North America in children by Nelson,[62] and by Johnston and Brown.[63] In the collective investigation of the Rockefeller Institute[64] 412 infants with diarrheal disease were studied and the dysentery bacillus found in 279 cases, only 29 being of the Shiga type. This is quite similar to the experience of Davison.[65] Agglutinins for the dysentery bacillus may develop in the blood of patients with ileocolitis.

It should be emphasized that other organisms than the dysentery bacillus also may be responsible for ileocolitis and, in fact, that there seems to be a variation from year to year in those causative of diarrheal conditions in the same locality (Kendall[66]). In some cases streptococci are found in predominant numbers in the stools, and agglutinins may develop in the blood

(Jehle[67]). The bacillus aërogenes capsulatus has been observed at times and presumed to stand in a causative relationship, as have the bacillus mucosus capsulatus and the bacillus pyocyaneus; and it has been held by some that the colon bacillus may assume pathogenicity. Concerning the pathogenic properties of the Morgan bacillus[68] there is still dispute. (See also Chronic Ileocolitis p. 594.)

Pathologic Anatomy.—The basic character of the disease is *inflammation,* this distinguishing it from the diarrheal disorders already described. The large intestine is the most frequent seat, the lower part of the ileum being much less affected. Even where most abundantly developed the lesions are not uniformly distributed, parts of the intestine being greatly involved and neighboring parts much less. In the **acute catarrhal form** the mucous membrane is congested and swollen, often covered with mucus, and the epithelium loosened in places. Small hemorrhages, usually scattered or in streaks, are seen on the surface especially upon the projecting portion of the folds, and superficial erosions may be found; and in severe cases these shallow ulcerations may be extensive, and the whole intestinal wall may appear much thickened. Both the solitary and the agminated follicles are generally swollen and the villi are elongated and prominent. Microscopically there is found an infiltration of small cells and of very numerous bacteria of different kinds in the mucous layer, penetrating even to the muscular layer in severe and long-continued cases. The lymph-follicles are infiltrated. In cases which recover the lesions disappear entirely. If the diseased process has advanced further, **follicular ileocolitis** is also found. There is here a more or less deep ulceration in the solitary follicles, and a moderate infiltration and ulceration of the submucous and muscular layers. Cases which recover do so with cicatrization of the ulcers. In the most severe form of the disease a **membranous ileocolitis** develops. In this there are regions in which the entire thickness of the intestinal wall becomes much swollen and stiff, with an obliteration of the usual folds resulting from the presence of fibrinous exudate and infiltration by round cells; and where the membranous deposit has become detached deep ulceration may be seen. There is no certain relationship in ileocolitis between the severity of the symptoms and that of the lesions. Cases with extensive ulceration, for instance, may sometimes exhibit but moderate fever and little or no blood in the evacuations, while catarrhal inflammation, although usually milder than other forms, may continue for some weeks and end fatally without any follicular ulceration having developed.

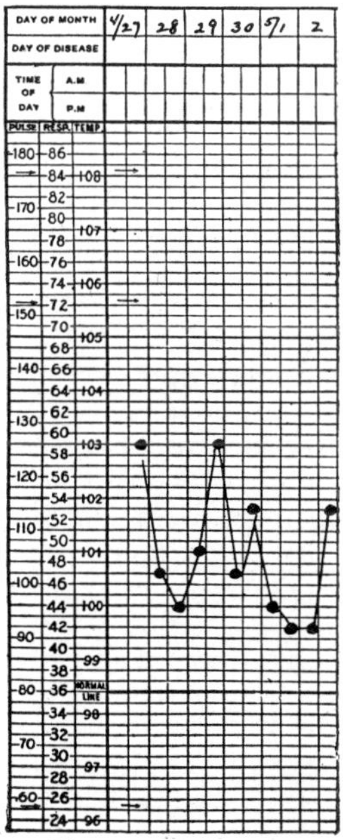

Fig. 138.—Acute ileocolitis of moderate severity. Mollie G., aged seven months. Bottle-fed. Apr. 27, been ill eleven days with mucus, blood and pus in the movements, very frequent, with straining, fever, prolapse of the rectum. Condition now apparently improving slowly. Temperature uncharacteristic.

Lesions of other regions are often observed, such as bronchopneumonia, swelling of the mesenteric glands, and degenerative changes in the kidneys, spleen, liver, and other organs.

Symptoms.—For the reasons pointed out a division of the disease into clinical types based upon pathologic and bacteriological findings is possible only to a limited extent. In an *average* case there may have been an earlier simple diarrhea or gastro-enteric intoxication, which gradually merged into or suddenly developed a condition of ileocolitis; or the disease may start abruptly as a primary affection, perhaps following an indiscretion in diet, with practically no prodromes. The onset cannot be distinguished with certainty from that of other acute intestinal disturbances. In the more acute cases there is fever of from 103 to 104 F. (39.4 to 40 C.); often vomiting, abdominal pain, and diarrheal movements containing undigested food. Promptly the stools become very frequent, small, are passed with straining efforts, and exhibit mucus either transparent or green in color, pus, fecal matter, and more or less blood. The abdomen becomes moderately distended and somewhat tender; the urine is scanty and may contain albumin. There are loss of appetite, coated tongue, thirst, decided prostration and rapid loss of weight. The tenesmus is not constant and the abdominal pain is colicky in nature; both symptoms developing or increasing at the time of evacuation of the bowels. Prolapse of the rectum is not uncommon. Cases may be *milder* than those in the condition described, with slower onset, symptoms less marked, and a larger amount of food in the stools. In *severer* forms the symptoms are exaggerated and there may be, in addition, various toxic manifestations, among them restlessness or apathy, great prostration, stupor, coma, or convulsions. The temperature in ileocolitis is very variable. (Fig. 138.) It is liable to rise rapidly in the primary and the severer cases and continue high; or to become less elevated than at the onset and more irregular in the milder cases; but this is open to numerous exceptions.

Course and Prognosis.—In very severe cases death may take place in from a few days to one or two weeks or longer, from exhaustion, a complicating pneumonia, or perhaps convulsions. In *catarrhal ileocolitis* of average severity the stools and intestinal symptoms may begin to improve after a week or two, the temperature gradually decline, and in four to six weeks recovery be complete. Relapses are, however, prone to occur. In *mild catarrhal* cases recovery may take place in two or three weeks. In *follicular ileocolitis* death usually results in three or four weeks, but in cases without extensive follicular ulceration recovery may take place after a tedious course of weeks and months, interspersed with frequent relapses. This form of the disease tends to run a more subacute course, the temperature after the onset not being very high, the stools not frequent, and tenesmus slight. The progressive emaciation is the worst feature.

In general the prognosis in ileocolitis is much graver if ulceration has developed. The clinical symptoms are of some value in determining this, and if there is no improvement in three or four weeks and blood still persists in the stools ulceration is probably present. The Shiga type of dysentery bacillus causes especially severe ileocolitis. Prognosis is also worse the younger the patient; with impaired health prior to the onset of the ileocolitis; under poor hygienic surroundings; in very hot weather; and with secondary cases as opposed to primary ones.

Complications and Sequels.—Bronchopneumonia is a frequent and serious complication, appearing generally late in the course of the case. Thrush or other forms of stomatitis may develop. Sepsis is a frequent and early cause of death in severe cases. Degenerative lesions of the kidneys are common. Purulent otitis, or furunculosis and other cutaneous suppurative conditions may occur. The most important sequel not infrequently following is a chronic ileocolitis. In other cases a persistent malnutrition may remain for months after the disease itself is over. Obstinate constipation is a not uncommon sequel.

Diagnosis.—The principal diagnostic symptoms of the disease are the tenesmus, abdominal pain and tenderness, fever, and frequent, small stools containing mucus and more or less blood. Bloody diarrhea should always lead to the suspicion of and the search for the dysentery bacillus. The mere discovery of the dysentery bacillus, ameba, or other micro-organisms or parasites in the stools is not, however, proof of their causative action. They may be found in other intestinal disturbances than ileocolitis, and even in normal children. The presence in the blood of agglutinins for the dysentery bacillus is of little value in diagnosis (Flexner[69]). As stated elsewhere (p. 579), blood in the stools without other characteristic symptoms of dysentery is no proof of the existence of this disease. When ileocolitis is preceded by *acute gastro-enteric infection* it is often impossible to determine at just what time the actual inflammation began, but the persistence of fever and pain and the constant occurrence of mucus and blood in the stools are suggestive of it. In *intussusception* there is more sudden onset without initial fever, complete lack of fecal matter in the stools, absence of the passage of gas from the bowels, more rapidly developing prostration, and the discovery of a tumor through the abdominal walls or by rectal palpation. *Typhoid fever* in infancy exhibits vague symptoms and often much resembles ileocolitis; and, indeed, the pathologic lesions are much the same. The onset in typhoid fever, however, is usually less abrupt and there is no tenesmus, while the Widal reaction and the roseola are characteristic. Some of the severer cases of ileocolitis with minor intestinal symptoms and marked cerebral ones may readily suggest *meningitis.* Although diarrhea of any degree is a contra-indication to the presence of this, yet this statement is by no means invariably true, and the diagnosis may be one of great uncertainty.

Treatment. Prophylaxis.—The same prophylactic measures are indicated as described under Acute Gastro-enteric Intoxication; namely, attention to general health, escape from excessively hot weather, guarding against indigestible or bacterially contaminated food, and the like. Any diarrheal disease present should be treated thoroughly and promptly. While the contagiousness of ileocolitis is uncertain, precautions must be taken against the possibility of its spread. There is a difference of opinion regarding the protective value of serum or vaccine. Wilkins and Wells[70] apparently secured some protection with a monovalent vaccine given hypodermically, but none by its oral administration although specific agglutinins were produced (Wilkins[71]). Flexner[72] stated that passive protection could be secured with dysentery-serum.

Treatment of the Attack. *Diet.*—Early in the attack milk should be withdrawn, even with breast-fed infants. There should be given fat-free broth and thin amylaceous decoctions, such as farina, rice, and arrowroot, frequently and in small amounts. Breast-feeding may be resumed in a day or two, but artificially fed infants should not receive milk until all acute symptoms have subsided. The strength of the food must now be gradually increased, giving cereal gruels, albumen-water, beef-juice, scraped beef, and broths, the last to be thickened with a starchy addition. Theoretically in cases due to the dysentery bacillus these protein foods should be given cautiously, since this organism is a protein-splitter. Practically, whatever the germ, it seems to be better to continue the cereal gruels, perhaps reinforced by lactose or dextrin-maltose sugars, for several days after the onset. If symptoms increase upon return to milk this must at once be withdrawn. Whey, skimmed and perhaps peptonized milk, and the acid milks, as buttermilk, acidophilus milk and the like, are often of value; trial determining which is best. Great wasting may result from the anorexia and the nourishment must not be too low in caloric value. There must be careful supervision of the diet perhaps for months, or relapses will be brought about. Particularly to be avoided are foods with much residue, as some of the cereals and green vegetables and the coarser fruits. Mention may be made here of certain special diets recommended for ileocolitis and other diarrheal conditions. Moro[73] uses for two or three days in children past the nursling age a diet consisting only of completely ripe, peeled, cored, and grated apples. From 500 to 1500 Gm. (17.5 to 52.5 oz.) are given daily. The caloric value of this diet is fairly high, and it is claimed that the apple-pulp is nonirritating, adsorbent, contains tannic acid, and, according to Schreiber,[74] favorably changes the intestinal flora. We have had some success with this dietetic measure. Fanconi[75] gives at first only fruit-juices or banana-pulp, then apples also after the second day for a few days.

Hygienic treatment is important and consists of fresh air, yet with the avoidance of chilling; rest; and, if possible and indicated, change of locality.

Medicinal and Local Treatment.—At the beginning of the attack a purgative such as castor oil, calomel, or a saline should be given and the bowels washed out with normal salt-solution. If there is continued high fever and probably irritating material retained in the intestinal tract, the purgative medication may be continued. In other cases bismuth, kaolin, or charcoal may be used. (See p. 589.) Intestinal lavage should not be continued if there are produced tenesmus and great disturbance of the patient. Normal salt-solution, starch-water, or 5 per cent soda bicarbonate-solution is suitable for the bowel-washings, using from one to two quarts of fluid. The addition of astringents to these, such as 0.5 per cent tannic acid or 0.1 per cent silver nitrate offers no advantage in our experience, and may increase the tenesmus. Pain, tenesmus, and continued frequent movements are treated with opium in sufficiently large doses, often repeated, after the bowels have been thoroughly evacuated by the initial purgatives and enemata. Later the administration of some tannic-acid preparation, such as tannalbin, tannigen, or the like is sometimes of service, as are acetate of lead, sulphate of copper, and silver nitrate. Emetine would appear to be a specific for amebic dysentery, the adult dose being 1 grain (0.065) hypodermically daily for eight days. Rectal enemata of quinine in solution of 1:5000 to 1:2000 are also used in this type. Jones and Turner[76] recommend highly an anti-amebic drug, iodoxyquinolin sulphonic acid. Certain arsenicals, such as carbarsone, have also been employed (Leake[77]). Digitalis, caffeine, and camphor may be given to sustain cardiac strength, and alcoholic stimulants in large amounts are often required. (For doses see p. 180.) Dehydration must be treated by hypodermoclysis and intraperitoneal and intravenous injections, and acidosis combated if present. (See p. 589.) Transfusions may be indicated.

Flexner[72] recommended antidysentery-serum as effective, but Josephs and Davison[78] and Wollstein[79] found it of little value, and this has been our own experience. Davison[80] secured no benefit in bacillary dysentery from the use of bacteriophage, although we feel that it is of some value.

During *convalescence*, in addition to the care of the diet there must be close observation of the general health, and avoidance of chilling and fatigue. Tonic remedies may be indicated, especially those suitable for the treatment of anemia.

CHRONIC ILEOCOLITIS. CHRONIC DIARRHEA

These two disorders are practically the same, any diarrhea which runs a chronic course being liable to be finally associated with inflammatory lesions.

Etiology.—A common cause is an attack of acute ileocolitis which passes into the chronic form. This is especially prone to happen with the amebic type. Other protozoa are sometimes found in chronic diarrhea, especially the flagellates, and a gram-positive diplostreptococcus has been observed (Bargen;[81] Horgan and Horgan;[82] Fradkin and

Gray[83]), believed to be the cause of chronic ileocolitis in many cases. On the other hand it has been claimed that this organism has been discovered in other conditions and even in normal persons. Other types of streptococci may be seen in some instances (Streicher and Kaplan[84]). These bacteria will be further discussed under treatment. In some instances ileocolitis develops insidiously in patients who have been suffering from a debilitating disease, especially when this has been complicated by chronic indigestion. Rowe[85] and others believe that certain chronic diarrheas are due to intestinal allergy.

Pathologic Anatomy.—Only a catarrhal condition of the mucous membrane may be present in some cases. To the naked eye there may be little alteration in appearance, but microscopically a decided cellular hyperplasia is discovered, with cellular proliferation and atrophy in the epithelial glandular tissue, and hypertrophy of the connective tissue. In the severer cases, especially those following severe acute ileocolitis, there may be decided thickening of the intestinal wall, with ulceration and with cicatricial tissue the result of the healing of ulcers. Associated lesions are pneumonia, degenerative alterations of the kidneys and liver, and enlargement of the mesenteric lymph-nodes.

Symptoms.—These consist largely of increasing debility and marasmus, combined with diarrhea and other digestive disturbances. The diarrhea is usually not severe, but is persistent or constantly recurring. The stools are looser than normal although not very thin; number perhaps two to six daily; are large in size; sometimes foamy; and always contain more or less mucus, with undigested food and sometimes pus in small amounts. Blood is not often present. The odor is generally very offensive; the color either dark-brown or light-brown, or sometimes greenish or greyish. The abdomen is commonly distended with gas. Prolapse of the rectum may take place. Vomiting is not common, fever is absent or occurs only in temporary outbreaks, and colic, abdominal tenderness, and tenesmus may be observed, but less often than in acute cases. The tongue is coated or sometimes dry and red; the appetite is often unaffected or is increased, but sometimes very poor. The child suffers from irritability or apathy, malaise, disturbed sleep, poor circulation, dry, rough skin, anemia, and emaciation which is sometimes extreme. There is a persistent whining cry. A marantic dropsy often develops.

Course and Prognosis.—The course is essentially chronic but is not uniform, there occurring periods of transitory improvement followed by relapse. In some instances a temporary disappearance of mucus from the stools may be attended by the development of fever. In cases which recover six months or longer may go by before convalescence can be said to be assured. The fatal cases exhibit improvement at times but grow rapidly worse in some one of the recrudescences, and the patient dies from exhaustion or from some complicating intercurrent disorder. A terminal extensive development of petechiae is not uncommon. The prognosis in general is always serious, and difficult to formulate for the individual case. If intestinal lesions are marked the outlook is very unfavorable; but inasmuch as the exact severity of these cannot be known during the life of the patient, an absolutely unfavorable prognosis must be given with reserve.

Complications and Sequels.—Bronchopneumonia is a common complication. Corneal ulcers are sometimes seen, as are purulent otitis, suppurative processes in the skin, thrush, and nephritis. Tuberculosis is a not infrequent sequel. As direct sequels to the intestinal involvement may be strictures, multiple polyposis, and perirectal abscess. Rarely sarcoma and other tumors may develop.

Diagnosis.—The milder forms with but little diarrhea cannot always be sharply distinguished from chronic intestinal indigestion in infancy, although the latter disease does not have large amounts of mucus in the stools, and seldom blood. It is important, too, to distinguish the nature of the cause, as far as possible, inasmuch as this has such an important bearing upon the prognosis. When the disease follows an acute ileocolitis it is probable that the case is one of the ulcerative type. If it has developed slowly in debilitated subjects or has followed a chronic intestinal indigestion, there is greater likelihood of it being catarrhal or follicular without ulceration. In the search for causative organisms cultures should be made from the ulcers through a sigmoidoscope. Helmholz[86] and others have found that in ulcerative colitis roentgenograms of the colon showed it to be thickened and contracted and without the normal sacculations; while proctoscopic examination reveals glazing of the mucosa, or, in severer cases, a granular appearance due to multiple ulcerations. The differentiation of chronic diarrhea from tuberculous enteritis is often difficult. As a rule, however, tuberculosis of the intestine is a later manifestation of this disorder already evident in other parts of the body, especially the lungs; the onset is slow; fever is present; there is more often blood in the stools; and there already exists decided involvement of the general health out of proportion to the severity and the duration of the intestinal symptoms.

Treatment.—In the matter of *diet* only trial can determine the food best suited to the patient, the examination of the stools being of aid in this. There may be tried peptonized-milk, skimmed milk, casein-milk, buttermilk or acidophilus milk. In many cases, however, milk in any form is always passed undigested and should be avoided, and broths thickened with a starchy addition are to be preferred. Dextrinized starchy foods are frequently better than unconverted starch. Beef-juice, scraped beef and white of egg are often serviceable, but sometimes an increase of the stools may result. The diet should contain a minimum of residue. Larimore[87] reported success, when other measures failed, with the use of vitamin-rich diets.

In the line of *hygiene*, rest combined with abundance of fresh air is important. Massage is of value. Precautions must be taken as far as possible against exposure to hot weather, by removing the child to the seashore or the mountains. Indeed, this decided change of air is often the most successful treatment. Large enemata of saline solution or of starch-water are useful for washing out the bowels when the stools are more abundant than usual, or should any temporary constipation occurring be attended by unfavorable symptoms. They should not be given routinely. Astringent enemata are probably of more service than in the acute cases, but are often irritating. (See p. 185.)

The giving of *drugs* is a minor part of the treatment. Their use is more fully discussed under the treatment of acute ileocolitis (p. 593). In the chronic forms purgatives may occasionally be administered, especially if the stools are very offensive or fever develops. The astringents are useful on occasions when the frequency and thinness of the stools are temporarily increased, and even opium may be necessary. In some cases the continued administration of cod-liver oil in small doses has proved of benefit. Improvement may follow the persistent employment of tincture of the chloride of iron. Haskell and Cantarow[88] found that calcium gluconate or calcium lactate was beneficial by causing healing of the ulcerations. Operative interference has been advised (Helmholz[86]) if there has been no improvement after several months. This consists in ileosigmoidostomy, with the establishment of a fecal fistula through which the colon can be irrigated, and the fecal stream temporarily short circuited. We have seen good results from this. If there is reason to suspect an allergic basis, testing with proteins and the elimination of certain foods may be tried (p. 486).

In regard to *vaccines*, these may be employed in addition to other forms of treatment, using those made from the organisms obtained from the patient's stools, or preferably by sigmoidoscope from the intestinal wall or from ulcers. Bargen[81] reports great benefit from vaccine treatment with the organism described by him. We have had moderate success with this in a few cases, but as much with other forms of streptococci recovered from the patient's stool.

CONSTIPATION

Although only a symptom, constipation is one of extreme importance and frequency at all periods of life. The term indicates evacuations which are either too infrequent, too small in amount, or too firm and dry. The title is, however, a relative one, applicable more to the character than to the frequency of the stools, unless the latter is much diminished, while always the individual habit is to be borne in mind. Some infants, for instance, of an age when two or three stools should occur daily, have regularly but one, and should not therefore be called constipated, if the evacuation is of sufficient size and of normal character. In other cases in older children, where but one movement daily is to be expected, there may be two or three, but these may be hard and small and constipation is present. There is, in fact, no absolute rule for the number of evacuations which should occur daily, or even for the emptying of the bowels every day, provided the health of the infant or child is perfect in every way and the stools of normal character.

Etiology.—The causes are various and numerous, and the etiological factors are not the same at different periods of life. Age appears to have little influence in determining the frequency. In the new-born entire absence of bowel-movements may depend upon atresia of the anus or imperforate rectum, or upon complete obstruction elsewhere. Other instances at this early age result from a lack of tone in the intestinal wall, combined with the fact that no food has been ingested. In other infants, or in older children, constipation may depend upon congenital dilatation of the colon; stenosis of the pylorus or of the intestine at some portion; gastro-enteroptosis; appendicitis; peritonitis; strangulated hernia; fissure at the anus which causes pain at stool and avoidance of effort; hemorrhoids acting in a similar manner; spasm of the sphincter; intussusception, or other forms of intestinal obstruction, including the blocking of the intestines by a foreign body or by a large, hardened mass of feces.

Other agencies, however, are far more often active than those mentioned. A predisposing cause in infants is the unusual length and tortuous course of the sigmoid flexure characteristic of this period, to which attention was called by Bednar[89] and especially by Jacobi.[90] The character of the diet is a frequent factor; constipation in infants being due to a deficiency in the quantity or strength of food. A breast-milk or a bottle-mixture poor in fat is liable to produce constipation; one poor in protein does to a less extent. Sometimes too fatty a food gives rise to constipated soap-stools. Boiling the milk is not as frequent a cause as is ordinarily supposed. We have often seen an infant who was constipated while taking raw milk cease to be so when the milk was boiled. In other infants cereal decoction or lime-water may occasion the trouble. It is largely a matter of individuality. After the age is passed where the diet should consist solely of milk, constipation may depend upon the persistence in the use of this as the chief food taken; or upon the limitation of the diet to foods which are too digestible and contain too little waste matter.

Perhaps the most frequent cause of constipation is a certain degree of atony of the musculature of the intestine and abdominal wall, produced by debility from rickets, anemia, or the like; convalescence from any disease, especially from diarrheal disturbances; lack of exercise; too frequent use of enemata or purgatives. This last is a fertile cause of lack of muscular tone. In all such cases the stools may be of normal consistency and there may be lacking only the expulsive power, but oftener the long continuance in the intestine has been followed by an absorption of the water and the feces are too firm. On the other hand, there is a spastic type of constipation caused by irritation of the bowel by constant use of cathartics, or the ingestion of excessive amounts of bran or other coarse food. The position of the body is also of importance, and a child may find it difficult to evacuate the bowels while recumbent. Nervous influences are of moment. The failure to observe regularity, and the ignoring of the sensation of a desire to evacuate the bowel, will soon develop a constipated habit. The hurry of the morning hour in school-children, haste or other disturbances during the time passed in the toilet, and many similar influences are effective. Heredity is also a nervous factor. With all instances of lack of muscular tone there is liable to be combined deficient secretion, and a consequent abnormal change of the bowel contents.

Symptoms.—Constipation may be either acute or chronic. The *acute form* may be congenital and persistent, while other severe acute cases may be dependent upon some of the organic causes mentioned, and attended by symptoms of these disorders. In the milder cases of later origin, symptoms other than the constipation may be lacking; or there may be evidences of indigestion, colicky pain, distention, and such symptoms as headache, torpor, fever, and similar manifestations, which often seem to be dependent upon the blocking of the bowel, and which not infrequently suggest the onset of some acute febrile disease. They have often been ascribed to the absorption of toxic substances formed in the bowel; but, as Alvarez[91] points out, inasmuch as they are almost immediately relieved when a stool occurs, they can hardly be produced in this way. Apparently some of them are reflex in nature and caused by the mechanical distention of the lower bowel. The bowel-movements in acute constipation are infrequent; there may be a desire to evacuate with inability to accomplish it; and when finally a stool is passed after straining efforts it is unduly hard, dry, large, and perhaps streaked slightly with blood and mucus. The condition may last several days with only unsatisfactory stools or with none at all. In *chronic* constipation there may be either a constant repetition of acute attacks with short intermissions, or the bowels may be persistently sluggish and the stools firm. Sometimes there is never an evacuation unless artificially obtained. Symptoms may be entirely lacking except the constipated condition, and the child appear in good health; but frequently there are abdominal pain and flatulence; loss of appetite; occasional fever; sometimes vomiting; anemia; high-colored, scanty urine containing indican; and less frequently various nervous symptoms, including headache, disturbed sleep, and, it is claimed, convulsions. Local disturbances may arise, such as fissures, prolapse of the anus, hernia, or hemorrhoids, and sometimes retained fecal masses may be felt as hard nodules through the abdominal walls, occasionally attaining tumor-like size and hardness.

Course and Prognosis.—In the *acute* cases relief is obtained in a few days when the disturbance is from acute indigestion and similar removable causes, while in those due to organic obstruction the prognosis is serious. In the *chronic* functional cases the course is indefinite and the general health sometimes suffers seriously. When dependent upon chronic dilatation of the colon the prognosis is more grave.

Diagnosis.—One is sometimes misled by the statement that a daily stool occurs, but investigation may show that this is insufficient and that much fecal matter is being retained in the colon. The nervous manifestations attending some of the acute attacks, or the exacerbations of the chronic condition, may simulate so closely the onset of acute infections, including meningitis, that difficulty in diagnosis may at first exist; removed later by the prompt recovery following the administration of a purgative. Fecal concretions in the colon discovered by palpation may readily suggest the presence of tuberculous peritonitis or of morbid growths. A careful examination combined with a study of other symptoms will generally remove all doubt.

The chief object of diagnosis is to discover the cause. In the acute cases this is imperative, since only surgical interference can avail for the relief of some of them; in the chronic cases it is necessary in order to select the proper treatment. In this connection the value in some cases of inspection of the anus and of digital and perhaps proctoscopic examination of the lower bowel must not be overlooked.

Treatment.—When *acute constipation* is complete and depends upon organic obstruction operative interference is required; when the result of other causes, the emptying of the intestine may be accomplished by enemata of soap and water. If the feces are very hard, 2 to 4 fl. oz. (59 to 118) of cotton-seed oil may first be injected and allowed to remain for a few hours; and if the mass is also large it may be broken up with the finger or with the smooth handle of a teaspoon. In many instances of brief duration a soap-stick is useful in the case of infants, or a glycerine suppository for older children. When evidences of indigestion accompany the constipation a cathartic is more serviceable, using calomel, castor oil, or milk of magnesia in infants, and in older children citrate of magnesia, calcined magnesia, castor oil, or rhubarb.

In the treatment of *chronic constipation* attention must be given to the cause, which is oftenest the *diet*. With breast-fed infants aid may occasionally be obtained by a modification of the mother's milk through attending to her own diet and hygiene, the effort being made to augment the supply and increase the total solids (see p. 80), if these are deficient. Apart from this, if the infant is in perfect health little treatment is required, since the apparent constipation may be simply relatively complete absorption; but if it seems advisable, olive oil, malt-extract, or the like may be used as for bottle-fed infants. In bottle-fed babies the amount of fat may be raised cautiously if this is found to be well-digested; although not infrequently a high fat-percentage is a producer of constipation. A high protein percentage appears sometimes to increase constipation, but it should seldom be reduced to less than 1.5 per cent or proper development may be interfered with. Change in the type of sugar used may be helpful, whether this be from lactose to malt sugar, or the reverse. In some instances the use of oatmeal-water or of bran-water as a diluent is of benefit. Increase in the amount of orange-juice is occasionally serviceable, but oftener of no avail. The administration daily of 1 to 2 fl. dr. (3.7 to 7.4) of olive oil or of a syrupy malt-extract is frequently effective.

In older children, and often in infants, food may be selected of a laxative nature suitable to the age. The quantity of milk should be diminished and that of solid food increased, but water should be given freely. Buttermilk and acidophilus milk may often be used with advantage instead of plain milk. Fruit-juices, and, later, fruits themselves, are excellent; especially to be mentioned here being prune-juice and sometimes apple-sauce. For older children, figs, prunes, apricots, and dates in moderate quantities do well if well-digested. Such green vegetables as spinach, beet-tops, lettuce, asparagus-tips, and string beans, and such flours as oatmeal, whole-wheat and Graham are of the laxative class, and should form a considerable part of the diet. Bran*-biscuits made at home are frequently serviceable. Increase in the amount of butter is often efficacious, and a piece of it may be given once or twice a day to a child of two years in addition to that used on bread and with vegetables. This is preferable to the giving of cream. Broth frequently exerts a laxative action through the salts contained in it, and dextrinizing the cereal porridges with a malt-extract (p. 100) may sometimes be done with advantage. In general those articles of diet which are largely digested and absorbed, such as the protein of milk and foods consisting chiefly of starch, should be restricted in amount, and those containing much waste, such as green vegetables, many fruits, and the outer coating of the grain, increased. It is important not to overdo this, or irritation of the intestinal tract may result, producing intestinal indigestion or the spastic type of constipation. When the constipation is one of the symptoms of chronic intestinal indigestion, food must be selected which is suitable for the digestive disturbance, and other means employed to relieve the constipation.

Training is of great importance at any age. Even when but a few months old a regular habit is favored by holding the infant on the nursery-chair at the same hours daily. Older children must attempt to empty the bowel at a fixed hour, at a time when the inclination is most strongly felt, and when there is nothing to cause hurry. Shortly after eating is generally a suitable time, since this increases the intestinal peristalsis and often produces the desire for an evacuation. The disposition of children is to resist this desire unless they are instructed not to do so. Hard straining is not to be encouraged; but a sufficient time, fifteen or even thirty minutes, allowed in the toilet will often be followed by a stool, even though at first no inclination is felt; and a child should be taught that it can do nothing in the way of play or other amusement until the bowels have been opened. A low seat in the nursery-chair or toilet may help when evacuation is difficult with a higher one.

Massage and *exercise* are valuable. The abdominal muscles should be kneaded daily to increase tone, and by a pushing movement with the flat of the hand along the course of the colon the intestinal muscles are reached and the fecal matter aided in its course through the gut. Abundant exercise is a decided aid. We have seen most obstinate chronic constipation, resistant to strong purgatives, promptly relieved by the removing of the patient to a hilly summer-resort, apparently through the greatly increased amount of exercise taken.

If constipation persists in spite of a proper diet and of careful training and exercise, *medicinal measures* and allied treatment must be employed to supplement these. They should, however, be used no oftener than necessary and discontinued as soon as possible. Suppositories are of service in this connection. These may be of soap, glycerine and soap, or gluten. Sometimes the introduction of the oiled thermometer-stem gives all the local stimulus that an infant requires. Glycerin suppositories are too irritating for constant use. In training to a daily habit suppositories may be used for several days, after which it is probable that this measure will be no longer required. Small enemata are also useful in emptying the bowels in chronic constipation, but, like suppositories, should not be employed as a routine measure. Those of cotton-seed or other bland oil are the least irritating and are employed to soften the feces; somewhat larger ones of well-diluted glycerine (1:10) are serviceable when there is lack of tone; and still larger

* Recipe for bran-biscuit: Mix 1 pint of bran, ½ pint of flour, and 1 level tablespoonful of baking soda. Mix ½ pint of milk and 4 tablespoonfuls of molasses. Add this to the bran-mixture and bake in gem-pans.

ones of normal salt-solution for infants, or of soap and water at this age or for older children, where there has been no passage for several days. Enemata are less serviceable than suppositories when only local stimulation is required, since they lose their effect and need to be constantly increased in size. A very successful course of treatment in chronic constipation is the giving nightly on retiring an enema of sweet oil of from 2 to 6 fl. oz. (59 to 177) or more, depending upon the age of the child and the tolerance of the bowel. In the morning the desire for an evacuation will probably be present and the softened stool passed without difficulty. In obstinate cases it may at first be necessary to administer a saline laxative in small dose before breakfast, but the need of this generally soon ceases. Stretching of the anal sphincter is occasionally serviceable for spasm of the muscle or when evacuation is evidently painful.

Treatment with drugs by the mouth, although often necessary, is to be deprecated. In infancy manna (5 to 10 grains) (0.32 to 0.65), phosphate of soda (5 to 20 grains) (0.32 to 1.3), or milk of magnesia ($\frac{1}{2}$ to 1 fl. dr.) (2 to 4) added to the bottle-food is of service. Castor oil, although laxative, commonly leaves constipation in its train, and, like calomel, should be reserved for times when distinct evidences of indigestion are also present. Some of the less bitter preparations of cascara in doses determined by trial are of great value. Senna, phenolphthalein, and the syrupy malt extracts are often efficacious. It is a good plan to continue no one of these substances, or indeed any other measure, without change. Thus the giving of a laxative may be replaced after a few days by the use of suppositories or by enemata. In this way the acquiring of a tolerance for the treatment is avoided as much as possible.

In older children the same internal remedies may be employed in larger amount and the same precautions taken as in infancy against the patient becoming accustomed to any one measure. Among some of the other remedies recommended for either infants or children are agar-agar and petrolatum liquidum which act mechanically. Dutcher, Ely and Honeywell[92] and Rowntree[93] point out that liquid petrolatum is a solvent of vitamin A. If, therefore, this substance is used vitamin A should be supplied abundantly. Children old enough to take pills may receive small doses of aloin or of podophyllin. Drugs which increase the tone of the intestinal or abdominal muscles are useful, especially to be mentioned being nux vomica. In spastic constipation belladonna may be given for its antispasmodic effect.

CHRONIC INTESTINAL INDIGESTION

This exceedingly common disorder affecting both infants and older children is frequently associated with gastric indigestion, but oftener occurs alone. It is, strictly speaking, a purely functional disturbance, yet in symptoms it may sometimes not be readily distinguishable from mild cases of ileocolitis. It is one of the most difficult diseases to treat, especially in infancy.

(*A*) Chronic Intestinal Indigestion in Infants

(Intestinal Dyspepsia; Decomposition)

Etiology and Pathology.—The disease is much oftenest seen in the first year of life and especially in the first six months. Poor hygienic conditions predispose, as does very greatly prematurity or a congenital constitutional debility. Among frequent causes are attacks of acute intestinal indigestion or acute ileocolitis. Of all etiologic factors, however, the continued employment of an unsuitable diet is the most influental and common.

In *breast-fed infants* the fault is sometimes too great a quantity of milk. In other instances the supply is insufficient and the infant's general health consequently suffers, until finally the intestinal functions are weakened. In still others—and these the most frequent of all—some of the constituents of the breast-milk are secreted in excess. Many times, however, analysis reveals nothing whatever to account for the persistent indigestion. It then appears to be some constitutional trouble with the mother, as for instance, a highly neurotic temperament, or ill health, although the way in which the milk is affected is not discoverable.

In *artificially fed infants* digestive difficulties are naturally much more common. The chemical differences in the proteins and fats make it impossible to prepare a milk-modification exactly like human milk, and there is also lack of similarity in the ferments, salts, and other bodies, the importance of which is still imperfectly understood. Often there is an evident and clearly recognizable fault with some one of the ingredients, an amount of this being given which the digestion cannot tolerate. In addition there comes prominently into play in bottle-fed babies the element of infection of the milk by germs of various sorts. (See Acute Gastro-enteric Intoxication, p. 583.) Finally it frequently happens in well-advanced cases that the infant comes under observation at a stage when no alteration of the diet has beneficial effect.

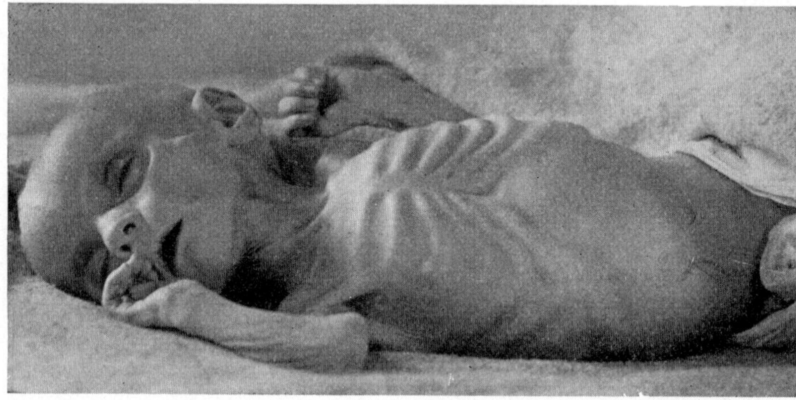

Fig. 139.—Chronic intestinal indigestion. Child of three and one-half months, in the Children's Hospital of Philadelphia. Great wasting; moderate fever; bowels loose; failure to improve under any treatment; death.

Just what the principal defects in the diet may be in bottle-fed infants is a matter much discussed and far from ultimately settled. This subject has already been considered to some extent. (See Action of the Different Food Elements in Digestion, pp. 24, 29, 77: Feces in Disease, p. 578.) Undoubtedly too much blame was formerly placed upon an excess of protein, and especially of casein; and the disposition to attribute indigestion solely to the whey, the carbohydrates, or the fat is likewise too dogmatic. Those who have seen good results from the use of whey hesitate to assign to it all the evil influences claimed by some observers. There is at any rate a very general agreement at the present time that the fat of the milk is one of the ingredients most difficult to digest. Less often the sugar causes trouble, but how much it acts synergetically with other elements of the food is still uncertain. The addition of amylaceous food to the nourishment aids digestion in many cases; and in others is certainly the cause of chronic intestinal indigestion. It must be recognized that the question is, to some extent, an individual one, and has to be determined largely for each child. Here may be again mentioned the fact that the trouble appears not always to be in the intestine itself, although perhaps primarily so, but in defective metabolism in the tissues of the body. This is more particularly true of infantile atrophy (p. 463).

Pathologic Anatomy.—In typical cases there are no lesions found, the disease being a purely functional disturbance. In advanced cases, however, complicating secondary lesions appear, among them inflammation of the intestinal mucous membrane. The disorder then has changed to a condition of chronic ileocolitis.

Symptoms.—In some instances there is constant diarrhea, the stools being watery, greenish, and containing curdy masses. The number is seldom large, they are passed without pain, and mucus is absent or in small amount. If later there is constantly a large amount of mucus present, it is probable that a chronic ileocolitis has developed. In other cases the stools are only occasionally diarrheal, or this may alternate with constipation, or there may be chronic constipation, the passages being pasty and white or grey in color and sometimes hard, either in small scybalous masses, or in larger form. In any event microscopical and chemical examination often reveals undigested food, especially fat; free, or in the form of soap. The odor is generally unpleasant or sour, and occasionally offensive if there is decomposition of protein. The buttocks may be reddened if the passages are diarrheal. Vomiting occurs occasionally, but is not a constant or troublesome symptom unless the disease is complicated by gastric indigestion. The abdomen is usually distended by gas and there is frequent colic if constipation is present, but less often so if diarrhea. The appetite is generally good; the tongue varies in appearance; there is often irregular fever alternating with normal or low temperature, or there may be more constant elevation, but only when symptoms of constitutional intoxication develop. The urine may show the presence of acetone bodies and increased output of nitrogen in the form of ammonia. In some patients there arises intolerance for cow's milk in any form, its administration being followed by an exacerbation of the symptoms, including sometimes cutaneous eruptions and disturbed nervous states.

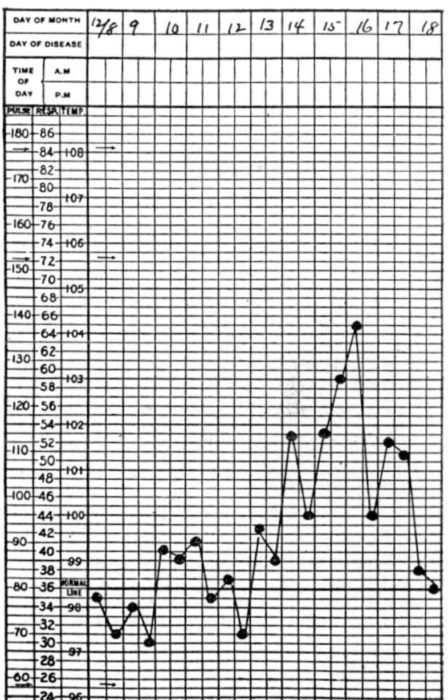

Fig. 140.—Exacerbation of symptoms in a case of chronic intestinal indigestion. George B., aged six months. In the Children's Hospital of Philadelphia for chronic intestinal indigestion. Weight 7 lb., 7 oz. (3374). Occasional vomiting; two to three slightly undigested and diarrheal stools daily; much emaciated. Dec. 12, suddenly developed apathy; toxemic symptoms; prostration; distended abdomen; five to seven diarrheal stools daily, greenish, with pus and mucus; increase of temperature. Final recovery.

The chief symptom, however, is *persistent increasing malnutrition*, with the symptoms already described under the heading of infantile atrophy (pp. 463, 552).

The children gradually waste more and more, and suffer from low temperature, feeble circulation, anemia, and increasing debility. They are usually constantly fretful in the early stage and often apathetic later. During this condition of malnutrition no positive evidences of indigestion may be discoverable. Yet diminishing the amount of food may increase the rapid loss of weight, while increasing the amount may have the same effect, often with attacks of diarrhea or sometimes of toxic symptoms of a dangerous nature.

Course and Prognosis.—The course and duration of the disease are very variable. At best it lasts for months. In some instances the loss of weight is constant and extreme (Fig. 139). In others there may be long periods during which the course is stationary or even shows temporary improvement. In still others, not too far advanced when coming under observation, there is eventually a more or less steady increase of weight and return to general health. In nearly all, however, there are liable to be exacerbations, and then often the symptoms of intestinal intoxication develop (p. 585), (Fig. 140).

The *prognosis* is always serious, especially in cases with active intestinal disturbance, or even without this if improvement in weight fails to take place no matter what change in diet is made. Death follows some complicating disorder, exhaustion, or intoxication, perhaps during an exacerbation. The earlier in the disease treatment is commenced the greater is the chance of recovery. On the other hand, an infant who has long tolerated the disorder may have acquired greater resisting power. Even apparently hopeless cases sometimes recover under proper treatment. When recovery does take place it is usually finally complete, and the condition of the child in the second or third year seems often no worse as a result of the illness in the first year of life. Some patients, however, continue delicate, or later suffer more or less from intestinal disturbances.

Complications.—These are largely those described under ileocolitis and infantile atrophy; consisting of thrush, erythema and intertrigo, furunculosis or other cutaneous suppurative processes, suppurating otitis, bronchitis, and atelectasis. The disease may readily pass into an ileocolitis of a chronic nature. Wide-spread petechiae, pneumonia, nephritis, or convulsions may be terminal processes.

Diagnosis.—The advanced cases are to be distinguished chiefly from *infantile atrophy* depending upon other causes, such as congenital asthenia, tuberculosis, and syphilis. The diagnosis is also to be made from mild, long-continued cases of chronic ileocolitis. Both diseases produce wasting and exhibit disturbances of the stools; but in indigestion these stools fail to show the constant large amount of mucus which is diagnostic of chronic ileocolitis. The recognition of the cause of chronic intestinal indigestion is diagnostically important but often difficult. A careful consideration of the earlier history of the case is of great aid, with special reference to the nature of the diet employed. Excess of carbohydrate produces colic and watery, irritating, acid movements, often with a penetrating odor suggesting acetic acid. Excess of protein may occasion either constipated or diarrheal stools with a putrefactive odor, and protein-curds may be present. Excess of fat may also result in either constipation or diarrhea. In the former the stools are of a gray or white color, are composed largely of insoluble fatty soaps, and may have an unpleasant smell. In the latter the stools may be pale-yellow, with a sour or offensive odor, be more or less glistening from the presence of fat, and reveal under the microscope fat-globules and crystals in excess; or they may be watery, mucous, greenish, and with numerous white, curdy masses. (See Feces in Digestive Diseases, p. 578.)

Treatment.—*Medicinal* treatment is purely symptomatic. Constipation is to be relieved by enemata or gentle laxatives; occasionally by free purgation if there are symptoms of acute gastric or intestinal indigestion. Diarrhea may be checked by appropriate means; colic by measures already referred to (p. 577). The strength must be sustained by stimulants; the body-temperature by external heat. During exacerbations, especially if toxic symptoms appear, brief starvation must be instituted and a purgative given.

In the line of *hygienic* treatment, care is required that there is plenty of fresh air, either indoors, or outside in suitable weather; especial care being taken that the infant's temperature does not become subnormal. In very hot weather the infant must be nearly unclothed and kept in the shade, or in a room as cool as possible. In very feeble infants rubbing the body under the covers with warm oil should replace the bath. In others a daily sponge-bath or tub-bath is of advantage, provided a good reaction follows.

By far the most important treatment, however, is *dietetic*, and this is frequently a most difficult problem. In *breast-fed infants* weaning must not be hastily advised. This cannot be insisted upon too strongly. Some infants in spite of apparent failure to digest breast-milk perfectly, continue to thrive in other respects, and in such it is certainly well to delay the withdrawing of breast-feeding, inasmuch as there is no surety that artificial feeding may not have a worse result. Sometimes a regulation of the mother's diet and method of life, or some alteration in the frequency of feeding the infant will suffice. In other cases the employment once or twice daily of an artificial food may answer, breast-milk being still the principal diet; since the giving of even a small amount of human milk seems frequently in some way to enable the infant to digest more satisfactorily a diet largely artificial. As a supplementary artificial food, one low in sugar and fat is generally to be preferred, protein-milk in some form being one of the best. The temporary withdrawal of the breast for twenty-four or more hours at a time may suffice in some cases. When, however, the indigestion is persistent and the child is losing ground in spite of faithful efforts to remove the difficulty, either the employment of a wet-nurse or the institution of weaning becomes necessary.

In the dietetic treatment of *artificially fed* infants there must be a minute study of the history, in the effort to determine what element of the food, or fault in the preparation, originally produced the disease or maintains it. Not only the character of the food must be considered, and the degree of digestion of this, especially by an examination of the stools, but the quantity given, the intervals of feeding, the rapidity of taking nourishment, the amount of dilution, and many other circumstances. If active symptoms are present, dietetic treatment may well begin with a moderate starvation for twenty-four hours or longer, giving a thin starchy decoction, as barley-water or arrowroot-water. After this there is a large choice of foods depending upon the dietetic cause and the character of the symptoms. They must at first be weak until digestive tolerance is established. If the study of the stools (p. 578) shows that the *fat* is especially difficult of digestion, as is true in the large majority of cases, milk-mixtures made from skimmed milk are suitable, or, still better, in our experience, those from buttermilk or acidophilus milk. (See pp. 105, 106.) Inasmuch as the caloric value of these foods is low, they may often be strengthened by the addition of carbohydrate in some form. If there is difficulty in the digestion of *sugar*, as shown, for instance, by acid diarrhea with irritation of the buttocks, buttermilk is of especial value on account of its low sugar-content. It frequently happens that a moderate amount of fat may be tolerated if the sugar-content of the food is low. Casein-milk in some of its forms is serviceable for the same reason, having a somewhat reduced amount of fat with a low percentage of carbohydrate, unless sugar has been added to it (p. 108). Sometimes certain sugars are tolerated better than others, and trial may be made separately of lactose, cane sugar, or dextrin-maltose preparations (p. 30).

In many conditions the addition of an insoluble carbohydrate, such as a cereal decoction or gruel, is of great advantage, its strength varying with the case (p. 112). It acts to a certain extent mechanically as a colloidal substance. It is for this reason that the giving of the various malt-soups is often more efficacious than the addition of sugar or of dextrin-maltose preparations alone (p. 113). The *casein* of the food is less frequently a source of indigestion, but can produce it, especially in the early months of life. The symptoms often consist in flatulence, colic, constipation, and an offensive odor to the stools; less often in the passing of casein-curds (p. 579). Under such conditions, whey is frequently a valuable remedy. Its caloric value is low; but in spite of this young infants will frequently thrive on it for a time. Its nutritional value may be increased by the addition of small amounts of strong cream, when no fat-indigestion is present. Where fat, too, is not tolerated, the whey should be made of skimmed milk, and white of egg may be added to it, and sugar also, preferably dextrin-maltose preparations, if found desirable. The employment of a malt-soup is sometimes useful here, inasmuch as it contains both soluble and insoluble carbohydrate. In still other cases the digestibility of casein may be increased by peptonizing, although generally only slightly. In many instances an intolerance for any form of milk develops, usually, however, only temporary. Here strong cereal gruels and albumen-water are often serviceable.

The methods described should be looked upon as temporary procedures, to be changed when the digestive disorder has been abated. So long as the strength is maintained, and the weight remains stationary or diminishes but little, the effort to cause a gain in this respect should be deferred until other symptoms are sufficiently relieved.

The dilution of the food and its frequency of administration must be considered. Some infants do better on a diluted food; others upon smaller amounts of a more concentrated one. Only trial can show which is to be preferred. As a rule, it is better to make the intervals of feeding longer than in health. A three-hour or four-hour interval in the early months of life may be better than one of two or two and one-half hours. The mutual influence which the different food-ingredients exercise upon each other is also important. For instance, the addition of a high carbohydrate-percentage may make both the protein and the fat more digestible, as seen, for instance, when malt-soup is employed; or in other cases fat may be tolerated if the whey is diminished in amount or if the sugar is reduced. (See pp. 29, 30, 113.)

The method of changing from any one of these substitutions mentioned to one containing the usual elements in more normal ratio is often a difficult matter which must be determined for the individual case. Thus an infant taking whey may have this fortified by egg-albumen, and later, in cases of casein-indigestion, after the symptoms have been relieved, by the gradual addition of peptonized milk; or if fat-indigestion has been present also, first of skimmed milk and then of whole milk. A baby with sugar-intolerance fed upon casein-milk may gradually have increased amounts of saccharose or dextrin-maltose added. One with fat-indigestion, fed upon buttermilk, may after a time have small amounts of cream added. There must be familiarity with the caloric strength of the foods employed, their method of preparation, and their percentage values, all of which are given in the appropriate sections. (See Index.) When additions or increases are to be made the percentage of fat, carbohydrate, or protein, as the case may be, should be calculated. (See pp. 92, 95.) Many cases are encountered in which no change in diet appears to influence the condition. Here nothing remains but to procure human-milk from some source, by purchase, or by securing a wet-nurse. Even this may be of no avail, especially if the mistake has been made of waiting too long. In advanced cases it may be necessary to dilute or skim the human milk for a time.

Reference must be made to the attempt to treat intestinal indigestion and diarrhea by direct modification of the intestinal flora. As pointed out by Kendall and Smith[94] and others, the multiplication of certain apparently harmful intestinal bacteria can be inhibited either by the direct administration of other germs, or by the giving of food which contains, or favors the increase of, the bacteria desired. It is especially the Bulgarian bacillus and similar lactic acid producing organisms and the bacillus acidophilus which are antagonistic to the proteolytic bacteria. Unheated buttermilk (fermented lactic acid milk) or acidophilus-milk is the preferable way to introduce large quantities of these. It has been shown that the administration of cultures and especially of tablets of these bacteria may be quite ineffective (p. 106). There is no doubt that the ingestion of large numbers of the organisms mentioned, or the administration of large amounts of lactose, which encourages the growth of lactic acid forming bacteria such as the acidophilus bacillus in the intestinal tract, is helpful in many cases of intestinal disturbance. Whether their effect is due to lactic acid or to the action of the organisms themselves is still to be determined. As we have pointed out elsewhere[95] Metchnikoff and his followers never proved that the Bulgarian bacillus was implanted in the intestinal tract; in fact, this implantation probably does not occur. Very likely the acidophilus bacillus, an inhabitant of the normal intestinal tract, can be implanted, as shown by Rettger and Cheplin[96] and others. At any rate its implantation is not necessary, since it produces lactic acid before and probably after ingestion when introduced in large numbers, and since milks made acid by chemical means possess similar beneficial action (pp. 106, 107).

(*B*) Chronic Intestinal Indigestion in Older Children

(Mucous Disease; Celiac Disease; Intestinal Infantilism)

This affection is common between the ages of three and ten years, although often beginning in the second. It may manifest itself in typical form, or give rise to symptoms which are confusing, and it may be combined with disturbance of the stomach.

Etiology and Pathogenesis.—A frequent factor is the continued ingestion of large amounts of carbohydrates, especially of starchy food and particularly potato. Other causes are too long continuance of milk as the chief article of diet; the giving of candies and other sweets in excess; eating between meals; excess of fat; insufficient mastication; and poorly prepared food or that of an indigestible nature. Debilitated health predisposes, and the disease may follow an acute diarrheal disturbance or other acute disease or parenteral infection. Apart from these factors the digestive power is at fault, even when the diet is not amiss. In the severe cases, often designated celiac disease, the exact pathogenesis is far from clear. It is usually stated that there is diminished ability to absorb fat, and there is certainly always an excess of it in the stools. It has also been suggested that there may be impaired action of the lipase of the blood and tissues. One of the older views, first sponsored by Cheadle,[97] was that the fat-indigestion depended upon cessation of secretion of bile; an "acholia," as named by him. Miller,[98] McCrae and Morris,[99] and others believe that there is a deficiency or disturbed function of bile-salts, and the last mentioned authors think, too, that a shift of the intestinal contents to the alkaline side also plays a rôle. The studies of Bauer[100] and of Parsons[101] failed, however, to show any abnormality in the bile or in lipase or trypsin. As had several others, Bauer found that the fat in the stools was greater than its intake, and also that the absorption of the fat was the same as in the normal child; and he concludes that the difficulty was not in the absorption of fat but in its transfer back into the intestinal tract. There is often in celiac disease digestive difficulty with carbohydrate, but when all the evidence, including the studies on sugar-tolerance curves and the respiratory quotient, is summarized, it does not appear proved that there is any metabolic fault in this connection or, if present, what its nature may be. A diminished secretion of gastric hydrochloric acid may occur, but is not an essential characteristic. An alteration of the intestinal flora was emphasized by Herter;[102] Brown, Davis and MacLachlan[103] and others as the cause of a certain type of case. (See p. 1088.) There can be no doubt that symptoms attributable to vitamin-deficiency, especially of vitamin C and the vitamin B complex, may develop in celiac disease, sometimes proceeding to the stage of scurvy or of beri-beri (Haas[104]), but this is probably the result of insufficient intake and absorption of vitamins rather than existing as a fundamental cause. Intestinal indigestion seems to develop more often in neurotic children, and there has also been made the unsupported suggestion that there is active an endocrine disturbance of some sort. Another hypothesis is that an imbalance of the vegetative nervous system exists; the only evidence for this being that Freise and Walenta[105] produced a condition somewhat resembling celiac disease in dogs and pigs by dividing the celiac plexus. There is no good reason to believe that celiac disease is identical with tropical sprue. In advanced cases there develop secondary disturbances of mineral absorption and metabolism. (See Intestinal Infantilism, p. 1088.)

It must be admitted that the most that can be said of the pathogenesis of the severer forms of chronic intestinal indigestion (celiac disease) is that there appears to be a faulty digestion and absorption of fat, but that even the latter is not universally admitted. There are, in fact, no positive data explaining the pathogenesis clearly.

Pathologic Anatomy.—The disease in a strict sense is a functional disturbance, no lesions of the intestine being present. Lesions of the liver or pancreas have not been found.

Symptoms.—In typical cases the symptoms come on insidiously and are finally characteristic. They are at first those rather of chronic toxemia than of local intestinal disturbance. There is a decided loss of flesh, the limbs especially being thin and the child having a delicate appearance, with an anemic or sallow complexion, dark rings or puffiness under the eyes, and perhaps a slightly yellow tint to the sclerae. The pallor is sometimes replaced for a time by a red flush of the cheeks, and on other occasions shows a great temporary increase, as though the child were faint or nauseated. It does not necessarily depend upon anemia, although this may sometimes be very decided. In some cases the skin is unduly dry; in others there is an urticarial or erythematous eruption. The appetite is variable and capricious and generally very poor. Eructation of gas is common, as is its passage from the bowel, and the abdomen is usually much distended and tympanitic, the gas being produced by the undue fermentation of the carbohydrates of the food. This abdominal distention is one of the characteristic symptoms and is dependent upon the dilated colon, as can be demonstrated by roentgenograms. Nausea and vomiting, bad breath, and coated tongue may occur if the stomach shares in the dyspeptic condition, but in some instances vomiting and headache appear to depend upon intestinal toxemia. It has seemed to us that the geographical tongue (p. 526) is particularly liable to be found in this disease. The bowels are generally constipated, or this may alternate with diarrhea, and the stools are as a rule of large size. Their color is usually pale and sometimes nearly white; at other times brownish, greenish or gray. They are frequently very offensive in odor, contain undigested food and a great excess of fat, and when loose are often frothy in appearance. Mucus is passed at times, perhaps in large amount. The mucus is mixed with the stool when this is loose, or coats it when formed. To that type in which unusually large amounts of mucus are passed Eustace Smith[106] applied the term "Mucous Disease." Abdominal pain is very variable and usually slight, being somewhat colicky and paroxysmal, and frequently accompanying an evacuation of mucus. The urine is not characteristic. At times it may show the presence of indican in considerable amount. The general health suffers and the children develop poorly in height and weight. There may, in fact, eventuate a condition of infantilism (see Intestinal Infantilism, p. 1088) or a severe degree of rickets.

The nervous symptoms are many and varied and always prominent manifestations of the disease. Although the child is often bright and even precocious, he is irritable, hypochondriacal, languid and easily tired. The hands and feet are cold, and the skin perspires readily. Sleep is nearly always restless, with frequent grinding of the teeth, outcries, dreaming, and not infrequently night-terrors and somnambulism. Wakefulness is not uncommon. In advanced cases there is stupor. Tetany or convulsions may develop, the first certainly being due to the low calcium content of the tissues consequent upon failure of absorption. These symptoms strongly suggest meningitis or other organic intracranial disease. Shortness of breath is sometimes witnessed, or the respiration may occasionally be sighing, or asthmatic symptoms may be present. There is usually little or no fever, or perhaps a constant subfebrile temperature; except during the occurrence of exacerbations when it rises considerably. Scurvy, beri-beri, and very rarely xerophthalmia may develop because of the faulty absorption of vitamins or their insufficient intake.

The symptoms as described are not seen in their entirety in every instance. In the milder cases, or those which have lasted but a short time, the disease is rather a series of acute attacks of moderate severity, with intervals of comparative health, and with but little disturbance of the general condition. In others there are symptoms of a severe type, with great wasting and much loss of fat in the pasty, white, offensive stools, and it is to these advanced cases that the title "Coeliac Disease," as used by Gee[107] is so often applied. An excellent recent discussion of this type is given by Parsons.[101]

Course and Prognosis.—Recovery is slow even under treatment, the disease often lasting for years. Only in mild cases can rapid improvement be expected. There is a tendency to acute exacerbations at irregular and often frequent intervals. Between attacks the evidences of indigestion may at first be slight, or even wholly absent; but it is not long before there is an increase in the intensity of the symptoms, until some of them are constantly present. The prognosis under treatment is on the whole good, except in the instances where little can be found wrong with the hygiene and diet, and where there seems to be a constitutional, or an early acquired and persistent, lack of functional intestinal power. In such cases death from exhaustion is liable finally to occur. There is always, too, the danger that the impaired general health may diminish the power of resistance to some intercurrent affection, such as bronchopneumonia.

Diagnosis.—The tympanitic condition in intestinal indigestion may be so great that we have known cases erroneously diagnosed as *idiopathic dilatation of the colon*, and have been able to prevent dangerous and unnecessary operative interference. The two conditions are quire distinct in their history and symptoms. The slight cough which may accompany the wasting can suggest pulmonary *tuberculosis*, but examination of the lungs fails to reveal any anomaly, unless there is coincidental tuberculous disease. The tuberculin reaction if negative would be of value. Tuberculous peritonitis exhibits tenderness, and either fluid or some evidence of deposit in or thickening of the abdominal walls, and there is also the absence of the frequent changing degree of distention which is commonly observed in intestinal indigestion. The presence of *intestinal worms* may produce abdominal pain, disturbed sleep and other nervous symptoms; but the administration of a vermifuge will reveal the cause and clear up the diagnosis. Convulsions in childhood may be considered to be a manifestation of *epilepsy*, but may actually depend upon chronic intestinal indigestion.

Treatment.—*Dietetic* treatment occupies the primary place. Carious teeth must be treated since they render mastication difficult. Hasty eating and improper mastication may sometimes be as harmful as the nature of the food taken at school-luncheons; and breakfasts, too, must not be hurried. Meals should be at regular intervals and no food eaten between them. The frequency of the feeding depends upon the case. In milder cases moderate restriction of fats and carbohydrates, or some simple regulation or limitation of the diet, depending upon the results of study in each case, may be all that is necessary. This individuality is a most important matter. In the severe cases there must be strict limitation of the fats, and the carbohydrates given with caution; the diet being largely a protein one. In the first stage of treatment fresh cow's milk is to be avoided, although dried milk and acid-milks (p. 104) of various types, particularly if skimmed, are better tolerated. Best is some form of casein-milk, prepared according to Finkelstein's method (p. 108) or some modification of it, or one of the proprietary protein-milks. The so-called "three-phase" diet, evolved by Howland[108] and used by Sauer[109] and many others with success, consists in giving only protein-milk for a few weeks; in the second stage of several months continuing this but adding beef-juice, scraped beef, egg and cottage cheese; and only in the third stage beginning carbohydrates, such as corn-syrup, zwieback, vegetables, and cereals and adding other meats such as lamb and chicken, and fish. In not all cases does carbohydrate need to be restricted so greatly, especially if fat be not too high, although its effect must always be carefully watched in the individual case. Taylor,[110] for example, found diluted corn-syrup could be given early, and Nelson[111] that dextrose in amounts of 200 Gm. (7 oz.) daily in 10 to 20 per cent, solution was well tolerated if given between meals. A carbohydrate much used and easily digested consists of banana, over-ripe and thoroughly mashed; several bananas being given daily. This was first strongly advocated by Haas[112] and since then by many others. When the skin has turned brown the carbohydrate of the fruit is composed of sucrose and invert-sugar with but little starch (Pease and Rose[113]). A powdered banana flour also has been employed by Haas.[114] Numerous other foods are suggested, which in most instances are high in protein. Ruhräh,[115] for example, used soy-bean flour and condensed milk, and Kerley[116] a combination of powdered casein, barley-flour, sugar, and water, of a caloric strength of 16 to the ounce.

In the early stages too much attention must not be paid to weight, provided there is no loss. In general, until several months have passed and convalescence is clearly progressing, vegetables and starchy foods are to be avoided. First may be tried water-crackers, oyster-crackers and the like, and zwieback, and later the less coarse starches, as rice, arrowroot and farina. Fruits may be allowed only later. Preferable vegetables are mashed and sieved string beans, spinach, squash, asparagus-tips, tomatoes, and lettuce. To be avoided until later, because of their carbohydrate or cellulose content, are lima-beans, peas, stewed celery, carrots, corn, beets, and parsnips. The possibility of vitamin-deficiency is to be borne in mind, although this is not likely after the vegetables can be added or when bananas are employed. Any new food must be given in small amounts, and the individual reaction to it ascertained.

Hygienic treatment is important. Conducive to general health are cool morning sponges if these are well borne, fresh air, sufficient sleep, the daily morning or afternoon recumbent rest, rest before and after meals, and the avoidance of mental and physical fatigue. Whether in the milder cases the child shall attend school, and for how many hours, must be carefully considered, balancing all the factors such as fatigue, lack of companionship, and the like. Clothing must provide warmth and avoid exposure without occasioning too free perspiration. Massage may be helpful. Change of climate is often most beneficial.

Medicinal treatment is a secondary consideration. Constipation should be overcome by oil enemata, or if necessary, by such mild laxatives as cascara, phenolphthalein, and the like. Any increase of laxative foods should be made with caution. It is sometimes beneficial to accomplish a mild purging once a week with calomel, castor oil, or citrate of magnesia. Saline douching of the bowel may be of service if much mucus is passed, but if long-continued may increase this condition. A malt-extract containing diastase may aid the digestion of starch. Nux vomica and gentian or small doses of an alcoholic tonic before meals may stimulate the appetite. In cases with diminished gastric acidity small doses of dilute hydrochloric acid may be given. To avoid rickets or to cure it, and, in any event, because of the low fat diet, cod liver oil should be administered. If this disagrees one of the active cod liver oil concentrates should be employed. Irradiated ergosterol (viosterol) is useful for its antirachitic effect. Ultra-violet irradiation from an artificial source may be given with care.

DILATATION OF THE COLON

This condition may be divided into: (*A*) Congenital Idiopathic Dilatation (Megacolon congenitum); and (*B*) Secondary Dilatation.

(*A*) Idiopathic Dilatation of the Colon.—Writing in 1899 we[117] were able to collect but 23 previously published cases which could be accepted with reasonable certainty. The number has greatly increased, and Finney[118] in 1908, collected 206 published articles upon the subject; Patel[119] collected 223 cases; and Porter and Weeks[120] found over 100 more. A bibliography from 1908 to 1916 is given by Cadwallader.[121] The disease was first described with care by Hirschsprung[122] and is often called by his name, but a number of well-characterized instances had been published earlier, as, for example, those by Parry,[123] Ebers,[124] Henoch,[125] Peacock,[126] and Hughes.[127]

Etiology.—The disease is three times more frequent in boys. That it is congenital is indicated by its presence in some cases soon after birth, and in one reported instance, according to Ladd,[128] in a seven-months fetus. The cause of the congenital tendency to dilate is unknown. It has been supposed by some to be neuromuscular; perhaps a paralysis of a region of the colon, with arrest of peristalsis; perhaps a spasm producing functional obstruction; perhaps due to a lesion of the sympathetic nervous system. The disease does not depend upon general muscular atony, since the children are healthy in other respects. The relatively great length of the colon and especially of the sigmoid flexure in infants, to which attention was called particularly by Jacobi,[129] undoubtedly aids in producing dilatation, but cannot alone account for it. Whether the hypertrophy of the wall is the cause, the attendant, or the result of the dilation is uncertain. In some fatal cases in the new-born both dilatation and hypertrophy have been found, so that in these instances at least the hypertrophy was not secondary. Generally, however, the latter appears to be secondary to the dilatation. That the dilatation and hypertrophy are both dependent upon a constriction in some lower portion of the gut has been maintained by Treves[130] and others. Search at necropsy has, however, failed to reveal any such constriction in the majority of cases, and any kinking or torsion of the colon discovered is probably the result of the hypertrophic dilatation rather than the cause. Cases in which dilatation is dependent upon mechanical obstruction belong to the category of Secondary Dilatation of the Colon.

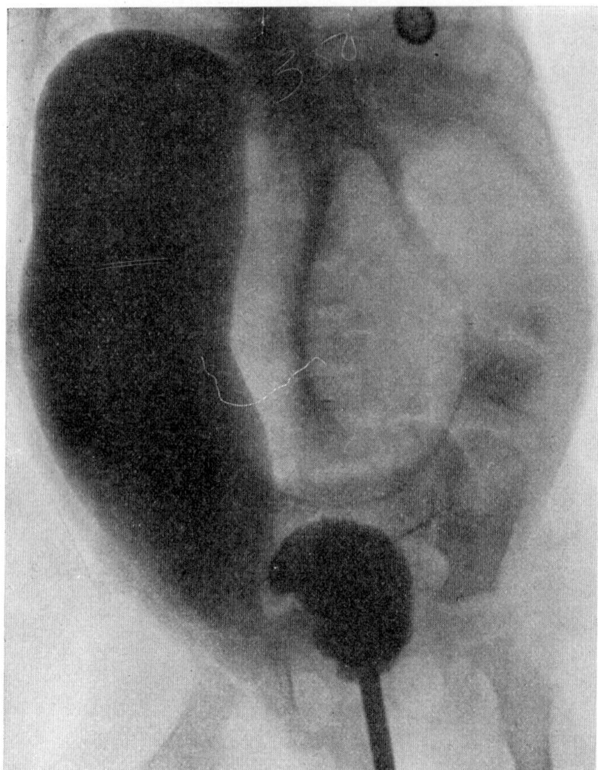

Fig. 141.—Roentgenogram of idiopathic dilatation of the colon. Boy of three years and four months. Girth 23 in. (57.5 cm.). Shows greatly distended colon partly filled with barium injected from the rectum.

Pathologic Anatomy.—The colon may be involved throughout, but much oftener the sigmoid flexure alone. Exceptionally the rectum and the lower portion of the ileum share in the dilatation, which is sometimes enormous (Fig. 141). There is usually also increase in the length of the colon, especially the sigmoid flexure. Hypertrophy of its wall, particularly of the muscular layer, is present in nearly all instances. The mesocolon may be longer or shorter than normal, and is sometimes thickened. In cases of long standing, inflammatory changes and even ulceration develop.

Symptoms.—These consist of obstinate constipation and of great dilatation of the colon (Figs. 142, 143). In the severer cases the constipation appears in the first few days of life. In others for some reason evidences of the disease come on more slowly, although still generally in the first three months of life, constipation being the first and dilatation developing later and increasing gradually. Occasionally dilatation has not appeared until the age of a year. Constipation is most obstinate, one or two weeks or more sometimes passing without a movement. Then under treatment an evacuation of enormous size takes place. The stools are rarely scybalous and may even be diarrheal, the difficulty of evacuation depending on the lack of expelling power. The degree of distention varies with the case, but is usually very great. In a child of two years and eleven months under our care, the girth

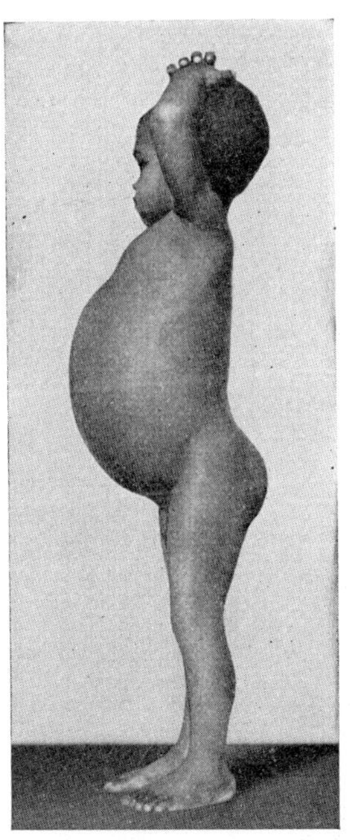

Fig. 142.

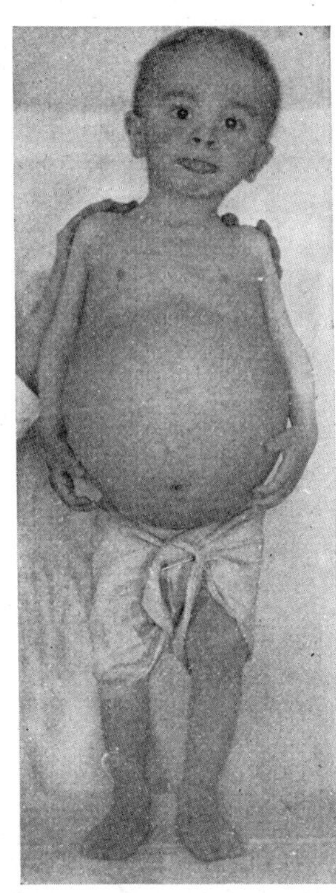

Fig. 143.

Fig. 142.—Idiopathic dilatation of the colon. Child of four years, patient at the Children's Hospital of Philadelphia. No discomfort in the abdomen, enlargement always present, constipation, maximum girth $27\frac{1}{4}$ in. (69.24 cm.).

Fig. 143.—Idiopathic dilatation of the colon. Child of two years and eleven months in the Children's Medical Ward of the Hospital of the University of Pennsylvania. Obstinate constipation from birth, sometimes a week without stool; distention. Began at five months. Maximum girth in hospital $28\frac{1}{2}$ in. (72.37). Right inguinal colotomy performed. Temporary relief was followed by failure of strength and death.

equalled $28\frac{1}{2}$ in. (72.37 cm.) (Fig. 143). The distention may be relieved to a considerable extent by a free evacuation of the bowels, yet not in every case. The health is liable gradually to suffer and emaciation to develop, but usually not for several years, and sometimes nutrition is only little affected. As a rule vomiting and pain are absent. Dyspnea may be produced by the pressure against the diaphragm. Peristaltic waves may be seen in the colon in cases without too much atony.

(*B*) Secondary Dilatation of the Colon.—The **etiology** of this condition varies. In some instances there is an intestinal stenosis or some other obstruction, either in the bowel itself or from without, as by the pressure of a tumor. Brennemann[131] reports 6 cases due to simple anorectal stricture. In other cases habitual constipation may finally be followed by dilatation, or an atonic state of the colon followed by dilatation may accompany tuberculous peritonitis, chronic indigestion, and debilitating diseases, as rickets.

The **symptoms** of secondary dilatation do not differ materially from those characteristic of the idiopathic variety. The distention in rachitis is not so great as in instances dependent upon other causes and is seldom productive of such obstinate constipation.

Course and Prognosis of Dilatation of the Colon.—The prognosis of congenital *idiopathic dilatation* is very unfavorable. Of our[117] 24 cases 18 were known to have died and in only 3 was recovery recorded. In 50 cases treated medically, collected by Löwenstein,[132] the mortality was 66 per cent while in 44 operated cases it was 48 per cent. In a later series of 110 cases subjected to surgical treatment, collected by Terry,[133] the mortality was 25 per cent. Ladd[128] reported on 118 cases. Of these 60 were treated medically with 41 deaths and 58 operated upon with 24 deaths. The majority of the patients rarely live to adult life. Most of them die before the age of five years of increasing inanition and debility, or some complication, as bronchopneumonia, cardiac failure, peritonitis from perforation, or chronic intestinal toxemia. There is not infrequently temporary slight improvement with recurrent exacerbations of the condition. The prognosis of the *secondary dilatation* following mechanical obstruction is unfavorable unless operative interference can effect a cure, although life may continue for years if the obstruction is not too great. That of dilatation associated with debilitated health depends upon the severity and the duration of the condition.

Diagnosis.—In idiopathic dilatation there is an absence of any discoverable obstruction, or evidence of previous bad health which might have produced intestinal atony. Secondary dilatation dependent upon rickets, chronic intestinal indigestion, or other debilitating disease, or upon tuberculous peritonitis, has a history and is associated with symptoms which usually make the recognition of the cause plain. The peristaltic waves of the congenital type are not found. Roentgenograms are occasionally helpful in differential diagnosis.

Treatment.—Cases in which the diagnosis of obstruction can be made demand operation; those the result of debility and digestive disturbance require treatment directed to these conditions. In idiopathic dilatation there should be employed massage of the abdomen, given gently since ulceration may be present; electricity; and measures for the improvement of the general health. With this may be combined the administration of strychnine. We have tried pituitrin without benefit. In all forms of dilatation the unloading of the bowel by purgatives and enemata is an unfortunate necessity. This should, however, be done as infrequently as possible, since it tends to weaken still more the muscular power of the colon; yet frequently enough to prevent overloading of the bowel and to allow the possibility for its contraction. Injections of large size are required, reaching well into the colon, and perhaps accompanied by abdominal massage. It has also been recommended to introduce a long, flexible tube into the rectum, leaving it in place for a day or more and repeating the procedure every few days. In anorectal stricture stretching and dilatation may be curative (Brennemann[131]). Puncture of the intestine with a small cannula has been practiced when the distention was great, but is a procedure attended by danger. The question of operative interference arises in all severe idiopathic cases which other treatment has failed to benefit. It should be done seasonably before weakness has become too great; but on the other hand the possibility for spontaneous recovery to occur should be permitted, inasmuch as the operation is in itself attended by decided danger to life. Resection of the colon is the usual procedure. The operation of lumbar sympathectomy was suggested by Bartle[134] and has been performed a number of times with satisfactory results and occasionally is followed by cure (Clarke and Miller[135]).

INTESTINAL OBSTRUCTION

A narrowing or complete obliteration of the lumen of the intestine, congenital or acquired, may occur in any portion of its course.

1. Congenital Stenosis or Atresia of the Small Intestine and Colon

Stenosis is found oftenest in the small intestine, and much less frequently in the colon. Davis and Poynter[136] in 1922 collected 401 instances of atresia of the intestine, not including the rectum. Baty[137] published 12 from the records of one hospital; and Webb and Wangenstein[138] estimated that about 450 cases of intestinal atresia had been reported. The duodenum is a portion of the gut involved with relative frequency, Garvin[139] finding 113 recorded cases of congenital duodenal occlusion or stenosis, and Kaldor[140] bringing this number up to 250. Good reviews of the literature are given by deSanctis and Craig[141] and by Weber.[142] We have records of 6 personal cases, in one of which torsion was present, while in 2 the occlusion was membranous. Garvin[139] intimates that there are from 35 to 40 reported cases of duodenal occlusion of this membranous sort. Other regions of the small intestine may be involved; sometimes one part, sometimes several. The lesion varies from a mere narrowing to, more commonly, complete atresia, and this may vary from involvement of a very small portion of the tube up to substitution of the entire small intestine by a fibrous cord. In some cases the portions above and below the affected region end blindly, the intervening portion having entirely disappeared. The intestine above an obstruction is much distended, that below is collapsed. Malformations elsewhere in the body may accompany the intestinal deformity.

Etiology.—The cause of congenital stenosis depends upon some pathological process or developmental defect arising during fetal life. Among those possible are fetal volvulus, peritonitis dependent upon syphilis or tuberculosis, intestinal ulceration, constriction by bands, arrested development, fetal intussusception, and constriction at the umbilical ring. In some instances obstruction is produced through pressure by a tumor, or constriction by a Meckel's diverticulum, or in other ways.

Symptoms.—These appear within a few hours after birth in obstruction high in the gut; somewhat later when it is lower. In atresia or great stenosis they consist of obstinate vomiting, colicky pain, complete constipation except for a few early mucous discharges, and distention of the abdomen, the seat and degree of this last depending to some extent upon the situation of the malformation. It occupies generally the umbilical region, leaving the flanks flattened. When the obstruction is in the duodenum or high in the jejunum there is distention in the epigastrium accompanied by visible gastric peristalsis. The higher the malformation is in the intestine, the sooner does vomiting begin. It may eventually be fecal if the obstruction is low. The general condition of the child is very serious. The face is pinched, the urine scanty or suppressed, there may be dyspnea from pressure of the gas against the diaphragm, and the temperature is low. If the intestinal stenosis is not complete, the symptoms are less severe.

Course and Prognosis.—The prognosis is always grave. Death results from collapse, asthenia, convulsions, or rupture of the bowel; the last particularly in low obstruction. In nearly all cases of high obstruction death occurs in less than a week; very occasionally not before several weeks or even months, if the intestinal stenosis has been less complete. In rare instances where the obstruction is but slight, as shown by necropsy, the patient has lived for some years and even reached adult life.

Diagnosis.—In stenosis of the *esophagus* the food is vomited almost at once, and the esophageal sound or the roentgenological examination will reveal the obstruction. *Pyloric stenosis* shows gastric peristalsis; a pyloric tumor may often be felt; distention is confined to the epigastrium; and the vomitus never contains bile as it does when the obstruction is below the ampulla of Vater. The course of the disease is more prolonged and the symptoms less severe than in cases of complete intestinal obstruction. In stenosis of the lower *ileum* or *colon* the vomiting is late in appearing and is eventually fecal. In all these conditions roentgenological studies may be of diagnostic value and may show the distended bowel and its location even when barium has not been given. *Idiopathic dilatation of the colon* cannot be differentiated with certainty from some of the rare instances of a moderate congenital stenosis of the colon. Stenosis of the *rectum* may be detected by local examination. The early and rapid development of the symptoms distinguishes congenital stenosis from most acquired forms.

The **treatment** is surgical. Operation should be done as promptly as possible. The results of this at the early age have been unpromising, yet correctible defects are sometimes found or anastomotic procedures can be performed.

2. Congenital Stenosis or Atresia of the Rectum or Anus

This is the most frequent variety of congenital intestinal obstruction, although still uncommon. Atresia is more common than stenosis. The developmental fault is failure of proper union between the infolding skin and the bowel. Most frequently there is complete closure of the anus with entirely normal intestine above this. In a second form the anus is closed and the rectum above it exhibits a varying extent of atresia. In a third variety the anus and the part of the rectum immediately above it are normal but are separated by a membrane from the patulous rectum farther up, and the presence of an accumulation of fecal matter beyond the separating membrane can sometimes be detected by the palpating finger introduced into the anus. Any one of the forms may be combined with anomalous communication with the vagina, bladder, or urethra, or exhibit a fistula into the perineum or elsewhere. Malformations in other regions of the body may also be present.

The **symptoms** are those of intestinal obstruction situated elsewhere, but coming on later than in this latter condition. Inspection or digital exploration of the anal and rectal region will disclose the malformation. Operation should be done as early as possible. This is easy where there is merely an occlusion of the anus or an obstruction of the rectum by thin membrane. Where, however, the rectum is obliterated to any extent an artificial anus must be made for temporary relief, leaving for a later period the more difficult plastic operation which will connect the rectal cul-de-sac with the anal region.

3. Acquired Intestinal Obstruction

This may be due to various **causes.** At any time of life there may be strangulation from a Meckel's diverticulum or a fibrous cord constituting its remainder. Congenital fibrous bands produced in other ways, as by a fetal peritonitis, and variously situated, may compress or even strangle the intestine; or it may be caught in retroperitoneal recesses or in abnormal openings in the mesentery. This may happen at any time of life. Volvulus may uncommonly occur in early life. We have seen it in an infant of two weeks of age; Ravdin[143] reports it in an infant thirty-six hours old; and Bruce[144] in one of fifteen days. Later in life peritonitis may cause obstruction, either by the production of fibrous bands, as seen especially in tuberculous peritonitis, or by paralysis of peristalsis and the accumulation of fecal matter. Appendicitis acts in a similar manner. Among other causes are foreign bodies in the intestine; inspissated meconium in the new-born; tumors of the bowel or pressing on it; rarely masses of ascarides in the intestine (Doberauer;[145] Perret and Simon;[146] Hoffmann[147]); and fecal concretions and incarcerated hernias. By far the most frequent agent in childhood is intussusception.

The **symptoms** usually develop suddenly and are similar to those described in congenital cases. Frequently the cause of the obstruction is in doubt until operation. Intussusception and hernia will receive separate consideration.

The cause of the toxic symptoms is a matter of dispute. It is known that there occurs, especially in high obstruction, an increase in the non-protein nitrogenous constituents in, and a concentration of, the blood, a fall in blood chlorides, and an alkalosis. This could be explained upon the basis of dehydration and consequent failure of renal excretion, upon the loss of chloride by vomiting, and the loss of electrolytes into the accumulated fluid in the bowel (Cooke, Rodenbaugh and Whipple;[148] Whipple and Cooke;[149] Haden and Orr;[150] Gamble and McIver;[151] McIver and Gamble;[152] Gatch, Trusler and Ayers;[153] Trusler,[154] and others). It has also been suggested that the absorption of a toxic body of the nature of histamin or of the class of proteoses, produced in the bowel or in the strangulated portion, might be responsible for some of the symptoms (Whipple, Stone and Bernheim;[155] Sweet, Peet and Hendrix;[156] Dragstedt et al,[157] and others). Proof of this or of the actual nature of the toxic body is lacking. Dehydration and loss of chloride would explain many of the symptoms, and it would seem likely that in certain cases, as those with strangulation and gangrene, the absorption of toxic bodies might also enter into the picture. The studies by Guest, Andrus, and their coworkers[158] indicate that in obstruction with strangulation the action is not that of a specific intoxication, but that histamin-like substances are absorbed and produce increased secretion of gastric juice, and therefore by vomiting its increased loss.

The **prognosis** depends upon the age of the patient the condition at operation, and the possibility of removal of the cause.

INTUSSUSCEPTION

Etiology.—This is one of the frequent forms of intestinal obstruction in children. Over ½ the cases occur in the first year of life and most of the remainder in the second, as shown by the statistics of Pilz,[159] Hess,[160] Kock and Oerum,[161] Harper,[162] and others. The condition is 2 to 3 times more common in males. In most instances it develops in those in perfect health, and is supposedly favored by the unusual mobility of the cecum and ileum and the hyperperistalsis which obtain in early life. Among predisposing factors sometimes operative are diarrhea; constipation; colic; abnormal conditions of Meckel's diverticulum (Griffith[163]); invagination of the appendix (Monsarrat,[164] Corner[165]); abdominal injuries; hemorrhage into or ulceration of the gut; foreign bodies, large fecal masses, or parasites in its lumen; polypi, papilloma or other tumors of the bowel (Lamb[166]); and swelling of the lymphatic tissue of the intestinal wall. These commonly act by producing an irregular hyperperistalsis occurring at the time of the expulsion of the feces. *Agonal intussusception,* encountered frequently in infancy, is caused by the irregular peristalsis which precedes death.

Pathology and Pathologic Anatomy.—The condition consists in an invagination of one portion of the intestine into another. The invagination is descending in form, an ascending invagination being very rare, except when agonal. The upper portion, the *intussusceptum,* slips into the lower, the *intussuscipiens,* pulling the mesentery with it. The intussusception thus consists of three thicknesses of intestinal wall, two mucous surfaces being in apposition, and two serous likewise (Fig. 144). The dragging upon the mesentery makes the intestine assume a curved, sausage-shaped form, with the concavity toward the mesenteric attachment to the spinal column. Although the bowel can remain patulous and the circulation of blood in it be preserved, this is usually not the case, but swelling promptly begins as a result of compression of the blood-vessels. This produces complete intestinal obstruction; incarceration of the intussusception, which later becomes irreducible through the adhesive inflammation between the adjacent serous surfaces; and finally strangulation with death of the part. In the fortunate cases the strangulated portion may become entirely separated by gangrene and discharged through the anus, and the lumen of the gut become reëstablished. The intussusception does not, however, become irreducible through adhesive inflammation for several days. The intestine above the intussusception is generally dilated; that below it contracted. Agonal intussusception shows no evidence of inflammation or swelling, and is without clinical significance.

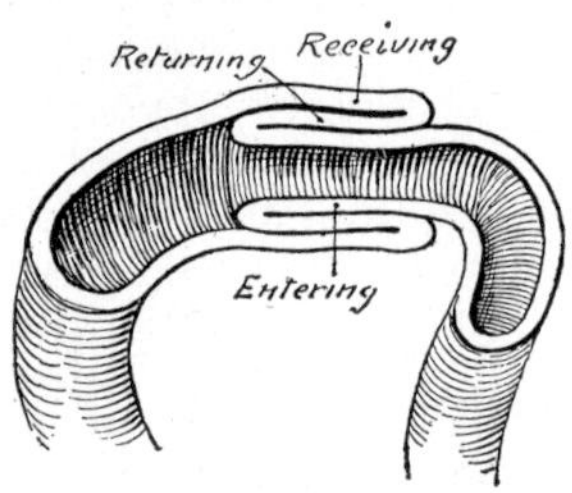

Fig. 144.—Diagrammatic representation of the production of intussusception. (*Kemp, Diseases of the Stomach, Intestines and Pancreas.*)

Intussusceptions are classified according to their situation:

1. Ileac (enteric) intussusception affects the small intestine in any part, and usually this only. It is less often seen than some other forms in early life, but is one of the more common after the period of childhood. This does not apply to the *agonal* variety which involves as many as from 6 to 12 different positions in the small intestine, being most frequent in the jejunum.

2. Colic intussusception may affect any part of the colon. It is one of the more common varieties, yet not as often seen as the ileocecal.

3. Ileocolic intussusception exhibits invagination of the ileum through the ileocecal valve. The cecum may then be invaginated secondarily, but the ileum remains as the most prominent protruding portion. This is the least frequent variety of intussusception.

4. Ileocecal intussusception is the form oftenest seen, and the younger the child the more likely is the invagination to be of this sort. In this the cecum with the ileum behind it passes into the colon, the valve continuing to be the apex of the projecting portion.

The relative statistical frequency of these different forms has been ably discussed by Leichenstern[167] and by Kock and Oerum.[161] Besides these types mixed forms of various sorts may occasionally occur, including double intussusception which is observed in less than 10 per cent of cases (Corner[165]). As time passes the intussusception of all varieties is prone to increase in size, the apex always remaining unchanged and the intussuscipiens invaginating more and more. As a result the ileocecal form may finally occupy all of the rectum, and the apex of the intussusception nearly reach the anus or even pass through it.

Symptoms.—In typical cases there is sudden onset with severe pain, vomiting, restlessness, and great prostration. The face is pinched, the eyes sunken, the pulse feeble and rapid, the urine scanty, the temperature normal or subnormal. The abdomen is at first soft; later distended and often tender. The fecal matter present in the colon and rectum is evacuated during the first day, but after this fecal movements are very small or oftener entirely absent, and little if any gas is passed by the bowel. Pain comes on in paroxysms, attended by straining efforts if the intussusception has reached the rectum, and by the frequent passage of small quantities of blood-stained mucus or even of blood in considerable amount. Blood generally appears in the first twelve hours, but sometimes not for one or two days. This condition of the bowel-movements is one of the most characteristic, but may be wanting in some cases. Absolute failure of evacuation of fecal matter and of gas is most common in enteric invagination in which, too, hemorrhage from the bowel may be later in appearing, or absent entirely. Vomiting is a less prominent symptom than in other forms of intestinal obstruction. It is usually worse at the beginning, or it may sometimes occur only a few times daily. It is most marked in enteric intussusception. Stercoraceous vomiting is seen in only a small proportion of cases, and generally not until late. The pain is sometimes intensely severe and causes loud outcries, or it may be evidenced only by the grunting sounds which attend the accompanying tenesmus. It is usually most intense early in the attack. In children old enough to describe it, it may be localized on the right side in the region of the beginning intussusception, or about the umbilicus. A tumor is discoverable in the majority of instances if examined before great distension has occurred. It may often be found very early in the disease, even on the first day, and may reach the anus by the second day, although usually later than this. It can very frequently be felt in the rectum even sometimes on the first day, and gives to the finger a sensation very like that of the vaginal portion of the uterus. Abdominal palpation reveals it on the left side in over one-half the cases, and in about one-third it may be discovered by rectal examination. During the paroxysm of pain rectal palpation shows the tumor temporarily increasing in size and approaching nearer to the anus. When protruding from the anus it may have the appearance of a rectal prolapse, or a polypus or hemorrhoid.

The symptoms described are those characteristic of most acute cases. At times, however, many symptoms are so little marked that the disease may be overlooked, if sufficient attention is not paid to the condition of the bowel-movements and the discovery of a tumor. Occasionally cases are more subacute in nature, the onset being more gradual, the pain and vomiting less severe, and constipation less complete. Yet other exceptional cases, well described by Still,[168] Beaven,[169] and others, and chiefly observed in children past the period of infancy, are of a more chronic nature, in which the occlusion is not complete and the circulation in the mesentery not entirely shut off. There is little pain or vomiting, no definite intestinal symptoms, and no bloody, mucous movements. Diarrhea may replace constipation. The symptoms may come in separate attacks, and suggest recurrences of catarrh of the large intestine. The general condition of the patient may suffer little, or there may be a gradual loss of strength, or symptoms of strangulation may suddenly occur.

Course and Prognosis.—If reduction has been accomplished, the tumor can no longer be felt, and all symptoms rapidly disappear. If this has not taken place the course of the disease is progressively onward to a fatal issue. A few exceptions are seen in which spontaneous reduction occurs, or in which gangrene and subsequent discharge of the invaginated bowel take place. Cicatricial stenosis may develop later in such instances.

Death is the result generally of the shock which the intestinal lesion produces. In the more subacute cases it follows from increasing exhaustion, sometimes with a final rise of temperature. Death from peritonitis is not common. The average duration of acute unoperated fatal cases ranges from one day up to two or three weeks. Chronic cases may last for months.

There is often seen a disposition for the intussusception to *relapse*, perhaps several times after successful reduction. This takes place with greatest frequency on the first day after reduction has been accomplished, but may be much delayed.

The *prognosis* is always grave especially in acute cases, although less so than formerly. The younger the patient the more serious the condition. Untreated cases are nearly always fatal. The probability of recovery varies, too, directly in proportion to the quickness with which the diagnosis is made and treatment instituted. In general it may be stated that the mortality of patients operated on the first day is about 35 per cent, by the second day 40 per cent, and rising rapidly to 75 per cent by the sixth day. In cases treated without operation the mortality is higher, according to most statistics.

Diagnosis.—The cardinal diagnostic symptoms are the sudden development of abdominal pain, vomiting, tenesmus and bloody stools without fecal matter, prostration, and absence of fever. Too much dependence, however, must not be placed upon the presence or absence of these symptoms. The diagnosis is made certain only by the discovery of a tumor. The bloody, mucous movements may be mistaken for *colitis.* Conversely colitis may be supposed to be intussusception, and operation urged accordingly. The earlier occurrence of diarrhea and the presence of fecal matter and especially fever, aid in the recognition of the inflammatory disorder. *Henoch's purpura,* if producing hemorrhage into the lumen and walls of the intestine, may strongly suggest intussusception, but the evidences of purpura elsewhere aid in distinguishing it. It is possible for purpura to be attended by intussusception. The protruding of an intussusception from the rectum, accompanied by straining and the passing of mucus, may sometimes strongly resemble *prolapse of the rectum.* As stated, the discovery of a tumor usually removes doubt, but as this is sometimes difficult, especially through the abdominal wall, in all uncertain cases a careful examination should be made under anesthesia. Enteric intussusception seldom has a discoverable tumor and there is no tenesmus, and these cases cannot with certainty be distinguished from instances of acute intestinal obstruction from other causes. It is to be remembered also that *appendicitis* is attended by the development of a tumor and often by constipation. There are, however, very rarely bloody stools and tenesmus, and the tumor occupies usually the region of the cecum, is more superficial, and of a different shape. *Meckel's diverticulitis* has the same distinguishing features as appendicitis, except that it not uncommonly is attended by bloody stools.

Even without the administration of barium roentgenograms may be of value by demonstrating the gaseous distension of the bowel (Guillaume[170]). If the picture is taken when the patient is erect the fluid level of the intestinal contents, and consequently the level of the obstruction, may be recognized (Kalbfleish[171]).

Treatment.—As soon as the diagnosis is made in cases which have lasted only one or two days it is possible to make efforts to reduce the intussusception by other than surgical measures. If this is determined upon the child should be anesthetized, the hips elevated, and the patient now and then held inverted. Injections should meanwhile be given of air, water, or oil. Air may be injected from a bulb-syringe or hand-bellows attached to a catheter. The anus must be compressed around the tube by the fingers, and the injection given slowly and carefully. In place of this, oil, or a warm normal saline solution, may be employed. The liquid should be in a fountain syringe which may be elevated not over 6 ft. (173 cm.) above the bed on which the child lies; the pressure being maintained for fifteen or twenty minutes. If successful, a rumbling sound can sometimes be heard; the tumor entirely disappears; the distention produced by the gas or liquid employed ceases to exist; the aspect of the child improves; vomiting stops; and a fecal stool may shortly occur. If unsuccessful, or if the result is uncertain, the liquid or air must be allowed to escape and the procedure tried once again. Retan[172] and Stephens[173] describe a method in which a barium enema is given and pressure made over the abdomen, the result being observed under the fluoroscope. Monard[174] favors a method with abdominal manipulation followed by injections of water, to be used for infants under two years of age and in early cases. The mortality was only 14 per cent with this procedure in 84 patients.

If there is no success with "medical reduction," operative aid must be had *immediately*, and the intussusception found and reduction accomplished by withdrawing the invaginated portion, if this is possible. In fact, owing to the frequent impossibility of determining accurately whether reduction has been accomplished, or of knowing what may be the condition of the intestinal wall, it is safer to regard all cases as purely surgical, and to proceed at once with operation for reduction, without attempting any medical treatment; and this is now the generally accepted course. In cases coming late to operation adhesion and swelling may prevent reduction; or the condition of the bowel may be such that enterostomy is necessary, and either an artificial anus must be made, or a resection of the intestine performed. Chronic cases are best treated by operation.

On account of the danger of recurrence of the trouble after either mechanical or operative reduction, peristalsis should be quieted as far as possible by small, repeated doses of an opiate. A purgative should never be administered. Shock and dehydration must be combated. This is best done by intravenous injections of normal saline and glucose solutions. (See p. 198.) A useful solution for this purpose is one containing 1 per cent of sodium chloride and 10 per cent of dextrose.

HERNIA

Hernia in children is of several varieties. Those deserving special mention are: (1) umbilical; (2) inguinal; (3) diaphragmatic, and (4) ventral. Of these the umbilical and inguinal are far the most frequent. Femoral hernia is so uncommon that further reference need not be made to it. The rare internal hernias other than the diaphragmatic will also be omitted. Some interesting statistics are given by Patterson and Gray,[175] who in 130,243 children up to five years of age found hernia in 1018, viz: 0.8 per cent. Of these 773 were inguinal and 214 umbilical; no femoral.

1. Umbilical Hernia

Hernia of the intestine at the umbilicus may be either (*A*) congenital or (*B*) acquired.

(*A*) Congenital Umbilical Hernia (*Hernia into the Cord*).—This is a very uncommon condition; of which we can recall seeing not more than 3 instances. Lindfors[176] in 20,735 births found it present in the ratio of 1:5184. The hernia forms a tumor, oval, round or conical in shape, and of the size of a walnut up to that of an orange or larger. The sac appears to be composed of the distended umbilical cord, its walls consisting only of peritoneum and of the amnion of the cord, and being of a greenish-white color and transparent character. The contents are usually coils of intestine, but sometimes the stomach, the spleen, Meckel's diverticulum, or all or part of the liver may be found in it. The color of these is readily distinguishable through the sac-wall. The size and tension of the mass increase with crying or coughing. The hernia can sometimes be reduced, sometimes not; and when of small size recovery may take place spontaneously with the process of the separation of the cord; reactive inflammation developing and leaving a cicatrix, but no navel. The **prognosis** is grave, and spontaneous healing is not common, but rather peritonitis, gangrene, or general sepsis develop. By far the larger proportion of patients died until the operative treatment was introduced and perfected, and even still the mortality is high. In the case of very large hernia, with the presence in the sac of a considerable portion of the abdominal contents, the continuance of the child's life is scarcely possible. In instances collected by Lotheissen[177] the mortality in 68 operated cases was 29.4 per cent, and in 23 unoperated cases 65.22 per cent. Somewhat similar statistics are given by Safford.[178] Sometimes the sac breaks during birth, leaving the child partly eviscerated. Often other malformations are present or the infants are premature or still-born. The **diagnosis** is readily made except in the case of small cylindrical hernias into the cord. Every child born with the cord decidedly swollen close to the body should be examined very carefully before a ligature is applied. **Treatment** consists, first of all, in the greatest care in handling a congenital hernia and in the use of every possible antiseptic precaution. The child must not be lifted into an upright position until the wound has completely cicatrized.

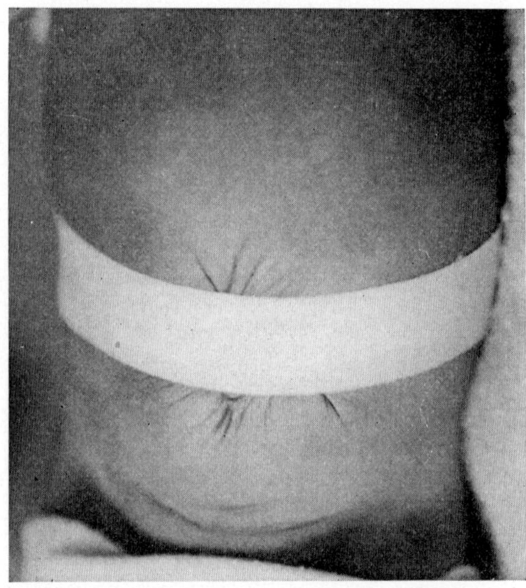

Fig. 145.—Umbilical hernia with adhesive strap applied in such a way that the folded skin closes the opening.

A much more successful plan of treatment, however, applicable also to the small, reducible hernias, is the performing of a radical operation a few hours after birth, and without any previous efforts at reduction having been made.

(*B*) Acquired Umbilical Hernia.—This is a common and seldom serious affection. It develops generally in the first few months of life, and oftenest in thin subjects, or those with flatulent distention from indigestion or other causes, or who cry greatly. The hernia appears oftenest as a small elastic tumor covered with skin, not sensitive to pressure, varying in bulk from a simple convexity of the navel to a tumor the size of a small marble, or occasionally larger, and globular or irregular in shape according to the width and form of the opening. It is always reducible unless the child is crying or straining. Strangulation very rarely occurs. The hernia consists of small intestine which protrudes through a portion of the umbilical ring, and is covered by the abdominal parietes. The **prognosis** is almost entirely favorable. The majority of cases will recover spontaneously if such causes as continuous abdominal distention or persistent straining efforts be removed. Preventive **treatment** is important. A firm compress should be worn under the abdominal band for the first few months, and all conditions liable to produce hernia should be removed. If a hernia is present it should be kept constantly reduced until the opening in the abdominal wall has had time to close. It is quite sufficient to cleanse the skin thoroughly and then draw it into two folds, one on each side of the hernia and meeting over it; holding these in place by straps of adhesive plaster crossing over the navel, or by a broad horizontal band of adhesive plaster reaching to the lumbar regions (Fig. 145). A little boric acid may well be powdered upon the navel before the plaster is applied. The dressing should be worn constantly, changing it from time to time as the old one loosens, and the hernia must not be allowed to protrude during the process of changing. The plaster must not be removed during the bath. From three to six months or more are required before the opening is permanently closed. The plaster sometimes produces considerable cutaneous irritation, especially in the first few months of life. In this event its application may be deferred for a while, and a closely fitting woollen or webbing bandage applied. In no case should any apparatus be used with a rounded surface which pushes the hernia inward, since this keeps the umbilical ring open.

In children older than a year the treatment described is usually unsuccessful, but it may, however, be tried. If cure is not progressing after several months, a radical operation is indicated.

2. Inguinal Hernia

This is much less frequent than umbilical hernia in the first few weeks of life, but more common when developing after this period. It may be congenital or acquired. The great majority of the acquired cases depend, however, on favoring conditions which are congenital in nature; viz. a patulous state of the funicular process of the peritoneum through which the testicle descends; the shortness and straightness of the canal, and the width of the inner ring. Omitting, then, the truly acquired hernia of later childhood, which is less often seen, we may divide the hernias of infancy into (*a*) **congenital hernia of the tunica vaginalis,** in which the funicular process of the peritoneum is completely open and the intestine descends to and often surrounds the testicle; (*b*) **funicular hernia,** in which the tunica vaginalis is closed above the testicle and the intestine fills the funicular process down to this closure, the intestine in this variety not enveloping the testicle; (*c*) **encysted or infantile hernia,** a rare form in which the internal ring has closed but the intestine pushes down a pouch of peritoneum to the side of this or into the patulous funicular process below the ring. Except for the anatomical differences mentioned, these various forms cannot with certainty be distinguished from each other unless at operation.

Etiology.—Apart from the anatomical causes mentioned, age is a strongly predisposing factor, the majority of cases in infancy occurring in the first year of life, but sometimes not until later, and sometimes seen immediately after birth. Heredity, too, plays some part. The great majority of instances are met with in boys. Distention of the abdomen by gas, excessive crying or coughing, straining at stool the result of diarrheal disturbances, the straining on urination caused by excessive phimosis or urinary concretions, impairment of the general health, and similar conditions may constitute the final active cause.

Symptoms.—The rupture is oftener situated on the right side, but not infrequently is double. The contents of the sac consist usually of small intestine only, perhaps with omentum; while sometimes the cecum occupies the sac, or rarely a Meckel's diverticulum, and occasionally an ovary. In a considerable number of cases the appendix is found within the hernial sac, either alone or with other portions of the intestinal tract (Jopson[179]). Reduction is generally easier than in adult cases, as the hernia is usually smaller and adhesions have not formed. It is only occasionally that a large rupture fills the scrotum (Fig. 146).

Prognosis.—Complete recovery usually follows the early application of a suitable truss; or if this does not succeed, operation gives excellent results. Strangulation is comparatively uncommon in early life. It is seen oftener in the first two years than in childhood after that period. Estor,[180] estimates that the likelihood of the development of this as compared with that of adults is only in the ratio of 1:131. Strangulation according to Moynihan[181] is more prone to occur in the first three months than after that period during the first year.

Diagnosis.—The only difficulty in diagnosis is in distinguishing the lesion from *hydrocele*. Hernia is usually opaque with transmitted light, and hydrocele translucent; but this is open to exceptions and hernia may also

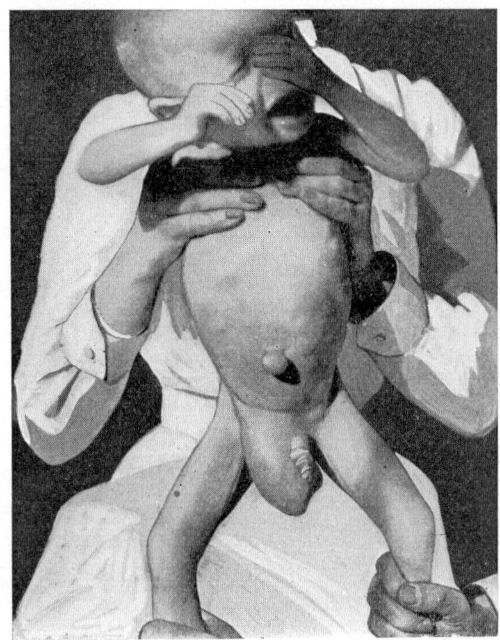

Fig. 146.—Large inguinal hernia. Infant of fourteen months, in the Children's Hospital of Philadelphia. Shows also small umbilical hernia.

sometimes appear translucent, if bowel only is present and is distended by gas without fecal matter. Hydrocele is dull on percussion and reduces slowly and often not at all. Hernia gives an impulse on coughing and reduces more quickly and often with the characteristic gurgling sound. The difficulty in diagnosis is increased by the fact that a hydrocele may occupy the tunica vaginalis and a hernia of the cord be situated immediately above this. Strangulation may in exceptional cases be readily confounded with severe *colic* unless the possibility of this occurrence is borne is mind and a systematic examination made. We have seen this error made.

Treatment.—This is very satisfactory, in that the majority of cases will recover completely under the application of a suitable truss and the removal of the exciting causes. A truss of hard rubber or a skein of woolen yarn must be worn constantly, and the mother impressed with the importance of never allowing the hernia to descend. The skin under the truss must be kept dry and clean. The constant wearing of a truss, applied soon after birth, will sometimes cure a rupture in three months, but even should this occur the truss should be worn as a precautionary measure for two years or perhaps longer.

3. Diaphragmatic Hernia

A distinction may be made between diaphragmatic hernia and diaphragmatic defect, both of them uncommon in children. In the former only the muscular layer of the diaphragm is wanting, and a layer of peritoneum and of pleura cover the herniating viscus. In true defect there is a complete absence of all the diaphragmatic tissue at the position of the opening. Not strictly speaking a hernia, yet similar in its results in that the abdominal viscera enter more or less into the thoracic cavity, is the condition properly designated **eventration,** in which there is a weakness and ballooning of one-half of the diaphragm. We have encountered 3 instances of this in infants born by breech delivery, who had apparently suffered from a birth-injury of the phrenic nerve in association with one of the cervical plexus, and these have been reported by Epstein,[182] Zeligs[183] and others. (See p. 982.) Hernia may also occur through the esophageal hiatus (Rito[184]). For practical purposes these various conditions may be denominated hernia and described together.

Omitting those cases which result from severe trauma, as from wounds of the diaphragm, diaphragmatic hernia is generally congenital; and even in the occasional acquired cases seems then dependent upon an already existing congenital lesion of the diaphragm. It is about 10 times as frequent on the left side as on the right. In well-marked cases the stomach and a large portion of the intestine have entered the thoracic cavity, with displacement of the lungs and heart, and with an abnormal sinking in of the abdominal walls. The percussion-note in the thorax is tympanitic, and the respiratory murmur absent. There are also dyspnea, cyanosis, and vomiting and other digestive disturbances. A roentgen-ray study will make the diagnosis clear. Occasionally subjects of this condition live until adult years, but more frequently life terminates in the first year, often within a few hours after birth, or death follows incarceration or strangulation with the usual manifestations. The prognosis as to the duration of life has been statistically reviewed by Latta.[185] Other general reviews are those by Hedblom,[186] Unger and Speiser,[187] Tuscherer,[188] and Greenwald and Steiner.[189] There is no treatment possible except an operative procedure, and this is not likely to be of avail, being especially difficult in large defects. According to Truesdale[190] the total reported number of patients operated on under ten years of age is 22, with a mortality of 41 per cent.

4. Ventral Hernia

This is not a very common form of hernia. It consists in the protrusion of a small portion of intestine either through a defect in the median line of the abdominal wall or in the lumbar region (*lumbar hernia*). The former is always small, sometimes multiple and is usually accompanied by umbilical hernia. The rare lumbar hernia may reach a much greater size. Treatment in either case is very similar to that recommended for umbilical hernia.

INTESTINAL ULCERATION

Reference is made elsewhere to various causes of ulceration in the intestinal tract, and only a few forms will be considered here in more detail.

1. Duodenal Ulcer

The round peptic ulcer, similar in method of production to the gastric ulcer, while uncommon in children, is more frequent than formerly supposed.

Theile[191] in an exhaustive review of the subject, collected 248 cases of gastro-duodenal ulceration, with 119 gastric, 125 duodenal, and 4 unstated. Schmidt[192] found duodenal ulcer in 1.9 per cent of 1109 necropsies on infants in the first year of life, and in 0.6 per cent of 2715 necropsies on older children. We[193] have elsewhere reported cases and reviewed the literature, and others have since published case-reports and reviews (Holt,[194] Veeder,[195] Bosányi,[196] Paterson,[197] Wright,[198] Kennedy,[199] Dickey[200]).

Among the assigned causes are thrombosis of a blood-vessel with subsequent auto-digestion of the mucous membrane, infectious processes of different sorts, and extensive cutaneous ulceration. Gerdine and Helmholz[201] believe that the disease may occur epidemically and be dependent upon the action of the streptococcus viridans. The lesion is oftenest seen in atrophic infants in the first year, especially between the ages of two and five months, and not unusually in relation with earlier digestive disorders. We have seen it, however, without previous digestive disturbance, the first symptom being bloody stools. It is relatively frequent in the new-born and constitutes a cause of melena. The ulcer is oftenest single, although two or more are not infrequently observed; possesses sharply defined edges, as in gastric ulcer; and is situated generally on the posterior wall of the duodenum and above the papilla. It may involve only the mucous membrane, or may extend to the serous layer and even perforate. Sometimes ulcers may be small and readily concealed by a fold of mucous membrane.

Symptoms.—In a large proportion of cases, these are entirely lacking and the condition is purely a post-mortem finding. In others there may be a sudden fatal collapse, indicating the possibility of a concealed hemorrhage or an intestinal perforation, but without such a diagnosis being possible. Melena in the new-born may, as stated, be due to duodenal ulceration, but there is usually no possibility of determining this with certainty, and the majority of cases of melena are probably not produced in this way, although Kennedy[202] regards duodenal ulcer as the usual cause. The only true suggestive symptoms indicating duodenal ulceration are hematemesis and the passage of blood by stool. The blood may be in large amount and bright-red, or appear as coffee-ground vomiting and as tarry evacuations. In older children there may exceptionally be pain and tenderness in the region of the duodenum just below the liver to the right of the median line. In a number of instances the symptoms have suggested pyloric stenosis, depending probably upon pylorospasm produced by a reflex irritation from an ulcer just below the pylorus. Such cases have been reported by Finney,[203] Torday,[204] Potter,[205] and others.

The **prognosis** is uncertain. Death may result promptly from hemorrhage, or a temporary improvement of symptoms may be followed by relapse. Recovery is probably not of frequent occurrence. A very real danger is that of perforation with death from collapse, or from subsequent peritonitis.

The **diagnosis** can be made only provisionally. The preponderance of the passage of blood by the bowel over hematemesis is suggestive. Careful exclusion must be made of entrance of blood into the stomach and intestine from outside sources, as from the nose or mouth or the nipple of the mother. In older children roentgenograms may show a characteristic appearance.

Treatment.—This consists in efforts to check hemorrhage or to prevent recurrence. (See Gastric hemorrhage, p. 566; Gastric ulcer, p. 566.)

2. Tuberculous Ulceration

(Tuberculosis of the Intestine)

Tuberculosis may be primary in the intestine, but is usually secondary to lesions in the lungs, and is nearly always combined with involvement of the mesenteric lymph-nodes. It may occur at any period of early life, but is most frequent in early childhood, yet less common than other forms of tuberculosis at this time. (See also Tuberculosis, p. 411.)

Pathologic Anatomy.—The lesions may be widely spread, but are located chiefly in the small intestine, especially the ileum near the ileocecal valve. Early in their course they consist of miliary nodules, but later these break down and form small erosions, and, by coalescence, large ulcers. The tuberculous ulcer is of irregular shape, with infiltrated edges which project above the level of the surrounding mucous membrane, while miliary tubercles cover the bottom. The largest diameter is usually transverse to the canal of the intestine. The smaller ulcers show a loss of mucous membrane only; the larger ones penetrate the submucous tissue as well, and even to, or sometimes through, the serous layer. If the case is long-continued some ulcers exhibit cicatricial changes, and a resulting contraction of the intestine at this position. Perforation is uncommon, because of involvement by the tuberculous process of the peritoneum adjacent to the ulcer, and consequent formation of adhesions.

Symptoms.—These are not characteristic, in the early stages. Small tuberculous ulcers frequently produce no symptoms whatever and are discovered only at necropsy. In other instances the symptoms are those of ileocolitis. That the lesions are tuberculous in such cases may be suspected from the chronicity of the case, and from the association of undoubted evidences of the infection elsewhere in the body, especially in the lungs. The stools are liable to be more watery than in ileocolitis, offensive, and to contain more or less blood, especially in older children. Abdominal distention and tenderness may be present; there is irregular fever; wasting is often great; anemia and debility decided; appetite is diminished; the pulse weak, and the abdomen tympanitic. In advanced cases the symptoms of tuberculous peritonitis are often present also, or deep palpation may reveal enlargement of the mesenteric lymphatic nodes.

Course and Prognosis.—The disease may run an irregular course and last for months, with a constantly increasing loss of health, or with temporary periods of improvement, diarrhea perhaps alternating with constipation. Although recovery is probably possible it is certainly very uncommon, and the majority of patients with the disease gradually fail in health and die from exhaustion, often with a terminal marantic edema. In other cases death may occur from some complication, such as profuse hemorrhage, peritonitis, or tuberculosis of some other region.

Diagnosis.—This depends chiefly upon the presence of tuberculosis elsewhere in the body, and the very slow development of symptoms. Discovery of tubercle bacilli in the stools means little, since these are present in patients whose sputum contains them. The occurrence of diarrhea in evidently tuberculous subjects is not positive proof that ulceration exists. Acute ileocolitis has a more sudden onset and a shorter course, and the chronic form gives often the history of an earlier acute attack. Hemorrhage of considerable size suggests tuberculosis rather than ileocolitis. Roentgenograms are of considerable diagnostic value.

Treatment.—Pain is to be relieved by hot applications to the abdomen, such as poultices or turpentine stupes, and if necessary by the internal administration of opiates. For the diarrhea bismuth and tannic acid preparations can be given, with or without opium. The administration of cod liver oil, orange juice, and tomato juice are highly recommended (Brown and Sampson[206]). Heliotherapy by sunlight or artificial means apparently is curative in some cases and greatly relieves the symptoms in others. The diet must be sustaining but nonirritating. Alcoholic stimulants are often required.

3. Ulceration of Other Nature

The **ulceration of ileocolitis** is a common condition in infancy. The ulcers are abundant and of sizes varying from minute erosions to larger, deeper lesions. (See p. 591.) **Typhoid ulcers** are, as a rule, not nearly so common or so large in early life as later. They may sometimes, however, be abundant and extensive even at this period, and perforation may take place. (See Typhoid Fever, p. 307.) **Syphilitic ulceration** of the intestine is a rare occurrence in children and infants. It is the result of gummatous or necrotic alteration affecting the intestinal canal.

INTESTINAL HEMORRHAGE

As this symptom is referred to in various sections treating of special diseases it will be mentioned here but briefly. Strictly speaking intestinal hemorrhage indicates blood arising from the intestine itself, but the term may be used to include any discharge of blood from the rectum. Thus in severe epistaxis the blood may be swallowed and later passed from the bowel, and hemorrhage originating in the stomach may reveal itself in like manner. Melena is the title applied to one of the earliest forms of intestinal hemorrhage seen. (See p. 220.) Another form occurring very early in life is that observed in the hemorrhagic disease of the new-born (p. 219), in which the loss of blood may be considerable. Intestinal hemorrhage also occurs in the ulceration of typhoid fever, intussusception, and ileocolitis, the last two exhibiting usually streaks of blood merely. The hemorrhage of tuberculous ulceration may be of the same streak-like character or may be of considerable size. Hemorrhage from the bowel may occur in leukemia, pernicious anemia, inflammation of Meckel's diverticulum, and occasionally in appendicitis. It is a common symptom of hemorrhagic purpura, and is sometimes seen in infantile scurvy. Bloody mucus or a few drops of blood with the stool are encountered in fissure of the anus and even in simple intense congestion of the intestinal mucous membrane, while ulceration of the rectum sometimes produces a considerable loss of blood, as may the hemorrhoids which occasionally occur in early life. Sometimes the hemorrhage depends upon the presence of a rectal polyp or other small papillomatous growths or a foreign body. The appearance of blood in streaks, or even to the amount of a fluidram or more, frequently attends in infancy the injury to the rectal mucous membrane done by the passing of a large, hard fecal mass.

The treatment of intestinal hemorrhage depends entirely upon the cause and is referred to under the separate headings where these causes are discussed.

APPENDICITIS

This title has in recent years supplanted the older ones of typhlitis, perityphlitis, and the like. Although abscess in the cecal region had been recognized at a much earlier date, the first recorded case proven to have been disease of the appendix appears to have been that reported by Mestivier in 1759 (Deaver[207]).

Etiology.—The disorder may occur at any period, yet it is most frequent in early and middle life and distinctly less under ten years of age, as shown by the studies of Hawkins,[208] McCosh,[209] Maguire,[210] Tasche,[211] Gerstley[212] and others. Probably from about 1.5 per cent to 2.5 per cent of operative cases at all ages occur under the age of five years. Writing in 1901 we[213] were able to collect but 14 cases from the literature occurring in the first two years of life, to which was added a 15th personal case in an infant of three months. Of the reported cases two (Pollard[214] and Goyens[215]) were in infants of six weeks of age. Other instances of the disease in infancy have been published since then, and Abt[216] has collected in all 80 cases of the disease in the first two years of life. One of the youngest appears to have been that of Gloniger[217] in an infant operated upon successfully when but forty-one hours old; while Jackson,[218] and Hill and Mason[219] record the lesion found at necropsy in infants aged respectively forty and fifty-five hours, and Corcoran[220] reported a ruptured (noninflammatory) appendix found at necropsy in an infant forty-eight hours old.

More males appear to be attacked than females (H. C. Deaver,[221] Alexander,[222] Edberg,[223] Tasche[211]). Digestive disturbances, especially constipation or diarrhea, are perhaps the most frequent predisposing causes in children. Infectious diseases sometimes predispose. This is especially true of tonsillitis, although observed also in typhoid fever, rheumatism, scarlet fever, pneumonia, and other respiratory infections. It may sometimes immediately follow tonsillectomy. Trauma seems sometimes to be a cause, and heredity is also not without influence, there being a distinct tendency for more than one member of a family to be attacked. Although foreign bodies, such as fruit-seeds, are sometimes, and fecal concretions often, found in the diseased appendix, there seems little reason to believe that these have any etiologic relationship except in occasional instances. In one of our collected cases a pin was discovered in the appendix, and occasionally the oxyuris and other parasites are found there.

As to the direct *exciting* cause little positive is known. The germs found most frequently are streptococci and colon bacilli.

Pathologic Anatomy.—The various divisions of appendicitis are only steps in the same anatomical process. As a result of kinking of the appendix or other cause obstructing its lumen, congestion, edema, inflammation, and round-celled infiltration of the mucous membrane and, especially, of the lymphatic follicles take place. The appendix is thickened, stiff and cylindrical, and may be much distended by the secretion, and a thick deposit of fibrin may be found on it and on the adjacent adherent coils of intestine. The condition produced is that denominated in its milder form *catarrhal appendicitis* or *appendicitis simplex;* or *diffuse appendicitis* when more severe. Entire resolution may take place, but often some remains of the inflammation persist, causing more or less constriction or the formation of adhesions. On the other hand, the process may advance further and may give rise either to a chronic inflammatory condition, or to suppuration. In the latter event *suppurative appendicitis* is spoken of when the pus is in the wall of the appendix, and perforates into the lumen; *perforative appendicitis* when it penetrates the serous layer; and *gangrenous appendicitis* when the tip, or all, of the appendix develops a gangrenous condition.

In cases of *chronic appendicitis* the appendix remains thickened and firm, perhaps with constrictions at one or more portions, while adhesions may connect it with other organs. A sudden, severe, acute attack may at any time develop upon the basis of a chronic disturbance. In other cases, especially infrequent in early life, a progressive involution of the appendix follows repeated mild acute attacks until the organ is much shrunken (*obliterative appendicitis*).

Symptoms.—These are sometimes very striking; sometimes recognized only with difficulty and uncertainty. In some instances they progress slowly and with no constitutional involvement; in others perforation producing a septic peritonitis comes almost as out of a clear sky.

Catarrhal appendicitis may be so mild that it is sometimes supposed to be a mere digestive disturbance. In general this form of the disease develops as a primary affection or consecutive to some digestive disorder, and is ushered in by colicky pain in the right iliac fossa or elsewhere in the abdomen, this constituting the principal symptom. With it are often combined nausea, vomiting, moderate fever, loss of appetite, coated tongue, and constipation or sometimes diarrhea. All these vary with the severity of the case. Palpation reveals tenderness, increased resistance in the cecal region, and often in one or two days an induration. Often, too, when there is a plastic exudate upon the serous surface of the appendix and the neighboring parts, a distinct tumor can be palpated.

Suppurative appendicitis is marked by the evident constitutional involvement, the rise of pulse-rate and perhaps of temperature, and other evidences of moderate septic infection. The inflammation may not pass beyond the serous wall, and no extensive induration may develop. In those nonperforative cases in which a localized plastic peritonitis has occurred palpation reveals a decided tumor. Fever may continue or may subside, and the symptoms are less severe than when a walled-in abscess forms about the appendix. In the latter event vomiting persists, tenderness and resistance are decided, pain is usually severe, and tympanites is common. The rapidity of the development of suppurative appendicitis varies greatly. In some cases the course is rapid from the beginning and the symptoms violent, with troublesome vomiting and pain, and in from two to three days undoubted abscess can be discovered. In others the early manifestations are all mild and vague, and evidences of abscess develop only after a number of days. In still others the early symptoms may be severe, but be followed by a period of comparative quiescence, lasting several days or even weeks, and then the signs of the formation of pus appear or perforation occur.

The constitutional symptoms of suppurative appendicitis depend not so much upon the local accumulation of pus as upon the degree of septic absorption. The temperature is not characteristic. Often the development of abscess is marked by a progressive increase of fever; while on the other hand the temperature may remain normal, or nearly so, even in cases which are clearly septic. In general, however, increase in the rapidity and weakness of the pulse and in the appearance of severe illness is in proportion to the degree of septic absorption.

Perforation into the peritoneal cavity may take place from a gangrenous appendix which has formed no adhesions, or from a periappendicular abscess which has finally burst the restraining wall. It is characterized by the development or increase of vomiting, severe abdominal pain, and profound collapse with the usual signs of rapid pulse, shallow thoracic respiration, and fall of temperature. The expression of the face is anxious and pinched, cold perspiration occurs, the abdomen is extremely tympanitic and the liver-dulness much diminished. Death may take place without any reaction, or the temperature may rise rapidly even to hyperpyrexia and septic peritonitis develop. The symptoms at this period may, however, be very deceptive, especially in children, there being sometimes only a moderate depression of temperature, with apparent improvement in the general symptoms attending the beginning of septic poisoning.

The symptoms of **gangrenous appendicitis** are very equivocal from the beginning. The early ones are not characteristic and are often no more severe than those of catarrhal appendicitis. Suddenly, after a few days illness, perforation takes place with the symptoms of this as described. In other cases of gangrene the local manifestations are severe from the onset with unusual tenderness, pain, and resistance of the abdominal walls.

Appendicitis in infancy exhibits symptoms which are liable to be very misleading, owing to the inability to determine with exactness the existence or position of pain and tenderness. Doubtless many cases are entirely overlooked at this age. The disease may exhibit a slow or sudden onset, troublesome vomiting, diarrhea or constipation, more or less fever, and finally peritonitis.

Recurrent and Chronic Appendicits.—There is a decided liability to the occurrence of repeated attacks of acute appendicitis. This depends on the persistence of kinking or narrowing, or of small, infected foci which at any time may precipitate an acute inflammation. Such recurrences may finally lead to a severe and fatal appendicitis; or the disposition to them may at last disappear, perhaps through obliterative inflammation of the appendix. Hawkins[224] estimates the liability to recurrence as at least 23.6 per cent as shown in the analysis of 250 patients of all ages. This condition of recurring attacks is one of the forms of *chronic appendicitis*. Sometimes the attacks are mild and very frequent, and supposed to be recurrent outbreaks of acute indigestion. Other cases may suggest chronic indigestion, with impaired general health, constipation or diarrhea, anorexia, and other indefinite digestive symptoms. Pain may be nearly constant, or irregular, or brought on by fatigue. It may be in the appendicular or umbilical region, or elsewhere, or diffuse. Attacks of recurrent vomiting have been claimed to be in some cases probably due to a chronic appendicitis (Comby[225]). Chronic appendicitis rarely occurs in children under five years of age (Mixter[226]).

A fuller consideration of the individual symptoms of acute appendicitis is of advantage.

Abdominal Pain.—This varies greatly in intensity; from severe and either continuous or paroxysmal, to pain which is hardly more than an uncomfortable sensation. As any movement increases the suffering the child lies quietly, perhaps with the right thigh drawn up on the abdomen, or walks leaning forward with the right thigh slightly flexed. There may sometimes be little pain even when an abscess is forming, or pain occurs only shortly before perforation takes place. The pain, at first often diffuse, is later confined to the right iliac fossa; but to this there are many exceptions, and it may be referred to various other regions, especially the umbilical and the epigastric, but depending upon the varying position of the appendix. According to Deaver[227] if the appendix lies beside or behind the cecum and is pointed upward the pain is in the region of the cecum or high in the loin. If in the true or false pelvis and pointed downward the pain is lower in the abdomen and usually on the left side. If below the apex of the cecum and pointing to the left the pain is in the region of the cecum. Sometimes there is pain during or before evacuation of the bowels; sometimes it is developed by traction on the testicle. The production of pain and tenderness in the appendicular region, produced by rectal insufflation (Bastedo's sign[228]) is a strong indication that appendicitis exists (Jerlov[229]). On the occurrence of perforation there is usually a sudden, severe, and diffuse abdominal pain.

Tenderness.—This is far from uniform, and depends to a certain extent upon the severity of the case, being but slight in catarrhal cases of the milder form. The occurrence of periappendicular inflammation is attended by increasing tenderness, and when abscess forms tenderness is great. The situation of the sensation is usually in the right iliac fossa, most marked at McBurney's point, but often above this in children. It varies in position, as does pain. It may be sometimes elicited by rectal palpation. In the examination of older children due regard must be given to the psychic element, the child either mistakenly maintaining that the symptom exists if the matter has been much discussed before him, or denying it if he has acquired a fear of operation. In younger children the attention must be carefully diverted. Slight, diffuse tenderness without increased muscular resistance is of doubtful import.

Increased Resistance of the Abdominal Walls.—This is very characteristic, and is nearly always present even in the mildest cases; and when tenderness is severe is so marked that a satisfactory examination cannot be made through the abdominal walls. The discovery, however, of either tenderness or increased resistance is often difficult or impossible, especially in young children or in older ones of nervous disposition.

Induration or Tumor.—In the milder cases of catarrhal appendicitis and in gangrenous cases there is no tumor, but it is present when the lumen of the appendix is distended by pus, or when plastic or purulent periappendicular inflammation occurs. Bimanual palpation with one hand in the loin often aids, and rectal examination should always be practised in doubtful cases, comparing with the finger in the bowel the condition of the two iliac regions. Yet palpation of any sort must be done always with great gentleness, lest any periappendicular abscess be ruptured. Percussion also is of aid in recognizing the tumor by the dulness of the sound produced. It should be done gently to avoid causing suffering. In cases of purulent perityphlitis the abscess which forms sometimes reaches large dimensions. The position of the induration or abscess corresponds to that of the pain, both varying with that of the appendix.

Tympanites.—When decided this is an evidence of suppurative appendicitis, probably with a mild grade of peritonitis. When very great, with disappearance of hepatic dulness, it indicates perforation.

Nausea and Vomiting.—These are symptoms seldom entirely absent except in the very mild cases, but they are prone to subside after the first day or two, except in the severe and rapidly developing attacks. Yet in many suppurative cases vomiting, like other acute symptoms, may lessen or disappear after the first few days, perhaps to return in force as the indication of the occurrence of a perforation. Stercoraceous vomiting is an evidence of absolute paralysis of peristalsis, as seen in wide-spread peritonitis.

Bowel-movements.—Diarrhea by no means excludes appendicitis in children, in whom it is more apt to occur than in adults. Generally, however, in severe cases, whether catarrhal suppurative or perforative, there is more or less paralysis of peristalsis, and constipation is decided and sometimes absolute.

Temperature.—Fever is so variable that few conclusions can be drawn from it. The mildest cases exhibit little or no elevation of temperature. Often there is some fever at the onset which may soon subside. In the severer attacks fever is liable to continue and reach a higher degree than in mild ones, although in septic cases the temperature may sometimes remain only slightly elevated. The temperature may fall to nearly normal in patients who are, in fact, not improving but developing abscess. A perforation may occur without premonitory return of fever; or renewed rise of temperature may indicate a rapid abscess-formation.

Blood.—A rapid increase of leukocytes to 20,000 or 30,000 per cubic millimeter, particularly of the polymorphonuclear cells, combined with the presence of other suggestive symptoms, is often an indication that the appendicitis is of a suppurative type. A diminution of a leukocytosis previously present is a favorable indication, if attended by improvement in other respects. On the other hand, little if any increase of the leukocytes is an equivocal sign. It may be present in catarrhal appendicitis or, conversely, in serious fulminating suppurative cases. A low leukocyte-count with threatening general symptoms is a bad indication. If the symptoms are severe, the higher the leukocyte-count and the greater the proportion of the polymorphonuclear cells the better is the prognosis. Some clinicians emphasize the value of the Schilling index (p. 1021).

Pulse.—The pulse is at first accelerated only in proportion to the degree of fever, or sometimes is slower than normal. If septic symptoms develop, and especially if perforation occurs, the pulse becomes rapid, weak and compressible.

Genito-urinary Symptoms.—These are sometimes decided. The urine is scanty and not infrequently contains albumin. Irritability of the bladder is sometimes great, and may easily be a misleading symptom. An acute nephritis may develop.

Course and Prognosis.—The total duration of *catarrhal appendicitis* is usually a week or less. In the milder cases the fever, pain, and vomiting disappear in one or two days. In the severer cases the general symptoms last somewhat longer and the indurated mass felt is very distinct. If the inflammation does not advance to a suppurative condition the prognosis of the individual attack is always good.

Should the inflammation advance to a *suppurative stage*, or be of this nature from the onset, the course varies. Periappendicitis may be produced and abscess result, and a mass may then often be outlined after two or three days. The duration of the attack in suppurative appendicitis has no well-defined limit. In some cases the course is rapid from the beginning and perforation may occur in two or three days, or suppuration be found if the case is operated upon. The ultimate termination in unoperated cases is very diverse. The pus, if in small amount, may eventually be absorbed, or it may extend in different directions and discharge spontaneously into the colon, the rectum, the bladder, through the abdominal wall, or into the peritoneal cavity. *Perforation* with general peritonitis occurs most frequently in cases of gangrenous appendicitis. This may happen even in the first two or three days of the attack. The great majority of fatal cases of appendicitis depend upon perforation with general peritonitis, which is especially liable to occur in early life. The prognosis in this condition is very grave, although cases of recovery under prompt operative treatment are not on the whole uncommon, particularly in infancy and childhood.

The general prognosis of appendicitis under *medical* treatment without operative interference is not unfavorable, owing to the large proportion of cases of catarrhal appendicitis. The prognosis of the individual case, however, is always uncertain, due to the absolute impossibility of predicating the possibility of peritonitis in any given instance. Those cases which perhaps appear the mildest, or to be on the road to recovery, not infrequently become suddenly and dangerously worse. The prognosis in the first two years of life appears to be unfavorable. This is probably dependent, in part, upon the difficulty in recognizing the disease at this age, the mildest cases never being discovered, and the fatal ones receiving a post-mortem diagnosis only. Peterson[230] places the usual average mortality in acute appendicitis in nurslings at over 70 per cent, and in children under six years at from 40 to 50 per cent. Recovery from an attack of appendicitis leaves the subject predisposed to later attacks, or chronic inflammation of varying degree may remain, or adhesions persist which give rise to symptoms. The pelvic organs in girls may be secondarily involved (Graves[231]). Location affects mortality; the prognosis when the appendix is in the pelvic region being more favorable than in the middle of the peritoneal cavity or near the diaphragm (Deaver[227]).

Under prompt *operative* treatment the general mortality in early life varies from 3 to 16.4 per cent in the series of H. C. Deaver,[221] Alexander,[222] and Riedel.[232] One of the dangers after operation is the development of intestinal obstruction from paralysis of peristalsis; and the formation of secondary abscesses is another. Even cases with a primary walled-off abscess of considerable size generally recover when operated upon. It is only where general peritonitis has developed that the mortality of operation is high.

Complications.—Abscess in various parts of the abdominal and pelvic cavities has been referred to. Pneumonia, hepatic abscess, phlebitis, and other evidences of sepsis may follow a septic peritonitis. Empyema may be the result of the penetration of a subphrenic abscess into the pleural cavity, or of the sepsis following perforation. Pleurisy, not of a purulent nature, is a not infrequent complication. Appendicitis may be complicated by hernia, and the inflamed appendix may be found in the hernial sac. (See Hernia, p. 623.) Appendicitis may be followed by intussusception, as in a child of five months reported by Rardin,[233] or an inflamed appendix may be found in the sac of a complicating hernia.

Diagnosis.—The principal diagnostic symptoms in typical cases are sudden onset; early vomiting and fever; and abdominal pain, tenderness, increased resistance, and later induration or tumor especially in the right iliac region. But the variations as already described are so great that diagnosis is often difficult. (See the detailed discussion of symptoms, pp. 631–633.)

A number of other morbid conditions are to be taken into consideration in reaching a conclusion. *Appendicular colic*, in which the contraction of the appendix in expelling retained secretion or fecal masses causes pain, is unproductive of fever, tenderness, leukocytosis, or the constitutional disturbance which appendicitis usually presents. *Umbilical colic* is situated more in the region of the navel, is more remittent, of longer course, and unattended by fever, tenderness, or leukocytosis. The diagnosis from mild chronic appendicitis is often, however, very difficult. *Intestinal colic* may cause peculiar difficulty in diagnosis if there happens to be a large fecal accumulation in the colon, particularly the cecum. It differs from the attack of pain due to appendicitis in that the latter is made worse by movement of the body. *Acute febrile indigestion* closely simulates many cases of appendicitis at the onset and diagnosis at first may be impossible. Generally, however, the pain is less intense and the constitutional symptoms less marked, except that the fever is often high. *Intussusception* might simulate appendicitis especially if tumor is found. The initial general symptoms are severe, but there is an absence of fever, and the tenesmus and bloody stools serve to distinguish it. *Ileocolitis* may resemble appendicitis and at first cause confusion through the early presence of vomiting and of abdominal pain; but the symptoms in general are so different that the diagnosis soon becomes clear. We have seen *acute tuberculous inflammation of the lymph-nodes near the cecum* resemble appendicitis so closely that operation for the latter was performed. Many similar cases are on record. The subject has been reviewed by Gage,[234] and others. Stout[235] finds that hyperplasia of lymphoid tissue in the appendix and cecum may simulate appendicitis. Abdominal pain due to *inflamed and enlarged mesenteric and retroperitoneal nodes*, not tuberculous in nature, may follow infections of the upper respiratory tract. The tenderness and rigidity are, however, not so marked in this condition, and the association of the pain with an infection of the throat, ear or nasal sinuses is a helpful differential point. We have seen a number of cases of this type since Brennemann[236] called attention to it. *Typhoid fever* may, at the onset, suggest appendicitis to a certain extent, through the vomiting and the tenderness in the right iliac region; but the course of the temperature, the absence of leukocytosis, and later the presence of the Widal reaction serve to differentiate. The diagnosis is, however, sometimes difficult and we have seen children with typhoid fever operated upon under the mistaken belief that appendicitis was present. The occasional referring by the patient of appendicular pain to the region of the right hip may cause the diagnosis of *hip-joint disease* to be made. Careful examination of the hip will prevent the mistake. *Ovarian disease* has likewise occasioned errors in some instances. *Urinary symptoms* may usher in appendicitis and cause confusion, but the presence of a vaginitis, or the examination of the urine, obtained by a catheter if there is retention, will aid in the diagnosis, although the not infrequent simultaneous occurrence of appendicitis and pyelitis must not be overlooked, and an inflamed retrocecal appendix, too, may cause some pus cells in the urine by irritation of the ureter. Unusual location of the appendicular abscess leads to mistakes later in the disease, and the possibility of a *psoas abscess* from spinal caries simulating a perityphlitic abscess must not be forgotten. Inflammation of *Meckel's diverticulum* has repeatedly been supposed to be appendicitis, and operation has been done for this condition; and there exists no certain differential diagnostic feature. Intestinal hemorrhage is common in diverticulitis, but rare in appendicitis. (See p. 637.) *Peritonitis* of a primary type due to the streptococcus or pneumococcus, in which there is no involvement of the appendix, presents difficulties in diagnosis, especially as it may develop without any apparent focus of infection. The error of believing a *pleurisy* or *pneumonia* to be an appendicitis is probably much more frequent than ordinarily supposed, and has repeatedly led to operation upon perfectly normal appendices. Writing in 1903 we[237] reviewed the subject with the report of a number of cases of what may be called "appendicular pneumonia" (see p. 734), and since then we have observed a number of additional instances, and know of some where surgeons of experience have operated. It is of common occurrence, especially in children, for the pain produced in the pleura to be referred through the intercostal and abdominal nerves to the region of the appendix. A mistake in diagnosis is to be avoided chiefly by careful examination of the lungs in every case of suspected appendicitis; by noting the increased rapidity of respiration in pneumonia; and by the fact that the abdominal resistance is generally relaxed during inspiration in this disease, but is maintained in appendicitis. The temperature and leukocyte count are liable to be higher in pneumonia, although these are not very reliable signs. The value of roentgenograms of the lungs should not be forgotten, since a pneumonia may be diagnosed in this way when the physical signs are still doubtful. We have seen a number of cases in which pneumonia and appendicitis occurred simultaneously, and the combination has been reported by others, as by Allan,[238] Feer,[239] Herrman,[240] and Greenebaum and Ransohoff.[241] Leiner[242] states that the lower abdominal reflex is absent in appendicitis, but present in pneumonia. Lastly in the case of older children especially, pain in the right iliac region may be *psychic* in nature, the result of the mental impression made by what the patients have heard regarding the disease. This is of common occurrence. The absence of fever and of tumor is suggestive, although a simulated tenderness of course is present.

Treatment.—In view, of the impossibility, already referred to, of determining whether a case is catarrhal, suppurative, or gangrenous, the only safe treatment is operative interference. This is especially true of infancy and childhood, at which time the danger of peritonitis is greater. If the patient is seen early, operation should be done at once. If an exudate has already taken place, the time for operation is to be determined for each individual case, it being sometimes better to delay until the abscess has become more distinctly localized; an occurrence, however, which is less likely to be seen in children than in adults. Under this condition, if symptoms subside and pus does not form, resolution may occur. But here again we are confronted with the possibility of sudden perforation in cases where it was supposed that no suppuration existed.

When for any reason early operation cannot be done, or when the diagnosis is uncertain, and in cases seen later in which operation is deferred by surgical advice, the patient must be kept at rest in bed, given a light diet, and an ice-bag be applied over the seat of inflammation. Vomiting may need to be controlled by the temporary abstaining from food, or the taking of it in very small amount, and the administration of appropriate remedies, such as the swallowing of ice, iced champagne, or the giving of lime water or bismuth. No saline or other purgative should be administered, and unirritating enemata should be employed if it is necessary to relieve constipation. Opium is better avoided if possible, since it obscures symptoms and increases constipation and tympanites. Cases where pain is very severe sometimes, however, make opium a necessity, and where operation cannot be done, there seems no remedy more certainly indicated than opium for the relief of this symptom.

Where there have been several attacks of recurrent appendicitis, even though slight, it is best to remove the appendix, as there is no predicating under what inopportune circumstances a severe or even fatal attack might occur. The operation is then conveniently performed in the interval between attacks.

DISEASES CONNECTED WITH MECKEL'S DIVERTICULUM

The omphalo-mesenteric duct passing in fetal life from the ileum to the umbilical vesicle remains after birth in from 1 to 2 per cent of all persons as what is known as "Meckel's diverticulum." This may exist only as a short patulous protrusion from the ileum, oftenest from its convex border and found at from 1 to 3 ft. (31 to 91 cm.) above the cecum; as a tube wholly or partially open; or as a cord merely, extending entirely or a portion of the way to the umbilicus, and in the latter event either free at its distal extremity, or attached to some other region, oftenest the mesentery. The organ is found much most frequently in males. Lesions are more likely to develop if the distal extremity is attached. As a rule the diverticulum gives rise to no symptoms whatever, yet it is oftener the cause of pathologic conditions than is usually supposed. Series of cases of such disturbances have been reported, and we[163] have reviewed the subject in a previous publication. Only a brief résumé can be given here.

1. Strangulation of the Intestine by the Diverticulum.—This is the lesion most frequently found. Of Wellington's[243] 326 cases of disease of the diverticulum, 144 were instances of constriction of the intestine by this organ or its remains. In 991 cases of intestinal strangulation from different causes collected by Halsted[244] 6 per cent were dependent upon the diverticulum. The majority of these cases occurred after the period of childhood. The symptoms of strangulation by the diverticulum are those of intestinal obstruction in general, with the exception of intussusception which has characteristic symptoms of its own.

2. Patulous Meckel's Diverticulum Opening at the Umbilicus.—This is an uncommon condition seen nearly always only in males, of which Strasser[245] could collect but 63 reported instances. Other cases have since been reported. We have met with it in but one instance. The mucous membrane of the diverticulum may protrude at the umbilicus, producing a small tumor covered by mucous membrane, and with a central fistulous opening. Should the entire wall of the intestine, as well as the mucous membrane of the duct, project through the diverticulum, the tumor is larger and with two lateral openings. Strangulation of the projecting portion may occur. When the diverticulum is open throughout its extent, feces and even intestinal worms may be discharged at the umbilicus; but if closed at its proximal extremity, only mucus is passed at the opening. The cases of fecal fistula usually terminate fatally. (See also p. 241.)

3. Invagination of the Diverticulum.—Of Wellington's cases 59 exhibited this lesion. Not only may the diverticulum be itself invaginated, but it may be followed by an intussusception of the ileum also. The accident takes place usually not before later childhood, this distinguishing it from ordinary intussusception, which is so much more common at a decidedly earlier age. The obstruction of the intestine is generally not complete, and the amount of blood discharged is small.

4. Volvulus of Meckel's diverticulum is a rare condition, either exceptionally of the diverticulum alone, or oftener of the ileum also, secondarily to this; or twisting of the ileum may depend upon the presence of the diverticulum but without any volvulus of the latter.

5. Hernia of the diverticulum is occasionally seen. Gray[246] collected 42 undoubted cases.

6. Diverticulitis.—This is an infrequent condition, one of the largest series of collected cases reported being that of Forgue and Riche[247] with 59 instances. Greenwald and Steiner[248] estimated the number at 51. About $\frac{1}{3}$ of the cases occur in children (Cahier[249]). The disease may be secondary to some other lesion of the diverticulum, or arise as a primary affection. It is much more common in males. The method of production and the pathological anatomy in this *primary* diverticulitis are usually entirely similar to those seen in appendicitis, and the different varieties are the same. In some instances, however, peptic ulcer occurs, there being islets of gastric mucosa in the diverticulum. The course may be acute or chronic. The symptoms strongly suggest appendicitis, and consist of abdominal pain, nausea, vomiting, often constipation, fever, leukocytosis, and the development of abdominal tenderness and resistance, with dulness on percussion. In a number of cases discharge of blood from the bowel has occurred. In a case under our care severe anemia was produced in this way. Attention to the occurrence of hemorrhage has also been called by Abt and Strauss,[250] Peterman and Seegar,[251] Meiss,[252] Smith and Hill,[253] and Tisdall.[254] In a case reported by Peterman and Seegar hemorrhage was in the peritoneal cavity as well as in the intestine. Perforation and septic peritonitis may take place; or in other instances intestinal obstruction may result from compression by the inflammatory mass, or in other ways. In *secondary* diverticulitis intestinal obstruction may first occur, and later the evidences of inflammation of the diverticulum be added. The diagnosis of diverticulitis from appendicitis rests chiefly on the localization of pain to the right of the umbilicus and somewhat higher than McBurney's point, or in some more distant region. Further suggestive of diverticulitis are the absence or slight degree of tympanites, and in some cases the presence of blood in the stools.

The only treatment of diseases of Meckel's diverticulum is operation. Indeed, should the organ in healthy state be discovered at any abdominal operation for other conditions, it is wise to remove it.

References

1. Wien. med. Wchnschr., 1915, **65**, 226. 2. Ztschr. f. Heilkund. Chir. Abt., 1904, **25**, 209. 3. München. med. Wchnschr., 1913, **60**, 2827. 4. Ztschr. f. ärztl. Fortbild., 1921, **18**, 486. 5. J. M. Soc. State of N. J., 1920, **17**, 279. 6. Nederlandsch. Tijdsch. v. Geneesk., 1923, **67**, 2378. 7. Brit. M. J., 1921, **1**, 1. 8. Am. J. Dis. Child., 1930, **39**, 1022. 9. Quart. J. Med., 1913, **6**, 242. 10. Quart. J. Med., 1920, **14**, 1. 11. Am. J. Dis. Child. 1928, **36**, 725. 12. J.A.M.A., 1926, **86**, 112. 13. Am. J. Dis. Child., 1927, **33**, 705. 14. Ztschr. f. Kinderh., 1926, **41**, 1. 15. Arch. Pediat., 1929, **46**, 637. 16. Am. J. Dis. Child., 1930, **40**, 27. 17. Bull. et mém. soc. méd. d. hôp., 1921, **45**, 1384. 18. Arch. Otolaryngol., 1925, **1**, 411. 19. South. Med. J., 1926, **19**, 157. 20. J.A.M.A., 1926, **87**, 220. 21. Arch. Otolaryngol., 1927, **5**, 39. 22. Mitchell, McCarthy, Leichliter and Seinsheimer, J.A.M.A., 1929, **92**, 970. 23. Jahrb. f. Kinderh., 1919, **89**, 298. 24. Monats. f. Kinderh., 1921, **22**, 273. 25. South. M. J., 1924, **17**, 552; Am. J. Dis. Child., 1925, **29**, 743. 26. Johns Hopk. Hosp. Rep., 1897, **6**, 159. 27. Seventeenth Cong. f. Inn. Med., 1899, 425; Escherich und Pfaundler, in Kolle and Wassermann Handb. d. pathog. Microörg., 1902, 433. 28. Am. J. Dis. Child., 1917, **14**, 354. 29. Am. J. Dis. Child., 1921, **22**, 284. 30. Am. J. Dis. Child., 1916, **11**, 309. 31. J.A.M.A., 1916, **67**, 1352. 32. Am. J. Dis. Child., 1917, **13**, 218. 33. Am. J. Dis. Child., 1918, **15**, 165. 34. Am. J. Dis. Child., 1920, **20**, 461. 35. Am. J. Dis. Child., 1921, **21**, 465. 36.

Am. J. M. Sc., 1925, **169,** 236. 37. Am. J. Dis. Child., 1928, **36,** 248. 38. Jahrb. f. Kinderh., 1928, **119,** 161. 39. Am. J. Dis. Child., 1929, **38,** 314. 40. Quart. J. Med., 1916, **9,** 164. 41. Proc. Soc. Exper. Biol. and Med., 1921, **18,** 101. 42. Proc. Soc. Exper. Biol. and Med., 1922, **19,** 323. 43. Arch. Int. Med., 1923, **31,** 297. 44. Jahrb. f. Kinderh., 1928, **120,** 162. 45. Am. J. Dis. Child., 1932, **43,** 1. 46. Mitchell, New York M. J., 1921, **114,** 155. 47. J. Pharmacol. and Exper. Therap., 1928, **32,** 437. 48. Monats. f. Kinderh., 1930, **48,** 481. 49. Am. J. Dis. Child., 1928, **35,** 557. 50. J. Exper. Med., 1929, **50,** 387. 51. Am. J. Dis. Child., 1929, **37,** 244. 52. Am. J. Dis. Child., 1931, **41,** 1347. 53. Am. J. Dis. Child., 1929, **37,** 683; 1930, **39,** 1346. 54. Am. J. Dis. Child., 1931, **42,** 291. 55. Virchow's Arch., 1875, **65,** 196. 56. J.A.M.A., 1930, **94,** 1. 57. Centralbl. f. Bakt., 1898, **23,** 599. 58. Bull. Johns Hopk. Hosp., 1900, **11,** 231. 59. Am. Med., 1902, **4,** 417. 60. Med. News, 1903, **82,** 289. 61. Ztschr. f. klin. Med., 1915, **73,** 81. 62. Am. J. Dis. Child., 1931, **41,** 15. 63. Canad. M. A. J., 1931, **25,** 417. 64. Bact. and Clin. Stud. of the Diarrh. Disorders of Infancy, 1904, 124. 65. Bull. Johns Hopk. Hosp., 1920, **31,** 225; Medicine, 1922, **1,** 389. 66. South. M. J., 1925, **18,** 120. 67. Jahrb. f. Kinderh., 1907, **65;** Ergänzunsheft, 40. 68. Brit. M. J., 1906, **1,** 908; Proc. Roy. Soc. Med., 1908–09, **2,** 133. 69. Bact. and Clin. Studies of Diarrheal Disorders of Infancy, Rockefeller Inst., 1904, 135. 70. J.A.M.A., 1924, **82,** 1599. 71. Am. J. Dis. Child., 1927, **33,** 711. 72. J.A.M.A., 1921, **76,** 108. 73. Klin. Wchnschr., 1929, **8,** 2414. 74. Med. Klinik., 1931, **27,** 1452. 75. Deutsche med. Wchnschr., 1930, **56,** 1949. 76. J.A.M.A., 1929, **93,** 583. 77. J.A.M.A., 1932, **98,** 195. 78. J.A.M.A., 1921, **77,** 1863. 79. Am. J. Dis. Child., 1923, **25,** 310. 80. Am. J. Dis. Child., 1922, **23,** 531. 81. J.A.M.A., 1924, **83,** 332; 1928, **91,** 1176; Arch. Int. Med., 1925, **36,** 818; 1929, **43,** 50. 82. J.A.M.A., 1929, **93,** 263. 83. J.A.M.A., 1930, **94,** 849. 84. J.A.M.A., 1930, **94,** 10. 85. J.A.M.A., 1931, **97,** 1440. 86. Am. J. Dis. Child., 1923, **26,** 418. 87. J.A.M.A., 1928, **90,** 841. 88. Am. J. M. Sc., 1931, **181,** 180. 89. Die Krankh. d. Neugeborenen, 1850, **1,** 64; 128. 90. Am. J. Obstet., 1869–70, **2,** 96. 91. Phys. Rev., 1924, **4,** 352. 92. Proc. Soc. Exp. Biol. and Med., 1927, **24,** 953. 93. J. Nutrition, 1931, **3,** 345. 94. Bost. M. and S. J., 1911, **164,** 306. 95. Mitchell and Lewis, Am. J. Dis. Child., 1921, **21,** 129. 96. A Treatise on the Transformation of the Intestinal Flora, etc., 1921; Arch. Int. Med., 1922, **29,** 357. 97. Lancet, 1903, **1,** 1497. 98. Arch. Pediat., 1923, **40,** 88. 99. Arch. Dis. Childh., 1931, **6,** 75. 100. Am. J. Dis. Child., 1928, **25,** 414. 101. Am. J. Dis. Child., 1932, **43,** 1293. 102. On Infantilism from Chronic Intestinal Infection, 1908. 103. Am. J. Dis. Child., 1925, **30,** 603. 104. Arch. Pediat., 1929, **44,** 567. 105. Monats. f. Kinderh., 1931, **50,** 1. 106. Wasting Diseases of Infants and Children, 2nd Am. Ed., 156. 107. St. Barthol. Hosp. Rept., 1888, **24,** 17. 108. Trans. Am. Ped. Soc., 1921, **33,** 11. 109. Am. J. Dis. Child., 1927, **34,** 934. 110. Am. J. Dis. Child., 1923, **25,** 46. 111. Am. J. Dis. Child., 1930, **39,** 76. 112. Am. J. Dis. Child., 1930, **39,** 76. 113. Am. J. Dis. Child., 1917, **14,** 379. 114. Arch. Pediat., 1931, **48,** 248. 115. Arch. Pediat., 1911, **28,** 841. 116. Arch. Pediat., 1930, **47,** 24. 117. Griffith, Am. J. M. Sc., 1899, **118,** 283. 118. Surg., Gynec. and Obstet., 1908, **6,** 624. 119. Toulouse méd., 1910, **12,** 282. 120. Am. J. Dis. Child., 1915, **9,** 283. 121. Arch. Pediat., 1916, **33,** 665. 122. Jahrb. f. Kinderheilk., 1888, **27,** 1. 123. Collect. from the Unpublish. Med. Writings of the late H. C. Parry, 1825, **2,** 380. 124. Hufeland's Journ. d. prakt., Arzneikunde, 1836, **83,** 62. 125. Beiträge z. Kinderh., 1861, 123. 126. Trans. Path. Soc. of London, 1872, **23,** 104. 127. Trans. Path. Soc. of Phila., 1887, **13,** 40. 128. Bost. M. and S. J., 1921, **184,** 81. 129. Am. J. Obstet., 1869–70, **2,** 96. 130. Lancet, 1898, **1,** 276. 131. J.A.M.A., 1927, **89,** 662. 132. Centralb. f. allg. Path., 1907, **18,** 929. 133. J.A.M.A., 1911, **57,** 731. 134. Am. J. M. Sc., 1926, **171,** 67. 135. Arch. Pediat., 1931, **48,** 553. 136. Surg., Gynec. and Obst., 1922, **34,** 35. 137. Am. J. Dis. Child., 1929, **37,** 591. 138. Am. J. Dis. Child., 1931, **41,** 262. 139. Am. J. Dis. Child., 1928, **35,** 109. 140. Ann. Surg., 1929, **89,** 6. 141. Am. J. Dis. Child., 1929, **37,** 818. 142. Monats. f. Kinderh., 1929, **45,** 208. 143. Am. J. Dis. Child., 1925, **29,** 518. 144. Am. J. Dis. Child., 1927, **33,** 949. 145. Prag. med. Wchnschr., 1914, **39,** 197. 146. J.A.M.A., 1917, **68,** 244. 147. Monats. f. Kinderh., Orig., 1918, **15,** 199. 148. J. Exp. Med., 1916, **23,** 717. 149. J. Exp. Med., 1917, **25,** 461. 150. J. Exp. Med., 1925, **41,** 107; 113; 119; 1927, **45,** 427. 151. J. Clin. Investig., 1925, **1,** 531. 152. J.A.M.A., 1928, **91,** 1592. 153. Surg., Gynec., and Obstet., 1928, **46,** 332. 154. J.A.M.A., 1928, **91,** 538. 155. J. Exp. Med., 1913, **17,** 286. 156. Ann. Surg., 1916, **63,** 720. 157. J. Exp. Med., 1919, **30,** 109. 158. J. Clin. Investig., 1932, **2,** 455; 475. 159. Jahrb. f. Kinderh., 1870, **3,** 1. 160. Arch. Pediat., 1905, **22,** 655. 161. Mitteilung. aus d. Grenzgeb. d. Med. u. Chir., 1913, **25,** 293. 162. Bost. M. and S. J., 1922, **186,** 700. 163. Griffith, J.A.M.A., 1914, **62,** 1624. 164. Liverpool Med.-Chir. J., 1901, **21,** 68. 165. Ann. Surg., 1903, **38,** 708. 166. Am. J. Dis. Child., 1929, **36,** 1017. 167. Prag. Vierteljahrschr. f. prakt. Heilk., 1873, 118–119, et. seq. 168. Arch. Pediat., 1921, **38,** 174. 169. Am. J. Dis. Child., 1929, **37,** 373. 170. Presse méd., 1922, **30,** 3. 171. Am. J. M. Sc., 1927, **174,** 500. 172. Am. J. Dis. Child., 1927, **33,** 765. 173. Am. J. Dis. Child., 1928, **35,** 61. 174. Acta paediat., 1926, **6,** 31. 175. Arch. Dis. Childh., 1927, **2,** 328. 176. Volkmann's Sammlung klin. Vorträge, 1893, n. s., 63; Gynäk., No. 26, 624. 177. Wien. klin. Rundschau, 1903, **17,** 757. 178. Phila. M. J., 1901, **7,** 393. 179. Univ.

Med. Mag., 1900, **13**, 94. 180. Rev. de chir., 1902, **25**, 249. 181. Lancet, 1897, **2**, 788. 182. Am. J. Dis. Child., 1927, **34**, 634. 183. J.A.M.A., 1928, **90**, 762. 184. J.A.M.A., 1930, **94**, 15. 185. Am. J. Dis. Child., 1922, **24**, 297. 186. J.A.M.A., 1925, **85**, 947; Ann. Surg., 1931, **94**, 776. 187. Am. J. Roentgenol., 1926, **15**, 135. 188. Jahrb. f. Kinderh., 1929, **124**, 307. 189. Am. J. Dis. Child., 1929, **38**, 361. 190. J.A.M.A., 1931, **96**, 847. 191. Ergeb. d. inn. Med. u. Kinderh., 1919, **16**, 302. 192. Berl. klin. Wchnschr., 1913, **50**, 593. 193. Griffith, New York M. J., 1911, **94**, 572. 194. Am. J. Dis. Child., 1913, **6**, 381. 195. Am. J. M. Sc., 1914, **148**, 709. 196. Jahrb. f. Kinderh., 1922, **97**, 182. 197. Lancet, 1922, **1**, 63. 198. Arch. Pediat., 1924, **41**, 646. 199. Am. J. Dis. Child., 1924, **38**, 694. 200. Am. J. Dis. Child., 1926, **32**, 872. 201. Am. J. Dis. Child., 1915, **10**, 397. 202. Am. J. Dis. Child., 1926, **31**, 631. 203. Proc. Roy. Soc. Med., 1908–9, Sect. Dis. Child., 67. 204. Jahrb. f. Kinderh., 1906, **63**, 563. 205. Arch. Pediat., 1930, **47**, 594. 206. J.A.M.A., 1932, **98**, 26. 207. Treatise on Appendicitis, 1900, 18. 208. Dis. of the Vermiform Appendix, 1895, 62. 209. J.A.M.A., 1904, **43**, 853. 210. Virginia Med. Semi-month., 1898–99, **3**, 400. 211. Am. J. M. Sc., 1931, **182**, 86. 212. Med. Clin. N. Am., 1930, **13**, 1175. 213. Griffith, Univ. of Pa. Med. Bull., 1901, **14**, 300. 214. Lancet, 1895, **1**, 1114. 215. Gaz. méd. Belge, 1900, **12**, 133. 216. Arch. Pediat., 1917, **34**, 641. 217. Kelly and Hurdon, The Vermiform Appendix, 1905, 453. 218. Am. J. M. Sc., 1904, **127**, 710. 219. Am. J. Dis. Child., 1925, **29**, 86. 220. Am. J. Dis. Child., 1930, **39**, 277. 221. J.A.M.A., 1910, **55**, 2198. 222. Penna. M. J., 1920, **24**, 135. 223. Acta chir. Scand., 1926, **60**, 397. 224. Dis. of the Vermiform Appendix, 1895, 113. 225. Arch. de méd. des enf., 1910, **13**, 401. 226. J.A.M.A., 1924, **83**, 967. 227. J.A.M.A., 1928, **90**, 1679. 228. Am. J. M. Sc., 1911, **152**, 11. 229. Acta chir. Scandinav., 1921, **54**, 145. 230. Ann. Surg., 1929, **89**, 48. 231. Arch. Surg., 1921, **2**, 315. 232. Münch. med. Wchnschr., 1907, **54**, 2365. 233. Virginia Med. J. Semi-monthly, 1901, **6**, 398. 234. Bost. M. and S., 1915, **173**, 301. 235. Am. J. Dis. Child., 1927, **34**, 797. 236. Am. J. Dis. Child., 1921, **22**, 493. 237. Griffith, J.A.M.A., 1903, **41**, 531. 238. Brit. J. Child. Dis., 1916, **13**, 207. 239. Pfaundler u. Schlossmann's Handb. d. Kinderh., 1923, **3**, 277. 240. Arch. Pediat., 1924, **41**, 208. 241. Am. J. Dis. Child., 1924, **28**, 76. 242. Med. Klinik., 1926, **22**, 1882. 243. Surg., Gyaec., and Obstet., 1913, **16**, 74. 244. Annals of Surgery, 1902, **35**, 471. 245. Med. Rec., 1903, **64**, 933. 246. Brit. M. J., 1907, **2**, 823; 1908, **2**, 909. 247. Le diverticule de Meckel, 1907. 248. Am. J. Dis. Child., 1931, **42**, 1176. 249. Rev. de chirurg., 1906, **34**, 338; 550. 250. J.A.M.A., 1926, **87**, 91. 251. Am. J. Dis. Child., 1928, **26**, 515. 251. Nederl. Tijdschr. v. Geneesk., 1928, **72**, 4020. 253. Arch. Pediat., 1929, **46**, 521. 254. Am. J. Dis. Child., 1928, **36**, 1218.

CHAPTER VII

DISEASES OF THE INTESTINE (Continued)

PROLAPSE OF THE RECTUM AND ANUS

Etiology.—This is a rather common affection of childhood, especially of the first three years of life, although not often seen in the first six months. It occurs oftenest where there has been repeated decided straining at stool or urination, and hence it is a frequent complication of ileocolitis or of diarrhea from other cause, chronic constipation, proctitis, stone in the bladder, phimosis or other urethral obstruction, thread-worms, rectal polypus, or other cause of tenesmus. It is also common in debilitated subjects in whom the sphincter ani has lost its tone, even without there having been excessive straining. Under these conditions it may be a complication of pertussis. The anatomical relationships of the rectum in early life favor the occurrence of prolapse, among them being its more vertical position and the less firm attachment to the neighboring parts. Sitting low when at stool and upon a vessel with a wide opening, as the ordinary chamber pot, is another predisposing factor.

Symptoms.—The condition suggests an invagination developing at the anus. The prolapse may be only partial and limited to the opening of the bowel (*prolapse of the anus*). In complete prolapse (*prolapse of the* *rectum*) there is a considerable portion of the rectum extruded including all the coats, and forming a sausage-shaped or more globular, soft, dark-red mass, somewhat furrowed, more or less coated with mucus, and often with slightly bleeding points especially if handled (Fig. 147). At the part farthest removed from the body is a small depression, indicating the much narrowed lumen of the gut. The presence of the tumor, if the case is an acute one, causes constant efforts at straining. As a rule the prolapse occurs only at stool, or when there is a straining effort from other causes; but sometimes, in severe and obstinate cases, even walking about the room may be sufficient to cause an extensive prolapse to occur, which may remain down with few subjective symptoms.

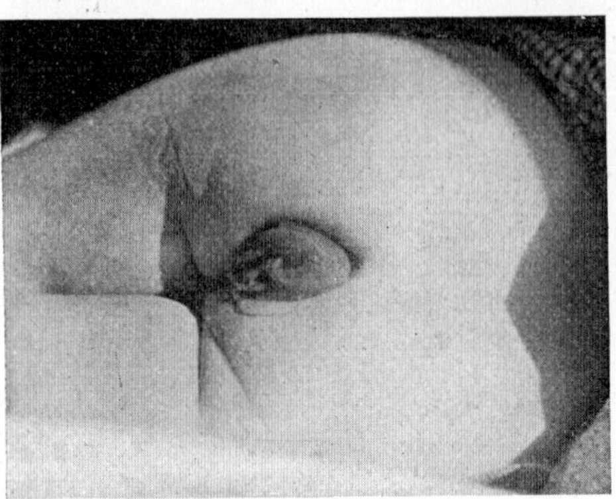

Fig. 147.—Prolapse of the anus. From a patient in the Children's Hospital of Philadelphia.

Course and Prognosis.—In mild prolapse, as of the mucous membrane only, the condition is self-reducing after defecation. In more severe cases the compression of the extruded gut by the anal sphincter causes swelling, and the prolapse persists unless reduced by treatment. The tendency to recurrence may be long-continued. Rarely necrosis of the mucous membrane may result from incarceration.

Diagnosis.—This is usually easy. A prolapsed rectal polypus is of firmer consistence and without a central opening. Ileocecal intussusception which protrudes from the anus may be recognized by the fact that the finger can be passed well upward between the sphincter and the protruding bowel.

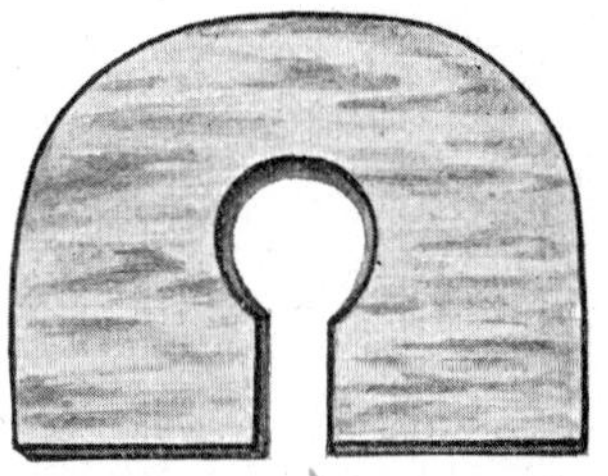

Fig. 148.—Toilet-seat for prolapse of the rectum. To be used over the seat of the ordinary nursery-chair.

Treatment.—The first indication is to replace the extruded bowel. The bowel and the hands of the physician are well oiled, and a steady, gentle pressure made until normal relations are obtained, reducing the central portion first. Should the oiled intestine slip too readily from the grasp of the fingers, a soft linen or similar cloth may be interposed. Inverting the child may be useful in some instances. In more obstinate cases the application of ice-cold compresses diminishes the swelling and renders reduction easier. It may be necessary to dilate the sphincter with the finger in cases where the prolapse has lasted some time.

To prevent recurrence some support must be given at the time of defecation, in such a way that the anal opening is narrowed. The child should lie on its back or side, the feces being passed into a wad of oakum or other soft material, the nates being meanwhile pressed together by the attendant. Older children may sit upon a seat especially constructed to support the tissues about the anus, which is placed over the ordinary infant's chair or toilet (Fig. 148). The seat should be sufficiently high from the floor to prevent undue flexing of the thighs, and the child should be prevented from leaning forward. When prolapse occurs very frequently efficient support may often be rendered by drawing the buttocks firmly together with a broad strip of adhesive plaster crossing them transversely. Constipation is to be prevented by gentle laxatives; diarrhea checked by appropriate remedies.

Frequent bathing of the anal region with cold water and the employment of tannic-acid suppositories help to contract the anus and give tone to the parts. Tonic measures of various sorts are also required. The rectal injection of solution of adrenaline chloride has been advocated, and good results claimed (Miserocchi[1]). Operative procedures are sometimes required.

PROCTITIS

Inflammation of the rectum may attend ileocolitis, and in that event the symptoms are in no way diagnostic. Only inflammation limited to the rectum will be considered here. Trauma is among the **causes;** such as is produced by too frequent employment of enemata, of the soap-stick or, still more, of glycerin-suppositories. A gonorrheal inflammation of the rectum may be produced by the extension from vulvovaginitis, or by the employment of an infected thermometer; or rarely in older children by rectal copulation. The presence of oxyuris may sometimes produce inflammation, and the disease may follow the infectious fevers or be a manifestation of tuberculosis. The **symptoms** are mainly local, and consist of rectal pain, tenesmus, and the discharge of bloody mucus. The last is often not mingled with the stool, but perhaps passed before the feces appear. Irritation of the bladder not infrequently accompanies proctitis, and rectal prolapse is common. When the inflammation is severe, ulcerative changes may take place and the discharge contain pus, and not uncommonly blood in small or even large amount. In some cases of a more continued nature, as in those due to tuberculosis, ulceration may be present with but little pain, and with no tenesmus unless the lesion is in the lower part of the rectum. Occasionally a pseudomembranous inflammation of the rectum is found, depending upon the action of the diphtheria bacillus or of the pneumococcus or streptococcus. The symptoms of this are those already described, with the addition of the discovery of the pseudomembrane in the stools, or by inspection of the bowel. The **course** of proctitis is usually acute and the **prognosis** favorable, the symptoms subsiding in a few days. Sometimes, however, the condition passes into a chronic form, and ulcerative cases are often very slow in recovering. A proctoscopic examination should be made in all patients in whom the symptoms do not abate. In the way of **treatment** in the acute condition the patient should be kept in bed and given injections of starch-water or normal saline or boric acid solution several times daily. The diet should be unirritating and the tenesmus relieved by opiates if necessary. Later a weak solution of tannic acid (0.5 per cent), or of silver nitrate (0.1 per cent), or stronger solutions of argyrol, protargol, or similar salt of silver are often of benefit. Suppositories of tannic acid may be serviceable.

FISSURE OF THE ANUS

Etiology.—This condition is by no means uncommon in early life, but seen probably oftener in infancy than in childhood. Among causes are congenital syphilitic ulceration, injury done by the use of a syringe, and the irritation produced by the oxyuris or by eczema. When occurring in older children the most frequent cause is constipation with the passage of large scybalous masses. Once formed the fissure is liable to be kept open by the feces passing over it, and by the alternate expansion and contraction of the anus which occurs during defecation. The **pathologic anatomy** consists in a linear break in the mucous membrane at or above the margin of the anus, and oftenest on the posterior wall. If of long duration its edges are indurated and the surface secretes pus and bleeds when touched. There may be a number of such fissures present. To reveal the lesion the child should be laid upon the side or back with the legs flexed as closely upon the abdomen as possible, and the buttocks should then be pulled apart firmly. A digital examination of the rectum for polypus should also be made, as this condition sometimes accompanies fissure. The **symptoms** consist in pain on and following defecation, and the discharge of a small amount of blood, which may streak the stool. The pain is often severe, and the patient abstains from defecation as long as possible. Sometimes reflex incontinence or retention of urine is observed, or pain may radiate to the legs, and may produce lameness and other symptoms strongly suggesting hip-joint disease. This has been emphasized especially by Svehla.[2] Various nervous symptoms occasionally develop. **Treatment** of the recent milder cases consists in keeping the stools soft, the rectum clean after defecation by the use of small enemata or of petrolatum on cotton; and the careful application of a 5 per cent solution of nitrate of silver, or of the solid stick, followed by a soothing ointment. Sometimes the employment of 1 to 2 per cent cocaine or novocaine ointment on the region of the fissure before defecation occurs anesthetizes the parts. The passage of a stool may then be produced by a small unirritating injection, as of oil or of normal salt-solution. In obstinate cases dilatation of the external sphincter and cauterization of the fissure under general anesthesia may be required.

ISCHIORECTAL ABSCESS

Ischiorectal abscess is not infrequent in early life, especially in infancy. It consists of an accumulation of pus in the cellular tissue about the rectum. It may result from trauma, deep fissures of the anus, phlebitis of the hemorrhoidal veins, or infection of the lymph-channels, and in about 20 per cent of the cases, according to Clarke,[3] the lesion is tuberculous. There develops fever without discoverable cause, since the abscess is often entirely overlooked for some time, owing to the impossibility of complaint by the youthful patient. Inspection often reveals an indurated or fluctuating area in the anal region, and digital examination a bulging of the wall of the rectum. Treatment consists in prompt, free incision. As a rule, the abscess heals readily, and only exceptionally does an anal fistula occur. Fistula is, in fact, of very rare occurrence in early life. According to Mitchener,[4] in 1500 cases of this operated upon in St. Thomas's Hospital only 12 were in children.

INCONTINENCE OF FECES

For this condition there are various etiologic factors. Lack of proper training may cause its persistence for some time after the control of the bowel should ordinarily have been attained. In greatly debilitated states and in the course of many severe acute diseases, fecal incontinence, similar to incontinence of urine, may be present until convalescence from the primary affection is under way. Incontinence of feces may depend upon some local condition of the lower rectum and the sphincter, such as dysenteric diarrhea, overdistention from chronic constipation, an old prolapse of the rectum, rectovaginal fistula, or earlier stretching of the sphincter for fissure. The most serious cases are those associated with diseases of the mind and the nervous system. Thus well-marked cases of idiocy may never learn to exercise control over the bowels, and there may be incontinence in the paroxysms of epilepsy, during severe chorea, or attendant upon spina bifida and different forms of myelitis. For many of these cases there is no relief possible, while in others recovery may take place after a time, the prognosis depending upon that of the primary disease.

Exceptionally fecal incontinence is a purely functional disturbance analogous to enuresis. We[5] have reported one such instance in a boy of eight years, and cases have been published by others, and the subject reviewed especially by Ostheimer.[6] In some instances incontinence of this nature has depended upon some reflex irritation; a vesical calculus in one of Ostheimer's cases, and apparently upon hypertrophy of the tonsils in an instance reported by Silvestri.[7] The incontinence may occur at night-time only, or in the waking hours as well. The disease is more common in boys, may date from birth, or may come on only when the patient is deteriorated in health or is undergoing some special nervous strain. It may yield readily, or may prove troublesome to cure. General treatment is required, including that of a tonic nature, such as cool bathing, outdoor life, and the administration of strychnine or arsenic. Sometimes belladonna and the bromides act favorably, as in enuresis.

HEMORRHOIDS

Hemorrhoids are very uncommon in childhood, although exceptionally they may be found very early in life. We have seen the disorder in an infant of twelve months. In rare instances it may be congenital (Milward[8]), but the condition is then not in reality a true pile, but a small benign neoplasm of a fibrous and fatty nature. Hemorrhoids may be either external or internal in nature, and are oftenest the result of chronic constipation. They may also be produced by sitting at stool upon a low wide-mouthed receptacle, as in the case of prolapse of the anus. Tonic remedies are usually indicated, since the children are frequently debilitated subjects. Other treatment is similar to that effectual in adult life; chiefly the employment of cold local bathing and a mild astringent ointment.

PRURITUS ANI

This annoying affection is not unusual in children, and is a symptom of many diverse conditions. Its most frequent cause is the presence of the oxyuris; but diabetes, eczema, hemorrhoids, constipation, indigestion from improper foods, and slight prolapse may produce it likewise. The treatment is that of the cause, and this must be sought for diligently. As palliative measures, application of cold water or of hot water is often serviceable, as are weak ointments of cocaine, novocaine, tar, carbolic aid or menthol, and the painting with compound tincture of benzoin, tincture of iodine, or a 5 per cent solution of oil of cade in flexible collodion.

FOREIGN BODIES IN THE INTESTINAL CANAL

The constant tendency of infants to put small objects into their mouths makes the swallowing of these a matter of great frequency; and even in older children the slipping of fruit-stones, pieces of bone, pins, and many other substances into the gullet and downward is not uncommon. The danger of these being arrested in the esophagus and stomach has already been referred to (pp. 549–568).

Symptoms.—In the intestine a foreign body causes, as a rule, little trouble, perhaps producing slight pain or abdominal discomfort or tenderness. Even if irregular and of rather large size, it generally advances steadily to the rectum and is expelled after from a few days to a week or longer. Occasionally foreign bodies in the intestines cause severe pain and intestinal irritation, and the passage of feces containing visible or occult blood; or they may even perforate the intestinal wall; or they may cause obstinate vomiting if the article is of a size and nature to produce intestinal obstruction. Rarely articles of small size become lodged in the appendix and may even be the cause of perforation there. In the *rectum* foreign bodies produce no symptoms in most cases, but sometimes may be the occasion of pain there or of tenesmus. Occasionally they enter the rectum through the anus, either by accident or having been inserted by the patient. In the class of foreign bodies are to be included large *fecal concretions* which, when in the colon, may attain a size readily felt through the abdominal wall and be the cause of obstruction; or, in the rectum, may be passed only with extraneous aid.

Diagnosis.—This is to be based upon an unquestionable history of the swallowing of an object. A careful watch should be kept upon all the passages from the bowel; the stools being thoroughly shaken with water until soluble, and then strained in the search for the article. The use of roentgenograms or the fluoroscope is invaluable in the case of substances opaque to the *x*-ray, to determine the position of the object, and whether or not it is passing downward in a normal manner. Sometimes palpation of the abdominal wall may reveal the presence of a body if favorably situated for this investigation.

As far as subjective symptoms are concerned, diagnosis is more uncertain. In children old enough to be influenced by suggestion, the alarm of and the questioning by the parents may readily elicit complaint of a purely hysterical nature. If the trouble is in the rectum there may be tenesmus.

Treatment.—The giving of starchy food, such as bread, arrowroot, oatmeal, and potato, tends to coat the body and render its passage through the intestine easier. In the case of fecal concretions repeated administration of purgative drugs in small dose may be needed, castor oil being one of the best of these. The occurrence of obstruction or of symptoms of peritonitis demands prompt operative interference, but this is seldom required. In the rectum the body may be removed by the finger or through a speculum.

MORBID GROWTHS OF THE INTESTINE

Rectal Polypus.—Not a common affection, this is oftener seen in childhood than at other periods of life, although rare in infancy. The growth is an adenoma, pea-size or larger, of a bright-red color, usually single, and situated upon the posterior, or sometimes the anterior, wall of the rectum, 2 or 3 in. (5.1 to 7.6 cm.) above the anus. There is generally a pedicle $\frac{1}{2}$ to 3 in. (1.3 to 5.1 cm.) in length, but occasionally the growth may be attached to the mucous membrane by a broad base. The chief **symptom** is hemorrhage, with or without the passage of mucus. If the pedicle is sufficiently long for the polypus to approach the anus, there are also discomfort or pain in the rectum, and tenesmus; and the tumor may be protruded through the anus during efforts at defecation. The **diagnosis** is to be made only from hemorrhage from other causes and from prolapse of the rectum; and careful examination, perhaps with the proctoscope, readily shows the differences. **Treatment** consists in removing the growth by operative measures. A return of the trouble is unusual.

Other Morbid Growths.—These are of great rarity in early life. Sarcoma may be either primary or secondary. Nobécourt[9] was able to collect but 13 cases. Fibroma, papilloma, angioma, lipoma, and cysts have also been found. The lymphoid growths of leukemia may also occur in this locality; and Zuppinger[10] has collected 12 instances of carcinoma, including one reported by himself. A diffuse polyposis of the colon and occasionally of the small intestine is an uncommon condition in children.

It shows a familial tendency, and is liable in early adult life to malignant degeneration. The subject has been reviewed by Kennedy and Weber.[11]

REFERENCES

1. Pediatria, 1905, **13,** 380. 2. Jahrb. f. Kinderh., 1906, **63,** 187. 3. Tubercle, 1926, **7,** 277. 4. Brit. J. Surg., 1914–15, **2,** 364. 5. Griffith, Arch. Pediat., 1899, **16,** 416. 6. Univ. Pennsylvania M. Bull., 1905, **17,** 405; J.A.M.A., 1907, **49,** 1115. 7. Gazz. d. osp., 1904, **25,** 46. 8. Lancet, 1907, **1,** 1489. 9. Traité d. mal. de l'enf., 1904, **2,** 257. 10. Wien. klin. Wchnschr., 1900, **13,** 389. 11. Am. J. Dis. Child., 1931, **42,** 69.

CHAPTER VIII

INTESTINAL PARASITES

All sorts of symptoms are attributed to "worms," but only the actual finding of the parasites or their ova justifies the diagnosis. The frequency of the occurrence of these varies with the locality and with the type of patient studied. Thus McLean[1] observed infestation in only 2.27 per cent of infants and children studied in New York; Rivas and Fife[2] in 26.5 per cent in Philadelphia; DeBuys and Dwyer[3] in 53.27 per cent in New Orleans; and Haughwout and Horrilleno[4] in 92 per cent in the Phillipine Islands. *Age* has a great influence in all types of intestinal infestation, infants under two years of age seldom being affected. In the subjects studied by McLean 119 were less than two years old, and in all of these the examination gave negative results. Similarly Peiser,[5] in 114 necropsies in subjects less than two years of age, found all were free from parasites. The occurrence of two or more varieties of parasites in the same case is very frequent.

ASCARIS LUMBRICOIDES

(Round Worm; Eel-worm)

This nematode worm is perhaps the most common intestinal parasite in children in this country, with the single exception of the hook-worm as encountered in certain districts. Its occurrence would appear to be most frequent at from five to ten years of age. It is rarely seen in infancy, perhaps the youngest recorded case being in an infant of three weeks, reported by Miller.[6] The total incidence of the disease is subject to wide variation with the geographical locality. A review by Lechler[7] showed a range of from 2.33 per cent to 43.33 per cent of the children examined. The worms occupy especially the small intestine, from which they may pass downward and be voided from the rectum, or they occasionally wander in other directions. Not infrequently they enter the stomach and may be vomited. They may also find their way into the larynx, causing asphyxia; the Eustachian tube and thence into the ear; the nose; tonsils; the trachea and thence into the lung; the bile-duct and thence the liver, where they have produced abscess; the pancreatic duct, producing acute hemorrhagic pancreatitis; the vermiform appendix, heart, hernial sacs, and Meckel's diverticulum, in the last perhaps being discharged from an umbilical fistula. Very rarely the worms may perforate ulcers in the intestine, or even the healthy intestinal or gastric wall, and enter the peritoneal cavity, causing peritonitis. Plew[8] has studied this occurrence, with the report of a case and a review of the literature. When in very large numbers they may occasionally produce intestinal obstruction (Hoffman,[9] p. 617). Frequently the presence of the parasites in the intestine can be shown in roentgenograms. This was first noted by Fritz[10] in 1922 and since then by others. The subject has been reviewed by Archer and Peterson.[11]

The round worm bears a close resemblance in form to the ordinary earthworm, but is of a pinkish color and of larger size, being from $\frac{1}{8}$ to over $\frac{1}{4}$ of an inch (0.32 to 0.64 cm.) in thickness, and the male from 4 to 8 in. (10 to 20 cm.) and the female from 7 to 12 in. (18 to 31 cm.) in length (Fig. 149). The eggs, which are produced by the million, are round or oval, brownish or yellowish in color, about $\frac{1}{500}$ of an inch (0.005 cm.) in the greatest diameter and with a nodular outer coat. If they are scanty they are best found by centrifuging a 1 to 100 dilution of the feces and examining the residue. The number of worms present in the intestine is usually not large, probably not exceeding from 5 to 20, but there may occasionally be hundreds, Pessôa,[12] for example, reporting the evacuation of 566 of them within less than forty-eight hours. The eggs enter the body through the mouth, having contaminated the drinking water or uncooked vegetables or fruits which have come into contact with human feces, perhaps in the form of manure. No intermediate host is necessary. The studies of Stewart[13] and of Ransom and Foster[14] have made the life-cycle clear. After the eggs have been swallowed they hatch into the larval form in the intestine. These larvae penetrate the intestinal wall and pass by way of the portal circulation to the liver; thence by the hepatic veins to the heart, and from there by the pulmonary artery to the lungs. In the lungs they migrate from the capillaries into the alveoli and thence through the bronchi and trachea to the pharynx, esophagus, stomach and intestines. Some of the larvae, however, may pass from the lungs back to the heart and be distributed to various parts of the body.

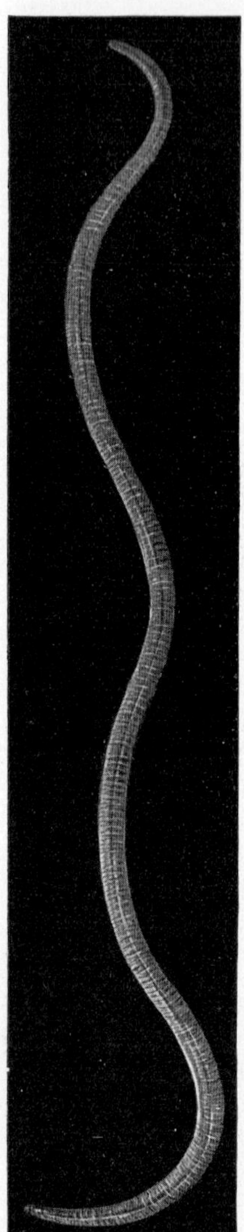

Fig. 149.—Ascaris lumbricoides. One-half natural size.

Symptoms.—As a rule there are none whatever and the diagnosis can be made only by the discovery of the worms or their ova in the passages. Sometimes there are produced irritability, restless sleep, grinding of the teeth, picking of the nose, colic, tympanites, and loss of appetite; but these are much more frequently dependent upon other causes than upon the presence of ascarides. Eosinophilia is generally present, but not marked. In three-fifths of Hille's[15] 85 cases it did not exceed 6 per cent. Brunner[16] believes that a cutaneous test with an extract of the ascaris will give a positive reaction to nematode worms. Brünning[17] and Cieszynski,[18] as well as Fülleborn,[19] after whom the reaction is named, do not believe that it has as yet any proven practical diagnostic value, although further studies are desirable. Various nervous manifestations are often attributed to the parasites, and are sometimes actually due to them when they occur in large numbers, as proven by the fact that their removal by treatment may be followed by cessation of the disturbance. It is probable that such nervous and other disorders are more likely to be caused by ascarides than by parasites of other sorts. This may possibly be through absorption of toxins produced by them. The larval form when in the lungs may give rise to pulmonary symptoms. Koino[20] demonstrated this experimentally upon himself, pulmonary involvement with expectoration of larvae in the sputum having followed ingestion of the eggs. The serious symptoms caused by the mechanical action of the worms when they have wandered into distant regions have been referred to (p. 645).

Treatment.—The most serviceable remedy is powdered santonin, combined with calomel or sugar, and given in doses of ½ to 1 grain (0.032 to 0.065) to a child four or five years of age, three times a day, for one or perhaps two days. The patient should be prepared for the treatment by short starvation or the use of a milk-diet for a day or two, and a dose of castor-oil or other purgative should be given after the course of santonin has been completed. When combined with calomel, ½ grain (0.032) of this to the dose, the castor-oil will probably not be required. It is important to obtain purgation after the administration of santonin in order to remove it from the system, or it may be absorbed and xanthopsia, or "yellow vision," result, with headache, vomiting, vertigo, and even convulsions. Another remedy sometimes employed is fluid extract of spigelia and senna, 1 fl. dr. (4) at four years of age, given three times a day for two or three days. Oil of chenopodium, 5 minims (0.31) on sugar at four years of age, administered three times a day, is also serviceable, as is also carbon tetrachloride in doses of 2 minims (0.123) for each year of age; in a single dose or divided. Caution with both of these drugs must be observed against an overdose. (See p. 512.) Lamson, Ward and Brown[21] recommend hexylresorcinol (0.6 to 1.0 Gm.) (9 to 15 grains) of the crystals in gelatin capsules; *not* in solution. A couple of weeks after treatment with any vermifuge the stools should be examined for ova and the treatment repeated if these are found to be present. In the way of prevention every possible precaution should be taken as to the cleanliness of the food and the proper disposition of the feces.

OXYURIS VERMICULARIS

(Thread-worm. Pin-worm. Seat-worm)

The oxyuris is a nematode worm found with greater frequency in children, but is by no means confined to this age. It is less often encountered in infants. A lack of cleanliness seems to predispose, but this does not appear to be essential. The frequency of occurrence is influenced by the locality and by other conditions; 30 per cent of the children examined in Munich (Trumpp[22]), 73.3 per cent in Halle (Japha[23]), 6.72 per cent in New Orleans (DeBuys and Dwyer[3]), 1.6 per cent in Rio Janeiro (Faria[24]). The parasites inhabit the rectum and large intestine, but appear to enter it from the small intestine, which seems to be their breeding place. They are not infrequently discovered in the vermiform appendix, and have occasionally been found in the stomach and even the mouth. Not rarely they wander into the vagina or under the prepuce, and occur in the groins, about the genitals, and in the folds about the anus.

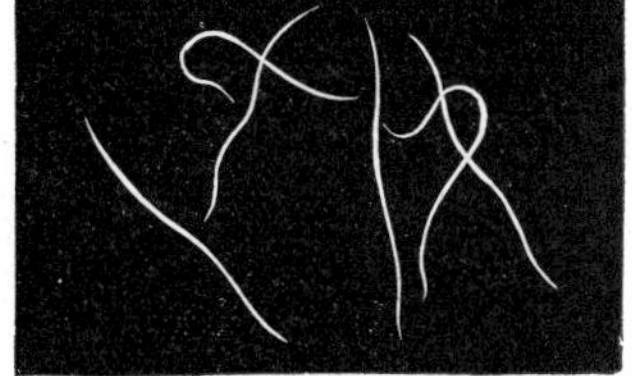

Fig. 150.—Oxyuris vermicularis. Natural size.

The oxyuris resembles a very short white thread (Fig. 150). The female measures from ¼ to ½ in. (0.64 to 1.27 cm.) in length and about $\frac{1}{25}$ in. (0.1 cm.) in thickness; the male not more than one-half or one-third of this size. In the intestines they are present in vast numbers, covering thickly the walls of the rectum, and being embedded in the mucus coating it. The eggs are produced in the bowel in large quantity, but are not always readily discovered in the stools. They are white in color, oval in shape but asymmetrical, with a smooth exterior, and measure approximately $\frac{1}{500}$ in. (0.005 cm.) in length and $\frac{1}{800}$ in. (0.0032 cm.) in diameter. The children constantly reinfect themselves and other children in the family by transmitting on their hands the eggs which have lodged under the finger-nails in the act of scratching at the anus; or the eggs may come into contact with raw food, toys, dust, and the like. Thus introduced they develop into fully matured worms in the small intestine, and these may be found in the feces in two to three weeks. No intermediate host is required. It has generally been believed that eggs produced in the intestine will not develop there until reintroduced by way of the mouth. This is, however, denied by Trumpp,[22] Goebel,[25] Heubner[26] and others.

Symptoms.—The principal symptom is intolerable itching at the anus, usually worse at night-time and interfering greatly with sleep. Examination may reveal the living and moving worms in small or in great numbers coating the stools, or within the anus if the mucous membrane be slightly everted, or even in the folds of the groin or about the genitals. The giving of an enema will often bring away large numbers of the parasites from the bowel. The scratching which the itching incites frequently produces a secondary eczema about the anus. If the worms have entered the vagina vulvovaginitis results, and the intense itching may induce masturbation. Other secondary symptoms often appear, among them being enuresis, frequent micturition, prolapse of the rectum from straining, and catarrhal inflammation of the colon and rectum with discharge of a large amount of mucus. More remote symptoms sometimes result from the irritation and the loss of rest, such as night-terrors, anemia, debility, and even convulsions. Eosinophilia is an uncertain symptom, present in one-half or less of the cases.

Course and Prognosis.—One great difficulty which often renders successful treatment a puzzling problem is the constant danger of reinfection when the worms are numerous and the itching severe and scratching frequent. Another obstacle to treatment is the firmness with which the worms are imbedded in the mucus covering the intestinal wall, as well as the fact that they penetrate into the intestinal follicles. The fact, too, that injections do not reach the upper colon satisfactorily, or the small intestine at all, renders the disease resistant to this treatment, and the course prolonged. Even the discovery of the worms or ova is not always easy, since the parasites are discharged often only periodically in cycles of from six to seven weeks, depending upon the development of a new generation of worms. Consequently any treatment employed should be repeated at intervals less than the full time for maturation, in order to kill the parasites before they have fully developed. There is no assurance of recovery until at least two months have passed without any evidence of the presence of parasites (Heubner[27]).

Treatment.—This consists in:

(*a*) Destruction of worms about to discharge eggs. For this purpose an enema of a 6 per cent infusion of quassia should be given as high as possible into the colon, with the hips elevated, using from a pint (473) to a quart (946) of liquid. This should be repeated every evening at bedtime for from seven to ten days. Success may be obtained also with large flushings with simple cold water or soap-water. Salt and water (1 oz.:1 pt.) (28:473), infusion of garlic, turpentine, vinegar, and corrosive sublimate (1:10,000) are also recommended. For worms or eggs in the vagina the bichloride injection may well be employed.

(*b*) Killing the worms situated higher in the bowel. To accomplish this santonin, spigelia, or chenopodium may be given by the mouth as for ascarides. Naphthalene has also been used, administering it in doses of $\frac{1}{2}$ to 1 grain (0.032 to 0.065) three or four times a day at two years of age, continuing for a week, and repeating the course after two weeks. Oily substances should be withheld while this drug is being employed. Carbon tetrachloride is recommended by McVail[27] and others. The dose is 2 minims (0.123) for each year of age, ingested at one time or in divided doses. (See p. 512.) Luzzatti[28] has found chloroform very effective, about 2 Gm. (0.068 fl. oz.) being given in castor oil, and the dose repeated every ten days for three courses. Loeper[29] and others obtained good results with bismuth carbonate given on each of two successive days in doses of 2 to 3 Gm. (0.068 to 0.10 fl. oz.) to infants and 4 to 5 Gm. (0.13 to 0.17 fl. oz.) to older children. Saline purgatives are excellent, citrate of magnesia often being taken readily by children. Any remedy administered is best given after a period of fasting. With regard to any treatment employed, either by the rectum or the mouth, what has been said above concerning the repetition of this at stated intervals should not be forgotten.

(*c*) Destruction of the eggs deposited on the skin of the ano-genital region. Preferably after every bowel movement, and certainly morning and night, the whole ano-genital region and surrounding parts should be bathed with a 1:10,000 bichloride solution. The bedding and night-clothes must be changed daily and thoroughly disinfected; the hands of the nurse and of the patient kept disinfected; the dirt beneath the child's finger-nails, where the eggs are so often embedded, removed carefully; and at night, and possibly in the day also, the hands mechanically hindered from contact with the anus and the mouth, as by the wearing of mittens or other protective covering, or of a pasteboard elbow-cuff which prevents flexion of the joint, or by dressing the child at night in close-fitting drawers. To relieve the itching and lessen the tendency to scratching, boric-acid ointment or mercurial ointment may be applied to the anus, especially at bedtime. This has the additional advantage of being destructive to eggs and worms. To cure any patient it is necessary that in the prevention of reinfection all those in the family who are infected must be treated.

TAENIA

(Tapeworm)

The cestode worms of this genus are of common occurrence in early life, their frequency probably equaling that in adults. To this statement infancy offers a decided exception, tapeworms of most species being found at this period only under unusual circumstances, perhaps dependent upon departure from the ordinary diet of milk. The youngest cases recorded in medical literature appear to be in two infants each five days old, reported by Müller[30] and Armor;[31] but with our knowledge of the life-history of the parasite such an occurrence seems scarcely credible. Taenia solium is reported by Pardo[32] in an infant of five months, and taenia saginata by Comby[33] in one of nine months, and by Grimm[34] in one of ten and one-half months.

The abode of the tapeworm is the small intestine, whence segments pass into the large intestine and are voided with the stools. The worm is of variable length, depending upon the species, and is composed of a series of flattened, white, opaque segments (*proglottides*) more or less rectangular in form and each sexually complete. The head (*scolex*) is the size of a small pin head, and is followed by a thread like neck, and this by the youngest segments, at first very small. These rapidly increase in size, until mature in from three to three and one-half months, when those toward the lower end of the worm separate and are discharged from time to time, singly or in short series, new segments being produced by the head The worm retains its position in the bowel by means of the hooks or the suckers with which the head is provided. The ripe segments, as passed, contain the eggs, which vary in size, shape and number with the species, and within which microscopic examination reveals the embryos. The number of tapeworms present varies with the species. Sometimes two or even three different species of tapeworm may occur simultaneously in the intestine, but this is unusual.

For reproduction the tapeworm needs an intermediate host, the species of animal depending upon the species of worm. The proglottides of the worm, after passing from the intestine, soften, and the eggs are discharged, or in the case of taenia solium the eggs may be thus set free before they leave the intestine. These are then swallowed by some animal, penetrate its intestine, and develop in the muscles and other tissues into the larval form of the worm; in the case of the *true* taeniadae, the *cysticercus*. The flesh of the animal after it is eaten by man sets free the larvae in the intestine, where they develop into tapeworms. The eating of the flesh containing these is not, however, absolutely necessary, since drinking water contaminated by them may rarely produce the disease. In the case of taenia elliptica infected insects are unconsciously eaten and the larvae ingested in this way.

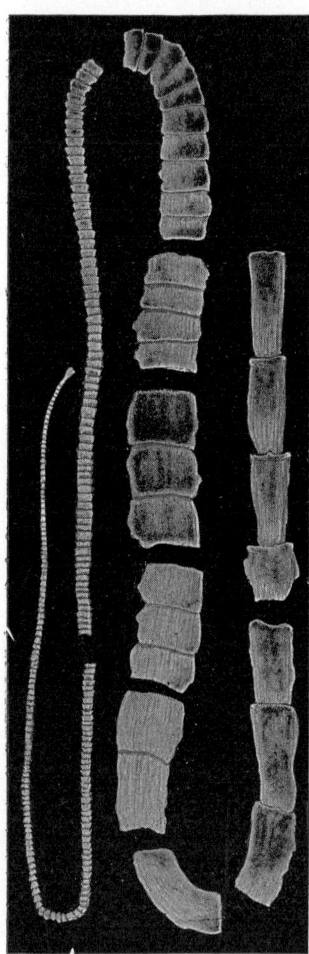

Fig. 151.—Taenia saginata. Different portions of worm. Natural size.

The tapeworms usually infecting human beings are as follows:

Taenia Solium; Pork-tapeworm; Armed Tapeworm.—This species has four sucking mouths and a double row of hooklets surrounding the probosis. The adult worm measures6 to 12 ft (183 to 365 cm.) in length, the segments averaging about $\frac{1}{2}$ in. (1.27 cm.) in length and $\frac{1}{4}$ to $\frac{1}{3}$ in. (0.64 to 0.86 cm.) in breadth. The ripe segments toward the end of the worm are longer and narrower. The proglottides contain in their interior the dendritic uterus with 8 to 12 rather thick lateral branches on each side. The eggs are brown, spherical, and about $\frac{1}{800}$ in. (0.0032 cm.) in diameter. This tapeworm is acquired by eating the raw or imperfectly cooked "measly" flesh of the hog. The eggs are often freed from the proglottides in the intestine and passed by stool, and patients may occasionally reinfect themselves by swallowing the eggs and in this way develop the cysticercus in various parts of the body. Taenia solium is very much less common in this country than is the taenia saginata, is smaller in size, and is quite infrequent in children. It occurs almost always only singly in the intestine.

Taenia Saginata; Taenia Mediocanellata; Beef-tapeworm (Fig. 151).—The head is larger than in the preceding species, pear-shaped, with four sucking mouths, but without hooklets or beak. This tapeworm measures 15 to 24 ft. (456 to 730 cm.) or more in length, the segments averaging $\frac{3}{5}$ to $\frac{4}{5}$ of an inch (1.5 to 2 cm.) in length and about $\frac{1}{3}$ in. (0.85 cm.) in breadth. Toward the middle of the worm the breadth is greater than at other parts. The uterus contains 20 to 25 slender branches on each side, and the eggs are oval and measure $\frac{1}{800}$ to $\frac{1}{600}$ of an inch (0.0032 to 0.004 cm.) in length by somewhat more than $\frac{1}{2}$ this in breadth. The worm is acquired by eating the affected "measly" flesh of cattle, which have themselves become diseased by ingesting the eggs of tapeworms upon vegetation that had come into contact with contaminated human manure. One or several worms may be present in the intestine at the same time. This species is very widely distributed geographically, and, although less common in the United States than in many other regions, it is by far the most frequent variety found, with the probable exception of taenia nana in some localities. It is rare in infants, but is occasionally acquired through the giving of scraped raw meat. We have observed the disease developing from this cause in several children under two years of age, one of whom first passed segments at the age of ten months.

Taenia Elliptica or Cucumerina; Dog-tapeworm (*Dipylidium caninum*).—This is a small tapeworm common in the dog and cat, but rare in the human race. Zschokke[35] collected 36 published cases, to which he added another; and Lins[36] raised the total number of reported cases to 68. The majority of instances of tapeworm of this variety have been observed in children and infants, over 65 per cent being in children over three years of age (Riley and Shannon[37]). Stuart and Augustine[38] report a case in an infant six months old. Usually the parasite occurs singly, but Lins[36] found from 20 up to 200 present at a time. The second host is the louse and the flea infecting dogs and cats, as well as the human flea. The close contact which play often brings with these domestic animals, and the natural tendency of the infants to put their hands to the mouth, leads to the swallowing of the infected insect and the subsequent later development of the tapeworm. This worm is slender and measures only 4 to 12 in. (10 to 31 cm.) in length. The head is armed with hooklets and a beak. The proglottides are from $\frac{1}{3}$ to $\frac{1}{2}$ in. (0.85 to 1.27 cm.) long and about one-third as broad. The eggs are about $\frac{1}{500}$ in. (0.005 cm.) in diameter, from 6 to 12 being contained in a common capsule.

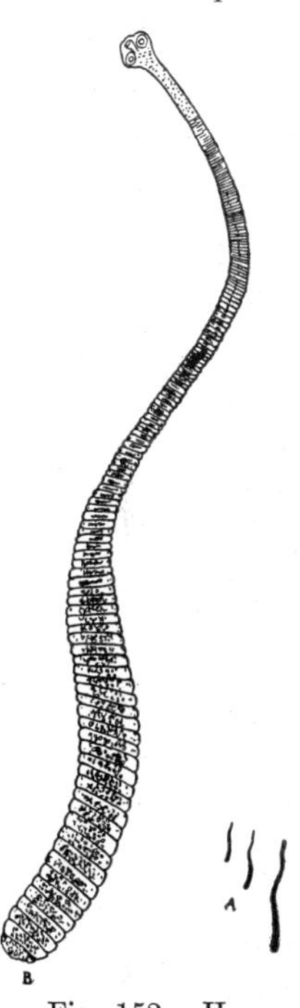

Fig. 152.—Hymenolepis nana. A, One-half actual size; B, enlarged; showing head and suckers. (*Schloss, Arch. of Pediat.*, 1910, **27**, 101.)

Taenia Flavopunctata; Rat-tapeworm (*Hymenolepis flavopunctata; Hymenolepis diminuta*).—This parasite is common in the rat and mouse. DeBuys and Dwyer[3] found it only once in 595 children. Riley and Shannon[37] collected 61 cases reported from all parts of the world. The age was not stated in 22 of these, but of the remainder 17 were in children.

Taenia Nana; Dwarf Tapeworm (*Hymenolepis nana*) (Fig. 152).—This is another variety of tapeworm which has been thought to be rare in this country, although more common in Italy. Ransom[39] collected 106 published cases occurring in man. The parasite is probably much more frequent than these figures represent, inasmuch as Greil[40] observed it in 5.75 per cent of children examined in Alabama; Schloss[41] in 6.08 per cent in New York; Narr[42] in 10 per cent in Philadelphia; DeBuys and Dwyer[3] in 9.25 per cent in New Orleans; Tsuchiya[43] in 0.84 per cent in St. Louis. The literature is reviewed to some extent by Tsuchiya and Rohlfing.[44] Its most frequent habitat is the small intestine of species of rats and mice. The parasite is only $\frac{1}{2}$ to 1 in. (1.27 to 2.54 cm.) long, and has a spherical armed head, and 150 or more short and broad proglottides each containing

80 to 100 eggs. It occurs chiefly in children and often in very large numbers in a single case. Even nurslings may be affected. The intermediate host is unknown, and it is possible that none exists, but that the larvae occupy the mucous membrane of the intestine and there develop into the perfect worm. This absence of intermediate host renders it possible for the spread of the disease from one child to another. There may, however, be cross-infection from man to rats and the reverse.

Dibothriocephalus Latus; Fish-tapeworm.—The head of this parasite is small, wedge-shaped, grooved on each side, and unarmed with beak or hooklets. The proglottides are broader than long, measuring $\frac{1}{2}$ to $\frac{3}{5}$ in. (1.27 to 1.52 cm.) in breadth and but about $\frac{1}{5}$ in. (0.51 cm.) in length. The sexual openings are on the surface of the proglottides instead of at the edge as in other varieties, and the uterus is rosette-shaped, instead of branched. The eggs are about $\frac{1}{400}$ in. (0.006 cm.) long and $\frac{1}{600}$ in. (0.004 cm.) broad, and are characterized by a lid-shaped closure at one end. After leaving the intestine the ova develop in water into a free-swimming infusorial organism, and then by way of the intestine enter the muscles of certain species of fish, where they remain as unencysted elongated larvae of perhaps several inches in length, suggesting the appearance of the fully developed worm. The eating of fish thus infected produces the sexually active parasite in the intestine of man. The worm is 25 to 30 ft. (762 to 915 cm.) or more in length. It is common in certain regions, as Switzerland and Scandinavia, but rare in the United States. Barron,[45] however, has observed 19 cases chiefly in adults, and Pilot and Levine[46] have collected, including 5 of their own, 21 cases in subjects from three to fifteen years of age. The disease occurs especially in the region of the Great Lakes, and seems to depend upon the habit of eating or tasting raw or partly cooked fish. We have observed the parasite once in an adult and again in a child of nine years.

Symptoms of Tapeworm.—As a rule, tapeworm produces no symptoms other than the passing of segments of the worm in the stools, and this constitutes the only positive diagnostic evidence. An eosinophilia is witnessed in rather less than one-half of the cases. In a small proportion there are various digestive disturbances present, such as occasional vomiting, abdominal pain or discomfort, excessive appetite, diarrhea, vertigo, headache, and the like, but it is doubtful in most of these whether the worm possesses any etiological relationship. This is equally true of the more distant reflex symptoms which have repeatedly been described, such as epileptiform and choreiform conditions. The dibothriocephalus and occasionally other parasites, however, can produce anemia of the pernicious type (p. 1028), and the cysticerci of taenia solium may be located in the cutaneous and muscular tissue, the eye, and the brain; in the last situation producing ataxia, bulbar palsy, psychic disturbances, or manifestations of cerebral tumor.

Course and Prognosis.—It is uncertain how long the presence of the worm may continue, but certainly this may even be for years. The danger to the patient is insignificant, barring the possibility of anemia or nervous symptoms referred to, and the chance of reinfection and the production of cysticercus in the case of the presence of taenia solium. Repeated efforts lasting over months are sometimes required before final relief is obtained.

Treatment.—In the way of **prophylaxis** care must be taken to prevent infection. All meat and fish eaten should be sufficiently well-cooked. Careful, frequent disinfection of the hands of little children, and the avoidance of too close contact with dogs and cats, are prophylactic measures against taenia elliptica.

For the actual **treatment** of the disease some vermifuge is required which will expell the head of the parasite. Should the head have remained in the intestine but the rest of the worm have been discharged, the elapse of about three months' time is required for the maturing of fresh segments. The child should receive a light dinner and still lighter supper, such as a bowl of broth or of bread and milk. On waking in the morning, an enema and a saline purgative should be given. Breakfast should consist of a cup of clear broth or beef-tea. After the action of the purgative, the vermifuge is administered in a single dose or divided doses, and followed in an hour by castor oil or a saline in sufficient amount to insure thorough emptying of the bowels. When the desire for an evacuation comes the child should be seated on a full vessel of water so that the nates are in contact with the fluid. Should, however, vomiting or depression be present, the child must remain recumbent in bed. No traction whatever should be made upon the worm but, if it ceases to pass easily, the nozzle of a syringe may be very carefully inserted into the anus and an enema given. After the passing of the stool and the parasite into the vessel of water, this latter should be rocked or stirred gently in order not to break the worm, the fecal matter poured off; then more water added and the process thus continued until the worm is clean; after which, still suspended in water, it can be examined with care for the head.

As the remedies for tapeworm are often nauseating and exhausting the child should be kept reclining in bed for a day or two after taking them, and the diet be light. Klein,[47] Margulis[48] and others advise giving medication through the duodenal tube. If the worm is not completely removed, another effort should be made after an interval of several weeks. The vermifuges recommended are supposed to have the property of killing, or at least numbing, the parasite and thus releasing the hold of its head on the intestine. One of the most effective is aspidium, or male fern (felix mas), of which the oleoresin or the freshly prepared ethereal extract may be administered in doses of ½ to 1 fl. dr. (1.8 to 3.7) to a child four or five years of age. This may be made into an emulsion or may be put into capsules holding 15 minims (0.92), administered every half hour until the complete amount is taken. Success has followed the employment of a very light diet for a day or two, combined with the repeated administration of turpentine; then finally the giving of the male fern in the manner described. It should be borne in mind that in exceptional cases felix mas is distinctly toxic for the patient. Consequently the briskly acting purgative is needed after the vermifuge, in order to prevent the latter from remaining long in the intestinal tract.

Another very useful remedy is a decoction of pomegranite (granatum), in doses of ¾ to 2 fl. oz. (22.2 to 60) for a child of from five to ten years of age. The taste is unpleasant, and the alkaloid pelletierine is to be preferred. We have had good results with a preparation of this (Tanret's) in some obstinate cases when male fern had failed. The drug is liable to produce vertigo, fainting, and nausea, and the child should be kept at rest, as already advised, whatever taenicide is chosen. Kousso is often an effective, but always a very disagreeable, remedy and one liable to cause vomiting. Pumpkin-seed is safe and not unpleasant to take, but is very uncertain in its effects. Sometimes a combination of anthelmintics may avail when a single one has failed. In 1 case where 33 unsuccessful attempts at removal of the head had been made over a period of five years, we obtained success with a combination suggested by Hare,[49] containing male fern, kamela, chloroform, croton oil, and castor oil.

Treatment for tapeworm should not be given to delicate children, or those suffering from digestive or other disturbances of moment, until the general health has been improved. In the anemia produced by dibothriocephalus, liver-feeding is claimed to be effective.

UNCINARIA

(Hook-worm. Ankylostoma. Necator Americanus)

Only two species of uncinaria have the intestine of man as their habitat. One of these is the uncinaria duodenalis (anchylostoma duodenalis), first described by Dubini[50] in 1838, and since then recognized as the cause of certain forms of anemia, seen especially in those working much in earth. It is very widespread in tropical and subtropical countries of the Old World, although much more frequent in certain regions, abounding, for instance, in Egypt. In the United States this species is of uncommon occurrence. Ashford[51] was the first to point out the seriousness of ankylos-

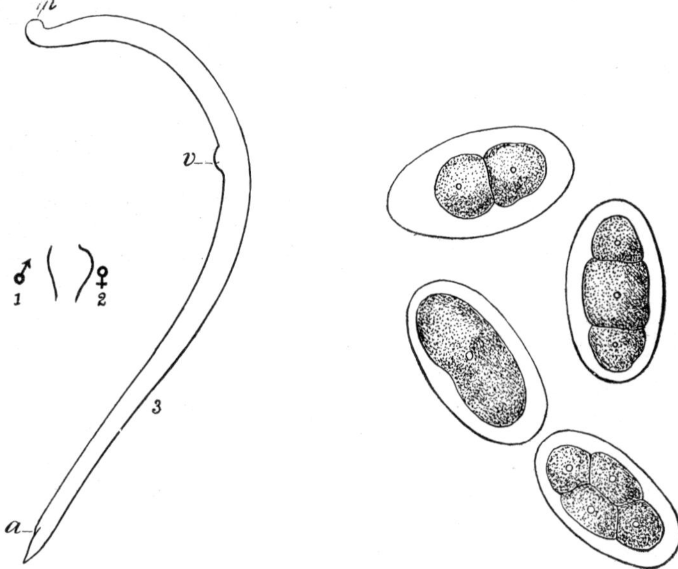

Fig. 153. Fig. 154.

Fig. 153.—New-world hookworm. (*Uncinaria Americana.*) Natural size: 1. Male; 2, female; 3, the same enlarged to show the position of the anus, *a*; the vulva, *v*; and the mouth, *m*. (*Stiles, 18th Ann. Report Bureau of Animal Industry.* 1901, 190.)

Fig. 154.—Four eggs of the new-world hookworm. Eggs exhibiting the one-, two-, and four-cell stages. The egg showing three cells is a lateral view of a four-cell stage. Greatly enlarged. (*Stiles, 18th Ann. Report Bureau of Animal Industry*, 1901, 193.)

tomiasis in this country; but Stiles[52] in May, 1902, reported that the hookworm of the United States differed from the European species. He named it Uncinaria Americana, and studies of recent years have shown that uncinariasis is one of the most frequent, widespread, and important diseases of the Southern States, the incidence ranging from 3 to 25 per cent of the population, varying with the locality. It prevails especially in rural districts where the soil is sandy, and it appears most common and serious in women and children. Although it affects especially the poor and dirty, it is by no means confined to these (Gage and Bass,[53] Greil,[40] Frick,[54] DeBuys and Dwyer[3]). It has been claimed that prenatal infestation is possible (Howard[55]).

Uncinaria Americana is a very small, thread-like nematode worm, the female being about $\frac{1}{2}$ in. (1.27 cm.) in length and the male slightly smaller (Fig. 153). Its buccal orifice is provided with a pair of cutting plates.

The numerous thin-shelled, segmented eggs are elliptical in shape and measure about $\frac{1}{400}$ to $\frac{1}{350}$ of an inch (0.006 to 0.007 cm.) in length and about one half as much in breadth (Fig. 154). The uncinaria duodenalis, or Old World hook-worm, differs in being a little longer and stouter, and in having the buccal orifice armed with teeth. The eggs are slightly smaller.

The life-history of the uncinaria duodenalis is known, and that of the uncinaria Americana is probably the same. The worm inhabits the small intestine, especially the duodenum and the jejunum, sometimes in enormous numbers. By its sucking apparatus it attaches itself to the intestinal mucous membrane and probably abstracts blood from it. The head, by turning backward, gives the parasite the form of a hook. In shifting its position the worm leaves minute bleeding points, and it is likely, too, that it produces a poisonous substance.

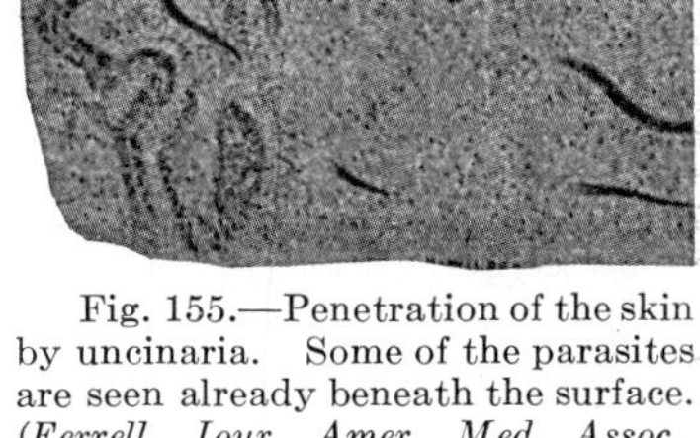

Fig. 155.—Penetration of the skin by uncinaria. Some of the parasites are seen already beneath the surface. (*Ferrell*, *Jour. Amer. Med. Assoc.*, 1914, **62**, 1941.)

The eggs will not mature within the intestine, but are passed with the feces, and enter moist ground or water where they promptly develop into the worm-like larvae. These remain alive, perhaps for months, until they again enter the alimentary canal, being conveyed by the hands soiled by earth, or through the swallowing of contaminated water or the direct eating of earth. In the intestine they finish their transformation, if sufficiently well-advanced, into the adult parasite. The larvae may also penetrate the skin directly from without (Looss[56]), (Fig. 155), thence by way of the circulation reach the pulmonary alveoli, then migrate along the bronchial tubes and trachea to the gullet, the esophagus, and finally into the stomach and intestine. No intermediate host is therefore needed. The worms very probably live in the intestine for years. A period of incubation of from four to six weeks is required from the time of the entrance of the larvae before maturity is reached.

Symptoms.—It is likely that a large number of parasites must be present to produce symptoms. After an initial gastro-intestinal disturbance, evidences of disease are entirely of a constitutional nature, and consist chiefly in the varied manifestations of anemia, this resulting from the direct loss of blood, from the poison entering the system from the mouth of the worm, or through the entrance of bacteria through the wounds. In well-marked instances the complexion grows pale and clay-colored, the expression is apathetic and of a peculiar dulness; the abdomen is much distended by gas and sometimes contains fluid; the liver and spleen are enlarged; the growth of the body is stunted; emaciation is present; and there may be edema, especially of the face. Pica, or the habit of eating dirt and the like, is a common symptom, probably oftener the result than the cause of the disease. The temperature may be subnormal or sometimes elevated. There is usually mental sluggishness or retardation, apparently proportional to the massiveness of the infestation. The blood exhibits marked reduction of the red blood-corpuscles and especially of hemoglobin, often to 20 or 30 per cent, and an eosinophilia, commonly of 8 or 10 per cent or more.

Prognosis.—Although many deaths occur, there is even greater disposition for the disease to last for years until terminated by some complicating affection. Many adults show a tendency to recovery, if reinfection does not occur. Under treatment the prognosis is favorable, except in the advanced cases with great debility and anemia.

Treatment.—**Prophylaxis** consists in hygienic precautions against infection in the districts where the disease prevails; these including especially the frequent washing and disinfection of the hands, the disinfection of the feces, the boiling of drinking water, and the forbidding of the children to run barefooted. In regions where the disease is endemic the correct construction, location, employment, and disinfection of privies should be insisted upon, and the disinfection of the ground about the dwelling-houses accomplished by the application of fire in some way.

Direct treatment is usually simple and efficacious. After a very light diet for twenty-four hours, thymol in emulsion or capsules may be administered to a total amount of ½ fl. dr. (1.8) in divided doses to a child of ten or twelve years, followed in two hours by a saline. No castor oil or other fatty substance should be given during the treatment. The feces should be examined for eggs after a week. If any are still found, the treatment must be repeated, or felix mas used as recommended for tapeworm. In weakly subjects the thymol should be administered in smaller and more frequent doses, since the drug is capable of producing dangerous symptoms. Oil of chenopodium is recommended by Levy,[57] Bishop and Brosius[58] and others as more efficacious and safer than thymol. The dose is one drop (0.062) on sugar every two hours for three or four doses for each year of the child's age. Some physicians believe that two such doses are all that should be given, owing to the toxic symptoms which sometimes develop. These consist of dizziness, vomiting, headache, and deafness; and in severe cases convulsions, stupor, paralysis and even death. The last dose of chenopodium should be followed in about two hours by castor oil. A saline laxative should be given on the day preceding the administration of the vermifuge. Hall and Foster[59] recommend chloroform as far superior to chenopodium. The adult dose is 2 to 3 cc. (33 to 49 minims) dissolved in castor oil. Carbon tetrachloride for the treatment of hookworm was brought into prominence by Hall,[60] and the drug has since been widely employed. The dose is about 2 minims (0.123) for each year of age, with a maximum dose of 60 minims (3.72) administered at one time or in divided amounts. (See p. 647.)

After the removal of the parasites by whatever method, tonic treatment directed to the anemia is required.

OTHER INTESTINAL PARASITES

Other animal parasites occurring in the intestine are of minor importance. Chief of them is the **trichocephalus dispar** (*trichuris trichiura*) or **whipworm,** a small slender nematode worm about 1½ to 2 in. (3.81 to 5.08 cm.) long, for two-thirds of its length very thin and thread-like, and then joined like a whip-lash to the thicker posterior portion, which in the male is rolled up like a spring (Fig. 156). The numerous eggs are lemon-shaped and of about the size of those of the oxyuris—$\frac{1}{500}$ in. (0.005 cm.) in length and $\frac{1}{800}$ in. (0.0032 cm.) broad—but with a plug-like closure at each end. The parasite, seldom in large numbers, inhabits especially the cecum. It is of very common occurrence in some countries, but was thought to be less so in the United States. Townsend,[61] however, discovered it in the feces of all of 16 children examined and DeBuys and Dwyer[3] in 595 persons studied found it in the stools in 35.1 per cent. Neumann[62] discovered the parasite in the feces of 13.9 per cent of 122 children of from one to sixteen years, and it is perhaps as often seen in adults. Christoffersen[63] in 200 autopsies of various diseases at all ages observed it in 29 per cent. It is often associated with other worms, especially the ascaris. The ova develop in water or damp earth, and are thence taken by accident into the stomach. There are generally no symptoms, except it may be diarrhea or anemia as reported in some instances. Treatment is, as a rule, unsatisfactory, but Lieb[64] had success with castor oil, low-residue diet, and kaolin by the mouth, combined with enemata of 0.5 per cent solution of monohydrated sodium carbonate; and Fernán-Núñez[65] has used with good results an extract made from the sap of the fig-tree. The **strongyloides stercoralis** is a round worm occasionally discovered. It was present in 6.72 per cent of DeBuys and Dwyer's[3] 595 examinations. Various **protozoa** are from time to time found in the intestinal canal in children, among them the *Amoeba coli, Entamoeba histolytica, Entamoeba nana, Dientamoeba fragilis, Cercomonas intestinalis, Trichomonas intestinalis, Balantidium coli* and the *Giardia intestinalis.* The last, also denominated *Lamblia intestinalis* and *Megastomum entericum,* would appear to be of more frequent occurrence than had been believed. In 304 children under twelve years examined at the Children's Hospital of Philadelphia by Noone, Waltz and Donnelly[66] Giardia was found in 16 per cent. Maxy[67] discovered it in 20 per cent, and several reports are published of others in different parts of the United States. The various protozoa are recognized by microscopic examination of the stools; but for details of their appearance reference must be made to works especially devoted to this subject. They ordinarily produce no symptoms, but it is to be noted that they appear to be more frequent in cases of diarrheal disturbance, and possibly have some etiologic connection with this condition. Giardia has been found in the gall-bladder. Treatment is generally unsatisfactory. For infestation by Giardia, Chantriot[68] has tried lemon juice or diluted hydrochloric acid by the mouth, and injections of arsenic and emetine. Among other remedies employed are gentian violet by mouth, in doses of 1 grain (0.06) three times a day; bismuth salicylate; Stovarsol (Pawan[69]), and gray powder (Arnozan[70]).

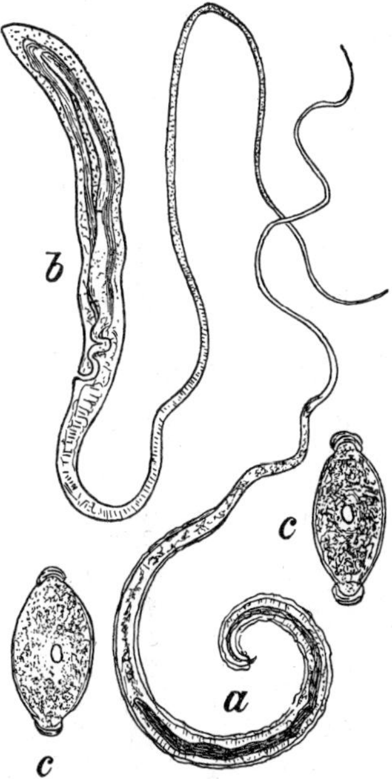

Fig. 156.—Trichocephalus dispar. *a,* Male; *b,* female; *c,* eggs. (*von Jaksch, Klinische Diagnostik,* 1887, 150, *Fig.* 54.)

References

1. J.A.M.A., 1920, **74,** 1774. 2. J.A.M.A., 1929, **92,** 624. 3. Am. J. Dis. Child., 1919, **18,** 269. 4. Phillip. J. of Sc., 1920, **16,** 1. 5. Med. Klinik., 1921, **17,** 722. 6. Jahrb. f. Kinderh., 1893, **36,** 319. 7. Arch. f. Kinderh., 1913, **62,** 49. 8. Arch. f. Kinderh., 1913, **62,** 11. 9. Monatschr. f. Kinderh. Orig., 1919, **15,** 199. 10. Fortschr. a. d. Geb. d. Roentgenstrählen, 1922, **29,** 591. 11. J.A.M.A., 1930, **95,** 819. 12. J.A.M.A., 1922, **78,** 1294. 13. Parasitology, 1916–17, **9,** 157; 1920, **13,** 37; Brit. M. J., 1919, **1,** 102. 14. J. Agric. Research, 1917, **40,** 395; U. S. Dept. Agric., 1920, Bull. No. 817; J.A.M.A., 1922, **79,** 1094. 15. Arch. f. Kinderh., 1928, **83,** 56. 16. J. Immunol., 1927, **15,** 83. 17. Monatschr. f. Kinderh., 1928, **39,** 81; Arch. f. Kinderh., 1927, **82,** 6. 18. Monatschr. f. Kinderh., 1928, **39,** 64. 19. Arch. f. Schiff. u. Tropen-Hygien., 1926, **30,** 732. 20. Japan Med. World., 1922, **2,** 317. 21. Proc. Soc. Exper. Biol. and Med., 1930, **27,** 1017. 22. Ztschr. f. Kinderh., Orig., 1913, **8,** 205. 23. München. med. Wchnschr., 1925, **72,** 473. 24. Arch. de méd. d. enf., 1913, **16,** 29. 25. Monatschr. f. Kinderh., 1921, **22,** 430. 26. Jahrb. f. Kinderh., 1922, **98,** 1; 1926, **114,** 127. 27. Indian Med. Gaz., 1922, **57,** 290. 28. Pediatria, 1924, **35,** 965. 29. Progrès méd., 1920, **35,** 339. 30. Ref. Barrier, Traité prat. d. mal. de l'enf., 1861, **2,** 99. 31. New York M. J., 1871, **14,** 618. 32. Soc. Ginec. Espan. Ref. Grimm. (Ref. 34). 33. Arch. de méd. d. enf., 1911, **14,** 525. 34. München. med. Wchnschr., 1914, **61,** 1780. 35. Centralb. f. Bact. u. Parasitenk., Orig., 1905, **38,** 534. 36. Wien. klin. Wchnschr., 1911, **24,** 1595. 37. J. Parasitol., 1922, **8,** 109. 38. Am. J. Dis. Child., 1928, **36,** 523. 39. Pub. Health and Marine Hosp. Service, U. S. Hyg. Lab., 1904,

Bull. No. 18. 40. Am. J. Dis. Child., 1915, **10,** 363. 41. Arch. Pediat., 1910, **27,** 100. 42. Arch. Pediat., 1919, **36,** 639. 43. Proc. Soc. Exper. Biol. and Med., 1931, **28,** 709. 44. Am. J. Dis. Child., 1932, **43,** 865. 45. J.A.M.A., 1929, **92,** 1587. 46. Am. J. M. Sc., 1931, **181,** 710. 47. Arch. f. Schiff. u. Tropen. Hyg., 1926, **30,** 250. 48. München. med. Wchnschr., 1929, **76,** 1510. 49. Practical Therap., 1912, 14th Edit., 115. 50. Annals universali di medicina, Milan, 1843, **106,** 5. 51. New York M. J., 1900, **71,** 552. 52. Amer. Med., 1902, **3,** 777. 53. Arch. Int. Med., 1910, **6,** 303. 54. Am. J. M. Sc., 1919, **157,** 189. 55. South. M. J., 1917, **10,** 793. 56. Centralb. f. Bakt. u. Parasit., 1898, **24,** 484. 57. J.A.M.A., 1914, **63,** 1946. 58. J.A.M.A., 1915, **65,** 1610. 59. J.A.M.A., 1917, **68,** 1961. 60. J. Agric. Research, 1921, **21,** 157; J.A.M.A., 1921, **77,** 1641. 61. Starr, Am. Text-Bk. Dis. of Child., 1894, 553. 62. Wien. klin. Rundschau, 1913, **27,** 387. 63. Ziegler's Beiträge z. path. Anat. u. allg. Path., 1914, **57,** 474. 64. Am. J. M. Sc., 1927, **173,** 523. 65. J.A.M.A., 1927, **88,** 903. 66. Atlantic M. J., 1927, **30,** 692. 67. Bull. Johns Hopkins Hosp., 1921, **32,** 166. 68. Clinique, 1932, **27,** 29. 69. Ann. Trop. Med., 1926, **20,** 197. 70. J. de méd. d. Bordeaux, 1926, **103,** 863.

CHAPTER IX

DISEASES OF THE LIVER, GALL-BLADDER AND PANCREAS

Anatomic and physiologic characteristics of the liver have been referred to elsewhere (p. 23). Functional and organic diseases of the liver are less common in early life than later.

TESTS OF HEPATIC-FUNCTION

These all need further study and have been little used in childhood. The different tests are intended to measure different hepatic functions; but the liver has such a large reserve capacity, and some of its activities are so closely associated with those of other tissues, that the results of tests must be interpreted with caution. Abel and Rowntree[1] found that the dye *phenoltetrachlorphthalein* was entirely excreted by the normal liver and eliminated in the stools. A number of modifications of this test have been proposed. In one about 50 mg. of the dye are injected intravenously after the insertion of a duodenal tube. The bile drops from this into white porcelain dishes containing 40 per cent of sodium hydroxide. In impaired ability of the liver to excrete the dye the appearance of this is delayed for thirty minutes or longer, and the two-hour excretion is less than 15 per cent. In another modification (Rosenthal[2]) 5 mg. of the dye per kilogram of body-weight are given intravenously. This should have completely disappeared from the blood in forty to sixty minutes, but may be present for many hours in hepatic disease. Other dyes employed are *indigocarmin* (Hatiéganu[3]); methylene blue (Bossert and Loers[4]); *rose-bengal* (Delprat;[5] Epstein, Delprat and Kerr[6]); and bromsulphalein (Rosenthal and White[7]).

MacLean and deWesselow[8] and others have shown that after the ingestion of 50 Gm. of levulose there occurs in hepatic disease an abnormal rise in blood-sugar, and a prolonged return of it to normal. If 40 Gm. of galactose are given to a healthy fasting adult not more than 1 Gm. should be excreted in the urine, but in icterus there may be as much as 2 Gm. and in hepatic cirrhosis 4 Gm. or more (Bauer[9]). A diminution in the fat-storing capacity of the liver is indicated by a rise in the lipase-content of the blood (Whipple[10]), and in some cases there is a rise in blood-fat. The cholesterol of the whole blood is increased in obstructive jaundice; normal in catarrhal jaundice, phosphorus poisoning, acute yellow atrophy of the liver and cirrhosis; decreased in hemolytic anemias (Shattick, Katayama and Killan[11]). When isotonic *hemoglobin* is injected intravenously in patients with faulty hepatic function, bilirubinemia occurs and jaundice may develop or be increased. In *Widal's hemoclastic crisis* test (Widal, Abrami and Iancovesco[12]) a leukopenia developing one-half to one hour after the ingestion of several ounces of milk is supposed to indicate hepatic disease. We[13] have shown, however, that decrease in leukocytosis frequently occurs in normal infants after the ingestion of food.

Bilirubin may be estimated in the blood by the spectrophotometric method or by the Van den Bergh test described below. Normally there is bilirubin in the blood varying between 0.1 and 0.2 mg. per 100 cc. In new-born infants even without visible jaundice it is higher. A diminished amount of bilirubin (hypobilirubinemia) may be found in secondary anemias, aplastic anemia, and in chronic arthritis. Clinical jaundice develops when over 2 mg. per 100 cc. persists for several days, because the bilirubin then diffuses through the blood capillaries and colors the skin and mucous membrane.

The principle of the Van den Bergh test (Van den Bergh and Snapper;[14] Van den Bergh[15]) is that bilirubin in the blood-serum reacts with Ehrlich's diazo-reagent in neutral or acid solution to give a red color. In aqueous solution the reaction may occur at once (*i. e.*, within thirty seconds), and is then called the *direct* reaction; or may develop slowly and then is called a *delayed* or biphasic reaction. A pinkish-violet color appearing promptly in alcoholic solution constitutes an *indirect* reaction. The direct reaction arises from bilirubin which has passed through the liver, the indirect from that which is formed by the reticulo-endothelial cells and has not passed through the liver. All sera giving the direct reaction will also give the indirect. The Van den Bergh test distinguishes between frankly hemolytic and frankly obstructive jaundice, but its value is slight as a means of differentiating icterus due to damage of the liver-cells from other types of jaundice. The *icterus index* (Meulengracht[16]) depends upon comparison of the color of the blood-serum with a standard. It is assumed that bilirubin is responsible for the color of the serum, although other substances such as carotin may also cause a yellow color. In this test the values for normal serum are below 5; clinical icterus occurs when the values are between 8 and 15; in marked icterus the values are above 30.

Reviews on the tests for hepatic function are given by Greene, Snell and Walters,[17] Mann and Bollmann,[18] Pierson and Rothman,[19] and Barron.[20]

Many have denied that a 25 per cent solution of *magnesium sulphate* introduced into the duodenum by tube will cause drainage of the gall-bladder, as claimed by Lyon.[21] Roentgenographic visualization of the gall-bladder may be obtained eight to twenty-four hours after the use of certain drugs (Graham and Cole,[22] Graham, Cole and Copher[23]). For this *sodium tetrabromphenolphthalein* or *sodium tetraidophenolphthalein* may be employed. For patients weighing over 115 lb. (52 kg.) the dose of the former is 5 Gm. dissolved in 40 cc. of distilled water. This is boiled fifteen minutes and injected intravenously in two doses one-half hour apart. The dose of the latter is 3.5 Gm. in 28 cc. of water, used in the same way. Both drugs may also be given by mouth.

FUNCTIONAL DISTURBANCE OF THE LIVER

(Biliousness; Bilious Indigestion)

A certain group of symptoms has long been attributed to functional hepatic disturbance, and to this applied the old designation "biliousness" or "bilious indigestion." In some cases the stools are constipated, or perhaps diarrheal, in character, and of too light a yellow color, or even whitish showing the absence of a normal amount of bile. In how far these and the various other dyspeptic symptoms present, such as loss of appetite, nausea, vomiting, malaise, flatulence, a bitter taste, sallow tint, headache, and the like, depend upon the liver, and to what extent upon other organs, especially the intestine, it is impossible to determine. The treatment is that for intestinal indigestion.

CONGESTION OF THE LIVER

This may be *active* or *passive*. The former sometimes occurs in acute fevers, from overeating, and from the ingestion of too rich a diet. Passive congestion is more frequent, and is seen in chronic diseases of the heart and lungs, chronic pleurisy, chronic malaria, or other causes which interfere with the normal venous circulation in the liver or in the system in general. The **symptoms** vary with the cause, and are not characteristic. The liver increases in size, both in an upward and a downward direction In the acute condition there may be pain and tenderness in the hepatic region and perhaps slight jaundice; in the chronic cases there may also be moderate jaundice, evidences of indigestion, and the symptoms characteristic of the cause. In cardiac cases partial rapid diminution in the size of the liver follows relief of the acute engorgement attendant upon improvement in the cardiac condition. The remaining enlargemant depends upon the damage to the hepatic tissue. In this connection it is well to bear in mind that the liver is often palpable in normal infants and children.

ICTERUS

(Jaundice)

This is a symptom due to many causes. That designated *icterus neonatorum* and that caused by *congenital obliteration of the bile-ducts* have already been discussed (pp. 223; 224).

The classification of the forms of jaundice is unsatisfactory. It is certain only that *obstruction* is the primary cause in some instances, *infection* in others, and *hemolysis* the prominent feature in the third group; but many cases cannot be classified with accuracy, and may, too, belong to more than one category. Rich[24] proposed a classification of "retention" icterus, including all cases with simple retention of bilirubin in the blood-stream, and "regurgitation" icterus, in which bilirubin, already excreted, reenters the blood-stream. Any classification can be but tentative.

1. Catarrhal Icterus

This form of icterus is often discussed under the title of *duodenitis* or *gastroduodenitis*. According to one theory the **cause** consists in an extension of catarrhal swelling of the mucous membrane of the duodenum to the opening of the common bile-duct, or into it. It may be, however, that the smaller bile-ducts are the ones involved, or that the hepatic cells are injured in some way and that the cause is of an infectious nature. In fact a tendency to the epidemic occurrence of this mild form of icterus is sometimes seen, and allies this variety very closely with that next to be described. The condition is comparatively infrequent in children, and uncommon in infancy. The only characteristic **symptom** is the yellow discoloration of the skin and mucous membranes and of the urine. Before the actual symptoms of jaundice are seen some degree of indigestion usually exists for a few days. Then slight icterus appears and increases, until in a day or two it is well-developed over all the visible mucous and cutaneous surfaces. The appetite is diminished or normal, the tongue coated, the breath heavy, and headache, fretfulness, and malaise are not infrequent. The urine is often dark-colored from bile, even before the yellow tint of the skin is apparent. The stools are more or less acholic, having a putty color. The abdomen is often distended with gas, and there may be tenderness in the hepatic region. Itching of the skin and slowness of the pulse may occur in the severer cases, but are not common. The bradycardia is due to increased tone of the vagus caused by the bile-constituents in the tissues. The liver is generally slightly enlarged and the spleen sometimes so. The **prognosis** is entirely favorable, but the course is sometimes somewhat prolonged, the icterus slowly fading but not disappearing completely for two or three weeks. The acute digestive symptoms generally cease in a few days after the onset. The **diagnosis** is seldom difficult. The association of the condition with dyspeptic disturbances is an indication of the cause, and the benign course and comparatively short duration remove doubt. When icterus has become evident the Van den Bergh reaction is direct, although before this it may be indirect. Occasionally in very early infancy the disease might be confounded with icterus neonatorum or other forms, but is distinguished by the greater degree of coloration and the large amount of bile in the urine; and from malformation of the bile-ducts by the course of the disease. In **treatment** fats should be reduced as far as possible, and starches should be given in somewhat diminished amount. Feeding with skimmed milk and broth free from fat is indicated; later with meat, when the acute febrile symptoms have disappeared. Water should be given freely, especially some alkaline water such as Vichy. Purgatives such as calomel and saline cathartics every day or every other day are of value. The employment daily or every other day of large enemata of tepid water is an aid in many cases. Such symptoms as abdominal pain, vomiting and the like require treatment especially directed to these. The administration of mineral acids has long been popular, but we have not found them of any special value. Some physicians have reported good results by using magnesium sulphate introduced through the duodenal tube after the method of Lyon. (See p. 659.) In the evaluation of any method of treatment it should be remembered that the condition is usually a self-limited one without much discomfort, and that treatment may be more disagreeable than the symptoms.

2. Icterus of Infectious or of Hemolytic Origin (see also p. 1049)

Simple catarrhal jaundice shades almost imperceptibly into the type now to be considered. This is of wide variety and may be made to include, for the sake of convenience, both those cases which are clearly infectious in origin, and those where it is known that hemolysis within the circulation has taken place; the latter condition being sometimes consecutive to the former; sometimes occurring independently of it. The probability is that all, or nearly all, instances of this form of icterus are in the final event and in the broader sense really obstructive. This may be the result in some cases of choking of the minute intrahepatic blood-vessels with released blood-coloring matter, or of the capillary bile-ducts with thick bile; both resulting from the hemolysis in process; or in other cases perhaps being caused by swelling of the biliary passages (angiocholitis), the product of the infectious process. There is no sharp differentiation possible between some of the cases believed with reason to be infectious and others of the obstructive catarrhal class; nor can we make a clear distinction between infectious and hemolytic icterus in all cases, inasmuch as the hemolysis very probably at times has an infectious origin. That true hemolytic icterus can occur without the necessity of obstruction in the liver seems very probable. Rich[25] appears to have demonstrated what has long been believed by many; that extrahepatic formation of bile-pigment can certainly take place.

Etiology.—The causes are various. The cases may develop in the course of any of the acute infectious diseases, such as malaria, typhoid fever, scarlet fever, pneumonia, and sepsis. Pernicious anemia is likewise a cause, the icterus being the result of the hemolysis which is occurring. The disease has also repeatedly been observed in local and sometimes widespread epidemics; a strong indication of its infectious origin. Doubtless more than one species of germ has the power to cause it. In some cases the bacillus paratyphosus, bacillus typhosus, or the colon bacillus has been isolated from the blood-stream. A large number of such outbreaks in England are quoted by Guthrie.[26] In the United States epidemics have been carefully studied by Blumer,[27] who found about 300 epidemic outbreaks of infectious jaundice occurring from 1920 to 1923. In 50 outbreaks, studied in more detail and involving approximately 3700 patients, 72 per cent took place in the autumn and winter, and 70 per cent of the patients were children or young adults. The severe form of icterus known as *Weil's disease* is also clearly of an infectious nature, in all probability being due to the Spirochaeta icterohaemorrhagica, an organism which has been discovered in the blood and various organs (Inada *et al.*[28]). Noguchi,[29] Jobling and Eggstein[30] and others have found the germ in rats, and believe that this animal may transmit the infection. Blumer's careful study of the subject does not, however, make it appear that any spirochete is the cause of the condition as usually seen in the United States.

Symptoms.—There is great variation in the intensity of the symptoms. In many cases the discoloration of the skin is less marked than in the catarrhal icterus previously described; the stools still contain bilirubin; the urine urobilin but no bilirubin; and there is an indirect Van den Bergh reaction. This is true especially of some of the cases of icterus resulting from septic poisoning. In other instances the jaundice may be intense, the urine exhibit bilirubin, and the Van den Bergh reaction be direct. The symptoms in general are little characteristic, and often overshadowed by those of the primary diseases. A slight albuminuria is not infrequent. In the severest cases of infectious icterus (*Weil's disease*) there are intense discoloration of the skin, enlargement of the liver and spleen, high fever, hemorrhage from the mucous membranes or into the skin, nephritis, delirium, and convulsions or coma. In the worst cases death may take place in the course of a few days. Instances of this sort are rare in children. In some cases of hemolytic icterus (Hayem[31] type), there are anemia, enlargement of the liver and spleen, and a chronic icterus with bile in the blood-serum but not in the urine, and no symptoms of obstructive jaundice are present. In none of Hayem's cases was there any familial history of icterus. The *prognosis, diagnosis* and *treatment* of forms of infectious and hemolytic icterus are those of the cause. (See also p. 661.) An excellent review of this and other forms of hemolytic icterus is given by Tileston.[32]

3. Icterus Gravis and Familial Icterus in the New-born

(Congenital Acholuric Jaundice; Congenital Hemolytic Icterus; Congenital Family Cholemia; Icterus Neonatorum Gravis)

Here may be grouped a class of cases characterized by the tendency to familial incidence usually seen, and the very early period at which the symptoms appear in some of them. Occasionally infants are born already jaundiced, or become so very promptly; have a very distinct familial history of the disease; are evidently much more ill than in the ordinary cases of icterus neonatorum, and exhibit a discoloration very persistent, although finally disappearing. We have seen a number of such cases, some with a distinctly hemorrhagic tendency. There must be excluded jaundice depending upon obliteration of the bile-ducts, congenital hepatic cirrhosis, or sepsis.

As to the familial incidence, some remarkable examples have been reported by Pearson,[33] Arkwright,[34] Hart,[35] Hutchison and Panton,[36] Hattesen,[37] Campbell and Warner,[38] Hoffmann and Hausmann,[39] Brühl and Bischoff,[40] deLange and Arntzenius,[41] and others.

It would appear certain that there are at least two conditions, entirely different in nature, to be included under the heading of familial icterus of the new-born. Minkowski[42] reported 8 cases occurring in the new-born through 3 generations, and drew attention to the fact that the icterus was of the acholuric variety, the urine exhibiting urobilin but no biliary coloring-matter. On the other hand, a very severe familial icterus has been described as occurring in the new-born, in which the urine contains biliary coloring-matter, and which in other respects differs from the acholuric hemolytic icterus. Such cases although not frequent, have been reported repeatedly, and critical studies have been made by Ylppö,[43] Abt[44] and others. Rolleston[45] collected reports of 25 family groups with 130 cases. Pfannenstiel[46] was one of the first to describe the disease in careful detail.

A brief account of the two forms may be given.

(*A*) Congenital Family Hemolytic Icterus (see also p. 1049)

This form of icterus is often referred to as the Minkowski-Chauffard type. It seems probable that there is a defect in the blood-forming functions of the body, and also that an increased destruction of the corpuscles takes place in the spleen. Other diseases seem to play no part. In older children chilling or over-fatigue has seemed in some cases to be the immediate cause of the development of the jaundice. Yet even although no jaundice may be present shortly after birth, the tendency to develop it appears to be a congenital one. The **symptoms** may be present at birth or appear soon after it, or develop only after the patient reaches childhood or even adult life. The degree of jaundice varies with the case, and even in the same individual from time to time. It is usually not great; and it is of an acholuric character, the urine, although dark-colored from urobilin, being free of biliary coloring-matter, or showing only at times a small amount, and the feces containing bile. As pointed out by Chauffard[47] there is increased fragility of the corpuscles, although this is not invariably present. Bile-pigment is generally present in the blood-serum, and the indirect Van den Bergh reaction is obtained. The spleen is always enlarged. There is anemia of moderate degree, with a few megaloblasts and normoblasts and many reticulated red cells, reaching even as high as 30 per cent of the erythrocytes. The number of leukocytes is not altered. There is sometimes seen a moderate tendency to hemorrhage. As the patient grows older the jaundice never entirely disappears but the general condition may be but little affected, except perhaps during the exacerbations, in which there may be digestive disturbances. There is no abdominal tenderness or pain. The **diagnosis** rests upon the family history; moderate jaundice; fragility of the corpuscles; absence of bile from the urine, but its presence in the feces; and the enlargement of the spleen. *The Hayem type of hemolytic icterus* is an acquired affection without familial history and occurs at any age. *Biliary cirrhosis* is of later development, generally without familial history, and there is a greater degree of jaundice. *Banti's disease* (p. 1048) is primarily a disorder of the spleen, the icterus is a later development, and no increased fragility of the corpuscles is present. The **treatment** for most cases is symptomatic. Splenectomy has met with some success but should not be performed unless the general condition of the patient is suffering.

(*B*) Familial Icterus Gravis in the New-born

Several infants in a family may exhibit the disease, but not always in succession. The direct cause is only surmised. Sepsis is suggested by Knöpfelmacher.[48] Ylppö[43] thinks it a persistence of the fetal condition of the liver. Buhrman and Sanford[49] observed in two cases extreme anemia and erythroblastosis (p. 246). Rolleston[45] found that of 130 cases the mother had been jaundiced during pregnancy in 15. Syphilis plays no part. The birth of the child is usually normal. The disorder is less apt to appear in the 1st or 2d child of the family than later. The **pathologic lesions** found vary. Extensive degeneration of the cells of the liver has been observed, as have fatty change and round-celled infiltration. Iff[50] described in some cases, possibly belonging in this category, miliary necrosis of the liver and other organs, perhaps from infection by way of the placenta. Cirrhosis of the liver has been reported (Mackay[51]). Increase of the iron content of the liver, phagocytosis of leukocytes, and erythroblastosis have been reported by deLange.[52] Hyperactivity of the reticulo-endothelial cells of the spleen has been mentioned (Klemperer[53]). The **symptoms** develop usually in the first forty-eight hours of life. The icterus at first suggests ordinary icterus neonatorum, but becomes progressively more intense. The stools are loose and yellow and sometimes exhibit blood; the urine contains urobilin and frequently bilirubin; hemorrhages take place from the skin and mucous membranes and the umbilicus; convulsions often occur, and death takes place in a few days. Of Rolleston's 130 collected cases only 30 survived. Spastic diplegia and idiocy may be sequels (Greenwald and Messer[54]). The **diagnosis** is to be made from *congenital obliteration of the bile ducts* by the absence of signs of obstruction, *i. e.*, the stools contain bile. From *familial hemolytic icterus* it is distinguished by the greater severity of the symptoms and intensity of jaundice, by the constant development of the icterus in the early days of life, and by the absence of characteristic changes in the blood. The **treatment** is entirely symptomatic. Klemperer[53] suggests administration of glucose to protect the liver by sustaining its glycogen reserve. Blood-transfusions may be tried. Hampson[55] claims that 17 of 18 cases recovered when injected with the mother's serum. Bernheim, Karrer and Grob,[56] in the case of a pregnant woman who had previously lost 5 children, gave boiled liver during the last ten days of the 6th pregnancy; and the 6th infant had only a slight icterus. This may have been coincidental.

4. Icterus from Other Causes

Jaundice appears in many other conditions than those mentioned. In some it is but a mild symptom; in some, although prominent, it is grouped with other features in such a way that a separate description of the complex is necessary. Typical obstructive jaundice, not of a catarrhal nature, occurs in childhood rarely from the presence of impacted gall-stones, the pressure of a malignant growth upon the bile ducts, or the wandering of a worm into these. Hemolytic icterus may be caused by snake-bite or by the ingestion of arsenic or phosphorus. Among other conditions in the course of which icterus may develop are cirrhosis of the liver, hepatic abscess, some forms of splenic enlargement or of anemia, acute yellow atrophy, and the acute infectious hemoglobinemia already described (p. 218).

5. Acute Yellow Atrophy of the Liver

This disease, uncommon at any time of life, is rare in childhood and infancy. Phillips[57] was able to collect 41 cases in children, including one of his own; Francioni[58] placed the number at 46, and a few additional ones have since been reported. One of the youngest on record was in an infant of four days (Politzer[59]). Twice as many boys as girls are attacked. We have seen 2 cases in later childhood, one of which, in a boy of seven years we[60] have previously reported. Matzdorff[61] and others report cases under the title of acute red atrophy of the liver, this being but a variety of yellow atrophy. The usual **pathologic lesions** are found at necropsy; the liver being shrunken perhaps to half size, with a more or less wide-spread parenchymatous degeneration present. Efforts at a reparative process in the liver have been discovered. The **causes** and **symptoms** are the same as in adult life. The former are unknown. The disease is ushered in by icterus of an ordinary type, which may last a few days or one or two weeks. After this there develop rapidly high fever, hemorrhages, vomiting, and such nervous symptoms as convulsions, delirium, or coma as in other forms of severe icterus. In addition there is a progressive diminution in the size of the liver with local tenderness, and death takes place in three or four days. The **diagnosis** rests upon the grave general symptoms, the presence of intense jaundice, the diminution in the size of the liver, and the occurrence of bile and of leucine and tyrosine in the urine. It is difficult to understand how patients with the serious alterations of the liver, which this disease shows at necropsy, could survive, and an element of doubt must attach to the few reported cases of recovery, although some appearing to be reasonably certain instances are on record. Fletcher[62] reports a case recovering after repeated hypodermoclysis.

Subacute Atrophy of the Liver.—Certain cases have been described under this title. Chisolm[63] details nine instances which he had collected from medical literature, Wegerle[64] reported 2 cases, Fraser[65] 1 case, and Spence and Ogilvie[66] 20 cases of which 5 were in children. The causes are probably different from those of the acute disease, vary with the case, and sometimes are discoverable at necropsy; cirrhosis, tuberculosis, and infection being among them. The symptom always present was jaundice; but in other respects the clinical manifestations were not characteristic. Spence and Ogilvie emphasize the nervous symptoms, such as mania, paralyses, and alteration in reflexes. Leucine and tyrosine were not found in the urine in any. The disease lasted several weeks. All of the cases reported have terminated fatally.

Enlargement of the Liver

Increase of the size of the liver is a symptom in a large number of diseased conditions. Among these may be mentioned rachitis; congenital syphilis; tuberculosis; congestion, especially from heart-disease; fatty and amyloid degeneration; tumors; hydatid cysts; cirrhosis; and certain diseases of the blood and the blood-making organs. The diagnosis of these various conditions is made by consideration of the symptoms exhibited by other organs. The remaining disorders of the liver to be described have enlargement as a symptom at some period of their course.

CIRRHOSIS OF THE LIVER

This is an uncommon disease in early life. We have seen but 3 cases, 2 being instances of alcoholic cirrhosis. Jones[67] in 17,891 necropsies on children gives cirrhosis an incidence of 0.185 per cent and Forbes[68] in 5500 necropsies 0.727 per cent. Collective studies in children have been made by Howard,[69] Edwards,[70] Jones,[67] Seitz,[71] Poynton and Wyllie,[72] Sutton,[73] Calvin and Saffro.[74]

Etiology.—The disease is more common in later childhood. In Seitz's series of 320 cases, 31 were in young infants, 72 in young children, and 217 in older children. Males are more frequently affected. It is evident that the causes of cirrhosis are numerous, and include such conditions as misuse of alcohol, infections, syphilis, obstruction to the biliary and circulatory systems of the liver, poisons such as copper, and unknown toxic agents. Alcohol seems to be the cause in childhood in about 10 to 20 per cent of the cases. A certain familial tendency is noted in some instances. Congenital biliary cirrhosis has already been referred to (p. 223). In some cases streptococci and colon bacilli are found in the liver at necropsy, and Opie's[75] experimental work might suggest that such agents as alcohol act by injuring the liver and preparing the ground for bacterial infection.

A special familial form of biliary cirrhosis in infants is reported as not infrequent in hot countries. Ghose,[76] Mukherji[77] and others found this common in India.

Pathologic Anatomy.—In *portal cirrhosis* (Laennec's cirrhosis) there is a diminution in the size of the liver, its surface is uneven, and section shows irregular distribution of connective-tissue hypertrophy compressing and penetrating the lobules. In *biliary cirrhosis* (Hanot's cirrhosis), there is hypertrophy of the liver and spleen, the former being greenish or yellowish in color, and on section showing interlobular overgrowth of connective tissue compressing the small bile-ducts. The misuse of alcohol causes the portal type. There is probably an unnecessary confusion of terms. Mixed forms occur, and the hypertrophic and atrophic types may simply represent respectively early and late stages of the disease (Sutton[23]). In syphilis there may be an interstitial hepatitis often combined with scattered gummata. In cardiac disease the passive congestion, combined with the moderate and unevenly distributed fibrosis of the capsule, may result in the so-called *nutmeg liver*.

Symptoms.—The early symptoms suggest digestive disturbance, with anorexia, and sometimes diarrhea and vomiting, followed later by progressive emaciation, sallow pallor, dilatation of abdominal veins, enlargement of the liver and spleen, and ascites. Splenomegaly is greater and occurs earlier than in adult cases. A complicating nephritis may produce albuminuria. Later, the liver may grow smaller than normal (*atrophic form*) or it may remain enlarged (*hypertrophic form*). As stated, the hypertrophic form may be a more recent and more severe inflammatory process, and the atrophic a final stage. Hemorrhages from the skin and mucous membranes are uncommon, with the exception of gastric hemorrhages, which are not infrequent; leukocytosis is often present; the temperature is irregular; there may be abdominal pain. In the hypertrophic form jaundice is often intense, the urine contains bilirubin, the stools are not acholic, the spleen is greatly enlarged, and ascites is less frequent. In the atrophic state jaundice is absent or slight and ascites is common.

A rare condition known as *hemochromatosis* is characterized by bronzing of the skin, symptoms of cirrhosis of the liver, and diabetes mellitus. There occurs a deposition of pigment in most tissues of the body, and destruction of hepatic cells and their replacement by connective tissue, the same process taking place in the pancreas. Two types of pigment are found; one iron-free (hemofuscin) and the other containing iron (hemosidirin). One cause, at least, of this disorder is ingestion of copper (Mallory[78]).

Course and Prognosis.—The course is more rapid than in adults, although the disease may last several years, with periods of improvement in the hypertrophic form followed by exacerbations. The child may die before the atrophic stage is reached. Prognosis is unfavorable, death taking place from exhaustion, often with diarrhea, delirium, coma, or convulsions. Pulmonary complications may be the direct cause of death. Growth of the body may be retarded in cases of long duration.

Diagnosis.—*Banti's Disease* (p. 1048) is distinguished by the leukopenia, the lesser degree of jaundice, and the predominating and early splenic enlargement. *Congenital hemolytic icterus* is recognized by the absence of bile in the urine, the lesser degree or absence of enlargement of the liver, and the increased fragility of red blood-cells. *Tuberculous peritonitis* may cause confusion until paracentesis of the abdomen has been performed, when the size of the liver may be determined. The occurrence of hemorrhage is a suggestive symptom of cirrhosis.

Treatment.—The diet should be as nonirritating as possible, milk being most useful. Syphilis should be treated if present. Purgatives may be of some value in removing edema, as may salts of mercury such as novasurol (see p. 826). Aspiration of fluid is sometimes necessary. Surgical measures to establish collateral circulation have succeeded in adults, and recovery followed in the case of a boy of six years with alcoholic cirrhosis reported by Grósz,[79] and Calvin and Saffro[74] observed improvement after drainage of the gall-bladder in a case of infectious origin.

FATTY LIVER

Fatty infiltration of the liver is common in early life, especially infancy. Freeman[80] found it in 40 per cent of 496 necropsies in children; oftener present in acute infections than in chronic wasting diseases, but without possessing any special relationship. Wollstein[81] recorded it in 45 of 67 patients dying from tuberculous disease. Kohn[82] described 4 fatal cases of acute fatty enlargement of the liver in infants under one year of age, one having ingested phosphorus and one arsenic. In **fatty infiltration,** which is the common form, the hepatic cells are infiltrated with fat but the cell-nucleus is unaltered. In **fatty degeneration,** the result of toxic or infectious processes, the cells and nuclei are degenerated. Apart from hepatic enlargement there are no special symptoms. The prognosis and treatment of fatty liver are those of the disorder producing it.

AMYLOID LIVER

This condition is associated with similar changes in other organs. Prominent among the **causes** are chronic suppurative processes, such as tuberculosis of the bone or lymph-nodes, bronchiectasis, and empyema. The disease may also attend rickets or syphilis. The **symptoms** are largely those of the causative primary disorder. There is a striking waxy pallor of the face; and emaciation, diarrhea, and digestive symptoms are common. Albuminuria and general dropsy are not infrequent, depending upon complicating amyloid kidneys or upon pressure of the very large liver upon the abdominal vessels. There is generally no icterus, abdominal pain, or tenderness. The much enlarged, smooth liver and spleen can be readily palpated. The course of the disease is slow, and the **prognosis** is unfavorable, although not invariably so if the causative disease can be arrested.

ABSCESS OF THE LIVER

(Suppurative Hepatitis)

This is an uncommon condition in early life. The disease at this period has been studied especially by Legrand[83] who collected 122 cases, and by Seitz[71] who refers to the number as 140. Even in tropical countries the first writer found abscess uncommon in early life. The youngest case we have seen was in an infant of four months of age, in whom there were three streptococcic abscesses of the liver apparently secondary to infection in the skin. Among the **causes** are trauma; suppurative processes of the skin, bones, appendix, peritoneum, etc.; the infectious diseases; dysentery; and pulmonary tuberculosis. In addition, in early life, abscess is due to the wandering of ascarides into the bile-ducts, and exceptionally to sepsis connected with the umbilical vessels. The abscess may be single, if traumatic; or oftener multiple, if of septic origin. Occasionally pus from a hepatic abscess collects between the diaphragm and the liver (*subphrenic abscess*). The **symptoms** of abscess consist of pain and tenderness in the hepatic region; enlargement of the liver either upward or downward; fever of a hectic type with chills and sweats; emaciation; loss of appetite and strength; vomiting; diarrhea; leukocytosis, and sometimes slight jaundice. In some instances the pain is referred to the chest, right shoulder, or abdomen.

There may be painful respiration and cough or shortness of breath if the disease is in the upper portion of the liver. When the symptoms described are associated with a history of an injury in the hepatic region, occurring perhaps some time before, the presence of solitary abscess is very probable; or, if following a suppurating focus, multiple abscess are more likely. Only a successful aspiration can make the diagnosis certain. The **course** generally covers one to two months. If in the case of single abscess the pus can be reached by operation, the chance of recovery is fair; less so if in the upper portion of the liver near the diaphragm. Multiple abscesses always give a most unfavorable prognosis. **Treatment** is entirely surgical; aspiration or incision being required.

MORBID GROWTHS OF THE LIVER

Tumors of the liver are not of common occurrence in early life. They have been studied especially by Steffen[84] who collected 39 cases of primary malignant growths. Carcinoma, adenocarcinoma, and sarcoma may be mentioned among these. Hepatoma, a primary epithelial tumor, is described by Wollstein and Mixsell.[85] In the majority of cases the growth is secondary to one elsewhere in the body, but in a considerable number it is primary. In early life carcinoma appears to be more frequent in the liver than in other localities. We[86] have observed 1 case of primary carcinoma in an infant of twenty-one months, and were able to collect in all, including this, 55 instances of primary carcinoma of the liver in early life. Rosenbusch[87] adds others. Nicolaysen[88] states that more than 100 cases of carcinoma of the liver have been recorded. Among nonmalignant growths are congenital multiple or unilocular cysts, acquired nonparasitic cysts, lipoma, fibroma, adenoma and angioma. Either of the last two may be multiple or single. Stoesser and Wangensteen[89] have reviewed the literature on nonparasitic cysts. Veeder and Austin[90] describe a case of multiple congenital hemangio-endothelioma, and refer to three others recorded in medical literature. These tumors may also be pedunculated and single (Spiegel[91]). Foote[92] also reports a case apparently of this type, which he designates hemangio-endothelio-sarcoma, occurring in a boy three months of age, and collects 10 others. The **symptoms** of growths of the liver consist in steadily increasing size of the organ, which often exhibits irregularly nodular masses; increasing debility; abdominal pain; and the various symptoms depending upon pressure. Yet ascites and icterus may be absent until, perhaps, the latest stages.

Among new-growths may conveniently be placed tuberculosis of the liver, always secondary to tuberculous lesions elsewhere. Only occasionally are large, cheesy masses found, but miliary tubercles are of common occurrence.

Of exceptional occurrence is *echinococcus of the liver* (Hydatids) due to the ingestion of eggs of the Taenia echinococcus. In North America reports of 14 such cases have been collected by Mills.[93] The condition may be recognized by the peculiar "hydatid fremitus" sometimes discoverable, and by the obtaining of the hooklets by aspiration. The prognosis is doubtful and the treatment surgical.

DISEASES OF THE GALL-BLADDER AND BILE-DUCTS

Conditions of this nature are very rare in early life. Congenital obliteration of the bile-ducts has already been described. Only exceptionally there exists a congenital absence of the gall-bladder. Several such reported cases have been collected by Eshner.[94] Occasionally a round worm penetrates into the bile-duct and sets up an inflammation there, and various protozoa in the intestinal tract may invade the gall-bladder and biliary passages. Acute cholangitis and cholecystitis are very infrequent conditions, but may occur after typhoid fever or from sepsis, or independently of these. Cholecystitis of a more chronic nature is probably not an infrequent sequel of typhoid fever. Tuberculosis of the gall-bladder is sometimes seen, and that of the bile-ducts is not uncommon, producing small nodules or cavities within the liver. Very exceptionally gall-stones are discovered. Kellogg[95] collected 44 reported cases including 1 observed by himself; Snyder[96] reports 1 instance and reviews some of the literature of gall-stones and of cholecystitis, and Skemp[97] reports gall-stones in an infant of seventeen months. According to Mohr[98] about 150 cases of gall-bladder disease of all types have been reported in children.

DISEASES OF THE PANCREAS

Organic disease of this organ plays a very minor rôle in early life. Syphilitic involvement is occasionally seen. Tuberculous nodules of considerable size, or an infiltration by many small nodules, may accompany a general tuberculosis, and amyloid degeneration may occur in conjunction with this change in other organs. Tumors also may involve the pancreas, being either primary, or secondary to morbid growths elsewhere. Among the former primary sarcoma has been described by Litten[99] and others. Cysts are occasionally found, oftenest of the class of retention cysts. Calculi and ascarides have been reported present in the pancreatic duct. An **acute pancreatitis** is occasionally seen as one of the manifestations of mumps (p. 371). Dependent upon other causes pancreatitis in early life is of great rarity, but may occur in the course of infectious diseases; as a result of the presence of round worms in the duct; by infection extending from the intestine; or be metastatic in origin. The inflammation may be either hemorrhagic or suppurative. Although abdominal pain and tenderness rapidly followed by collapse occur as symptoms, these are not distinctive. A **chronic pancreatitis** is distinctly more common, producing a fibrosis of the organ. The most frequent cause is hereditary syphilis, although the disease may also accompany gastro-enteritis. It is seen also in diabetes mellitus. It is possible that some of the cases of fatty stools depend upon this form of pancreatitis. In hemochromatosis (p. 666) the pancreas is involved and there is produced "bronzed diabetes." In deLange's[100] case the cirrhosis of pancreas and liver were supposed to be caused by toxic disturbance of the mother during pregnancy.

How often a *functional* disturbance of the pancreas may account for difficulty in digestion is not known, but it is very probable that some of the instances of fat-indigestion may be due to this. Some cases of infantilism are believed to be associated with disturbance of the functions of the pancreas (p. 1088). Soecknik and Thoenes[101] described a case of steatorrhea as an instance of familial insufficiency of the pancreas.

A few cases have been reported in which with tumors, or with overaction or hypertrophy of the islands of Langerhans, there is persistent hypoglycemia ("hyperinsulinism"). Gray and Feemster[102] reported such a case in an infant born of a diabetic mother.

References

1. J. Pharmacol. and Exper. Therap., 1909–10, **1,** 231. 2. J.A.M.A., 1922, **79,** 2151. 3. Ann. de méd., 1921, **10,** 400. 4. Jahrb. f. Kinderh., 1924, **107,** 291. 5. Arch. Int. Med., 1923, **32,** 401. 6. J.A.M.A., 1927, **88,** 1619. 7. J.A.M.A., 1925, **84,** 1112. 8. Quart. J. Med., 1921, **14,** 103. 9. Wien. med. Wchnschr., 1906, **56,** 2538. 10. Bull. Johns Hopkins Hosp., 1913, **24,** 357. 11. Am. J. M. Sc., 1928, **175,** 103. 12. Presse méd., 1920, **28,** 893. 13. Mitchell. Am. J. Dis. Child., 1915, **9,** 358. 14. Deutsch. Arch. f. klin. Med., 1913, **110,** 540. 15. Die Gallenfarbstoff im Blute 1918. 16.

Deutsch. Arch. f. klin. Med., 1920, **132,** 285; 1921, **137,** 38. 17. Arch. Int. Med., 1925, **36,** 248. 18. Arch. Path. and Lab. Med., 1926, **1,** 681. 19. J.A.M.A., 1928, **91,** 1768. 20. Medicine, 1931, **10,** 77. 21. Nonsurgical Drainage of the Gall-Tract, 1923. 22. J.A.M.A., 1924, **82,** 613. 23. J.A.M.A., 1925, **84,** 1175. 24. Bull. Johns Hopkins Hosp., 1930, **47,** 338. 25. Bull. Johns Hopkins Hosp., 1925, **36,** 233. 26. Brit. J. Child. Dis., 1913, **10,** 1. 27. J.A.M.A., 1923, **81,** 353. 28. J. Exper. Med., 1916, **23,** 377. 29. J. Exper. Med., 1917, **25,** 755. 30. J.A.M.A., 1917, **69,** 1787. 31. Presse méd., 1898, **5,** 121. 32. Medicine, 1922, **1,** 355. 33. Underwood's Dis. of Child., 1842, 101. 34. Edinburgh M.J., 1902, **54,** 156. 35. Canad. M.A.J., 1925, **15,** 1008. 36. Quart. J. Med., 1909, **2,** 432. 37. Mittheil. a. d. Grenzgeb. d. Med. u. Chir., 1924, **37,** 293. 38. Quart. J. Med., 1926, **19,** 333. 39. Monatschr. f. Kinderh., 1926, **33,** 193. 40. Ztschr. f. Kinderh., 1926, **40,** 702. 41. Jahrb. f. Kinderh., 1929, **124,** 1. 42. Verhandl. d. Kong. f. inn. Med., 1900, **18,** 316. 43. Ztschr. f. Kinderh., 1918, **17,** 334. 44. Am. J. Dis. Child., 1917, **13,** 231. 45. The Practitioner, 1920, **104,** 1. 46. München. med. Wchnschr., 1908, **55,** 2169; 2233. 47. Semaine méd., 1907, **27,** 25. 48. Ergeb. d. inn. Med. u. Kinderkr., 1910, **5,** 205. 49. Am. J. Dis. Child., 1931, **41,** 225. 50. Beitr. z. path. Anat. u. z. allg. Path., 1931, **86,** 83. 51. Lancet, 1927, **1,** 1183. 52. Jahrb. f. Kinderh., 1926, **114,** 15. 53. Am. J. Dis. Child., 1924, **28,** 212. 54. Am. J. M. Sc., 1927, **174,** 793. 55. Lancet, 1929, **1,** 429. 56. Ztschr. f. Kinderh., 1931, **50,** 672. 57. Am. J. M. Sc., 1912, **143,** 177. 58. Riv. di clin. pediat., 1914, **12,** 653. 59. Jahrb. f. Kinderh., 1860, **3,** 40. 60. Griffith, Arch. Pediat., 1899, **16,** 330. 61. Monatschr. f. Kinderh., 1929, **43,** 262. 62. Garrod, Batten and Thursfield, Dis. of Children, 1913, 210. 63. Brit. J. Child. Dis., 1914, **11,** 397. 64. Frankfurter Ztschr. f. Path., 1914, **15,** 89. 65. Am. J. M. Sc., 1916, **152,** 202. 66. Arch. Dis. Childh., 1927, **2,** 41. 67. Brit. J. Child. Dis., 1907, **4,** 1. 68. Trans. Path. Soc., London, 1906, **157,** 354. 69. Am. J. M. Sc., 1887, **94,** 350. 70. Arch. Pediat., 1890, **7,** 502. 71. Pfaundler u. Schlossmann, Handb. d. Kinderh., 1924, **3,** 359; 362. 72. Arch. Dis. Childhood, 1926, **1,** 1. 73. Am. J. Dis. Child., 1930, **39,** 141. 74. Am. J. Dis. Child., 1932, **43,** 914. 75. J. Exper. Med., 1910, **12,** 367. 76. Lancet 1895, **1,** 321. 77. Indian M. Rec., 1929, **49,** 43. 78. Arch. Int. Med., 1926, **37,** 336. 79. Ref. Monatschr. f. Kinderh., 1903, **2,** 386. 80. Arch. Pediat., 1900, **17,** 81. 81. Am. J. M. Sc., 1902, **123,** 817. 82. Am. J. Dis. Child., 1924, **27,** 376. 83. Arch. de méd. d. enf., 1906, **8,** 129. 84. Malign. Geschwülste im Kindersalter, 1905, 77. 85. Arch. Pediat., 1919, **36,** 269. 86. Griffith, Am. J. M. Sc., 1918, **155,** 79. 87. Virchow's Arch. f. path. Anat., 1926, **261,** 326. 88. Norsk. Mag. f. Laegevidensk., 1924, **85,** 719. 89. Am. J. Dis. Child., 1929, **38,** 241. 90. Am. J. M. Sc., 1912, **143,** 102. 91. Arch. Pediat., 1929, **46,** 188. 92. J.A.M.A., 1919, **73,** 1042. 93. Surg., Gynec. and Obst., 1926, **42,** 585. 94. Med. News, 1894, **64,** 548. 95. Ann. Surg., 1923, **77,** 587. 96. J.A.M.A., 1925, **85,** 31. 97. J.A.M.A., 1931, **96,** 108. 98. Am. J. Dis. Child., 1931, **42,** 372. 99. Deutsche med. Wchnschr., 1888, **14,** 901. 100. Am. J. Dis. Child., 1927, **34,** 372. 101. Jahrb. f. Kinderh., 1927, **115,** 315. 102. Arch. Path. and Lab. Med., 1926, **4,** 348.

CHAPTER X

DISEASES OF THE PERITONEUM

ACUTE PERITONITIS

The great majority of cases of peritonitis are secondary to a lesion elsewhere. What appears to be an acute primary peritonitis does, however, sometimes occur, although much less frequently than the secondary form.

Etiology.—Age exerts a decided influence. The disease may occur before birth, sometimes as a result of hereditary syphilis, or produced by various malformations, rupture of the intestine (Fischer[1]), or other causes. In the new-born peritonitis is not uncommon, depending upon septic infection usually from the umbilicus, at times on placental transmission, or occasionally on rupture of the intestine during labor; or being a complication of imperforate bowel. In infants after this period it is rare, and becomes frequent only with the increasing incidence of appendicitis. This last condition is much the most common cause of a secondary peritonitis in childhood.

Very rarely in early life perforation of a gastric or duodenal ulcer, or the rupture of an abscess in some other abdominal organ, gives rise to secondary peritonitis. We have seen it, for instance, consecutive to perforation of a duodenal ulcer, to diverticulitis, and in a number of instances to perforation in typhoid fever. In other cases peritonitis may be produced by the rupture of an empyema, or of an abscess resulting from spinal caries or from inflammation about the kidney. Strangulation of the intestine, as in hernia and intussusception, may likewise cause the disease, as may also forms of enteritis. Trauma and exceptionally exposure to cold are sometimes followed by a primary peritonitis. Acute infectious diseases may produce a peritonitis dependent upon the infection. Here especially are to be mentioned erysipelas, grippe, scarlet fever, typhoid fever, diphtheria, pleurisy, and pneumonia.

The streptococcus is the most frequent micro-organism found in cases depending upon sepsis in the new-born, or upon scarlet fever, tonsillitis, erysipelas, and some other infectious diseases. In some instances a streptococcic peritonitis appears to be primary. The pneumococcus is capable of producing a primary peritonitis, or that consecutive to pneumonia or pleurisy. In primary peritonitis after the new-born period the pneumococcus is perhaps the germ oftenest found. This variety is about twice as frequent in early as in adult life. Barling,[2] McCartney and Fraser,[3] Heiman,[4] Salzer,[5] and Fricke[6] give reports and analyses of collected cases, and Mouriquand, Bernheim and Rendu[7] describe an abortive and recurrent type. In pneumococcic peritonitis the infection is probably oftenest through the blood-channels, although Annand and Bowen[8] would assign the majority of cases to infection from the intestinal tract. The fact that the larger number of cases is in girls has led to the belief that the pneumococcus may gain access to the peritoneal cavity through the Fallopian tubes. In perhaps the greater number of instances of secondary peritonitis the bacillus coli is found, frequently in combination with some other species. Other cases exhibit the staphylococcus aureus, the bacillus pyocyaneus, the proteus vulgaris, meningococcus (Moeltgen[9]), or other germs. The gonococcus is only exceptionally the cause of peritonitis, and oftenest in cases following vulvovaginitis.

Pathologic Anatomy.—The lesions, as in adults, consist of the formation of a serous, fibrinous, or purulent exudate, with the production of more or less firm adhesions. In all varieties of the disease the lesions may be general, or be limited to certain regions, as the pelvis, appendix, or neighborhood of some intestinal lesion elsewhere. In localized purulent peritonitis a walled-off abscess of some size may result.

Symptoms.—In typical cases of **general peritonitis** the onset is usually sudden and severe, with vomiting, high fever, abdominal pain and tenderness, constipation, or frequently diarrhea. The face has a pallid, strained, sunken aspect, with sharpness and coldness of the nose, hollowness about the eyes, and dryness of the teeth and tongue. The pulse is rapid, small and compressible, and the breathing is shallow and rapid on account of the pain which abdominal respiration produces. The temperature usually continues high, but may be normal or subnormal. The abdomen is rigid, tympanitic, and even meteoric. The patient lies on the back with the legs drawn up on the abdomen; the extremities are often cold and cyanotic; the mind is clear; vomiting may cease or may continue troublesome; hiccough may be present. The urine is often scanty, or there may be dysuria necessitating catheterization. The blood generally exhibits a decided polymorphonuclear leukocytosis, especially in perforative cases; except in the very severe instances where no reaction can take place, and where even a leukopenia may be found. Later in the disease evidences of fluid in the abdominal cavity may appear.

The most frequent form of **localized peritonitis** is that associated with appendicitis (p. 628). Peritonitis is also to be suspected whenever a child with gonorrheal vulvovaginitis suddenly develops fever with abdominal pain, tenderness, and distention. We have, however, seen this very infrequently, and it occurs usually only in late childhood. Rarely in children the inflammation is localized just below the diaphragm (*subphrenic abscess*). This is generally secondary to affections of the liver, or often to pneumonia or pleurisy, and the symptoms simulate closely those of empyema. (See p. 756.)

Acute peritonitis in infancy may exhibit symptoms so obscure that no diagnosis is made. Vomiting may be absent and the temperature little if at all elevated. On the other hand, it may be high, especially in the new-born. The abdomen is distended and rigid; but distention of and pain in the abdomen in infancy are so common from other causes, such as colic, that the symptom is of little value. Abdominal tenderness is characteristic when present, but is often absent. In many cases, however, the symptoms are sufficiently like those of childhood to make the diagnosis clear.

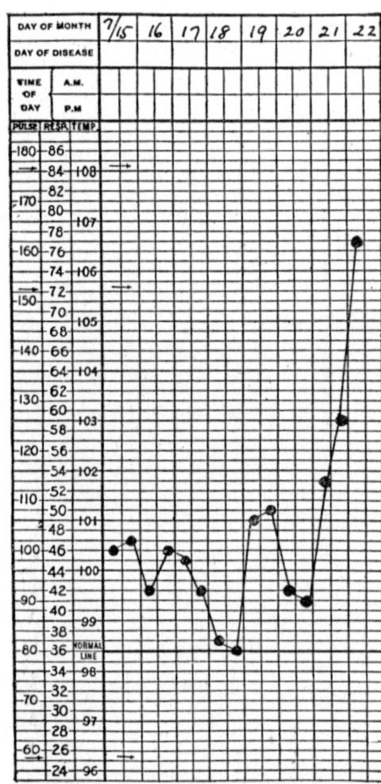

Fig. 157.—Septic peritonitis. John W. Entered the Children's Hospital of Philadelphia, July 15, aged four days. Increasing weakness, distended abdomen, moderate, irregular temperature, chiefly subfebrile until the last day. Laparotomy July 21. Post-mortem examination showed thick plastic exudate. A diplococcus, streptococcus and an undetermined bacillus were found in the fluid.

Course and Prognosis.—Infants with acute fetal peritonitis are born dead, or almost invariably die within a few days. In the new-born and in later infancy the ending is generally fatal. Apart from the influence of age, the disease is always a serious one, the final issue depending largely upon the localization, the nature of the pathologic lesions, and, to some extent, the specific cause. In the most severe cases of wide-spread **general purulent peritonitis** the course is short and death is liable to occur in three or four days or less; or in less severe cases in from one to two weeks. General peritonitis dependent upon intestinal perforation runs a rapid and fatal course, unless perhaps checked by prompt operative interference. Peritonitis of a septic nature is nearly always fatal. Fibrinous peritonitis gives a better prognosis than the purulent form and serous cases are still more favorable.

In localized peritonitis the prognosis is better in proportion as the area involved is small; and depends, too, on the nature of the lesion. A small fibrinous area following upon inflammation of some neighboring region disappears with the recovery of the original lesion. There is always a danger, however, that the localized inflammation may become a general one. Purulent peritonitis may be entirely localized and may end in recovery by discharging into the rectum, the kidney, or through the umbilicus. The cavity remaining heals by granulation as does any other abscess-cavity. The danger of extension to the general peritoneal cavity is greater in a localized purulent peritonitis than in the fibrinous form.

The nature of the germ exerts an influence upon the course and prognosis. In **streptococcic peritonitis** the course is severe and rapid to a fatal termination (Fig. 157) although an occasional case may recover when operation is performed. **Pneumococcic peritonitis** (Fig. 158) may be preceded or attended by some affection of the lungs or pleura, but frequently develops independently of this as a primary disorder. It often presents certain definite characteristics. After the sudden onset and early severe symptoms a remission may take place in from six to eight days, but diarrhea and abdominal distention persist and often suggest the diagnosis of typhoid fever. In about two weeks fluid collects in the abdominal cavity. The general symptoms may remain favorable, or there may be emaciation, fever, and a condition suggesting tuberculous peritonitis. The pus produced in this form of the disease shows a decided tendency to encapsulation, and after several weeks may be spontaneously discharged in some direction.

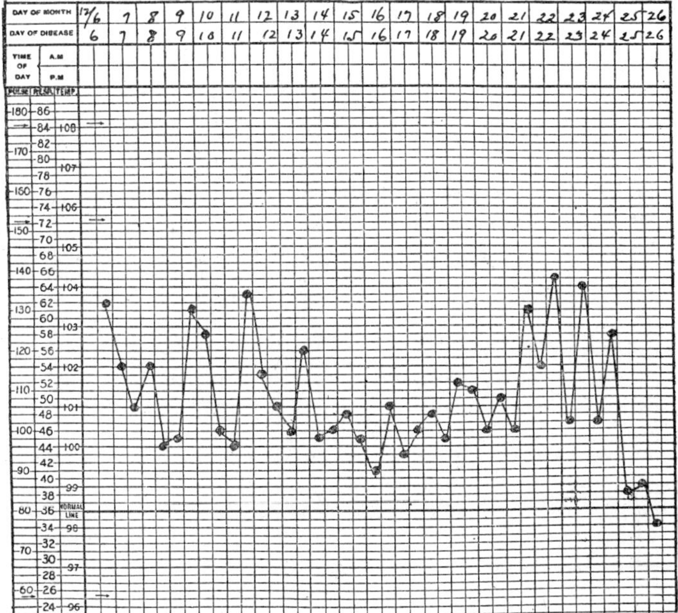

Fig. 158.—Pneumococcic peritonitis; followed by phlebitis and empyema. Margaret K., aged five years. Sudden onset Dec. 1 of apparently acute gastric indigestion, with vomiting, diarrhea and fever. Seemed convalescing in less than a week; Dec. 6, developed severe abdominal pain, fever, and diarrhea; by Dec. 17, symptoms had moderated, but physical signs of fluid in lower part of abdominal cavity had appeared. Signs of pleuropneumonia developed, and child much more ill. Abdominal condition grew worse. Operation for peritonitis done Dec. 23. One and one-half quarts (1420) pus removed, containing pneumococci. Gradual improvement. Pulmonary signs cleared up. Dec. 29, phlebitis left leg, with fever; Jan. 7, empyema has developed, operated upon today; Jan. 16, convalescing. Chart shows very moderate fever even shortly before peritoneal cavity opened.

In many instances, however, the inflammation finally becomes widespread; or the course may be very short from the beginning, no remission occurs, the inflammation becomes general, and the prognosis is unfavorable; the worst cases dying in a few days from the onset. The mortality in the pneumococcic cases is much less than in those dependent upon the streptococcus.

Gonococcic peritonitis develops oftenest by an extension from a vulvovaginitis. It rarely may be general in nature, but usually, although the onset may be threatening, the symptoms soon abate, the inflammation is localized in the pelvic region, and, as a rule, resolution occurs. When gonococcic peritonitis is generalized the course, prognosis and termination are the same as in other severe forms.

Diagnosis.—In typical cases this presents little difficulty and rests upon the sudden onset; peculiar expression of the face; obstinate initial or continued vomiting; prostration and collapse; abdominal tenderness and distention; and, later, the discovery of a general or localized collection of fluid. As, however, the disease is subject to many variations the diagnosis is often obscured. *Typhoid fever* with abdominal pain and distention often resembles it closely. The matter of greatest importance is to recognize the occurrence of perforation and consequent peritonitis in this disease (see p. 311). The absence of leukocytosis may be of value in excluding peritonitis, but is not trustworthy. *Intussusception* or other obstruction of the bowel may, like peritonitis, cause vomiting, tympanites, and constipation. The last is, however, more obstinate in intestinal obstruction, and in intussusception the passage of bloody mucus with straining, and the discovery of a tumor, aid in its recognition. In intestinal obstruction there is usually no fever. *Acute ileocolitis* may strongly suggest localized peritonitis due to an appendicular inflammation; and when peritonitis develops as a sequel to acute enteritis, it may be with difficulty differentiated from the primary disease. *Pneumonia* and *pleurisy*, with their well-recognized tendency in some cases to develop pain referred to the abdomen, may readily simulate peritonitis. There is, however, no real abdominal tenderness in these conditions, and a careful examination of the thorax will generally serve to make the diagnosis certain (p. 730). Pneumococcic peritonitis, when in the stage of effusion, is to be distinguished from *tuberculous peritonitis* by the more sudden and severe onset. It is to be differentiated from *appendicitis* by the absence or slight development of localized rigidity in the appendicular region. When peritonitis in infancy does not exhibit typical symptoms it can hardly be recognized with certainty. In the diagnosis of the disease and in differentiating the type present, the obtaining of some of the fluid by the method of Denzer[10] is often useful.

Treatment.—The treatment for acute general purulent peritonitis involves surgical interference. When the diagnosis is in doubt, or when for any reason operation cannot be performed, palliative and symptomatic medical treatment must be employed. The patient should be at absolute rest, with the head of the bed elevated, and the peristalsis and pain held in control by opiates, best administered hypodermically. Purgatives should not be given. Owing to the obstinate early vomiting and the danger of exciting peristalsis it is often inadvisable to administer any food by the mouth at first, fluids being given by the bowel or parenterally. Later broth, skimmed lactic acid milk, and albumen-water may be allowed in small amounts frequently repeated. The application of ice-bags to the abdomen is to be recommended, or, if this fails to relieve the pain, warm compresses or turpentine stupes may be employed. For the prostration strychnine, camphor, or adrenaline may be given hypodermically. In streptococcic and pneumococcic peritonitis the specific sera may be employed intravenously.

In cases of localized peritonitis, the need for prompt surgical aid is not always so great, depending largely upon the cause. When secondary to appendicitis, although not certainly purulent, undoubtedly the safest procedure is early operation. When the peritonitis is gonorrheal, operation is rarely indicated and the medical treatment prescribed is to be preferred. Whenever peritonitis can be determined to be pneumococcic in nature, the waiting for encapsulation or local manifestation is to be advised. It is, however, always to be borne in mind that the large majority of cases of peritonitis, except in infancy, are dependent upon appendicitis, and that the prompt operative treatment as recommended for this is to be employed, unless it is certain that appendicitis is not the cause.

Subphrenic Abscess

This condition, which may be regarded as a localized secondary peritonitis, is uncommon in children. Jopson[11] could find but 22 cases under fifteen years of age in a total of 247 reported in medical literature. It may be due to pneumonia, empyema, abscess of the liver, tuberculous cavities, or appendicular abscess. The most frequent situation is above the liver; much less commonly above the spleen. The symptoms are similar to those of empyema but the fluoroscope and roentgenograms may show immobility and increased height of the diaphragm and other diagnostic differences. Occasionally the abscess contains air also, and then simulates a pyopneumothorax. The treatment is operative.

NONTUBERCULOUS CHRONIC PERITONITIS

The **lesions** and **symptoms** of this condition vary with the cause. A chronic, localized purulent peritonitis may follow the acute form. In other cases there is a diffuse fibrinous inflammation, sometimes chronic from the beginning, with extensive adhesions. This may be localized especially about the spleen or the liver, or may involve the coils of the intestines, and the fibrous bands produced may result in intestinal obstruction. Fetal peritonitis may be chronic from the beginning, or may have become so by the time of birth and numerous firm fibrous adhesions may be found post-mortem. These may be productive of malformations of the intestine, although perhaps oftener the peritonitis has been the result rather than the cause of these.

Chronic Ascitic Peritonitis.—This is a somewhat characteristic form of chronic peritonitis so closely resembling the tuberculous variety that many claim it is identical. Henoch[12] and others, however, maintain its independence. The condition is uncommon, seen generally in later childhood, and the cause is unknown, although trauma may have an influence, and cases have been reported after measles. There is, in addition to a fibrinous inflammation with adhesions, a large amount of serous effusion. The **symptoms** resemble those of tuberculous peritonitis in the gradual failure of health, loss of appetite, weakness, and abdominal distention with evidences of fluid free in the peritoneal cavity. They differ from them, however, in the absence of nodular masses discoverable on palpation, the moderate degree or even lack of abdominal tenderness, the normal or but slightly elevated temperature, and the absence of that degree of emaciation usually seen in the tuberculous variety. In fact the chief symptom is ascites for which no discoverable cause can be found. If the tuberculin-reaction is negative, and if inoculation of guinea-pigs with the fluid procured by aspiration gives a negative result, the disease is probably not tuberculosis. The disorder is to be distinguished from simple ascites through the lack of any evidence of disease of the liver, kidneys or heart. The course and **prognosis** are usually favorable, the fluid being gradually absorbed. In some cases chronic peritonitis may be combined with a chronic pleurisy with serous effusion, mediastinitis, or a serous pericarditis; the condition then being in fact a *polyserositis* of a nontuberculous variety.

Treatment consists in rest, the administration of diuretics (p. 826) and of saline purgatives in moderate amount, the maintaining of the general health by tonic measures, and eventually aspiration or even laparotomy if recovery does not take place without these.

TUBERCULOUS PERITONITIS

The majority of the cases of chronic peritonitis are of this nature, and the disease may also develop acutely as a part of miliary tuberculosis. Its incidence as a clinically recognized disease is about 0.1 to 0.25 per cent of sick children (Schmitz,[13] Cassell[14]). At necropsy it is found frequently (about 18 per cent, Biedert[15]) in tuberculous children, in many cases only a few tubercles being present.

Etiology.—In the study of cases with clinical manifestations, *age* is prominent among the predisposing causes. According to the statistics of Osler,[16] Faludi,[17] Fletcher,[18] Ashby,[19] and Giaume,[20] the disease is rare under one year, but quite common in early childhood from two to six or eight years, and Osler believed that adults are as frequently attacked as children. Weill and Pehu[21] could collect only 100 cases with clinical manifestations occurring in nurslings. It may, however, even be congenital (Charrin[22]). The disease is about equally divided between the sexes. Exceptionally it may appear to be incited by such causes as trauma of the abdomen, or one of the infectious diseases. The process may develop apparently simultaneously in the peritoneum and elsewhere in the body, as in the pleura; or may be secondary to lesions in the lungs, intestine, bones, or the mesenteric or other lymphatic glands, or be one of the evidences of a general miliary tuberculosis. Oftenest, from a purely clinical standpoint, the peritonitis seems to be the primary or sole manifestation of tuberculosis, although actually it is usually secondary to some small or perhaps undiscovered remote tuberculous lesion. Tuberculous peritonitis is probably one of the most frequent forms of tuberculosis dependent upon the bovine bacillus. The bacilli may reach the peritoneum either through the general circulation, as in cases of widespread acute tuberculosis; from the intestinal tract by way of the lymphatic vessels and the mesenteric glands, with or without a discoverable primary intestinal lesion; or, still oftener, from other regions of the body. Indeed, the combination of tuberculous peritonitis with intestinal tuberculosis is often absent.

Pathologic Anatomy.—Gray miliary tubercles are disseminated over the involved portion of the peritoneum. These may disappear if the case recovers, or may become confluent into larger, centrally caseous masses. The serous membrane exhibits fibrinous exudate, and always present is a varying amount of effusion; serous, sero-purulent, or, infrequently, hemorrhagic. The omentum is usually thickened with large tuberculous nodules, or shrunken, or rolled up into a firm mass. The relative amount of the fluid and of the fibrinous exudates respectively varies with the type of the disease. In the ascitic form fluid predominates and adhesions are few, scattered, and easily torn apart. In the fibrous there is comparatively little fluid, but fibrinous exudate is abundant, and firm adhesions are produced, binding the coils of intestines together and to neighboring tissues and organs. Most cases, however, show both conditions in varying degrees, and no sharp division into types can be made. With either, large caseous masses may develop, and these may become encapsulated, or may finally produce pus, which may discharge through the abdominal wall, especially at the navel, or by ulceration into the intestine.

Symptoms.—As just indicated, no clear-cut distinction of forms can be made, since so many intermediate ones exist, but the following classification may be utilized as a matter of convenience: (1) *The ascitic form.* (2) *The fibrous, adhesive, or plastic form.* (3) *The caseous, or ulcerative form.*

In addition there is the development of miliary tubercles upon the peritoneum attending cases of acute general miliary tuberculosis, but producing no certain clinical manifestations, and not considered here.

1. The Ascitic Form.—The development of symptoms may be insidious, or be marked by gradually increasing loss of health, vague or slight abdominal pain and tenderness, and irregular fever of moderate degree. There may be vomiting, but this is not characteristic, and the bowels may be constipated, diarrheal or unchanged. There is nothing on which to base a diagnosis until finally attention is called to the gradually increasing distention of the abdomen, which may, indeed, be the first symptom noted. The abdomen is at first tympanitic, but later exhibits fluid free in the peritoneal cavity, with fluctuating dulness in the flanks, a shifting with change of position, upward displacement of the diaphragm and of the hepatic dulness, flattening or pouting of the umbilicus, and dilatation of the abdominal veins. When the fluid is in small amount careful examination may be required to show its presence, and the distention is principally tympanitic. Sometimes the thickened omentum or enlarged lymphatic glands can be palpated. The fluid is usually chiefly serous and straw-colored or slightly brownish.

In exceptional cases the inflammation may begin much more suddenly and severely, and may strongly suggest appendicitis if the pain and other evidences of the tuberculous disease are at all marked in the appendicular region.

2. The Fibrous Form.—The presence of a relatively large amount of fibrinous exudation, in combination with more or less ascitic fluid, constitutes probably the most frequent form of the disease. A strictly dry, fibrous peritonitis is uncommon. The early symptoms are very similar to those described, but the onset is even more gradual and the development slower. Fever is still less prominent and is often absent (Fig. 159). Enlargement of the abdomen is usually found to be tympanitic in nature. Careful palpation may reveal nodules, or areas of dulness on percussion which are not limited to the flanks and which do not alter with change of position of the patient. These depend upon tuberculous deposits or upon localized encapsulated collections of fluid. The abdomen may be globular in shape, as in the ascitic form; or irregular in outline dependent upon the presence of adhesions. Some fluid may be found in amounts varying with the case. Abdominal pain and tenderness are absent or slight. The formation of tuberculous masses or of firm contracting adhesions may proceed so far that secondary symptoms result, due to pressure upon various regions. Among these are edema from interference with the circulation; digestive disturbance from pressure upon the intestine or stomach; intestinal obstruction; and abnormal urinary conditions. Fibrous peritonitis may be such from the beginning, or may be a sequel to the ascitic form first described.

3. The Caseous or Ulcerative Form.—This severe type may be a sequel of the others described, or may less commonly exhibit its peculiarities from the beginning. Its chief characteristic is the formation of large tuberculous masses and smaller nodules which undergo caseation and often produce pus. Owing to this and to the fact that tuberculosis in other parts of the body is also generally present the symptoms early become severe. There is more constant and greater elevation of temperature, which often assumes a hectic type (Fig. 160); diarrhea is frequent; there are abdominal pain and tenderness; and emaciation, anemia and loss of strength are progressive and decided. The abdomen becomes distended, but, although fluid, which is often purulent, may be present in considerable quantities, the matting of the intestines and the presence of the large tuberculous masses frequently prevents the discovery of this by percussion or palpation. The abdomen may give a characteristic doughy sensation on palpation.

Course and Prognosis.—These vary with the nature of the lesion. In favorable cases of the *ascitic* form the effusion varies but little in amount from time to time, or may exhibit periods of temporary diminution or increase; but finally it gradually disappears completely, while fever lessens, the general health improves, and recovery takes place. The gray tubercles, and even the larger masses, may disappear entirely, but some adhesions

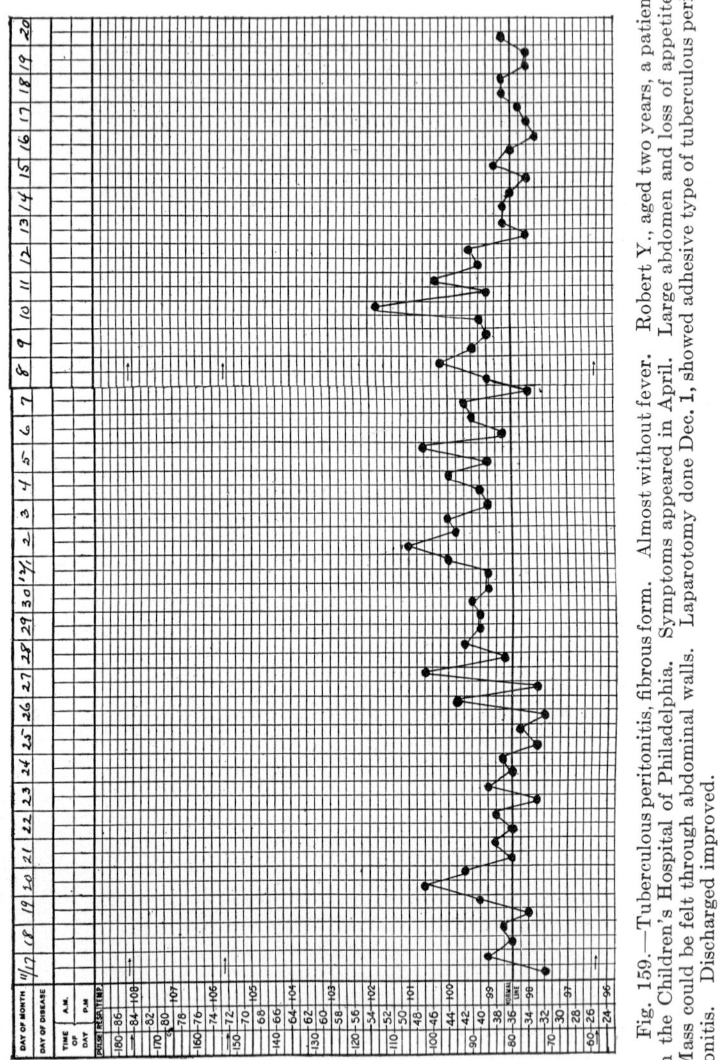

Fig. 159.—Tuberculous peritonitis, fibrous form. Almost without fever. Robert Y., aged two years, a patient in the Children's Hospital of Philadelphia. Symptoms appeared in April. Large abdomen and loss of appetite. Mass could be felt through abdominal walls. Laparotomy done Dec. 1, showed adhesive type of tuberculous peritonitis. Discharged improved.

are likely to remain. In other cases relapse may later occur, or tuberculosis make its appearance in other parts of the body. In the more unfavorable cases emaciation increases, and death takes place from exhaustion or following tuberculosis of some other organ; or the case passes into the fibrous or the caseous type.

In the *fibrous* form the course is slower, lasting several months or even a year or more. It may then slowly undergo recovery, but leaves firm adhesions remaining, even after apparent cure; and there is a decided tendency to relapse. This variety may prove fatal by gradually exhausting the patient, may pass into the caseous form, or may be followed by the development of tuberculosis elsewhere in the body. The *caseous* form is of shorter duration than the two just described, lasting usually only a few months after evidences of the breaking down of the lesions show themselves. The duration is influenced considerably by the course of the tuberculosis usually present in other parts of the body.

The prognosis of tuberculous peritonitis in general is determined by various circumstances, such as the inherent strength and resisting power of the patient; the type of the disease; the age of the child; and the presence or absence of tuberculosis in other regions. The younger the patient, the worse is the prognosis. The ascitic form has the most favorable prog-

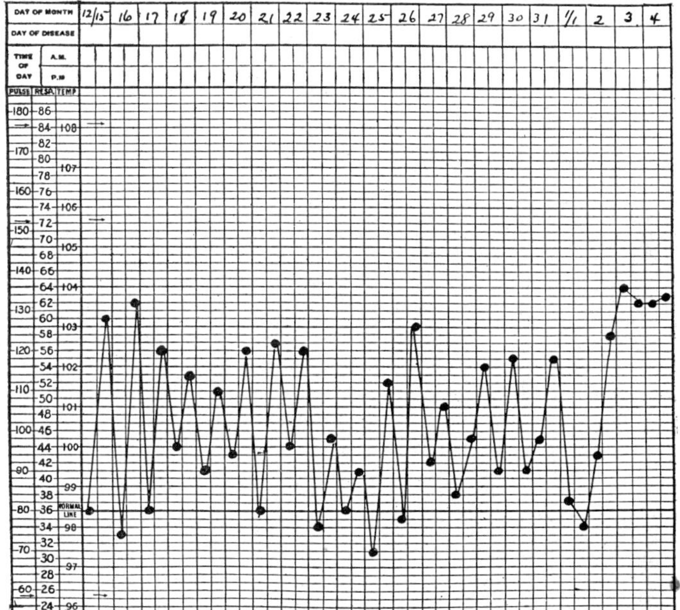

Fig. 160.—Tuberculous peritonitis, caseous form, with hectic type of temperature. Elizabeth R., aged eleven years. Said to have been taken ill in June. Admitted to the Children's Hospital of Philadelphia, Dec. 15. Operation Dec. 29, showed fibrocaseous tuberculosis of the peritoneum. Died the following March. Principal symptoms, progressive loss of health, with fever.

nosis; the caseous the worst. No patient should be considered as having recovered until at least two years have elapsed without symptoms.

It would appear from a study of statistics that operative treatment has not the vogue which it once possessed, and does not accomplish all that was once expected; but there seems also no question that it is followed by excellent results in many instances.

Complications.—These are principally the occurrence of manifestations of tuberculosis elsewhere in the body, as the pleura, pericardium, meninges, lungs, intestine, and mesenteric glands. The genital organs are only occasionally attacked secondarily in children. To be noted also are septic processes from a collection of pus, amyloid changes in the liver and spleen, and intestinal obstruction or other pressure-symptoms of various sorts produced by fibrous adhesions.

Diagnosis.—Early in the attack this is usually difficult. It rests principally upon slow failure of health; irregular fever without discoverable cause; slight abdominal pain and tenderness; and finally decided abdominal enlargement with the discovery of fluid, or of evident thickening of the abdominal wall and the presence of masses beneath it. The existence of tuberculosis elsewhere in the body is suggestive. The employment of the tuberculin-test is of value if negative, but it must be remembered that severe cases may have lost the power to respond. A positive reaction is equivocal. There is an absence of the leukocytosis characteristic of most inflammatory conditions.

Ascites of tuberculous nature is to be distinguished from that due to other causes. That dependent upon *cardiac* or *renal disease* is accompanied by dropsy elsewhere, and other characteristic symptoms are present. *Atrophic cirrhosis* of the liver gives diminution in the size of this organ, and icterus may attend. In doubtful cases examination of the fluid obtained by puncture will probably show in tuberculosis an increase in the number of lymphocytes, and inoculation-experiments will produce tuberculosis in animals. Puncture is, however, a procedure not without danger of perforation of the intestine. It may be performed after the method of Denzer.[10] Tubercle bacilli are not often discovered microscopically. *Chronic nontuberculous peritonitis* is distinguishable by the absence of discoverable nodular masses and of so decided a degree of emaciation and loss of health. The presumption should always be that chronic peritonitis is tuberculous unless certainly proven otherwise. Chronic *enteritis* with diarrhea, abdominal distention, and wasting may resemble tuberculous peritonitis, but the history of the case and continued observation will generally remove any doubt. Tuberculous peritonitis with masses discovered through the abdominal wall is to be distinguished from *abdominal tumors* of other nature, as well as from fecal accumulations in the colon. The existence of other symptoms characteristic of tuberculosis is of service here. That the disease is of the caseous type is rendered probable, when, in addition to the presence of the tuberculous nodules discovered by palpation, there are decided abdominal pain and tenderness, tympanitic distention, and severe constitutional symptoms.

Treatment.—The medical treatment consists in the employment of all hygienic and other measures which will aid the patient to overcome a tuberculous process of any nature (p. 424). The diet should be digestible and abundant, unless contraindicated by digestive disturbance, and there is no reason to abstain from a highly nitrogenous regimen because fever is present. Alcoholic stimulants may be given as required. Exposure of the abdominal walls to the direct rays of the sun has been recommended. Indeed, heliotherapy offers one of the best means of treatment. (See p. 204.) Much benefit can be obtained from the employment of ultraviolet rays from an artificial source, and excellent results have been reported by Meyer,[23] Gerstenberger and Wahl,[24] and others. Exposure to the roentgen-ray has also been successfully used, especially in the fibrous form of the disease. If employed in the ascitic variety the fluid should first be removed, as otherwise the rays will be absorbed by it. Tonic remedies may be needed, including cod-liver oil if it is well tolerated, and such treatment also as complications demand. In general, however, the chief dependence is to be placed upon hygiene, diet, and heliotherapy. There is some reason to believe that tuberculin-treatment is of more value here than in some other forms of tuberculosis, but further experience is needed.

Operative interference in the form of laparotomy should be recommended in all cases of the ascitic type, if thorough medical treatment has been without influence. In the purely fibrous form without tuberculous masses recovery may take place spontaneously; but even here laparotomy may do good and can do little harm, although less is to be expected than in the ascitic type. Cases where a small localized or more generalized accumulation of pus can be discovered require operation. The reason for the beneficial effect of operation in ascitic cases is not understood. It seems to depend in some way upon the entrance of air, since good results have been obtained by the injection of air and of oxygen.

TUMORS OF THE PERITONEUM

These are of occasional occurrence in early life and may be either malignant or benign in nature; primary or secondary. Cysts of various sorts are sometimes found, including dermoid, hydatid, chylous and serous. They are oftenest in the mesentery. Carcinoma is very rare even when secondary. Sarcoma, fibroma, angioma and lipoma may occur. The last has sometimes attained a large size.

ASCITES

By this title is designated an accumulation of serous fluid in the general peritoneal cavity. The condition is but a symptom dependent upon various causes. The fluid may be entirely clear and either colorless or of a yellowish tint; or more or less hemorrhagic or contain flakes of lymph and other evidences of inflammation. Microscopically it may show either few cellular elements when it is a transudate, or many when the cause is a local inflammatory condition. If the inflammation is a tuberculous peritonitis, the lymphocytes are in excess; if an acute peritonitis dependent upon other germs, the polymorphonuclear cells predominate. Among the **causes** may be mentioned peritonitis of various sorts, including polyserositis; cirrhosis of the liver; obstruction to the portal circulation from other sources, such as pressure of a tumor or of an enlarged lymphatic gland; great anemia; and renal or cardiac disease. These last two are the most common causes. It may also develop without discoverable agency and be associated with hydrothorax and anasarca. Ascites may in rare cases be congenital, is uncommon in infancy, somewhat less so in early childhood, and is observed oftener in later childhood. The **symptoms** are similar to those seen in adult life. The abdomen is distended; there is often flattening or pouting of the umbilicus; fluctuation on palpation, with a distinct wave-like impulse obtained by sharp tapping with the hand; and dulness on percussion, which shifts with change of position unless the amount of fluid is very large. The course, prognosis and treatment depend entirely upon the cause.

CHYLOUS ASCITES.—This is an uncommon form of ascites at any time of life. Schall,[25] adding 2 instances to the list of reported cases in the first three years of life published by Cowie,[26] could collect but 11 observed during this period. An additional case is reported by Bruchsaler.[27] In the instances of true *chylous* effusion there has been an injury to, or pressure upon, the thoracic duct or some of its tributaries, as a result of which the chyle has entered the abdominal cavity. The fluid has the appearance of milk and contains fat-cells in very large numbers. In other cases the fluid is *chyliform* only, and the condition depends upon tuberculous or nontuberculous chronic peritonitis, and the color appears to be the result of degeneration of the inflammatory products. Chylous ascites has also been produced by the rupture of a mesenteric cyst. The prognosis is, as a rule, unfavorable; yet recovery after operative interference has been reported (Huber and Silver[28]).

REFERENCES

1. Am. J. Dis. Child., 1928, **36**, 774. 2. Practitioner, 1912, **88**, 557. 3. Brit. J. Surg., 1922, **9**, 479. 4. Arch. Pediat., 1921, **38**, 677. 5. Deutsche Ztschr. f. Chir., 1928, **208**, 226. 6. Am. J. Surg., 1930, **8**, 48. 7. Arch. de méd. d. enf., 1926, **29**, 572. 8. Lancet, 1906, **1**, 1591. 9. Centralbl. f. Chir., 1917, **44**, 94. 10. Arch. Pediat., 1922, **39**, 720. 11. Arch. Pediat., 1904, **21**, 120. 12. Vorlesung. ü. Kinderkr., 1895, 539. 13.

Jahrb. f. Kinderh., 1897, **44,** 316. 14. Deutsche med. Wchnschr., 1900, **26,** 596. 15. Jahrb. f. Kinderh., 1884, **21,** 178. 16. Johns Hopkins Hosp. Rep., 1890, **2,** 67. 17. Jahrb. f. Kinderh., 1905, **62,** 304. 18. Garrod, Batten and Thursfield, Dis. Childr., 1913, 242. 19. Brit. M. J., 1923, **2,** 863. 20. Pediatria, 1926, **34,** 1. 21. Arch. de méd. d. enf., 1909, **12,** 415. 22. Lyon méd., 1873, **13,** 295. 23. Jahrb. f. Kinderh., 1918, **87,** 126. 24. J.A.M.A., 1924, **83,** 1631. 25. Monatschr. f. Kinderh., 1922, **23,** 34. 26. Arch. Pediat., 1911, **28,** 595. 27. Monatschr. f. Kinderh., 1929, **45,** 439. 28. Am. J. Dis. Child., 1914, **8,** 50.

SECTION V

DISEASES OF THE RESPIRATORY SYSTEM

THESE are among the commonest of the disorders of early life, being exceeded in infancy only by digestive disturbances, and in early childhood even surpassing these in number. Some forms of disease belonging in part here have already been described elsewhere, such as adenoid growths of the nasopharynx and membranous laryngitis dependent upon diphtheria.

CHAPTER I

COUGH

A SHORT review of the causes and indications of this symptom is of importance. (See also p. 165.)

Cough is an expulsive effort of respiration of such force and suddenness that the characteristic sound is produced. It is incited by a pathologic stimulation of the respiratory terminals of the pneumogastric nerve, or reflexly through irritation of other branches of this or of other cranial nerves. Along these afferent filaments the sensation is conducted to the medulla and the expulsive effort set going from this center through the action of the muscles concerned in respiration. In some cases this appears to depend upon irritation of the nerve-centers solely, without peripheral disturbance, as seen, for instance, in a hysterical or a habit cough. The distribution of the pneumogastric and communicating nerves being so wide and diverse, the causes of cough may be extremely varied. In some instances it results from direct stimulation by secretion resting upon the respiratory mucous membrane in some part of its course or in the pharynx, or from the presence of a foreign body in the respiratory tract. It is then a real effort to expel a removable offending substance, and is of a serviceable nature. With this exception cough is generally unproductive and useless.

The following conditions may be mentioned in which cough occurs:

In *bronchitis* it is at first frequent, severe and unproductive. Later it is loose and sometimes only relieved when the secretion is expelled. It may be severe enough to cause vomiting, and often produces soreness in the muscles of the chest and abdomen. *Tracheitis*, when occurring alone, produces cough of a similar nature. In *catarrhal laryngitis* it is at first dry, and later loose as in bronchitis. The accompanying hoarseness serves to distinguish it. *Spasmodic laryngitis*, on the other hand, occasions a loud, barking and ringing cough. This is not paroxysmal, but comes on especially at night with the symptoms of croup. *Diphtheritic laryngitis* gives rise to a cough very like that of catarrhal laryngitis, although with more of a croupy character. In *pneumonia* and *pleurisy* the cough is usually short, suppressed, and evidently painful; sometimes frequent and harassing. Pleural effusion may produce a persistent and troublesome, short, dry cough without the element of pain.

Pharyngeal irritation is one of the most common causes, giving rise to a cough which is very frequent and hacking, especially at night, and with a constant sensation of tickling in the throat. It may be due to the reflex irritation arising from adenoid growths of the nasopharynx or of the base of the tongue, or develop in the pharynx itself through the accumulation of secretion on the posterior pharyngeal wall, or be brought about by the tickling sensation caused by an elongated uvula. It is often troublesome and resistant to treatment. An *ear-cough* sometimes arises from the presence of foreign bodies or of wax in the auditory canal or the existence of an external otitis.

Cough of a peculiarly paroxysmal character is heard in *pertussis*, but may sometimes occur also in severe tracheobronchitis, or accompany pressure by *enlarged bronchial glands* or an *abscess* produced by spinal caries. The condition often described as *spasmodic nocturnal cough*, or *periodic night-cough*, heard frequently in older children, may be due to enlarged bronchial glands or abscess, or to adenoid growths or an unrecognized rhinitis. There is also in many cases a strong nervous element combined with the causes mentioned, or acting alone. The cough occurs in paroxysms, chiefly or solely about the middle of the night or soon after going to bed; or the attacks may repeat themselves several times during the night and occasion much loss of rest. The disease may extend over months.

"*Stomach-cough*" is a term too indiscriminately used. There are, however, cases in which cough accompanies indigestion and disappears when this ceases. In some this is probably dependent upon the frequent complicating pharyngeal irritation. In others it appears to be a direct reflex from the stomach. This latter type is heard, for instance, in some infants who suffer from cough when the stomach is over-distended from nursing. A short stomach-cough may also be observed at times just before an attack of vomiting occurs.

Cardiac cough is produced chiefly by the passive congestion of the lungs. It is hard and usually dry in character.

Finally there is to be considered the *nervous* or *hysterical cough* encountered especially as puberty is approaching. It is dry, noisy, harsh, forced, frequent, usually not paroxysmal, does not occur during sleep, and is increased by excitement. It may disappear for months if the general nervous state of the child improves, but reappears readily with the return of nervous disturbance or with the development of anemia.

In this connection may be mentioned the infrequency with which sputum is expectorated in infancy and early childhood (see p. 421) and the comparative rarity of **hemoptysis** in early life. This latter is seen occasionally in pneumonia and tuberculosis, oftener in pertussis, and may be severe in gangrene of the lung. Fatal hemoptysis is exceedingly uncommon. Magruder[1] refers to 33 cases collected by Meusnier[2] and adds 5 others including 1 of his own. The condition has since been studied by Rolleston and Robertson-Ross.[3] We have seen an instance of fatal hemoptysis in an infant of fourteen months. (See p. 415.)

Treatment of Cough.—The treatment of these different varieties of cough is that of the original cause. To be said here is only that when the symptom is dependent upon acute inflammation of the larynx, trachea, or bronchi sedatives are often of value, but usually after the first few days those remedies are indicated which favor secretion. In cases of other nature expectorants are of no benefit. Nasopharyngeal or pharyngeal irritation is always to be searched for, and local treatment of these conditions, including remedies to diminish the size of an elongated uvula, will often promptly relieve cough over which sedatives have practically no control. Inhalations of water-vapor, plain or medicated (p. 187), often give relief. In the periodical nocturnal cough and in the nervous day-cough the general health is to be cared for, the pharynx kept from becoming dry at night-time, and such sedatives as bromides administered. In some cases of very persistent cough quinine has proved of benefit.

REFERENCES

1. Arch. Pediat., 1908, **25**, 520. 2. Thèse de Paris, 1892. 3. Brit. J. Child. Dis., 1914, **11**, 407.

CHAPTER II

DISEASES OF THE NOSE

MALFORMATIONS

Deviations of the septum nasi are usually the result of injury or of faulty development of the adjacent structures. **Perforation of the septum** may occur in syphilis and tuberculosis, or from trauma. **Depression of the bridge** of the nose may be a congenital peculiarity or be the result of injury or of the destructive action of hereditary syphilis. **Stenosis** of the nasal passages or even entire **closure** of these may be of congenital origin; manifesting itself, if bilateral, by difficulty or inability on the part of the infant to suck. Examination with the sound will reveal the obstruction, which may be membranaceous, but is oftener bony in nature. We have seen one instance of infantilism associated with complete bony obstruction of the nares. Among other deformities to be mentioned are the broadening of the bridge in *ocular hypertelorism;* the broad nose combined with the upward tilt of the nostrils seen in *cretinism;* and the narrow nasal fossae, small nostrils, and pinched appearance of the nose often present in *adenoid growths.*

The treatment of nasal deformities consists chiefly in operation which, if indicated, should be done early lest malformations of the chest, palate, jaws, or even of the skull develop.

ACUTE RHINITIS

(Coryza)

Etiology.—The tendency to develop "cold in the head," one of the most common affections seen in children, may begin promptly after birth and continue active throughout life. It has been estimated that at least 75 per cent of children have one or more colds each year (McLean[1]). In certain individuals there is a special predisposition, which may sometimes be hereditary or familial in nature, and the exudative diathesis is also to be mentioned here. Other agents, likewise, are operative more as predisposing factors, such as insufficient fresh air and ventilation, adenoid hypertrophy (see p. 543), rickets, or other debilitating diseases. Many diverse influences, however, are the more active agents. Especially to be mentioned is local chilling, as from draughts from playing on the floor, wet feet, or either too much or too little clothing; this acting especially after over-heating of the body from exercise, warm baths, and excessive perspiration. Inhalation of dust and other irritants is likewise a directly active cause.

Coryza is most likely to develop in autumn and spring, with their sudden changes in temperature; and the damp raw weather and high winds of winter are determining causes. The local chilling, or other operative first cause, probably initiates a congestion of the mucous membrane, and this, in most instances, permits of the action of micro-organisms. That several members of a family may be attacked in quick succession would indicate that the common cold is undoubtedly contagious. The fact must be remembered that all the members of a family, or scholars of a class, may have been exposed simultaneously to other factors than contagion, such as changes in the weather; and conclusions as to the universality of microbic action in producing colds must be drawn with caution. Certainly many colds would appear to be allergic in nature, such as those seen in hay-fever. The extreme promptness with which a severe rhinorrhea may develop after short exposure to cold, or after the getting of wet feet, and yet disappear in a few hours after the body has become warmed, would indicate that in such cases microbic action can be eliminated; and the condition considered as a purely vasomotor disturbance.

Rhinitis is a constant attendant upon certain diseases, such as grippe, measles, and nasal diphtheria, and follows also the ingestion of such drugs as iodides. Among the various germs associated with rhinitis are the streptococcus, staphylococcus, pneumococcus, micrococcus catarrhalis, influenza bacillus, and bacillus rhinitis (Tunnicliff[2]). No one of these is constantly found in pure culture or in predominance. Very rarely the gonococcus may cause rhinitis. The specific forms accompanying grippe, measles, or diphtheria may be produced by the causative agents of the disease, perhaps acting alone, or perhaps in combination with other germs. It has been maintained by a number of observers that colds may be produced by a filterable virus, which stimulates into greatly increased activity any potential pathogen which happens to be present (Kruse;[3] Foster;[4] Olitsky;[5] Shibley et al.;[6] Dochez et al.;[7] Long et al.,[8] and others). In some of these studies a minute filter-passing germ was seen, termed by Olitsky, Bacterium pneumosintes.

Symptoms, Course and Prognosis.—Following the congestion of the mucous membrane there occurs an augmented thin secretion from the nose. In the milder cases this may subside in a few hours and the attack be over, or it may last two or three days. In other more severe ones the congestion grows greater, there is frequent sneezing, the discharge is irritating and reddens the edges of the nostrils and the upper lip, respiration through the nose becomes almost or quite impossible, and the general condition is one of extreme discomfort. The compulsory breathing through the mouth dries the throat and produces a sensation of soreness; and in the case of infants mechanically interferes with the taking of food, since the child cannot suck and breathe through the mouth at the same time. The temperature is seldom more than slightly elevated except in young infants. After a day or two the discharge becomes more seropurulent, and finally of a green mucopurulent character, perhaps more or less tinged with blood. The entire course lasts a week or ten days. Attending the rhinitis, or sometimes preceding it, there are, in the severer cases, lachrymation and slight conjunctivitis. The inflammation may spread through the Eustachian tube to the ear, and otitis, often purulent, develop. Not infrequently the process attacks simultaneously, or in sequence, the nose, pharynx, larynx, trachea and bronchi. Bronchopneumonia may develop. In many cases pharyngitis is the first manifestation and rhinitis appears subsequent to this. Even repeated attacks of rhinitis do not seem to confer immunity, perhaps because the different attacks are due to different germs or because they are not the type to produce antibodies.

Diagnosis.—The persistence of high temperature renders one always suspicious that the coryza is not a primary disorder, and the possibility of grippe or measles will be entertained. The discharge of nasal diphtheria early becomes bloody and very irritating to the lips, is unattended by the complicating conjunctivitis or other symptoms of simple acute rhinitis, and is longer continued. Examination of the nose may reveal a pseudomembrane, but in suspicious cases cultures should be taken promptly. Vincent's infection may attack the nose with a resultant ulceration, the causative germs being found on examination. (See p. 537.)

Treatment. **Prophylaxis.**—Particular attention should be given to this. Contact with infected persons must be avoided, especially in the case of infants. When repeated attacks of rhinitis occur, predisposing causes must be diligently sought for, and hygienic conditions improved on the lines discussed under etiology. Careful attention must be given to the details of exercise, pure air in the sleeping room, proper clothing, house-temperature, and out-door life. Some rearrangement is necessary when the routine of bathing, feeding and the like interferes with the daily airing. Moreover, it is not essential that the day be perfectly clear to permit the taking of the infant out of doors. High, cold winds and a temperature below freezing are, however, to be avoided. The sheltered side of a veranda offers a suitable place under such conditions, or the young infant may be dressed in its outdoor clothing and put in a room with the windows open. Older children should be accustomed to go out properly protected in almost any sort of weather. More children are dressed too warmly than the reverse. It is better to have the arms and legs always covered except in hot weather, but the clothes should be of only moderate weight, and an outside wrap of some sort may be worn when necessary.

Every means must be taken to improve the general health. A cool bath given before breakfast and followed by brisk friction will be found an excellent measure to harden a child. Tonic treatment may be required. Yet it must be observed that in the extensive study of Jordan, Norton and Sharp[9] on 1600 students, so-called "resistance-building" measures had little effect on the frequency of colds, and Barrows[10] could find no relation to different types of heating or ventilation. Finally the effect of removal of adenoids may be tried, and any infection of the sinuses be treated. Nasal polyps should be removed or deviated septum corrected if either is present. Exposure to lamps emitting *ultraviolet* rays is being widely employed in the attempt to reduce the incidence of colds. We have not been impressed with its value. There are studies, such as those of Manghan and Smiley,[11] which apparently indicate good results, and others as those of Barenberg, Freeman and Green[12] which show a greater incidence of respiratory infections in the group which had been treated. There is no clear-cut clinical evidence that the administration of *vitamins* lowers the incidence. (See Vitamins p. 134.) Cod liver oil, while often employed, has no certain specific effect in reducing the susceptibility. Many clinicians believe that *vaccines*, especially the autogenous, are helpful in prophylaxis or at least diminish the severity of colds. Their value is not yet established.

Treatment of the Attack.—When seen early, the patient should be given a warm general bath or a hot mustard foot bath, and be kept in bed in the effort to produce a sweat. Purgation is employed if indication for it exists. Later the child should be kept quiet and in an evenly heated, rather warm room, and in the winter off of the floor. The air, however, must be fresh. The diet should be restricted, particularly if there is fever. The salicylates or small doses of the coal-tar derivatives may make the patient more comfortable. Menthol and camphor with liquid petrolatum (grain $\frac{1}{2}$ to 1: oz. 1) (0.003 to 0.006:30) as a spray are serviceable, or an ointment containing them may be used. If there is much obstruction to breathing great relief may be obtained by instilling a few drops of a 1 per cent solution of ephedrine. Synephrin tartrate in $2\frac{1}{2}$ per cent solution may be employed for the same purpose. Inhalation of vapor from hot water is also serviceable (p. 187). Cold cream or a boric acid ointment should be applied to the upper lip and the edges of the nostrils. Internally small doses of atropine are of value in checking the discharge and relieving the congestion, especially in the earlier stage. Occasionally quinine seems to have a special power in curtailing or aborting an attack. In the later stages, a spray or gentle douch of warm diluted liq. sod. boratis comp. (Dobell's solution), or of warm normal saline solution, employed three or four times a day, is useful for cleansing purposes, followed by the instillation of a few drops of a solution of argyrol or some similar silver-preparation in 10 per cent strength. In all local treatment it should be remembered that the nasal mucous membrane possesses a self-disinfecting power, which should not be interfered with too greatly. Antiseptics sufficiently strong to kill germs would also cause local injury.

Membranous Rhinitis.—There is rarely seen a condition similar to diphtheria but due to the streptococcus, staphylococcus, pneumococcus, or pseudodiphtheria bacillus. The local symptoms are like those of diphtheritic rhinitis; and even the failure to discover the diphtheria bacillus does not make it certain that this is not the condition present. (See p. 346.)

Sinusitis

The older medical literature emphasized the infrequency of disease of the sinuses in early life. Kelly,[13] for example, could collect but 16 cases of empyema of the antrum occurring in infants, and Õnodi[14] only 53 instances of any disease of the sinuses developing before ten years of age. Both Phelps[15] and Skillern[16] stressed the rarity of sinusitis in infancy and early childhood, owing to the imperfect development of the sinuses at this period. (See p. 35.) Recently more attention has been directed to sinusitis and, in fact, the term is too often applied to almost any nasal infection. It is obvious that most if not all cases of rhinitis are likely to have involvement by continuity of any sinuses sufficiently developed. Among the many who have written of sinus-disease in children are Dean and Armstrong;[17] Pfaunz;[18] Cleminson;[19] Strachan;[20] Davis;[21] Dean;[22] Jeans[23] and Ruskin.[24] Collet[25] collected 6 and reported 1 instance of maxillary sinusitis in infants from three days to five weeks of age.

The **symptoms** of acute sinusitis in addition to those of rhinitis are fever, localized pain and tenderness and possibly edema over the affected sinus, and headache. The last can be elicited better in older children, and may be of assistance in localization; being in sphenoidal sinusitis in the suboccipital region; in anterior ethmoidal sinusitis in the temples and over the eyes; in posterior ethmoidal sinusitis over the distribution of Meckel's ganglion especially about 2 inches posterior to the external auditory meatus. Nasal discharge is present unless there is blocking of the opening of the sinus. Local examination of the nose will show pus escaping from the sinuses. Suction may be employed to confirm the diagnosis. The roentgenogram may or may not demonstrate opaqueness due to pus in acute cases, and, furthermore, any cloudiness discovered may be caused by thickened membrane rather than fluid. Goodyear[26] and others have found it advantageous to inject or insufflate the sinuses with lipiodol before the roentgenograms are taken. Transillumination or puncture of the sinuses may be helpful in diagnosis, but the latter is not without danger and perhaps too freely employed. **Treatment** is that for rhinitis, puncture of the sinuses being seldom indicated.

Chronic Sinusitis.—The acute condition may pass into a chronic form, especially in children with poor nutrition and in unfavorable hygienic surroundings. The general symptoms are much the same as in the acute form, but less marked. Fever is of a low grade, or only occasionally present. Sneezing is a rather frequent symptom. The nasal discharge is more or less constant, purulent or mucopurulent, and may be unilateral. The general health may suffer from the absorption of purulent material, and arthritic affections develop. Loss of vision may follow infection of the ethmoidal sinus, as pointed out by White[27] and others; or orbital abscess and exophthalmos appear. Persistence of nasal discharge after removal of infected adenoids should lead to the suspicion of sinus-disease. The treatment is that for chronic rhinitis, operative procedures being a last resort.

Hay Fever

This title designates a form of acute rhinitis of an allergic nature recurring at the same season of each year, but oftenest in the summer and autumn. It is brought about by the action of various local irritants, such as the pollen of numerous varieties of plants; the odor of roses, violets, peaches, etc.; and the emanations from certain animals, as the cat or dog, and especially the horse. Abnormalities of the mucous membrane of the nose may be a predisposing cause. An individual susceptibility is necessary and the patients are generally of a highly nervous temperament. Inheritance is frequently observed. The disease is not common until after three or four years of age. The **symptoms** come on suddenly after exposure, and increase in severity if this continues. They consist of severe coryza; conjunctivitis; intense itching in the nose and eyes; profuse watery nasal discharge; frequent violent sneezing; lachrymation, and photophobia. As the patient grows older and the annual attacks have been repeated, asthma is liable to be associated with the rhinitis, and sometimes even largely to replace it. The **prognosis** for ultimate recovery is poor. The **treatment** is largely prophylactic. When possible the child should be removed before the season of danger to a region which experience shows renders him free from the disease. For the direct treatment of the disorder little can be done except the employment of palliative measures, as recommended for ordinary severe acute rhinitis. Adrenaline or ephedrine locally may give some relief. The patient may be kept in a room without draughts, and, if possible, the air filtered to remove pollen or other irritants. The value of immunizing against the specific pollens responsible, as determined by skin-testing, is uncertain, but a trial of it is to be recommended. (See also Asthma, p. 713; and Allergy, p. 484.)

CHRONIC RHINITIS

Chronic rhinitis may assume one of several forms, and may be consequently divided into: (1) Simple Chronic Rhinitis; (2) Hypertrophic Rhinitis; (3) Atrophic Rhinitis; (4) Syphilitic Rhinitis.

1. Simple Purulent Chronic Rhinitis

(Chronic Nasopharyngitis; Post-nasal Catarrh; Chronic Nasal Catarrh)

This common disorder may follow repeated attacks of acute coryza, or be the result of the introduction of foreign bodies into the nose, deviations of the septum, adenoids, or the presence of the exudative-lymphatic diathesis. (See p. 841.) Rarely larvae of flies may be harbored in the nose. Often the children appear to be in perfect health in other respects. The **symptoms** consist of a more or less constant discharge from the nose of a secretion which is mucous, or oftener mucopurulent or purulent, and sometimes bloody, especially when foreign bodies are the cause. Children old enough to blow the nose remove the secretion readily, but it soon reaccumulates. Redness and excoriation of the upper lip and edges of the nostrils are common and eczema may develop here. There is a frequent association of redness of the eyelids and of eczema, perhaps dependent upon the exudative diathesis. The **course** varies. Cases due to foreign bodies are usually promptly cured by removal of these. When from other causes the disease may continue indefinitely, even extending over years; perhaps being better in summer and returning in winter. If long-continued the atrophic form of chronic rhinitis may develop. Otitis, pharyngitis, or enlargement of the glands of the neck may occur as complications. In **diagnosis** the chief indications are search for a foreign body, and the differentiation from specific rhinitis caused by syphilis, tuberculosis, or diphtheria. In the way of **treatment** the *prophylaxis* already outlined under Acute Rhinitis is to be carried out to prevent the recurrence of the acute attacks to which the chronic form may be a sequel. In the *treatment of the attack* foreign bodies, adenoids, and polypi should be removed if present, and any septal deviation or infection of the sinuses relieved. The nasal passages must be kept as free as possible of secretion, by the employment twice daily or oftener of douching or spraying (see p. 189) with some warm, alkaline antiseptic solution, such as liq. sod. borat. comp. (Dobell's solution) or a teaspoonful of bicarbonate of soda and ½ teaspoonful of salt to 8 oz. of water. This cleansing should be done cautiously without undue pressure, and may be followed by a spray of some gentle astringent, such as diluted fluid extract of hamamelis, a solution of sulphocarbolate of zinc (grains 2 to 5:oz. 1) (0.13 to 0.32:30), 0.5 per cent mercurochrome, or some of the silver preparations (p. 688); and then by a final spraying of liquid petrolatum. Sometimes good follows the application within the nostril of an ointment of calomel grain 1 (0.07) and petrolatum dr. 1 (3.9). *Constitutional treatment* is often even more important than local measures. It is frequently only after the general health has been improved by appropriate remedies or climatic change that relief of the local condition can be expected.

2. Hypertrophic Rhinitis

This disease is not common in children, and in early childhood is almost unknown. It is usually preceded by numerous attacks of acute rhinitis; is frequent in cold damp climates; may result from continued inhalation of dust; and is oftenest associated with chronic nasal obstruction, particularly from deviated septum. The chief **symptom** is persistent, more or less complete obstruction to respiration on one or both sides, varying from time to time, with which is associated nasal discharge which is mucopurulent but not abundant. The secretion is often chiefly postnasal and drops into the throat. Many secondary symptoms of stenosis arise, such as mouth-breathing, with constant irritation of the throat and pharyngeal cough; attacks of asthma or of croup; bronchitis; deafness; alteration of the voice; disturbance of sleep; nervousness; restlessness; headache; and mental backwardness. These symptoms are similar to those resulting from the presence of adenoids; which lesion, with enlargement of the faucial tonsils, is often combined with hypertrophic rhinitis. Examination of the nose shows the covering of the turbinated bones greatly thickened, pink in color, and very resistant to pressure. The accessory sinuses are little, if at all, involved. The **treatment** of the local condition and of the general health is similar to that for other forms of chronic rhinitis but with a greater employment of astringent applications, such as sulphocarbolate of zinc (grains 5:oz. 1) (0.32:30), or a combination of iodine (grains 5) (0.32), potassium iodide (grains 24) (1.56) and glycerin oz. 1 (30). The local treatment had better be in the hands of a rhinologist. It may be necessary to correct a deviated septum, remove polps and perhaps tonsils and adenoids, or cauterize or remove hypertrophied turbinates.

3. Atrophic Rhinitis
(Ozena)

In some cases this may be a sequel to simple long-continued purulent rhinitis, or succeed the hypertrophic form of the disease, or appear to be a primary process. It is rarely seen before later childhood and is more frequent in females. Such conditions as anemia and especially glandular tuberculosis exert a powerful causative influence, and that of heredity is sometimes observed. The chief **symptom** is the excessively offensive character of the nasal secretion. The patient's sense of smell is impaired. Rhinoscopic examination shows abnormally wide nasal passages, with atrophy of the mucous membrane and the presence of numerous crusts, with underlying ulceration. In advanced cases there is broadening of the nose, and the atrophy within spreads to the pharynx and nasopharynx. The disease lasts an indefinite time, with no tendency to spontaneous improvement. Mild cases may have further progress arrested by systematic, long-continued treatment, but atrophy which has developed cannot be cured. In the line of **diagnosis** syphilitic rhinitis is to be distinguished by the extent of the deep ulceration present, the absence or slight degree of atrophy of the mucous membrane, and the presence of syphilitic symptoms elsewhere. As regards **treatment,** *prophylaxis* is to be sought in the prompt and thorough treatment of a simple chronic or of a hypertrophic rhinitis, which might be the precursor. In the *direct treatment* of the atrophy already present the methods of cleansing recommended for other forms of rhinitis are to be employed. The atomization of peroxide of hydrogen diluted with three parts of water is serviceable in softening the crusts. If these are firmly attached forcible removal of them with cotton on an applicator will be necessary. This and, in fact, all local and operative treatment of the disease is best carried out by a rhinologist. Anemia and other evidences of impaired health must receive appropriate remedies. Polyglandular therapy, using thyroid, pituitary, epinephrine, and the like, has been recommended by Beck[28] on the ground that lowering of the basal metabolism has been found in some cases.

4. Syphilitic Rhinitis

This variety of chronic rhinitis has been considered to some extent in the chapter upon Syphilis (see pp. 431, 434). The principal early symptom is the chronic rhinitis producing the characteristic "snuffles." The nose is greatly obstructed, making respiration and feeding difficult, and there is an abundant serous or mucopurulent discharge, often slightly blood-tinged. The upper lip becomes excoriated and sometimes fissured. In the late form of the disease, apart from the deformities which may result, there is a free discharge of pus, often with a very offensive odor if destruction of the bone is going on. Obstruction to respiration may be produced by the pressure of gummata or by cicatrizing processes. In other cases the nasal passages are left unduly wide and the formation of crusts readily occurs. The **prognosis** is good in the early cases, so far as the nasal condition is concerned, and the disorder readily yields to antisyphilitic treatment. Some permanent alteration of the mucous membrane or even of the shape of the nose may perhaps be detected in later years. In advanced cases the destruction which has already taken place cannot be repaired. In the way of **diagnosis** the early cases are recognized by the continuance of the condition for a longer period than is usual in acute simple rhinitis, and by the presence of other evidences of inherited syphilis. Vincent's infection and that of diphtheria are to be thought of in differential diagnosis. Rhinitis occurring as a late symptom of syphilis can scarcely be confounded with any other affection in early life. The **treatment** consists in the usual cleansing methods suitable for simple chronic rhinitis and in antisyphilitic medication.

EPISTAXIS

Etiology.—Nose-bleed is a symptom of varied significance deserving separate consideration. It is rare in the new-born and in infancy, common in childhood, and decreases after puberty. In the new-born it is generally dependent upon syphilis. It is especially frequent in school-life, induced perhaps by overheated, dry rooms; faulty position of the body producing congestion; and the like. Coryza, coughing, or such traumata as blows upon and forcible blowing or picking of the nose may be exciting causes. Adenoids, or varicosities on the mucous membrane of the septum are frequent agents in producing recurrent attacks. Rhinitis is a common cause especially when due to syphilis, diphtheria or Vincent's infection. Foreign bodies in the nose, nasal polypi, mental excitement, the strain of physical exercise, or sometimes the mere bending over of the body, may be sufficient to occasion it. Various diseases are liable to produce it, prominent among these being affections of the heart, lungs or kidneys, resulting in passive congestion; and it may occur, too, in severe anemia of any form, leukemia, purpura, scorbutus, and hemophilia. Certain infectious disorders may also be accompanied by it, chief among these being typhoid fever, in which epistaxis is an early symptom. It is frequently brought on by the passive congestion attending the paroxysms of pertussis, and may occur also in the course of diphtheria, scarlet fever, measles, grippe, and malaria. Toward the development of puberty it is not infrequent in girls, and may then be viewed as vicarious menstruation. Previous to this time it is more common in boys.

Symptoms.—Usually the hemorrhage comes on without warning and flows slowly from one nostril. Exceptionally it may be in large amount especially in some constitutional diseases, and may even prove fatal. In some cases it occurs at night, the blood being swallowed and the diagnosis made only by the vomiting of blood or its passage in the stools, or by rhinoscopic examination. Generally an attack of epistaxis stops of itself in ten to twenty minutes or less, but not uncommonly it occurs every few days and produces a decided anemia.

Treatment.—Firm pressure against the jaw in the region just below the nose will often control the bleeding. Ice inserted into the nostril or applied to the bridge is of service, or placed on the nape of the neck may aid through the reflex contraction of the nasal vessels. Compressing the alae between the thumb and finger is also useful. The child should keep as still as possible, remain erect in a sitting position, have the clothing around the neck loosened, and refrain from blowing the nose. An excellent remedy is the introduction on cotton of a few drops of a solution of epinephrine (1:1000), perhaps with 2 per cent of cocaine added. Should none of these measures avail, it may be possible to detect the bleeding area and to touch it with a caustic of some sort. Packing the nares must be resorted to if this fails, but is seldom required. Internal medication may be tried in severe cases. For this purpose ergot, calcium lactate, or oil of erigeron, may be used. In obstinate cases the hypodermic injection of horse serum is often efficacious, giving 20 or more cc. (0.676 fl. oz.). Autocoagulants may stop the hemorrhage. Among these is fibrinogen, administered by mouth or hypodermically in doses of 1 to 2 cc. (0.034 to 0.068 fl. oz.), or thromboplastin may be used hypodermically. If these measures are of no avail, 10 to 20 cc. (0.338 to 0.676 fl. oz.) or more of human whole blood should be injected intramuscularly or intravenously.

In cases with a disposition to frequent epistaxis examination should be made for ulceration or varicose condition of the septum, and cauterization should be employed. Hygienic and other measures should be used to improve the general health and remove anemia. The clothing about the neck should be worn loose and the position of the child in sitting should be one which does not favor congestion of the nasal mucous membrane. It may be necessary to avoid the hot, dry air of the school-room, and to pass more time out of doors. Violent blowing of the nose must be forbidden.

MORBID GROWTHS OF THE NOSE

Nasal Polypi.—These growths are not common in children and are especially rare in infancy and early childhood. The most powerful predisposing factor is hypertrophic rhinitis, or other cause which produces persistent nasal stenosis with retention of secretion. The polypi are sessile or pedunculated; multiple; of color varying from gray to red; and either myxomatous or oftener fibromyxomatous in nature. They are situated especially upon the middle turbinate bone, and generally in both nostrils. They become larger in damp weather or when the patient has an attack of acute rhinitis. The **symptoms** consist of stenosis or complete obstruction of the nasal passages; mucous or mucopurulent discharge of moderate amount; and mouth-breathing and its natural results. Secondary symptoms are those common to obstruction. Among them are headache; dulness of hearing, taste and smell; reflex cough; sneezing; and asthmatic attacks. Rhinoscopic examination will reveal the presence of the growths. **Treatment** consists in removal of the growths, combined with attention to the chronic rhinitis or other obstruction.

Other Nasal Growths.—These are all rare in early life. Among those of a benign nature may be mentioned fibroma, papilloma, glioma, and chondroma. They occupy the nasopharynx and, if not removed, may grow to large size. Of malignant growths sarcoma is the form oftenest encountered, although unusual.

FOREIGN BODIES IN THE NOSE

The introduction of foreign bodies of various sorts into the nose is of common occurrence in early childhood. Among these are peas, beans, shoe-buttons, cherry-stones, beads, and the like. The object is situated at first well forward, but unskillful efforts of the patient or others to remove it often push it farther in. Frequently the child says nothing of the occurrence, either through fear or forgetfulness. The early symptoms are only obstruction to respiration, pain, and perhaps sneezing from the local irritation. If the object is smooth and hard and not of a nature to swell by absorption of liquid it may sometimes remain weeks or months without producing other symptoms. Generally, however, evidences of increasing irritation soon develop, with free purulent nasal discharge, swelling of the mucous membrane, and increased obstruction. Ulceration may later take place and the discharge become bloody and offensive. The fact that the affection is always unilateral strongly suggests the presence of a foreign body, and examination with a probe and speculum will generally reveal it. Removal is usually easy. Forcible blowing of the nose with the healthy nostril compressed is sometimes effective.

References

1. Arch. Pediat., 1931, **48,** 145. 2. J. Infect. Dis., 1913, **13,** 283; 1915, **16,** 493. 3. München. med. Wchnschr., 1914, **61,** 1547. 4. J. Infect. Dis., 1917, **21,** 451. 5. Medicine, 1930, **9,** 387. 6. J.A.M.A., 1930, **95,** 1553. 7. Proc. Soc. Exper. Biol. and Med., 1931, **28,** 513. 8. J. Exper. Med., 1931, **53,** 447. 9. J. Infect. Dis., 1923, **33,** 416. 10. J.A.M.A., 1926, **87,** 920. 11. Am. J. Hyg., 1929, **9,** 466. 12. J.A.M.A.,

1926, **87,** 1114. 13. Edinburgh M. J., 1904, **58,** 302. 14. Jahrb. f. Kinderh., 1915, **81,** 159. 15. Arch. Pediat., 1917, **34,** 520. 16. J.A.M.A., 1917, **69,** 895. 17. Am. J. Otol., Rhinol., and Laryngol., 1919, **28,** 452. 18. Jahrb. f. Kinderh., 1920, **93,** 313. 19. J. Laryngol., Rhinol. and Otol., 1921, **31,** 505. 20. Canad. M. A. J., 1923, **13,** 807. 21. Therap. Gaz., 1924, **48,** 1. 22. J.A.M.A., 1925, **85,** 317. 23. Am. J. Dis. Child., 1926, **32,** 40. 24. Am. J. Dis. Child., 1928, **36,** 1020. 25. Arch. intern. de laryngol., 1922, N. S. **1,** 1041. 26. J.A.M.A., 1930, **95,** 1002. 27. J.A.M.A., 1920, **74,** 1510. 28. Applied Path. in Dis. of Nose, Throat and Ear, 1923, 137.

CHAPTER III

DISEASES OF THE LARYNX

ACUTE LARYNGITIS

Any classification of laryngitis is to an extent arbitrary and to be used only as an aid to study. The disease may be divided into: (1) Catarrhal Laryngitis; (2) Spasmodic Laryngitis; (3) Subglottic Laryngitis; (4) Pseudomembranous Laryngitis.

1. Acute Catarrhal Laryngitis

The disease is seen perhaps oftener in later childhood than earlier. It may be secondary to various other diseases, such as rhinitis, pharyngitis, scarlet fever, grippe and especially measles, or be an exacerbation of a more chronic condition; or it may be primary, brought on by exposure to chilling or other defective hygienic conditions, as in acute rhinitis; or by the irritation of the larynx by excessive crying or shouting, or the inhaling of irritating substances, such as coal-gas, dust, steam, and the like. The chief **symptoms** are hoarseness of the voice and a dry, hoarse, and, later, loose cough without the peculiar barking character of croup. In the lighter cases the general condition is usually unaffected, the appetite good, and there is little or no fever. The hoarseness may vary in degree up to complete aphonia in severe cases. There is no dyspnea. Rhinitis nearly always occurs in conjunction with or antedates the laryngitis, and involvement of the trachea is frequent. The **course** is usually short, equaling from three to eight days, the cough growing gradually looser and the hoarseness lessening. The **prognosis** of the disease itself is entirely good, but such complications as pneumonia or bronchitis may develop, or the disorder may be a precursor of the more severe form of laryngitis to be described (subglottic laryngitis).

Treatment.—The same general methods of treatment are indicated as in acute rhinitis. The most important is rest of the larynx, and talking should be avoided. The child should be kept in a room well ventilated but rather warmer than usual, preferably with the air moistened with water-vapor. (See p. 187.) If there is any fever, a purgative and a hot bath should be given, the patient kept in bed and salicylates perhaps administered. The continued application of warm or cold compresses over the larynx is useful in many cases. In other instances counter-irritation over the larynx may be employed, using weak mustard-plasters, camphorated oil, soap-liniment, etc. If cough is troublesome sedatives may be required.

2. Spasmodic Laryngitis

(False Croup; Spasmodic Croup; Stridulous Laryngitis)

In this disease there is sometimes great spasm and little or no catarrhal inflammation, or in other cases chiefly the latter with only slight tendency to croup. Thus catarrhal and spasmodic laryngitis shade into each other by many gradations. The same causes operate as in simple catarrhal laryngitis. In addition are seen certain other etiologic factors. Croup is especially frequent between the ages of two and four years. There is a decided individual and family predisposition, some children showing a great proneness to recurrences on very slight causes, and may continue to do so even through later childhood. Rachitis, adenoids, and a neurotic disposition are among the predisposing causes. In some cases the attacks appear to be produced by acute indigestion. The **symptoms** of the attack are often preceded by some hours of moderate coryza and hoarseness, the latter perhaps coming on only in the late afternoon; or the child may have been put to bed apparently entirely well. In still other cases there had been decided laryngitis with fever and a somewhat croupy cough. Then, usually early in the night, either after gradually increasing slight dyspnea and some cough or quite suddenly, the child wakens with a characteristic barking, metallic cough and noisy stenotic inspiration. It sits up in bed struggling for breath and evidently frightened, and often grasps at the throat where the feeling of oppression and impending suffocation is located. The face is congested and has an anxious expression; the lips and extremities are cyanotic; the nasal alae and the accessory muscles of respiration move with each noisy, stridulous inspiration. The voice is hoarse, the pulse accelerated, the skin perspiring; there is moderate or no elevation of temperature and more or less prostration. The dyspnea increases with any excitement or without discoverable reason. After several hours, or a much shorter time, the severity of the spasm and the other symptoms diminish. By the following morning no evidence of stenosis is present and perhaps only slight hoarseness and loose cough; or the child seems quite well. Occasionally a second attack occurs later in the night.

This is the description of the condition as seen in severe cases. In the milder ones there may be a croupy cough and a moderate degree of stenosis and dyspnea, perhaps sufficient to arouse the child. In well-developed cases, another attack is liable to occur upon the next night unless prevented by treatment, and still another may take place upon the third night, or even rarely upon later ones. These later seizures are usually less severe, and in the milder cases an attack occurs generally upon one night only. During the daytime the child is apparently in perfect health or has perhaps slight hoarseness and a loose cough, which may persist for several days. The **prognosis** is good and recovery may be expected in practically every uncomplicated case. The **diagnosis** from *diphtheritic laryngitis* is made by the very abrupt onset, the short duration of the paroxysms, the usual prompt relief under treatment, the cessation of symptoms during the day, the absence of constitutional involvement, and the history of former occurrences of spasmodic croup. It is only when one is called at the height of the first attack that the diagnosis between the two diseases is uncertain. In true croup (diphtheritic laryngitis) the onset is gradual, the hoarseness and stenosis slowly becoming worse; there are more constantly fever and decided depression of strength, and the cough is not so barking. Most instances of diphtheritic croup are accompanied by evidence of diphtheria in the pharynx or nose. If a membrane is seen by direct laryngoscopic examination, diphtheria should be diagnosed. Of 344 patients suffering from croup who were admitted to the Willard Parker Hospital, 126 had catarrhal laryngitis (Tolle[1]). *Laryngismus stridulus* exhibits no fever whatever and no hoarseness or cough. The attacks are of momentary duration and are repeated many times during the daytime. Moreover, this is a spasmophilic disorder confined almost entirely to infancy, and is often associated with symptoms of rickets or of tetany. The diagnosis from *subglottic laryngitis* will be considered under that heading.

Treatment.—**Prophylactic** treatment should be given when a child known to be subject to attacks of spasmodic croup develops hoarseness or a suspicious cough during the daytime. For this purpose a combination of ipecac and opium may be given, using enough of the former to bring the patient to the verge of vomiting, and enough of the latter to cause a moderate drowsiness. The addition of sodium bromide or of antipyrine is often of service. The child should be kept in a warm room with the air slightly moist for several days until all threatening symptoms are gone. To prevent attacks of croup in the future all the hygienic measures should be adopted which have been outlined for the prophylactic treatment of rhinitis, such as outdoor life and sleeping in airy rooms, as well as cold sponging of the region of the neck or general cool baths. All possible determining causes, as rhinitis, adenoids and the like, must be sought for and removed, not forgetting the frequent influence of acute indigestion.

For the **treatment of the attack** relaxation of spasm should be sought by giving an emetic of a teaspoonful of syrup or wine of ipecac and putting the patient into a warm bath. If emesis does not occur in twenty minutes the dose may be repeated. Warm or cold compresses to the neck are also often of service. An additional useful remedy to insure relief for the balance of the night is the surrounding of the child with water-vapor, often best applied in a croup-tent. (See p. 188.) Sedatives may also be given. Many physicians administer preparations of calcium. In very urgent cases a slight inhalation of chloroform may be employed. It is rarely if ever that intubation is necessary in undoubted cases of spasmodic laryngitis.

3. Acute Subglottic Laryngitis

(Severe Laryngitis; Severe Form of Spasmodic Laryngitis; Inflammatory Edema of the Glottis; Submucous Laryngitis)

This variety of acute laryngitis occurs much less frequently than those already described. It is observed chiefly in infancy and early childhood, and is usually secondary to a catarrhal laryngitis or to some infectious disease, especially measles and grippe, although occasionally it appears to be primary.

Symptoms.—Evidences of acute rhinitis or of mild catarrhal laryngitis may be present for several days, or the attack may start with vigor almost from the beginning, or may be consecutive to an attack of croup. In well-marked cases there is fever up to 103 or 104 F. (39.4 or 40 C.), loss of appetite, thirst, prostration, rapid pulse, hoarseness, and a persistent, painful, hoarse, croupy cough. There are tenderness and pain in the larynx and a constant annoying tickling sensation there. The dyspnea in some instances is moderate, in others extreme with all the attendant symptoms of suffocation. It may be paroxysmal to a certain extent, but with only partial relief between times, or gradually increase from the beginning. Unlike spasmodic laryngitis, the stenosis is present in the daytime, although usually worse at night. There is practically always an accompanying tracheitis, and not infrequently bronchitis or pneumonia develops. Laryngoscopic examination reveals a marked degree of redness and swelling of the mucous membrane of all parts of the larynx, but the most characteristic feature is the swollen, deep-red subglottic mucous membrane, projecting beneath the vocal cords and being the cause of the stenosis.

The **prognosis** is on the whole favorable, but in individual cases is often doubtful, and especially so when the disease accompanies infectious disorders. Severe symptoms may last for two or three days, or even occasionally a week or more, before decided improvement begins. In other cases the stenosis persists and the child dies in a few days from obstruction to the respiration, or later from a complicating pneumonia. In one unusual case under our observation, which seemed to belong more to this affection than any other, symptoms lasted for two and one-half months, during a portion of which the wearing of an intubation tube was necessary.

Diagnosis.—The disease is distinguished from *spasmodic laryngitis* by the persistence of the stenosis to some extent during the daytime, the greater duration of the whole attack, the more decided elevation of temperature, and the general constitutional disturbance. Occasionally pressure by an enlarged *thymus* gland may produce a stenosis which bears a superficial resemblance to that of subglottic laryngitis. The slower onset of the thymic affection, the more protracted course, the absence of fever and particularly of hoarseness, and the roentgenological examination will usually exclude laryngeal involvement. The differentiation from *diphtheritic laryngitis* is the most difficult unless evidences of diphtheria of the nose or pharynx are discoverable. In subglottic laryngitis there is a greater tendency to paroxysmal increase of stenosis, and less often the steady augmentation of the dyspnea from a gradual beginning, as seen in diphtheria. Inspiration is more affected than expiration. The condition is usually worse during the night-time and the fever is often higher than in diphtheria. To all this there are, however, so many exceptions, and the symptoms may be so like those of diphtheria, that diagnosis may be impossible except by bacteriological and laryngoscopic examination. Even a negative bacteriological finding is not an absolute proof, although a very probable one.

Treatment.—Prompt treatment should be employed to abate the laryngeal inflammation. A purgative should be given if the case is seen early, and a warm bath be followed by putting the child to bed in blankets in the attempt to induce free perspiration. The repetition of warm baths or warm packs during the attack often gives great relief to the dyspnea, as may hot, wet compresses over the larynx. Internally the administration of ipecac and opium is useful as in spasmodic laryngitis; combined often with citrate of potash and tincture of aconite root. Antipyrine and the bromides may also be of value if the element of spasm is decided. Of all remedies the inhalation of water-vapor (p. 188) is the most useful. The child should be kept in a croup-tent for twenty minutes at a time, and the treatment repeated every hour or less often according to the requirements and the effect produced. Benzoin, menthol, or turpentine may be added to the water. Too long continuance in the tent at one time is sometimes exhausting, and there is also often an insufficient supply of fresh air. Inhalation of oxygen may be combined with the treatment. When the child is out of the tent the air of the room should be kept as moist as possible by water-vapor medicated or otherwise. In the severest instances intubation may be required, even though the disease has been proven not to be diphtheria. Inasmuch as the diagnosis is so often doubtful, the administration of diphtheria-antitoxin should be employed in all suspicious cases.

4. Pseudomembranous Laryngitis

While usually diphtheritic in nature, yet cases of membranous laryngitis are reported in which no evidence of diphtheria could be found. Such a condition may be a primary affection of the larynx, or secondary to some of the infectious fevers, or be produced by irritating vapors or liquids. The streptococcus, pneumococcus, influenza bacillus or other germ may be discovered in the pseudomembrane in place of the diphtheria bacillus. The symptoms do not differ from those of diphtheritic laryngitis, as described elsewhere, and every case of pseudomembranous laryngitis must be considered diphtheritic until proven not to be such.

CHRONIC LARYNGITIS

This disorder is a comparatively uncommon one in early life. It may be a sequel to acute laryngitis; may be primary; may remain a symptom for some weeks after such affections as measles; or may attend a chronic pharyngitis or rhinitis, or adenoid hypertrophy. Hereditary syphilis may be a cause in infancy, and much more rarely in childhood. Tuberculosis is an unusual cause of chronic laryngitis in early life, especially in infancy and early childhood, although reported by Barthez and Sanné,[3] Rheindorff,[4] Heubner,[5] and Demme.[6] The chief **symptom** is a chronic hoarseness, perhaps with a severe laryngeal cough. In tuberculous cases there may be mucopurulent expectoration, together with blood and containing tubercle bacilli. In syphilitic laryngitis, in addition to the hoarseness and cough, some degree of stenosis or even severe suffocative attacks may occasionally be present. The **prognosis** of chronic syphilitic laryngitis is to an extent unfavorable through the possibility of fatal stenosis occurring, and on account of the advanced condition of ulceration and cicatrization which may be present before treatment is commenced. If treatment is begun early, recovery may eventually take place. This is certainly true of the catarrhal laryngitis which occurs as an early manifestation of hereditary syphilis, but the late forms are very resistant. Tuberculous ulceration of the larynx is generally overshadowed by advanced pulmonary disease to which death will probably be due. Simple chronic catarrhal laryngitis will usually disappear under treatment. The **diagnosis** between tuberculous and syphilitic ulceration is not easy by laryngoscopic examination. The symptoms of one or the other of the two disorders elsewhere in the body serve to differentiate. With neither of these diseases present, the recognition of chronic laryngitis and its differentiation from the hoarseness due to papillomata or other cause is to be made by the laryngoscope. **Treatment** should be directed especially against the primary cause. Such procedures as spraying, inhalations or counterirritation are seldom necessary and often inefficacious. The cure of the pharyngitis or the rhinitis, the removal of adenoids, or the instituting of hygienic measures to prevent repeated attacks of acute laryngitis will usually suffice. Syphilitic laryngitis is to be treated by specific medication. If stenosis occurs intubation is indicated.

PERICHONDRITIS OF THE LARYNX

Etiology.—This disease is uncommon at any time of life, although a case is reported by Blechmann and Peignaux[7] occurring as early as the age of three weeks. It depends oftenest upon the acute infectious diseases, but is also caused by syphilis, tuberculosis, and sepsis, and may be the result of injury by intubation or trauma of other nature. The inflammation attacks any portion of the larynx, but oftenest the cricoid and arytenoid cartilages, and may advance to the production of abscess (*suppurative perichondritis*). The seat of the abscess, however, may sometimes be in the areolar tissue rather than in the cartilage. In other cases the process is necrotic in nature and in still others productive of connective tissue. The **symptoms** consist of pain and tenderness in the laryngeal region, dysphagia, hoarseness, stridulous cough, and sometimes dyspnea. The temperature is usually high, but if the condition complicates one of the acute infectious fevers this symptom is equivocal. If an abscess forms and points within the larynx entire obstruction results unless relief is given. If it points externally it is readily recognized by inspection and palpation. The **course** will be rapid if the condition is an acute pyogenic process; otherwise it may be slow, especially if no abscess develops. It is chronic in tuberculosis and syphilis. The **prognosis** is always serious on account of the danger of suffocation from obstruction by an abscess or by acute edema, abscess within the larynx being oftenest dependent upon a suppurative perichondritis. In other cases deformity of the larynx from cicatricial processes is liable to remain, with permanent alteration of voice or interference with respiration. The prognosis is best in syphilis, since the course is slower and the disease often more amenable to treatment. In **treatment** local applications are indicated to reduce the swelling, such as ice-bags to the neck, leeching, and the like. Any abscess developing must be opened. In cases depending upon syphilis energetic constitutional treatment is required. Tracheotomy or intubation may be necessary to avoid suffocation.

EDEMA OF THE GLOTTIS

Under this heading are frequently included two distinct forms. The *serous*, uncommon in early life, depends upon constitutional causes, especially acute or chronic nephritis. It may also be caused by diseases of the heart; pressure by tumors, or any other condition which interferes with the circulation in the larynx; angioneurotic edema; or the ingestion of potassium iodide. *Inflammatory* edema, allied to subglottic edema, is secondary to catarrhal or ulcerating inflammation of the larynx or of neighboring parts. Among the **causes** are erysipelas or abscess in the neck, retropharyngeal abscess, and the trauma produced by foreign bodies or by the entrance into the larynx of steam or other irritating or corrosive substance. The **symptoms** are much the same in each variety. There occurs a more or less sudden inspiratory laryngeal dyspnea with the general characteristics already described in considering spasmodic laryngitis. A sudden suffocative attack may be the earliest manifestation of a general edematous condition of the body about to occur in chronic nephritis. There is no fever in the serous form unless dependent upon the primary disease. In the inflammatory variety there are pain and swelling, tenderness on pressure, high fever, cough, hoarseness, often difficulty in swallowing, enlargement of the cervical lymph-nodes and severe constitutional symptoms. Apart from the danger of death in a few hours, especially present in the serous variety, the **course and prognosis** depend upon the nature of the cause of the edema. The majority of cases recover, but the prognosis is always doubtful. The **diagnosis** can usually be made by exploration with the finger or the laryngoscope, the great swelling of the laryngeal tissue being characteristic of the disease. Even mere depression of the tongue may reveal this condition. The serous form exhibits but slight redness. The differentiation of the inflammatory form from diphtheria is not always easy. However, in this latter disease there are usually a slower onset and evidences of diphtheritic membrane in the nose or pharynx. In edema depending upon nephritis energetic **treatment** must be employed to promote diaphoresis and diuresis. (See p. 826.) In inflammatory cases localized antiphlogistic measures are required, such as leeching of the neck, the application of ice over the larynx, and the like. Purgatives may also be employed, remembering, however, that the strength is already often much depleted. Scarification of the larynx is recommended. If suffocation is impending tracheotomy must be done, intubation often being difficult on account of the swelling, and also dangerous from the trauma produced.

MORBID GROWTHS OF THE LARYNX

Malignant growths of the larynx are very uncommon in early life. Occasionally as a result of chronic laryngitis small fibromatous nodules of a benign nature develop on the vocal cords and produce a roughening of the voice. Small granulomata may follow intubation and tracheotomy, and angiomata may rarely be found. The most common morbid growth of the larynx is the papilloma.

Papilloma of the Larynx.—This may be congenital, or be the result of repeated laryngitis. It may occur at any period in childhood, but oftenest between three and four years of age, and in boys. The growths are usually multiple, may vary in size, are whitish in color, may be sessile or have a peduncle, and may occupy any part of the larynx, but usually are attached to the vocal cords. The **symptoms** are chiefly hoarseness or even loss of voice, and a proxysmal cough with more or less stenosis and dyspnea if the tumors reach a considerable size, or if a catarrhal condition is present. The growth is usually slow. Sometimes the neoplasms retrograde of themselves, in other cases they require removal. Recurrence is very liable to take place. Sudden death from suffocation may occur. The **diagnosis** is to be made only by laryngoscopic examination, which serves to distinguish the condition from chronic laryngitis of any form. The **treatment** should be entirely in the hands of a specialist. It is a disputed question whether the growths should be removed, or be let alone and tracheotomy be performed if the symptoms are threatening, since after rest of the larynx is obtained in this way for a number of months the tumors may disappear of themselves.

FOREIGN BODIES IN THE LARYNX

The penetration of foreign bodies into the larynx is not uncommon in early life, about ⅔ of the cases of the presence of such bodies in the air-passages occurring in children (Graham).[8] They generally consist of the small objects which children are liable to put into the mouth, as well as of articles of food which are being masticated. Fortunately the rapid closure by the epiglottis of the opening into the larynx renders the accident far less frequent than it would otherwise be. It is especially liable to occur during the sudden, deep inspiration attending crying, coughing, sneezing, or laughing, and it may follow operative procedures, as, for instance, the discharge of pus after the opening of a retropharyngeal abscess, or the dropping into the larynx of an excised tonsil. Exceptionally bodies may enter the larynx from other regions than the mouth, as in the cases where ascarides have made their way into it. The chief **symptom** is a sudden attack of suffocation, with violent laryngeal cough. In the majority of instances the foreign substance is immediately driven out by the cough, although the sense of irritation may not disappear so promptly. If the object is of sufficient size and is not at once expelled, death may immediately follow from suffocation. If this accident does not happen and the object is not displaced, paroxysmal cough persists, and there are suffocative attacks, bloody expectoration, hoarseness, pain, and other evidences of severe acute laryngitis. If the object is small and smooth the acute symptoms may subside and only hoarseness and moderate paroxysmal cough remain, but at any time an acute fatal attack of suffocation may occur through closing of the glottis by the foreign body, aided by the swelling of the mucous membrane which has taken place. Should the body remain sufficiently long in the larynx ulceration is liable to follow, perhaps with hemorrhage as a result of erosion of vessels. The **prognosis** is uncertain, and is in accord with the character, size and position of the object. Ultimate recovery depends upon the possibility of the removal of the body. After its long presence with ulceration, cicatrices develop which may cause persistent stenosis to a greater or less degree. In many cases the object passes from the larynx into a bronchus and occasions pneumonia or abscess. The **diagnosis** is usually easy. The suddenness and severity of the attack and the absence of fever are characteristic. The laryngoscope may sometimes be of service, or even digital examination may disclose the body. Roentgenography may aid in locating it. **Treatment** at the onset consists in inverting the child in the hope of aiding cough to expel the body. If suffocation is impending the only procedure is immediate tracheotomy. Should the case not be so urgent and the object be still present surgical aid in the removal must be sought at once.

CONGENITAL LARYNGEAL STRIDOR

Although described earlier this condition was first brought prominently into attention by Lees.[9]

Etiology and Pathology.—It occurs in the new-born or in early infancy. The theory of Lees and others, based upon postmortem examinations, is that there exists a congenital alteration of the shape of the larynx, perhaps due to a degree of atony, in which the edges of the epiglottis as well as the aryepiglottic ligaments approach each other too closely, leaving only a rhomboidal or slit-like fissure at the entrance of the glottis, with consequent obstruction to inspiration. Thomson[10] attributed this to a spasmodic incoördination of the respiratory muscles of the nature of a neurosis. The deformity which is observed was shown by Thomson and Turner[11] to be a secondary matter, the result of a functional disturbance acting upon the normal soft, collapsible tissue of the infant's larynx. It would appear, however, that a number of different causes are operative in producing cases which have been included in this category, and that the condition may not be an entity. Hochsinger[12] claimed to have demonstrated by roentgenograms that enlargement of the thymus gland can produce the symptoms, and this has been supported by others. However, Weill-Halle and Dreyfus-See[13] performed thymectomy without sufficient improvement following to permit assigning the symptoms to this cause. Brecely[14] has seen the symptom attend pseudodiphtheritic involvement of the palate; Shukowsky[15] observed it with cleft palate; Meyers[16] found it in a case caused by pressure from an anomalously placed left pulmonary artery; we have observed the condition due to a cyst at the base of the tongue, and similar instances are reported by Thomas[17] and others. Bagg[18] reports 7 cases with the symptom-complex, but with a varying assortment of pathologic conditions. Wernstedt[19] observed an instance of the disease in which at necropsy nothing abnormal was discovered, and he suggests that at least in some instances the disorder may be purely a functional laryngological disorder, thus agreeing with Thomson and Turner. We likewise have seen an instance with normal larynx at necropsy, but in which during life laryngoscopic examination revealed the collapsible condition of which Thomson and Turner wrote.

There seems to be no doubt that there does occur a congenital stridor in which deformity of the larynx is present, at least during life; and it might be better to limit the term "congenital laryngeal stridor" to such cases; the broader term "respiratory stridor" including these and all others.

Symptoms.—These appear at birth or within a few weeks and consist chiefly of noisy inspiration which varies in intensity from time to time and is made worse by excitement. It is more or less continuous, is always less when the respiration is quiet, and there are times in the milder cases when it is temporarily absent. It may entirely or nearly disappear during sleep. The sound does not resemble that of spasmodic croup, but suggests, according to Thomson, the crowing sound made by a hen. Expiration is generally entirely quiet and there is no urgent dyspnea, although some sinking in of the episternal fossa, intercostal spaces, and epigastrium is present. There is, as a rule, no cyanosis, the voice is unaffected, and cough is uncharacteristic, if present. The general health of the infant is usually good. In rare severe cases attacks of asphyxia may occur.

Course and Prognosis.—The prognosis is usually favorable in cases without definite discoverable cause, or when an evident cause is removed. The symptoms persist or even increase in severity for several months, but gradually disappear entirely between the ages of one and two years. Occasionally, however, death may occur, but this is rare and generally from some complication, especially from respiratory infections, or perhaps from asphyxia.

Diagnosis.—All intratracheal and extratracheal causes of obstruction and pressure must be sought for. The discovery of an enlarged thymus does not necessarily prove that this is causative of stridor. The absence of cyanosis is said to be characteristic, but we have seen one very persistent case, where the cyanosis was decided, but in which the symptoms finally disappeared completely. Croup is a disease of later infancy or childhood, and is sudden in onset and of short duration. Papilloma of the larynx produces hoarseness, and develops at a later period of life. Adenoid growths occurring in very early infancy may give rise to diagnostic difficulty. The noisy breathing in this condition is, however, worse during sleep, and there is evident interference with nasal respiration present.

In view of the usual favorable prognosis **treatment** is scarcely required, other than the effort to overcome any malnutrition present or to remove a cause of pressure or obstruction. If the thymus is enlarged radiologic treatment of it may be tried. Iglauer[20] removed the epiglottis in one instance.

STENOSIS OF THE LARYNX

In the broader sense this constitutes a narrowing of the larynx from any cause, and the number of such causes is considerable. Of those acting within the larynx itself may be mentioned pseudomembranous laryngitis; edema of the glottis; subglottic laryngitis; foreign bodies in the larynx; the alteration in shape seen in congenital laryngeal stridor; very rarely malformations of the larynx of other sorts; syphilitic or tuberculous ulceration; abscess; and spasm of any kind, as in spasmodic croup and laryngospasm, and the rare cases of spasm from other causes, as in some cases of apnea from spasm of the larynx occurring in the new-born. Rarely there may be found a congenitally imperforate larynx, as in the case reported by Sieg.[21] New[22] records a case of congenital angioma of the larynx. Produced by causes acting outside of the larynx, stenosis may follow pressure by enlargement of the thyroid gland; abscess; enlarged lymphatic glands, and tumors.

The **symptoms** consist briefly of inspiratory dyspnea, with the energetic action of the respiratory muscles naturally resulting; cyanosis; and in some cases suffocation. It is to be distinguished from tracheal stenosis by the altered voice and the characteristic cough often present. The treatment depends upon the etiological factors operating.

References

1. Am. J. Dis. Child., 1930, **39,** 954. 2. Griffith, Arch. Pediat., 1902, **19,** 183. 3. Mal. d. enf., 1891, **3,** 1048; 1053. 4. Jahrb. f. Kinderh., 1892, **33,** 71. 5. Lehrb. d. Kinderh., 1911, **2,** 245. 6. 20. Bericht ü. d. Thätigk. d. Jenner'schen Kindersp. in Bern., 1882; Ref. No. 4. 7. Nourrisson, 1922, **10,** 187. 8. Am. J. Dis. Child., 1920, **19,** 119. 9. Trans. Path. Soc. of London, 1883, **34,** 19. 10. Edinburgh M. J., 1892, **38,** Pt. 1. 205. 11. Brit. M. J., 1900, **2,** 1561. 12. Wien. med. Wchnschr., 1903, **53,** 2106. 13. Bull. de la soc. de pédiat., 1926, **24,** 15. 14. Jahrb. f. Kinderh., 1904, **59,** 54. 15. Jahrb. f. Kinderh., 1911, **73,** 459. 16. Nederland. Tijdschr. v. Geneesk., 1928, **72,** 1.B., 2800. 17. Ztschr. f. Kinderh., 1929, **47,** 168. 18. Monatschr. f. Kinderh., 1929, **45,** 102.

19. Nord. Med. Ark., 1914, **2,** H 1–4, No. 22. 20. Laryngoscope, 1922, **32,** 56. 21. J.A.M.A., 1922, **78,** 628. 22. J.A.M.A., 1923, **81,** 63.

CHAPTER IV

DISEASES OF THE TRACHEA, BRONCHI AND LUNGS

FOREIGN BODIES IN THE TRACHEA AND BRONCHI

A FOREIGN body entering the larynx (see p. 700) may either be expelled immediately, remain impacted, or pass into the trachea or into one of the bronchi. Approximately three out of four foreign bodies in the bronchi are situated upon the right side.

Symptoms.—A foreign body in the trachea may promptly cause death if of sufficient size to interfere seriously with respiration. If smaller it may remain in position indefinitely, producing more or less stenotic dyspnea, possibly a characteristic sound on auscultation caused by the slight moving up and down of the body, and attacks of violent coughing during one of which the object may perhaps be driven upward against the glottis and cause suffocation, or even through it into the mouth and thus be gotten rid of. If the body is immovable there are no paroxysmal suffocative attacks. Ulceration may occur and produce sanguino-purulent expectoration and finally cicatricial contraction with increasing stenosis.

If the object enters a large bronchus the lung supplied by it soon collapses if the obstruction is complete. There are cyanosis and great dyspnea, with violent attacks of coughing, and with pain in the chest. The physical signs consist in the absence of breath-sounds over the whole lung, or a large portion of it, although early in the condition the percussion resonance is unimpaired. Later there is perhaps dulness, or hyperresonance from emphysema of the neighboring pulmonary tissue, and still later tympany from the production of an abscess-cavity. Râles may be present in the opposite lung. In partial obstruction there is likewise dyspnea, and auscultation may perhaps give a loud whistling respiratory murmur on the affected side with feeble respiration, and there is somewhat diminished vocal fremitus with normal percussion-sounds. Yet even in partial obstruction the fremitus may be absent, due to the filling of the lung with secretion, the so-called "drowned lung." A wheezing sound may be heard when the stethoscope is placed over the patient's mouth (Jackson[1]). If the obstruction is limited particularly to expiration the lungs instead of collapsing become over-distended. Small bodies, after the initial suffocative and spasmodic symptoms, may cause no signs until after a latent period of several weeks or months. The symptoms produced by foreign bodies may vary with their nature. Exceedingly fine râles (tissue-paper râles) may be heard at times over the position where a metallic body is lodged (McCrae[2]). Diffuse purulent bronchitis with excessive secretion of mucus occurs especially after the aspiration of such objects as peanut-kernels (arachidic bronchitis) (Jackson and Spencer[3]). Inhalation of infant-powders, particularly of zinc stearate, may produce almost complete asphyxia with early death, or a bronchopneumonia may follow. (See p. 718.) The entrance of oils and fats into the lungs leads to an infectious pneumonic process (Pinkerton[4]). Additional valuable contributions to the subject of foreign bodies in the air-passages have been made by Jackson;[5] Jackson, Spencer and Manges,[6] Rowland,[7] and others.

Course and Prognosis.—Escaping immediate suffocation, there is always the danger that this will occur in some attack of coughing and dyspnea, if the object is loose in the trachea. Later, if the body is in a bronchus, ulceration takes place, and there is great danger of the development of symptoms of recurrent or chronic bronchopneumonia, or those of bronchiectasis or pulmonary abscess. Sometimes bronchopneumonia develops in a day or two after the entrance of the body and rapidly advances to a fatal septic condition. Yet a patient may live for months with abscess or bronchiectasis due to a foreign body in a bronchus, and in fortunate cases the object be finally ejected and recovery take place. The general outcome is, however, unfavorable unless the object can be removed.

Diagnosis.—Without the knowledge that a foreign body has entered the respiratory tract diagnosis is difficult, especially in cases where the symptoms develop late. Among the most suggestive symptoms are the sudden onset, the later recurrence of dyspnea and violent paroxysmal cough, and the absence of breath-sounds on one side if a bronchus is involved. Roentgenograms and the fluoroscope may give conclusive evidence, even when the foreign body is nonopaque to the ray. Thus, in an early stage, there may be depression of the diaphragm, transparency on the affected side from obstructive emphysema and displacement of the mediastinum to the unaffected side. If complete obstruction develops there is the picture of collapse of the lung (p. 746). The bronchoscope also should settle the diagnosis in some cases. Later in the course the development of an abscess, or a chronically recurring bronchopneumonia especially in the right lower lobe, is a suspicious indication of a foreign body.

Treatment.—The inversion of the patient combined with striking him upon the back is a dangerous procedure if an object has passed below the larynx, lest it be thus made to obstruct the glottis from below. Tracheotomy should be first performed or all preparations for it made. The employment of the bronchoscope, as brought into prominence by Jackson,[8] has rendered the removal of foreign bodies more readily possible than was formerly the case.

STENOSIS OF THE TRACHEA AND LARGER BRONCHI

This is a result of various **causes,** and may even rarely be congenital. Of the conditions situated within the tube the most frequent is diphtheritic inflammation. Fibrinous bronchitis (p. 710) and foreign bodies also may produce it. In the walls of the tube itself are to be enumerated strictures of various sorts, such as those depending upon cicatricial growths after tracheotomy, or resulting from syphilitic or other ulceration. Compression of the trachea or bronchus from without may be caused by an enlarged thymus (p. 1076), hypertrophied bronchial and mediastinal glands, mediastinal tumors, an enlarged thyroid gland, and retro-esophageal or other abscess in the neck or within the thorax. The **symptoms** may develop suddenly or slowly, according to the nature of the acting agent. They consist in dyspnea especially during inspiration, which is often attended by a peculiar characteristic noisy whistling sound; often more or less cyanosis; and vigorous action of the respiratory muscles. Cough is not infrequent. It is dry, barking and somewhat paroxysmal. When a bronchus is involved the physical signs are those described under Foreign Bodies in the Bronchi (p. 703). In tracheal stenosis the respiration is usually more noisy than when a bronchus is involved, and there is no difference between the physical signs of the two lungs. Prognosis and treatment depend entirely upon the nature of the cause.

MALFORMATIONS OF THE TRACHEA

Tracheal **fistula** has already been described under Diseases of the Esophagus (p. 547). Very rarely an opening may form from the trachea into the esophagus as the result of trauma with subsequent ulceration. **Tracheocele** is an unusual condition in childhood, although it has been observed at birth. It consists in a hernial opening in the trachea, oftenest situated posteriorly. Upon laughing or straining, a tumor-like swelling of the neck develops, which is tympanitic on percussion, shows bronchial respiration and voice-sounds on auscultation, and an impulse on coughing. The subject has been reviewed by Orgel.[9] The tumor is to be distinguished from pneumatocele, emphysema of the neck, and transitory congestive enlargement of the thyroid gland.

ACUTE BRONCHITIS

(Acute Tracheobronchitis)

Tracheitis seldom occurs alone, but is generally combined with laryngitis and inflammation of the bronchi. It will be grouped with bronchitis for consideration.

Etiology.—The disease is exceedingly frequent and may be either primary or secondary. Among the causes of the secondary form are the infectious diseases, as measles, typhoid fever, pertussis, grippe, rubella, diphtheria and scarlet fever. Bronchitis is also a common attendant on or sequel to laryngitis, rhinitis, pharyngitis, pneumonia, pleurisy, rickets, the exudative diathesis, malnutrition, cardiac disease, and passive congestion of the lungs. Primary acute bronchitis is usually the result of chilling brought about by the various causes mentioned under Rhinitis (p. 685). Early age is a powerful predisposing factor. In the first three years of life, except the first six months, it is a very common affection; but after this period it decreases steadily in frequency. The agency of micro-organisms such as the pneumococcus, streptococcus, micrococcus catarrhalis, influenza-bacillus, and the staphylococcus is positive, but their exact action uncertain. The relationship between these and other causes is probably similar to that suggested for rhinitis (p. 685). Family and institutional outbreaks of bronchitis are not infrequently seen, and it seems probable that the virulence of the germs may be sufficient to produce the disease without the operation of any other factor.

Pathologic Anatomy.—The process affects the bronchi of both lungs, although not uniformly. A localized bronchitis is generally secondary to some other pulmonary lesion. In older children the trachea and larger bronchi are involved, except in the severer cases where the middle-sized bronchi share in the process. In young infants there is a greater tendency to inflammation of the smaller and even the smallest bronchioles. The term "capillary bronchitis" is best avoided; this process always being accompanied by inflammation around the bronchioles, and being in fact a bronchopneumonia.

Symptoms.—The symptoms vary greatly in intensity. In the *mild form* the onset may be either acute or quite gradual, and is very commonly preceded by the symptoms of rhinitis, pharyngitis, or laryngitis. Cough begins or, if already present and laryngeal in character, becomes frequent, sometimes paroxysmal, and dry. It is often more distressing at night and is frequently excessively annoying soon after the child is put to bed. Older children often complain of a sense of soreness or discomfort in the chest. Constitutional involvement of any sort is absent or slight; and there is little or no elevation of temperature in older children, and only moderate fever in infants. In from one to two days, as secretion becomes established, the cough grows looser and less racking, and in children over six or seven years of age expectoration begins. This is at first of transparent or whitish mucus only; later it is greenish or yellowish. In young children the secretion is swallowed, or reaches only as far as the larynx and returns again to the bronchial tubes. Sometimes vomiting is induced by the violence of the cough, or by the choking caused by the large amount of secretion in the throat.

The physical signs vary with the stage of the disease. At first there are only a few rhonchi audible, or none at all. Later coarse, moist râles can be heard over the entire chest, but especially at the bases behind. If the disease is limited to the trachea and the largest bronchi there may be only rhonchi. The fremitus produced by the râles can often be felt on palpation, or the sound heard at a distance from the chest. The percussion-note is not affected. The number of râles, provided these are coarse in character, appears to bear no necessary relationship to the severity of the symptoms in general. Numerous coarse râles may occur in children with only moderate bronchitis, while an adult, with an acute bronchitis exhibiting fewer râles, would probably suffer from decided constitutional disturbance.

Severe bronchitis owes its character chiefly to the fact that the smaller bronchi are involved. In infancy the fever is higher than in the milder form, reaching 101 to 103 F. (38.3 to 39.4 C.); the cough more constant and distressing, or feeble and ineffective; and there are acceleration of respiration, dyspnea, sometimes slight cyanosis, and often prostration. In older children also the onset may be with such decided constitutional symptoms as headache, chilliness, and high fever. After secretion becomes established the temperature ceases to remain high in uncomplicated cases. The physical signs of severe bronchitis are similar to those of the milder form except for the presence also of fine râles, often in large numbers, in the smaller tubes, combined in infancy with feebleness of the respiratory murmur from the obstruction to the passage of air.

Complications and Sequels.—Bronchitis is so often a secondary disease that it is liable to be associated with other morbid conditions. The complications are those of the respiratory tract, such as rhinitis, laryngitis, pneumonia, and temporary enlargement of the tracheobronchial glands. Recurrent attacks of bronchitis can be followed by the chronic form. Tuberculosis of the lungs may date from an attack of bronchitis.

Course and Prognosis.—The duration of acute bronchitis is from one to two weeks in mild cases not occurring in conjunction with other diseases. The severer cases are prone to last from two to four weeks before recovery is complete. In all cases there is a great disposition to relapse, and under unfavorable environment a child may suffer from recurring attacks for months. The prognosis as to the duration is, therefore, always somewhat uncertain; that as regards recovery is generally good except in severe attacks in infancy, where bronchopneumonia and atelectasis are liable to develop. Especially in quite young infants, or in those older who are debilitated or who possess decided rachitic deformity, severe bronchitis may cause death owing to difficulty in clearing the bronchial tubes of secretion (*Suffocative bronchitis; Suffocative catarrh*). In such cases cyanosis, rapid and shallow respiration, feeble cough and cry, feeble pulse, stupor, and perhaps subnormal temperature develop unless relief is obtained.

Many influences affect the duration and severity of the disease and the tendency to a fatal ending. The factor of age has been mentioned. Bronchitis secondary to typhoid fever or pertussis runs a long course. That associated with measles is often severe, but seldom of long duration; that with grippe is frequently obstinate. In debilitated health bronchitis is dangerous, as mentioned above, or recovery is likely to be slow. This is especially true of rickets, in which deformity of the chest may also be an unfavorable factor. (See also Recurrent Bronchitis, p. 712.)

Diagnosis.—The disease most difficult of differentiation from bronchitis is bronchopneumonia; and many cases supposed to be the former are in reality mild attacks of the latter. In general, temperature which continues high for longer than one or two days, or a rate of respiration decidedly out of proportion to the temperature or the other symptoms, is an indication that something more than bronchitis is present. Râles of moderate size limited to a small area may indicate tuberculous consolidation. Cases with a loose or a harassing, tickling cough and no râles or only coarse rhonchi may depend upon tracheitis or upon bronchitis of the larger tubes, but may, on the other hand, be the result of pharyngitis. The first stage of pertussis is often very confusing. As a rule, early in this disease there are few if any râles, the cough is more paroxysmal and is more troublesome at night, the condition grows worse in spite of treatment, and a lymphocytosis may be present. In some cases of bronchitis, however, the cough is of a very hard paroxysmal character, and few râles are heard, and pertussis cannot be positively eliminated.

Treatment. **Prophylaxis.**—This is of utmost importance. All possible causes likely to produce bronchitis must be sought for and avoided, and all hygienic and other measures followed which will tend to strengthen the child and prevent susceptibility to attacks. These have been discussed under etiology and prophylaxis of Rhinitis (pp. 685–687). To be emphasized is the importance of keeping the child much of the time in the open air; of avoiding too much or too little clothing, and the playing on the floor on cold winter days; of giving cool morning baths; and of sleeping in a well-ventilated bedroom not necessarily cold. In addition, energetic treatment must be at once employed for rhinitis, pharyngitis, or laryngitis already developed, because of their tendency to spread to the bronchi. Precautionary measures are even more indicated in the case of rickets or of delicate children with a tuberculous tendency. For the latter, residence in a warmer climate may be of great benefit in the winter season. Tonic remedies are often needed.

Treatment of the Attack.—At the onset the disease may sometimes be aborted by giving a full dose of a purgative, a warm general bath or hot mustard foot-bath and a hot lemonade, and covering the patient warmly in bed in the hope of producing sweating. The child should be confined to bed in a warm room upon the following day, and as much longer as fever lasts. In some cases the administration of quinine in full doses is efficacious. Much can be accomplished for the developed disease, especially in the early stages, by the administration of syrup of ipecac (4 to 8 minims) (0.25 to 0.49) in combination with deodorized tincture of opium ($\frac{1}{8}$ to 1 minim) (0.008 to 0.064) every two to three hours at two years of age, or in older children an opium-alkaloid. In spite of the apparently opposing action of these drugs, and although there has been much written against the use of each of them, our own experience has often shown that they may give prompt relief of the troublesome cough. When secretion is well-established opium is usually contra-indicated, since it diminishes this and especially the power of emptying the bronchial tubes. It is particularly to be avoided in infants with abundant secretion and diminished expulsive power. In many severe cases in infancy atropine has decided value, as it both stimulates respiration and diminishes secretion. Enough should be given to stop just short of producing flushing of the face, probably $\frac{1}{2000}$ to $\frac{1}{1000}$ of a grain (0.00003 to 0.00006) every three hours at from one to three years of age. It should not, of course, be combined with an expectorant. For cases where there is much dyspnea, and especially when there are any asthmatic symptoms, the injection of epinephrine or the administration of ephedrine is often of great benefit. After secretion has begun but has not become excessive in amount it is sometimes advantageous to give expectorants such as squills, chloride of ammonium, terpene hydrate, iodide of potassium, or citrate of potassium, with the intention of favoring and thinning the secretion. In the choice of these two plans one is guided toward that of checking secretion by the fineness and number of the râles with the presence of dyspnea or perhaps cyanosis; and toward the favoring of secretion by the coarseness of the râles and the absence of any alarming symptoms.

In older children expectorants are oftener indicated, the treatment with atropine being less frequently needed. Even in the stage of secretion, however, the cough is sometimes so frequent and disturbing that more benefit is obtained from the administration of opiates, provided no contra-indications are present. In many cases of severe frequent cough, relief can be secured by the bromides, luminal, or other sedatives without the use of opiates. Apomorphine and antimony are to be avoided. In the severest cases where fever is present such remedies as phenacetin or the salicylates may well be added to the treatment. Emetics are seldom needed, being required only in unusual cases where the secretion is very abundant and cannot be expelled satisfactorily. If there is much debility, alcoholic stimulants should be employed.

In all cases *hygienic* treatment is of great value. Older children with fever should be confined to bed; those without fever may be up and dressed, but guarded from draughts. Their afebrile state renders increase of the bronchitis by exposure easy. Playing upon the floor on cold winter-days readily prolongs the attack. All infants with bronchitis should be in bed and be turned frequently, as well as taken up at times and held in the nurse's arms. In dangerous cases in young infants, relief is sometimes obtained by suspending the patient for a moment by the feet and allowing the secretion to flow from the mouth. The room, although well-ventilated with access of abundance of fresh air, should be of a uniform temperature, about 70 F. (21.1 C.). This plan of treatment is open to exceptions. We have seen afebrile cases, for instance, where the attack was lasting a longer time than usual, in which prompt improvement followed the exposure of the child, well-protected, to fresh out-door air near the open window.

External applications are often of benefit. Rubbing with amber oil, camphorated oil, and the like is usually not very efficacious. The best method is the application of a mustard plaster every three hours (p. 190). The wearing of a cotton jacket (p. 195) does not, in our opinion, serve any good purpose. Dry cups aid in severe cases in older children. A strong mustard-pack (p. 193) or a hot tub-bath (p. 191) is sometimes remarkably efficacious in young infants with failing circulation, or with respiratory obstruction caused by retained secretion. Their chief action is the rousing of the infant and the consequent crying and deeper respiration which follow. For the same purpose alternate hot and cold douches or flagellation is useful, as employed in atelectasis of the new-born.

Inhalations of water vapor (p. 187), alone or medicated with benzoin, turpentine, or menthol, are frequently beneficial. In severe attacks these should be given in a croup-tent. With cyanosis and dyspnea inhalations of oxygen may be employed.

Should cough persist after other evidences of the disease have disappeared, or should the attack pass into the subacute form, treatment suitable for chronic bronchitis and other measures are indicated, such as those described for the prophylaxis of acute rhinitis (p. 687).

CHRONIC BRONCHITIS

Etiology.—This not uncommon condition is the result of repeated attacks of acute bronchitis, between which the intervals are short and finally cease entirely. The predisposing factors are those mentioned under acute bronchitis (p. 705) and acute rhinitis (p. 685). Important factors are living in damp, hot, and poorly ventilated dwellings; local chilling after being overheated; improper feeding especially with an excess of carbohydrates; chronic heart-disease; and nasal obstruction with its consequent mouth-breathing. Other disorders of the lungs, such as asthma, emphysema, tuberculosis, and chronic pneumonia, are liable to be attended by bronchitis. Chronic bronchitis is occasionally a sequel of measles, and frequently of pertussis. Apart from all these, there is a tendency in some children, otherwise healthy, to the persistence of a slight cough and a few coarse râles in the chest especially in the winter season. In a few cases Vincent's infection of the lungs is responsible.

Symptoms.—In milder cases seen especially in infancy and early childhood, the chief symptom is moderate chronic cough, the general health being not at all affected. In the more prolonged and severer cases, which are commoner in later childhood than earlier, the cough is troublesome and often paroxysmal, especially in the morning, when the bronchial tubes are being freed of accumulated secretion. In other cases it is either dry or loose, but without dislodging the mucus, and it is sometimes distressing throughout the night, or may be sufficiently severe to cause vomiting. Usually the secretion is not profuse unless there is a complicating bronchiectasis. Children with chronic bronchitis often learn to expectorate at an earlier age than others. The sputum may be mucoid or mucopurulent. There is usually little dyspnea and the constitutional involvement is seldom great. Physical examination reveals coarse râles or rhonchi, with rhonchial fremitus on palpation. These may disappear after coughing; or nothing abnormal may be found at any time.

Complications.—Prominent among these are bronchiectasis, atelectasis, emphysema, and enlargement of the tracheobronchial lymph-nodes.

Course and Prognosis.—The symptoms may consist in a series of exacerbations; or no improvement may occur until warm weather, and the disorder recur again with the advent of autumn. Prognosis is favorable so far as life is concerned, but uncertain as to duration of the disease, which is usually prolonged. Complete recovery can take place if serious structural pulmonary lesions do not develop, or if no incurable cause such as chronic heart-disease is operative.

Diagnosis.—The disease is to be distinguished from cough depending upon reflex causes, pharyngeal irritation, adenoid growths, and the like. Pertussis may cause confusion. Tuberculosis of the lungs gives more or less fever, and a greater constitutional debility. A negative tuberculin-reaction is an aid, but roentgenography and examination of the sputum may be required in doubtful cases. Moreover chronic bronchitis often attends tuberculosis. The symptomatology of bronchiectasis is not always characteristic, and roentgenography and lipoidal injections are frequently necessary in the differential diagnosis from bronchitis. In some cases Vincent's infection of the lungs will be discovered by examination of the sputum.

Treatment. All causes should be removed. Rickets and valvular disease of the heart, if present, should receive attention. Climatic treatment for general debility is often indicated. Prophylactic measures along the lines indicated for acute bronchitis (p. 707) should be carried out. The diet should be studied especially for determining any influence of an excess of carbohydrate. Vaccine treatment may possibly be of benefit. In the way of internal medication cod liver oil is highly esteemed, with iron and copper or arsenic for any attendant anemia. Direct modification of the bronchial mucous membrane is not very satisfactory, the best remedies probably being iodide of potassium, the turpentine derivatives, eucalyptus, creosote, and preparations of tar. Inhalation of such drugs as eucalyptus, oil of pine, and benzoin may well be tried. Opiates should be employed only if unavoidable.

FIBRINOUS BRONCHITIS

(Plastic Bronchitis)

The most frequent **cause** is extension of diphtheria from the larynx or trachea. Fibrinous bronchitis occasionally attends croupous pneumonia, cardiac disease, tuberculosis, asthma, or one of the acute infectious disorders. Rarely it is primary, the cause then being uncertain, but various organisms have been found associated with it, oftenest pneumococci and streptococci. It is the nondiphtheritic disorder to which attention is given here. The **lesions** consist of pseudomembrane in either large or small bronchi. The **symptoms** of the *acute form* are similar to those of ordinary bronchitis, but much more severe. Auscultation may reveal râles, and also a fluttering sound if the membrane is loose. The most important diagnostic signs are the troublesome cough, the severe dyspnea, and the expectoration of fibrinous casts, the last temporarily relieving the dyspnea. The duration is from one to several weeks, death being more common than recovery. In the *chronic form*, which is more frequently seen although still not common, there are recurring attacks lasting a few days at a time, with short or long intervals; the disease extending possibly over years. Acute constitutional symptoms are absent, and the physical signs are those of chronic bronchitis or of asthma. The diagnosis from the latter is made by the expulsion of large or small casts and the failure to respond to adrenaline or ephedrine. The chronic form, while persistent, is usually not dangerous. **Treatment** is unsatisfactory. In the acute form, inhalations, stimulating expectorants and emetics are of some value. In the chronic form there may also be tried the administration of iodides. Bronchoscopic treatment is to be considered.

ASTHMA

(Asthmatic Bronchitis. Bronchial Asthma)

Nature.—This disease may show itself in several forms. Its nature is two-fold;—a catarrhal bronchitis, and a respiratory neurosis; one or the other predominating according to the case. In addition to any exciting cause or "trigger mechanism" it is evident that there must be some underlying hereditary or acquired predisposition, in the presence of which the initiating factor acts. (See Allergy p. 484.) One hypothesis is that there is a constitutionally labile vegetative nervous system (vagotonia), this being based partly on the fact that stimulation of the vagus is followed by constriction of the bronchioles. Comby[10] believes that asthma is but an expression of a respiratory neurosis. It has been thought also that in some cases an etiologic connection with endocrine disturbance, such as hyperthyroidism, existed but there is little evidence to support this belief. A number of authors, as Reisman and Mason,[11] claim that asthma is due to sensitization to tuberculin in subjects infected with tuberculosis; but this would not account for the majority of cases and there is no conclusive proof of such an association.

Etiology.—Typical attacks of asthma are usually not seen before the beginning of late childhood, according to many authors. On the other hand asthmatic bronchitis is not infrequent in early childhood, and even in infancy. We have observed a number of patients with their first attack of asthma beginning at this period, and Peshkin[12] found that the onset was most frequent at one year; that as the age of ten years was approached the incidence became progressively less; and that onset after the age of ten years was uncommon. Heredity plays an important rôle, the family history often showing that members of it had suffered from asthma or other allergic conditions. Statistically this family incidence is seen in from 40 to 80 per cent of the cases. Asthmatic subjects have had eczema as infants in approximately 10 per cent of the cases, and they often suffer from hay-fever (p. 689).

The immediate *exciting causes* are many. Among them should be mentioned exposure to high wind; dampness; rapid changes in temperature, either heat or cold; the occurrence of infection of the upper or lower respiratory tract; acute febrile diseases; an attack of indigestion; psychic disturbances; and fatigue. In the allergic cases the usual initiating factor is exposure to proteins of some sort, one or more of which act specifically in an individual case. This is most likely to be an inhalation-sensitivity to animal hair or emanations, feathers and the like, such as horse hair or dander, goose or chicken feathers, and quite frequently rabbit hair; perhaps to the pollen of certain flowers and grasses; and less frequently to ingested proteins such as egg-albumen, beef, etc. Any one of a large number of proteins, however, may be responsible. (See Diagnosis, p. 713.) We[13] have been impressed with the frequency with which there seems to be an association of asthmatic bronchitis or even true asthmatic attacks with sensitivity to bacteria carried in the patient's nose and throat. In some cases there seems to be an etiologic connection with disease of the nasal sinuses, but there is apparently little association with diseased tonsils and adenoids. At times the first attack follows an acute infection, and notably the contagious diseases; or repeated attacks of bronchitis have first occurred, perhaps with a consequent enlargement of the tracheobronchial lymph-nodes. On the other hand an interesting fact is that the occurrence of some acute febrile disease, as pneumonia, may sometimes bring about a cessation of the attacks perhaps for months.

Etiologically asthma can be divided into two classes; *viz.* the protein-sensitive and those apparently not reacting to protein, the latter group constituting about 10 per cent of the cases (Peshkin[14]).

Symptoms.—Clinically the disease may be divided into (1) Asthmatic bronchitis and (2) Bronchial asthma. The two conditions, however, shade into each other by intermediate forms.

1. Asthmatic Bronchitis.—In this form the attack nearly always begins as an ordinary respiratory infection, but soon distinct asthmatic symptoms (p. 712) due to the element of spasm develop. The fever generally disappears in a few days, but the other symptoms continue. There is moderate cough and usually no expectoration. The respiratory rate is increased. The expiration is somewhat prolonged and often noisy, with more or less dyspnea. The general condition is undisturbed. Examination shows undue distention and hyperresonance of the thorax, the expiratory excursion limited, the diaphragm depressed, the cardiac dulness diminished or absent, and dry coarse râles and rhonchi audible especially with expiration. The attack may last for a few days up to two to four weeks. Occasional wheezing and slight dyspnea, with the hyperresonance of emphysema, may persist between the attacks, or symptoms may be absent. Sometimes only one attack occurs, but frequently there are recurrent attacks brought on by exposure to cold or by allergic disturbance. These often follow each other with such short intervals that the condition seems to be

almost continuous, especially during the winter. It is particularly in such cases that there is sensitivity to the bacteria of the nose and throat.

Recurrent Bronchitis.—Under this title there is a condition described by a number of writers, which borders closely on the one hand on acute bronchitis and on the other on asthmatic bronchitis. It consists of frequent repeated attacks of bronchitis, sometimes with asthmatic symptoms, recurring every few weeks, and believed by Rachford[15] and Kerley[16] to be in origin allied to recurrent vomiting. The disease would appear to be probably a mild form of asthmatic bronchitis.

2. Bronchial Asthma.—This is the variety in which the nervous element predominates. The attack comes on suddenly, generally without any warning and often at night. It begins with wheezing respiration and dyspnea, this growing worse until there is orthopnea, the patient being obliged to sit up in bed with the head thrown back and the shoulders elevated in the effort to place the body in the most favorable position for breathing. There is vigorous action of the accessory respiratory muscles with inspiratory retraction and moving of the alae nasi. The mouth is open; the expression anxious, and the face pale, moist and cyanotic; the respiration very noisy, difficult and wheezing, with expiration much prolonged; the pulse rapid, feeble and small; there is no fever. The thorax exhibits little respiratory excursion, and auscultation shows very numerous loud wheezing râles of all sorts with feeble respiratory murmur. Percussion is tympanitic, with the cardiac dulness obliterated and the hepatic dulness diminished. As the paroxysm gradually subsides the râles in the chest grow coarser and there is some cough and more or less expectoration, the latter being clear or frothy, perhaps with numerous eosinophilic cells and possibly Charcot-Leyden crystals. Exhaustion and sleep follow. The attack lasts usually only a few hours but may be longer. It may be repeated daily or not for weeks or months. In the intermission there are no symptons, unless the paroxysms are frequent and severe, in which event more or less complicating emphysema and bronchitis may be constantly present and the general health may suffer. In cases dependent upon sensitivity to some certain protein the symptoms develop with the greatest suddenness after exposure to these.

Complications.—A permanent emphysema with resultant thoracic deformity may develop in severe asthma, and during the attack some degree of emphysema is always present. Other allergic manifestations such as eczema and urticaria are liable to occur in asthmatic subjects. A rare complication is massive pulmonary collapse (Peshkin and Fineman[17]).

Prognosis.—The majority of cases of *asthmatic bronchitis* cease to exhibit symptoms as the predisposition to respiratory infections disappears with increasing age. In *bronchial asthma* the prognosis is not so favorable. The younger the child at the onset, the better the outlook for ultimate recovery. If the exciting cause can be removed or the patient guarded against it, attacks may cease even though the underlying predisposition remains. Sometimes, too, the patient may cease to be sensitive to certain factors which had been exciting causes. Death may very rarely take place during an attack.

Diagnosis.—*Asthmatic bronchitis* is distinguished from the ordinary catarrhal bronchitis by the presence of more or less of the nervous spastic element, the existence of some degree of dyspnea, the prolonged expiration with noisy moist râles, and the evidences of hyperdistention of the lungs. The dyspnea of typical *bronchial asthma* more resembles that of obstruction of the larynx or trachea, but the disease is recognized by the combination of prolonged expiratory dyspneic respiration without involvement of inspiration; asthmatic râles; and the evidences of an acute emphysema. The difference between asthmatic bronchitis and bronchial asthma is largely one of degree. In the former there is initial fever and the catarrhal element greatly prevails, with a greater number of moist râles in the chest; in the latter the spasmodic symptoms predominate. Intermediate forms cannot be assigned with positiveness to either category.

In asthma of any kind there is usually a decided eosinophilia of 10 to 20 per cent. Cutaneous tests likewise may give a positive reaction in either clinical variety if the cause is of an allergic nature. In this connection is to be remembered the importance of dust, which may chance to contain protein material of various sorts, such as dandruff, hair, orris root, bacteria, and molds or other fungi. Yet a positive reaction of the skin is not proof that the asthma is dependent upon the protein used, and, on the other hand, a person may react clinically to certain proteins by developing asthma, when his skin is not sensitive to them. Weltz[18] claims it is characteristic of the roentgenogram in asthma to find arch and furrow formation of the diaphragm most noticeable on deep inspiration.

Treatment.—The most important **prophylactic** consideration is the removal of the exciting factor, if this is possible. Impaired health, anemia, rickets, and repeated attacks of bronchitis should receive appropriate treatment. There is no specific effect of ultraviolet irradiation from an artificial source. An outdoor life and avoidance of excitement and mental and physical fatigue are important. Obstruction in or infection of the upper respiratory tract, particularly the sinuses, should receive careful attention; remembering, however, that tonsillectomy and adenoidectomy offer little chance in themselves of curing asthma. Attention to the general state of digestion, as well as the avoidance of proteins to which the patient is sensitive, are an important part of prophylaxis, and cutaneous tests should be made to determine these. It has been claimed by Bray[19] that asthmatic children have a diminished acidity of the gastric juice, and that the administration of hydrochloric acid and pepsin is of benefit. Qsman[20] believes that abundant sugar in the diet is helpful. Peshkin and Fineman[21] report improvement obtained through ketogenic diets (p. 867). Change of environment and locality is sometimes curative when all other methods fail. When this is indicated a warm, dry situation should first be tried, but the seashore or the mountains have a better effect in certain cases. High elevations are not suitable for subjects who have developed asthma. Climatic treatment started early is more helpful than when commenced later, and, if possible, the child should remain in the beneficial surroundings until the tendency to recurrence has disappeared. Filtered air which is dust-free may be obtained in rooms by means of mechanical devices (Cohen[22]). The room in which the asthmatic child sleeps should be as clean and free from dust as possible. The floor should be oiled frequently, and only essential furniture allowed to remain, and the pillows and mattresses should not be stuffed with animal hair or feathers. These measures should be observed as precautionary procedures, even though there is no known sensitivity to dust or animal emanations. Occasionally a child will be sensitive to cotton or kapok used in pillows and mattresses (Brown[23]). All precautions should be observed when an asthmatic patient receives injections of animal serum (p. 487).

In the **treatment of the attack** a number of remedies are in vogue. The selection depends upon the symptoms. Hypodermic injections of 3 to 5 minims (0.19 to 0.31) of 1:1000 solution of epinephrine may give immediate relief to severe spasm, or the oral administration of ephedrine in doses from 15 to 50 mg. (0.23 to 0.77 grains) may act in the same way (Piness and Miller;[24] Munns and Aldrich,[25] and others). These drugs may be repeated every three or four hours. Atropine is often serviceable. Weiss and Magassy[26] employ epinephrine by inhalation with a special apparatus. Göppert[27] claimed that calcium salts were beneficial, and phosphorus preparations have been found useful by Sterling.[28] Counter-irritation of the chest is an aid, and a hot bath or hot pack may relieve the spasm. The inhalation of oxygen can be tried if the dyspnea is great. Antipyrine or acetylsalicylic acid given at bedtime sometimes seems to prevent a seizure. Iodide of potassium and lobelia have been used for the same purpose. Serviceable in some cases during an attack is the inhalation of fumes from burning saltpeter, combined with stramonium leaves, given in a croup-tent or by some other measure which insures inhalation. An old formula consists of powdered stramonium 1 oz. (31), powdered anise fruit ½ oz. (16), potassium nitrate ½ oz. (16), bruised tobacco 30 grains (2). From 10 to 30 grains (0.64 to 2) of this should be placed on a plate and ignited. Blotting paper which has been moistened with a 1:15 solution of potassium nitrate and dried may be burned. Water-vapor, perhaps medicated with menthol or eucalyptus, may be helpful. Among other remedies which may give relief are chloral, nitroglycerin, and morphine, guarding against habit-formation with the last.

It seems occasionally indicated to attempt to immunize the patient with minute doses of the proteins to which he is sensitive, this applying particularly to cases of food-allergy. The procedure should be carried out with care, as alarming symptoms may develop. We[13] have been favorably impressed with the value of vaccines prepared from micro-organisms carried in the patient's nose and throat, to which he is skin-sensitive. Good results have been claimed for the injection of peptone (Auld[29]) or autoserum (Widal et al.[30]); and autogenous defibrinated blood has been tried with success by Kahn and Ensheimer.[31] Radiologic treatment of the chest and spleen has been reported as successful. (For review, see Waldbott.[32])

BRONCHIECTASIS
(Bronchiolectasis)

Etiology.—This is more common in early life than ordinarily supposed. Rarely it is a congenital condition. Grawitz,[33] Heubner,[34] Peiser,[35] and Carr,[36] and Vogt[37] have published cases observed in the first two years of life. Reports of the disease in childhood have been made by Findlay and Graham,[38] Thorpe,[39] and others. Temporary dilatation of the bronchial tubes may attend many acute pulmonary disorders. Chronic bronchitis or bronchopneumonia, especially when developing after measles, pertussis or grippe, may readily produce a more permanent bronchiectasis, and that of a local nature may occur after chronic interstitial pneumonia, pleurisy, pulmonary abscess, and foreign body. Recently there has been stressed the importance of chronic disease of the sinuses as an etiologic factor. There is some evidence that there exists a hereditary tendency. The condition appears more common in institutional children, perhaps because of the frequency of pulmonary infections in them and, in the case of infants, due also to the greater time spent in the horizontal position in institutions and consequent poor bronchial drainage. The micro-organisms found in the material obtained by bronchoscopy are diphtheroids in practically all cases, often streptococci, and in some cases the micrococcus catarrhalis, pneumococcus, fusiform bacillus, spirochetes, and influenza bacillus. In general bronchiectasis requires for its development a chronic pulmonary affection in which there is sclerosis of the lungs.

Pathologic Anatomy.—The bronchial dilatation may be cylindrical, fusiform, or sacculated, the last being most common, and sometimes its connection with the bronchus closing and a cyst resulting. The dilatations are multiple, oftener unilateral, range in size from that of a pea to a hen's egg, and are most frequent in the lower lobe. In the condition of *bronchiolectasis* there are innumerable minute cavities, apparently dilatations of the bronchioles, producing the "honeycomb-lung."

Symptoms.—The disease generally comes on slowly, although its presence may be early suspected if the physical signs, especially the occurrence of coarse râles, are most marked in one locality. Fully developed bronchiectasis requires several months for its evolution. There is then a paroxysmal loose cough, more marked in the morning or on change of position; productive in older children, with the expectoration of a somewhat large quantity of thin, mucopurulent secretion. This is sometimes streaked with blood, and in some cases decided hemoptysis may take place. Hours may pass without any cough whatever, or even several days before an emptying of the cavity occurs. The odor is not as offensive as in gangrene of the lung, yet some odor is nearly always present on the breath, even when the expectoration is swallowed. The sputum may on standing separate into the three layers often described as characteristic; an upper, thin and frothy; a middle, thin and clear or slightly turbid; and a lower, thick and purulent.

Examination of the lungs reveals decided physical signs only in cases of unusually large bronchiectatic cavities. Then numerous râles may occur on some occasions, and on others bronchial respiration and bronchophony or even amphoric respiration; while the percussion-note may have a tympanitic quality, or at other times be impaired. Signs of cavity are, however, uncertain in character. The alteration in the physical signs from time to time depends upon whether or not the dilatations have been emptied of their contents. Decided dyspnea is not a usual symptom of the disease, and when present depends upon other causes. Yet in some cases the patient may be obliged to sit upright all night or assume some other position, because any except this produces violent coughing. The general condition is good, the appetite not impaired, and there is no fever when the cavities are kept well emptied. Otherwise fever, sometimes of a hectic type, may occur, and emaciation and loss of general health follow. Fever in other cases may be dependent upon a complication. Decided clubbing of the fingers (*pulmonary osteoarthropathy*) is not uncommon in long-continued cases (p. 998).

Complications.—The diseases of which bronchiectasis is a complication or sequel have been mentioned. In addition intercurrent attacks of bronchitis or of bronchopneumonia can occur from time to time in cases of bronchiectasis. Pulmonary gangrene, pericarditis, peritonitis, nephritis, nephrosis, or pleurisy, generally purulent, may develop, or metastatic abscesses in the liver, brain, spleen or elsewhere, or amyloid changes result from the long-continued suppuration.

Course and Prognosis.—In acute temporary bronchiectasis the lesion disappears with the primary disease. In the more permanent condition the course perhaps extends over years, with little immediate danger to life except from complications. Eventually, however, the general health is liable to fail. The best prognosis is in the cases dependent upon a foreign body in the bronchus, if this is removed fairly early.

Diagnosis.—This rests chiefly upon the periodic attacks of cough with profuse expectoration, and on the discovery of localized coarse râles and sometimes of tympanitic percussion with bronchophony and bronchial respiration. When these signs are not well developed, difficulty may arise in distinguishing the disease from encapsulated empyema, and even exploratory puncture may mislead. Tuberculous cavities are attended by severe constitutional symptoms, and tubercle bacilli may be found in the sputum. Many cases at first thought to be tuberculosis are probably in reality instances of bronchiectasis. Chronic bronchitis with profuse expectoration may not be distinguishable from bronchiectasis unless physical signs of the latter can be found, although the paroxysmal discharge of a large amount of sputum at one time, with long intervals of freedom from coughing, is suggestive of bronchiectasis. The perforation of an empyema into a bronchus may at first suggest the emptying of a bronchiectatic cavity, but the much larger amount of pus evacuated on the first occasion and the much smaller amount later make the diagnosis of empyema clear. Pulmonary gangrene runs a more acute course with severe constitutional symptoms, and the expectoration and the breath possess a gangrenous odor. Pulmonary abscess communicating with a bronchus may give the physical signs of a large bronchiectatic cavity. The history and the other symptoms present aid in coming to a conclusion. The differential diagnosis in all these conditions is often made clear only by injection of lipiodol or similar substances into the bronchial tree. (See p. 153.)

Treatment.—The general health must be supported by all those measures discussed in detail under the etiology and prophylaxis of rhinitis (pp. 685, 687), with especial emphasis on life in the open air, and, if possible, in a dry climate at not too high an elevation. Inhalation of vapor containing turpentine, eucalyptus, or creosote is of some use in modifying the secretion, and the same class of remedies may be tried internally as in chronic bronchitis, but possess no established value. Autogenous vaccines may be of some benefit, using the micro-organisms obtained from the bronchial secretion. Postural drainage, with the foot of the bed raised and the patient on the abdomen, assists in clearing the bronchial tubes. Lipiodol injections in themselves may have a therapeutic value, and good results may be obtained by the employment of the bronchoscope and the removal of pus by suction or by bronchial washings. Operation is too dangerous to be recommended, except possibly for large localized bronchiectasis with increasing general symptoms.

References

1. Am. J. M. Sc., 1918, **156,** 625. 2. Am. J. M. Sc., 1920, **159,** 313. 3. J.A.M.A., 1919, **73,** 672. 4. Am. J. Dis. Child., 1927, **33,** 259. 5. Am. J. M. Sc., 1921, **161,** 625; 1923, **165,** 313. 6. Am. J. Roentgenol., 1920, **7,** 277. 7. Am. J. Dis. Child., 1924, **28,** 183. 8. Bronchoscopy and Esophagoscopy 1922. 9. Am. J. Dis. Child., 1925, **29,** 41. 10. Arch. de méd. d. enf., 1925, **28,** 729. 11. N. Y. State J. Med., 1929, **29,** 919. 12. Am. J. Dis. Child., 1928, **36,** 98. 13. Mitchell and Cooper, Arch. Pediat., 1931, **48,** 75. 14. Am. J. Dis. Child., 1926, **31,** 763. 15. Arch. Pediat., 1914, **31,** 488. 16. Arch. Pediat., 1914, **31,** 741. 17. Am. J. Dis. Child., 1931, **42,** 590. 18. München. med. Wchnschr., 1932, **79,** 216. 19. Quart. J. Med., 1931, **24,** 181. 20. Lancet, 1929, **2,** 1187. 21. Am. J. Dis. Child., 1930, **39,** 1240. 22. J. Lab. and Clin. Med., 1928, **13,** 963. 23. J.A.M.A., 1929, **93,** 370. 24. J.A.M.A., 1927, **89,** 515. 25. J.A.M.A., 1927, **88,** 1233. 26. Orvosi hetil., 1927, **71,** 1326. 27. Med. Klin., 1914, **10,** 1003. 28. J. Lab. and Clin. Med., 1928, **13,** 997. 29. Brit. M. J., 1918, **2,** 49. 30. Presse méd., 1914, **22,** 525. 31. Arch. Int. Med., 1916, **18,** 445. 32. Arch. Int. Med., 1928, **41,** 683. 33. Virchow's Arch. f. path. Anat., 1880, **82,** 217. 34. Lehrb. d. Kinderh., 1911, **2,** 286. 35. Monatschr. f. Kinderh., 1910, **8,** 602. 36. Practitioner, 1891, **46,** 87. 37. Jahrb. f. Kinderh., 1911, **74,** 627. 38. Arch. Dis. Childhood, 1927, **2,** 71. 39. Am. J. M. Sc., 1929, **177,** 759.

CHAPTER V

DISEASES OF THE LUNGS (Continued)

PNEUMONIA

Pneumonia is one of the most common and serious diseases of infancy and childhood. It is described under several forms, the two chief varieties being (1) *Bronchopneumonia* and (2) *Croupous Pneumonia.* In addition reference must be made to (3) *Chronic Interstitial Pneumonia* and (4) *Hypostatic Pneumonia.* The first two were clearly differentiated from each other in 1838 by Rilliet and Barthez.[1] Although in typical cases the distinction is now firmly based on anatomical, clinical, and roentgenological findings, there are numerous instances in which the last two are far from conclusive, and others which even at necropsy may be found to be hybrid forms. The anatomical differences consist in a fibrinous exudate into the vesicles, chiefly in a circumscribed form, in the case of croupous pneumonia, and a peribronchitis and perialveolitis in bronchopneumonia, with exudation of cells into the alveoli, the process being more scattered and lobular in character. Yet a pneumonia which is fibrinous in its histologic character may sometimes have a lobular distribution; and, on the other hand, a bronchopneumonia may involve all or a large portion of one lobe and be confined to this. The terms "lobar" and "lobular" are consequently misleading. We[2] have discussed this matter elsewhere.

This unavoidable uncertainty in diagnosis explains the great variation in opinions and in statistics concerning the relative frequency of the two forms. The figures given show a ratio of croupous to bronchopneumonia, in children in the first two years of life, varying from 1:0.5 to 1:17 (Comby,[3] Dunlop,[4] Holt and Howland,[5] Morse,[6] Smith,[7] Heiman,[8] Lyon,[9] Somerville,[10] McNeil and Alexander,[11] Manace[12]). As far as figures can be trusted, bronchopneumonia is decidedly the more common disorder during the first two years, and its mortality is certainly much greater than that of the croupous form; while after the age of four years the latter becomes constantly more frequent, and the former exceptional. In our own opinion croupous pneumonia in infancy is probably more common than many statistics indicate.

ACUTE BRONCHOPNEUMONIA

(Catarrhal Pneumonia; Lobular Pneumonia; Capillary Bronchitis)

As a disease which involves both the alveoli and the bronchial tissues, and in which bronchitis is always present, this affection is properly denominated "bronchopneumonia." The title "lobular" used as a synonym should, as stated, be avoided, and "catarrhal" does not fully express the pathologic changes. Pathologically it is difficult, and clinically it is impossible, to separate "capillary bronchitis" from bronchopneumonia.

Etiology.—The influence of age is decided, 75 per cent or more of the cases occurring before the age of two years. It is very common in new-born and, especially, in premature infants. In some of these cases it appears to be antenatal in origin, due to premature rupture of the membranes and consequent infection of the child. After the fourth year it appears to be infrequent, except as a complication of the infectious fevers. Sex has little influence. Hygienic conditions are factors, crowding and unsanitary surroundings increasing the susceptibility. Season predisposes, much the greater number of cases occurring during the winter and spring. Hill[13] found the frequency increased both in warm and rainy and in abnormally cold and dry weather. The coexistence of other diseases is of great importance. Consequently, bronchopneumonia is conveniently divided into the *primary* and the *secondary* forms. In the former the disease develops independently of the condition of health. Especially in these instances local chilling of the body appears often to be the sole acting cause. In the secondary form, which is from two to three times as frequent, apart from the influence of chilling bronchopneumonia occurs as a complication of typhoid fever, scarlet fever, sepsis, or other infectious disorder, and especially of measles, pertussis, grippe, and diphtheria; or it develops in children debilitated by syphilis, rickets, or gastro-intestinal affections. Bronchopneumonia secondary to bronchitis might with propriety be called primary, since it is but a further extension of the bronchitic process. In severe digestive disturbance bronchopneumonia is a common terminal manifestation. The majority of primary cases appear to occur in the first two years of life, whereas half or more of the secondary cases are seen after this age (Dunlop[4]).

In early infancy some cases are caused by the entrance of food into the air-passages after vomiting, or during efforts at swallowing;—the so-called "deglutition" or "aspiration" pneumonia; and in childhood the accident may happen during unconscious or greatly debilitated states, or be the result of the entrance of a foreign body into a bronchus. A number of cases are reported due to the aspiration of stearate of zinc intended as a dusting-powder (Bass,[14] Boehme,[15] Heiman and Aschner[16]).

The **exciting cause** is infection by a germ. The pneumococcus of Fränkel is probably that most frequently present in cases of primary bronchopneumonia. In secondary forms the streptococcus, staphylococcus, or pneumococcus is perhaps oftenest seen; or the colon bacillus, micrococcus catarrhalis, diphtheria bacillus, pneumobacillus of Friedlander, influenza bacillus, or typhoid bacillus may occur. The tubercle bacillus is present in combination with other germs in the very frequent cases of tuberculous bronchopneumonia. In all forms of bronchopneumonia the infection is very often a mixed one, the germs being associated in a varied manner, sometimes one species being most in evidence and sometimes another. (See bacteriologic studies by Netter,[17] Dürck,[18] Pearce,[19] Lyon,[20] Cecil,[21] Liston,[22] and Ellison.[23])

With regard to the incidence and influence of the pneumococcus, the investigations of Dochez and Gillespie,[24] Cole and Dochez,[25] and others have shown that Types I and II are those most frequently found in croupous pneumonia of adults; Type III being infrequent but producing the greatest mortality. The so-called "Group IV," which has recently been subdivided into at least 21 different types, is found in about 25 per cent of cases, in these the mortality being low. Studies of pneumococcus types in children have been made by Pisek and Pease,[26] Wollstein and Benson,[27] Mitchell,[28] Westlund,[29] Neumann and Happe,[30] Sakamoto,[31] Trask et al.;[32] and Raia, Plummer and Shultz,[33] most of the series including both croupous and bronchopneumonia. Group IV seemed to be more common in early life and in bronchopneumonia, although in croupous pneumonia at any time of life Types I and III may be found. It is a matter of discussion whether bronchopneumonia is contagious. The primary form is so rarely if at all. In the secondary form, especially as associated with the infectious fevers, a certain degree of contagiousness would appear to exist. Pneumococci of various types are frequently present in cultures from the nose and throat in normal persons. Increased prevalence of the fixed types in cultures is not accompanied by increased incidence of pneumonia (Powell, Atwater and Felton[34]). Probably the germs in the mouth and nasopharynx remain harmless until the general resisting power of the mucous membranes is lowered in some manner. It is likely that the germ makes its way directly from the nasopharynx to the lung, or perhaps in some cases enters the blood-vessels through the affected mucous membrane of the nasopharynx. The latter view is supported by the fact that blood-cultures taken early in the disease are frequently positive for pneumococci.

Pathologic Anatomy.—The basic lesion in bronchopneumonia is an inflammation with a small-celled infiltration into the walls of the bronchi, the peribronchial connective tissue and the surrounding air-vesicles. The exudate may contain fibrin, but in small amount. The pathologic process produces scattered foci, at first small, with thickened bronchioles as the center. The confluence of neighboring foci results in larger areas of varying size, rather firm and projecting on section, and in color at first red and later

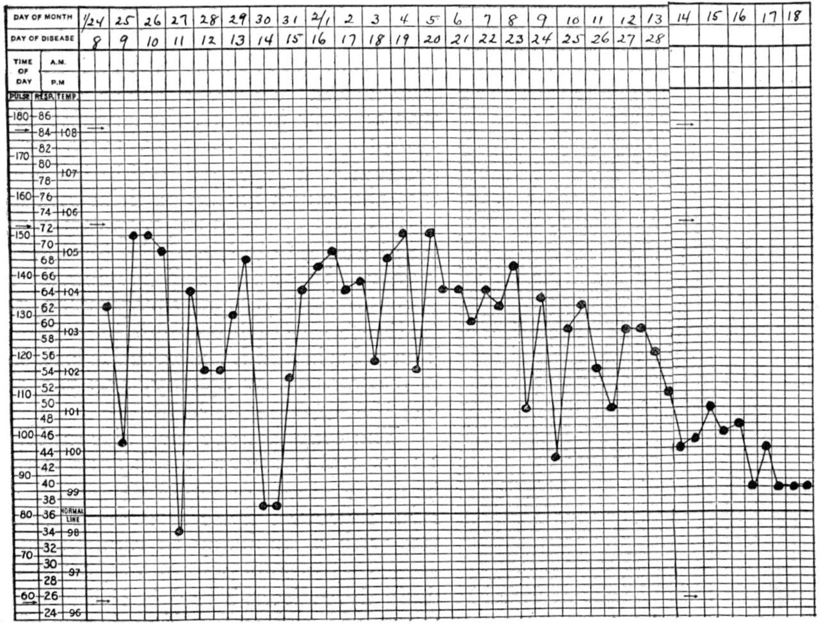

Fig. 161.—Acute lobular bronchopneumonia. High temperature, severe case, long course. Pearl L., aged twenty months. Admitted to the Children's Hospital of Philadelphia, Jan. 24, approximately eighth day of disease. Cough for a week, vomiting, fretful. While in hospital had many scattered coarse râles throughout lungs, fine râles over consolidated areas situated chiefly in right side and to a less extent on the left, cyanosis, dyspnea, stuporous, toxemic state, pulse 160–170, respiration 40–50 +, leukocytes 21,000 to 23,000, systolic pressure 103, diastolic 80. Recovery.

of a grayish or yellowish tint. The portions of uninvolved pulmonary tissue between the consolidated areas are soft, edematous, congested, and often atelectatic or sometimes emphysematous. The disease spreads slowly and not to any great extent in cases of short duration, but in those lasting longer it gradually invades most of the lung, particularly the bases, and oftenest on both sides, and a characteristic mottled appearance is produced. As a rule the external portion of the lung is that chiefly involved. In many cases the extension has been largely in one region, and the confluent foci have produced a consolidated area, sometimes occupying the greater part of a lobe (*pseudolobar bronchopneumonia*). In cases much prolonged the section is gray in color, and minute or larger abscess-cavities may be found. Gangrene is uncommon. Resolution in bronchopneumonia takes place by gradually progressing absorption following the gradual spread of the disease, and different parts of the lung show different stages as compared with each other. In protracted cases there may take place overgrowth of connective tissue in the alveolar septa, bronchial tubes, and pleura. (See Chronic Pneumonia, p. 743.)

In addition to the changes in the lung, pleurisy is a frequent attendant; a small amount of serum may be present in the pleural cavity and occasionally pus; and enlargement of the bronchial glands is always found.

Symptoms.—No exact classification of bronchopneumonia is possible, since the clinical symptoms and the anatomic lesions are not always in accord. The first of the following varieties is the most frequently seen.

1. Acute Lobular Bronchopneumonia.—In well-marked cases the symptoms begin acutely, perhaps after some days of preceding nasal and pharyngeal catarrh or of tracheobronchitis. There is then a sudden rise of temperature accompanied often by vomiting and sometimes ushered in by a convulsion. In cases where bronchitis was already present, the severity of the symptoms may increase more or less gradually, with or without initial vomiting, the cough becoming drier and more suppressed and painful, respiration more rapid and labored, and the temperature higher. In any well-developed case there are rapid dyspneic respiration, prostration, more or less cough, and cyanosis. The pulse is rapid, the appetite lost, there is restlessness or apathy, and the child has the appearance of illness.

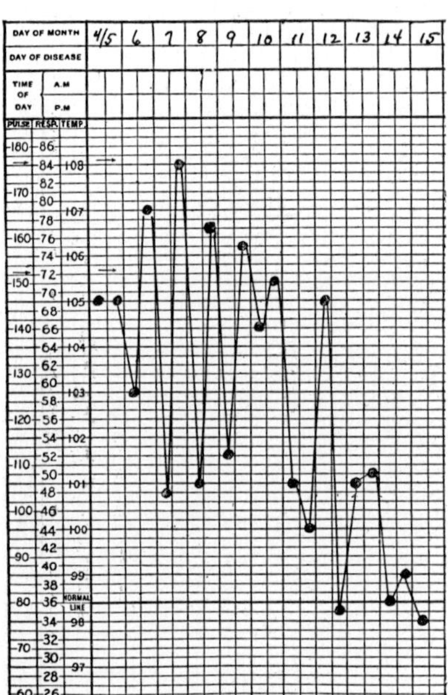

Fig. 162.—Acute lobular bronchopneumonia with very high and irregular temperature. Muriel D., aged two and one-half years. Chart begins approximately on the fifth day. Gradually increasing consolidation of both lungs, principally of left apex and right base. Some degree of delirium, cyanosis and cardiac weakness. Respiration only moderately accelerated. Short course. Recovery.

The **temperature** may rise rapidly to 104 or 106 F. (40 or 41.1 C.) and remains in many cases continuously high. As a rule, however, there is a more gradual rise with a tendency to remittance not seen in croupous pneumonia, often with daily drops from 3 to 4 F. (1.6 to 2.2 C.) (Figs. 161 and 162). The degree of elevation is no necessary indication of the severity of the disease. Although in the mildest cases the temperature is more likely to be lower, some of the more severe ones may never exceed 101 to 102 F. (38.3 to 38.9 C.). Sometimes a hyperpyrexia of 107 F. (41.7 C.) or over occurs just before death; but we have seen this high temperature in cases which recovered (Fig. 162). In debilitated subjects, especially in young infants or the new-born, the temperature may occasionally remain afebrile or even subnormal throughout. The fall of temperature is nearly always by lysis. Not infrequently there is a fall followed by another rise; often indicating the spread of the pneumonic process to other parts of the lungs.

The **respiration** is always accelerated and the lack of proportion of this to that of the pulse is often striking, the ratio reaching sometimes 1:2 instead of the normal 1:3 or 4. The rate is generally over fifty and one of seventy or eighty per minute is not uncommon, and it may sometimes decidedly exceed this.

Dyspnea is a constant symptom except in new-born infants, where it may be absent. In the mildest cases at later periods of infancy it may be insignificant and shown only by slight moving of the alae nasi when the child is excited or exerts itself. Moving of the alae cannot alone be taken as a certain sign of pneumonia, since it may occur even under the mere influence of nervous excitement. In well-marked cases, however, the alae nasi dilate with each inspiration; there are episternal and epigastric retraction, inspiratory retraction of the sternocleidomastoid muscles and of the attachment of the diaphragm, and sinking in of the costal interspaces. A moaning or grunting cry,—the "expiratory moan,"—may accompany many of the expirations, but loud crying is uncommon, owing to the difficulty in getting breath. In mild cases, however, the cry may be vigorous. Not infrequently the respiratory rhythm is altered, the pause coming after inspiration instead of expiration as in normal breathing.

Cough is a variable symptom. Often it is dry, painful, harassing and causing much loss of rest. In other cases there may be little cough. This may occur in either mild or severe cases and in the latter is an unfavorable symptom, indicating that the patient has not sufficient power to relieve the bronchioles of secretion. There is no expectoration in infancy and early childhood; the secretion being swallowed or drawn back into the lung.

The **circulatory system** exhibits always accelerated pulse, but in average cases generally of good strength and regular. In bad cases it grows weak and thread-like. The tension is usually lowered, except in the beginning. The pulse-rate may reach even two hundred per minute in young subjects with severe attacks of the disease. Cyanosis may show itself only in a slightly bluish tint of the lips and fingers and of the flush of the cheeks. In a severe attack the whole surface of the body may be pale and bluish; in fact in many severe cases pallor may largely replace cyanosis. The sudden development or increase of cyanosis may indicate a congestion or collapse of some portion of the lung previously unaffected. It may be attended by a sudden increase of dyspnea.

Prostration is observed to some extent in all cases, and in serious ones may be very great and be attended by much loss of weight.

Digestive symptoms are common in infants and of great importance. Tympanites is of serious import, inasmuch as it adds to the difficulty in breathing. It is seen oftenest in rachitic subjects. Vomiting frequently ushers in the disease and is not uncommon later. It may occur only occasionally, or repeatedly and be resistant to treatment. Diarrhea is sometimes troublesome, especially in summer-time. Both vomiting and diarrhea usually depend upon the debilitated digestive power attending the pneumonia, rather than upon a true enteritis. Both are oftenest met with in the first two years of life. The appetite is usually greatly diminished, and dyspnea, too, may interfere with the taking of food.

Nervous symptoms are frequent especially as the disease advances. Convulsions may usher in the attack. Occurring later they are of serious import. In some cases there is great restlessness, particularly if the respiratory symptoms are severe, when jactitation from air-hunger may develop. Delirium may occur, or the patient be unusually excitable. Oftener, however, there are fretfulness and sleeplessness; or a decided degree of apathy and even a stuporous state; and sometimes complete unconsciousness. In all well-developed cases the children appear ill and frequently lie with half-opened eyes.

The **blood** exhibits early a leukocytosis especially of the polymorphonuclear cells. The number of leukocytes usually equals 20,000 or decidedly more per cubic millimeter. In many severe cases, especially when associated with grippe, there may be no leukocytosis whatever. The **urine** shows only the ordinary changes characteristic of febrile diseases.

Physical Signs.—Generally the physical signs develop somewhat slowly and may not be discovered until the case is well advanced. The first signs are usually the presence of fine râles, combined frequently with coarser ones, limited to some small area or areas, or most marked there. These areas are oftenest in the posterior part of the lower lobe or in the intervertebral spaces. They may be too small to permit of any alteration of the percussion-note. Later the râles become more widespread, and change of the respiratory murmur is present, but this may be of a degree only sufficient to be classed as bronchovesicular, and is characterized chiefly by a harsher expiration heard if the patient breathes deeply, the respiration at other times being often feebler than normal. Increased vocal resonance also is now audible, although perhaps only at the time of a cry, or consisting in the more clearly ringing character of the râles at the affected spot and in their apparent nearness to the ear. There may by this time be very slight dulness elicited if percussion is done gently. In many cases, however, the voice-sounds are feeble and respiration so superficial that no positive auscultatory change can be discovered, and a slight dulness on percussion may be the only suggestive sign. Sometimes the percussion-note over the affected region is at first fuller and more hyperresonant than normal, owing to the presence of neighboring areas with distended vesicles. Often the emphysematous free border of the lungs in front diminishes the normal hepatic and cardiac percussion-dulness. Vocal fremitus generally gives unsatisfactory signs owing to the high-pitched and less resonant voice of the child. As the case advances no further change in the physical signs may occur; or in other instances there slowly develops decided consolidation over larger areas, and the usual loud bronchial respiration, bronchophony, and dulness on percussion observed in the croupous pneumonia of adults are discoverable. Always, however, there is a large admixture of coarse and fine râles, and friction sounds may sometimes be heard. In some instances physical signs suggesting cavities are present, whether or not these actually exist. The pneumonic process is seldom limited to only one region in typical cases, but eventually scattered areas of the disease are usually present in both lungs, especially in the lower lobes.

Always bronchopneumonia is characterized, at least early in the disease, by the lack of correspondence between the severity of the symptoms and the degree of the development of the physical signs. In many cases percussion-dulness remains absent throughout or until late in the attack, and auscultatory signs are often not discovered at all, or only if the child is made to cry, and the diagnosis must consequently rest upon the symptoms and not the physical signs.

2. Acute Toxemic Bronchopneumonia. (*Acute Congestive Form.*) In some extremely severe cases of bronchopneumonia, especially as seen at times in early infancy, and either primary or secondary in nature, the process may not go beyond the stage of widespread intense congestion of the lungs, and the general symptoms appear to be dependent upon the toxemic condition. There are hyperpyrexia, great prostration, cyanosis, rapid respiration, and nervous symptoms consisting of delirium, stupor, or terminal convulsions. Râles may be entirely absent and no physical signs of any sort discoverable. There may be a painful, frequent cough, or none at all. The symptoms are like those of some malignant cases of any of the acute infectious fevers. Death may occur in one or two days. In other instances the intensity of the symptoms diminishes and recovery is rapid; or the case may develop the symptoms and run the ordinary course of bronchopneumonia as usually seen.

3. Acute Disseminated Bronchopneumonia.—There occurs in this form, which is seen oftenest in infancy, in addition to the involvement of the alveoli a widespread involvement of the finer bronchioles throughout much of both lungs, with filling of these with secretion. The title "capillary bronchitis" has often been applied to this variety. After a short period of mild respiratory catarrh, there is a rapid development of moderate fever, accelerated respiration, extreme dyspnea, decided cyanosis, and severe cough. Numerous râles of all sorts are widespread throughout the chest, but there are no signs of actual consolidation. The percussion-note may even be hyperresonant from the presence of emphysema. Life is threatened especially by the suffocative condition.

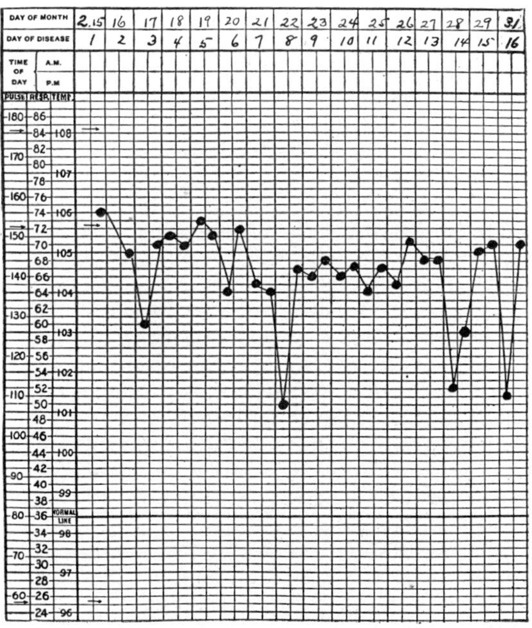

Fig. 163.—Primary bronchopneumonia, pseudolobar type. Andrew R., aged two and one-half years. Sudden onset with convulsions on Feb. 15. On next day physical signs of consolidation in the right lung, extending thence over the entire upper part of the right lung in lobar form. No physical signs in left lung. Restlessness, delirium, at times opisthotonos, persistent high temperature with few remissions, increasing prostration, cyanosis. Many attacks of profound collapse. Death Mar. 1. Necropsy and microscopic examination showed pseudolobar bronchopneumonia of right lung, left lung free.

4. Pseudolobar Form of Bronchopneumonia.—This differs little in symptoms from the form first described, except for a greater tendency to a persisting high temperature. The physical signs, on the other hand, resemble closely those of croupous pneumonia. That the condition is a bronchopneumonia is to be suspected if at the onset separate smaller areas were distinct from each other, and if later small areas may be found as well in other parts of the chest. Often, however, the development of the condition is so rapid that a diagnosis from croupous pneumonia is impossible (Fig 163).

5. Latent Form of Bronchopneumonia.—This is seen in very young infants, in older ones suffering from severe gastro-enteric diseases, and in still older children unconscious and much debilitated in the course of some serious disorder. The onset is insidious. Fever due to the pneumonia may be thought to be dependent on the primary condition, or there may be no fever whatever, no cough or dyspnea, and nothing in fact to draw

attention to the lungs. As a rule, the disease is discovered only by accident or not until necropsy.

6. PROTRACTED FORM OF BRONCHOPNEUMONIA.—The protracted form is to be distinguished from the chronic interstitial form presently to be described in that the last is a sequel of pneumonia. It is seen principally in weakly infants or children, or occurring secondarily to the infectious diseases, especially pertussis, diphtheria, and measles. It at first resembles the ordinary lobular or the pseudolobular form in symptoms and physical signs; but the former fail to ameliorate and the latter increase in extent and may become suggestive of cavitation. There may sometimes be temporary remissions in the severity of the symptoms, but, on the whole, loss of strength and weight is progressive until an extremely cachectic state is reached.

7. ASPIRATION PNEUMONIA.—This occurs in conditions of great cachexia, in coma or stupor, or after tracheotomy or intubation, and is the result of the entrance into the lung of food or other material or, in the case of the new-born, the aspiration of amniotic liquid. The exudate in the lungs in these cases is more purulent than in other forms. If the accident does not produce abscess or gangrene, there results a bronchopneumonia of the lobular type. (See also p. 718.)

8. TUBERCULOUS BRONCHOPNEUMONIA.—The very common form of pneumonia associated with the tubercle bacillus may occur as a primary disease or be secondary to other disorders, especially measles and pertussis, or to tuberculous processes elsewhere in the body. The pathologic lesions and clinical symptoms have already been described (p. 414).

9. BRONCHOPNEUMONIA SECONDARY TO OTHER DISEASES.—Occasionally the pneumonia appears with the symptoms of invasion in the infectious diseases. With *measles*, it may occur at any time in the course of the disease, but oftenest in the stage of eruption or as it fades. Any of the types described may be observed, but the disseminated and protracted forms are frequent. The process may be simple or tuberculous. In *pertussis* bronchopneumonia is prone to make its appearance after the disease has reached its height or is in the stage of decline, and is most commonly of the disseminated or the protracted type, or frequently tuberculous. The onset is often insidious. The paroxysmal cough of pertussis may to a large extent be replaced by the nonparoxysmal cough of pneumonia. In other instances the onset is more abrupt; but in any event there is a change from comparative health to decided illness. In *scarlet fever* the development of bronchopneumonia is much less frequent than in measles or pertussis. It may be attended by purulent pleural effusion. As a complication of *grippe* pneumonia is common, and may be either of the ordinary or the pseudolobar form. The onset may be sudden and the existence of grippe entirely overlooked; or the process may develop during the height of or as a sequel to the primary disease. The predisposition to the development of empyema as a sequel to the pneumonia is noteworthy. *Diphtheria* of the larynx is not infrequently complicated by bronchopneumonia. In other instances of diphtheria it is secondary to the septic condition. In intubated cases the diagnosis is difficult, since the presence of the tube greatly alters the auscultatory signs. In *gastro-enteric disease* pneumonia is often of the latent type. *Rachitis*, when severe, is liable to be complicated by a bronchopneumonia of a protracted form, sometimes with little fever.

Complications and Sequels.—Pleurisy as a pathologic lesion attends most cases of bronchopneumonia, but as a recognizable clinical condition it is not as frequent as in croupous pneumonia. Empyema may follow, and is oftener seen in certain epidemics, notable those associated with grippe. Purulent otitis media and diarrhea are common. Tuberculosis may be a sequel, but many cases exhibiting lesions of this nature probably began as tuberculous bronchopneumonia. In protracted cases bronchiectasis and emphysema may persist as sequels, and various purulent inflammations of the skin may develop. Less common or rare results are gangrene of the lung, pneumothorax, pyopneumothorax, nephritis, purulent arthritis, osteomyelitis, meningitis which is generally serous but may be purulent, and pericarditis which is perhaps purulent.

Relapse and Recurrence.—Fresh extensions of the pathologic process are almost a part of bronchopneumonia, and true relapses are also common. These may take place in a part of the lung previously unaffected, or in one where resolution has been practically completed. Recurrence is not infrequent. Indeed, an attack of bronchopneumonia appears to a certain degree to favor subsequent ones. Relapse or recurrence may be either more or less severe than the first attack.

Course and Prognosis.—These vary greatly with the type of the disease. The duration of the average case of lobular bronchopneumonia is two to three weeks, milder cases lasting often decidedly less than this, and severe ones considerably longer. *Acute toxemic* cases usually die in from one to two days. In the *disseminated* form the course is short and death may occur from asphyxia or heart-failure on the third or fourth day, often with a terminal hyperpyrexia. In patients who recover the symptoms may rapidly ameliorate or may change into those of the ordinary type. The *pseudolobar* form does not differ from the ordinary type in its course. In the *latent* form the symptoms remain uncharacteristic throughout and the duration is, therefore, uncertain. The prognosis is extremely unfavorable. In the *protracted* form death takes place after five to ten weeks, or recovery may finally occur, the symptoms and physical signs changing slowly, and general ill-health persisting for a long time. More cases die than recover.

The *prognosis in general* is always doubtful. Statistics are misleading for the reasons previously stated (p. 717). The mortality may be placed at 10 to 25 per cent in private practice and much higher in institutions. It is influenced by many conditions. Secondary cases are more unfavorable than primary ones, varying with the nature of the primary disease. In diphtheria nearly all the cases of bronchopneumonia die; in measles the mortality is also high, and in pertussis likewise. Cases due to the pneumococcus in practically pure culture are more favorable than others, and the type of pneumococcus has an influence. (See p. 718.) The mortality is higher in the first two years of life than later, and in the first year half or more of the cases die. Unfavorable hygienic conditions increase the danger.

Various *individual symptoms* have prognostic significance. Among unfavorable signs are persistent hyperpyrexia, early appearance of cyanosis, marked pallor, great dyspnea, decided irregularity of respiration, extensive involvement of the lung, persistent excessive tympanites, disappearance of cough in patients not otherwise improving, great prostration and emaciation, persistent diarrhea, prolongation of the attack over four weeks, repeated convulsions, and evidence of tuberculosis elsewhere in the body. Failure to develop leukocytosis is an unfavorable sign. Meyer[35] in studies on both croupous and bronchopneumonia in children found the mortality inversely proportionate to the number of leukocytes, except when the latter was over 50,000 per cubic millimeter.

Diagnosis.—The diagnosis of bronchopneumonia from the *croupous* form will be discussed later (p. 737). From *bronchitis* bronchopneumonia is distinguished by the greater severity of symptoms rather than by a difference in physical signs, since the latter may be late in developing. *Tuberculous bronchopneumonia* in theory is differentiated from nontuberculous forms by the lower temperature, tendency to attack the upper lobe, and the slower course. Practically the only certain diagnosis is the discovery of the tubercle bacilli; especially as the protracted cases of nontuberculous bronchopneumonia may run a very long course. In young infants and in those with rachitic chest-deformities the diagnosis of bronchopneumonia from *atelectasis* may occasion difficulty. In the latter condition there would be absence of high fever and of rapidly developing prostration. The possibility that *Vincent's infection* of the lung may occur should not be overlooked.

Roentgenograms are of service in recognizing consolidated areas in the lung, but their value must be judged in connection with symptoms and physical signs. The intensity of the shadow can not by itself be relied upon. We[36] have discussed the subject elsewhere. In general the picture of bronchopneumonia shows a more scattered and less well-defined shadow than that of croupous pneumonia, but the pseudolobar type of the former may produce an intense and uniform shadow. The shadows produced by tuberculous bronchopneumonia may not at first be distinguishable from those of the nontuberculous type.

Treatment.—This will be discussed in connection with Croupous Pneumonia (p. 739).

CROUPOUS PNEUMONIA

(Lobar Pneumonia. Fibrinous Pneumonia)

Etiology.—For the reason stated (p. 717) it is difficult to estimate the influence of age on the incidence of croupous pneumonia. The disorder is certainly one of the most common affections of early life, and even cases of intra-uterine pneumonia have been reported (Netter,[37] Levy,[38] Gordon and Lederer[39]). From our own experience, and the figures given by the authors quoted in the section upon the Etiology of Bronchopneumonia, croupous pneumonia is less often observed than is bronchopneumonia in the first two years of life, and especially in the first year, but it then increases in frequency; more cases occurring from two to six years than at any other period of infancy and childhood. Rather more males appear to be attacked. The greatest number of cases develop in the colder months and most of all in the spring, but not a few cases are seen in the summer. The disease is less common in the tropics than in the temperate zone. Direct irritation of the respiratory mucous membrane is an important etiologic factor, here being especially exposure to chilling, as also sometimes trauma of the chest, and the administration of an anesthetic, particularly ether. The previous state of health predisposes only to a limited extent. The majority of cases are *primary* in origin, and while debilitated health, tracheobronchitis, the infectious fevers, and the like may be accompanied by croupous pneumonia, these usually are predisposing causes of bronchopneumonia. There is sometimes an individual predisposition to recurrent attacks, or this may be familial. Epidemics of croupous pneumonia have been reported, but ordinarily its contagiousness is slight (p. 739).

Exciting Cause.—The first germ intimately associated with it in medical literature was the pneumobacillus of Friedländer,[40] but it has since been proven that the usual agent is that designated the diplococcus lanceolatus (diplococcus pneumoniae), or pneumococcus, earlier described by others but claimed to be the cause of pneumonia by Fränkel[41] and by Weichselbaum.[42] With this may be associated the streptococcus, staphylococcus, influenza bacillus, typhoid bacillus, colon bacillus, pneumobacillus, or other germs; and exceptionally the Friedländer bacillus acting alone would appear to produce the disease. The method of entrance of the pneumococcus and the incidence of the various types have been discussed in the section on Bronchopneumonia (p. 718).

Pathologic Anatomy.—The basis of the process is a fibrinous inflammation occupying the alveoli and bronchioles. In the first stage, that of *congestion,* lasting only a few hours, there is an exudation of serum and round cells into the alveoli, and the lining epithelium is swollen. In the second stage, that of *red hepatization,* lasting from several days to one or two weeks, the affected pulmonary tissue is hard, swollen and on section cuts and looks like liver, but with a coarsely granular surface. The alveoli and bronchioles are filled with an exudation of fibrin, epithelial cells, pneumococci, and red and white blood-corpuscles. There is usually a pneumococcic fibrinous exudate of varying thickness upon the pleura. In the third stage, that of *gray hepatization,* the lung becomes more moist and paler, because of less congestion and the increase of the exudation of white blood-cells which have undergone fatty degeneration. The pleural inflammation persists and serofibrinous and seropurulent fluid may be found in the pleural cavity. In the fourth stage, that of *resolution,* the lung becomes softer and again contains air. The change is brought about by the liquefaction of the inflammatory products. Resolution lasts but a few days as a rule; but sometimes is considerably delayed (p. 736). It generally begins with the fall of temperature to normal. The bronchial lymph-nodes are swollen and the mucous membrane of the trachea and larger bronchi is generally reddened. Occasionally pericarditis, peritonitis, meningitis, arthritis, parotitis, or general pneumococcic septicemia may be found.

Portions of the Lung Involved.—According to the statistical studies of Barthez and Sanné,[43] Comby,[3] Dunlop,[4] Koplik,[44] Cunningham,[45] Jurgensen,[46] Holt and Howland,[47] and others the disease appears to be localized oftenest either in the right upper or the left lower lobe. In approximately 5 to 10 per cent of cases portions of both lungs are involved.

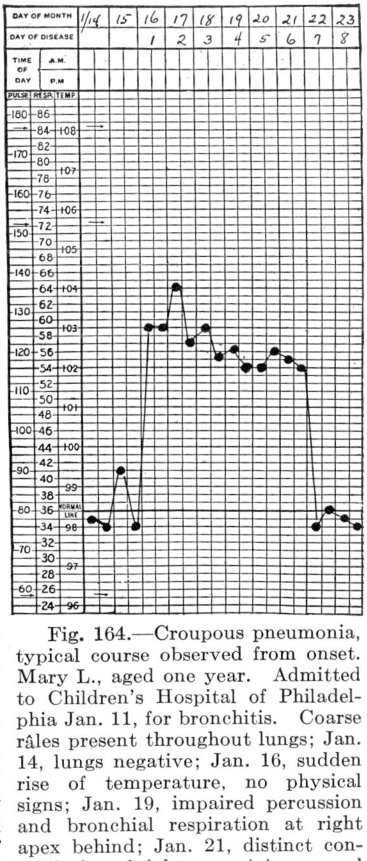

Fig. 164.—Croupous pneumonia, typical course observed from onset. Mary L., aged one year. Admitted to Children's Hospital of Philadelphia Jan. 11, for bronchitis. Coarse râles present throughout lungs; Jan. 14, lungs negative; Jan. 16, sudden rise of temperature, no physical signs; Jan. 19, impaired percussion and bronchial respiration at right apex behind; Jan. 21, distinct consolidation of right upper lobe, general condition good, pulse been 140 to 150 and respiration 50 to 65; Jan. 22, crisis.

Symptoms. (1) Typical Course.—In typical cases the disease begins suddenly, usually with vomiting, accompanied by sudden rise in temperature and sometimes diarrhea. In infancy there is often an initial convulsion, which replaces the chilliness of early childhood and the rigor occasionally seen in later childhood. The patient appears and feels ill. There are headache, prostration, flushed face, accelerated respiration and pulse, thirst, loss of appetite, and often pain referred to the chest or abdomen. Cough may be frequent, dry, harassing and painful, or may be trivial. As the disease progresses the symptoms continue in force; the fever remains high; the tongue is coated; respiration may become more dyspneic, with moving of the alae of the nose and a moaning expiration; the face is flushed; there is a slight cyanotic tint to the cheeks, lips and finger-tips; and later may follow more or less delirium, especially or solely at night, or stupor. No change takes place for the better, although often for the worse. The dyspnea perhaps grows greater, the pulse more rapid, and the strength less, with a decided degree of prostration and apathy; but by the end of from five to seven days the temperature falls rapidly by crisis to normal, perspiration occurs, respiration becomes easy, all unfavorable symptoms promptly disappear, and convalescence is rapid. In some cases the fall of temperature is accompanied by profuse sweating, feeble pulse, coldness of the extremities, pallor, decided prostration, drowsiness, and sometimes signs of undoubted collapse. In cases which terminate fatally without crisis the respiration becomes more labored, and often finally shallow and

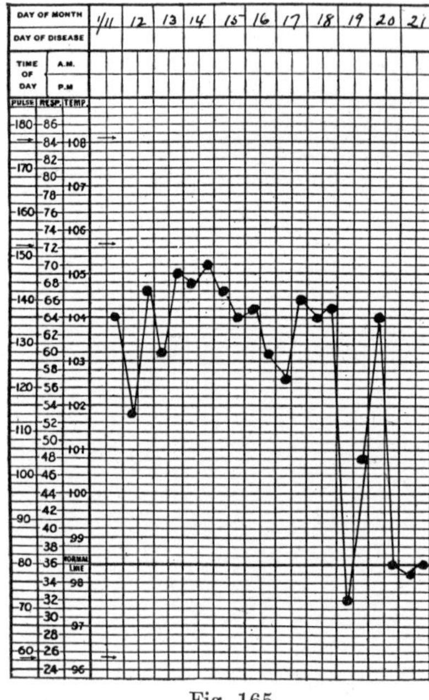

Fig. 165.

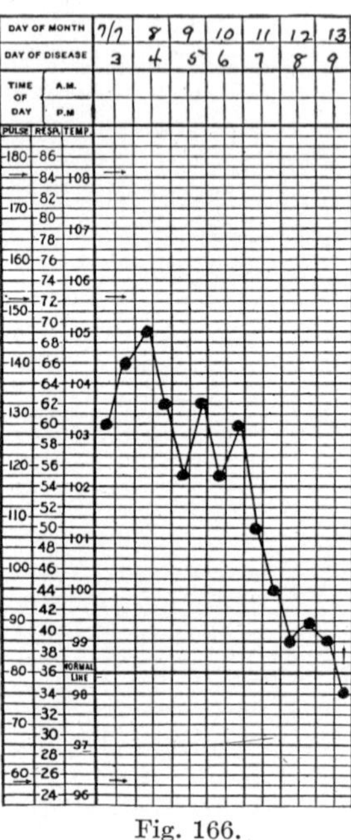

Fig. 166.

Fig. 165.—Croupous pneumonia, pseudocrisis and crisis. Rosie L., aged three years. Previous duration of the disease uncertain. Been suffering from cough, fever, loss of appetite and occasional vomiting. Entered Children's Hospital of Philadelphia Jan. 11. Examination showed bronchial respiration and dulness on percussion over the upper part of the right lung posteriorly; Jan. 16, some extension of the process in the right lung, respiration 40–60; Jan. 19, pseudocrisis; Jan. 20, no change in general condition, many râles at right base; Jan. 21, crisis.

Fig. 166.—Croupous pneumonia, fall by lysis. Walter E., three years old. Admitted to the Children's Hospital of Philadelphia, July 7. Illness began three days ago with vomiting. Dry cough on second day of disease. On admission delirious, toxic, apparently very ill; dulness, bronchial breathing and bronchophony right upper lobe. Severe symptoms began to ameliorate when the fall of temperature commenced.

very rapid; coldness of the extremities develops; there are cyanosis, rapid, feeble pulse, and increasing stupor and prostration.

A more detailed study of the characteristics usually met with is necessary:

Onset.—As a rule prodromal symptoms, such as headache, malaise, and chilliness, are absent or overlooked. An actual rigor is the exception even in later childhood. In infants marked pallor and coldness may usher in the disease. The initial convulsion is frequent in infancy; less so in early childhood. Vomiting is one of the most common symptoms of the onset.

Fever.—The rise of temperature is rapid, reaching 103 to 105 F. (39.4 to 40.6 C.) within a few hours (Fig. 164). There then follows little change in the elevation, the morning temperature being perhaps 1 or 2 F. (0.6 or 1.1 C.) less than that of the evening. The final fall is generally by a distinct crisis, a drop often of 6 or 8 F. (3.3 or 4.4 C.) to normal or below it occurring within the course of from twelve to twenty-four hours. In exceptional instances the fall of temperature may be so great that symptoms of collapse develop, and rarely even terminate fatally. The crisis takes place oftenest anywhere from the fifth to the ninth day, sometimes a day or two earlier or later. Not infrequently shortly before the final disappearance of fever a *pseudocrisis* occurs (Fig. 165); the temperature dropping to normal and giving the impression that the disease is over. A return to high fever does not necessarily indicate an extension of the process in the lung. For some days after the crisis the temperature may remain subnormal. In infants or even in older children it not infrequently runs a more irregular course throughout the attack, with greater daily differences exhibiting almost a remittent type; and a decline by lysis is frequently seen, the temperature descending gradually, requiring three or four days to reach normal (Fig. 166), and sometimes showing irregular elevations later. A decided and more persistent return of fever after the decline renders one always suspicious of some complication, especially purulent pleurisy (p. 758, Fig. 178). Fall by lysis occurs in approximately 10 per cent of cases. In fatal cases hyperpyrexia is not uncommon. However, a continued fever of 105 or even 106 F. (40.6 or 41.1 C.) is not in itself in children an unfavorable symptom. Recovery may follow even after a temperature reaches as high as 109 F. (42.8 C.) (Cough[47]) or 110 F. (43.3 C.) (Parkinson[48]). A similar case was observed by us, the temperature dropping in twelve hours from 109 F. (42.8 C.) to nearly 97 F. (36.1 C.) (Fig. 167). It is to be noted in this connection that croupous pneumonia, typical in other respects, may uncommonly run an entirely afebrile course.

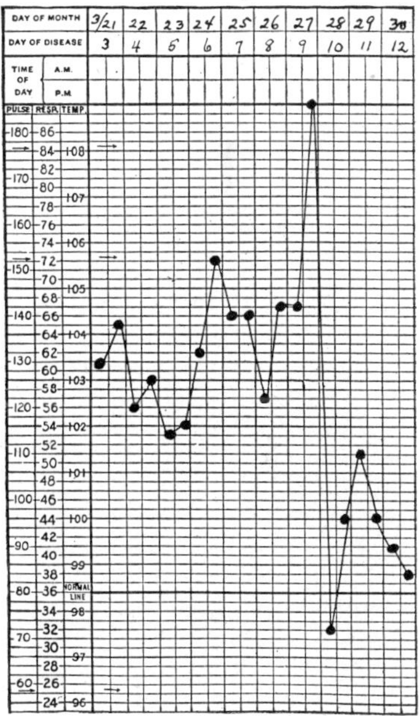

Fig. 167.—Croupous pneumonia with great hyperpyrexia. Fall of temperature of nearly 12 F. in twelve hours. Nathan M., aged five and one-fourth years. Typical croupous pneumonia upper portion of right lung. What appeared to be crisis occurred on the tenth day, with a drop of nearly 12 F. (6.7 C.) in twelve hours, with profound prostration, delirium and sleeplessness. This was followed by a slight extension of the lesion to the lower part of the right lung and moderate brief return of fever, the upper part of the lung having meanwhile cleared. Recovery.

Respiration.—The respiration is always increased in frequency, reaching from forty to eighty per minute. A certain degree of dyspnea is nearly always present, shown perhaps as mere irregularity and jerkiness in breathing. In the mildest cases it may be discoverable by placing the hand upon the abdomen, or by noticing the moving of the alae of the nose. Generally there is inspiratory retraction of the costal interspaces, with more or less tugging of the sternocleidomastoid muscles, and sinking in of the epigastrium and the episternal notch. The expiratory moan or grunt accompanying respiration is a characteristic symptom when present. The ordinary rhythm of respiration may be altered, the pause which normally follows expiration being transferred to the moment after inspiration.

Pulse.—This is always accelerated. In serious cases the tension is lowered and the pulse becomes more rapid, weak and running. A pulse-rate of 140 to 180 is not infrequent in infants and young children, and is in itself not unfavorable if the character remains good.

Pulse-temperature-respiration Ratio.—In pneumonia the pulse reaches a greater rapidity than in adult life, but, allowing for the normally higher rate in a state of health at this time of life (pp. 38; 162; 163), it does not increase with any greater ratio to the increase of temperature (10:1) than in adults. The respiration on the other hand departs from the normal ratio to the pulse, and frequently equals that of 1:2½ or even 1:2. During convalescence the pulse regains its normal rate, or is even for a time slower and irregular. This irregularity is not an unfavorable symptom.

Cough.—Repeatedly cases occur in which there is little or no cough. Generally, however, it is present and occasionally is distressing, and may be debilitating through the resulting lack of rest. The cough is dry, short, and often painful; consequently the patient makes an effort to suppress it, and a facial expression of pain, or a short cry, follows an attack. After convalescence begins the cough becomes looser through the establishing of secretion.

Expectoration.—In children beyond the age of seven or eight years, although not always then, sputum is expectorated having the characteristic rusty or blood-stained appearance and containing pneumococci. In infancy and early childhood there is rarely any expectoration, unless perhaps expelled as a result of the straining efforts attending vomiting.

Pain.—Thoracic pain is often present on coughing and often, too, independently of this. Not infrequently the pain is referred to the abdomen, and when in the region of the appendix may cause great diagnostic difficulty. (See p. 635.)

Cry.—It has been claimed that children with pneumonia cry little owing to the dyspnea present, with inability to sustain a prolonged sound. In milder attacks in infancy, however, the cry is often loud and continued.

Blood.—A prominent characteristic of pneumonia is the marked increase in the number of leukocytes, especially of the polymorphonuclear cells which reach 15,000 to 25,000 or more to the cubic millimeter, 50,000 or 60,000 being sometimes observed. Only in mild cases, or in those unfavorable ones in which there is no resisting power, is there little increase seen. The leukocytosis appears early and grows steadily greater until a day or two before the temperature falls. After the crisis the count decreases rapidly or slowly in proportion to the rapidity of the fall of temperature. If the temperature descends quickly and the leukocytosis persists it is probable that a pseudocrisis has occurred. A slow decline in the number of leukocytes with a persistence of high fever indicates delayed resolution or the development of complications. There is a retention of nonprotein nitrogenous constituents of the blood during the active stage of the disease, and the blood-chlorides are low.

Digestive Symptoms.—The initial vomiting seldom continues after the first day or two. The appetite is greatly diminished or lost, although thirst may sometimes obscure this fact in the case of infants; milk being taken in place of water in order to satisfy this. The tongue is coated, but seldom dry except in severe cases; the throat is not often involved; constipation is frequent, diarrhea common. Unusual tympanitic distention is of unfavorable prognostic import, indicating the lack of resisting power of the muscles and adding greatly to the dyspnea.

Urine.—This is high-colored, of high specific gravity, scanty, and loaded with urates, as is febrile urine from other causes. The sodium chloride is markedly diminished, but becomes of normal amount at the time defervescence occurs. A febrile albuminuria with a few hyaline casts is not uncommon, but nephritis is unusual. The presence of acetone in small amounts is a matter of no moment.

Nervous Symptoms.—The occurrence of initial convulsions has already been referred to. Headache and pain in the limbs may also be observed as early symptoms. There may be delirium, perhaps only at night or while the temperature is increasing; but infants and young children do not often in average cases exhibit more disturbance than a degree of apathy and somnolence, or perhaps sleeplessness or great restlessness. The last may reach active jactitation, especially if the dyspnea and consequent air-hunger are excessive. An unusual development of nervous symptoms is seen in cerebral pneumonia (p. 734). The severity of nervous symptoms depends more upon the height of the temperature, the intensity of the infection, and the general constitutional disturbance than upon the part or amount of pulmonary tissue involved. The patellar reflex is frequently absent (Pfaundler[49]).

General Condition.—In many instances the decision against the presence of pneumonia can almost be made by merely observing the patient, who does not look sufficiently ill. A child with pneumonia has no desire to be out of bed, and takes little, if any, interest in his surroundings. Placing him in the sitting position for examination causes evident fatigue. The prostration is, however, only temporary, for as soon as defervescence occurs strength is rapidly regained.

Skin.—Flushing of the cheeks is generally present, sometimes one more than the other; but this difference is without significance as indicating the portion of lung involved, unless the redness is due to the child lying more upon the cheek of the affected side. Cyanosis may develop, but in cases of moderate severity is slight, and seen only as a faint purplish tint to the flushed cheeks or a slight blueness of the hands or feet. This degree of cyanosis is not a sign of immediate danger, but a warning that the respiratory or circulatory power is not entirely sufficient for the work demanded. Increasing cyanosis is a distinctly threatening condition, especially if combined with pallor. Herpes of the lips, face, or other region of the body appearing about the third or fourth day is frequent.

Physical Signs.—Early in the attack the most characteristic physical signs are very fine râles at the end of inspiration, and slight localized impairment of the percussion-note; or in some cases a tympanitic note in the region which will later reveal dulness. Truly crepitant râles, however, are seldom discovered, the sounds being rather of a subcrepitant nature. If the physician's ear is placed close to the patient's open mouth a soft, fine crepitation may be heard (Burghard[50]). Auscultation of the chest may show only slight prolongation of expiration with a suspicion of a bronchial character, and slight increase of vocal resonance; or, on the other hand, feebleness of respiration over the affected area (possibly due to choking of the bronchus with secretion), with exaggerated breath-sounds over the healthy lung which is doing compensatory duty. As the consolidation increases and the affected portion becomes airless, perhaps by the second or third day, the respiration is distinctly bronchial; there is bronchophony; any mucous râles present are of coarse quality and appear to be close to the ear; friction sounds may be heard; and the dulness on percussion is decided, although not often as great as in pleural effusion. The surrounding healthy region may exhibit a hyperresonant note on percussion. If much of the lower part of the lung is involved the affected side of the chest shows diminished expansion and lessened depression of the interspaces with inspiration. Palpation may reveal increased vocal fremitus, but the feebler, higher-pitched voice of children usually renders this sign of little value.

As resolution begins râles become more numerous and there is a disappearance of the evidences of consolidation. This disappearance is sometimes remarkably rapid, and even in average cases all or nearly all evidences have vanished in two or three days. Sometimes, however, a much longer time is required.

The employment of roentgenograms will not infrequently reveal consolidation before it is discoverable by physical signs. This method of examination has apparently disproved the existence of central pneumonia, or certainly has demonstrated its rarity. Weill and Mouriquand[51] and Mason[52] have shown with roentgenograms that pneumonia begins at the periphery, the early shadow being triangular in shape with the base on the pleura. It is only when the apex of the consolidated portion has extended

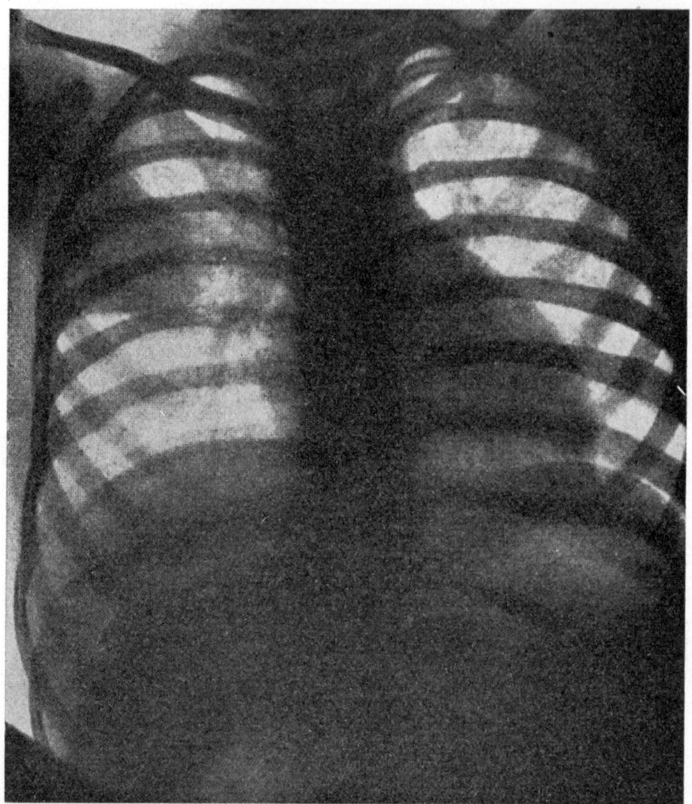

Fig. 168.—Lobar pneumonia. Fifth day of the disease. No dulness and no bronchial voice or breathing. Roentgenogram shows cone-shaped consolidation beginning at the periphery and not reaching the root of the lung. (*Mason, Am. J. Dis. Child.*, 1916, **11**, 189.)

to the hilus of the lung that bronchial breathing and bronchophony develop (Fig. 168). Earlier than this only a slight impairment of percussion-resonance and feebleness of respiratory murmur may be discovered, or often nothing whatever abnormal. Roentgenography has shown that a moderate displacement of the heart to the affected side may take place in cases of pneumonia. We[53] have observed this repeatedly, and it has been reported also by Thoenes,[54] Wahlgren,[55] Jones,[56] and Tallerman and Jupe.[57]

Significance of and Variation in Physical Signs.—One of the great characteristics of pneumonia, particularly in infancy and early childhood, is the tendency to variation, and the frequent lack of correspondence between the severity of the symptoms and the degree of development of the physical signs. In fact, at least early in the disease, the symptoms may clearly indicate the existence of a pneumonia while the signs are inconclusive. The dulness on percussion is often absent during the whole of the attack, and signs of any nature may be discovered only just before or at the time of defervescence. The hyperresonant or tympanitic note frequently heard may denote either the existence of healthy pulmonary tissue doing compensatory work, or that consolidation is about to develop in this region. In the latter event the percussion is often deep and full; not the high-pitched Skodiac tympany. Later tympany is commonly replaced by dulness. When a tympanitic note is heard under the clavicle it often signifies that consolidation is to be looked for posteriorly at the base or elsewhere on the same side. The superficial breathing of children with pneumonia frequently renders auscultation deceptive. A lung may appear normal until the child, as a result of crying, coughing, or other cause, draws a deep breath, when the bronchial character of the respiration may become evident. In other cases a slight roughening of the breath-sounds or a little prolongation of expiration may be all that can be detected. In many instances the auscultation at the time of crying is of far more value than that of respiration; bronchophony being perhaps revealed by it in a small area otherwise without physical manifestations. In fact the crying of the patient during the examination is sometimes to be desired, since during it vocal resonance may be studied to advantage, and after it the character of the following deep inspiration may be observed. In other instances the persistence of localized râles is sufficient, with the general symptoms of the disease, to make the diagnosis of consolidation certain; and this is especially true if the râles appear to be very near the ear; *i. e.*, there is *increased vocal resonance of the râles.* Fine râles are much less common in early life than in adults, being replaced by those of a more moist character.

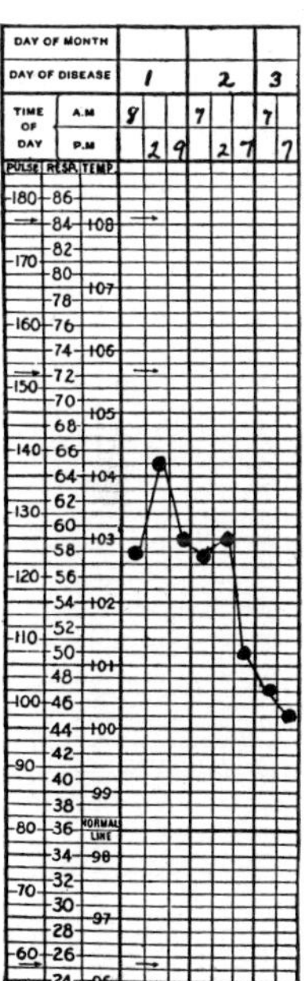

Fig. 169.—Croupous pneumonia, abortive type. A. A., male, one year old. Sudden onset, with cough, evidently severe illness, respiration dyspneic, from 60 to 70. Rapid, short course, child convalescing on second day. No certain physical signs found until several days after attack was over.

A frequent mistake is the diagnosis of pneumonia upon the wrong side of the chest. This is the result of comparing feeble respiration of the affected side with the exaggerated breathing of the other side, the incorrect conclusion being drawn that the latter is bronchial in character. Another mistake easily made is that of diagnosing a double pneumonia, when the sounds heard upon one side of the spinal column are merely those transmitted from the thoroughly consolidated lung upon the other side; the small size of the chest in early life readily lending its aid to this error.

It is often necessary to examine the lungs carefully day after day before a diagnosis based upon physical signs can be made; not forgetting careful examination of the apices in front and of the axillary regions. In these cases the lesion must be either small or so situated that it cannot be recognized by the ordinary methods. The importance of light percussion in pneumonia cannot be too strongly insisted upon, since by forcible tapping all abnormal percussion-signs are concealed by the general vibration of the whole resilient chest characteristic of the child.

Variations from the Type.—Certain of the variations from the normal course are so characteristic that they constitute distinct varieties of the disease.

2. Abortive Pneumonia.—In this not infrequent form the symptoms are well-developed, but the process terminates abruptly after only three or four days illness, or even less, and in cases of very short duration the physical signs may not become evident. A case lasting but eight hours is reported by Conrad,[58] with typical symptoms but no physical signs, the diagnosis being confirmed by roentgenograms. Among the abortive cases are to be included many of those called "congestion of the lungs," the pathologic process reaching only this stage; and very probably belong here many other instances of high fever of short duration in childhood, in which the diagnosis was entirely unsuspected. Usually in abortive pneumonia there is a rapid disappearance of the physical signs of consolidation, although sometimes they are more persistent. A number of interesting instances of this type have been detailed by Kerr,[59] and we[60] have witnessed the condition repeatedly (Fig. 169).

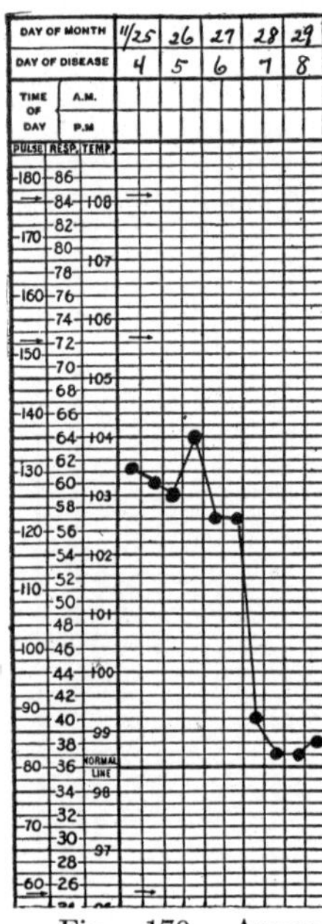

Fig. 170.—Appendicular pneumonia. Walter E. C., aged eleven years. Admitted to Children's Hospital of Philadelphia, Nov. 25. Taken ill acutely Nov. 22, with vomiting, headache, and pain at McBurney's point. This very severe and continuous until admission. Case pronounced appendicitis by two prominent physicians, one a surgeon. *Examination in Hospital.*—Respiration 40 to 45, fever, pulse 95 to 130, well-developed croupous pneumonia at base of right lung, pain had shifted to right hepatic region, epigastrium and right shoulder.

3. Cerebral Pneumonia.—This well-recognized variety is characterized by an unusual prominence of cerebral symptoms, present from the onset or developing during the course. Convulsions occur as an initial manifestation, and may be repeated. In other cases there may be unusually severe headache, squinting, rigidity, opisthotonos, persistent active delirium, coma, repeated vomiting, or other symptoms suggesting meningitis. A serous meningitis actually is present in many of these cases, the cerebrospinal fluid showing an increase of pressure, and the number of cells being above normal. In many others, however, the condition is purely a toxemic one. (See Meningismus, p. 918.) There seems to be no good ground for the formerly prevalent belief that pneumonia of the apex is particularly prone to exhibit cerebral symptoms.

4. Gastro-intestinal Pneumonia.—In this variety the digestive apparatus appears especially involved. The tongue is coated, the appetite lost, diarrhea is common, and vomiting occurs early and may be persistent without the presence of cerebral symptoms to suggest meningitis as the cause. Many such cases continue for days without physical signs, and give reason to believe that the attack is due to a digestive disturbance.

5. Appendicular Pneumonia (Fig. 170).—The characteristic of this variety is the unusual degree of pain and tenderness in the appendicular region, while symptoms pointing to respiratory disorder are but little marked. Many such cases have been diagnosed as appendicitis, and operations have repeatedly been performed. We[2] have previously reported a number of instances of the disease and reviewed the published cases, and since then an extensive literature has accumulated. (See p. 635.) Adams and Berger[61] found the diagnosis of appendicitis wrongly made in 17.8 per cent of 145 cases of croupous pneumonia in children. The combination of pneumonia and appendicitis is perfectly
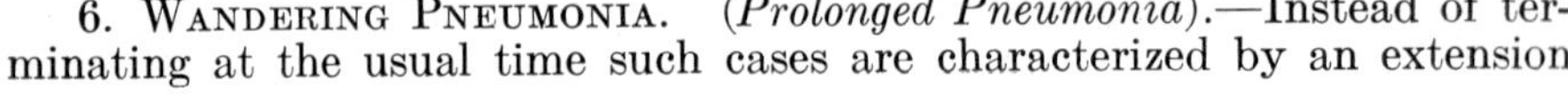
possible, although not often encountered. We have observed several cases of this nature.

6. Wandering Pneumonia. (*Prolonged Pneumonia*).—Instead of terminating at the usual time such cases are characterized by an extension

of the pneumonic process from one portion of the lung to another. The temperature may be persistently elevated, or there may be repeated remissions, or even a crisis, to be followed immediately by a renewed elevation marking the development of the disease in a fresh location. In the meanwhile resolution may take place in the part first affected and the physical signs disappear there.

7. PLEUROPNEUMONIA.—The title pleuropneumonia is applied to those cases in which a decided degree of a complicating pleurisy modifies the complex of symptoms. The constitutional manifestations and the pain in the thorax are often more marked than in ordinary pneumonia. The physical signs are a combination of those of pneumonia and of pleurisy.

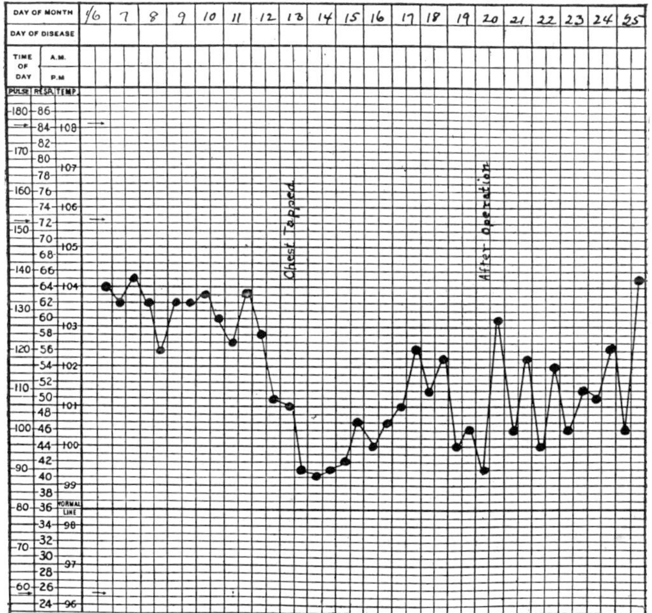

Fig. 171.—Pleuropneumonia. Chas. E., aged three years. Admitted to Children's Hospital of Philadelphia, Jan. 6, on the sixth day of the attack, with well-marked physical signs of pneumonia in the upper part of the left lung in front and over the whole left side posteriorly; Jan. 10, whole left side very dull, expansion, fremitus and breath-sounds diminished, heart displaced; Jan. 13, aspiration gave 285 cc. (9.64 fl. oz.) of straw-colored fluid containing staphylococci, temporary relief of symptoms with fall of temperature followed; Jan. 20, temperature soon rose again, general condition grew worse, very toxic, evident pressure-symptoms, exploratory puncture on 19th gave somewhat thicker and whiter fluid which deposited some sediment of pus-cells; transferred to surgical ward, and resection with drainage done; Jan. 25, been a profuse discharge of fluid, never of the characteristic appearance of empyemic pus as usually seen. Condition grew worse and death on this date.

Ordinarily the pleuritic condition does not go beyond the deposit of a large, thick, plastic exudate with small localized foci of pus (Fig. 176), but empyema is liable to develop (Fig. 171). Pneumococcic meningitis or peritonitis may be present also. (See also Pleurisy, p. 752.)

Complications and Sequels.—By all odds the most frequent complication of pneumonia is *pleuritis*. A moderate degree of dry pleurisy is, in fact, a nearly constant attendant upon all cases of pneumonia; or there may be a small amount of serous effusion. Large serous effusions are uncommon complications in early life, and particularly until childhood is well advanced, but the development of an *empyema* is a sequel especially to be feared before this period. This condition is much more frequent in children than in adults, occurring in approximately 5 to 10 per cent or more of cases. (See Pleurisy, p. 756.) Pyopneumothorax is rare (Johnson[62]). *Bronchitis* is frequent as a precursor or complication of pneumonia. *Otitis* is also common, seen oftenest in infancy and early childhood, and observed in about 15 per cent of the cases. *Endocarditis and pericarditis* are unusual. The latter is either fibrinous or purulent, and occurs oftenest in infants. *Peritonitis*, often of a pneumococcic nature, may develop in combination with pneumonia and perhaps accompanied also by pneumococcic empyema. We have seen a number of such cases. A *pneumococcic meningitis* is sometimes encountered and ends fatally. It develops usually late in the course of the pneumonia and is ushered in by convulsions, repeated vomiting and high fever, and the discovery of the pneumococcus in the spinal fluid obtained by puncture. This appears to be much less common than pneumococcic meningitis occurring alone. A *serous meningitis* is oftener seen, and systematic lumbar puncture in cases with meningitic symptoms might show it to be quite frequent. *Nephritis* occurs in occasional cases and perhaps more frequently than ordinarily believed; and *pharyngitis* is also encountered and may be pseudomembranous. Among rare complications reported may be mentioned arthritis, parotitis, hemiplegia and other paralyses, multiple neuritis, osteomyelitis, subcutaneous emphysema, gangrene of the lung, pulmonary abscess, and general pneumococcic infection.

Relapse and Recurrence.—True relapse may take place in another part of the lung, or there may be a redevelopment of the process in the portion which has just completely recovered. One attack of pneumonia offers no protection against following ones; in fact appears rather to predispose to their development (p. 726).

Course and Prognosis.—Croupous pneumonia in children past infancy as a rule terminates favorably. After the fall of temperature, resolution of the lungs takes place quickly, but where any decided degree of pleurisy has been present the impairment of percussion-resonance may be long in disappearing. Not infrequently, too, *delayed resolution* is observed and the patient, usually past the age of infancy, may continue to show both symptoms and physical signs of consolidation much longer than the usual time. Sometimes the latter continue with little change for weeks or months after the general symptoms have disappeared.

The recovery of the general health and strength in most cases of pneumonia is very rapid. In fatal cases death takes place often from cardiac weakness with secondary failure of respiration, but not frequently from interference with respiration by the extent of the pneumonic infiltration. If cyanosis is marked and combined with pallor and rapid, weak pulse, the outlook is unpromising. In cases nearing a fatal termination there are in addition to these signs coldness of the extremities; rapid, shallow, labored breathing; numerous coarse râles in the chest, and great prostration. Mere rapidity of the pulse is in itself not of moment. Great abdominal distention is also a distinctly unfavorable sign, as is a low leukocyte-count. While low blood-pressure is claimed to be an unfavorable symptom, it is by no means always so, as has been shown by the investigations of Porter and Newburgh,[63] Lambert,[64] and others. (See p. 739.) Early vomiting is a matter of no consequence, but this or diarrhea occurring later in the attack diminishes the chance of recovery. The mere existence of high temperature is not in itself an unfavorable prognostic indication in uncomplicated cases, provided hyperpyrexia is not persistent. Its continuance beyond the time when resolution should take place points to a wandering pneumonia or to complications. Severe nervous symptoms early in the disease will probably be of temporary duration; occurring later they are of more serious prognostic import, since they may depend upon a meningitis. The presence of pneumococci in the blood adds to the gravity of the case. The existence of any complication increases the danger. Pneumococcic meningitis is usually fatal; peritonitis is very serious; empyema serious especially in young infants.

The prognosis is influenced to some extent by the type of the disease. Abortive pneumonia terminates favorably, as its name indicates. Pleuropneumonia is always serious. There is in it a great liability to the development of empyema, or occasionally of chronic pneumonia. In pleuropneumonia in infancy death is very liable to occur even early in the course. Wandering pneumonia is dangerous on account of the long duration and necessarily greater exhaustion produced. The development of pneumonia in the course of other acute diseases or in those enfeebled by imperfect hygienic or chronic diseases naturally adds to the danger. Among other prognostic influences are the type of infecting micro-organisms (p. 718) and the character of the epidemic, the malignancy of the disease being decidedly greater at some times than at others. The influence of age is very decided. The greater majority of fatal cases in early life are in subjects under three years, and especially under one year of age. The extent of the lesion bears some relationship to the prognosis; but only to a certain degree.

In general the mortality figures of croupous pneumonia in early life are surprisingly low. The usual mortality in children, including infancy, according to a number of statistical calculations, is from 3 to 5 per cent, some series being decidedly over this. This is in sharp contrast to the high mortality for adults. The figures for the first two years of life, however, are distinctly higher, even reaching in some exceptional series approximately 25 per cent in hospital practice. In private practice the mortality is lower. In uncomplicated pneumonia of an undoubtedly croupous nature in healthy subjects in childhood the patient almost always recovers, and even in infancy the mortality is low. Many cases reported as fatal have been in reality instances of bronchopneumonia. A small number recover from the acute attack, but suffer from abscess or gangrene of the lung, interstitial pneumonia, or tuberculosis as sequels.

Diagnosis.—The diagnosis in general rests upon the sudden onset with a convulsion or chilliness and, not infrequently, vomiting; the rapid rise of temperature, its persistence at a high elevation, and its final rapid fall; the increased rate of respiration with the ordinary signs of usually moderate dyspnea; the possible slight cough; the suppressed cry or expiratory moan in infants; the aspect of decided illness; and the physical signs as described.

Owing, however, to the irregularity in symptoms and in the appearance and character of the physical signs, mistakes in diagnosis are easily made. The disease is to be differentiated especially from simple or tuberculous *bronchopneumonia.* The chief distinguishing features of bronchopneumonia consist in its frequent existence as a secondary disease; slower and more insidious onset; slower development of physical signs, which are oftener in diffuse lesions with scattered mucous râles due to the attendant bronchitis; involvement generally of both lungs, especially the bases; slower rise of temperature and a more irregular temperature-curve with frequent remissions at uncertain times; decidedly greater degree of dyspnea; longer course, and more gradual disappearance of symptoms and physical signs. But frequent failure, on the one hand, of croupous pneumonia to run a typical course and, on the other hand, the not uncommon occurrence of pseudolobar forms of bronchopneumonia, as well as other deceptive symptoms, make the diagnosis often one of the greatest difficulty. (See p. 723.)

The next most frequent cause of difficulty in diagnosis is *pleurisy.* The principal differential diagnostic marks of pleurisy in typical cases, after effusion has taken place, are the slower development; greater degree and extent of dulness on percussion combined with feeble voice and breath-sounds; absence of vocal fremitus; absence or feebleness of bronchitic râles; a percussion-dulness shifting with change of position; fullness of the intercostal spaces and increased resistance there on palpation; greater diminution in the respiratory expansion of the affected side; displacement of the apex-beat in lesions of the left side of the chest; feebleness of the voice and breath-sounds even if these are of a bronchial character. The dulness is most intense in the lower part of the chest and posteriorly. In spite of these characteristics the diagnosis is often uncertain and frequently only the employment of exploratory puncture can settle it, and this examination should always be made in doubtful cases. In pleuropneumonia the diagnosis is, of course, rendered doubly difficult, and here even exploratory puncture may give no positive results, owing to the exudate being largely plastic.

Delayed resolution in pneumonia is to be distinguished from a *slowly disappearing plastic or serous pleurisy* by the presence of decided auscultatory signs of consolidation with the absence of those of pleurisy; although the evidences from percussion may be equivocal. *Chronic interstitial pneumonia* may exhibit physical signs not readily distinguishable in some respects from those of delayed resolution; but differs in the history of the case, the character of the symptoms, the presence of evidences of contraction of the lung or of bronchiectasis, and in the fact that there is not, as in delayed resolution, a final disappearance of all symptoms and physical signs.

Cerebral pneumonia suggests often the possibility of the presence of *meningitis* of some kind. Leukocytosis occurs in both conditions. The employment of lumbar puncture will be of service early in the attack; while later the development of the physical signs of pneumonia renders the diagnosis clear, except in those cases where pneumonia and meningitis are combined. Cerebral pneumonia exhibits its nervous symptoms usually at the beginning of the attack and these persist, as a rule, but a short time. Meningitis occurring as a complication of pneumonia comes on later in the disease when physical signs of the pulmonary disorder are already present.

Grippe at its onset often closely resembles pneumonia. There may be a convulsion followed by sudden, rapid rise of temperature, cough, and rapidity of respiration. Only after several days can pneumonia be excluded by the failure of characteristic symptoms and physical signs to appear.

Scarlet fever is sometimes suspected on account of the initial vomiting and high fever. This is true also of cases of *gastro-intestinal disturbance*. In some instances of pneumonia with few constitutional manifestations it is only the existence of a respiratory rate out of proportion to other symptoms which distinguishes the condition from an attack of indigestion with fever. Appendicular pneumonia so closely resembles the onset of *appendicitis* that operations for this condition have repeatedly been needlessly performed. (See Appendicitis, p. 635.) The only safeguard is a careful repeated examination of the lungs, and perhaps a roentgenogram before operation is done.

Massive collapse of the lung is to be distinguished by the displacement of the heart toward the affected side; the high position of the diaphragm as shown by the roentgen-ray; the mildness of constitutional symptoms, and the presence of an exciting cause which would have acted by bringing about immobilization of the diaphragm or respiratory muscles. As already stated (p. 732) however, moderate cardiac displacement to the affected side may occur in some cases of pneumonia. We[53] have observed this repeatedly.

The mistake of overlooking a pneumonia is much more common than that of wrongly considering it present. Consequently every child with sudden development of high temperature should have its chest carefully examined as a routine measure, and the examination repeated frequently as long as the diagnosis is not entirely beyond question; but in doing this it must never be forgotten, as already pointed out, that the diagnosis of pneumonia in early life rests more upon the symptoms than upon the physical signs, and that pneumonia cannot be excluded solely because no physical signs are discovered.

Treatment of Bronchopneumonia and of Croupous Pneuomnia.—It is more convenient to consider together the therapeutic measures for the two diseases.

Prophylaxis.—In general those prophylactic procedures are to be followed which are recommended for preventing any inflammation of the respiratory tract (pp. 685–687), and prompt treatment given for any respiratory infection, especially in infancy. As indicated, primary cases are unlikely to be contagious, but the secondary forms of bronchopneumonia, particularly those following the infectious fevers, may possibly be so. At any rate isolation should be carried out, and especially in hospital wards pneumonic patients should be separated from those with other respiratory diseases or with infectious fevers. In institutions or wherever large groups of persons are in close contact, or in recurring attacks of pneumonia, polyvalent pneumococcic vaccines have been employed with apparent success in prevention (Cecil,[65] Neumann and Happe[36]).

Treatment of the Attack.—It is of great importance to remember that croupous pneumonia in children is a self-limited disease which runs a short and usually favorable course. Apart from hygienic and analogous measures the best medicinal treatment of the average case frequently is the absence of it. Skillful nursing and watchfulness by the physician are the important matters, with a prompt but not officious assistance when required. In the case of bronchopneumonia, however, symptomatic treatment is more frequently indicated.

Hygiene.—The child should be confined to bed, but its position changed frequently, laying it now on the abdomen, now on one side or the other, in order to prevent hypostatic congestion. Infants may be held upright for short periods and dyspnea possibly relieved in this way, or older children may be helped by extra pillows or a back-rest; but in the main they may be allowed to choose the position most comfortable to them. The extremities should be kept warm, and the bed-covering usually light, but of a weight in accord with the sensation of the patient. There is practically no danger from chilling of a pneumonic patient with fever. The open cold-air treatment, with the child thoroughly wrapped up, is undoubtedly of benefit in properly selected cases. There are, however, many exceptions to this, especially with very young infants, and in those with bronchopneumonia who have abundant bronchial secretion. Here the best results, in our experience, are obtained by placing the patient in a croup-tent or in a room with warm, moist air. This often gives surprising relief to the cough, dyspnea, cyanosis, and general distress. Careful judgment must be exercised in selecting the treatment for the case. The cold-air treatment seems to make the child more comfortable, but it appears to be based upon an observation which has not been substantiated, namely, that it increases blood-pressure and that this is beneficial. The observations of Freeman,[66] Morse and Hassman,[67] and others indicate that blood-pressure bears no relationship to the temperature of the surrounding air; and it has been shown by others that it has little relationship to prognosis. The matter illustrates the fact that no routine treatment of this or any other sort exists, and that sometimes only trial can determine the selection. The croup-tent should not be used continuously, since the air becomes overheated and stale. Under all conditions the air in the room must be fresh and pure. A fire in an open fireplace is one of the most satisfactory means for obtaining this, or ventilation may be secured from another room.

Diet.—Milk is probably the best food, but the appetite is so diminished that there can be given any digestible liquid or semi-liquid nourishment suitable to the age, which the patient can be induced to take. The caloric intake should especially be watched in bronchopneumonia, since the disease may be long-continued and exhausting. Sometimes milk of any sort, even diluted, is not well tolerated and causes or increases tympanites. Water should be supplied abundantly, and if not enough is ingested a daily enteroclysis may be given, or hypodermoclysis employed. Intraperitoneal injections may be serviceable unless there is already abdominal distention.

Counterirritation.—This is of little value in croupous pneumonia, but may be beneficial in bronchopneumonia with a large bronchitic element, or for pleuritic pain. Mustard-plasters every three or four hours are helpful under these circumstances. Poultices are rarely useful and their weight may interfere with respiration. The cotton-jacket is of little value. Dry cupping is advantageous in severe cases of bronchopneumonia. When crisis occurs in croupous pneumonia external heat may be useful if the fall of temperature is excessive.

Inhalations.—These are serviceable in relieving cough, especially in bronchopneumonia. Benzoin, menthol, and the like may be used in the water employed in the moist-room treatment, or given from a croup-kettle. Inhalations of oxygen, or of oxygen and carbon dioxide, not too continuously employed, are of great value in cardiac or respiratory failure, and should be given before these are too far advanced. Efforts should be made to administer oxygen in from at least 35 to 50 per cent concentration. In the ordinary crude inhalation-method only about 5 per cent of it reaches the lung, although even this gives some symptomatic relief. Effective concentration may be secured under the croup-tent or by means of special tents and oxygen-chambers. We have had excellent results by administering it through a catheter strapped in place as a nasal tube, and the effectiveness of this has been shown by Barach.[68] The catheter should be a No. 10 French, the terminal inch should be perforated by six small holes, and it should be employed in conjunction with a high pressure oxygen tank. Prolonged use of the nasal catheter causes irritation of the pharyngeal mucous membrane. The gas can be administered for a few minutes every half hour or hour, or can be given more or less continuously when urgently needed. Oxygen has been given subcutaneously in doses of 200 to 400 cc. (Kirk,[69] Montford[70]). In the prevention of postanesthetic pneumonia inhalations of oxygen and carbon dioxide are recommended by Henderson, Haggard and Coburn,[71] and Henderson.[72]

Hydrotherapy.—Treatment of this sort is needed in croupous pneumonia only if hyperpyrexia is present, or with more moderate fever to relieve nervous symptoms and to increase the sensation of comfort of the child; since it is not the high temperature but the accompanying nervous manifestations which may need control. In bronchopneumonia, however, with its longer course, hydrotherapy fills a more important place. Infants may be given a warm tub-bath every three hours if the temperature exceeds 103 F. (39.4 C.) or if there are decided nervous manifestations. It often produces fall in temperature, stimulates the circulation, relieves restlessness and dyspnea, and induces sleep. In patients with feeble circulation or in those with bronchopneumonia and low temperature, brief plunging into the hot bath with or without mustard is sometimes helpful. The tepid pack is often successful in the reduction of fever. Sponges and packs may be more tedious and trying to the child and less efficacious than the tub-bath. (For technique of these various procedures, see pp. 190–195.)

Most infants and many older children do not tolerate cold water well, and sponges or tubs with water of 70 F. (21.1 C.) are seldom more efficacious and generally more depressing than those with warmer water. Symptoms indicating circulatory weakness are a special warning against the use of cold water. Always hydrotherapy in any form must be adapted to the case. It is often not well borne.

Internal Medication.—Drugs should be given only when really needed, and with due consideration of possible digestive upset. Particularly in croupous pneumonia there is a disposition to overdose. Moderate stimulation is advisable in many instances, and it is easier to sustain the strength of the patient than to restore it. While alcohol has been used too frequently and much has been written against it, it is our clinical experience that in some way it does good in many cases. The initial dose may be 15 to 30 minims (0.92 to 1.8) of whiskey or its equivalent every three hours for a child of two years. Mild cases do not need it. The value of digitalis in pneumonia is a subject of much controversy. We believe that it should certainly be given where there is auricular fibrillation; or where myocardial weakness is known to have existed previously, or the symptoms show that it is developing. It seems to us that it has value in bronchopneumonia, but it is better to start it early, and that digitalization be brought about before the onset of cardiac failure. (For dosage of digitalis, see p. 795.) In the average case of croupous pneumonia it is seldom required. For rapid stimulation in cases of cardiac or respiratory failure there may be given, to an infant of one year, hypodermic injections of 2 to 4 minims (0.12 to 0.25) of camphor and oil (1:10), caffein sodium-benzoate ($\frac{1}{8}$ to $\frac{1}{4}$ grain) (0.008 to 0.016), or epinephrine [(2 to 4 minims) (0.12 to 0.25) of a 1:1000 solution]. Nitroglycerin hypodermically, $\frac{1}{200}$ grain (0.0003), is often valuable in relieving an overburdened heart. Atropine, $\frac{1}{2000}$ to $\frac{1}{1000}$ grain (0.00003 to 0.00006) every three or four hours is a serviceable respiratory stimulant, and useful where there is a large amount of secretion. Strychnine is used, but offers no advantage over the drugs mentioned and may induce nervous excitability. We feel that it is often employed too frequently. Its dose is $\frac{1}{300}$ grain (0.0002) every three or four hours at one year. The sedative of most value is opium if there are no contraindications, and it is certainly one of the most helpful means to support the heart. It does not appear to be frequently required for cough or restlessness in croupous pneumonia, but in bronchopneumonia seems sometimes almost indispensible. In place of it symptoms may often be controlled by a barbital derivative, antipyrine, or phenacetin. Such drugs should be given at frequent intervals in small doses.

Special Symptoms and Complications.—The treatment of these has been outlined in part, but the subject may be reviewed briefly. Cyanosis and pallor demand medicinal stimulation and the use of the hot pack or bath and oxygen. Judicious bleeding may be of great value in older patients with dilatation of the right side of the heart. Moderate fever requires no treatment except hydrotherapy. Should this not be well tolerated, small doses of coal tar derivatives may be given if necessary. Excessive bronchial secretion is best treated by counterirritation and atropine, and occasionally by emetics. Expectorants of any sort are of doubtful value, and not indicated at all for the fibrinous exudate of croupous pneumonia. Cough is often relieved by inhalation; if not, and if it is frequent and weakening, sedatives may be given, including opiates if necessary. Nervous symptoms are best treated by hydrotherapy or the administration of small repeated doses of sedatives. Tympanites is to be relieved by the rectal tube, douching the intestine with saline solution, the application of turpentine-stupes or mustard-plasters to the abdomen, and the rectal administration of milk of asafetida. In severe cases not responding to these measures, a hypodermic injection of eserine, $\frac{1}{500}$ grain (0.00013) to a child of two years, often gives relief. Its depressing action must not be forgotten. Pituitrin has been used for this condition, but is of little value in our experience. Diarrhea and vomiting, and also tympanites, may demand a change in diet, especially withdrawal of milk. Douching of the bowel and mild purges are also of benefit for these symptoms. Convulsions require bromides, chloral, and other sedatives; and in certain cases where there is increase of intracranial pressure lumbar puncture is indicated. There is a theoretical danger in this procedure in that the relief of intracranial pressure may favor the passage of micro-organisms from the blood-stream into the subarachnoid space. We have on two occasions seen pneumococcic meningitis develop after spinal puncture in cases of pneumonia.

There has been discussion regarding the advisability of administering alkalies in croupous pneumonia to prevent a possible acidosis (Means and Barach;[73] Killian;[74] Haden;[75] Binger, Hastings and Sendroy;[76] Darrow and Hartmann[77]). With the favorable course run by the great majority of cases of croupous pneumonia in children, there seems no good reason for any medical interference of this sort. The same is true of the routine administration of quinine preparations.

Miscellaneous Methods.—Diathermy has been used in the treatment of pneumonia and good results with it in children have been reported by Forbes.[78] Ibrahim and Duken,[79] Coghlan,[80] and others have used artificial pneumothorax during the acute stage of pneumonia. W. J. Freeman and his coworkers[81] employed mercurochrome intravenously in both croupous and bronchopneumonia, giving 0.005 Gm. per kilogram (0.03 grain per pound) of body weight. Particularly in prolonged bronchopneumonia where there is anemia favorable results may be obtained from blood-transfusions (Bass[82]). As recommended by Quimby and Quimby,[83] Krost,[84] and others radiologic treatment may hasten cure in delayed resolution in croupous pneumonia, and we have found this of value in some instances. Nonspecific protein therapy has likewise been employed, injecting such substances as sodium nucleinate.

Specific Treatment.—Various therapeutic sera and vaccines have been used, but much more widely in adults than in children. The best results are obtained with antiserum for Type I pneumococcus. A serum has also been developed for Type II, but none which are satisfactory for Types III and IV. These sera can be of relatively little value in children, since Type I pneumococcus is so seldom found. (See p. 718.) Huntoon and his coworkers[85] have prepared a serum or antibody solution, and Felton[86] a similar solution. These are concentrated and refined so that inert and deleterious chill-producing substances are largely removed, and it is claimed that they lower the mortality in pneumonia due to Types I and II pneumococcus. Treatment with convalescent's serum is said to be helpful (Gundel[87]). Favorable results with vaccine therapy have been maintained by many, among them Wynn[88] and Lambert.[89] Pneumococci alone may be used, or the vaccine contain the streptococcus, staphylococcus, micrococcus catarrhalis, and other germs. Nobécourt and Paraf[90] claim favorable results in infants from injection of autoserum into the consolidated lung. Berger and Montgomery[91] have given chicken blood, or the serum, intravenously or intramuscularly to children with pneumonia, on the ground that it contains protective bodies.

It must be admitted that, as far as children are concerned, no form of so-called "specific therapy" offers uncontested evidence of value.

Convalescence.—Cases of croupous pneumonia generally convalesce rapidly. No treatment is needed, and a full diet may be resumed promptly. The patient should be kept in bed until evidences of consolidation have disappeared, a matter of a week or ten days or less. An exception exists in the cases with physical signs of delayed resolution, yet without symptoms. Such children may be cautiously taken from bed despite the physical signs. The slow and irregular pulse rate often observed after pneumonia is usually unimportant.

With bronchopneumonia tonic treatment is often required. Particular attention should be paid to the improvement of the general health, and if there is much anemia or debility change of climate is often beneficial.

CHRONIC PNEUMONIA

(Interstitial Pneumonia)

Etiology.—The title "chronic pneumonia," which in no way applies to the delayed resolution of croupous pneumonia, properly designates the long persistence of constitutional symptoms and physical signs, which, in the large majority of cases of chronic pneumonia, occurs as a sequel to bronchopneumonia. It is rarely seen after the ordinary croupous form; somewhat oftener after a pleuropneumonia; and exceptionally after chronic bronchitis, chronic passive congestion of the lungs, or chronic pleurisy. It is likely that hereditary syphilis is a factor in some cases, as in those reported by Smith.[92] It is especially liable to develop when there have been repeated attacks of the acute form, or when this has occurred in connection with the infectious diseases, particularly measles, pertussis, and grippe, or has depended on the presence of a foreign body in a bronchus. Some cases, especially when associated with bronchiectasis, may be continued, if not initiated, by chronic infection in the upper respiratory tract. Chronic pneumonia is sometimes tuberculous, either primarily or by later secondary infection. The disease is more common in childhood than later, and especially in late infancy and early childhood; the period when bronchopneumonia is more often observed.

Pathologic Anatomy.—In fully-developed cases there are bands of connective tissue passing in different directions through the lungs, starting from the pleura, which in itself thickened. The alveoli are obliterated by organizing infiltration, their walls as well as those of the small bronchi are much thickened, and in many places these bronchi are dilated. The process is irregularly distributed, healthy areas being adjacent to those diseased. The lesions are most marked about the bronchi, and in advanced cases decided bronchiectasis is observed. Usually only a part of one lobe is involved, and the lower part of the lung is more often attacked, except in tuberculous cases. In cases which have lasted over a year no trace of healthy pulmonary tissue may be discoverable in the parts involved, and sections show only much dilated bronchial tubes filled with mucopus.

Symptoms.—After a severe and long continued attack of bronchopneumonia the symptoms may finally disappear, except perhaps a certain degree of debility and anemia, with moderate cough and shortness of breath. Examination, however, shows some traces, or even more decided evidences, of physical signs of consolidation remaining. In other cases the physical signs are first found after an attack of pertussis in which no acute bronchopneumonia had been discovered; or they develop in the course of a prolonged gastro-intestinal disturbance; or in still others the initial disease was considered to be a plastic pleurisy only. After a variable time there may be a second attack of pneumonia with slow convalescence; or without this there may develop more or less fever of a remittent type, and there is eventually a progressive loss of weight and strength; troublesome cough; increasing dyspnea; and sometimes pain in the chest, sweating, clubbing of the fingers, and diarrhea. Fever may be absent for days and return again.

As the disease advances the physical signs become characteristic. Evidences of decided shrinking of the lung appear. If this is at the apex there will be depression of the supraclavicular fossa. If in the region of the heart an abnormally large cardiac dulness and unusually distinct pulsation are observed. There are also decided dulness on percussion, diminished expansion of the affected region, and very commonly a peculiarly feeble respiratory murmur. Sometimes bronchial respiration and bronchophony are found, if not present earlier; and over large bronchiectases or numerous associated smaller ones there may be a somewhat tympanitic note on percussion and a respiratory murmur suggesting the existence of a cavity. The diaphragm may be drawn upward on the affected side, and eventually there may develop decided deformity of the chest. The intensity of all the signs depends upon the extent and degree of pulmonary change which has taken place. They may vary, too, from day to day. If only a partial consolidation exists, the respiration may be merely bronchovesicular or enfeebled, with slight impairment of percussion resonance. Bronchitic râles are a variable element, present only at such times as an attack of bronchitis coexists. When bronchiectasis is well-developed and has become a prominent lesion, there is usually abundant mucopurulent secretion of a more or less offensive odor. Hemoptysis sometimes occurs.

Course and Prognosis.—Until decided shrinking of the lung has taken place, complete resorption is possible, yet it may take months for this to be accomplished. After this shrinking has occurred the passing of the physical signs is impossible; but this by no means precludes recovery from the majority of the symptoms. In many cases the course of the disease is typically chronic, with exacerbations at times, and with a tendency to gradual involvement of a whole lung. The general health may be excellent for a long time, but eventually suffers, and finally death may occur after months or years of increasing emaciation, anemia, and exhaustion. Death may occur in a recurrent attack of pneumonia. Many of the cases, if not tuberculous at the onset, finally become so.

Diagnosis.—This rests chiefly upon the history of the case and on the presence of persistent physical signs of consolidation after a pneumonia. *Delayed resolution* of a pneumonia is to be distinguished by its association with the croupous form of the disease, the absence of the symptoms of chronic pneumonia as described, and the final recovery after a much shorter time than the duration of chronic pneumonia. *Pleural effusion* is to be excluded by its more widespread and absolute dulness on percussion, the presence of egophony, and the absence of vocal fremitus. The last sign is, however, equivocal, since the thickening of the pleura seen in chronic pneumonia may readily diminish vocal fremitus. The employment of the exploring needle is the surest diagnostic method between the two conditions, but is not without some danger if the disease is an interstitial pneumonia. The most important and the most difficult diagnostic question is between the *simple* and the *tuberculous* forms of chronic pneumonia. Tuberculosis affects more often the apex; simple chronic pneumonia the base. The tuberculin-reaction, if negative, indicates the simple form of the disease. Repeated examination of the sputum even with final positive findings, does not prove that the affection was primarily tuberculous. In any case of chronic nontuberculous pulmonary disease, especially if the signs are localized in one lung, the possibility of the presence of a *foreign body* should be borne in mind.

Treatment.—This is essentially tonic in character. The administration of cod-liver oil is one of the best methods, and iodide of potassium is to be recommended in some cases. Any chronic infection in the upper respiratory tract should be treated. The clothing and the habit of life in general should be such that exacerbations of the disease are prevented. Cool morning baths are of service if well tolerated. Abundant digestible nourishment is necessary. Change of climate and life in the open air are among the best of remedies. Pulmonary gymnastics are of service in expanding the diseased lung if the condition has not advanced too far. When there is decided bronchiectasis the treatment recommended for this condition is to be employed (p. 716).

HYPOSTATIC PNEUMONIA

This is the result of prolonged passive congestion from various causes. It may attend, for instance, severe typhoid fever, or occur in any marantic state such as seen in the chronic gastro-enteric diseases of infancy. Lying long in one position may favor its development. The **lesions** consist of a low-grade inflammation of the pulmonary tissue beginning in the lower portion of the lung. They differ from mere congestion in the presence of an exudate of epithelium, and of red and white blood-cells. The process is lobular and affects only the more dependent portions of the lungs, generally on both sides. The **symptoms** are uncharacteristic. There is neither dyspnea nor fever, unless dependent upon the primary disorder. The physical signs consist principally in slight dulness on percussion, feeble respiratory murmur, and the presence of moist râles. In the way of **prognosis** the condition is only a sign of the influence which the primary disease is exerting, and, while it increases the danger, is not in itself the real cause of death. The **treatment** is preventive, consisting in that of the primary affection, in sustaining the general and circulatory strength, and in frequent change of position.

PULMONARY EMPHYSEMA

Emphysema, always a secondary affection, may be either *acute* or *chronic*. The former is common and is seen oftener in childhood than at any other period. It may be produced by any condition which increases the air-pressure in the lung. Thus it may be a *compensatory* process in pneumonia, atelectasis, or in pleural adhesions which interfere locally with expansion of the lung. In other cases it is *obstructive* and follows forcible coughing, such as occurs in pertussis and bronchitis, or results from obstruction to breathing, as in diphtheria of the larynx. The more chronic form is less common in early life, and seen then chiefly in later childhood. It is liable to follow long-continued dyspnea, as in rachitic deformities, tuberculosis, chronic pneumonia, asthma, chronic bronchitis, adenoids, and tracheobronchial adenitis; or it may persist after severe acute bronchopneumonia or pertussis. The **lesions** in *acute vesicular emphysema* consist merely in the distension of the vesicles. It may be generalized, but is more frequently limited to certain regions, as the anterior border of the lungs, especially of the upper lobe, or may be scattered among areas of consolidation or atelectasis if these are present. The affected portion is paler and more prominent than normal, and does not collapse readily. In *chronic emphysema*, which also may be generalized or partial, there is permanent loss of elasticity, and many of the alveoli are ruptured and communicate with each other, producing distended saccules up to the size of a pea or larger. As a further result of the rupture, air may enter the interstitial pulmonary tissue (*interstitial emphysema*), or accumulate between the lobules (*interlobular emphysema*), or even under the pleural surface or about the root of the lung or in the mediastinum, from whence it may find its way into the subcutaneous tissue (*subcutaneous emphysema*). (See p. 1093.) Mediastinal emphysema has been studied especially by Stransky.[93] The **symptoms** are not definite, being masked by the attendant primary disease. Physical examination shows marked hyperresonance on percussion, perhaps with obliteration or diminution of the cardiac dulness and depression of the upper border of the hepatic dulness, and accompanied by feeble respiratory murmur and diminished vocal fremitus. The only certain clinical evidence of the interstitial form is the rare occurrence of subcutaneous emphysema, appearing first in the neck. The **prognosis** depends upon the primary disease. In cases attending acute conditions, emphysema disappears following recovery from the primary disorder. In chronic cases, as in asthma, hyperresonance is persistent, the chest becomes barrel-shaped, and the expiratory excursion is limited. Emphysema adds to any dyspnea and cyanosis which the primary disease may produce. The **treatment** is that of the primary affection.

ATELECTASIS

Atelectasis as occurring in the new-born has already been discussed (p. 233). One of the principal **causes** in infancy is unusually well-developed rickets, which favors its production by the deformity and lowered resiliency of the chest-wall, and the diminished muscular power. Other deformities, as from caries of the spine, also predispose to it, as does any debilitating disease. Consequently it is frequent in atrophic and debilitated states in infancy, the tendency to it being increased by the weakened force of the cough at this time and the feeble respiratory power. It is produced also by the pressure of intrathoracic tumors, pericardial effusion, pneumothorax, and especially pleural effusion. A common cause is severe bronchitis or bronchopneumonia, in which collapse of the vesicles follows obstruction of a bronchus by mucus. Acquired atelectasis is thus an attendant upon numerous affections, but is not a primary disease. The **lesions** consist of regions in the lung which are airless, congested, deep-red in color, hard, and depressed below the neighboring healthy or emphysematous lung. The distribution is in the form of scattered lobules, but in some cases a considerable portion of a lobe is involved by coalescence. When dependent upon local compression, as by a pericardial or pleural effusion, or a deformed chest, the distribution corresponds with these conditions. When of long duration the lung shrinks from connective-tissue changes. The **symptoms** are gradual in onset. There are rapid shallow respirations, dyspnea with inspiratory recession of the thoracic wall, rapid feeble pulse, normal or subnormal temperature, and cyanosis. On physical examination there is a feeble respiratory murmur with moist râles, and perhaps slight dulness on percussion. Both symptoms and physical signs are often masked by the primary disease. In other cases the disease cannot be distinguished clinically from hypostatic pneumonia. The **prognosis** depends upon the cause and upon the age. Cases due to pleural effusion recover when this is removed, unless adhesions remain. In rickets the prognosis is unfavorable because of the persistence of chest-deformity. In all chronic debilitated conditions, and in disorders obstructing respiration, prognosis is unfavorable, especially under the age of two years, and the collapse of the lung greatly increases the danger already existing. **Treatment** consists in frequent change in position, stimulating hot baths, hot mustard-packs, maintaining the body temperature, fresh air, inhalation of oxygen, and the like.

MASSIVE COLLAPSE (MASSIVE ATELECTASIS) OF THE LUNG

(Apneumatosis)

Attention was first directed to this condition by W. Pasteur,[94] occurring in his cases in children. The **etiologic** factor is often one which brings about immobilization of the diaphragm or respiratory muscles. Thus it may follow general or local anesthesia, particularly in operations on the upper abdomen, although also consecutive to those for hernia or appendicitis. Postdiphtheritic paralysis of the diaphragm may be a cause, as may trauma of the thoracic wall and occasionally of the pelvic region. Affections of the central nervous system, such as poliomyelitis and meningitis, may be operative. Any obstruction in a bronchus brought about by a foreign body, chronic inflammatory products, asthma, or tuberculosis; or pressure as by tumor, pericardial effusions and the like constitutes another group of causes. Experimentally the condition has been produced in dogs by the injection into their bronchi of material removed from the bronchi of human cases,

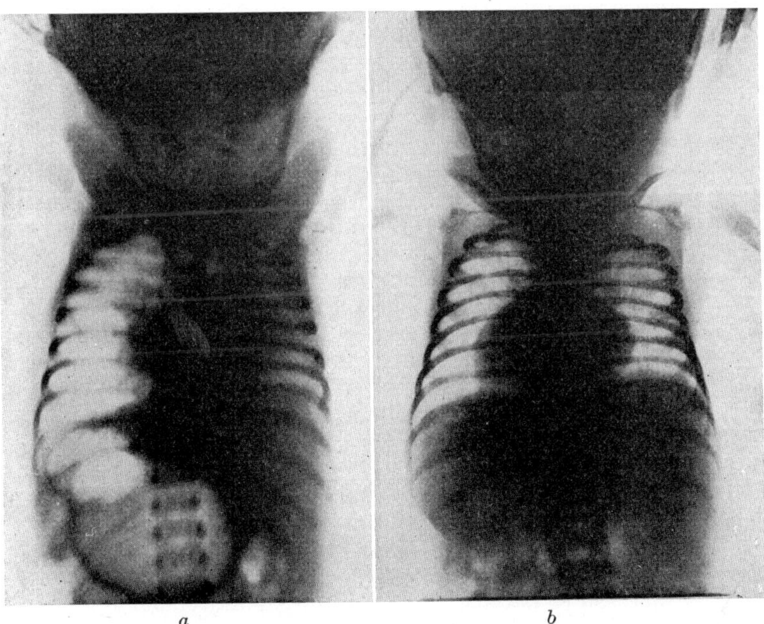

a *b*

Fig. 172.—Massive pulmonary atelectasis (massive collapse of the lung). Marie R., aged three weeks. Very slight cough; regurgitation of food through nose while feeding with probable entrance of it into the trachea. Dulness over right side with bronchial respiration and bronchophony. Roentgenogram (*a*) showed a dense shadow over the entire right lung, with high stand of the diaphragm and heart entirely to the right. A week later roentgenogram (*b*) showed the heart returning to the normal position, the right lung clearer, and auscultation and percussion revealed no evidences of consolidation.

as also by the injection of solution of acacia after the cough-reflex has been abolished (Lee, Tucker, and Clerf[95]). Coryllos[96] and others believe that in the postoperative type the dominant factor is occlusion of the bronchial tree. The **symptoms** develop suddenly within a few hours to several days after the exciting cause. There are moderate fever, increased rate of the respiration and pulse, and cough. The general symptoms are usually mild, but there may be cyanosis and dyspnea in cases with extensive involvement. On physical examination there are immobility, narrowing of the intercostal spaces, and dulness or flatness on percussion upon the affected side. Breath-sounds and voice-sounds are usually increased, and there is bronchial breathing and bronchophony, the bronchial character being present even in cases where the breath-sounds are diminished. A friction-rub may or may not be present, and râles occur later when expansion takes place. The heart and mediastinum are displaced toward the affected side. The lower lobes are more frequently affected. If the collapse is in the upper lobe, or if there is much fluid in the air passages ("drowned lung"), the cardiac displacement is less marked. In bilateral cases there will be no cardiac displacement. Roentgenograms show the collapse of the lung with elevation of the dome of the diaphragm on the affected side, and the cardiac and mediastinal displacement toward the affected side, as indicated especially by the deviation of the trachea (Fig. 172). The **prognosis,** while depending on the exciting cause, is usually good, and expansion takes place in a week or earlier if pneumonia or pleural effusion does not complicate the process. The differential **diagnosis** from pneumonia is based on the mildness of the general symptoms, the displacement of the heart toward the affected side, and the high position of the diaphragm, these last two signs also helping in the differentiation from pleural effusion. It should be stated, however, that displacement of the heart to the affected side is not a positive proof of the existence of massive collapse, since it may occur at times in pneumonia. (See p. 732.) In the *preventive* **treatment** the encouragement of deep breathing after operation is to be thought of. Scott and Cutler[97] have found that the incidence was apparently reduced by hyperventilation with 70 per cent oxygen and 30 per cent carbon dioxide at the close of operation, combined with raising the head of the patient's bed 15 or 20 inches. Hyperventilation by the same means may be used in *treatment of the attack*, some clinicians employing only 5 per cent CO_2 in oxygen. Forced coughing (or in children, crying) with the patient lying on the unaffected side may be helpful. Aspiration through a bronchoscope may allow expansion of the lung (Jackson and Lee[98]). Sante[99] recommends rolling the patient back and forth on the unaffected side. It must not be forgotten that many cases recover spontaneously without treatment, and also that relapse is not infrequent.

PULMONARY EDEMA

This is an unfavorable symptom, not common in childhood, which may be seen in various disorders, as valvular disease of the heart, rickets, nephritis, bronchopneumonia, eruptive fevers, and cachectic conditions. There are present increase of percussion-dulness in the lower portion of the chest without bronchial respiration, numerous moist râles, cyanosis, cough, and dyspnea. In the rapid severe cases dry cupping, free cardiac stimulation, atropine and at times morphine, purgatives, and hot mustard-packs are to be used in the treatment.

PULMONARY ABSCESS

Multiple pulmonary abscesses, usually small, may attend sepsis (Fig. 173) or severe bronchopneumonia; or larger ones may be seen in tuberculosis. A single nontuberculous abscess of any size is exceptional in early life. It may result from a foreign body or a disintegrating consolidation in croupous pneumonia; or may be secondary to an infectious disease, a suppurating bronchial gland, or to an operative procedure such as tonsillectomy. Recent reports indicate that pulmonary abscess is on the increase, or possibly the recognition of it through the wider employment of roentgenography. While surgical procedure of any kind may be a cause, many of the cases follow tonsillectomy or other operations on the upper respiratory tract (Fig. 174). General anesthesia has been used in the majority of these, but in a smaller number local anesthesia. Moore,[100] who collected 202 cases in patients of all ages following operation on the upper respiratory tract, estimates that abscess occurs once in every 2500 to 3000 tonsillectomies. The subject is also reviewed by Fischer,[101] Apfel,[102] and others.

Clinical and experimental evidence seems to show that in the production of such abscesses aspiration of infected material and micro-organisms is the important cause, but that embolic abscesses do occur. Cutler,[103] who has studied the subject extensively, suggests that embolism from a septic field produces the original lesion, and that it becomes a chronic abscess only when secondarily infected by the ever-present mechanism of aspiration.

The **symptoms** are uncharacteristic. In some instances the condition is not suspected unless there is sudden rupture of the abscess into a bronchus and a discharge of pus containing elastic fibers and sometimes possessing an offensive odor. Generally no such sudden rupture is observed, although communication with a bronchus is not infrequent. The principal clinical features consist of fever of an irregular and often hectic type, with increasing debility and anemia, a high leukocyte-count, and at times a troublesome cough. When the abscess is large and there is free communication with a bronchus the physical signs suggest those of a tuberculous or a large bronchiectatic cavity. If no such communication is present, there are dulness on percussion and feeble respiratory murmur over the consolidation, and a localized empyema is suspected. If the abscess discharges at intervals only, a corresponding alteration in the physical signs is observed. In cases of distinct localization the exploratory needle may reveal pus; but is apt to fail to do so owing to the smallness of the accumulation. Even when pus is found, the diagnosis of localized empyema is often erroneously made. Roentgenograms may aid greatly in the diagnosis (Fig. 174). Small, deep-seated abscesses may present no physical signs whatever. A characteristic symptom of abscess, although not pathognomic, is decided clubbing of the fingers. The abscesses following tonsillectomy usually develop in about a week, although sometimes not for two or three weeks.

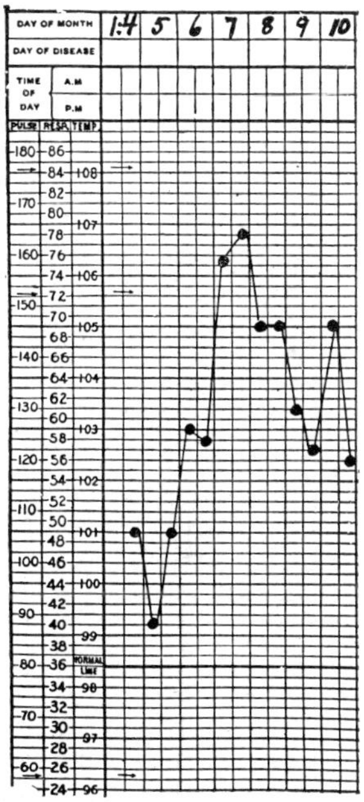

The **prognosis** is uncertain. The abscess may rupture into a bronchus, and perhaps be followed by healing. This is especially true if the original cause was a foreign body which had been expelled or removed. In other cases the abscess may continue to discharge, with progressive loss of strength and the usual symptoms of prolonged suppuration. If the **diagnosis** can be made surgical **treatment** may be employed. Aspiration may be followed by cure, or resection of a rib and drainage may be required. In recent years the employment of the bronchoscope in skilled hands has been of aid both in diagnosis and treatment.

Fig. 173.—Multiple pyemic abscesses of the lungs following cervical adenitis. Rose T., aged five years. Illness began a week before admitted to the Children's Hospital of Philadelphia, on Jan. 4, with inflammation of the tonsils and of the cervical gland on the left side; Jan. 5, incision of abscess in neck; Jan. 7, child toxic, delirious, general condition poor; Jan. 10, numerous râles have been present in both lungs. No other positive physical signs, except slight bronchial respiration in the lower part of right side. General condition grew worse. Death on this date. Necropsy showed numerous scattered pyemic abscesses, size of walnut, throughout both lungs. Pus in pleural cavity on both sides.

PULMONARY GANGRENE

Etiology.—This is not common in early life and is always secondary. It is oftenest seen in connection with bronchopneumonia especially after measles; croupous pneumonia; tuberculosis of the lungs and bronchial glands; typhoid fever and other acute infectious diseases; aspiration-pneumonia, as produced by foreign bodies or especially by necrotic or gangrenous tissue entering the lung in the case of diphtheritic or gangrenous stomatitis; septic embolism or thrombosis of the pulmonary vessels resulting from suppurative processes elsewhere in the body; and gastro-enteritis. Any greatly debilitating agent predisposes to it. As a result of some of these causes inflammation and consequent interference with the circulation

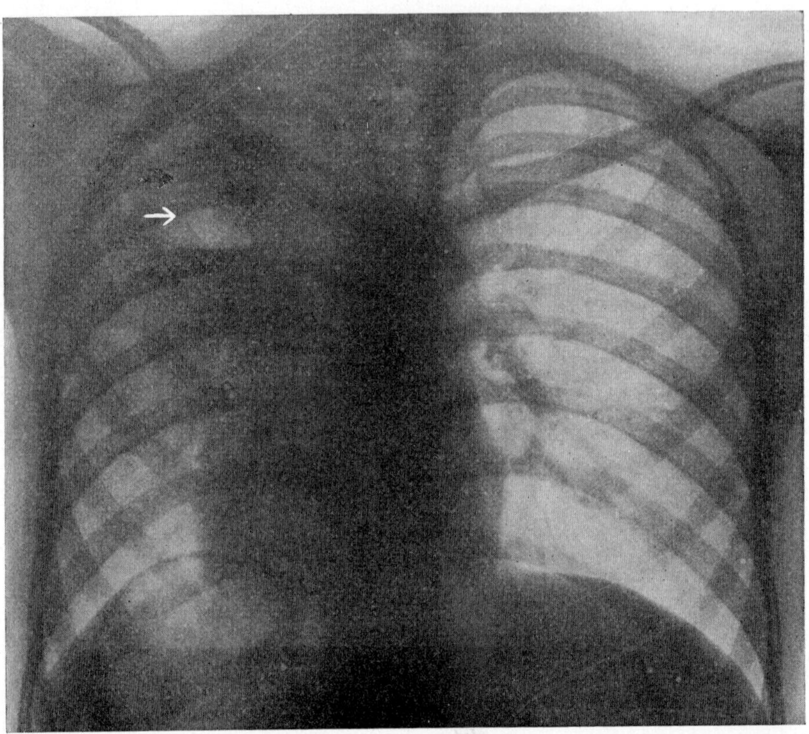

Fig. 174.—Abscess of the lung following tonsillectomy. G. C., boy aged nine years. Admitted to Children's Medical Ward of the Hospital of the University of Pennsylvania March 13th. Tonsils had been removed eighteen days previously; four days later developed cough, pain in left shoulder, expectoration, and fever. *Examination.*—Expansion diminished over left upper lobe; percussion impaired except for a tympanitic note under clavicles; whispered pectoriloquy; breath-sounds absent over affected area. Leukocytes 31,400. Irregular febrile temperature. *March 14th*—Roentgenogram shows consolidation with cavity containing fluid. *March 18th*—Expectorated a large amount of pus, and bronchial breathing now heard over affected area. Later bronchoscopic treatment and cure.

in the lung take place; but in order to have a gangrenous process follow there must be the presence of micro-organisms capable of producing putrefaction. These may enter the lung either by way of the respiratory tract or through the blood-vessels. According to the investigations of Veillon and Zuber,[100] these germs are anaerobic putrefactive bacteria of various sorts, but spirochetes and bacilli similar to those observed in Vincent's angina have been found in pulmonary gangrene by Rona;[105] Fishberg and Kline;[106] Kline and Blankenhorn;[107] Spano,[108] Kline and Berger;[109] Lewis and Barenberg[110] and others, and are evidently causative. The **lesions** are usually multiple and sometimes are present in both lungs, but oftener in the right only; are of variable size, and situated oftenest in the lower lobe and near the surface. The affected region is blackish or greenish in color, moist, and later it either still contains a slough or exhibits a cavity filled with pus.

Symptoms.—In well-developed cases there is a horribly putrefactive odor to the breath and to the expectoration, the latter consisting of dirty, greenish material, containing gangrenous pulmonary tissue and sometimes blood in large amount; pallor; high remittent fever; rapid feeble pulse; and profound prostration (Fig. 175). There may be but little cough. The symptoms, however, are by no means always typical in children, since the gangrenous area may not communicate with a bronchus. Odor to the breath is probably oftener absent than present in early life. The physical signs suggest those of a lobular pneumonia or of a cavity, according to the case; or of a pyothorax or pneumothorax if the gangrene has perforated the pleura.

The **course** is often rapidly fatal in from one to three weeks. Gangrene due to the presence of a foreign body offers perhaps the best hope; but even this is slight.

Diagnosis is necessarily usually difficult owing to the frequent absence in children of the characteristic symptoms. Even if an odor to the breath is present the possibility of fetid bronchitis, bronchiectasis, pulmonary abscess, anthrax, and actinomycosis (p. 763) of the lung, or of gangrenous or ulcerative stomatitis must be taken into account. Strongly stimulating and supporting **treatment** is indicated. Efforts should be made at pulmonary disinfection by the inhalation of antiseptic substances such as thymol, creosote, turpentine and eucalyptus. Operation is indicated if the gangrene is localized and situated near the surface of the lung. If the infection has been found to be with the Vincent's organisms, vigorous, intravenous arsenical treatment should be given, using somewhat smaller doses and at more frequent intervals than generally employed in the treatment of syphilis (pp. 838–839).

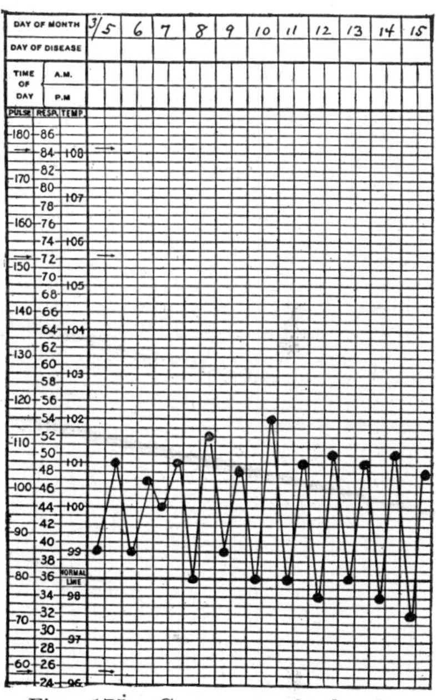

Fig. 175.—Gangrene of the lung. James S., aged eight years. Seen Mar. 4, had grippe eleven weeks previously, followed by pneumonia. Signs of consolidation said to have cleared rapidly. About four to five weeks before seen developed daily fever, failing strength, violent paroxysms of coughing, with purulent expectoration and sometimes vomiting. Examination showed numerous râles at the lower part of right side posteriorly. Excessive weakness prevented further study. Odor of breath and of expectoration horribly offensive. Death Mar. 21.

References

1. Malad. d. enf., 1838. 2. Griffith, Med. News, 1896, Dec. 5. 3. Traité d. mal. de l'enf., Grancher, 1904, **3**, 399. 4. Brit. M. J., 1908, **2**, 367. 5. Dis. of Inf. and Child., 1922, 479. 6. Arch. Pediat., 1904, **21**, 641. 7. Personal Communication. 8. Am. J. Dis. Child., 1920, **20**, 119. 9. Boston M. and S. J., 1921, **185**, 189. 10. Arch. Dis. Childhood, 1928, **3**, 194. 11. Edinburgh M. J., 1928, May. 12. Canad. M. A. J., 1929, **20**, 609. 13. Boston M. and S. J., 1927, **197**, 93. 14. Arch. Pediat., 1919, **36**, 185. 15. Med. Rec., 1919, **96**, 364. 16. Am. J. Dis. Child., 1922, **23**, 503. 17. Arch. d. méd. exper., 1892, **4**, 49. 18. Deutsche. Arch. f. klin. Med., 1897, **58**, 368. 19. Boston M. and S. J., 1897, **137**, 562. 20. Am. J. Dis. Child., 1922, **23**, 72. 21. Arch. Int. Med., 1927, **40**, 253. 22. Arch. Dis. Childhood, 1929, **4**, 283. 23. Arch. Dis. Childhood, 1931, **6**, 37. 24. J.A.M.A., 1913, **61**, 727. 25. Trans. Assoc. Am. Phys., 1913, **28**, 606. 26. Am.

J. M. Sc., 1916, **151,** 14. 27. Am. J. Dis. Child., 1916, **12,** 254. 28. Mitchell, J. Pa. State M. Ass., 1917, **20,** 343. 29. J. Infect. Dis., 1926, **38,** 514. 30. Monatschr. f. Kinderh., 1929, **45,** 141. 31. J. Pediat., (Tokyo), 1929, No. 344, 153; Ref. Am. J. Dis. Child., 1929, **38,** 175. 32. J. Clin. Investig., 1930, **8,** 623. 33. Am. J. Dis. Child., 1931, **42,** 57. 34. Am. J. Hyg., 1926, **6,** 510. 35. Am. J. M. Sc., 1931, **181,** 245. 36. Griffith, J.A.M.A., 1928, **91,** 1331. 37. Soc. de biol., 1889, **1,** 187. 38. Arch. exper. Path. u. Pharm., 1889, **26,** 155. 39. Am. J. Dis. Child., 1928, **36,** 764. 40. Fortschr. d. Med., 1883, **1,** 715. 41. Verhandl. III Kong inn. Med., 1884, **3,** 17. 42. Wien. med. Jahrb., 1886, 483. 43. Traité de. mal. de l'enf., 1884, **1,** 712. 44. Boston M. and S. J., 1905, **152,** 741. 45. Boston M. and S. J., 1916, **174,** 753. 46. Ziemssen's Handb. der spec. Path. u. Therap., 1874, **5,** 50. 47. Brit. M. J., 1896, **2,** 1212. 48. Brit. J. Child. Dis., 1919, **14,** 112. 49. München. med. Wchnschr., 1902, **49,** 1211. 50. Arch. f. Kinderh., 1926, **77,** 306. 51. Ann. de méd. et de chir. inf., 1913, **17,** 275. 52. Am. J. Dis. Child., 1916, **11,** 188. 53. Griffith, Med. J. and Rec., 1926, Jan. 26; Am. J. M. Sc., 1927, **174,** 448. 54. Monatschr. f. Kinderh., 1922, **22,** 353. 55. Acta paediat., 1922, **3,** 81. 56. Proc. Roy. Soc. Med., 1928, **21,** 1327. 57. Arch. Dis. Childhood, 1929, **4,** 230. 58. Am. J. Dis. Child., 1917, **14,** 296. 59. New York Med. Rec., 1910, **77,** 701. 60. Griffith, J.A.M.A., 1903, **41,** 531. 61. J.A.M.A., 1922, **79,** 1809. 62. Am. J. Dis. Child., 1927, **33,** 740. 63. Boston M. and S. J., 1914, **170,** 125. 64. J.A.M.A., 1911, **57,** 1827. 65. New York State J. Med., 1930, **30,** 210. 66. Am. J. M. Sc., 1916, **151,** 1. 67. Am. J. Dis. Child., 1916, **12,** 445. 68. J.A.M.A., 1929, **93,** 1550. 69. Brit. M. J., 1928, **2,** 195. 70. Brit. M. J., 1929, **2,** 757. 71. J.A.M.A., 1921, **76,** 672. 72. J.A.M.A., 1929, **93,** 96. 73. J.A.M.A., 1921, **78,** 1217. 74. Proc. N. Y. Path. Soc., 1922, **22,** 72. 75. Am. J. M. Sc., 1927, **174,** 744. 76. J. Exper. Med., 1927, **45,** 1081. 77. Am. J. Dis. Child., 1929, **37,** 323. 78. Arch. Pediat., 1927, **44,** 349. 79. Arch. f. Kinderh., 1928, **84,** 241. 80. Lancet, 1932, **1,** 13. 81. Am. J. Dis. Child., 1924, **28,** 310; Arch. Pediat., 1926, **43,** 694. 82. Am. J. Dis. Child., 1925, **29,** 318. 83. New York M. J., 1916, **103,** 681. 84. Am. J. Dis. Child., 1925, **30,** 57. 85. J. Immunol., 1921, **6,** 117; 123; 185. 86. Boston M. and S. J., 1924, **190,** 819; Bull. Johns Hopkins Hosp., 1926, **38,** 33; J.A.M.A., 1930, **94,** 1893. 87. Klin. Wchnschr., 1931, **10,** 728. 88. Lancet, 1922, **2,** 493. 89. Trans. Ass. Am. Phys., 1926, **41,** 224. 90. Presse méd., 1920, **28,** 593. 91. Arch. Int. Med., 1924, **34,** 867. 92. Am. J. Syph., 1928, **12,** 177. 93. Monatschr. f. Kinderh., 1928, **39,** 104. 94. Am. J. M. Sc., 1890, **100,** 242. 95. Ann. Surg., 1928, **88,** 6; 15. 96. J.A.M.A., 1928, **93,** 98. 97. J.A.M.A., 1928, **90,** 1759. 98. Ann. Surg., 1925, **82,** 364. 99. J.A.M.A., 1927, **88,** 1539. 100. J.A.M.A., 1922, **78,** 1279. 101. Am. J. M. Sc., 1928, **176,** 253. 102. Arch. Pediat., 1929, **46,** 231. 103. Am. J. Dis. Child., 1929, **38,** 683. 104. Arch. de méd. exper. et d. anat. path., 1894, **10,** 517. 105. Arch. f. Derm. u. Syph., 1905, **74,** 171. 106. Arch. Int. Med., 1921, **27,** 61. 107. J.A.M.A., 1923, **81,** 719. 108. Am. J. Dis. Child., 1925, **29,** 621. 109. J.A.M.A., 1925, **85,** 1452. 110. Am. J. Dis. Child., 1929, **37,** 351.

CHAPTER VI

DISEASES OF THE PLEURA

PLEURISY

THIS is a common disorder in early life, occurring nearly always as a secondary affection. The disease may be divided into: (1) the *dry or plastic form,* (2) the *serous or serofibrinous form* and (3) the *purulent form,* or *empyema.* A plastic pleurisy may later produce a serous exudate, or a serofibrinous pleurisy become purulent.

Etiology.—*Age* is a decided factor. In the new-born pleurisy is uncommon, at least in a clinically recognizable form, but cases are reported and the subject studied by Hervieux,[1] Steele,[2] Mace,[3] Roger,[4] Glaser and Epstein,[5] and Corcoran.[6] It appears at this period oftenest to be purulent and bilateral, and always secondary. After this age plastic pleurisy is frequent in both infants and children and empyema is more common than in adult life; up to the age of five years the large majority of pleural effusions being of this nature [51 purulent out of 54 effusions under two years in the Children's Hospital of Philadelphia (Miller[7])]. In later childhood serous effusion is decidedly the more frequent. The youngest case of serous effusion we have seen was in a premature infant of five weeks whose tuberculin reaction was negative. (For further statistical studies see Israel,[8] Netter,[9] Reano,[10] Nasso,[11] and Mazzeo.[12]) Pleurisy develops oftener in the colder season and occurs rather more frequently in boys than in girls. Trauma is an uncommon cause. Exposure to cold is a factor in later childhood, and unquestionably some cases of serous or plastic pleurisy are related to rheumatism. The purulent form may occur as a complication of scarlet fever, measles, grippe, typhoid fever, and sepsis; the last particularly in the new-born. In adults about 20 to 25 per cent of the cases of tuberculosis develop pleurisy in some form as one of the lesions, generally consecutive to involvement of the lungs or bronchial lymph-nodes. Just this relationship does not obtain in later childhood, at which time tuberculous pleurisy is generally serous or serofibrinous rather than purulent, and apparently a primary affection, not associated with discoverable disease of the lungs. In fact, pleurisy of this nature, developing at this period of life and apparently primary, should be considered as tuberculous until this is disproved. We have seen cases, however, in which tuberculosis could be excluded by all methods of examination made at the time and later.

Some cases of empyema come on insidiously without previous illness, but much the most common factor is extension from a pneumonic process usually of the croupous variety. According to various statistics from about 5 to 12 per cent of cases of croupous pneumonia develop empyema, and about 1.5 to 3 per cent of bronchopneumonias; and approximately 70 to 90 per cent of all the cases of empyema occur as a complication of pneumonia. (See statistical studies by Gossage,[13] Dunlop,[14] Churchill,[15] Farr and Levine,[16] Spence,[17] Glenn-Ravdin,[18] and McNeil, MacGregor and Alexander.[19])

The *exciting cause* in empyema is usually the pneumococcus, this being found in about 75 per cent of the cases (Netter,[9] Dunlop,[14] Sillitti,[20] Downes[21]). The next most frequent germ is the streptococcus, often of the hemolytic variety, and at times of epidemics of influenza this may be especially frequent. Less often found are nonhemolytic streptococci, staphylococci, colon bacilli, influenza bacilli, typhoid bacilli, etc. Naturally cases following pneumonia are associated with the pneumococcus, alone or with other germs. Those occurring with sepsis and the infectious fevers usually show the streptococcus or the staphylococcus. Blood-culture may not infrequently be positive for pneumococci or other germs. In the plastic and serofibrinous forms so few pyogenic germs may be found that their causative relationship is uncertain. Most frequently, however, in these the tubercle bacillus is present, perhaps discovered only after the material obtained by puncture has been inoculated into animals.

1. Plastic Pleurisy

Pathologic Anatomy.—In mild cases only the visceral pleura over the affected lung is involved, but in others the process is extensive and the parietal layer also attacked. The pleura is rough, dry, and lustreless, and in advanced cases covered with fibrin, which may exist in shreds, or may form a thick yellow-green layer (Fig. 176). On recovery the exudate is absorbed, but adhesions usually remain between the pleural surfaces. In tuberculous pleurisy tubercles may sometimes be seen and the pleura becomes much thickened.

Symptoms.—These are indefinite and perhaps obscured by the primary disease. Pain over the affected region, or perhaps referred to the abdomen or sometimes to the neck, and worse with deep breathing or coughing is the chief manifestation, but may be complained of only by older children. The cough is short, frequent, and harassing; there are usually fever and local tenderness on pressure. A pleuritic friction rub is heard, sometimes difficult to distinguish from the crepitant râle of pneumonia. It accompanies both inspiration and expiration. Distinction must be made from epidemic pleurodynia (p. 357) by the absence in the latter of physical signs and cough, and by its epidemic occurrence. The tuberculous nature of plastic pleurisy is to be suspected especially when not occurring with an acute disease.

Course and Prognosis.—It is only exceptionally in children that dry pleurisy is chronic, such cases probably being tuberculous. There is often a decided tendency to recurrence. Generally the prognosis is good unless the pleurisy goes beyond the plastic stage.

Treatment.—Apart from the treatment of the primary disease, measures should be taken to relieve pain. An ice-bag to the affected region may afford relief, and some one of the salicylates or phenacetin or other coal-tar derivative may be given, or even opiates if necessary. A bandage around the chest, or strapping with adhesive plaster aids in preventing pain. Rest in bed in the position most comfortable to the patient is needed. There is little if any value in counterirritation applied to the chest in the attempt to control inflammation.

2. Serofibrinous Pleurisy

Pathologic Anatomy.—The early stages of this are the same as in the plastic form. Soon, however, and sometimes from the onset, an exudation of serum takes place, which may be situated in small or large pockets of an extensive thick exudate, or may be free in the pleural cavity. The process is nearly always unilateral. The fluid is sometimes almost clear, sometimes quite turbid, depending upon the amount of fibrin and leukocytes. Tuberculous fluid is usually quite clear and the cells may be predominantly lymphocytes. The exudate may be gradually absorbed, but adhesions and thickening of the pleura persist to a varying extent. In some cases, especially the nontuberculous forms, a purulent character may develop. A *hemorrhagic exudate* is very uncommon in early life, and accompanies oftenest cases associated with rheumatism, tuberculosis, or malignant neoplasms.

Symptoms.—Those characteristic of plastic pleurisy (p. 753) are at first present, with perhaps a greater degree of fever, but without the evident constitutional impression of pneumonia. Fluid is effused in two or three days, or usually longer, and if the exudate is in considerable quantity pain and cough grow less, and often fever likewise; dyspnea becomes decided, and there may be orthopnea and cyanosis. In many cases the onset is insidious, the patient does not complain of illness, and the disease is discovered only on physical examination. In uncomplicated cases leukocytosis is moderate.

On *physical examination* in cases with considerable effusion, inspection shows fullness of the interspaces, diminished expansion, and broadening of the costosternal angle. Palpation reveals diminished or absent vocal fremitus; distinct fullness and resistance in the intercostal spaces; and displacement of the heart to the side opposite the effusion, more pronounced in left-sided effusions. To percussion there is entire flatness with increased resistance in very large effusions. In less marked effusion the lower portion of chest gives a flat note, while above this is only dulness, or skodaic tympany, and at the apex in front possibly hyperresonance. Posteriorly on the healthy side there is usually found a narrow triangular area of dulness (Grocco's triangle) with its apex upward and about on a level with the upper layer of the dulness on the diseased side. There is some doubt as to the reliability of this sign. If the effusion is on the right side, the lower border of liver dulness may be depressed; if on the left, the normal cardiac

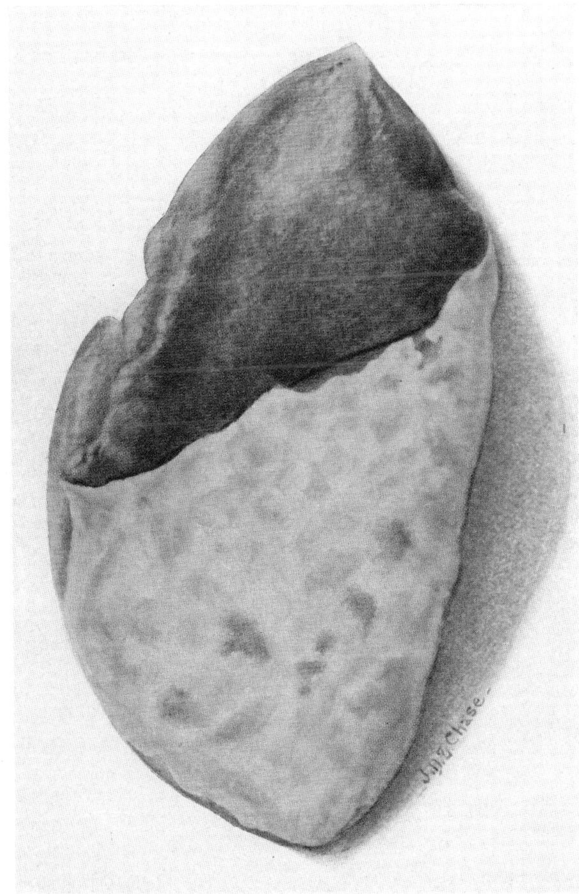

Fig. 176.—Plastic pleurisy with pneumonia. Child of sixteen months with symptoms of pleuropneumonia. Illustration shows the dense layer of plastic exudate found at autopsy. About 2 oz. (59) of yellow serous fluid in the pleural cavity.

dulness is displaced to the right of the sternum, and in Traube's semilunar space dulness replaces gastric tympany. Percussion-dulness may shift with change of position. Auscultatory signs vary considerably. Theoretically there should be absent or feeble respiration and diminished vocal resonance or egophony, and these are, in fact, the signs present in many cases. In others in children there is bronchial respiration and bronchophony, of an intensity which readily leads to the suspicion of pneumonia. In still others, even with considerable effusion, breath-sounds and voice-sounds may show little alteration. Not uncommonly râles may be transmitted through a layer of fluid sufficiently thick to produce dulness on percussion. Friction-sounds may perhaps be heard above the effusion. When the fluid is free and the patient in a sitting position, the greatest amount of it will be found at the base, a thinner layer spreading up over the lung behind and in the axilla, and to the lower part of the thorax in front. Roentgenograms and the fluoroscope will show a uniform shadow in the region of the fluid, and, with an effusion of any considerable size, depression of the diaphragm and cardiac displacement. When there is not encapsulation the movability of the fluid can be demonstrated by the fluoroscope. When adhesions encapsulate the fluid the signs will be correspondingly changed.

Course and Prognosis.—In many instances the fluid does not become excessive and is gradually absorbed in two or three weeks, or often considerably lònger in tuberculous cases. With slow absorption there may develop debility, anemia and irregular fever,—these being symptoms of the pleurisy or of the underlying condition. Sometimes aspiration of a portion of the fluid, perhaps repeated a few times, will hasten its absorption; in other cases reaccumulation repeatedly occurs. In all cases adhesions remain, but if these are not extensive may leave little final residual difficulty, although evidence of them may remain for months. Pleurisy associated with tuberculosis by no means indicates a severe or rapid form of this disease. Particularly in cases secondary to pneumonia the effusion is likely to become purulent. Only exceptionally is the amount of serous effusion so great as to endanger life by pressure upon intrathoracic organs.

Diagnosis.—The symptoms and the physical signs of fluid in the chest have been sufficiently discussed. The differentiation of effusion of any kind from other intrathoracic conditions will be considered later (p. 759). In cases admitting of any doubt the exploratory needle should be used to determine the diagnosis. (For puncture of the pleural cavity, see p. 150.) It is important to distinguish between a serous and a purulent effusion because of the therapeutic implications. (See Empyema, p. 759.) Armand-Delille[22] calls attention to the value of injecting lipiodol into the pleural cavity to detect interlobar pleurisy.

Treatment.—In the early stages this is similar to that required for dry pleurisy (p. 754). After the acute symptoms are over and the amount of fluid has become decided, measures should be taken to promote absorption. Painting the skin of the thorax with iodine or the use of other counter-irritants is a favorite method with older children, but of problematic value. Internally salicylates and calcium preparations have been recommended, and the administration of diuretics and laxatives is useful to a limited extent. The combination of free purgation with diminution of fluid-intake is efficient, but distressing and perhaps harmful. The patient should be kept in bed and sudden sitting up forbidden, since fatal syncope sometimes follows abrupt movement. In effusion of less amount, in which recovery is delayed, the patient may be placed in a chair and taken into the open air. Indeed, the fluid is often so slow in disappearing that all possible measures must be adopted to improve the general health. Iodides internally are sometimes of value in long-continued cases. Danzer[23] claims good results from the administration of thyroid extract. Tonic remedies are indicated, iron often being needed for the anemia. Lassen[24] found ultraviolet light beneficial.

Thoracentesis is needed only in cases where a rapid increase of the exudate threatens life, or where the amount remains unchanged in spite of other treatment. Sometimes in such cases removal once or several times of a small quantity of fluid appears so to alter the conditions that the remainder is absorbed. Incision and drainage have occasionally been performed, but are certainly less often required than aspiration. For the latter a Potain aspirator is satisfactory, with a small trocar and cannula. The child should be in a sitting position; the skin, instruments and the hands of the operator sterilized in the usual manner, and the needle inserted by preference in the 7th interspace in the posterior axillary line, or elsewhere if the fluid is unusually situated. The fluid should be withdrawn slowly, and if the chest is very full, no attempt should be made to remove the entire amount, or faintness may develop. In cases with less fluid the aspiration may continue until the flow ceases or troublesome coughing occurs, although this completeness of removal is not necessary. The needle is then withdrawn and the puncture closed by antiseptic gauze or by cotton and collodion. After recovery from long-continued serous effusion with firm adhesions and diminished expansion of the lung pulmonary exercises are useful, including such as swinging from a horizontal bar, vigorous horseback riding, and the like, and the blowing exercises discussed later (p. 760). In one instance we found benefit come from having a country-child pump water for the household.

3. Purulent Pleurisy

(Empyema)

Pathologic Anatomy.—The lesions differ from those of serofibrinous pleurisy in that large numbers of pus-cells are present in the fluid. When the staphylococcus or the streptococcus is causative the fluid may be purulent from the beginning, contains less fibrin, is thinner and of a greenish-gray color, and separates into layers on standing. In the cases due to the pneumococcus the pus is thick, tenacious, green, does not separate on standing, and contains a large amount of fibrin. Sometimes it is at first apparently serofibrinous and more or less rapidly becomes purulent. These distinctions between the two varieties of pus are not, however, absolute. Not uncommonly the purulent fluid is more or less tinged with blood (*hemorrhagic empyema*). At first the effusion is encapsulated by adhesions, and may remain so; but if the amount is large these give way and the thorax fills on the affected side, which is oftenest the left. *Bilateral empyema* is exceptional, but is recorded by Blaker,[25] Hellin,[26] Fabricant,[27] Koplik,[28] and Ladd and Cutler.[29] We have seen it very rarely.

When the fluid of an empyema is free a layer extends upward over the back of the lung, and often still higher in the axilla, and to a less extent in front, gradually diminishing in thickness the higher its position. When the amount is large the lung is compressed in the direction of its root and becomes almost airless (Fig. 177). The other organs are affected as in serous effusion. Sometimes small encapsulated effusions contain only 2 to 4 oz. In other instances the quantity may equal several pints. In cases in which recovery takes place under proper treatment adhesions will remain, but give no trouble except where the duration has been long; in which event contraction of the chest may occur. This happens much oftener than with serous effusion.

Symptoms.—In the large majority of cases, in which the disease follows upon a pneumonia (*metapneumonic empyema*), the temperature of the primary affection falls to normal and may remain so for several days, and then begins to rise again, exhibiting an irregular course (Fig. 178). Sometimes no distinct intermission occurs between the pneumonia and the empyema, and in some of these cases the development of the empyema is coincident with that of the pneumonia (*parapneumonic empyema*). This is much less common than the metapneumonic form, especially in pneumococcic infection. Where there has been no preceding pneumonia, as for instance after the infectious diseases or in the primary cases, the

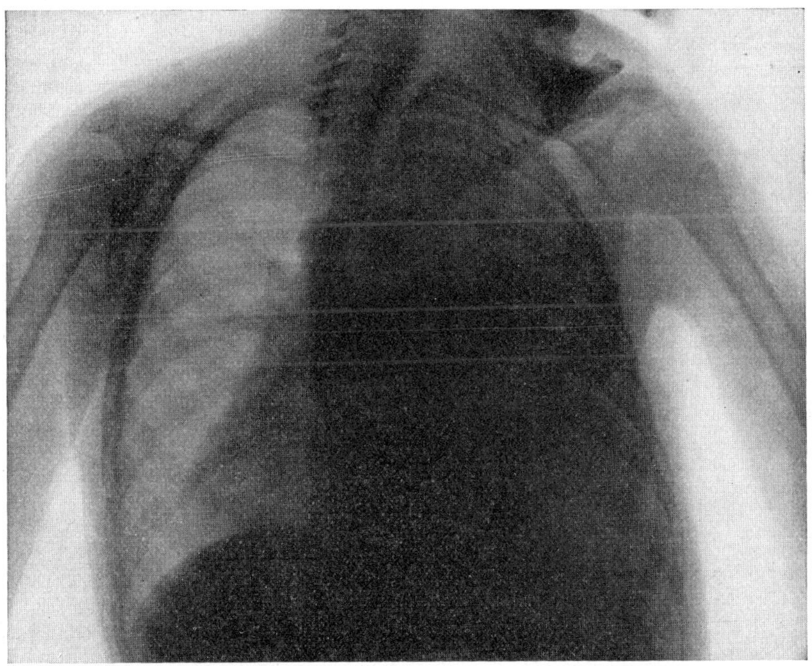

Fig. 177.—Roentgenogram of purulent pleural effusion. Jessie G., aged six years. Admitted to the Children's Medical Ward of the Hospital of the University of Pennsylvania, June 2. Had suffered from cough for two weeks, pain in right side. *Examination.*—Moderate prostration, decided dyspnea, right side of chest shows obliterated interspaces and diminished expansion and breath-sounds, percussion flat below 4th rib, leukocytes 21,000, exploratory puncture gave yellow pus. Viewed from behind.

onset is marked by the development of irregular fever, increased rapidity of the pulse and respiration, dyspnea, cough, debility, anemia, loss of appetite, emaciation, and a decided leukocytosis. Diarrhea may occur, especially in the cases dependent upon the streptococcus. As a rule the fever is higher than in serous effusion.

After a varying time the acuteness of the symptoms is prone to subside, but there is little if any improvement in the general condition; while the dyspnea, anemia, debility, sweating, and signs of general cachexia persist. In long-continued cases there may be enlargement of the spleen and liver, albuminuria, enlargement of the terminal phalanges, and general edema. The unusual condition denominated *pulsating empyema* has occasionally been observed in children;—in Wilson's[30] series of 68 cases 5 occurred in the first ten years of life. The effusion in purulent cases generally develops rapidly, and the physical signs then do not differ from those characteristic of serous effusion (p. 754). When localized it may be near the apex; between two of the lobes of the lung; between the lung and the diaphragm; or in the mediastinum.

Complications.—Purulent pericarditis may develop in the cases of left-sided pleural effusion; or an abscess of the lung form; or meningitis, arthritis, peritonitis, or other manifestation of septic involvement extend from the pleura as a center. A pneumothorax sometimes forms if the pus communicates with a bronchus. Bronchopneumonia may occur and be a serious complication.

Prognosis and Course.—In the majority of cases not relieved by treatment the course is progressively towards a fatal ending. The debility, anemia and prostration continue to increase and fever persists, unless the

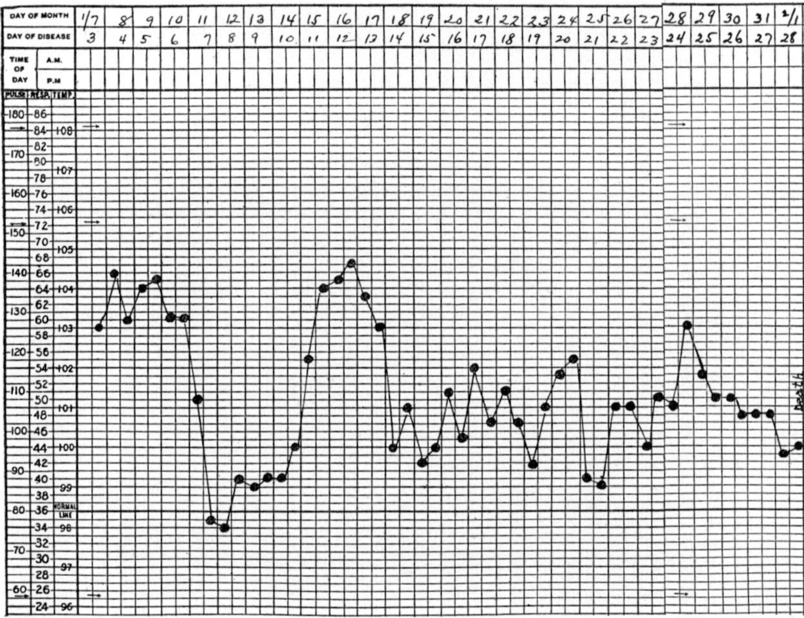

Fig. 178.—Empyema, following pneumonia. Fannie B., two years old. Admitted to the Children's Ward of the University of Pennsylvania Hospital, Jan. 7. Croupous pneumonia, with crisis on the seventh day. Rise of temperature began on the tenth day. Aspiration showed pus on the eleventh day, and operation done on the following day. Gradual failure of strength, and death on the twenty-eighth day.

pus finds a way out by perforating a bronchus, or oftener by breaking through the chest-wall (*empyema necessitatis*). When about to perforate externally a fluctuating, red swelling appears between the ribs, usually in front near the nipple. In other instances the pus perforates the diaphragm and enters the peritoneum.

The duration of the disease before death occurs is indefinite. It is possible in infancy for a chronic empyema to exist unsuspected for many months, the case having the appearance of marasmus, or being attributed to tuberculosis. In a case in the Children's Hospital of Philadelphia reported by Hand[31] the disease had lasted eighteen months, and the child of three and one-half years weighed but 8 lb. 14 oz. (4026). It happens very occasionally that a small purulent exudate is absorbed and recovery follows without treatment. Under surgical intervention the prognosis is influenced by various circumstances. In infancy the mortality is high even when operation has been done and other conditions are favorable. In statistical studies the mortality under one year varies from about 65 to 75 per cent. In some reports, as in Nathan's,[32] it was almost 100 per cent, 45 of 46 patients dying. In the second year of life the mortality is usually given as between 50 and 60 per cent. After the third year it declines rapidly and the mortality in childhood is about 10 to 15 per cent, after eight or ten years being still less. (For statistical studies see Wightman,[33] Nathan,[32] Netter,[9] Hellin,[26] Holt,[34] Dowd,[35] Spence,[17] Ladd and Cutler,[36] Alexander and Sherk,[37] Downes,[21] Farr and Levine,[16] Rienhoff and Davison,[38] and McNeil, MacGregor and Alexander.[19])

Streptococcic empyema at any time of life is less favorable than the pneumococcic variety, according to most studies. The prognosis of bilateral empyema is unfavorable, and left-sided empyema is more serious than right-sided. Tuberculosis, the cause of many fatal cases of purulent pleurisy in adults, is exceptionally the active agent in early life. Naturally the previous state of health, the condition at the time of operation, and the presence of complications, have all prognostic significance. The prognosis would also appear to depend upon whether the pleurisy is metapneumonic or parapneumonic, being much more unfavorable in the latter. Of 34 parapneumonic cases in the first two years of life reported by Cameron and Osman[39] all died, while of 12 metapneumonic cases all recovered.

The final recovery from empyema in children, if operated on sufficiently early and successfully, is usually remarkably complete, the lung expanding fully and little if any deformity of the chest remaining. If operation is unduly delayed, there is the danger of unyielding adhesions persisting, with failure of the lung to expand and contraction of the chest wall resulting. The duration of the disease after operation is about six to eight weeks in favorable cases with recovery, but may be much longer.

Diagnosis.—First to be determined is that an effusion exists. The recognition of this depends upon the presence of the diagnostic physical and roentgenological signs already discussed under serofibrinous pleurisy (p. 754). In many cases the diagnosis presents difficulties. The fluid may occupy the same region as a preceding pneumonia, be situated in the middle or upper portion of the chest instead of at the base, or be interlobar and small. Exploratory puncture (p. 150) should be performed in every case admitting of the slightest doubt. Not only the presence of fluid but its type must be established early in order to determine whether operation is indicated. Many times when the effusion is small or unusually located, repeated punctures may be needed to establish its existence. The distinction between an empyema and a serofibrinous effusion is of great importance therapeutically and prognostically. Empyema is the form nearly always present in infancy; the serofibrinous after five years. Fever continuing after a pneumonia, or returning after the crisis, denotes a probable empyema, and a high leukocytosis does the same. The evidences of ill health are greater in empyema. All these, however, are suggestive only, and inasmuch as the physical signs of the two conditions are the same, exploratory puncture of the chest should invariably be performed.

Pleural effusion either serous or purulent is to be distinguished from *pneumonic consolidation.* This has already been discussed elsewhere (p. 737). In *pleuropneumonia* the plastic exudate modifies the signs of croupous pneumonia and suggests effusion. Yet no displacement of the organs occurs, and there is less fulness of interspaces and diminution in the expansion of the chest-wall than accompanies effusion. Nevertheless, in pleuropneumonia, as also in pneumonia with delayed resolution, only exploratory puncture may exclude empyema. *Hydrothorax* is recognized by the existence of causes sufficient to account for it, together with the abnormal presence of fluid elsewhere; the absence of symptoms of inflammation in the chest; and the fact that both sides of the thorax are involved. Fluid obtained by puncture is of low specific gravity, and the few cells present are endothelial rather than leukocytic. *Massive collapse of the lungs* gives rise to dulness on percussion, feeble respiration, the diaphragm is high on the affected side, and the heart displaced toward the affected side (p. 748). *Pericardial effusion* if large may simulate pleural effusion of the left side. We have seen dulness reach so far to the left that puncture in the axillary region revealed serous fluid, only later found to be derived from the pericardium. *Chronic adhesive pleurisy* produces dulness and feeble respiration suggestive of effusion, but there is retraction rather than distention of the chest-wall. Yet many cases are so doubtful that exploratory puncture should be done.

Treatment.—Apart from general tonic remedies, sustaining diet, stimulants, and the like, the treatment of empyema consists in the removal of the pus. It is advisable to aspirate as often as need be in cases associated with pneumonia, until the pneumonic process is over and the acute symptoms have subsided, and such adhesions have formed as will limit the size of the post-operative pneumothorax. Sometimes simple aspiration is done, while certain clinicians recommend intrapleural instillation of such substances as genitan violet (Major[40]), sodium taurocholate (Cocchi[41]), or ethyl hydrocupreine hydrochloride (Leitner;[42] Lowenburg[43]). After the acute symptoms are over there exists the choice of several procedures. There is no doubt that merely repeated aspirations may be used with success in some cases, especially in infancy, and a trial of this should be made. The more radical surgical procedures consist of simple incision between the ribs followed by insertion of a short drainage tube; resection of a rib and drainage of the same sort; and the so-called "closed method," in which syphonage is instituted at the time of the incision, by means of a long tube passing into a vessel of water, thus preventing any ingress of air, and avoiding the shock from a suddenly collapsed lung. Personally we prefer the last method, but the selection must vary somewhat with the case.

If after operation fever continues or returns, it is usually an indication that drainage is not sufficient or that some complication is present. In a few cases we have been able finally to stop drainage by injection of bacteriophage into the pleural cavity. Irrigation with a sodium hypochlorite or other solution is often used. Perhaps autogenous vaccines may be of value in the final healing of the wound. To facilitate expansion of the lung in cases where decided adhesions have formed, the patient may be taught to employ forced expiration, as by blowing soap-bubbles, or by driving colored fluid with the breath from one bottle into another connected with it by tubing. Occasionally it is necessary to perform the Estlander's operation of removing a considerable portion of several ribs.

HYDROTHORAX

This symptom consists in the accumulation of liquid which is noninflammatory in character; a transudate in contradistinction to an exudate. It is of somewhat lower specific gravity than the fluid of serofibrinous pleurisy, more watery, contains much less albumin, no bacteria or leukocytes, and does not form a fibrin-clot on standing. Hydrothorax is nearly always bilateral, although commonly greater on one side than the other; and is usually accompanied by the accumulation of fluid in the peritoneum, pericardial cavity, subcutaneous tissues, and other regions. Its most frequent cause is disease of the heart or kidneys, although it occasionally occurs in combination with other effusions in cases where no cause whatever can be discovered; and in that event may finally disappear completely and permanently. Rarely it may be produced by pressure upon the veins. Fever, cough, pain, and friction-fremitus are absent; and any symptoms present are produced by the primary disease, with the exception of those the direct result of the mechanical interference by the fluid. Dyspnea and cyanosis are prominent among these, although they may be caused chiefly by the primary affection. The physical signs are those of fluid found in the pleural cavity, with ready shifting of the level of dulness by change of position. The treatment is that of the primary disorder. In addition aspiration may be necessary if the symptoms produced by pressure are threatening.

CHYLOTHORAX

This rare condition has been studied especially in childhood by Sherman,[44] who analyzed 11 cases, including 1 of his own, and later by Hussy,[45] who did not extend the number beyond 12, his list not entirely duplicating that of Sherman. Stewart and Linner[46] report the disease in a new-born infant. It depends upon the escape of more or less chyle from the thoracic duct or its branches into the thoracic cavity. This is probably oftenest produced by trauma with subsequent rupture, but apparently may sometimes be a transudation, brought about by pressure of enlarged bronchial glands upon the duct, or in other ways. The effusion may be unilateral or rarely bilateral. In certain cases a *chyliform* milky fluid is obtained which is due to a fatty degeneration of formed elements, and not to a true effusion of chyle. Effusions of this kind do not clear when shaken with alkalies or ether, and contain numerous leukocytes.

The symptoms and physical signs are those incident to the presence of fluid in the thoracic cavity. The characteristic of chylothorax is the discovery by puncture of a chylous effusion containing fat. There may also be present sugar, albumin, cholesterin, lecithin and a few lymphocytes. The prognosis is grave. Aspiration may be needed to relieve the pressure, and may be attended by permanent relief.

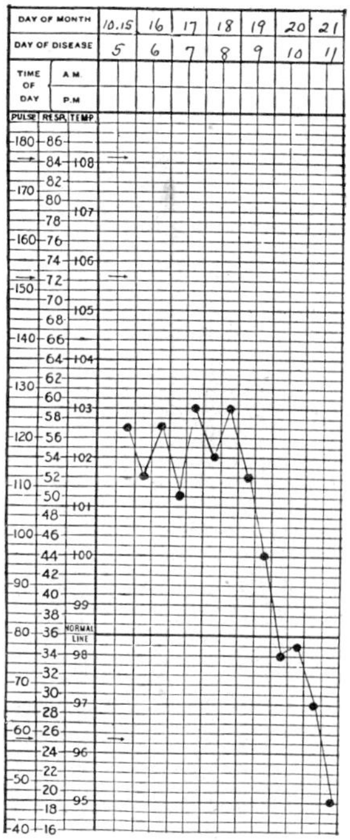

DAY OF MONTH	10.15	16	17	18	19	20	21
DAY OF DISEASE	5	6	7	8	9	10	11

Fig. 179.—Pneumothorax following croupous pneumonia. Annie G., aged three and one-half years. Crisis of pneumonia began on the tenth day, at which time typical physical signs of pneumothorax were discovered. Child failed and died on twelfth day. Necropsy showed croupous pneumonia, a fibrinous patch on the pleura, and a small perforation here passing into a small bronchus and producing a pneumothorax.

PNEUMOTHORAX

This is comparatively uncommon in early life, but cases are recorded by West,[47] Bovaird,[48] Steffen,[49] Benjamin,[50] Johnson,[51] Bashinski,[52] Stransky,[53] Rogatz and Rosenberg,[54] and Stoloff[55] who tabulates 84 spontaneous nontuberculous cases in addition to 3 of his own. We have seen a number of instances, one in a new-born infant. The condition may occur congenitally (Stein[56]). Tuberculosis is rarely the active agent in children. It is seen after pneumonia (Fig. 179), pertussis, measles, diphtheria, or emphysema, in which coughing ruptures a vesicle into the pleural cavity; or it occurs in connection with empyema, abscess or gangrene of the lung, bronchiectasis, or foreign body in, or infarct of, the lung, where a rupture through the pleura has taken place. Trauma of the chest with fracture of a rib may be the cause, as may naturally any operative procedure allowing the introduction of air into the pleural cavity. This last condition is not considered here.

The lung collapses toward its root, unless adhesions already present prevent this. The entrance of germs is liable soon to cause a pyopneumothorax, or perhaps only serous fluid may be found. **Symptoms** and physical signs may be difficult to recognize in early life. If the pneumothorax is limited in extent displacement of intrathoracic organs does not occur, and the development of the condition may be quite insidious. In other

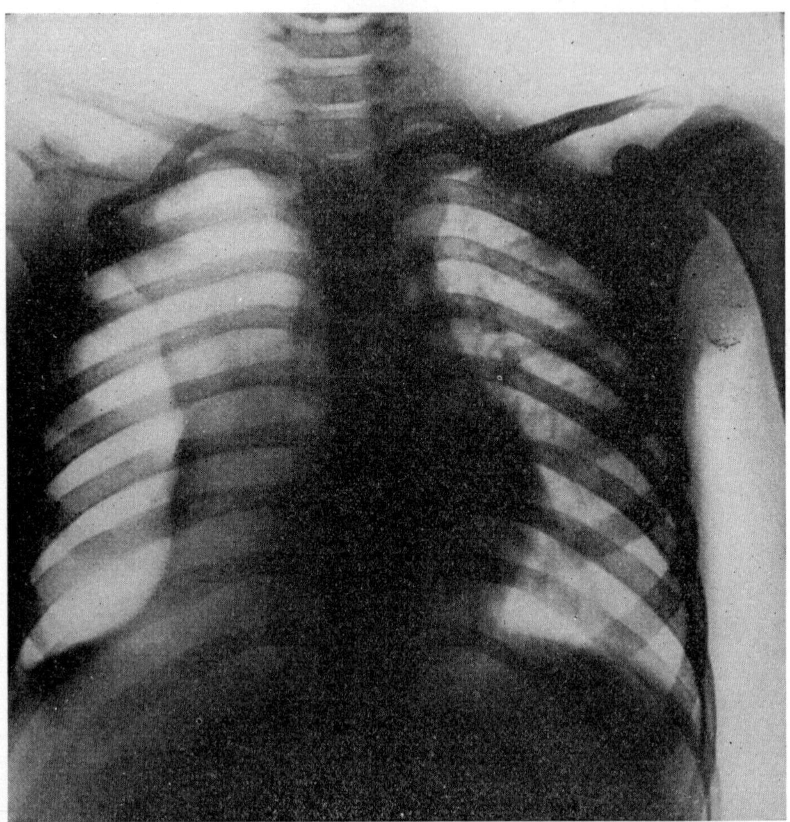

Fig. 180.—Roentgenogram of pneumothorax following empyema. Anna Z., aged six years. Children's Hospital of Philadelphia. Percussion showed hyperresonance over almost entire left side except toward the base posteriorly. Heart displaced to the right; breath-sounds nearly absent; egophony; decreased expansion of left side.

Roentgenogram shows the left side of thorax half filled with air and the lung collapsed.

cases, however, there are sudden dyspnea, prostration, cyanosis, widespread tympany, faint amphoric breathing, bell-percussion, and perhaps a positive coin-test. The physical signs and symptoms vary, depending upon the amount of fluid which may be present. Pneumothorax is to be **diagnosed** from emphysema; resembling it in the tympanitic resonance and feeble respiration, but differing in the amphoric breathing. Emphysema, too, is bilateral. A high situation of a dilated stomach may on examination suggest pneumothorax, and this may also readily be simulated by large phthisical cavities. In these, however, the amphoric breathing and the breath-sounds are generally louder. Roentgenograms of the chest are very characteristic (Fig. 180). The **prognosis** depends upon the cause. When this is not one which occasions repeated entrance of air into the chest, or which is productive of pus, simple pneumothorax will usually recover with the resorption of the air. **Treatment** other than symptomatic is only needed when the pressure of air is sufficient to cause great embarrassment of respiration, or when a pyopneumothorax exists. In the former, aspiration is necessary, in the latter surgical treatment for empyema.

MALFORMATIONS, PARASITES, AND MORBID GROWTHS OF THE LUNGS AND PLEURA

Absence of one lung is a very unusual defect. Levy[57] was able to assemble a total of 21 reported instances to which he added 1. He found in addition reports of 4 cases in which it was probable that a **rudimentary lung** covered an imperfectly developed primary bronchus. **Hernia** of a portion of the lung through a defect in the thoracic wall is a rare congenital anomaly. It presents an elastic tumor covered by skin and pleura, gives a resonant percussion-note and is reducible by mild pressure. **Congenital cysts** may be found. Koontz[58] collected 108 cases and others have since been reported by deLange,[59] Swanson, Platou and Sadler,[60] Gibson,[61] Wolman,[62] and Parmelee and Apfelbach.[63] **Hydatid cysts** are unusual and found mostly in regions where this parasite is encountered. Morquio[64] records 112 cases in children. **Actinomycosis** is exceptional, but a few cases in children have been reported from North America (Halpern and Levinson,[65] Christison and Warwick,[66] Johnson and Kernan[67]). Nobécourt and Kaplan[68] give a review of the subject. The symptoms suggest neoplasm or empyema. In addition to large doses of potassium iodide, treatment by injections of iodized oil through a bronchoscope has been advised. **Anthrax** may be encountered rarely. A case in a child is reported by McKitterick and Pearson.[69]

Malignant neoplasms, especially sarcoma, are sometimes seen as secondary developments in the lung or pleura, or very exceptionally primarily there. **Bronchomycosis** or fungus infection of the lung, may occur with various types of these organisms, such as Monilia albicans (Stokes, Kiser and Smith[70]). Among the rarer infecting ones may be mentioned the Sporotrichum (Forbus[71]), and the Torula histolytica (Hirsch and Coleman[72]).

References

1. Journ. f. Kinderkr., 1864, **42,** 371. 2. Phila. M. J., 1898, **2,** 557. 3. L'Obstetrique, 1900, **5,** 7. 4. Thèse de Paris, 1902. 5. Am. J. Dis. Child., 1931, **41,** 110. 6. Am. J. Dis. Child., 1926, **31,** 439. 7. Arch. Pediat., 1911, **28,** 28. 8. Thèse de Copenhagen 1882. Ref. Netter Ref. No. 9. 9. Grancher: Traité de mal. de l'enf., 1904, **3,** 644; 674. 10. Pediatria, 1913, **21,** 588. 11. Pediatria, 1922, **30,** 841. 12. Pediatria, 1926, **34,** 1292. 13. Proc. Roy. Soc. Medicine, 1907–08; Med. Sec. 63. 14. Edinburgh M. J., 1914, **13,** 4. 15. Bost. M. and S. J., 1919, **181,** 87. 16. Surg. Gynec. and Obst., 1928, **46,** 79. 17. Am. J. Dis. Child., 1920, **20,** 545. 18. Am. J. M. Sc., 1922, **163,** 246. 19. Arch. Dis. Childh., 1929, **4,** 270. 20. Pediatria, 1923, **31,** 577. 21. M. J. Australia, 1927, **2,** 109. 22. Am. J. Dis. Child., 1926, **32,** 497. 23. Ann. Clin. Med., 1927, **5,** 959. 24. Ugesk. f. Laeger., 1928, **90,** 220. 25. Brit. M. J., 1903, **1,** 1200. 26. Berl. klin. Wchnschr., 1905, **42,** 1415. 27. Deutsche Ztschr. f. klin. Chir., 1910–11, **108,** 584. 28. Dis. Inf. Child., 1910, 652. 29. Am. J. Dis. Child., 1921, **21,** 546. 30. Trans. Assn. Am. Phys., 1893, **8,** 195. 31. Arch. Pediat., 1910, **27,** 26. 32. Arch. f. Kinderh., 1903, **36,** 252. 33. Lancet, 1895, **2,** 1357. 34. Amer. Med., 1913, **19,** 381. 35. New York State J. Med., 1914, **14,** 342. 36. Surg., Gynec. and Obst., 1924, **39,** 429. 37. Atlantic M. J., 1926, **29,** 602. 38. Arch. Surg., 1928, **17,** 676. 39. Lancet, 1923, **1,** 1097. 40. Am. J. M. Sc., 1921, **162,** 405. 41. Riv. di clin. pediat., 1927, **25,** 410. 42. Jahrb. f. Kinderh., 1928, **119,** 227. 43. J.A.M.A., 1929, **93,** 106. 44. Arch. Pediat., 1907, **24,** 646. 45. Jahrb. f. Kinderh., 1918, **87,** 491. 46. Am. J. Dis. Child., 1926, **31,** 654. 47. Lancet, 1884, **1,** 791. 48. Arch. Pediat., 1903, **20,** 817. 49. Arch. Pediat., 1926, **43,** 50. 50. Arch. f. Kinderh., 1926, **77,** 241. 51. Am. J. Dis. Child., 1927, **33,** 740. 52. South. M. J., 1929, **22,** 525. 53. Monatschr. f. Kinderh., 1930, **46,** 109. 54. Am. J. Dis. Child., 1931, **41,** 1104. 55. Am. J. M. Sc., 1928, **176,** 657. 56. Am. J. Dis. Child., 1930, **40,** 89. 57. Am. J. M. Sc., 1920, **159,** 237. 58. Bull. Johns

Hopkins Hosp., 1925, **37,** 340. 59. Acta paediat., 1927, **6,** 352. 60. Am. J. Dis. Child., 1928, **35,** 1024. 61. Am. J. Roentgenol., 1929, **22,** 155. 62. Bull. Ayer Clin. Lab. Penna. Hosp., 1930, **2,** 49. 63. Am. J. Dis. Child., 1931, **41,** 1380. 64. Arch. de méd. d. enf., 1926, **29,** 5. 65. J.A.M.A., 1928, **91,** 13. 66. J.A.M.A., 1927, **89,** 1043. 67. Am. J. Dis. Child., 1928, **36,** 508. 68. Arch. de méd. d. enf., 1930, **33,** 391. 69. Am. J. Dis. Child., 1929, **38,** 1252. 70. J.A.M.A., 1930, **95,** 14. 71. Am. Rev. Tuberc., 1927, **16,** 599. 72. J.A.M.A., 1929, **92,** 437.

SECTION VI

DISEASES OF THE CIRCULATORY SYSTEM

CHAPTER I

INTRODUCTORY

The characteristics of the anatomy and physiology of the heart and blood-vessels in early life, including the arrangement of blood-vessels in the fetus, have already been discussed. (See p. 36.) There remain to be considered the diagnostic indications of circulatory symptoms, and also the changes occurring in the circulation after birth.

INDICATIONS DERIVED FROM THE PHYSICAL EXAMINATION OF THE HEART IN EARLY LIFE

The fact that the percussion-dulness of the heart is relatively greater in early life than in adults (p. 36) is important in making a diagnosis of pathologic conditions. Equally important is the knowledge of the normal position of the apex-beat at this period. Thus in infancy an apex-beat found in the fifth interspace is abnormally low by one interspace, and it is only after the seventh year that it is discovered nearly always in this position. Normally, too, the apex-beat is farther to the left than in adult life, and a situation beyond the mammillary line is not an evidence of enlargement (p. 36). It is particularly in early life, owing to the yielding character of the thoracic framework at this time, that cardiac enlargement is so often productive of decided precordial bulging. Irregularity of the cardiac rhythm is a normal feature of infancy and to some extent of early childhood, especially during sleep. As a pathologic manifestation it may occur during convalescence from infectious disorders; in toxic conditions from intestinal and other sources; in intracranial affections, and in maladies of the heart itself. Reduplication of the heart-sounds observed at this period is frequent, and is likewise not necessarily an indication of disease. Slowness of the heart's rhythm is often pathologic. It may be due to various toxic agents, as seen, for instance, in jaundice and diphtheria; and is observed also in endocarditis, diseases of the brain, and heart-block; but is also not uncommon in convalescence from fevers and often possesses no special significance. (See pp. 37; 801.) Increased rapidity, on the other hand, is of such frequent occurrence that by itself it possesses little pathologic meaning. It may result from fear, nervous excitement, or the action of certain drugs and poisons; and in one form is compensatory to a reduced cardiac output. Among auscultatory phenomena, of most importance is to remember the normal accentuation of the pulmonary second sound, which is louder in early life than is the aortic. This is especially true during infancy and early childhood. The first sound of the heart is always louder than the second during the first four or five years of life and in the first year is very valve-like, the rhythm suggesting the ticking of a watch. This, so serious a sign of great cardiac weakness in adults, is therefore of no pathologic importance at this earlier period. The diffusion of murmurs, as well as of the normal sounds, is often extensive. This is dependent upon the small size of the chest and the comparatively large mass of the heart. Naturally, therefore, fewer inferences can be drawn from this diffusion than is the case in adult cardiac disease. The accidental cardiac murmurs so common in adult life are claimed to be less often heard in children, and rarely in infancy. (See p. 802.) In our experience they occur, on the whole, not at all infrequently, especially as the result of anemia; or they may be cardiopulmonary in nature. The anemic murmurs are often loud, systolic, and suggestive of a valvular lesion. In addition to these murmurs there may be others audible in the arteries and veins, especially of the neck. Those in the arteries are usually merely transmitted from a heart affected by valvular disease. Care must be taken not to exert too great a pressure with the stethoscope, or a murmur by compression may be produced. This is, in fact, true even of the heart itself, where firm pressure in rachitic subjects may readily give rise to a systolic murmur. Venous murmurs are common in cases of anemia at all ages. They are oftenest heard in the neck, but sometimes over the front of the thorax also, and may be developed over the manubrium of the sternum when the head is thrown back. It is to be noted, however, that a venous murmur may occur in individuals not anemic (p. 804). The employment of roentgenography is of service in the examination of the heart for the purpose of confirming or amplifying the results of the examination by percussion. The polygraph and electrocardiograph have been purposely omitted from consideration; largely because much special training is required for their satisfactory employment and for the interpretation of the results obtained.

FETAL CIRCULATION AND THE CHANGES AT BIRTH

The fetal circulation (Fig. 181) has an intimate relationship to the production of congenital diseases of the heart. During intra-uterine life the smaller, pulmonary circulation is not in action, since aeration takes place through the placenta. The blood enters the right auricle from: (1) the superior vena cava, which carries blood of a wholly venous character; and (2) the inferior vena cava, in which the blood is of a mixed quality, being composed, namely, of the venous blood from the body of the child and the oxygenated blood brought from the placenta by the umbilical vein. The greater part of the blood from the umbilical vein circulates through the liver before entering the inferior cava; the smaller quantity enters the cava directly from the umbilical vein. After entering the right auricle the partly oxygenated blood from the inferior cava passes to a large extent, according to the generally accepted view, through the foramen ovale into the left auricle and thence to the left ventricle and into the aorta. The wholly venous blood from the superior cava, on the other hand, passes from the right auricle into the right ventricle and thence into the pulmonary artery, whence it goes partly, although in but small amount, to the lungs, but chiefly through the ductus arteriosus into the aorta. According to Patten[1] it is probable that the volume of blood circulating through the lungs at the close of fetal life is adequate to care for respiration in the new-born as soon as the lungs are properly ventilated. Since the ductus arteriosus joins the aorta beyond the point of origin of the innominate and the left carotid and subclavian arteries, it follows that these vessels are supplied with blood oxygenated to a greater degree than it is after the entrance of the purely venous blood from the ductus arteriosus has taken place. The blood of the body returns from the general circulation to the placenta by way of the umbilical arteries.

With the cessation at birth of circulation in the umbilical arteries and vein, and the simultaneous beginning of the respiratory function, the pressure in the right heart is much diminished, and, as a result, blood ceases to pass through the foramen ovale and the ductus arteriosus, and both of these close. Christie[2] found the foramen ovale closed prior to twelve weeks in 87 per cent of 509 normal infants up to one year of age, and the ductus arteriosis before eight weeks in 88 per cent of 558 infants. Sometimes the

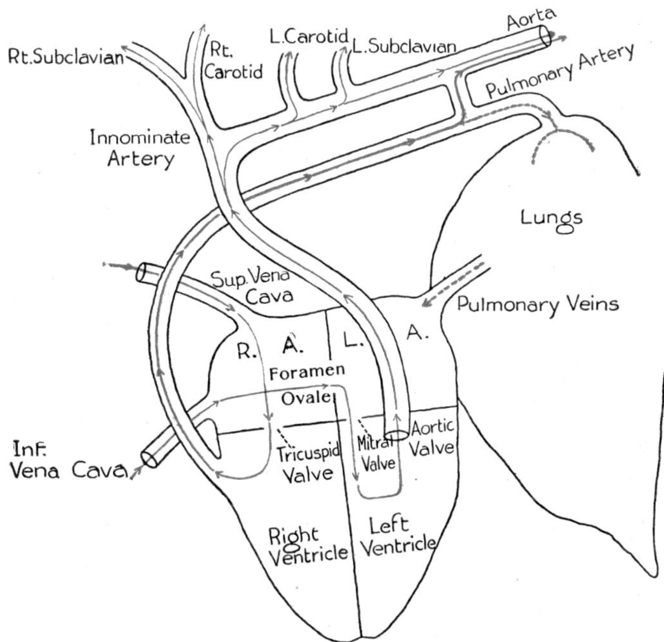

Fig. 181.—Diagram illustrating the course of the blood-currents in the fetal circulation. *Red*, partly arterial blood; *blue*, venous blood.

foramen ovale remains as a small opening throughout life (20 per cent (Patten[1])).

References

1. Am. Heart J., 1930–31, **6,** 192. 2. Am. J. Dis. Child., 1930, **40,** 323.

CHAPTER II

CONGENITAL CARDIAC DISEASE

This condition while encountered repeatedly is less frequent than acquired disease of the heart. Norris[1] in 1272 collected cases of cardiac disease found 7.6 per cent to be congenital. It is observed oftenest in early life, since many of the patients die before reaching maturity. In 1000 necropsies on children under thirteen years of age, Epstein[2] recorded cardiac anomalies in 4 per cent. In 2792 sick children under ten years of age, Still[3] found symptoms of congenital heart-disease in 0.57 per cent. Of 500 patients two to twenty years of age coming to a heart-clinic, 11.2 per cent had congenital cardiac defects (Wilson[4]). These various figures do not for the most part include the frequent instances of small patulous foramen ovale found only at necropsy.

Etiology.—This is not clearly understood. The effect of constitutional disease of the parents is questionable. The percentage of children with congenital heart-disease who have syphilis, and the percentage of congenital syphilitics who have congenital heart-disease, is slightly if any greater than in any average group. That any cause influencing harmfully the health of the parent might be a predisposing factor is indicated by the frequent coincident occurrence of other developmental defects, such as atresia of the anus, harelip, idiocy, polydactylia, and the like. Old age of the parents, although claimed by some authors to be a factor, does not seem to be proven so. A familial tendency has sometimes been observed, as in the cases reported by de la Camp[5] and by Sprague, Bland and White,[6] but this is not usual. There appears to be a preponderance of cases among males and first-born infants. We have suspected that there is frequent association of light complexion and, especially, red hair with congenital heart-disease, but cannot prove this statistically.

Many cases are due to *interference with the normal process of development*, although the reason why this took place is not clear. Here, for example, can be included defects of the interventricular septum. Other forms may be due to a *fetal endocarditis*. In this category belong cases of stenosis of the valvular orifices, at least in part; others probably being produced by arrested development. Most defects depending upon any inflammatory process must make their appearance before the third month of intrauterine life (Owen and Kingsbury[7]). Still other instances depend upon *failure of closure after birth of normal prenatal openings*, this being the result of some other diseased condition of the heart. In this category are patulous ductus arteriosus and patulous foramen ovale. In some cases there is *faulty insertion* or *insufficient rotation of fetal vessels*, as in anomalies of the great vessels; or *vessels may be absent*. It is to be remembered that endocarditis may develop as a secondary lesion in extrauterine life, or in intrauterine life be secondary to an arrested development.

Pathologic Anatomy.—The usual lesions of congenital cardiac disease may be divided into: (1) Anomalies of the septa between the chambers of the heart; (2) anomalies of the vessels or their valves; (3) anomalies in the size or position of the heart. In tabular arrangement the subdivisions of these chief classes are as follows:

TABLE 68.—CLASSIFICATION OF FORMS OF CONGENITAL CARDIAC DISEASE

1. ANOMALIES OF THE SEPTA		Patulous foramen ovale Perforate septum ventriculorum
2. ANOMALIES OF THE VALVES AND VESSELS	(*a*) Valves	Pulmonary stenosis Pulmonary insufficiency Aortic stenosis Aortic insufficiency Mitral stenosis Mitral insufficiency
	(*b*) Vessels	Patulous ductus arteriosus Stenosis of pulmonary artery Dilatation of pulmonary artery Narrowing of aorta Dilatation of aorta Hypoplasia of aorta and vessels Transposition of great vessels
3. ANOMALIES IN THE SIZE AND POSITION OF THE HEART		Transposition of heart chambers Dextrocardia Congenital hypertrophy Ectocardia

The figures shown on p. 769 are abstracted from the statistical table of Abbott[8] based on 850 cases.

The tendency is for more than one lesion to exist at a time, and many varied combinations are met with. In the list given the great majority are combined with other cardiac defects. Most of the lesions mentioned are uncommon and present no diagnostic symptoms by which they can be recog-

TABLE 69.—FREQUENCY OF DIFFERENT FORMS OF CONGENITAL CARDIAC DISEASE

Variety.	No. of Cases.
Defects of the interauricular septum	312
(258 of these being patent foramen ovale)	
Defects of the interventricular septum	269
Patulous ductus arteriosus	235
Pulmonary stenosis and atresia	173
Stenosis (coarctation) of the aorta	140
Anomalies of the semilunar cusps	124
Transposition of arterial trunks	88
Anomalies of the heart as a whole	69
Anomalous septa or chordae	52
Complete defects of cardiac septa	52
Hypoplasia of the aorta	52
Tricuspid and mitral stenosis	45
Defects of aortic septum	44
Displacement of the heart	40
Aortic stenosis and atresia	34
Anomalies of the pericardium	32

nized during life. Those of most importance are defects in the interauricular septum; defects in the interventricular septum; stenosis of the pulmonary orifice; patulous ductus arteriosus.

1. **Congenital Defect in the Interauricular Septum.**—This is a relatively common lesion, but usually of no great clinical importance. In fact, a slightly patulous condition of the foramen ovale was found in 44 per cent of 300 necropsies reported by Wallmann.[9] Fisher[10] observed slight patency present in over 25 per cent of post-mortems on adult subjects. (See also p. 36.) Generally the opening is small, and in such cases, if occurring alone, it can hardly be called pathologic. When large enough to constitute an abnormal condition it is present oftenest in combination with other congenital cardiac defects. In Abbott's[8] 850 cases of congenital heart-disease there were 112 of persistence of the foramen ovale of a size which could be called pathologic, and in 32 of these it was the only lesion present. Much more rarely the lower portion of the interauricular septum may exhibit defective formation, showing one or more apertures, or the septum may even be entirely wanting.

2. **Congenital Defect in the Interventricular Septum.**—This is among the most frequent of congenital cardiac lesions. It occurs usually in association with anomalies in the condition of the large vessels or orifices; and probably the most common condition with clinical manifestations seen in congenital cardiac disease is the combination of this with pulmonary stenosis, and often with patulous ductus arteriosus. It is found alone in a very much smaller number. The opening is situated at the upper part of the septum in the large majority of cases and may be very small, but is generally big enough to admit the tip of the little finger. Sometimes it is larger than this, and even the entire septum may be absent, thus producing a heart with two auricles and one ventricle; the *cor triloculare*. If the auricular septum is also absent the *cor biloculare* results.

3. **Stenosis or Atresia of the Pulmonary Ostium.**—This is one of the most common of congenital lesions of the heart, and the most important of those which permit of the continuance of life. It was present in 173 of Abbott's series of 850 cases. Peacock[11] reported atresia or stenosis in 119 of 181 cases of congenital heart-disease; *i. e.*, 65.75 per cent; and in patients surviving at the age of twelve years it was observed 38 times in 45 cases; *i. e.*, 84.44 per cent. Hochsinger[12] estimated it at about 60 per cent of all cases. The narrowing of the pulmonary ostium may be of various degrees. Complete atresia is less common than stenosis. Vierordt[13] found 83 collected cases of stenosis and 24 of atresia; a ratio of 3.46:1. The contraction is sometimes in the ostium alone, but in the large majority of cases the conus

arteriosus is also involved. The semilunar valves may be more or less movable or may be stiffened into entire immobility. Pulmonary stenosis generally occurs in combination with other congenital cardiac diseases; in fact is a cause of them in many instances, they existing as an attempt at compensation to admit of the better passage of blood from the right side of the heart. Consequently stenosis is present in combination with defect of the interventricular septum more frequently than it occurs alone. In Vierordt's 83 cases of stenosis, 71 (85.5 per cent) had also septum-defect; and in the 24 cases of atresia, 14 (58.3 per cent) had this lesion. In 192 cases of pulmonary stenosis collected from medical literature Rachfuss[14] noted 171 with combined defect of the ventricular septum, and only 21 without this. This association is especially true of patients over one year of age, inasmuch as stenosis occurring alone usually does not permit of a long continuance of life. A patulous foramen ovale is a very frequent attendant upon pulmonary stenosis. Küssmaul[15] reported the foramen open in 39 out of 53 cases (73.6 per cent). The ductus arteriosus is also patulous in many instances. According to Küssmaul this was true in 9 out of 39 cases (23.1 per cent) of stenosis and in 14 out of 17 cases (82.53 per cent) of atresia.

4. Patulous Ductus Arteriosus.—This, like patulous foramen ovale, is not a malformation but the persistence of a fetal condition normally present at birth. It is common in association with other lesions, especially pulmonary stenosis and perforate ventricular septum; but is infrequent alone. Vierordt collected but 26 uncomplicated cases from medical literature. Abbott's list contains 84 instances. It is usually a secondary lesion, oftenest to those of the septum and pulmonary artery, and is then compensatory, offering a means for the unoxygenated blood to reach the lungs. In other cases it is the result of early pulmonary atelectasis. When of small lumen, as of a size sufficient to admit only a probe, it has no clinical significance and is probably quite common.

Other Congenital Disorders of the Heart.—These are either less common or have no special clinical significance. Congenital *disease of the tricuspid orifice* is not common, and rarely occurs except in combination with other cardiac lesions; and that of the *mitral orifice* is still rarer. J. Hess[16] was able to collect but 8 reported cases of uncomplicated atresia of the tricuspid orifice, to which he added another. Stenosis or atresia of the *aortic ostium* likewise is infrequent. It may or may not be associated with perforate septum or with patulous foramen ovale. In rare instances a subaortic stenosis has been observed (Thursfield and Scott[17]). There may be an *anomalous origin of the vessels* leaving the heart. This is a not uncommon condition. Various forms may be seen, as when both vessels arise from one ventricle, or the aorta from both; or both vessels from one trunk, or an incomplete separation of the aorta and pulmonary artery exists, or there is complete absence of the arch of the aorta, of which anomaly Gödel[18] could find but 8 instances including one of his own. One of the most interesting forms is complete transposition, in which the pulmonary artery arises from the left ventricle and the aorta from the right (Fig. 182). This occurred in 58 of Abbott's series. Kato[19] records 5 cases of transposition of the great vessels and collected published reports of a number of others. All these anomalies are associated with other cardiac malformations. Congenital *narrowness* or *dilatation of the pulmonary artery* may occur, the former oftenest in combination with stenosis of the pulmonary orifice. Dilatation of the pulmonary orifice is uncommon existing alone, but often seen in combination with other lesions. It is associated oftenest with defect in the interventricular septum or with patulous ductus arteriosus. A not uncommon condition is *stenosis of the isthmus of the aorta* near the origin of the ductus arteriosus. This is of two types, as described by Bonnet;[20] the infantile, in which there is a diffuse narrowing of the isthmus of the aorta, slight or severe, which is generally accompanied by a patulous ductus arteriosus; and the adult type, which is produced in the process of closing of the ductus, and results in a narrow constriction of the aorta between the ductus and the left subclavian artery. The infantile type is associated with numerous other cardiac malformations. It is not often encountered after the period of infancy. The other, more frequent form, called also

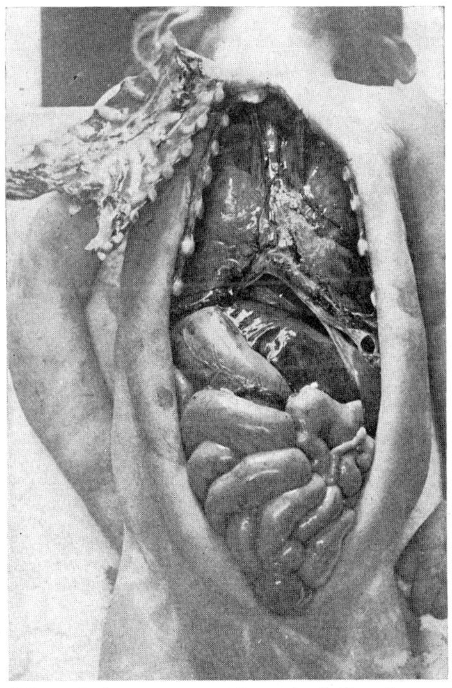

Fig. 182.—Transposition of the great vessels and of the viscera in a case of congenital cardiac disease in a male infant of eight months. Cavae emptied into the left auricle, pulmonary veins into the right. Aorta arose from right ventricle and descended on right side of the spinal column. Pulmonary artery arose from left ventricle, small, orifice stenosed. Upper part of ventricular septum deficient. Right lung 2 lobes, left lung 3. Stomach, liver, spleen, and cecum transposed. (*Griffith, Univ. Med. Mag.*, 1899, *Aug.*)

coarctation of the aorta is accompanied later by extensive development of the collateral circulation. A general *hypoplasia of the aorta and arterial system*, with smallness of the heart, is sometimes seen. Finally in rare cases a congenital cardiac hypertrophy may occur (p. 798), or the apex of the heart points to the right (*dextrocardia*); or its *chambers are transposed*, often in combination with transposition of the abdominal viscera; or the heart may project through an opening in the diaphragm into the abdominal cavity, or from the body through an abnormal aperture in the chest-wall (*ectocardia; ectopia cordis*). This uncommon condition usually has congenital absence of the pericardium associated with it. Numerous other congenital defects and anomalies are described in medical literature but possess only academic interest.

General Symptomatology.—There are certain manifestations which, when present, render the existence of congenital cardiac disease very probable. Among these are especially the following:

Cyanosis.—This condition, indicating oxygen unsaturation, is observed usually soon after birth, and may be very intense and distributed over the entire surface of the body, including the mucous membranes especially of the mouth. In other cases it is limited to the fingers, toes, lips, nose, cheeks, and ears; may be evident only after crying, or, in older children, after exercise or excitement; or may appear especially during some pulmonary disorder. In still other instances cyanosis does not develop until the child is some months or even years of age, and then may be general or limited; continuous or intermittent. In well-marked cases the skin is of a bluish-red or of a slate color and the mucous membrane of the mouth is purple-red (Figs. 183, 184, 185). In long-continued cases dilatation of the veins and of the cutaneous capillaries occurs, and the retinal vessels may be distended and tortuous.

The cause of the cyanosis has been much disputed and the question is by no means settled. One view is that it is due to a mixture of arterial and venous blood, and another that it depends upon imperfect oxygenation of blood from a passive congestion in the general venous system and in the pulmonary circulation. Holman[21] after a careful study of several cases concludes that it is due to admixture, but only when the venous blood flows through abnormal openings into the arterial circulation, *i. e.*, a shunt from right to left. This subject is especially well discussed by Lundsgaard and Van Slyke.[22] The absence of cyanosis by no means proves the absence of congenital cardiac disease. It may be absent even with severe cardiac malformation where, although admixture is beyond question, as in two-chambered hearts, cyanosis is only a terminal symptom; and it has been stated that with a hemoglobin content of the blood as low as 30 per cent cyanosis does not develop, but pallor may be present. This is seen oftenest in cases of pulmonary stenosis. The nature of the malformation is the deciding element in the production of the cyanosis, pulmonary stenosis occupying perhaps the chief position here. Transposition of the great vessels is a less frequent cause. On the other hand, the presence of congenital cyanosis is not of itself proof that congenital malformation of the heart exists, since it may be well-marked in cases of congenital atelectasis and in other conditions with deficient arterial circulation.

Blood.—With the cyanosis there are characteristic alterations of the blood. The amount of CO_2 present is augmented and the number of red blood-cells is decidedly above normal, reaching frequently as high as 7,000,000 or 8,000,000 to the cubic millimeter or sometimes even well over this. The percentage of hemoglobin is usually increased proportionately.

Clubbing of the Fingers.—This is a very characteristic symptom seen in severe cases and always associated with cyanosis, although developing somewhat later. The whole terminal phalanx of the finger or toe is enlarged (Figs. 184, 185), either from involvement of the soft parts only, or dependent as well on an osteoperiostitis. A similar condition, although without cyanosis, may be seen in chronic pulmonary diseases. (See also p. 999, Fig. 237.)

Other Symptoms.—Among other symptoms observed is dyspnea, which, with increased rapidity of respiration, is present in all cases of cyanosis. It may be slight or occur only on exertion; or there may be in bad cases in infants and young children severe suffocative or anginoid attacks, during which the cyanosis becomes intense and death seems imminent. The attacks may be accompanied by unconsciousness or by epileptiform convulsions. Hemorrhages from the mouth or nose occasionally occur. Edema is not a common manifestation except as failure of compensation becomes marked. Palpitation is sometimes troublesome. The temperature is usually subnormal, the extremities cold, and the patient complains of chilli-

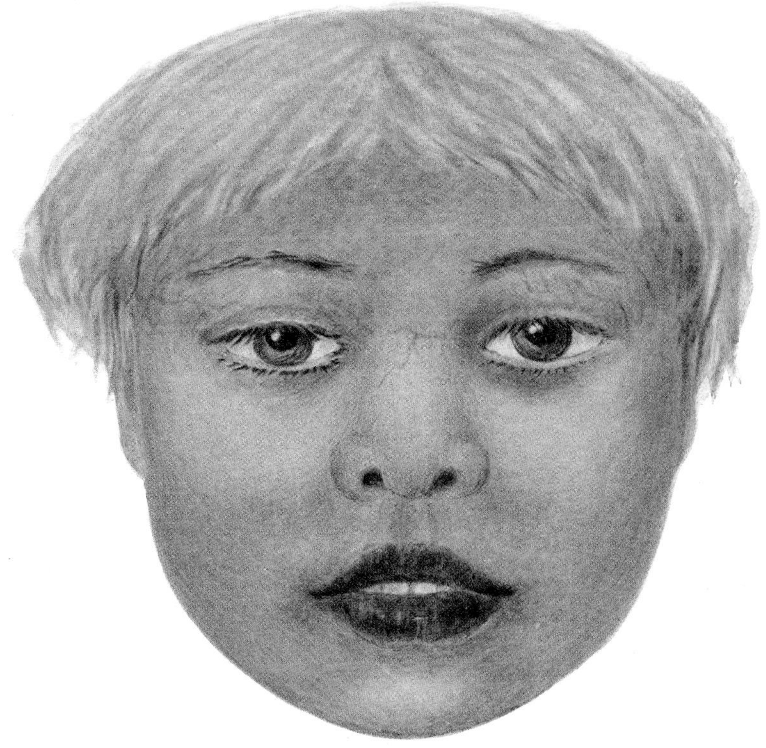

Fig. 183.—Congenital disease of the heart. Boy, aged three years. Intense, wide-spread cyanosis; attacks of syncope and severe dyspnea. No murmur. Red blood-cells 9,040,000; hemoglobin 120 per cent. Roentgenogram showed decided enlargement of the heart to the left. Condition presumably anomalous origin of the great vessels.

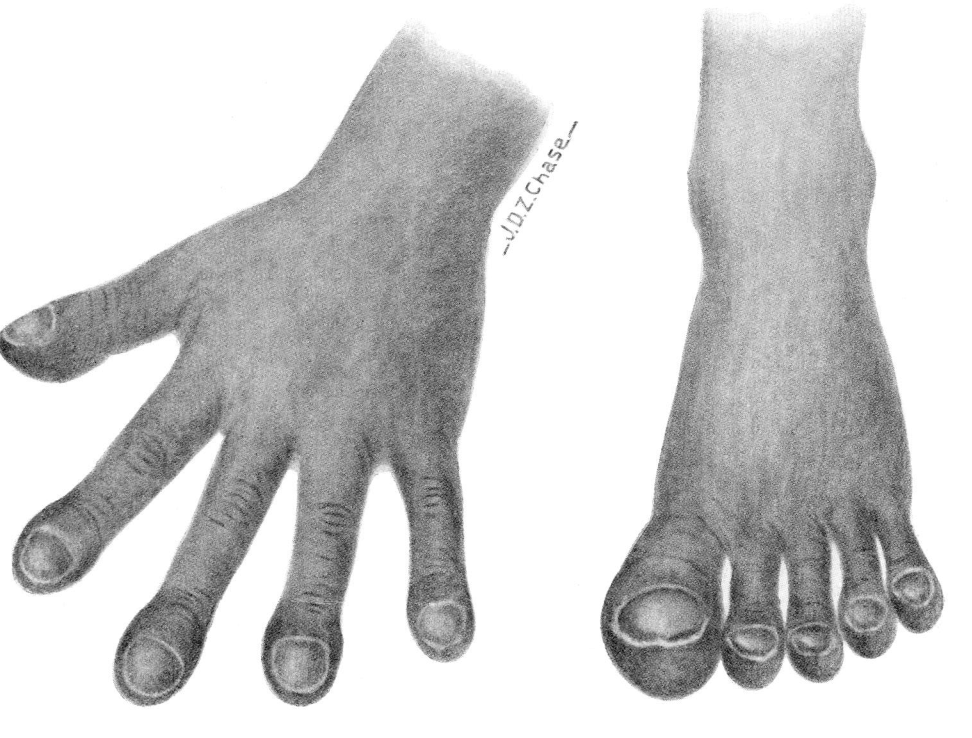

Figs. 184 and 185.—Clubbing of fingers and toes in congenital heart-disease. (Same case as in Fig. 183.)

ness. The pulse generally is rapid; exceptionally is slow. Bodily and mental development are retarded in well-marked cases, the general nutrition suffers, and a condition of infantilism may follow.

Cardiac Examination.—There are generally a loud widely diffused murmur; precordial thrill; often an accentuated pulmonary second sound; and but little cardiac enlargement, at least early in the case. The physical signs will be discussed in detail in connection with the different forms of congenital cardiac disease.

Diagnosis.—The diagnosis in general rests upon the data already given. A patient in the first two or three years of life, with cyanosis, thrill, a loud murmur, and only moderate enlargement of the right side of the heart, usually not in proportion to the cardiac symptoms and physical signs, is probably suffering from congenital cardiac disease. As a rule the murmur is loud, rough, and sometimes musical, and heard best at the mid-sternum or to its left; and the apex-beat is weak or at least not increased in strength. Yet the diagnosis is often difficult and sometimes impossible; especially as grave cardiac lesions may exist without in some cases producing any murmur whatever, or in other cases any cyanosis. Postnatal lesions depending upon endocarditis exhibit the symptoms and physical signs characteristic of the variety present; and the position of maximum intensity and the nature of diffusion of the murmur vary with the lesion and are quite different from those observed in the congenital cases. Cyanosis in acquired disease of the heart is a later symptom, edema usually developing first. There is generally, too, the history of an antecedent rheumatism or some other cause.

The diagnosis of congenital murmurs from those of an accidental nature is sometimes difficult. The latter are either functional, and then of a softer, less diffused nature; or are dependent upon anemia, and then are transmitted into the vessels of the neck and are attended by evidences of anemia but not of enlargement of the heart. The cyanosis of congenital heart-disease is to be distinguished likewise from that due to other causes; notably atelectasis in infants; and later from the cyanosis with polycythemia and enlargement of the spleen described by Vaquez,[23] and which is known by his name (p. 1022).

The diagnosis of the different forms of congenital disease of the heart from each other is, as a rule, a matter of great difficulty. The variety of combinations which may occur is great, and, moreover, the physical signs may not be those which could be expected from the mechanical difficulties present. Furthermore, lesions may be found at necropsy in patients who had exhibited no positive evidence of cardiac disease during life. Nevertheless, the effort should always be made to diagnose the condition present; especially as the prognosis varies with the type of the lesion. The following symptoms and physical signs are to be expected:

Defect in the Interauricular Septum.—It is questionable whether patulous foramen ovale or other defect of the septum is productive of any symptoms, especially when occurring alone, unless the defect is a large one. When associated circumstances greatly disturb the relative intracardiac pressure in the two auricles, cyanosis may develop and a diastolic murmur over the upper part of the sternum may be heard in some instances. Such disturbing conditions are, however, usually due to the presence of other congenital cardiac malformations, and these obscure the diagnosis of interauricular defect.

Defect in the Interventricular Septum.—Perhaps of all the varieties this gives the most characteristic symptoms and physical signs; yet it is possible for it to exist without any evidence whatever during life. Occurring alone it has been described especially by Roger[24] and is often named for him,

"Maladie de Roger." In this form cyanosis and dyspnea may be absent or present, varying with the case and due to factors not well understood but probably dependent on the size of the defect; since naturally a small defect and the greater pressure in the left ventricle would allow little if any venous blood to flow into the arterial circulation. The presence of other complicating lesions, such as pulmonary stenosis, usually results in cyanosis; and the absence of this symptom generally indicates the absence of such a lesion. In Abbott's[8] series cyanosis was observed in less than half of the uncomplicated cases. Examination of the heart generally reveals a loud systolic murmur over the whole precordium, with maximum intensity at the mid-sternum or in the third interspace just to the left of the sternum. The murmur is generally less loud at the apex and is widely diffused, being audible even in the back, but in uncomplicated cases not conducted along the large vessels. All the valve-sounds are audible. The murmur is produced in cases of simple perforate septum by the blood passing from the left ventricle into the right. This necessarily increases the pressure in the right side, normally less than on the left, and the pulmonary second sound is consequently accentuated to a moderate degree. In cases combined with pulmonary atresia or well-developed stenosis the blood passes in the other direction; *i. e.*, through the perforate septum from the right side to the left, as this is often the only sufficient method of exit; and in some such cases, the murmur, being produced by whirls of blood just beneath the opening of the aorta, may be transmitted along this vessel into the carotid and subclavian arteries.

The loudness, or even the presence, of the murmur is not in proportion to the size of the defect in the septum. Even large openings may sometimes be unattended by murmur, and if the septum is completely wanting no murmur can be produced. A distinct systolic thrill is sometimes felt, but is not a necessary accompaniment. If the case is long-continued, enlargement of the right side of the heart will develop, but in earlier cases is not discovered, especially when the septum-defect occurs alone.

Uncomplicated defect of the interventricular septum is to be distinguished from pulmonary stenosis by the lower situation of the murmur; its wider diffusion; the more frequent absence of cyanosis; and the presence of valvular sounds when cyanosis does exist. Very important in uncomplicated cases of each condition is the auscultation of the pulmonary second sound. In perforate septum the sound is accentuated; in pulmonary stenosis it is weaker than normal. In the numerous cases in which septum defect is combined with pulmonary stenosis the diagnosis can be made only by a careful consideration of all the symptoms. Auscultation alone is hardly sufficient.

The diagnosis of septum-defect from early acquired mitral regurgitation is often difficult. However, in mitral disease the symptoms and signs develop after the first few years of life; there is enlargement of the left ventricle; the murmur is heard usually loudest at the apex; the first sound of the heart here is obscured; there is usually no thrill; edema generally develops before cyanosis, and there is not the decided retardation of general development.

Stenosis or Atresia of the Pulmonary Orifice.—This may exist uncomplicated, or much more frequently combined with other lesions. Cyanosis is present in the majority of cases, usually seen immediately or soon after birth. Sometimes its appearance is delayed, and not infrequently it is replaced by pallor. With the cyanosis are the other symptoms usually accompanying this, namely polycythemia, clubbing of the fingers, palpitation, dyspnea, suffocative attacks, etc. Enlargement of the right side of the heart is a valuable diagnostic sign often well marked in older children, or earlier in life in cases of uncomplicated pulmonary stenosis. Frequently the enlargement of this chamber seems but slight, inasmuch as the tension on the ventricular walls produced by the stenosis is relieved by the so common presence of septum-defect. A systolic thrill is sometimes felt, but is oftener absent.

Auscultation usually reveals a systolic murmur with maximum intensity over the pulmonary cartilage to the left of the sternum or in the second left interspace. It is conducted well to the left, but its intensity diminishes rapidly toward the right. Cases may occur, however, in which no such murmur is audible. This is true, for instance, of complete uncomplicated atresia of the pulmonary orifice, or when the opening is very small. In many cases the exact localization of the murmur is rendered most difficult by the presence of other murmurs, especially that of defect of the septum. When the two are associated the combined murmur is loudest in the second or third interspace to the left of the sternum, and may be conducted along the carotids. Sometimes in such cases it is possible to observe that there are two areas in which the murmurs are respectively of different quality and pitch.

The condition of the pulmonary second sound is of great diagnostic importance. In uncomplicated pulmonary stenosis, at least in young subjects, the sound is always weaker than normal. This is the necessary result of the small amount of blood which enters the pulmonary artery and the consequent diminished diastolic pressure there. Later in life the weakness of this sound may be removed through decided hypertrophy of the right ventricle; or in complicated cases the tension within the right ventricle may be increased by the existence of a septum-defect which allows the greater power of the left ventricle to exert a direct influence. In either of these ways a second sound of normal strength may be produced. When, however, there exists a patulous ductus arteriosus and the pulmonary leaflets are freely movable the pulmonary second sound is very much accentuated, owing to the increased direct pressure in the pulmonary artery which is the natural result of communication with the aortic system.

In brief, the diagnosis of pulmonary stenosis and of atresia rests upon the presence of decided cyanosis and accompanying symptoms, and, in the case of stenosis, of a systolic murmur to the left of the sternum in the second or third interspace. A feeble pulmonary second sound indicates simple stenosis; a normal pulmonary second sound an accompanying septum-defect; and an accentuated one the presence with these of a patulous ductus arteriosus. When there is little if any hypertrophy of the right ventricle it is probable that a communication exists between the auricles or the ventricles respectively. The presence of pallor instead of cyanosis, combined with the murmur at the pulmonary orifice, may readily lead to the mistaken diagnosis of a persistent, severe anemia with a murmur of functional origin. This is, according to Hochsinger,[25] particularly true of moderate stenosis of the conus arteriosus, in which murmurs may come and go from time to time, exactly as in the case of anemic murmurs. Very important, too, in the differentiation between simple and complicated pulmonary stenosis is the fact that very few cases of the former, if at all well marked, are encountered after the end of the first year of life.

Patulous Ductus Arteriosus.—In the very exceptional cases of uncomplicated open ductus there are no characteristic symptoms. There are two types to be found;—in the first, part of the blood flows directly from the pulmonary artery into the aorta without passing through the lungs; and in the other some of it may flow from the aorta into the pulmonary artery and through the lungs, with consequent diminution in the amount going through the systemic circulation and the right heart. Cyanosis is usually absent, but to this there are exceptions, as shown in the 4 cases reported by Variot and Bouquier[26] in which, with uncomplicated patulous ductus, cyanosis was decided and permanent. It is in the first type, *i. e.*, where much venous blood may be in the systemic circulation, that cyanosis may be present. Hypertrophy of the right side of the heart is frequent in the first type; hypertrophy of the left side in the second, in which, too, there may be a low diastolic blood-pressure and other signs which generally accompany aortic insufficiency. A small area of percussion-dulness has been found in the first and second interspaces to the left of the sternum. There is a loud systolic murmur heard over the pulmonary cartilage and conducted into the vessels of the neck, but not downward, and often uniting with a diastolic murmur and producing a continuous rumble ("*humming-top murmur*"). The diastolic murmur depends upon insufficiency of the pulmonary orifice. There is often a systolic thrill in the second left interspace and the pulmonary second sound is much accentuated. This accentuation is a diagnostic sign of great importance, and is the natural result of the diastolic action of the combined aortic and pulmonic pressure upon the pulmonary leaflets. An enlargement of first the right and then the left side of the heart is of especial diagnostic significance, since no other congenital cardiac lesion recognizable during life will produce this. The blood may flow either from the aorta into the pulmonary artery or vice versa, as previously stated. In 16 of 28 collected uncomplicated cases analyzed by Holman[27] the blood appeared to flow from the pulmonary artery and in 9 from the aorta.

When patulous ductus arteriosus occurs in combination with other lesions the symptoms observed are largely those of these latter, and those of the former may be modified. If there is atresia of the pulmonary artery, a murmur is usually not audible, at least at the ductus arteriosus, as apparently both the pulmonary artery and aorta must supply blood in order to produce it. The coexistence of pulmonary stenosis and patulous ductus will produce a murmur the localization and nature of which possess the character of the murmur of each of these, which cannot then be separated one from the other. When these two are associated a defect in the septum is present in the large majority of cases. The existence of the combination is suggested by the presence of cyanosis, the marked accentuation of the pulmonary second sound usually present, the harshness and loudness of the murmur, and the existence of thrill.

Other Congenital Lesions.—Other lesions possible in congenital heart-disease are for the most part either of very uncommon occurrence, or not susceptible of clinical recognition. Anomalous origin of the pulmonary artery and aorta, or even transposition of these, although a comparatively frequent form of disorder, exhibits no certain symptoms. Suggestive of transposition is the complex of symptoms pointed out by Hochsinger,[25] viz., cyanosis with much accentuated pulmonary second sound and enlargement of the heart, but without any murmurs whatever. Dilatation of the pulmonary artery produces of itself no diagnostic symptoms. That of the orifice gives rise to a diastolic murmur. Congenital narrowness of the aortic orifice is not common. Its symptoms would probably not differ from those of the lesion acquired later in life; characterized especially by enlargement of the left ventricle, displacement of the apex-beat, and a systolic murmur carried into the vessels of the neck; but the duration of life is so short that a diagnosis could hardly be made. Atresia of the aortic orifice causes no murmur whatever even when a patulous ductus arteriosus is present. In such cases the blood must reach the aorta by way of a perforate septum taking the blood from the left ventricle, and a patulous ductus arteriosus transmitting it from the pulmonary artery. There is intense congestion of the lungs and life continues for only a few weeks.

Stenosis of the aorta in the neighborhood of the entrance of the ductus arteriosus (coarctation of the aorta; stenosis of the isthmus) is seen more frequently. It may exhibit no evidences of its presence until childhood is passed; or there may be early symptoms consisting of a systolic murmur at the upper part of the sternum and to its right, extending to the neck, where pulsation can be detected, and conducted into the vessels there. The left ventricle is hypertrophied. The pulse in the vessels of the lower extremities is weaker than in those of the upper and of the neck. In subjects reaching adult life with considerable stenosis of the isthmus there develops a very distinct establishment of collateral circulation through the upper intercostal and internal mammary arteries connecting with the epigastric arteries and lower intercostals. The surface of the thorax and abdomen may show the branching, much dilated vessels. This is the result of the effort to furnish blood to regions below the situation of the stenosis. Congenital hypoplasia of the general aortic system has no typical cardiac symptoms, except that early in life the heart is abnormally small. There is some hypertrophy later in a considerable number of cases. The general symptoms are those of anemia and debility with retarded development of the genital organs. Unassociated disease of the tricuspid or mitral valve is rare. Although in uncomplicated cases the symptoms should be those of the acquired condition, inasmuch as these lesions nearly always occur only in combination with others the differential diagnosis is usually impossible. In a case of tricuspid insufficiency described by Hotz[28] the symptoms were very typical, including pulsation in the veins and in the liver. In this connection may be mentioned a combination of defects associated with cyanosis and clubbing of the fingers known as the *tetralogy of Fallot*[29] in which there are pulmonary stenosis; defect of the interventricular septum; dextro-position of the aorta so that it over-rides the septal defect and receives blood both from right and left ventricles; and marked hypertrophy of the right ventricle. This is claimed to be the most common cardiac abnormality in patients with congenital cyanosis who reach adult life.

A brief review of the principal diagnostic features differentiating some of the various lesions follows:

1. *Cyanosis decided, without murmur,* suggests transposition of the large vessels without other complicating lesions. Corroborative of this is accentuated pulmonary second sound and cardiac enlargement. Yet the studies of Reuben and Steffen[30] on the findings at necropsy in a series of 25 collected cases would indicate that the symptom depends more frequently upon other malformations, especially complete atresia or great stenosis of the pulmonary artery with defect of the interventricular septum and patent foramen ovale.

2. *Cyanosis with systolic murmur in the second left interspace* suggests pulmonary stenosis. The stenosis is uncomplicated or only with patulous foramen ovale if the pulmonary second sound is feeble. It is combined with septum-defect if the pulmonary second sound is normal or somewhat accentuated. If the second sound is much accentuated it is probable that patulous ductus arteriosus is also present.

3. *Systolic murmur loudest over mid-sternum or in the third left interspace, without cyanosis,* suggests probable simple septum-defect. The murmur is then not conducted along the large vessels.

4. *Systolic murmur very loud and harsh over the second interspace or upper part of the sternum and carried into the vessels of neck, with great accentuation of the pulmonary second sound,* indicates the presence of patulous ductus arteriosus with pulmonary stenosis. The existence of patulous ductus arteriosus is corroborated by enlargement of the left side of the heart as

well as of the right side. Either patulous foramen ovale or ventricular septum-defect will also be present. The absence of cyanosis might indicate that the patulous ductus was an isolated lesion.

5. *Systolic murmur over upper part of the sternum and to its right and carried into the vessels of the neck, with hypertrophy of the left ventricle,* suggests stenosis of the isthmus of the aorta. It is corroborated later in life by visible collateral circulation.

6. *Diastolic murmur* usually suggests pulmonary insufficiency; sometimes the existence of patulous foramen ovale.

As earlier stated, however, owing to the great variation of the symptoms observed and the many possible combinations, the diagnosis of the forms of congenital heart-disease present can seldom be more than provisional. The electrocardiogram may show those characteristics which demonstrate preponderance of the right ventricle when this is present (*S.* marked in Lead I; *R.* highest in Lead III). It is not, however, of practical value, since right ventricular preponderance can generally be readily recognized in other ways.

Prognosis.—In general prognosis is unfavorable. More than half of the cases die during the first five years of life. Many live but a few days or weeks, the nature of the lesion preventing a longer existence. Others die in the early years, either through the development of lack of compensation, or from the occurrence of complicating diseases. On the other hand, some reach adult life, either with manifest symptoms or sometimes without any of moment. It is also possible for infants with evidences of congenital cardiac disease to lose both the symptoms and the physical signs later, either temporarily or permanently.

As regards the relationship of *complicating conditions,* there is a tendency to the development of pulmonary disease, and such an occurrence is always serious. Pertussis is borne very badly. Rachitis influences the patient unfavorably, as do gastroenteric affections. Tuberculosis is liable to develop in those passing the years of childhood. The acute exanthemata are generally fairly well tolerated. The frequency of a superimposed bacterial endocarditis seems to be great, according to Abbott.[31] In a total of 555 cases of congenital cardiac disease of clinical significance, endocarditis developed in 98 cases (17.6 per cent). The subject is also well discussed by Gordon and Perla.[32]

As far as the indications from the symptoms go, the prognosis seems to be to a large extent unfavorable in proportion to the degree of cyanosis; and of the dyspnea, palpitation and the like which are liable to accompany this. Infants born with intense cyanosis generally die very soon; those without it, or who soon lose it if present at first, give the best prognosis, as a rule.

Viewing the prognosis from the standpoint of the *individual lesion* the following analysis may be made:

Defect in the interauricular septum, uncomplicated or producing no symptoms, affects in no way the duration of life. If other lesions are present or develop later, the septum-defect may affect life by producing overfilling of the right auricle.

Defect in the interventricular septum, if uncomplicated, often permits of life into adult years. It is, however, prone to be complicated at this period or earlier by endocarditis affecting the neighborhood of the opening or other part; and this, or the presence of other lesions of a congenital nature, may modify the prognosis and shorten life.

Pulmonary atresia, occurring alone, usually causes death in a few weeks. If compensated by perforate septum with patulous ductus arteriosus, life is longer. Yet the average duration of life in all cases of atresia, according to the calculations of Vierordt,[13] based on Rauchfuss'[14] statistics, is only 3.27 years.

Pulmonary stenosis gives a better prognosis; yet fully 50 per cent of the cases die before the age of ten years, and 75 per cent of them before that of fifteen years. Vierordt reckons the average duration of life of pulmonary stenosis, based on Moussous' cases, as twelve to thirteen years; or, based on Rauchfuss' collection, as 9.36 years; and cases without compensatory septum-defect are still less favorable. On the other hand, many patients with pulmonary stenosis live to adolescence or even adult life. An unfavorable termination is attended by increasing loss of cardiac compensation, with general passive congestion and edema.

Patulous ductus arteriosus occurring alone has on the whole a not very unfavorable influence upon the duration of life. Of the 26 cases collected by Vierordt over half lived to adolescence or adult life. In fatal cases there is progressive failure of compensation, perhaps due to a secondary endocarditis. A patulous ductus arteriosus associated with pulmonary stenosis acts rather as a compensatory lesion.

Anomalous origin of the great vessels gives a prognosis varying with the exact nature of the condition. Some of these do not permit of life at all, while in others adult life is exceptionally attained. Cases of transposition of the vessels seldom live beyond the second year. In 75 cases collected by Vierordt only 9 were over five years of age.

Stenosis of the aortic ostium presents a very unfavorable prognosis, most cases dying in the first week; only 1 of 33 cases collected by Rauchfuss passing the first month of life.

Stenosis of the isthmus of the aorta at the position of the ductus arteriosus gives a much better prognosis. The course is chronic and the patient frequently reaches adult life with but few symptoms. The fatal ending comes probably from heart-strain during middle age, with evidences of failing cardiac compensation.

Treatment.—This can be but symptomatic, and often the nature of the lesion renders even this valueless. The greatest care to sustain and advance the state of the nutrition; the guarding against chilling and especially against over-exertion; and, in general, exact attention to hygienic and dietetic management are the only means open to us. Respiratory diseases are especially to be prevented, since patients with congenital cardiac disease are particularly liable to contract them and bear them very badly. In some cases the continued administration of nitroglycerin appears to be of benefit, probably through relieving the strain on the heart by dilating the peripheral vessels. In others, subject to sudden attacks of intense cyanosis and cardiac pain, the hypodermic injection of nitroglycerin or of morphine or the inhalation of nitrite of amyl is of value during the attack. Inhalations of oxygen have been tried to relieve dyspnea and cyanosis, but have little if any effect on the latter. If syncope occurs, hypodermic injections of camphor or caffeine may be given.

References

1. Arch. Pediat., 1906, **23,** 509. 2. Am. J. Dis. Child., 1931, **41,** 1363. 3. Common Disorders and Dis. of Childhood, 1909, 472. 4. Am. Heart J., 1928, **4,** 164. 5. Allg. med. Central-Zeit., 1902, **71,** 665. 6. Am. J. Dis. Child., 1931, **41,** 877. 7. Brit. J. Child. Dis., 1924, **21,** 161. 8. Osler and McCrae, Modern Med., 1927, **4,** Chap. 21. 9. Prager Vierteljahrsschrift f. d. prakt. Heilk., 1859, **16,** 2, 20. 10. Rep. Brit. Soc. Dis. in Child., 1902, **2,** 263. 11. Malformations of the Heart, 1866, 193. 12. Pfaundler und Schlossmann Handb. d. Kinderheilk., 1910, **3,** 506. 13. Nothnagel, Spec. Pathol. u. Therap., 1901, **15,** 2, 77; 83; 104; 128; 164. 14. Gerhardt's Handb. d. Kinderkr., 1878, **4,** 1, 69; 134. 15. Ztschr. f. rationale Med., 1865, **26,** 161. 16. Am. J. Dis. Child., 1917, **13,** 167. 17. Brit. J. Child. Dis., 1913, **10,** 104. 18. Arch. f. Kinderh., 1921, **69,** 337. 19. Am. J. Dis. Child., 1930, **39,** 363. 20. Rev. de méd., 1903, **23,** 108. 21. Arch. Int. Med., 1925, **36,** 516. 22. Medicine, 1923, **2,** 1. 23. Le bull. méd., 1892, **6,** 849. 24. Bull. de l'acad. de méd., 1879, Ser. 2, **8,** 1074. 25. Die Auscultation des kindlichen Herzens, 1890, 155; 168; 178. 26. Arch. de méd. d. enf., 1920, **23,** 292. 27.

Bull. Johns Hopkins Hosp., 1925, **36,** 61. 28. Jahrb. f. Kinderh., 1923, **102,** 1. 29. Marseille méd., 1888, **25,** 77; 138; 207; 270; 341; 403. 30. Arch. Pediat., 1922, **39,** 811. 31. Ann. Clin. Med., 1925, **4,** 189. 32. Am. J. Dis Child., 1931, **41,** 98.

CHAPTER III

PERICARDITIS; ENDOCARDITIS; MYOCARDITIS

ACUTE PERICARDITIS

THE statements regarding the incidence of acute pericarditis are somewhat at variance, but on the whole it appears to be less common in infancy and early childhood, especially the latter, than later. The statistics of Baginsky,[1] which include all forms of pericarditis, record an unusually large number (20 per cent) occurring in the first year, and Poynton,[2] dealing with suppurative cases, found 84 per cent of them in patients in the first four years of life. According to Cnopf[3] and Haas[4] the disease is observed in about 4 or 5 per cent of necropsies in children, which is only about half the number found in necropsies in adults (Weill[5]). It is not until the beginning of later childhood that the influence of rheumatism in the production of pericarditis becomes prominent. The disease is never primary, except possibly as an initial evidence of tuberculosis (Blatt and Greengard[6]) or as a first or only manifestation of rheumatism, but in both of these conditions it is possible that other localizations have been unrecognized. Among other causes are the various infectious diseases, nephritis, and septic processes in other parts of the body. Inflammation may spread to the pericardium by extension in cases of pneumonia and pleurisy, and also in inflammatory disease of the abdominal structures, bronchial glands, thymus, esophagus, or the bony framework of the thorax. Trauma constitutes a local cause in some instances.

The relative frequency of these agents depends upon the age of the patient. Rheumatism is rarely a cause under the age of five years, but in later childhood is by far the most frequent source, the pericardial involvement being generally combined with endocarditis. It happens oftener than in adult life that a rheumatic pericarditis, usually also with endocarditis, develops without or before any arthritic involvement is seen. It may be a complication of chorea or, as in the case of arthritis, appear before there has been an attack of this disorder. Septic conditions and especially pneumonia are the most common forerunners of pericarditis in infancy and the first portion of early childhood. Tuberculosis is an infrequent cause in the first two years of life, and after this time is less often seen than in adults. The other infectious disorders are factors chiefly in later childhood. Extension of inflammation from neighboring diseased tissues may occur at any period of early life.

Pathologic Anatomy.—Either the visceral or the parietal layer or both may be involved. In *plastic* (dry) pericarditis the pericardium is injected and dry, or in severer cases is covered by a more or less thick deposit of fibrin containing pus-cells. In the *serofibrinous* form there is an effusion of serum containing cellular elements and flakes of fibrin. The fluid may be clear or somewhat turbid, or perhaps bloody. Cellular infiltration and a varying degree of degeneration of the cardiac muscle may be present in severe cases. The amount of fluid is usually small, but sometimes it is so large that errors in diagnosis are readily made. In *purulent* pericarditis the conditions are as in the serofibrinous form, except for the presence of large numbers of pus-cells. The exudate may be purulent from the beginning or become so only later. Adhesions may develop between the layers of the pericardium in all of the forms of pericarditis, and these may remain after recovery, and sometimes later occasion complete obliteration of the pericardial sac.

The variety of pericarditis found depends upon the nature of the cause and the character of the germs present. Rheumatism produces generally a plastic or serofibrinous inflammation and endocarditis is frequently combined with it. Any of the pyogenic germs may be producers of purulent pericarditis, but by much the most common is the pneumococcus (Poynton[7]). Tuberculosis may give rise to any of the forms and is a frequent cause also of *mediastinitis*, in which, with a pleuritis, the external layer of the pericardium as well as the inner is involved.

Symptoms.—These vary greatly in severity and depend to some extent upon the form of pericarditis present. Frequently the diagnosis is made only accidentally. The earliest of the characteristic *physical signs* is a rough and superficial friction-sound, best heard over the upper part of the precordial region, but sometimes loudest over the apex. A distinct fremitus can often be felt. Although synchronous with the heart's action the sound has, in typical cases, little of the character of an endocardial murmur; is usually more circumscribed; more irregularly continuous; heard with both systole and diastole; not transmitted; and varies much in character from time to time. Sometimes it is purely systolic in time. If effusion takes place friction-sounds may disappear, unless loose adhesions in certain locations still permit a friction to develop. Even, however, with effusion of considerable size a friction-sound may quite commonly still be heard, since the fluid gravitates to a position behind and at the sides of the heart, at the apex, or about the great vessels. In other cases disappearance of the friction depends upon a close adhesion of the opposing roughened surfaces of the pericardium. A friction-sound may sometimes be made more distinct by firm pressure with the stethoscope, or by placing the patient in a sitting position inclined slightly forward. Pericardial friction is encountered chiefly in the cases dependent upon rheumatism and uncommonly in suppurative cases.

Alteration of the cardiac percussion-dulness is important. A small amount of exudate does not change this perceptibly. Larger amounts may produce the well-known triangular dulness, the apex of this being in the second or third left interspace; the right side extending below to 1 inch (2.5 cm.) or more beyond the sternum, and the left side reaching beyond the nipple-line. Sometimes, however, the dulness does not assume the triangular form but is more circular, and its outline is influenced by gravity, depending on whether the child is reclining or sitting. In the case of very large effusions the dulness may extend well into the left axilla and to the right as far as the nipple. Physical signs suggesting pneumonic consolidation may sometimes be found posteriorly over the lower part of the left side. This depends probably upon the pressure on the lung exercised by a large pericardial effusion or by a dilated heart. Dulness to the right of the sternum in the fifth interspace and the rounding out of the cardio-hepatic angle are also considered valuable signs by many. Both of these, however, are often absent. It is noteworthy that the apex-beat, when still palpable, is not displaced to the left of the normal position unless a complicating cardiac dilatation exists. With large effusion the apex-beat can be felt only with great difficulty if at all, and the impulse is diffuse and may occupy a position above the normal one. Having the child lean forward may cause the apex-beat to become again discoverable. Large effusion also alters the character of the heart-sounds, making them weak or scarcely audible; and the precordial region is distinctly too prominent and changes less with respiration. Another sign of importance is that the strength of the radial pulse is out of proportion to that of the apex-beat. The roentgenogram bears out the results obtained by percussion, the shadow showing the triangular or the circular form. It reveals, too, that in small effusions the fluid accumulates either around the sinus at the base of the heart or along the lower margin and above the apex (Morris and Bader,[8] Williamson[9]). This may be discoverable before effusion becomes evident by percussion. With the fluoroscope it is not possible to differentiate the pulsations of the auricle from those of the ventricle, the impulse, contrary to the normal condition, being diffuse over the entire cardiac area. This sign may be present with either effusions or adhesions (Holmes[10]). In rare instances the effusion may be encapsulated (Wessler and Fried[11]).

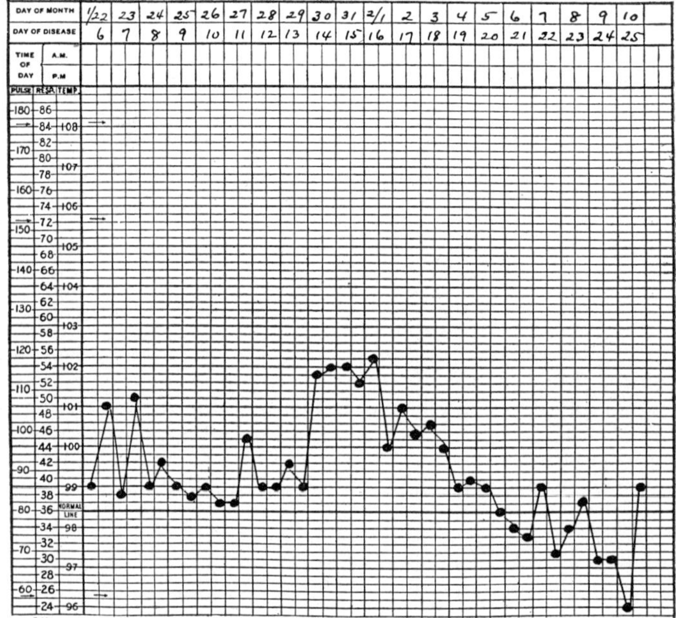

Fig. 186.—Plastic pericarditis, followed by endocarditis, dilatation of the heart and pleuropneumonia. Beckie C., aged six years. Five days previously had pain in the abdomen, and vomited at times after this; insomnia. Entered the Children's Hospital of Philadelphia, Jan. 22. Examination showed typical pericardial friction-sounds over the base of the heart, no dyspnea, general condition good; Jan. 29, apical systolic murmur developed; Feb. 2, very decided dyspnea, evidence of fluid in the left pleural cavity, with bronchial respiration and râles, aspiration in the axillary line gave clear, straw-colored fluid, containing the pneumococcus, signs of increasing mitral regurgitation and of cardiac dilatation appeared. Child grew steadily worse and died Feb. 10.

The *general symptoms* of pericarditis are not characteristic. Dyspnea or even orthopnea, and palpitation or irregular and rapid cardiac action are often witnessed. Pain and tenderness may be present, but are not necessary symptoms. Sometimes there are vomiting, cough, and cyanosis. More or less fever usually attends the disease in the early stages. It is of the remittent type in cases of purulent effusion. Rarely in large effusions unusual pressure-symptoms may occur, such as paralysis of the recurrent laryngeal nerve. In patients already suffering from other diseases the possibility of the development of pericarditis is to be considered when symptoms rapidly appear referable to the heart and not explainable by the pre-existing condition.

Complications.—Endocarditis is a very frequent complication in cases of rheumatic origin. Pneumonia or pleurisy, especially of the left side, is often associated with pneumococcic pericarditis (Fig. 186). Myocarditis and cardiac dilatation are frequent in severe cases. Compression of the lung is a natural result of large effusions.

Course and Prognosis.—The *course* varies with the form of the disease. The inflammation may remain plastic throughout, or physical signs of effusion may soon develop. Death may occur in one to two weeks, or recovery be under way by this time; but in the cases which escape an early fatal termination the convalescence is often much prolonged, and many patients are left with chronic and finally fatal lesions. Acute pericarditis may rapidly have dilatation occur, and cyanosis, edema, albuminuria, enlargement of the liver, and hypostatic congestion of the lungs appear; or pneumonia may develop and be the immediate cause of death. In subjects of chronic valvular heart-disease the occurrence of an acute pericarditis may fatally destroy the compensation. The *prognosis* in children is in general unfavorable. Death may take place suddenly, or be preceded by evidences of failing compensation. Other cases recover from the acute symptoms but die later from sequels depending upon pericardial adhesions. Many of the milder cases of plastic pericarditis recover completely, at least so far as any immediate danger is concerned. The prognosis of the suppurative cases due to the pneumococcus or other germ is unfavorable, although recovery may follow operative interference. Cases end fatally in which pyopericardium is only one of the symptoms of general sepsis.

Diagnosis.—Owing to the insidiousness of the onset and the presence of other diseases the diagnosis of pericarditis is often difficult. It is to be recognized by the study of the symptoms and physical signs as described, including in all but plastic cases the discovery of fluid in the pericardial sac. The differential diagnosis of fibrinous pericarditis is to be made especially from *plastic pleurisy.* It is possible, but infrequent, for a dry pleurisy with inflammation of the external layer of the pericardium to produce a friction-sound which suggests that of pericarditis, although the sound is more systolic than of the irregular type heard in pericarditis, and is influenced by respiration. Pericardial effusion of moderate degree may closely simulate cardiac *dilatation.* The peculiar shape of the dull area, the presence of dulness in the fifth interspace to the right of the sternum, and the extension of the dulness to the left beyond the position of the apex-beat are characteristic of effusion. Change of position, too, produces in pericardial effusion a great alteration in the shape of the precordial dulness and of the intensity of the apex-beat on palpation; provided always that adhesions are not present which fasten the heart to the pericardial sac to a certain extent. The apex-beat is often displaced upward in effusion, and is moved downward and to the left in dilatation. A rapid increase in the precordial dulness points to dilatation rather than to effusion. The shape of the heart in the roentgenograms may be helpful, as may the greater pulsation of the cardiac shadow in dilatation, as seen in the fluoroscope. The diagnosis from dilatation is often, however, very difficult, especially as both conditions may be present. A large exudate may simulate a *pleural effusion* of the left side. Careful study of the patient in different positions aids in the differentiation. The apex-beat of the heart is displaced to the right in pleural effusion. The severity of the general symptoms in large pericardial effusion is much greater than in pleurisy. Yet in cases of large effusion the diagnosis is often difficult, and exploratory aspiration may be necessary. We have seen the pericardial sac tapped from the axillary line under the impression that the condition was pleural effusion. The difficulty in diagnosis is increased when both pericardial and pleural effusions are present. A small purulent pericardial effusion may sometimes be present without any physical signs, although the symptoms are severe.

From *acute endocarditis* a plastic pericarditis is to be distinguished by the jerking, intermittent, and superficial character of the murmur, which does not keep exact time with the impulse. The murmur is also not conducted in any definite direction as it is in endocarditis, and it is often influenced by change of position or by pressure with the stethoscope. At times, however, a pericardial friction is soft in character or is heard only during systole, and the diagnosis is then extremely difficult. In still other cases there exists the combination of an endocardial and a pericardial murmur. In such the diagnosis is best made by observing the differences in character over different portions of the precordium. Should pericardial effusion be combined with acute endocarditis, there is added to the murmurs of the latter an enfeebling of the apex-beat out of proportion to the strength of the pulse. *Hydropericardium* resembles pericardial effusion in the signs elicited by percussion, but is readily distinguished by the accompanying conditions, such as hydrothorax or generalized edema.

Treatment.—A patient with rheumatism should promptly receive antirheumatic treatment with the hope that this might help to prevent involvement of the pericardium, and rest in bed should be insisted upon. If a plastic pericarditis has already developed the same treatment should be employed, although it is questionable whether medication is of benefit. In all cases absolute rest in bed is imperative. The diet should be light and easily digestible if fever is present. Pain is to be relieved by the application of an ice-bag over the precordium and the administration of opium in sufficient dose. The same drug is useful in quieting cough. Evidence of cardiac weakness should be treated by suitable stimulation. Digitalis is objected to by some clinicians, and caffeine, strychnine and camphor are often to be preferred, sometimes best given hypodermically. For rapid cardiac action the ice-bag is often serviceable. Blisters over the precordium are to be avoided. In cases of large effusion the presence of threatening cyanosis and dyspnea may necessitate aspiration, but this should be deferred until actually imperative. Many of the cases of rapidly increasing pericardial dulness are in reality dependent upon dilatation, and the difficulty of reaching a positive diagnosis makes the chance of wounding the heart a very real one. The method of procedure has been described elsewhere (p. 151). In cases possibly purulent aspiration is indicated for diagnostic purposes, but incision of the pericardial sac is the therapeutical procedure to be preferred. In tuberculous pericarditis Emil-Weil and Loiseleur[12] and others recommend the injection of air after aspiration of the sac, and Oppenheimer[13] injects nitrogen or oxygen.

In the cases of pericarditis which recover every care must be taken to maintain the general and the cardiac strength, since dilatation is so likely to be present or pericardial adhesions to remain. Continued rest in bed is necessary long after recovery from the acute condition. Even when the patient is out of bed there must be precaution against over-exertion.

CHRONIC PERICARDITIS

(Chronic Obliterative Pericarditis. Adherent Pericardium)

Etiology.—More or less adhesion between the opposite layers of the pericardium remains in probably every instance of acute rheumatic pericarditis, and this may be found at necropsy when unsuspected during life. Another form is that associated with a chronic mediastinitis. Adherent pericardium does not often follow purulent pericardial effusion, and the most common causes are rheumatism and tuberculosis, the former being very much the more frequent in early life. Pericardial adhesion was found by Lees and Poynton[14] in 113 of 150 fatal cases of rheumatic cardiac disease, and in 77 it completely closed the sac. It may occur at any age, but is much less often seen in infancy than later, and probably is oftenest found in later childhood, although perhaps not recognized until after this period.

Symptoms.—When there is but partial adhesion limited to a small area symptoms may be absent, and it is even possible for complete obliteration of the pericardial sac to take place unattended by clinical manifestations. As a rule, however, some evidences of the disease are present, particularly in the frequent cases in which adhesions have also formed between the external pericardial layer and other tissues in the anterior mediastinum. The symptoms largely depend upon the interference with the development of the heart, and upon the myocardial changes which the thickened, adherent pericardium produces. Consequently they may appear only months or years after recovery from acute pericarditis. Prominent among them are dilatation of the heart with increased percussion-dulness; bulging of the precordium; and, frequently, systolic retraction of the whole region, or limited to the apex-beat or the epigastrium. This last is a characteristic symptom, but is observed only where there exists also an adhesion of the external layer of the pericardium to the chest-wall, a condition developing oftenest when tuberculosis is the cause. The systolic retraction is followed by a visible diastolic expansion. There may be in these cases of *anterior mediastinitis* diastolic collapse and inspiratory swelling of the jugular vein, together with the pulsus paradoxus, in which the radial pulse becomes almost imperceptible during inspiration. The heart does not change its position by altering that of the patient. Another valuable sign is that described by Broadbent,[15] consisting in systolic retraction of the chest-wall on the left side posteriorly, between the 11th and 12th ribs. The pulse is rapid and later weak, and the apex-beat is often feeble. Cardiac systolic murmurs may be present, since organic valvular lesions are almost always associated with the pericardial disease. As the case advances the usual evidences of failing compensation develop.

Prognosis.—The prognosis is always bad in patients with extensive adhesions. The duration, however, is variable. Death may take place suddenly in cases where the disease was not suspected; or in others the fatal ending may come on suddenly or slowly after months or years.

Diagnosis.—When symptoms of adherent pericardium follow shortly upon an acute pericarditis the diagnosis is rendered easier, but in the majority a positive recognition of the disease is difficult or impossible. The diagnosis rests upon the evidences of failing circulation and cardiac dilatation, combined with the systolic apical retraction if this is present. The disorder is often confounded with chronic valvular disease, and not suspected when combined with this. Some of the more chronic cases of pericardial adhesion show a resemblance in symptoms to cirrhosis of the liver. Dieuaide[16] has found diagnostic aid in the electrocardiogram.

Treatment.—Operative interference, with the purpose of freeing the heart of adhesions, was suggested by Brauer,[17] and Rehn[18] reported 4 successful cases in children. According to Marvin and Harvey[19] only 6 cases so treated, none occurring in children, had been reported in the United States up to the year 1924.

ACUTE ENDOCARDITIS

Etiology.—This is a frequent disorder in early life. Weill[20] places it as forming 5 per cent of all diseases at this period, but this is a high figure. In 16,120 sick children admitted to two hospitals in Philadelphia and one in Boston the incidence of cardiac disease was 1.4 per cent (Norris[21]), and

Dusch[22] found chronic valvular disease in but 0.17 per cent of 52,281 collected cases of sick children in various German hospitals. Among the predisposing causes age occupies a position of importance. In fetal life endocarditis may be the cause of some of the cases of congenital heart-disease. It is uncommon in infancy, but cases in the first year are reported by Steffen,[23] Sutiagin,[24] Skinner,[25] Dible,[26] White,[27] Sansby and Larson,[28] and Loffredo.[29] Geiger[30] collected 108 reports in children up to four years of age. In infancy the cases are oftenest of a septic nature. Denzer,[31] however, reported three patients under two years of age in whom the disease seemed to be of rheumatic origin. Certainly from the age of six to ten years the disease is as frequent as at any later period of life, if not more so. After puberty the incidence declines. It occurs rather more often in females than in males in the ratio of about 6:4. Endocarditis may develop in the course of any of the infectious fevers, especially scarlet fever, or be associated with pneumonia or septicemia; but by far the most common cause is rheumatism. About $\frac{3}{4}$ or more of cases have a history of rheumatic disease (Weill,[20] Wilson et al.,[32] Reid[33]). As already pointed out in discussing rheumatism (pp. 472–474), endocarditis may follow promptly upon some other manifestation of the basic disease, such as arthritis, chorea, torticollis, and tonsillitis (p. 473); or may itself be the first and perhaps the only evidence of rheumatism. In this sense we may speak of endocarditis as being in some instances a primary affection. The younger the patient the more liable is rheumatic arthritis to be followed by endocarditis, either in the first or in later attacks (Church[34]). (See also p. 474.)

Although the disease seems to be without doubt an *infectious process* no one germ is invariably present, and usually no micro-organisms whatever can be discovered in the endocardium or cultivated from the blood. Most frequently found are the pneumococcus and forms of staphylococcus and streptococcus, but various other organisms have been observed. The relationship of disease of the tonsils to endocarditis has been much discussed. These organs have been regarded as a portal of entry for the infectious agent of rheumatism and endocarditis; or, on the other hand, tonsillitis has been considered as one of the rheumatic manifestations. The subject has been considered at length elsewhere (pp. 540, 541). There would appear to be two forms of acute endocarditis viewed etiologically; that to which in most cases the title rheumatic may be applied, and in which no bacteria can, as a rule, be found; and that depending upon a discoverable germ. In many of the latter cases, with a course not very acute, the streptococcus viridans appears to be the usual causative agent. (See p. 789.)

Pathologic Anatomy.—The lesions developing in antenatal endocarditis are situated oftenest at the pulmonary orifice. In cases arising after birth the left side is oftener attacked, especially the mitral leaflets. There takes place an increase of connective tissue near the surface of the valve or extending more deeply, with the formation of new blood-vessels and the growth of granulation-tissue producing small vegetations (*verrucose endocarditis*). These vegetations may be completely absorbed and recovery follow, or they may be transformed into cicatricial fibrous tissue with shrinking of the valve leaflets. In other, but infrequent, cases the granulation-tissue may break down and an ulcerative process follow (*ulcerative endocarditis, malignant endocarditis*), extending to the papillary muscles and even to the muscular tissue of the cardiac wall. In either condition clotting of blood may take place upon the leaflets and minute portions of this, or of the vegetations themselves, may be detached and carried into the circulation, thus producing emboli in various parts of the body. Pericarditis, myocarditis, and dilatation are quite generally found. Hypertrophy may also be seen in cases which have passed into the chronic stage.

Symptoms and Course.—Two forms of endocarditis may be recognized clinically: (*A*) Simple Endocarditis and (*B*) Septic Endocarditis.

(*A*) Simple Acute Endocarditis.—Apart from the murmurs and the **symptoms** characteristic of the various chronic valvular lesions respectively, the evidences of acute endocarditis are not characteristic. The onset is more or less acute, with fever and general indisposition; sometimes vomiting and cough; restlessness; precordial pain; dyspnea; and rapid and irregular action of the heart (Fig. 187), which varies little during the twenty-four hours. Rapid, irregular heart-action is one of the most suggestive signs in doubtful cases when no murmur is as yet audible. If the disease develops

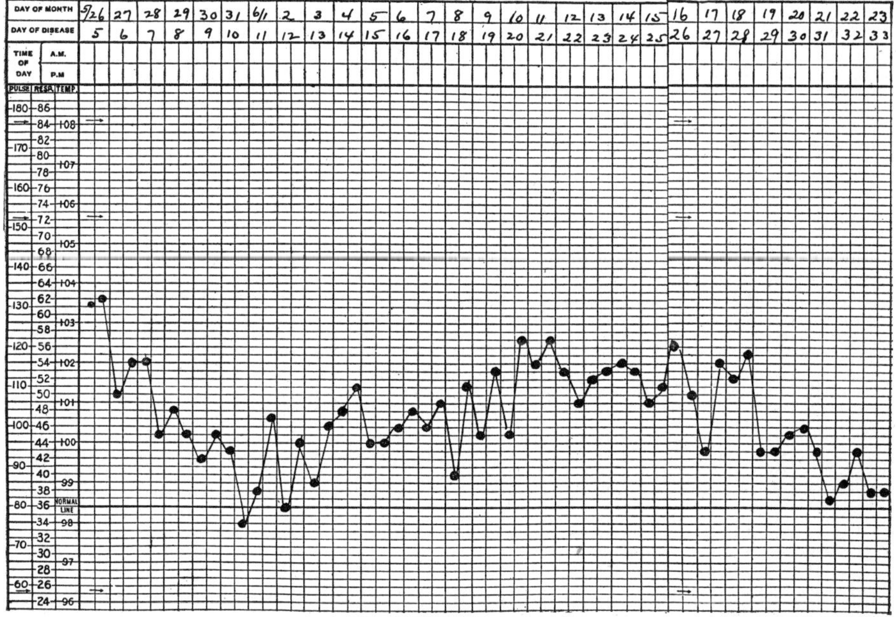

Fig. 187.—Acute mitral endocarditis following old lesion, gradual development of aortic lesion. Eva C., aged eleven years. Rheumatism four years previously. Been indisposed to active exercise. Taken ill four days before with vomiting, headache, fever, backache, marked dyspnea, praecordial pain, and diarrhea. Entered Children's Ward, University of Pennsylvania Hospital, May 26. *Examination.*—Evidently seriously ill, nervous, restless, respiration 45–60, cardiac action rapid and irregular, loud, harsh systolic murmur over whole precordium, slight arthritis lower extremities, no edema; June 2, general condition gradually improved, but an aortic regurgitant murmur is developing; June 14, evidences of cardiac dilatation on percussion, dyspnea persisting, aortic regurgitant murmur harsh and louder; June 23, fever gone, slight dyspnea, mitral and aortic murmurs present.

in the course of other febrile disorders the recognition of endocarditis is difficult, unless there has been constant observation of the heart. If repeated examinations are made the gradual development of a murmur may be discovered. This is usually soft, and is oftenest situated in the mitral area and accompanied by accentuation of the pulmonary second sound. Sometimes increase in the percussion-dulness of the heart can be demonstrated; in other cases no such change can be detected.

The **duration** of the acute stage is from two to four weeks, by the end of which period in favorable cases the subjective symptoms have disappeared, and sometimes all traces of murmur as well, and recovery is complete. The **prognosis** for entire recovery is not so favorable and permanent valvular lesions remain, but usually no marked disturbance of compensation is seen until later. In occasional instances failure of compensation immediately follows and persists, and death takes place in a short time. Rheumatic subcutaneous nodules, if present, constitute a bad prognostic sign according to some authors (p. 473). **Complications** are common and influence the prognosis unfavorably. Pericarditis occurs not infrequently. Cardiac dilatation is present in all fatal instances, and some degree of myocarditis is common in severe cases. Death is not infrequently due to pneumonia, and occasionally to embolic processes in the brain. (See p. 932.) Usually, however, the prognosis of endocarditis is good as far as recovery from the acute attack is concerned; but it is not possible to determine early in the course how much permanent damage will remain, and there is always the probability that later attacks will occur.

The **diagnosis** depends upon the evidence of disturbance of the cardiac action as described, combined with the physical signs of cardiac disease. Acute endocarditis is to be distinguished carefully from the *functional murmurs* which are so commonly heard in the course of febrile affections or at other times in children. (See p. 802.) Functional murmurs are usually soft; more distinct in the pulmonary area and at the base of the heart than at the mitral orifice; not transmitted so loudly to the axilla; and without cardiac hypertrophy or undue accentuation of the pulmonary second sound. Functional murmurs which are loud and diffuse are usually accompanied by decided anemia. Acute endocarditis is further to be distinguished from *pericarditis*. (See p. 784.)

(*B*) Septic Endocarditis.—This condition is distinguished pathologically from simple endocarditis by the uniformity of bacterial involvement of the valves and mural endocardium, and the destructive process which follows. Different varieties of micro-organisms have been observed; streptococci and pneumococci predominating. Clinically, it is a quite distinct affection. It has been considered rare in early life, only 47 cases having been collected from medical literature by Adams,[25] which occurred in subjects under fourteen years of age. Other cases have since been reported including some in the first year of life. (See also p. 786.) We have seen several instances of the disease in older children. The heart of a case under our observation is shown in the illustration (Fig. 188). It may develop suddenly in the midst of health; occur in the course of an infectious malady; complicate chronic valvular disorder; or be associated with rheumatism instead of the ordinary simple form. The **symptoms** and physical signs are somewhat similar to those seen in acute simple endocarditis, but in general are indefinite, variable and puzzling. The temperature may be continuously high or very irregular and intermittent (Fig. 189) and accompanied by the general evidences of sepsis. Septic emboli may occur in different regions with the varying symptoms characteristic of the locality, such as paralysis in different parts of the body, hematuria, intestinal hemorrhage, petechiae, and enlargement of the spleen. In other cases diarrhea, tympanites, fever, petechiae, sweating, and the development of the typhoid state may mark the typhoidal form. Sometimes the rapid production of cardiac dilatation and insufficiency, with murmurs heard oftenest over the mitral area but perhaps widely diffused, may aid in forming a diagnosis. In cases where the lesion is on the walls of the heart and not at the valve no murmurs may be audible. The **duration** of the disease is variable, the range being from a few days to several weeks. The **prognosis** is very unfavorable, although there were three reported recoveries in Adams' 47 cases. The **diagnosis** rests upon the combination of the grave symptoms described with subjective and objective evidences of cardiac disease. The condition is to be distinguished from typhoid fever by the sudden onset, presence of leukocytosis, absence of the Widal reaction, irregularity of the fever, and possibly by the discovery of pyogenic germs in the blood.

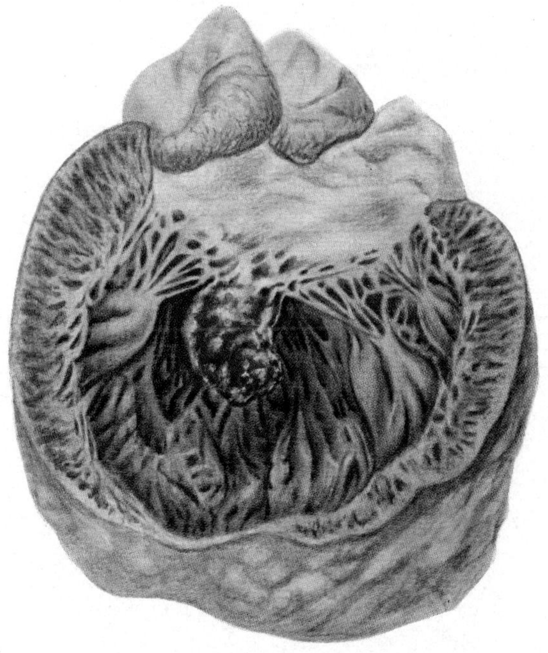

Fig. 188.—Malignant endocarditis. Same case as in Fig. 189. Shows large mass of vegetations attached to the mitral valve.

Subacute Bacterial Endocarditis (*Endocarditis lenta*).—This is a form of septic endocarditis of a more chronic nature, and with a somewhat better prognosis. In the literature it is sometimes difficult to distinguish the reports from the more acute septic form. The subacute variety, however, constitutes a distinct group. The physical signs are those of ordinary endocarditis, but the course is more prolonged and the temperature more variable. Crops of petechiae frequently occur, and the spleen is usually enlarged and tender. There is often a pallor (*café-au-lait color*), and tenderness of the pads of the fingers and toes (*Osler's nodes*). Hemorrhage from the bowel, into the retina, and into the brain may occur, the last causing hemiplegia

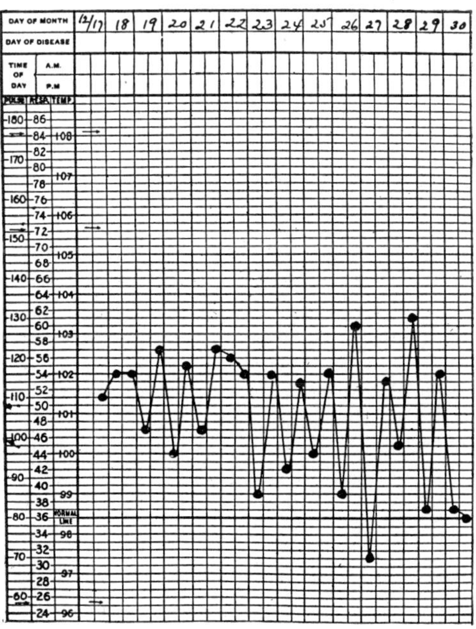

Fig. 189.—Malignant endocarditis. Eileen K., aged thirteen years. Gradual onset during four weeks, with malaise, drowsiness, fever; bed four days ago. Entered Children's Ward, University of Pennsylvania Hospital, Dec. 17. *Examination.*—Somewhat emaciated, general condition fair, scattered spots on body suggesting petechiae, no edema, loud systolic murmur and thrill, moderate cardiac enlargement; Dec. 19, negative Widal, leukocytes 36,400, presystolic murmur also now audible; Dec. 29, general condition somewhat better, but abdominal pain and tenderness below liver; Dec. 30, became unconscious, developed right hemiplegia, pulse 160, weak and irregular, leukocytes 91,000, respiration moderately accelerated, lungs negative, liver enlarged, blood-culture gave streptococcus mitis. Death. Necropsy showed acute malignant vegetative mitral valvulitis, chronic vegetative aortic valvulitis, beginning bronchopneumonia, hemorrhagic nephritis with septic infarcts, degenerative changes in other regions. (See Fig. 188.)

or other types of paralysis. Blood-cultures usually reveal the streptococcus viridans, although in a few cases the influenza bacillus, the meningococcus, or the gonococcus has been found. The course may last several months. Recovery has taken place in a few instances, as reported by Warren and Herrick,[36] Graham et al.,[37] Libman[38] and others. The subject is well reviewed by Blumer.[39] Cases due to the meningococcus are more favorable than others. A healed rheumatic endocarditis or a congenital heart lesion seems to predispose to subacute bacterial endocarditis, and Sprague[40] believes that patients with simple mitral regurgitation are more predisposed than when stenosis is combined with this. Rost and Fischer[41] have collected reports of 64 cases in children, and add 12 of their own. (See also reports by Leech,[42] Gordon and Perla,[43] Boysen,[44] Nedelmann,[45] and Schlesinger.[46])

Treatment of Acute Endocarditis.—In the way of prophylaxis a patient with rheumatism should be treated and kept at rest in bed. In the attack of endocarditis itself the chief element of treatment is likewise absolute rest in bed in the recumbent position while the acute symptoms are present, in order to prevent dilatation or to relieve it if present. All excitement and exertion of any sort should be avoided. Even after acute symptoms are over, rest in bed should continue for several weeks until the temperature and pulse are normal and activity does not cause an increase in temperature or a sustained increase in pulse-rate. The diet should be light and easily digestible. An ice-bag should be kept constantly over the precordium. This is useful in quieting the action of the heart and in relieving precordial pain and distress. Hydrotherapeutic measures may be of service to control fever.

As regards internal medication, it is a question whether any direct benefit is obtained by the use of the salicylates, but they may be tried if the digestion tolerates them. Pain may be relieved, when severe, by opiates, and restlessness by bromides or other sedatives. Digitalis or other cardiac tonics are needed only in cases where there seems danger of compensation being lost. It is better to defer their employment, if possible, until the acute febrile stage is over.

The treatment of malignant endocarditis is symptomatic, like that of the simple form, but is usually valueless. The necessity of supporting the strength is great, transfusion being useful for this. Vaccine treatment with cultures of germs obtained from the blood may be tried, as may anti-streptococcic sera. Trial also has been made with some success of sodium cacodylate, best given subcutaneously or intramuscularly in doses of 1 to 2 grains (0.065 to 0.13) daily. Benefit has also appeared to follow intravenous injections of gentian violet, acriflavine, and mercurochrome. (For dosage see p. 198.)

CHRONIC VALVULAR DISEASE OF THE HEART

Etiology.—The sequel of acute endocarditis is chronic valvular disease, which follows in the large majority of cases, either after the first or after some later attack. Sometimes the primary attack has been mild and overlooked and the first symptoms noticed are those of chronic valvular affection. Some of the sclerosing causes operative in adult life, such as arteriosclerosis, diabetes, tuberculosis, acquired syphilis, etc., are not noteworthy etiologic factors in childhood. While pathologic changes can be found in the heart and blood-vessels in cases of congenital syphilis (Matusoff and White[47]) there is no evidence that the disease causes clinical cardiac disorder during childhood (Previtali et al.,[48] Givan,[49] McCulloch[50]).

Pathologic Anatomy.—The lesions consist of thickening, hardening, shrinking and later calcification of the leaflets, sometimes with adhesions connecting them. The change involves also the papillary muscles and the chordae tendineae. There results either inability of the leaflets to close the orifice (*insufficiency*), or narrowing of the orifice (*stenosis*), or both. Consequent upon these conditions develop hypertrophy of the cardiac muscle in different regions, and, later, myocardial change and dilatation. Dilatation with failing compensation in chronic valvular disease, although common, is oftener deferred until later childhood or adolescence. The valve affected in childhood is the mitral in the great majority of cases, and next the aortic, according to most studies (Lees and Poynton;[14] Dunn;[51] Still;[52] Poynton;[53] Priestley;[54] Seham, Shapiro and Hilbert[55]). In a large proportion more than one valvular lesion is present.

Symptoms.—The symptoms of valvular disease vary to some extent with the lesions, but depend for the most part upon the state of compensation; *i. e.*, the maintenance of an adequate circulation. Children with complete compensation may long show no general symptoms whatever, and be about and indulge in active exercise without distress. In other cases with somewhat less complete compensation there may be moderate shortness of breath on exertion; sometimes palpitation, cough, epistaxis, indigestion and headache. Commonly there is an anemia which is resistant to treatment, and a characteristic disposition of the patient to indulge in quiet games rather than active ones. The children make no complaint, not realizing that their inactivity is abnormal; and it may be only by accident, or induced by the observation of these symptoms, that the physician makes an examination and discovers the valvular disease. The duration of this

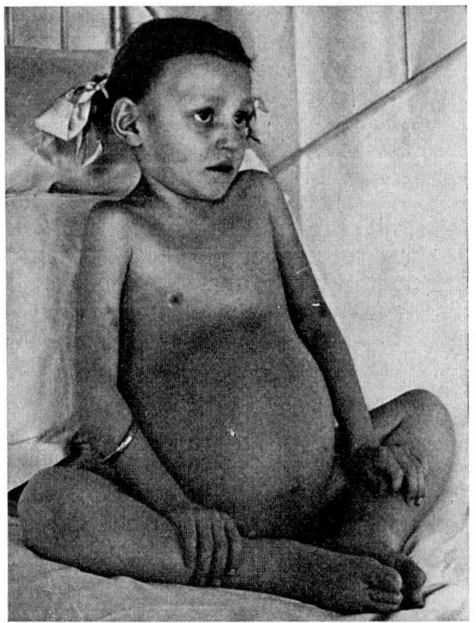

Fig. 190.—Edema of cardiac dropsy. Child of six years in the Children's Hospital of Philadelphia. Ill three years with cardiac disease. Edema and ascites. Much improved later under treatment.

period of compensation is variable. It may be almost continuous for years until puberty is approached, when the increased rapidity of bodily growth may occasion its loss. Sometimes it is more or less intermittent; some temporary impairment of health or unusual physical exertion disturbing it. Prominent among the causes of loss of compensation are recurring attacks of acute endocarditis. With failure of compensation there develop the general symptoms of venous stasis. There are cough; orthopnea; sometimes hemoptysis; epistaxis; dropsy (Fig. 190), first in the feet and then widespread and involving the serous cavities; enlargement of the spleen and liver; cyanosis; distention of the superficial veins; disturbances of digestion; albuminuria and urobilinuria with diminished secretion of urine. The heart is dilated, the apex-beat diminished in strength, and the radial pulse small. All these symptoms are the result of the stasis which the loss of compensation produces, but not all of them need be present at any one time, and they vary slightly with the lesion which exists; and all may disappear if compensation is restored.

Clinical Forms and Physical Signs.—The physical signs vary with the valve affected:

Mitral Insufficiency.—This is by far the most frequent of the chronic cardiac lesions (241 of Still's[52] 250 cases); in from about $\frac{1}{3}$ to $\frac{1}{2}$ of the cases being combined with mitral stenosis. The principal physical signs are a systolic murmur with maximum intensity oftenest at the apex, but widely transmitted to the axilla and the back; accentuation of the pulmonary second sound; and hypertrophy, and later dilatation, of the right side of the heart and finally of the left as well. This latter is indicated by displacement of the apex-beat to the left, and downward as far as the 5th or 6th interspace. In children in whom the disease has lasted for some time there is often a visible bulging of the precordium, and the broadened cardiac dulness reaches from the right of the sternum to the left anterior axillary line. Until decided dilatation has occurred there is a forcible impulse of the whole precordium and especially at the apex. With dilatation the impulse grows feebler and the murmur less distinct and even absent. Among the special symptoms are chiefly those of passive congestion of the pulmonary and of the general circulation, the latter dependent upon the regurgitation of blood through the dilated tricuspid orifice.

Mitral Stenosis.—This occurring alone is not common in childhood. It is found oftenest in combination with mitral insufficiency in cases where this disease has been of rather long continuance. Characteristic of it are the diastolic (mid-diastolic, presystolic) murmur limited to the usual small area in the neighborhood of the nipple, accentuation of the pulmonary second sound, enlargement of the right side of the heart, and diastolic thrill. The murmur is usually rough and ends abruptly with the first sound of the heart or ceases before this occurs, and sometimes occupies only the first portion of the diastole. Accompanying it is rarely the *Graham-Steell*[56] early-diastolic blowing murmur, heard along the left border of the sternum and due to an associated functional pulmonary insufficiency. The left side of the heart does not hypertrophy in uncomplicated cases. There are few symptoms, the most characteristic being evidences of pulmonary congestion, such as cough, attacks of bronchitis, dyspnea, and hemoptysis; and sometimes precordial pain, rapid pulse, and palpitation. General edema does not occur unless the tricuspid orifice dilates. Auricular fibrillation is more common in mitral stenosis than in any other form of heart-disease.

Aortic Insufficiency.—As stated this is a much less common affection in childhood; found chiefly in subjects approaching puberty. This certainly, at least, applies to cases in which it can be recognized clinically. As a post-mortem finding in cardiac disease the lesion is probably more frequent (Lees and Poynton[14]). Exceptionally it is the only lesion present. The physical signs consist of a loud, widely diffused, diastolic murmur with maximum intensity near the second right costal cartilage, and transmitted down the sternum or toward the apex. There are absent or enfeebled aortic second-sound, decided hypertrophy of the left ventricle, often bulging of the precordium, displacement of the apex-beat downward, strong but quickly receding radial pulse (*Corrigan's*[57] *pulse; trip-hammer pulse*), and throbbing in the carotids. A double murmur may be heard over the large vessels such as the femoral in the groin when partial pressure is made with the stethoscope (*Duroziez's sign*[58]); and *Traube's*[59] *pistol-shot sound* may be heard, this consisting of a short systolic shock followed by a fainter second-sound, diastolic in time. No pressure should be made by the stethoscope in eliciting the latter sign. The diastolic blood-pressure will be low or even absent and the systolic pressure high. A capillary pulse may often be seen in the finger-nails or the lips. The right chambers are not enlarged, unless mitral disease is a complication; or until, through failing compensation, general cardiac dilatation occurs, when a dynamic insufficiency of the mitral and tricuspid valves may develop. Cases in which aortic regurgitation is the only or the predominating lesion exhibit certain characteristic symptoms, among these being headache, dizziness, syncope, flashes of light before the eyes, precordial pain, anemia, epistaxis, and sometimes hemoptysis.

Aortic Stenosis.—This condition is generally considered to be even more uncommon in children than is the last. Poynton[53] encountered it in only 2 of 500 cases of heart-disease in children, and Schlesinger[46] in 2 of 550 cases. Nobécourt and Toni,[60] however, claim that evidence of it was found in 39 per cent of 33 cases of endocarditis, most of which were rheumatic in origin. We have seen 2 instances confirmed by necropsy. A systolic murmur heard at the aortic orifice must be determined only with great caution to be evidence of stenosis. The murmur is heard loudest at the aortic cartilage and is transmitted into the vessels of the neck. The aortic second-sound is weak or is replaced entirely by the diastolic murmur of an accompanying aortic regurgitation. Because of the delayed output of blood from the left ventricle the arterial pulse tracing shows the maximum rise to be in the latter part of systole (*pulsus tardus*). The left ventricle is hypertrophied and later dilated, as in aortic insufficiency. The symptoms are few, unless compensation is lost, when dyspnea, syncope, and precordial pain are liable to develop, and as dilatation advances there is relative insufficiency of the mitral valve with the accompanying symptoms.

Tricuspid Insufficiency.—This is a condition practically always secondary in post-natal endocarditis; there being no disease, but only a dilatation, of the tricuspid orifice. It is seen most often accompanying mitral insufficiency, but is capable of developing in any disorders of the heart which produce dilatation of the right ventricle, among these being interstitial pneumonia, asthma, and emphysema. There is a systolic murmur heard loudest over the lower part of the sternum, and the jugular veins are dilated and sometimes show pulsation. The so-called *positive venous pulse* occurs only when there is failure of the right auricle to contract properly. The lesions following passive congestion are found in the liver, spleen, and kidneys, and ascites is present.

Tricuspid Stenosis.—This is uncommon, and nearly always only secondary. In the analysis of 128 cases by Ashton and Stewart[61] there were none younger than eleven years of age. It can scarcely be distinguished by physical signs and symptoms from mitral stenosis. There is dyspnea, but without evidence of pulmonary congestion unless from an accompanying mitral disease.

Course and Prognosis of Chronic Valvular Disease.—To a great extent the prognosis of any valvular lesion depends upon the condition of the myocardium. A number of tests have been devised to determine the functional efficiency of the heart-muscle, and studies made by Barringer[62] have been applied to children by Wilson,[63] Seham and Seham,[64] Epstein,[65] Wallace,[66] and others. Normally after gymnastic or other exercise short of fatigue, such as the use of dumb-bells, climbing stairs, or the like, the immediate increase in the pulse-rate, as well as the rise of systolic pressure, which follows within thirty seconds, should return to normal in about two or three minutes. In cardiac weakness the return to normal pulse-rate is delayed and the systolic pressure both increases and decreases more slowly, or in more severe cases shows a primary fall. As already stated a large number of cases developing in early life exhibit for a long time no functional disturbance; or only at such times as some accidental cause produces temporary loss of compensation. The occurrence of any severe acute disorder is liable to bring about a more serious disturbance of compensation and to affect the prognosis unfavorably, and acute dilatation takes place readily in early life. So, too, any condition producing a chronic impairment of the general health, such as insufficient food, unsuitable hygiene, and the like, is liable to exercise a harmful influence. Especially to be mentioned here is an undue amount of exercise. Under some of these influences, or from the development of recurrences of acute endocarditis to which children are especially predisposed, or as the result of complicating pericarditis or pericardial adhesion (p. 784), there is a tendency to a gradual increase in the severity of the condition; and towards puberty, owing to the rapid growth of the body and the increased strain which this puts on the heart, decided disturbance of compensation becomes more common and persistent. As regards the influence of recurring attacks of cardiac inflammation Fineberg and Steuer[67] found that of 100 children with an apical systolic murmur, followed for an average time of six years, 30 developed serious complicating cardiac conditions, such as mitral stenosis, aortic insufficiency, or both. On the other hand, there is a remarkable ability in early life for compensation to be regained. Not many deaths occur until well on in later childhood; but after this the course is liable to be unfavorable in those children who have severe cardiac lesions, and not many of them reach adult life. When the lesion is but slight and well-compensated and the general health is good the chances are better. If such cases reach puberty with few if any signs of loss of compensation, the prognosis is not unfavorable; and it must not be forgotten that complete and final recovery with disappearance of all symptoms and physical signs may exceptionally occur, even in those children who have exhibited earlier what appeared to be positive evidences of chronic valvular disease lasting through several months or years. That this may take place more frequently than is commonly supposed is shown by the important study by Morse.[68] Of 100 persons who had acute endocarditis as children from ten to thirty years before, 37 of those who were alive and well had normal hearts.

The prognosis in general, as to the duration of life and the symptoms which may develop, is influenced to some degree by the nature and extent of the lesion. Uncomplicated *mitral insufficiency* is readily compensated in childhood but less satisfactorily later. In cases of moderate mitral insufficiency, which escape later attacks of endocarditis or pericarditis, a permanent compensation is not infrequently attained. *Mitral stenosis*, if uncomplicated, is of slow course and long in producing evidences of disturbed compensation. When, as is so frequently the case, it is associated with mitral insufficiency, the prognosis becomes that of the latter lesion. *Aortic insufficiency*, if alone or the predominating lesion, is capable of continuing for a long time with few symptoms and patients may reach a useful adult life. It may produce sudden death in later years, or finally be attended by dilatation of the left ventricle and failure of compensation; oftener from the frequently complicating mitral insufficiency. On the whole its prognosis is unfavorable. *Aortic stenosis* offers often a favorable prognosis for the duration of life. Eventually dilatation of the left ventricle is liable to occur with mitral leakage and loss of compensation; but it is probable that in many of the cases of apparently secondary mitral disease the mitral valve was attacked at the same time as the aortic.

Death in chronic valvular disease may sometimes be the result of cerebral or pulmonary embolism or of sudden cardiac paralysis. Oftener it results from some intercurrent disorder especially of the pulmonary apparatus or of the kidneys. Usually it is brought about by gradual loss of compensation due to myocardial changes and cardiac dilatation. Auricular fibrillation is a bad prognostic sign.

Diagnosis.—On account of the slight development or absence of symptoms so frequently observed in children, the diagnosis is often only to be made by examination of the heart of every child with any signs of illness. The nature of the lesion is to be decided from the character of the physical signs, and these have already been considered. In addition to other methods roentgenograms may be employed to determine alterations in the shape of the heart, and teleoroentgenograms to show the size. The electrocardiogram may be helpful, but is not necessary in the diagnosis of the type of cardiac lesion. The differentiation from congenital cardiac disease has already been discussed (p. 773). The distinction between organic and accidental murmurs is often difficult, unless positive evidences of loss of compensation are present. (See Accidental Murmurs, p. 802.) This is especially true if decided anemia exists. It is important to avoid a hasty conclusion as to the existence of valvular disease based upon murmurs alone, particularly if they are systolic; and even the evidence of cardiac enlargement may be inconclusive. Repeated observations extending over a considerable time may be needed in some instances. Never to be forgotten, too, is the normal accentuation of the pulmonary second sound which is characteristic of childhood, since it is impossible to base upon this the diagnosis of engorgement of the pulmonary circulation due to valvular disease, unless the accentuation passes the limit which may be called physiologic. It should be mentioned, too, that Duroziez's and Traube's signs are not positive proof of the existence of aortic regurgitation, since they may be heard in severe anemias and in some cases of open ductus arteriosus (p. 776).

Treatment.—**1. Treatment for decompensation** is guided more by the degree of this than by the nature of the lesion. Absolute rest unaided may restore the compensation. Whether a cardiac tonic, especially digitalis or a substitute, is needed must be determined for the individual case. It is better avoided if possible, should an acute inflammatory relighting of the old cardiac condition be present. When urgently demanded full doses should be given. To digitalize a patient there is required about 0.145 cc. (2.32 minims) of the tincture per pound (453) of body-weight (Eggleston[69]), or 0.015 Gm. (0.23 grain) of the powdered leaf; or, better still, the strength of the preparation should be known in cat-units (the amount of drug calculated per kilogram of cat just sufficient to kill), and 0.15 cat units be given per pound of body-weight (Sutton and Wyckoff[70]). Of this dose, $\frac{1}{3}$ to $\frac{1}{2}$ may be administered at once, followed in from four to six hours by $\frac{1}{4}$ to $\frac{1}{3}$ of the total dose, the remainder being given in a few doses at intervals of four to six hours. Some clinicians have advised pushing the dose of digitalis until nausea and vomiting occur, but Schwartz and Schwedel[71] believe that this is not practical, since sinus-bradycardia and the appearance of nausea and vomiting show no relationship. The signs of overdose of digitalis are nausea and vomiting, premature contractions, auriculoventricular block, and alterations in the T-wave of the electrocardiogram. In this connection it may be mentioned that in cardiac failure from digitalis the blood-pressure usually is normal or increased, because of constriction of the peripheral vessels. Often when digitalis begins to show its effect the blood-pressure, if previously increased, will fall to normal. Strychnine is not a particularly valuable cardiac tonic. Camphor is helpful, although it is a circulatory rather than a cardiac stimulant. Caffeine or epinephrine may be needed for rapid stimulation, or employed while the slower action of digitalis is being reached. Strophanthin is probably the best substitute for digitalis. The patient having been digitalized, the daily maintenance dose (*i. e.*, the rate of elimination) is about 1.5 cc. (24 minims) of the tincture, or 0.15 to 0.2 Gm. (2.3 to 3 grains) of the leaf. Digitalis may be given hypodermically in somewhat smaller doses than those suggested, employing one of the numerous preparations on the market. However, nausea and vomiting are due to a central action of the drug and not to a local one, and these symptoms do not necessarily demand hypodermic medication (Eggleston and Wyckoff[72]). It is important to be sure that a reliable form of digitalis is employed, and all preparations should have been freshly prepared and physiologically tested. Smaller doses of digitalis are not without value, especially in the milder ambulatory cases of heart-disease, and it should be remembered that there is a wide margin between the minimum dosage necessary to produce therapeutic effect and the maximum that can be tolerated (Gold and DeGraff[73]).

Certain symptoms require special therapeutic measures:

Dyspnea and *orthopnea* are aided by propping the patient semi-erect with pillows or a back-rest. The origin of the dyspnea is to be sought, since, in addition to cardiac asthenia, there may be hydrothorax, pressure from a distended abdomen, etc. *Edema* of the cardiac type will be helped by the administration of digitalis, and it may be that the mercurial diuretics (novasurol, salyrgen) may be beneficial. Some of the edema may be due to the secondary action of the disease on the kidney and in these cases the caffeine diuretics (diuretin and theocine) should be tried. (See also Treatment of Nephritis, p. 826.) If edema is continued probably a salt-poor diet is advisable, or one of the high carbohydrate diets advised in nephritis may be employed (p. 825). The Karell[74] diet for cardiac dropsy is really one consisting of milk, the patient receiving 200 cc. (6.76 oz.) of milk four times a day and no other food or liquid. After about a week other food is gradually added, beginning with eggs and toast. Large *pleural* or *abdominal effusions* should be aspirated. *Cyanosis* is sometimes benefited by the combination of nitroglycerine with digitalis; although it is to be remembered that the arterial pressure is seldom greatly increased in children. *Vomiting* depending on passive congestion from cardiac weakness may be improved by digitalis and other cardiac stimulants, although it may be necessary to treat it symptomatically. *Tumultous cardiac action* is quieted better by opiates than by digitalis, although the two drugs may be combined. *Restlessness* and *sleeplessness* may need sedatives including opiates. In fact, the rest obtained by morphine is one of the best therapeutic measures when properly used. *Precordial pain* requires the application of an ice-bag, and perhaps opiates or nitroglycerine. As improvement begins, rest in bed should continue, and cardiac tonics gradually diminished in dosage. Resumption of exercise must be made cautiously, and with careful watching of the effect on temperature, cardiac rate, production of fatigue, and other symptoms.

2. Maintenance of compensation is easier to compass than is the restoration of it when lost. The patient should always be under medical supervision, even although the general health appears to be perfect. The whole method of life should be arranged in detail; yet refraining from creating the idea of invalidism, unless the natural carelessness of the patient or the degree of restraint needed compels this. The time should be spent largely in the open air; the hygiene of the dwelling carefully regulated with avoidance of confinement to close, dark, or illy ventilated rooms; the clothing should be warm in winter, preferably of wool, and in summer not of a nature to permit of sudden chilling or of overheating. The diet should be abundant and digestible with the avoidance of coffee, tea and cigarettes. Mental over-work and undue excitement must be guarded against. The child should retire early and obtain an abundance of sleep.

Not every child who exhibits physical signs of valvular disease need be forbidden active games and sports. It is as imperative to keep the cardiac muscle in good condition by sufficient exercise as it is to avoid weakening it by over-exertion. It is particularly those exercises which throw long-continued, severe strain on the heart, or those involving sudden violent strain, which are to be avoided; but all other forms are to be encouraged in suitable subjects. Everything, in fact, depends upon the individual case, and only by a tentative increase of exercise under careful supervision can the proper limit be determined. In other words, the load which the circulation can carry must be determined in each case. Whenever the slightest indication of cardiac over-strain appears, a few days or a week in bed is advisable; and in many instances a serviceable prophylactic procedure is the systematic resting recumbent for an hour in the middle of the day.

The possibility of the contraction of any of the acute infectious diseases is to be shunned as far as possible, since they are so liable to disturb the compensation; and the avoidance of rheumatism by the seeking of warm climates in winter and spring is equally important. Respiratory infections are especially to be avoided. It may be stated that attacks of decompensation are more common in children whose tonsils have not been removed, and this indicates that the operation of tonsillectomy and adenoidectomy may be performed when favorable conditions for this are present. (See also p. 541.) This is a matter entirely different from the removal of tonsils during acute decompensation, which some clinicians recommend, but which we believe both unnecessary and perhaps harmful. About the time of puberty, with the increase of physiologic strain put upon the heart by the rapid growth, precautions must be taken against over-exertion, either bodily or mental. During adolescence the selection of a future occupation often becomes a matter of moment. When possible, one is to be chosen which combines fresh air with moderate exercise but without undue exertion.

As regards medication no digitalis or other cardiac tonic is required in cases of fully established compensation. They are indicated only for cardiac failure, not cardiac disease. The practice of giving such drugs simply because a murmur is heard is to be condemned. Great care, however, must be taken to watch for and treat promptly the anemia which is so common in chronic valvular disease.

MYOCARDITIS

Myocarditis is rare as a primary affection in childhood, but common as a secondary disorder in the acute infectious diseases, particularly diphtheria; in acute endocarditis and pericarditis; and in chronic valvular disease and chronic adhesive pericarditis, especially as a final fatal complication. In rheumatic inflammation of the heart it is practically always present. Syphilitic and tuberculous myocarditis may also occur, and exceptionally there is seen a septic variety due to pyogenic bacteria. The disease may occur in a *parenchymatous form*, much the more frequent, which is circumscribed or oftener diffuse, and with degenerative rather than inflammatory lesions; or in an *interstitial form* which in septic cases advances to the formation of minute abscesses; or in the chronic interstitial variety produces opaque, indurated areas in the cardiac wall, which may later give rise to cardiac aneurysm. We[75] have seen an instance of this in an infant of nineteen months. Syphilis may cause this form, but with extreme rarity in childhood. The **symptoms** are those of cardiac weakness as described for failing compensation (p. 791). The **prognosis** is grave, but depends upon the cause and upon the degree with which the structures of the heart are otherwise involved. The mild myocarditis following infectious fevers usually terminates in full recovery. The severer cases may end in sudden death. This is particularly true of diphtheria. The myocarditis accompanying chronic inflammation of the heart may slowly advance to a fatal termination. The **treatment** is prophylactic in nature, and is largely that used during slow convalescence after any severe febrile disease. In the form associated with diphtheria strychnine is apparently sometimes of service, but digitalis of little if any value (p. 350). The treatment is in other respects that for failing compensation. (See p. 795.)

HYPERTROPHY AND DILATATION OF THE HEART

Enlargement of the heart by increase of the thickness of its walls (*hypertrophy*) commonly results as a compensatory process, and is in that sense salutary and not to be looked upon as a disease. With the augmentation in size of muscle-fibers the strength of muscle is increased and more work is possible. The heart may hypertrophy as a whole, or only the musculature of certain chambers, depending upon the type of cardiac lesion. Unfortunately, associated with hypertrophy there is often myocardial change which offsets the advantage of the former. Enlargement of the cavities of the heart (*dilatation*) is always a pathologic condition. It may occur with or without thickening of the cardiac walls. To a certain extent dilatation may be favorable or compensatory, because it has been shown that a lengthening of muscle-fibers enables them to develop greater energy. The boundaries of the normal heart have already been considered (p. 36).

Among the frequent **causes** of dilatation is myocarditis, produced by toxic or other influences arising in the course of acute rheumatic inflammation of the heart or of acute infectious fevers; but it results also from pericardial adhesion, and chronic valvular disease is uniformly attended by it in cases with failing compensation. Nephritis and, very rarely in childhood, arteriosclerosis lead to hypertrophy which may eventually have dilatation follow. Anemia, pertussis, general malnutrition, and chronic pulmonary diseases, especially chronic bronchopneumonia, are often attended by a moderate degree of dilatation. In all these conditions there is either insufficient blood-supply to the cardiac muscles (*imperfect oxygenation*) or the possibility that toxic substances injure the myocardium. Overexertion is not a frequent cause in early life, except in the presence of an abnormal heart.

Dilatation may be acute or chronic; the former being seen especially in rheumatic carditis and in infectious diseases, or in diseased hearts when the load of work is suddenly increased over the capacity of the muscle; the latter consequent upon chronic valvular disease and pericarditis. The **symptoms** consist of those characteristic of failing cardiac compensation (p. 791), since dilatation is the accompaniment of this condition. The *physical signs* on percussion vary with the cause. Usually both sides of the heart are involved, with corresponding increase in cardiac size, although the right side is generally the first to suffer. Auscultation reveals a weakened, short first-sound and an accentuation of the second-sound; and a soft systolic murmur is not uncommon, this depending upon the incomplete closure of the widened orifices. The **prognosis** of acute dilatation is always grave. Chronic dilatation is often removable if sufficient compensatory hypertrophy can be established. When moderate and dependent upon conditions other than pericarditis or valvular disease the prognosis is usually good. The **diagnosis** of dilatation from pericardial effusion is often extremely difficult, especially as the conditions may be combined. (See p. 783.) When dilatation is dependent upon chronic valvular disease, the **treatment** for this latter is indicated. The moderate dilatation which results from anemia or similar conditions is to be treated by remedies directed to the primary disease. Acute dilatation requires the management indicated for failing compensation (p. 795).

Idiopathic Hypertrophy of the Heart in Infants and Young Children.—A condition of hypertrophy of the heart without discoverable cause occurring in quite early life has been described by Bednar,[76] Simmonds,[77] Obendorffer[78] and others, and the subject reviewed by Howland[79] in 1919, who added 5 cases and estimated that there were not more than 20 in all recorded. Riesenfeld[80] reported 5 cases and reviewed the subject. Other probable cases are those recorded by Rieder,[81] Carrington and Krumbhaar,[82] Savage,[83] Mouriquand et al.,[84] Krstulovic,[85] Scott and Zeiler,[86] Abt,[87] Stoloff[88] (who thinks that only 17 of the reported cases can be accepted); and Steiner and Bogan[89] who make the number 21. Abbott[90] in 850 cases of congenital heart disease lists 13 as instances of primary hypertrophy.

The age of the reported cases runs from a few months to four years, some being still-born. Riesenfeld[80] found lymphatism in all his cases and believes, with certain others, that this may possess an influence. In some instances there has been noted a familial tendency to cardiac defects. In others the condition appears to have been a rhabdomyoma as in those reported by Farber.[91] Abbott[90] also lists 13 cases of congenital rhabdomyoma. Postmortem examination shows that hypertrophy and dilatation involve sometimes the whole heart, sometimes one ventricle more than another. There is no myocardial degeneration or infiltration, and no disease of the valves or lesions of congenital cardiac disorder. The **symptoms** are those of a final complete loss of compensation, often not coming on for two or three years after birth; but the severe terminal symptoms develop rather abruptly, and the duration to a fatal termination is then comparatively short. Dyspnea is at this period the most marked condition; cyanosis and edema being sometimes observed, sometimes absent. There may be a soft, blowing systolic murmur, or this may be absent. The physical signs and roentgenograms confirm the diagnosis of enlarged heart. No **treatment** appears to be of any avail.

References

1. Berlin klin. Wchnschr., 1898, **35**, 1053. 2. Brit. M. J., 1921, **2**, 583. 3. München. med. Wchnschr., 1889, **36**, 357. 4. J.A.M.A., 1921, **77**, 1969. 5. Traité d. mal. de l'enf., 1904, **3**, 773. 6. Am. J. Dis. Child., 1928, **35**, 631. 7. Quart. J. Med., 1907–8, **1**, 225. 8. J.A.M.A., 1917, **69**, 450. 9. Arch. Int. Med., 1920, **25**, 206. 10. J.A.M.A., 1925, **83**, 1745. 11. Am. J. M. Sc., 1928, **175**, 331. 12. Bull. et mém. soc. méd. d. hôp., 1916, **40**, 1715. 13. J.A.M.A., 1924, **82**, 1685. 14. Med.-Chir. Trans., 1898, **81**, 445; 449. 15. Lancet, 1895, **2**, 200. 16. Arch. Int. Med., 1925, **35**, 362. 17. München. med. Wchnschr., 1902, **49**, 1072. 18. Arch. f. Kinderh., 1920, **68**, 179. 19. J.A.M.A., 1924, **82**, 1507. 20. Grancher, etc., Traité d. mal. de l'enf., 1904, **3**, 808. 21. Arch. Pediat., 1906, **23**, 508. 22. Gerhardt's Handb. d. Kinderkr., 1878, **4**, 1; 362. 23. Klinik d. Kinderkr., 1889; 3; Ref. Lempp, Monatschr. f. Kinderh., 1907–8, **6**, 78. 24. Dissert. Zürich, 1904, Ref. Lempp, Monatschr. f. Kinderh., 1907–8, **6**, 78. 25. Lancet, 1922, **1**, 1147. 26. J. Path. and Bact., 1919–20, **23**, 196. 27. Am. J. Dis. Child., 1926, **32**, 536. 28. Am. J. Dis. Child., 1930, **39**, 1261. 29. Pediatria, 1930, **38**, 311. 30. Ztschr. f. Kinderh., 1925, **40**, 370. 31. J.A.M.A., 1924, **132**, 1243. 32. Am. Heart J., 1928, **4**, 164. 33. New England J. Med., 1928, **199**, 139. 34. St. Bartholomew's Hosp. Rep., 1887, **23**, 269. 35. Trans. Am. Pediat. Soc., 1902, **14**, 160. 36. Am. J. M. Sc., 1916, **151**, 556. 37. J.A.M.A., 1924, **82**, 1721. 38. Am. Heart. J., 1925, **1**, 25. 39. Medicine, 1923, **2**, 105. 40. J.A.M.A., 1930, **94**, 1037. 41. Am. J. Dis. Child., 1928, **36**, 1144. 42. Am. J. M. Sc., 1930, **180**, 621. 43. Am. J. Dis. Child., 1931, **41**, 98. 44. Am. J. Dis. Child., 1932, **43**, 143. 45. Arch. f. Kinderh., 1927, **81**, 106. 46. Brit. J. Child. Dis., 1928, **25**, 33. 47. Am. J. Dis. Child., 1927, **34**, 390. 48. Am. Heart J., 1930, **6**, 128. 49. Am. Heart J., 1930, **6**, 132. 50. Am. Heart J., 1930, **6**, 136. 51. Am. J. Dis. Child., 1913, **6**, 107. 52. Common Disorders and Dis. Childhood, 1909, 432. 53. Garrod, Batten and Thursfield, Dis. of Child., 1913, 447. 54. Brit. J. Child. Dis., 1916, **13**, 356. 55. Am. J. Dis. Child., 1931, **42**, 503. 56. Med. Chronicle, 1888, **9**, 182; 1895, **3** (new ser.), 409. 57. Edinburgh M. and S. J., 1832, **37**, 225. 58. Arch. gén. de méd., 1861, **17**, 417. 59. Berlin. klin. Wchnschr., 1872, **9**, 573. 60. Presse méd., 1921, **29**, 733. 61. Am. J. M. Sc., 1895, **109**, 177. 62. Arch. Int. Med., 1917, **20**, 829. 63. Am. J. Dis. Child., 1920, **20**, 188. 64. Am. J. Dis. Child., 1923, **25**, 1; **26**, 554. 65. Arch. Pediat., 1924, **41**, 625. 66. Am. J. Dis. Child., 1924, **29**, 282. 67. Am. Heart J., 1932, **7**, 553. 68. Am. J. Dis. Child., 1932, **41**, 735. 69. Arch. Int. Med., 1915, **16**, 1. 70. Am. J. Dis. Child., 1931, **41**, 801. 71. Am. J. Dis. Child., 1930, **39**, 298. 72. Arch. Int. Med., 1922, **30**, 133. 73. J.A.M.A., 1930, **95**, 1237. 74. Arch. gén. de méd., 1866, **8**, 513. 75. Mitchell and Speckman, Am. Heart J., 1927, **2**, 331. 76. Krankh. d. Neugeb. u. Säugl., 1850, **3**, 160; Kinderkrankh., 1856, 319. 77. München.

med. Wchnschr., 1899, **46,** 108. 78. Verhandl. d. Gesellsch. f. Kinderh., 1906, 181. 79. Contrib. to Med. and Biol. Res., Osler Testimonial Volume, 1919, **1,** 582. 80. Jahrb. f. Kinderh., 1917, **86,** 419. 81. Jahrb. f. Kinderh., 1922, **97,** 9. 82. Am. J. Dis. Child., 1924, **27,** 449. 83. Lancet, 1930, **2,** 348. 84. Arch. de méd. d. enf., 1926, **29,** 83. 85. Monatschr. f. Kinderh., 1926, **33,** 113. 86. Am. J. Dis. Child. 1926, **31,** 31. 87. Am. J. Dis. Child., 1926, **31,** 448. 88. Am. J. Dis. Child., 1928, **36,** 1204. 89. Am. J. Dis. Child., 1930, **39,** 1255. 90. Osler and MacCrae, Modern Med., 1924, **4,** Chapt. 21. 91. Am. J. Path., 1931, **7,** 105.

CHAPTER IV

FUNCTIONAL AND MECHANICAL CARDIAC DISEASES, MORBID GROWTHS, AND DISEASES OF THE BLOOD-VESSELS

FUNCTIONAL AND MECHANICAL DISEASES

THE tendency to disturbed cardiac function increases as the subject enters the period of later childhood. Among the various causes are anemia; the existence of a febrile affection; general malnutrition; indigestion; various neuroses; an irritable heart-muscle or nerves; over-work at school; fright or other psychic disturbance; the use of tobacco, tea or coffee. However, in many cases of bradycardia, heart-block or angina, included here as a matter of convenience, an actual lesion of the heart-muscle or vessels, or of the conducting mechanism, is the cause.

Symptoms.—There exist great differences in the nature of the disturbances. Some of the more important of them may be enumerated:

Tachycardia.—This may be paroxysmal or more continuous. In the *paroxysmal* form, if severe, the attack is characterized by rapid action of the heart, oppression, pallor, weakness, sweating, dyspnea and even orthopnea, perhaps slight cyanosis, and the child appears ill. Sometimes, however, there are few symptoms except the rapid pulse, which may reach a rate of 200 or over. The seizure may last several hours or but a few minutes, and some degree of dilatation may develop. It may occur at any age, but the frequency in childhood is not great. Among reports in children are those by Hutchinson and Parkinson;[1] Koplik;[2] O'Flyn,[3] in an infant of eight months; Colgate and McCulloch;[4] Frank, Wolfgang and Wiener;[5] Willius and Amberg;[6] Van Cleve;[7] Essig;[8] who tabulates 35 cases in addition to one of his own; Shookhoff, Litvak and Matusoff,[9] who state that the total number of cases reported under fifteen years of age is 40; and Werley,[10] who saw the condition in an infant of four days. The more *continuous* form may last several days, the principal symptom being the rapid pulse without marked disturbances of other nature. The difference between the two forms is, however, only one of degree. The disease in either form comes on in repeated attacks, the whole extending sometimes over several years.

A few cases are reported (Hochsinger[11]) in which tachycardia had been continuous without intermission for over a year, the cause being probably a compression of the vagus by enlarged bronchial glands. Rarely in children continued tachycardia may be an early sign of hyperthyroidism. There are cases, too, in which a continuous tachycardia appears to be an individual and familial peculiarity and cannot be considered pathologic, since it is unaccompanied by any other evidence of faulty cardiac action or circulatory disturbance.

Palpitation.—Palpitation is the perception by the patient of an uncomfortable, disturbed cardiac action which is often rapid, but which may be simply irregular or forcible. In addition to the consciousness of the disturbed rhythm, there is a feeling of oppression; sometimes shortness of breath or perhaps even orthopnea; and in some cases dizziness, paleness and profuse perspiration.

Bradycardia.—This is often seen during convalescence from some of the infectious fevers, particularly typhoid fever, and without there being reason to believe that it depends upon a myocarditis, although this latter disease is a frequent cause of bradycardia of organic origin. It may sometimes occur also in dyspeptic conditions. It is common after grippe and diphtheria, and in the latter disease probably is due to myocarditis. It often occurs, too, during tuberculous meningitis and with other conditions of increased intracranial pressure, and in jaundice. The pulse may fall to 50 or 60 or less per minute. The condition may last for a number of days. Arrhythmia is usually combined with it.

Heart-block. Stokes-Adams-Syndrome.—This is not usually a strictly functional disturbance, but depends, at least in some cases, upon actual pathologic changes of certain of the muscular fibres of the heart,—the bundle of His. The attack is paroxysmal in nature and presents the complex of slow pulse; a disturbed cerebral state, such as syncope, vertigo, or convulsions; and auricular contractions more rapid than those of the ventricle, the former perhaps being visible in the veins of the neck. The disease is one of adult life, but has been reported in childhood. Recent reviews on this are those by Yater[12] and Leech,[3] the former author accepting 31 of the cases as of congenital origin. It has been shown by Butler and Levine,[14] Chamberlain and Alstead,[15] and others that heart-block may persist for months after diphtheria, and Jones and White[16] suggest that an earlier occurrence of diphtheria may be responsible for some cases. (See also Diphtheria, p. 343.) Other cases have been associated with trauma, congenital heart-disease, rheumatism, cardiac tumor, or acute infections, as grippe, measles and sepsis.

Angina Pectoris.—This is an uncommon disorder in children, yet Stolkind[17] has seen 4 cases, and has collected and carefully reviewed 25 others, the youngest in a child of six years. The causes and pathogenesis are the same as in adults; organic, including valvular disease, in many cases; probably functional in others. The symptoms likewise are similar. There is generally no cyanosis or true dyspnea, which aids in distinguishing the disease from various other forms of cardiac pain, such as may occur in pericarditis or at times in severe cases of endocarditis with cardiac decompensation.

Arrhythmia.—Sinus-arrhythmia (respiratory arrhythmia) in early life should be regarded as physiologic (p. 37), and its absence, especially in older children, points to myocardial damage. Sinus-arrhythmia may be exaggerated during convalescence from acute febrile diseases; it may be abolished by the administration of atropine or digitalis. Less commonly extrasystoles (premature contractions) may give rise to arrhythmia in children. As isolated phenomena and without other signs of heart-disease they have no significance. They may occur with the administration of digitalis. *Auricular fibrillation* may be encountered in childhood (Ogden,[18] Resnik and Scott[19]). Schwartz and Weiss[20] found it in 10 of 60 children with rheumatic heart-disease. Cookson[21] in 1164 cases of auricular fibrillation recorded 30 under seventeen years of age. The condition is most often associated with mitral stenosis and may occur with adhesive pericarditis (Holt[22]).

In this connection it may be stated that sometimes there seems to be an unusually small heart, as though its growth had been arrested. The symptoms are fatigue, arrhythmia, and palpitation. Sometimes there is an associated retardation of general growth. (See Talquist.[23])

Syncope.—Fainting attacks, less common than in adults, are not often associated with any actual weakness of the heart; in fact, children with organic cardiac disease do not often have syncope. Syncope and vertigo are usually the result of anoxemia of the cerebral centers brought about by fall in blood-pressure. The attacks are liable to occur in nervous, debilitated, anemic children, and particularly in girls. They are ushered in by yawning, pallor, dizziness, and feeble pulse, and end in partial or complete loss of consciousness. The disorder is to be distinguished from some of the milder attacks of petit mal, and from the rare cases of the Stokes-Adams syndrome.

Accidental Cardiac Murmurs.—These are frequently present in early life in cases of marked anemia or in acute febrile diseases; but often found where explanation is entirely lacking. Some of them are perhaps cardiopulmonary in nature, produced by the impulse of the heart against the border of the lung (Hochsinger[24]). Another view attributes them to obstruction of the blood-flow by angulation or rotation of the heart and blood-vessels; another to the thin character of the blood if anemia is present; and still another to relaxation of the pulmonary muscles and temporary widening of the mitral or tricuspid orifice.

The accidental (functional) murmur is of frequent occurrence, observed in from 65 to 70 per cent of children, according to some studies (Lüthje,[25] Hamill and LeBoutillier[26]). It is nearly always systolic in time; is often heard best over the base of the heart; is most evident at the end of expiration, and while the patient is recumbent; disappears during full inspiration; and is not loudly transmitted to the axilla and seldom to the back. In cases of severe anemia, however, it may be widely diffused and audible in the carotid and subclavian arteries, and accompanied by a venous hum in the neck. Corrigan's pulse, Duroziez's murmur, and Traube's pistol-shot sound may be present in severe anemia without cardiac disease being discovered (p. 792). In accidental cardiac murmurs there should be no symptoms or signs of organic cardiac disease.

Prognosis.—The prognosis of functional cardiac disorders is usually good in most of the conditions described. Paroxysmal tachycardia, unless frequent and severe, is not necessarily serious. Bradycardia usually indicates a myocarditis with an unfavorable prognosis; except when it occurs as an individual peculiarity or follows some infectious fever, such as typhoid or grippe, without there having been reason to believe that myocarditis exists. Of the 21 instances of heart-block collected by Eyster and Middleton[27] seven were known to have died, as did 10 of the 31 cases mentioned by Seham.[28] Angina dependent upon organic causes finally terminates fatally. Accidental cardiac murmurs have no significance, but it is often difficult to distinguish between these and the murmurs of organic cardiac disease.

Treatment.—For many of the disturbances mentioned in this section rest of body and mind is the best treatment, combined with a search for and management of the cause. Digitalis should probably not be given in partial heart-block, but may be tried in the complete form. It is to be used in auricular fibrillation, and for this condition, as well as other cardiac irregularities, quinidine may be employed. Partial heart-block may also respond to the hypodermic injection of epinephrine or the oral administration of ephedrine (Wood[29]). An attack of angina requires morphine and the nitrites.

MORBID GROWTHS OF THE HEART

These are of extremely uncommon occurrence. The most frequent form is lymphosarcoma extending to the heart from a primary growth in the mediastinum. The symptoms produced are those of pericarditis with effusion, and the fluid withdrawn is commonly blood-stained. Syphiloma of the heart has also occurred in children, and echinococcus-cyst has been reported. Anderson[30] published a case of rupture of the heart in a five-year-old girl, apparently dependent upon syphiloma. A case of tuberculous aneurysm of the heart with rupture, secondary to tuberculosis of the bronchial glands, is reported by Korybut-Daszkeiwicz,[31] and Laves[32] reported an aneurysm of the heart, probably syphilitic, in an infant of six months. We have seen one remarkable instance of large tuberculous growths in the heart.

DISORDERS OF THE BLOOD-VESSELS

None of these are common in early life, including even those of a congenital nature (pp. 776, 777). **Arteriosclerosis with atheroma** is rare, yet probably more common than ordinarily supposed. Although it has been found even in the fetus, the most frequent period in childhood is shortly before puberty. It may be associated with the unusual cases of chronic interstitial nephritis occurring in childhood (p. 820); is sometimes a result of congenital syphilis; or may occasionally occur after rheumatism or infectious diseases. Stumpf[33] in a long series of examinations found it common, especially following chronic disorders of different sorts; much less often after acute infections. The subject has been exhaustively reviewed by Fremont-Smith[34] and Saltykow.[35] The latter thinks that the small yellowish spots found at times on the aortic valve in early life are the beginnings of the same process. Zeek[36] has been able to collect only 98 cases of juvenile arteriosclorosis recorded since 1829. **Acute arteritis** of the peripheral vessels may occur as the result of various infectious diseases, syphilis, and rheumatism, and produce narrowing or occlusion of the lumen. It may also follow the formation of a septic thrombus or embolus, and a secondary aneurysm may result. An **aortitis** may very exceptionally occur with rheumatism, syphilis, or some infectious process (Marfan[37]). Levy-Franckel[38] collected 35 instances of chronic aortitis and atheroma, including some of his own, occurring up to the age of seventeen years. Thoenes[39] reports a number of instances in the new-born, and reviews cases published by others.

Aneurysm of the aorta is of rare occurrence in early life. LeBoutillier[40] made a careful review of the published cases, equalling, with one of his own, 16 not over twelve years of age, including one developing in fetal life reported by Phänomenow.[41] The youngest, excluding this last, was in a child of two years. The causes are various, among them being syphilis, rheumatism, and trauma, but oftenest the origin is obscure. The thoracic aorta is the portion oftenest involved, Calvin[42] having collected 31 instances of this, besides two of his own. Only 21 of them, however, occurred under the age of twelve years. **Aneurysm of the peripheral vessels** is also uncommon. V. Koos[43] collected reports of 14 cases of aneurysm of vessels in different parts of the body. It is dependent oftenest upon syphilis; sometimes on sepsis. Roeder[44] reported 2 cases of aneurysm of the ductus arteriosus, Hutchison[45] 1, and Guggenheim[46] 1; and 1 of the carotid in a child of eleven months in which the symptoms suggested retropharyngeal abscess is recorded by Vas.[47]

Embolism is uncommon in early life. It is sometimes seen in acute endocarditis as a result of small thrombi leaving the heart and being carried by the blood to the brain or other parts of the body. We recall two typical instances of cerebral embolism attending acute endocarditis in children of eleven and thirteen years respectively. **Thrombosis** of the arteries is uncommon. It may form in severe cases of infectious fevers, pneumonia, from atheroma, or in conditions of great debility. We have seen gangrene of the leg produced by thrombosis of the artery in diphtheria, and again in a case of exhaustion resulting from unusually severe recurrent vomiting. Large thrombi are not infrequently found in the heart at necropsy upon greatly debilitated subjects or those with infectious or cardiac diseases. They form usually just before or after death. Very rarely thrombosis of the aorta may develop at an earlier period. Thrombosis of the veins is more common. It may occur as a result of an infectious **phlebitis** in acute infectious fevers; or in anemia, pneumonia or conditions of great debility; or from pressure. Any of the large venous trunks of the body may be affected, oftenest those of the lower extremities. David[48] reported an instance of double phlebitis of the lower extremities in a new-born, following umbilical infection. **Thrombosis** of the superior or inferior vena cava has been observed repeatedly, the cause being marantic conditions, mediastinitis, or the pressure of intra-abdominal growths or of enlarged tracheobronchial glands. The jugular veins are also sometimes affected. The most frequent seat is the venous sinuses of the brain. (See p. 933.) *Coronary thrombosis* may occur in late childhood, cases being reported by Dreschfeld[49] and Benda,[50] and it has been recorded in infancy (Ramsay and Crumrine[51]). A case of *thrombo-angiitis obliterans* (Buerger's Disease) is reported in a child of two years of age by Cahill.[52] **Raynaud's disease** is infrequent in childhood. In 168 cases analysed by Cassirer[53] there were 22 under five years of age and 8 between five and ten years. Potter and Silverman[54] report a case in a child of six months; and 1 in a child of four and one-half months was observed in the Children's Hospital in Philadelphia. Hand and Reilly[55] saw a case in a child of five years, which we had an opportunity of studying. **Nodular periarteritis** (Kussmaul's disease) may rarely occur in children (Debré et al.[56]).

Arterial hypertension in infancy and childhood is almost always an accompaniment of diseased conditions in which increased blood-pressure might be expected. Among these are certain types of acquired heart-disease; congenital heart-disease, such as coarctation of the aorta with the increased pressure confined to the upper part of the body; increased intracranial pressure; and chronic nephritis. In a few cases it exists without any explanation, and then may be classified as essential hypertension, such cases having been reported by Amberg,[57] Siegel and Thomas,[58] and others.

Dilatation of the veins, not of the nature of varicosities, is of very common occurrence in early life. It is seen in rachitis or in other conditions attended by anemia or debility. Situated in the veins of the scalp it is sometimes very marked in hereditary syphilis. Dilatation of the veins of the abdominal walls often attends abdominal tuberculosis or morbid growths. Dilatation of comparatively small groups of vessels is seen in nevi and the like. (See Diseases of the Skin, p. 1110.) An extensive and excessive congenital or developmental dilatation of the arteries and veins is a rare condition, associated with hypertrophy of the limb in which it is situated. The subject has been reviewed by Parkes Weber.[59] A case of congenital varix of the jugular vein is reported by Forst,[60] who could find but 17 recorded cases. Lereboullet[61] reported a case of congenital varix of the leg. Congenital varices in other parts of the body occur more frequently.

Symptoms.—The symptoms of the various lesions of the blood-vessels vary with the situation and do not for the most part differ from those seen in adult life. Reference may be made to the frequency of a venous hum heard in the jugulars or beneath the upper part of the sternum. Landis and Kaufman[62] found it present in 84 out of 99 children examined, and could discover no special relationship to anemia. They believe it is present in the majority of children. In adults the murmur was much less frequently heard, and generally in connection with anemia. This confirms the observations of Sawyer[63] and of Coombs.[64] (See also p. 766.) The murmurs which may be heard in the arteries of the body, occurring in connection with valvular diseases of the heart or anemia, have been described elsewhere when considering these affections. A cephalic systolic bruit is not infrequently audible at the open fontanelle in infancy. More interesting is a similar murmur heard after the fontanelle is closed and during early childhood, but rare after this time. It is frequently audible to the child himself. This condition has been discussed especially by Still.[65] In a case in a perfectly healthy child under our own observation this systolic murmur was distinctly musical, and could be heard while the observer was merely standing close to the child.

References

1. Brit. J. Child. Dis., 1914, **11,** 241. 2. Tr. Ass. Am. Physicians, 1917, **32,** 533. 3. Brit. M. J., 1925, **1,** 507. 4. Am. Heart J., 1926, **2,** 160. 5. Ztschr. f. Kinderh., 1928, **46,** 676. 6. Am. J. Dis. Child., 1929, **38,** 551. 7. J.A.M.A., 1930, **94,** 1758. 8. Monatschr. f. Kinderh., 1930, **48,** 288. 9. Am. J. Dis. Child., 1932, **43,** 93. 10. Arch. Pediat, 1925, **42,** 825. 11. Pfaundler und Schlossmann, Handb. d. Kinderh., 1910. **3,** 489. 12. Am. J. Dis. Child. 1929, **38,** 112. 13. Am. J. Dis. Child., 1930, **39,** 131, 14. Am. Heart J., 1930, **5,** 529. 15. Lancet, 1931, **1,** 970. 16. Am. Heart J., 1927, **3.** 190. 17. Brit. J. Child. Dis., 1928, **25,** 1. 18. Am. J. Dis. Child., 1925, **29,** 767. 19, Am. J. Dis. Child., 1926, **31,** 357. 20. Am. J. Dis. Child., 1928, **36,** 22. 21. Lancet, 1929, **2,** 1139. 22. Am. J. M. Sc., 1929, **178,** 615. 23. Finska Läk.-sällsk. Handl., 1921, **63,** 335. 24. Arch. f. Kinderh., 1913, **60–61,** 377. 25. Med. Klin., 1906, **2,** 404. 26. Am. J. M. Sc., 1907, **133,** 55. 27. Am. J. Dis. Child., 1920, **19,** 131. 28. Abt's Pedia. trics, 1924, **4,** 333. 29. J.A.M.A. 1932, **98,** 1364. 30. Lancet, 1915, **1,** 647. 31. Arch-de méd. des enf., 1922, **25,** 150. 32. Wien. klin. Wchnschr., 1929, **42,** 1469. 33. Beiträg. z. path. Anat. u. z. allg. Path., 1914, **59,** 390. 34. Am. J. M. Sc., 1908, **135,** 199. 35. Correspondbl. f. Schweiz. Aerzte, 1915, **45,** 1057. 36. Arch. Path., 1930, **10,** 417. 37. Semaine méd., Paris, 1901, **21,** 97. 38. Arch. d. mal. du coeur., 1912, **5,** 637. 39. Ztschr. f. Kinderh., 1928, **33,** 113. 40. Am. J. M. Sc., 1903, **125,** 778. 41. Arch. f. Gynäk., 1881, **17,** 133. 42. Am. J. Dis. Child. 1921, **21,** 327. 43. Jahrb. f. Kinderh., 1916, **83,** 471. 44. Arch. f. Kinderh., 1900, **30,** 157. 45. Brit. J. Child. Dis., 1922, **19,** 85. 46. Frankfurt. Ztschr. f. Path., 1930, **40,** 436. 47. Jahrb. f. Kinderh. 1916, **83,** 493. 48. Arch. de méd. d. enf., 1913, **16,** 615. 49. Practitioner, 1890, **44,** 28. 50. Arch. f. path. Anat., 1925, **254,** 600. 51. Am. J. Dis. Child., 1931, **42,** 107. 52. South. M. J., 1928, **21,** 105. 53. Die vaso-motorisch-tropischen Neurosen, 1901; Ref. Garrod, Batten and Thursfield-Dis. of Child., 1913, 504. 54. Arch. Pediat., 1920, **37,** 744. 55. Atlantic M. J., 1923, **26,** 740. 56. Arch. de méd. d. enf., 1928, **31,** 325. 57. Am. J. Dis. Child., 1929, **37,** 335. 58. Arch. Pediat., 1930, **47,** 473. 59. Brit. J. Dis. Child., 1918, **15,** 13. 60. Frankfurt. Ztschr. f. Path., 1915, **17,** 137. 61. Bull. soc. de pédiat. de Paris, 1926, 76. 62. Arch. Pediat., 1912, **29,** 88. 63. Brit. J. Child. Dis., 1910, **7,** 310. 64. Brit. J. Child. Dis., 1911, **8,** 109. 65. Brit. J. Child. Dis., 1921, **18,** 13.

SECTION VII

DISEASES OF THE GENITO-URINARY SYSTEM

CHAPTER I

DISORDERS OF URINARY SECRETION

It is advisable to make a routine examination of the urine at stated intervals in presumably well infants and children, in every febrile disease, and in any condition in which the diagnosis is not clear. The method of procuring the urine in infancy has been discussed (p. 148), and also the physiologic characteristics of the normal secretion of the kidneys (p. 42).

DISTURBANCES IN THE QUANTITY OR THE METHOD OF THE EXCRETION OF URINE

1. Anuria (*Ischuria; Oliguria*).—This is the failure to excrete urine in normal amount, if at all; in a narrower sense it indicates the latter condition only. It may be divided into (*a*) retention, and (*b*) suppression.

(*a*) **Retention of Urine; Dysuria.**—Here the amount of urine is normal, but there is failure of the bladder to expel it. In the new-born this may be due to malformation of the urinary tract, such as great phimosis, or atresia of the labiae; or to obstruction by abnormal folds of mucous membrane, uric-acid crystals, or a calculus. A balanoposthitis, vulvovaginitis, or inflammation of the meatus may cause retention through the pain which urination produces. Disturbances in the innervation of the bladder, and various reflex or direct inhibitions are factors, as in meningitis, rectal irritation, myelitis, spasm of the vesical sphincter, hysteria, and the debility attending fevers.

(*b*) **Suppression of Urine.**—In this form urine is secreted in small amount, or temporarily not at all. This may be a normal condition in the first twenty-four hours of life (p. 41). Among other causes of diminution or suspension of secretion are acute nephritis, profuse watery diarrhea, lack of fluid intake, prostration after operation, and hysteria.

2. Polyuria.—This consists in a large increase in the amount of urine, as seen in diabetes mellitus and diabetes insipidus. It is observed also after the fall of temperature following acute febrile diseases, in nephrosclerosis, after convulsions, when a large amount of fluid is imbibed, and during the reduction of edema. Nervous excitement and chilling of the body-surface may produce a temporary increase in urinary secretion.

3. Frequent Urination (*Pollakiuria*).—This is normal in the first two years of life (p. 42). It also attends polyuria, is present in cystitis, occurs from reflex stimulation by renal calculi, and is seen with nervous excitement. A highly concentrated, acid urine causes it by irritation of the bladder (p. 839).

4. Incontinence of Urine.—Apart from enuresis, which may be considered a neurosis, (p. 840) this depends upon a variety of causes. It is observed in marked phimosis, cystitis, impaction of a calculus in the urethra, paralytic conditions of the bladder resulting from disease of the brain or spinal cord, including spina bifida, and in profound exhaustion or coma.

The bladder becomes over-distended until there is persistent overflow, or sometimes an intermittent expulsion of urine without the patient's knowledge. Malformations, such as exstrophy of the bladder, abnormal openings of the ureters into the vagina, persistent urachus, and absence of the vesical sphincter, allow the urine to flow constantly. Incontinence is a characteristic symptom in many idiots, being then really a form of enuresis.

ALTERATIONS IN THE CHARACTER OF THE URINE

1. Albuminuria. (*a*) **Physiologic or Benign Albuminuria.**—Many studies, as those by Hamill and Blackfan,[1] Moor,[2] Calvin, Isaacs and Meyer,[3] Hench,[4] Ashburn,[5] Palmer,[6] and others, have shown that children and young adults, who do not exhibit or later develop any evidence of nephritis, often have albumin in the urine. The subject is reviewed by Fishberg.[7] Delicate tests show albumin in the majority of persons. In these benign albuminurias the proteins found include euglobulin, nucleo-albumin, and mucin. Casts are seldom present. The incidence is higher in girls. Small amounts of albumin may sometimes be found following violent exercise, overeating, and cold bathing. Some authors have considered this benign albuminuria as a phenomenon of growth.

(*b*) **Orthostatic Albuminuria.** *Postural, Cyclic, Lordotic Albuminuria.*—This form of albuminuria, early described especially by Pavy,[8] is in a sense physiologic, since it has no organic renal change as its basis.

Etiology.—The frequency of orthostatic albuminuria is difficult to determine, because of the differences in terminology employed in many studies. Probably some of the causes included in this category in the literature belong in the group of physiologic or functional albuminurias described. Perhaps the incidence could be placed at about 5 per cent of children examined (Palmer,[6] Götzky[9]). It is seen particularly in later childhood; with equal frequency in males and females; and a familial tendency has been noted. There are various theories concerning its cause. One attributes it to circulatory disturbance produced by change in position from the recumbent to the upright (postural albuminuria), associated with an alteration of blood-pressure, which, according to Erlanger and Hooker,[10] consists in a rise in diastolic pressure and a corresponding decrease in pulse-pressure. Bass and Wessler,[11] however, found that the blood-pressure in these cases differed little from the normal. Jehle[12] denominated the condition *lordotic albuminuria*, believing pressure was exercised upon the renal vessels by the spinal curvature in cases of lordosis. In support of such a view is the observation that the left kidney, which would naturally be more subject to compression, is the one which excretes the albumin (Sonne[13]). It must be stated, however, that faulty posture is not present in many of the patients who have this type of albuminuria, and conversely that not all cases of lumbar lordosis exhibit albuminuria; and Saito[14] consequently assumes other influences also to be at work, such as a vasomotor instability. Samuels[15] suggests that lack of calcium may affect protein metabolism and be in this way the main cause of albuminuria, and Rieser and Rieser[16] would attribute it to pressure exerted by the great vessels on the left renal vein.

Among the *symptoms* is the characteristic that albumin appears in the urine secreted during the daytime, but not in that which has accumulated in the bladder during the night. Thus the urine passed on first rising contains no albumin, while that excreted in the afternoon shows its presence. In some instances a posture which will increase the lordosis increases also the amount of albumin, and Hempelmann[17] found that this produced in addition a retardation in phenosulphonephthalein elimination. Serum-albumin may or may not constitute a part of the protein substance excreted. The general health may be perfect, or oftener there may be faulty nutrition, anemia, fatigability, and various nervous symptoms. Pallor may be present without real anemia. In the line of *course and prognosis* there may be intermissions during which albumin is absent for weeks or months, and there is a tendency for the disorder to disappear after adolescence. If nephritis later develops, it is always questionable whether the albuminuria may not have been a symptom of this condition rather than simply of the orthostatic or functional type. The *diagnosis* is to be made especially from nephritis, and prolonged observation may be necessary. No other signs or symptoms of nephritic disease should be present in orthostatic albuminuria. The occurrence and persistence of granular casts, or even of hyaline ones, should lead to a suspicion of nephritic changes. The *treatment* consists in an improvement of the general health, a defect in which so often underlies the condition. Protein need not be restricted in the diet. A moderate amount of exercise may be helpful, although that of a violent sort is to be forbidden. Rest in bed during a portion of the day in a position which would tend to straighten the lordotic curve is helpful, and perhaps also postural gymnastic treatment. Samuels[15] found that fasting until noon prevented the albuminuria. The wearing of braces to correct the position seems to do little good, and the same is true of any mechanical apparatus devised to relieve ptosis of the kidney. Nassau[18] observed that the administration of an alkali prevented the appearance of albumin in the urine.

(*c*) **Febrile Albuminuria.**—This disorder is of the nature of a cloudy swelling or degeneration of the kidney, and probably should not be classed as a real inflammation. Most cases of acute infectious disease with continued fever, or in fact with elevation of temperature from any cause, are liable to exhibit albuminuria, which disappears on the cessation of the fever. The urine is high-colored; concentrated; contains a small amount of albumin, chiefly nucleo-albumin; and occasionally a few hyaline or epithelial casts.

(*d*) **Adventitious Albuminuria.**—The presence in the urine of blood, bacteria, or pus from any source will produce an albuminuria.

(*e*) **Albuminuria from Organic Renal Disease.**—This variety will be considered elsewhere under the respective headings of the different diseases of the kidney.

2. Pyuria.—This is characterized by the appearance of pus-cells in the urine. Normally there may be found as many as 4 to 6 leukocytes to every high-power (4 mm. ($\frac{1}{6}$ in.) objective) field of uncentrifuged urine, and up to 10 or 12 in girls. Our[19] studies have indicated that when the number of cells (counted in an ordinary blood-counting chamber) is over 40 to the cubic millimeter there is probably infection in the genito-urinary tract. Mere concentration of urine by fever or dehydration will seldom increase the number over this figure. If the pus is in considerable amount it may readily be recognized by its appearance in the test tube, and the urine shows the presence of albumin. Pyuria may be produced by many causes. In vulvovaginitis the pus is usually in small amount and mixed with mucus and many epithelial cells. Pyuria may arise from inflammation of the urethra. In cystitis there is usually an admixture of mucus and the urine is either acid or alkaline. The most common source is pyelitis (p. 833) where the urine is often acid, contains clumps of pus-cells, and the few epithelial cells present are of the small, round, renal type. Pus may also be present in tuberculosis of the kidney, pyonephrosis, renal calculus, acute nephritis, or when abscess without the kidney ruptures into the urinary tract.

3. Bacteruria. Bacilluria.—Numerous micro-organisms usually accompany pyuria from any cause, but there is a form to which the title is properly applied, in which bacteria are excreted in unusual numbers without the presence of pus, and often without constitutional symptoms. The urine may be cloudy from the great number of germs present, which are

usually colon bacilli. The condition was discussed by Mellin[20] and Ramsey;[21] but since then bacilluria appears to be oftener recognized and is probably not uncommon, Schwartz,[22] for example, finding bacilli in the urine in more than 50 per cent of 63 infants with gastro-intestinal disorders, and in 21 per cent in sufficient number to apply the title bacilluria.

4. HEMATURIA.—This may vary from blood-red to brown-red urine to the finding of red blood-cells only under the microscope. Sometimes the urine has just enough blood to produce a characteristic "smoky" appearance. The **causes** are various. In infancy hematuria may be evidence of the hemorrhagic disease of the new-born, acute nephritis, scurvy, renal tumors, sepsis, or uric acid infarction. Later it is a symptom of urinary calculus; hemorrhagic forms of acute infectious disorders; nephritis; neoplasms; tuberculosis of the kidney; renal congestion; blood-dyscrasias, as hemophilia, leukemia and purpura; malaria; renal angioma; trauma; the action of irritant poisons; echinococcus-disease, and bilharzia. An idiopathic hematuria of unknown origin, but apparently associated with nephritis, has been observed in rare instances in children. It seems in some cases to be familial in nature (Guthrie,[23] Hurst[24]). Large hemorrhages are generally renal, but blood appearing only at the beginning or the end of micturition is probably from the lower urinary tract. Blood-casts are proof that hematuria is of renal origin. Cystoscopic study or ureteral catheterization may be necessary to determine the site of the hemorrhage. Bleeding in the new-born must be distinguished from the brick-red staining sometimes caused by urates. The **treatment** depends on the cause, but with any hemorrhage the patient should be kept at rest in bed, given a light diet, and hemostatic measures employed, as injections of horse-serum, whole blood, or the like, if the bleeding is severe. In certain cases of idiopathic hematuria radiologic treatment of the kidney has been beneficial (Hager[25]), done cautiously so that roentgen-ray nephritis will not be produced.

5. HEMOGLOBINURIA.—Here the urine exhibits hemoglobin, but with few if any erythrocytes. Albumin is present in small amount, and hyaline and granular casts are usually found. The urine is red or reddish-brown in color and sometimes almost black; and the granular pigment is seen under the microscope. The pigments are oxyhemoglobin, methemoglobin, and occasionally hematin. Sometimes the urine is rose-colored due to the pigment uro-erythrin, probably derived from hemoglobin (Namba[26]). Hemoglobinuria may occur in severe infectious diseases; burns; parasitic diseases, as malaria; poisoning, as with carbolic acid, potassium chlorate, oxalic acid, arsenic, phosphorus, carbon monoxide, chloroform, and quinine; and in transfusion with incompatible blood. In fact, hemoglobin appears in the urine whenever the amount of free hemoglobin is more than $\frac{1}{60}$ of the total hemoglobin content of the body (Ponfick[27]). Hemoglobinuria of the new-born has been described (p. 218).

Paroxysmal hemoglobinuria may occur in children. Herrman[28] collected 24 cases in children, others have since been reported, and at times several children in the same family are affected. Puris[29] reviews the subject and states that the condition is as frequent as in adults. The cause of this variety is not known, but the action is a hemolytic one taking place at the time of the attack. Reiss[30] discovered the resistance of the red cells diminished. Donath and Landsteiner[31] found that the blood contained a lysin which united with the cells only at a low temperature, and that with increase of temperature there was destruction of the cells, setting free the hemoglobin. Puris[29] and others believe that syphilis is a probable underlying factor, and Mackenzie[32] claims its presence in over 90 per cent of the cases. There seems to be a very close relationship to Raynaud's Disease.

Chilling of the body-surface appears to be a very prominent cause, and the attack may be produced, for instance, by immersing the feet in ice-water for three-quarters of an hour (Rosenbach[33]). Sometimes over-exertion or emotional stress produces an attack. With the passing of the hemoglobin there may be fever, prostration, slight jaundice, pain in the lumbar region, and such vasomotor symptoms as cyanosis, pallor, urticaria and coldness of the extremities. Some cases show no symptoms except the urinary ones. The erythrocytes in the blood diminish in number during the attack, but later rapidly return to normal, and there may be a slight polymorphonuclear leukocytosis, a diminished coagulation-time, and an indirect van den Bergh reaction. The discharge of hemoglobin may last for from a few hours rarely up to one or two days, and attacks occur at irregular intervals but oftener in the winter season.

The **prognosis** of hemoglobinuria depends on the cause. The paroxysmal type is not dangerous. **Treatment** consists in rest and warmth, and, in the paroxysmal type, perhaps residence in a warm climate and vigorous antisyphilitic treatment.

6. Glycosuria. (*Lactosuria, etc.*).—Sugar of some sort may be found in small amounts in the urine of healthy infants in the early months of life (p. 43). Eagle[34] states that the reducing substances frequently present in presumably normal persons are not glucose. It has been claimed that gastro-intestinal disease in infants increases the permeability of the intestinal wall for lactose, but Schloss[35] found that in such cases the sugar was usually glucose, and suggests that it may be of metabolic origin. Feeding large amounts of saccharose to normal infants may produce saccharosuria, sometimes with the elimination of glucose and levulose as well (Gaujoux,[36] Aschenheim[37]). The term *alimentary glycosuria* is employed when small amounts of glucose are excreted by healthy children given excessive quantities of it. *Transient glycosuria* may result, too, from the action of poisons, as mercury, carbon dioxide, or opium; may occur in febrile diseases or in disorders interfering with respiration, as pertussis and pneumonia; or may attend such nervous maladies as convulsions, meningitis, brain-tumor, or brain-injury. A continued glycosuria without any symptoms and with a low renal threshold for sugar is sometimes seen, in which there is a hereditary tendency. In the so-called *renal diabetes* (normal glycemic glycosuria) there is simply a glycosuria, but the blood-sugar is normal, the sugar-tolerance-curve normal, and the amount of the glycosuria little influenced by the amount of carbohydrate taken. In *diabetes innocens* there is normal fasting blood-sugar but the response to the carbohydrate tolerance test shows an abnormally high blood-sugar and glycosuria (Powelson and Wilder[38]). The most common cause of continued glycosuria is *diabetes mellitus.* It should always be remembered that other substances besides glucose will reduce copper solutions, among them being salicylic acid, and that the diagnosis of diabetes depends upon the fermentation or the phenylhydrazine test, or on examination with the polariscope. The blood-sugar, too, must be examined, and the response to the ingestion of glucose. (See Glucose Tolerance, p. 154.)

An uncommon condition is *pentosuria.* This form of sugar will reduce copper slowly but is not fermentable. It is said to occur sometimes after the ingestion of certain fruits, as pears, plums, cherries and strawberries. While rare it is more common in males and in Jews, but is uncommon at any age. Usually it is not an ingestion-pentosuria, but a metabolic disorder. Cases in children are reported by Aron,[39] Schippers,[40] Rossen,[41] Margolis,[42] and Fischer and Reiner.[43]

7. Lithuria.—A certain amount of uric acid is always excreted in the urine, even during complete starvation. The amount is augmented in

conditions of indigestion, or of increased destruction of tissue, as in leukemia, anemia, lead-poisoning, pneumonia; and also by an increased amount of purine bases in the diet. It is relatively increased in concentrated urine. In infancy it may form a whitish or reddish deposit upon the diaper. Uric acid may be precipitated in the bladder when the urine is highly acid, and give rise to pain on micturition. In the new-born there may be uric acid infarctions of the kidney, producing attacks of abdominal pain, but not possessing any special significance. The mere discovery of urates or an excess of uric acid in the urine has no particular indication. If necessary to treat the condition, water should be given freely and the urine alkalinized.

8. Indicanuria.—Indican is usually present in small amounts in artificially fed infants. It is increased in digestive disturbance and with putrefaction of proteins in the intestinal tract, or with decomposition of protein in other parts of the body. It is a frequent attendant upon constipation.

9. Lipuria.—Fat in the urine may depend upon an excess of it in the food or upon fatty degeneration of the kidneys. In **chyluria** there is sufficient fat to give the urine a milky appearance, and there may be albuminuria and red blood cells as well. The course of chyluria is chronic and the prognosis uncertain. Some cases are due to filaria. Nonparasitic chyluria is rare in early life, but cases have been reported by Hymanson,[44] Goebel,[45] and others.

10. Acetonuria.—The acetone bodies, acetone, aceto-acetic acid and β-oxybutyric acid may occur in small amounts in the urine of healthy infants. An excess indicates disturbed carbohydrate metabolism, but not necessarily an acidosis. (See page 489.) Acetonuria is seen especially in diabetes and in recurrent vomiting, but accompanies also starvation, acute digestive diseases, and acute febrile disorders.

11. Urobilinuria.—Urobilin in the urine in small amounts has no special significance, and may occur in normal bottle-fed infants. It is increased in quantity in intestinal disturbance, acute febrile diseases, hemorrhagic disorders, certain anemias (especially pernicious anemia), scurvy, and congestive heart-failure. In icterus its presence indicates a hemolytic form of this rather than an obstructive one.

12. Alkaptonuria.—This appears in early infancy and lasts indefinitely; is sometimes familial; and has no influence on the general health. It may be associated with pigmentation of the skin, and in later life may be followed by chronic arthritis. The urine becomes brown or deep-black on exposure to the air, and yields a reddish-black precipitate when treated with copper solution. This depends upon the presence of homogentesic acid or allied substances.

13. Cystinuria.—It has been supposed that this is an anomaly of metabolism in which the sulphur-containing amino-acids are not properly oxidized. Lewis and Lough,[46] however, suggest that the origin of cystine may be largely endogenous. The condition is rare, usually congenital, and often hereditary. Cystine is found in the urine and occasionally may form a calculus in the bladder, but except for this there is no effect on the general health.

14. Porphyrinuria (Hematoporphyrinuria).—This very rare condition may be congenital and persistent. Toxic symptoms may be absent, or they may occur and be combined with attacks of abdominal pain. The condition may also follow the continued administration of sulphonal or trional. There is great sensitiveness of the body to light, and an eruption (hydroa vacciniforme) may develop on exposed parts, which becomes markedly pigmented, and perhaps leaves permanent scarring. Pigmentation of the teeth and the bones may also occur; blindness sometimes develops, and tuberculosis is frequent. The color of the urine is like port

wine. (See Rothman;[47] and for a review of this, as well as alkaptonuria, cystinuria, and pentosuria consult Garrod.[48])

15. The Diazo Reaction.—This is found particularly in measles, typhoid fever, and tuberculosis, but may occur in other infectious disorders.

16. Abnormally Colored Urine.—In addition to, or as a synopsis of, what has already been mentioned some of the abnormal colorations of the urine may be referred to. A red tint may be due to blood, hemoglobin. porphyrinuria, the ingestion of beets (anthocyaninuria) or of certain dyes, Urates produce a reddish precipitate. Bile may produce a reddish yellow color. A green or blue urine may be caused by the ingestion of methylene blue; purple by fuchsin; magenta by phenolphthalein; red with a greenish fluorescence by eosin; black by ingestion of carbolic acid, alkaptonuria, or the presence of melanin; bright yellow by the ingestion of carotin-containing foods. Some of these colorations may follow the ingestion of certain artificially colored candies.

17. Ammoniacal Urine.—If ammonia appears in the urine a considerable time after exposure to air, this is of no significance; but if it develops rapidly and strongly, there is probably increased excretion of ammonia due to a disturbance of metabolism, depending upon disturbance of the acid-base balance (p. 488), or the excessive ingestion or malassimilation of fat. The condition can be prevented by the administration of alkalies and the regulation of the diet.

References

1. Am. J. Dis. Child., 1911, **1,** 139. 2. Brit. M. J., 1921, **1,** 671. 3. J.A.M.A., 1926, **86,** 1820. 4. J.A.M.A., 1926, **87,** 8. 5. J.A.M.A., 1928, **90,** 535. 6. J.A.M.A., 1931, **96,** 1559. 7. Hypertension and Nephritis, 1930. 8. Lancet, 1885, **2,** 706. 9. Jahrb. f. Kinderh., 1910, **71,** 427. 10. Johns Hopkins Hosp. Rep., 1904, **12,** 145. 11. Arch. Int. Med., 1914, **13,** 39. 12. Die lordotische Albuminurie 1909. 13. Ztschr. f. klin. Med., 1920, **90,** 1. 14. Am. J. Dis. Child., 1921, **22,** 388. 15. Am. J. Dis. Child., 1929, **37,** 367. 16. J.A.M.A., 1922, **78,** 644. 17. Am. J. Dis. Child., 1915, **10,** 418. 18. Ztschr. f. Kinderh., 1922, **33,** 158. 19. Friedman and Mitchell, Am. J. Dis. Child., 1928, **35,** 201. 20. Jahrb. f. Kinderh., 1903, **58,** 40. 21. Am. J. Dis. Child., 1922, **24,** 218. 22. Arch. Pediat., 1918, **35,** 1. 23. Lancet, 1902, **1,** 1243. 24. Guy's Hosp. Rep., 1923, **73,** 368. 25. J.A.M.A., 1930, **94,** 762. 26. Deutsch. Arch. f. klin. Med., 1927, **156,** 272. 27. Ueber Hämoglobinämie und ihre Folgen, 1883. 28. Arch. Pediat., 1903, **20,** 105. 29. Am. J. Dis. Child., 1929, **37,** 1027. 30. Jahrb. f. Kinderh., 1913, **78,** 723. 31. München. med. Wchnschr., 1904, **51,** 1590. 32. Medicine, 1929, **8,** 159. 33. Berl. klin. Wchnschr., 1880, **17,** 132; 151. 34. J. Biol. Chem., 1927, **71,** 481. 35. Am. J. Dis. Child., 1921, **21,** 211. 36. Ann. de méd. et chir. inf., 1913, **17,** 129. 37. Monatschr. f. Kinderh., 1921, **22,** 302. 38. J.A.M.A. 1931, **96,** 1562. 39. Monatschr. f. Kinderh., Orig., 1913, **12,** 177. 40. Nederl. Maandschr. v. Geneesk., 1928, **15,** 285. 41. Arch. Pediat., 1929, **46,** 46. 42. Am. J. M. Sc., 1929, **177,** 348. 43. Am. J. Dis. Child., 1930, **40,** 1193. 44. Am. J. Dis. Child., 1916, **11,** 455. 45. Arch. f. Kinderh., 1921, **70,** 122. 46. J. Biol. Chem., 1929, **81,** 285. 47. Am. J. Dis. Child., 1926, **32,** 219. 48. Inborn Errors of Metabolism, 2d ed., 1923.

CHAPTER II

DISEASES OF THE KIDNEYS

TESTS OF RENAL FUNCTION

VARIOUS tests have been devised to determine the functional capacity of the kidney, but none of them gives exact information. They are more valuable in determining prognosis than in recognizing nephritis or in differentiating its type, since conditions nonnephritic in nature, as anhydremia and febrile states, may cause temporary functional insufficiency of the kidney. Certain of the most useful of these tests will be described.

PHENOLSULPHONEPHTHALEIN TEST.—This was first recommended by Rowntree and Geraghty,[1] and is widely employed. We[2] found that infants and children excrete the dye at about the same rate as do adults. Three milligrams of phenolsulphonephthalein (one half the amount used in adults) are injected intramuscularly or intravenously. Except in children old enough to void, catheterization should be performed at the end of sixty or one hundred twenty minutes, or both. Normally 40 to 60 per cent of the dye will be excreted by the end of the first hour, and 60 to 85 per cent by the end of the second; slightly higher values being found after intravenous injection. Values as low as 30 or 40 per cent in two hours indicate a moderate degree of functional impairment; 20 per cent serious impairment; and 5 or 10 per cent a marked insufficiency. Functional failure of one kidney can be determined by ureteral catheterization.

URINE CONCENTRATION TESTS.—The most valuable of these is the determination of the specific gravity, proposed by Hedinger and Schlayer.[3] In carrying out this test on children, Hill[4] recommends the following adaptation of Mosenthal's[5] technique: The child is put on a full, normal diet containing a considerable amount of protein especially with the noon-meal. A capsule holding 1 Gm. (15.42 grains) of salt and a pill of 2 grains (0.12) of caffeine sodiobenzoate are given with each meal, to take the place of the tea or coffee used in the adult test-diet. There results a diet containing a considerable amount of salt, protein and diuretic material, all of which will stimulate the kidney to its maximum efforts. Exactly 10 oz. (295.74) of fluid is given with each meal, and no fluid or food whatever between meals. The urine is collected in two-hour periods from 7 A. M. to 7 P. M., the amounts passed being kept separate, and the night-urine in one specimen from 7 P. M. to 7 A. M. The specific gravity of each specimen of urine is recorded. The normal response shows a wide variation in gravity between the different specimens, at least eight or ten points between the highest and lowest. Normally the night-urine is small in amount and almost always has a specific gravity of 1020 or over. Not over 300 cc. (10.14 fl. oz.) of urine should be voided during the night by the normal child. The child with damaged kidneys, on the other hand, is unable to vary the concentration of the urine and the specific gravity of the individual specimens may differ only one or two points. In the nephritic the night-specimen will be large in amount and of a low specific gravity.

BLOOD-CHEMISTRY AND THE RENAL FUNCTION.—The normal values of certain blood-constituents are given elsewhere (p. 41, Table 26). The ability of the kidney to eliminate some of these substances is impaired when its functional capacity is limited. When the urea-nitrogen rises to 30 or 40 mg. per 100 cc. with the uric acid 6 to 8, a moderate impairment of renal function is indicated. With values such as 80 to 100 for urea-nitrogen and 12 to 15 for uric acid there is serious insufficiency. Increase of creatinine over 4 mg. is of unfavorable prognostic significance, and values of 8 to 10 indicate that a fatal ending is immediately impending. At present it is thought that creatinine studies are more reliable than those of urea-nitrogen in estimating prognosis. As pointed out by Patch and Rabinowitz[6] substances supposedly creatinine may not be this. There may be at least 50 per cent impairment of renal activity before these nonprotein nitrogenous constituents begin to accumulate in the blood. Their increase is often termed *azotemia*. High values have less prognostic significance in acute nephritis, where they may be temporary, than in chronic nephritis. The so-called *urea clearance test* is of distinct value in determining renal function (Van Slyke et al.[7]). In chronic nephritis there may be an increase in the inorganic phosphorus above the normal of 4 to 5 mg., and also, according to Wakefield, Power and Keith,[8] above the normal of $2\frac{1}{2}$ to 5 of the inorganic sulphates. With edema the blood-chlorides are increased over the normal of 500 to 600 mg. (as NaCl). In nephrosis the total lipoids of the blood may exceed the normal 600 to 700 mg., and the cholesterol the normal 140 to 170 mg. In nephrosis, when edema is present, the total protein of the serum, which is normally about 7.5 to 8.5 per cent, falls below 5.5 per cent and the albumin, normally averaging 4.3 to 6.5 per cent, falls below 2.5 per cent. In this disease there is also a relative increase in the globulin (normally 1.2 to 2.5 per cent) as compared with the albumin.

Salt-solution Test.—As proposed by Aldrich and McClure[9] this is performed as follows: 0.2 cc. of an 0.8 per cent aqueous solution of sodium chloride is injected intradermally. Duplicate injections are made about 2 cm. apart, either on the flexor surface of the forearm or the inner surface of the calf. The wheal produced normally disappears in about sixty minutes, but coincident with or preceding the development of edema the disappearance-time is definitely decreased.

Roentgenography of the Urinary Tract.—Flat roentgenographic plates may reveal urinary calculi, remembering, however, that uric acid stones cast no shadow. Fifteen to forty minutes after the intravenous injection of iodine-containing drugs satisfactory visualization of the urinary tract may be had on the roentgenogram. Such preparations as iopax, skiodan, and merbaphen are injected in about 30 per cent solution, employing from 25 to 60 cc. depending upon the age and weight of the patient. These may also be injected through the ureteral catheter in 10 to 20 per cent solution and roentgenograms subsequently taken. Iodochloral when taken orally in doses of 1 to 2 Gm. is said to be excreted by the kidney and to give visualization of the urinary tract. McKhann,[10] Campbell[11] and others have shown that simple cystograms are often helpful in revealing abnormalities of the bladder and sometimes of the ureters. A 5 per cent solution of sodium iodide or a 12.5 per cent solution of potassium iodide is used for the contrast medium, or one of the other iodine preparations mentioned. The solution is introduced until the bladder is full, or (in small infants) under slight hydrostatic pressure, and later washed out.

MALFORMATIONS OF THE KIDNEYS

The lobulated condition characteristic of fetal life may persist into childhood, but has no clinical significance. Both kidneys may be absent; or that upon one side, especially the left, may be absent or imperfectly developed, the other being correspondingly enlarged. The kidneys may be fused, causing the so-called "horseshoe-kidney." When the kidney is absent the suprarenal gland may still be present and normal. Malformations of the ureters frequently accompany those of the kidneys, or exist independently. They consist of constriction, absence, dilatation, and duplication. Pressure upon the ureter may be due, among other things, to unusual origin or course of the renal blood-vessels. The anomalies of the genito-urinary tract have been reviewed and studied by Rolleston,[12]

Bigler,[13] Hurt,[14] Campbell and Lyttle,[15] and others. The incidence discovered at necropsy appears high, and, according to various studies, ranges from 2.3 to 13 per cent. Obstructive malformation of the ureters may eventually lead to hydronephrosis and destruction of functional renal tissue, and all the signs and symptoms of nephrosclerosis, including the osseous changes (p. 821). Minor degrees of obstruction may be the basis of persistent pyuria.

Congenital Cystic Kidney.—In this condition the parenchyma of the kidney is occupied by small or larger cysts, often numerous. The kidneys may be hypoplastic or more frequently greatly enlarged, and generally both are involved. A familial incidence is sometimes observed, Fuller[16] reporting 9 affected of 27 individuals in four generations of one family. Other anomalies are frequently present elsewhere in the body. In cases of large cystic kidneys the principal early symptom is the increased size of the abdomen. The patient may die in early infancy of uremia, or may live to adult life, all the signs and symptoms of nephrosclerosis eventually developing, including the osseous changes and renal infantilism (pp. 821, 822). Removal of the kidney is contraindicated unless it is proven that the condition is unilateral.

Hydronephrosis.—This is not uncommon in early life, and may be either congenital or acquired. In the latter event it is not, strictly speaking, a malformation. It depends upon obstruction which may be anywhere along the urinary tract, and which results in dilatation of the pelvis of the kidney and often of the ureter, with more or less destruction of the renal parenchyma. Responsible for the obstruction are impacted calculus, congenital or acquired stenosis, external pressure, extreme phimosis, congenital valves or hypertrophied folds in the urethra, and the like. The cause is not always discovered at necropsy, and such cases may have depended upon defective co-ordination of the muscular and nervous control of the excretory apparatus (Thomson[17]). Trauma sometimes appears to be a factor, Aldibert[18] having collected 17 such instances. In unilateral hydronephrosis, if of large size, the presence of a tumor becomes apparent, or perhaps local signs of pressure develop. In the bilateral form the functional insufficiency of the kidney soon leads to symptoms of chronic nephritis (p. 820), or infection of the kidney occurs. In the way of treatment it is possible at times to relieve some of the forms of obstruction or to dilate strictures. Nephrectomy is sometimes indicated in unilateral cases.

DISPLACEMENT OF THE KIDNEY

Dystopia.—Accompanying or independent of some of the malformations described, the kidney, especially the left, may occupy a position lower and nearer the midline of the body than normal. On palpation this may cause confusion with such conditions as intussusception, fecal accumulation, appendicitis, and undescended testicle. There may be no symptoms, or the bending of the ureter may cause pain and dysuria, and lead to hydronephrosis.

Movable Kidney.—This may occur in the new-born or in older children and, although not common, has been reported by Comby,[19] Dupoux,[20] Phillips,[21] and others. The acquired form is seen oftener in later childhood in girls, and may result from pressure by tumors or corsets, or from trauma. **Symptoms,** if present, consist in a sensation of pressure or dragging in the abdomen or lumbar region, and attacks of renal colic. General splanchnoptosis may also be present. Hydronephrosis may develop from kinking or twisting of the ureter. In the diagnosis it should be remembered that it is often possible to palpate the lower pole of the kidney in normal children. The **treatment** consists of efforts to retain the kidney in position by a pad or bandage, the avoidance of violent exercise, and attention to general health and nutrition; surgical aid seldom being required.

Congestion, Degeneration and Inflammation of the Kidneys

A large number of classifications have been proposed to clarify this subject, but these have often accomplished the reverse of this. They have been based on conceptions of etiology, pathologic changes, or symptomatology, or on combinations of these. There is little justification for complicated terminology in the present state of knowledge of nephritis and allied conditions. We have adopted a simple classification to which clinical symptoms can be linked and which is as follows: (1) Congestion of the kidneys; (2) Acute degeneration of the kidneys; (3) Acute glomerular nephritis; (4) Acute diffuse nephritis; (5) Acute interstitial nephritis; (6) Chronic nephritis; and (7) Nephrosis. Undoubtedly the different classes shade one into the other to a large extent; and this applies especially to the pathologic lesions of the different types of nephritis.

(1) CONGESTION OF THE KIDNEYS

Acute congestion may occur in the early stage of nephritis; or be a result of fever, exposure to cold, over-exertion, surgical operation, trauma, or the irritation caused by such substances as turpentine and cantharides. The kidneys may be swollen and congested, but show no evidence of other change. The urine is diminished in amount; may contain albumin, red blood-cells and casts; and the phenolsulphonephthalein elimination may be diminished. The course is short, and the diagnosis from nephritis is made by this and by the absence of other symptoms of that disease. The *treatment* consists chiefly of rest in bed, with the patient kept warm, the bowels kept open, and the administration of plenty of fluid. If there is great diminution in the secretion of urine, measures recommended for this under the discussion of nephritis should be employed (p. 825).

Passive congestion results from any disorder producing general venous stasis, as chronic heart-disease or pressure on the kidney or its vessels. It may be part of a nephritic process. The kidneys are enlarged, of a deep red color, and the blood-vessels are everywhere dilated and engorged. Degenerative and inflammatory changes eventually follow as sequels, unless the condition is relieved. The symptoms are chiefly those of the primary or causative disease. The urine is diminished in quantity, concentrated, and may contain a few red blood cells and an occasional hyaline cast. The *diagnosis* from chronic nephritis is made by the presence of a cause for passive congestion, the absence of any symptoms of nephritis, and the minor degree of albuminuria and cylinduria. The differentiation is not always easy, especially as sclerosis of the kidney may eventually develop.

(2) ACUTE DEGENERATION OF THE KIDNEYS

Acute degeneration of the kidneys is a term sometimes applied to the cloudy swelling of these organs which occurs in severe febrile diseases. The condition is designated "larval nephrosis" by some writers. It is in all respects similar to the febrile albuminuria already described (p. 808).

(3) ACUTE GLOMERULAR NEPHRITIS

(Acute Hemorrhagic Nephritis)

Etiology.—This is much the most common form of nephritis in childhood. Age is not an important factor, and, although infants are less often attacked than older children, congenital or fetal nephritis has been reported (Arnold;[22] Jacobi;[23] Widakoivich and Dutrey[24]). Nephritis may occur in the early weeks of life (Jacobi,[23] Ashby,[25] Mensi[26]), and its presence in later periods of infancy has been reported by Holt,[27] Goulkewitch,[28] and others. In many of these, however, it is not clear as to what type of nephritis was present, and probably not all of them were of the acute glomerular variety (Mitchell[29]). Congenital syphilis is rarely the cause of acute glomerular nephritis. (See also p. 819.) The possible influence of heredity will be discussed in the section on chronic nephritis (p. 820). Acute glomerular nephritis occasionally appears in epidemic form. In the majority of cases it is a complication of infections which are known or suspected to be streptococcic in origin. There need only be mentioned here the studies of Steiner and Neureutter,[30] Hill,[31] James,[32] Boyd,[33] Allison,[34] Clausen,[35] Blackfan,[36] Longcope et al.,[37] Gray,[38] and others which demonstrate that in children such conditions as tonsillitis, scarlet fever, respiratory infections (including otitis media, sinusitis, pneumonia and bronchiectasis), pyogenic infections, purpuric disease, burns, and impetigo contagiosa and other cutaneous infections, are quite frequently direct antecedents of acute glomerular nephritis. Among less frequent apparent causes may be mentioned gastro-enteritis, pleurisy, typhus fever, typhoid fever, grippe, varicella, mumps, variola, vaccination, meningitis, pertussis, and appendicitis. Measles may occasionally be the cause. We[39] have seen a number of instances of this, 4 of which have been reported, and others have been recorded by Steiner and Neureutter,[30] Henoch,[40] Aronade,[41] Ernberg,[42] and Heubner.[43] We have seen acute nephritis several times follow operations on the tonsils and adenoids and upper respiratory tract. Certain poisons, such as phenol, turpentine, cantharides, and potassium chlorate, may produce an acute renal irritation of the nature of acute glomerular nephritis. Chilling or exposure to cold and dampness, or to heat, seems to act as the sole cause in some cases, but in what manner is not clear. Sometimes the condition appears suddenly without any discoverable cause, the designation "primary" then being applied.

It is probable that infection is the real basis of practically all cases of acute glomerular nephritis. In cases following infections the direct cause may be the toxin produced by the bacteria, or perhaps the bacteria themselves. The possible methods of production have been reviewed by Cabot and Crabtree,[44] Gray,[38] Longcope,[37] and Bell and Clawson.[45]

Pathologic Anatomy.—The typical large red kidney of acute glomerular nephritis shows enlargement of the cortex, with the pyramids unusually red and the Malpighian bodies standing out as dark, red points. Microscopically the glomeruli exhibit swelling, with alteration in the cells of the tufts and of Bowman's capsule. The capsule may be filled with albuminous exudate, leukocytes, and erythrocytes. A certain amount of swelling and degeneration of the cells of the tubules may be present, and perhaps some involvement of the interstitial tissue; these tubular and interstitial changes becoming more marked if the condition has been at all prolonged.

Symptoms.—These vary with the extent and degree to which the glomeruli are involved, with the primary disorder which the nephritis complicates, and with the age of the patient. In typical cases the onset is sudden, with fever and perhaps vomiting, headache, and frequency and urgency of urination. (See Fig. 191.) Edema may be absent, or, if present, is, as a rule, not very extensive or of great degree. Anemia develops rapidly. Signs of impaired renal function, such as increased blood-pressure, increased nonprotein nitrogenous constituents in the blood, and decreased phenolsulphonephthalein elimination may occur, but often in mild cases are absent, or present only for a few days. The urine is usually somewhat diminished in amount, concentrated, and contains albumin in varying quantity, and an amount of blood ranging from sufficient to give a gross hemorrhagic appearance to that which can be discovered only by microscopical examination. Hyaline and blood-cell casts are usually found.

In infancy especially the symptoms may be obscure and overlooked, edema may not occur, and only an examination of the urine may reveal the nature of the malady. In severe cases with many of the glomeruli involved all the symptoms of renal insufficiency occur, such as suppression or great diminution of urinary output, increased blood-pressure, retention of non-protein nitrogenous constituents in the blood, and the development of uremia. With the last there may be convulsions, which in a few instances may be the initial symptom. The cause of these is not always clear, but they appear to depend on increased intracranial pressure.

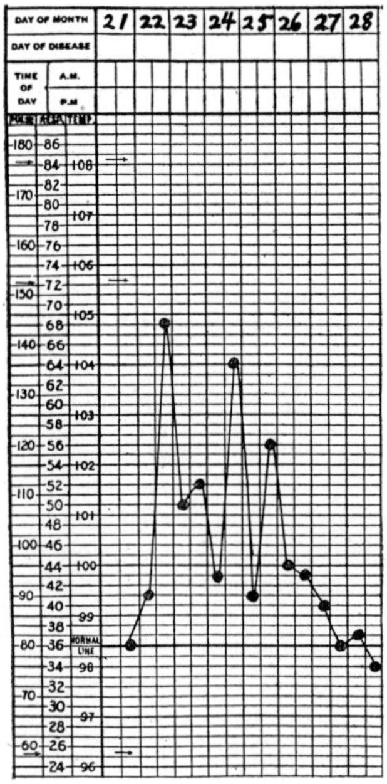

Fig. 191.—Acute nephritis. Katie G., four years old. Taken ill Feb. 19, edema of feet, face and arms. Entered the Children's Hospital of Philadelphia, Feb. 21, face much swollen, could not open right eye, urine very much diminished and contained hyaline and granular casts, red blood-cells and leukocytes, nothing found in lungs, respiration somewhat accelerated, gradual improvement.

Course and Prognosis.—In favorable cases fever and other symptoms lessen in a few days, and in a few weeks the urine becomes free from albumin and casts. Complete recovery without any apparent residual damage to the kidneys frequently follows. Prognosis is influenced by age; the younger the patient the more serious being the condition. The cases complicating scarlet fever seem to vary distinctly in severity and likelihood of recovery in different epidemics of this disease. Uremic symptoms and the associated finding in the blood of retention of nonprotein nitrogenous constituents are unfavorable, but the latter has not the same prognostic importance as in chronic nephritis. Some cases pass into the chronic stage, producing a chronic glomerular nephritis, this perhaps eventually leading to a generalized nephrosclerosis. Studies by Lyttle and Rosenberg,[46] Levy,[47] Guild[48] and others show that the mortality during the acute stage is seldom more than 4 or 5 per cent, although figures as high as 18 per cent are occasionally given; and that 10 to 15 per cent pass into a subacute or chronic stage.

Complications and Sequels.—Here are to be mentioned pneumonia, pleurisy, endocarditis, pericarditis, peritonitis, septicemia, edema of the glottis, pulmonary edema, acidosis, and the accumulation of fluid in serous cavities. The sequel most to be dreaded is chronic nephritis.

Diagnosis. Distinction must be made between febrile albuminuria and acute nephritis. There are no nephritic symptoms in the former, while red blood-cells found in the urine are diagnostic of a true renal irritation. A number of authors, such as Elwyn[49] and Fishberg,[50] classify as a distinct group the so-called *focal glomerular nephritis*. The cause of this is subacute bacterial endocarditis, and there occurs an infarction of the glomeruli with the streptococcus viridans.

(4) ACUTE DIFFUSE NEPHRITIS

This variety is sometimes designated acute edematous nephritis, and in some classifications would be termed the acute parenchymatous form. Its pathologic designation should be acute glomerulo-tubular nephritis.

Etiology and Pathologic Anatomy.—Acute diffuse nephritis may occur as a primary disease following the same types of infection as are operative in acute glomerular nephritis, or it may be a subacute stage of this. It represents an acute inflammation in which the parenchyma of the kidney is more generally involved than in the ordinary glomerular type, and in which the damage to the tubules may predominate. It is the form especially well-marked early in severe cases of diphtheria, and is that oftenest seen in gastro-enteric diseases in infancy.

Symptoms and Diagnosis.—The chief clinical feature distinguishing it from typical cases of acute glomerular nephritis is the presence of decided and widespread edema. There is variation in the symptoms and signs, depending upon the relative degree of involvement of glomeruli and of tubules respectively, either one of which may predominate over the other. If the glomeruli are much affected there will be such symptoms as high blood-pressure, retention of nonprotein nitrogenous constituents in the blood, uremia, and the like. On the other hand extensive tubular degeneration may cause marked edema, with but few other signs of renal insufficiency, and in such cases the hematuria may be slight and inconstant.

(5) ACUTE INTERSTITIAL NEPHRITIS

This form of nephritis was defined by Councilman[51] as an acute inflammation of the kidney characterized by cellular and fluid exudation into the interstitial tissue, accompanied by, but not dependent on, degeneration of the epithelium. The exudation is not purulent in character, and the lesions may be diffuse or focal. It accompanies septic states and may follow diphtheria, scarlet fever, smallpox, and measles. The diagnosis is often a post-mortem one, since such symptoms as edema and increased blood-pressure are usually absent, and the urine may show little except decrease in amount, and the presence of albumin. In fact it is questionable whether the condition is renal disease *per se*, since similar exudation and infiltration may be found in other parts of the body as well as in the kidney (Fishberg[50]).

(6) CHRONIC NEPHRITIS

(Chronic Glomerular Nephritis. Chronic Diffuse Nephritis. Chronic Interstitial Nephritis. Nephrosclerosis)

Etiology.—Chronic nephritis is much less common than the acute type. It is usually the result of an acute glomerular nephritis of a severe form which has failed to heal, and often of several attacks of this. The condition which caused the acute nephritis may disappear, but in some cases persisting foci of infection seem to be causative. Certain chronic poisons, such as alcohol and lead, are seldom operative in producing chronic nephritis in children. It does not seem clear just how these act, but presumably they cause vascular injury with secondary action upon the kidneys. The so-called *arteriosclerotic* and the *arteriolosclerotic* types, in which the injury is primarily in the vessels of the kidneys, are not often met with in childhood. Newburg et al.,[52] and Polvogt, McCollum and Simmonds[53] claim that high protein diets may cause nephritic changes, although this is denied by McCann[54] and others. From a practical standpoint protein can seldom be a cause in childhood. It would appear that syphilis, while theoretically a disease which can injure the kidney, is seldom actually a cause of nephritis in early life. We[29] have found that in the majority of reported cases of chronic nephritis in children there is offered no clinical or serological evidence of syphilis.

We[29] have gathered also much clinical data to show that there is an inherited tendency, or "tissue-predisposition," to renal disease. In some cases this is linked to a tendency to arterial disease to which the renal involvement is secondary. It must be noted, however, that this hereditary predisposition is not a necessary factor, since quite regardless of it certain chemical or bacteriological poisons have a specific effect in causing the injury. A number of cases of chronic nephritis have been reported as being congenital in origin (Sawyer,[55] Baginsky,[56] Mitchell[29]).

Pathologic Anatomy.—The glomeruli become hyalinized and some of them obliterated in whole or in part. Many of the tubules are destroyed, the arteries show thickening, and the interstitial tissue is increased in quantity. Eventually the kidney becomes much smaller than normal and granular. Some measure of amyloid degeneration is a frequent attendant. The nature and degree of the changes vary greatly with the case (see p. 821), and intermediate forms of all sorts occur; but in all which have lasted a considerable time both parenchymatous and interstitial alterations are found.

Symptoms and Course.—At first there may be few symptoms, but examination discloses albuminuria with occasional hematuria. These have persisted after an attack of acute nephritis, or may occur without the patient's knowledge that there has been acute renal involvement. There may be headache, malaise, and variable edema which is usually slight and consists perhaps simply of puffiness under the eyes, or scarcely noticeable swelling of the ankles. If there is increase in blood-pressure or retention of nonprotein nitrogenous constituents in the blood, these are of slight degree. After a period of months or even years, perhaps interspersed with attacks of acute nephritis, or exacerbations of the chronic condition, the urine becomes increased in amount and its specific gravity lowered and more or less fixed (p. 813). Albumin, casts, and red blood-cells are found in varying quantities; and the phenolsulphonephthalein elimination is reduced. There may be polydipsia combined with the polyuria. There occurs increase in the nonprotein nitrogenous constituents of the blood, the degree of this changing from time to time; the blood-pressure, while variable, is constantly elevated over the normal; and the heart becomes hypertrophied. Edema is a prominent feature in most cases. It varies in degree with the case, and also from time to time in the individual patient. Sometimes it is evidenced mainly by a slight swelling of the face and ankles; sometimes by general anasarca (Fig. 192), together with dropsy of the serous cavities. With edema there is retention of both sodium and chlorine and a high plasma chloride content, unless chlorides are reduced by vomiting (Boyd et al.[57]). Headache and other manifestations mentioned, together with anorexia, gastro-intestinal disturbances, drowsiness and dyspnea, are all symptoms which may be present, and may be exaggerated by any intercurrent infection or complication, during which, too, uremia may develop. Anemia may be marked and persistent, and usually parallels the amount of nitrogen retention. It appears to be due to disturbance of blood-formation (Brown and Roth,[58] Becher[59]). A yellowish discoloration of the skin often develops, ascribed by Becher[60] to the change produced by the action of light on the chromogens of the urinary pigments stored in the skin. Finally, after perhaps a number of years, all these symptoms and findings are exaggerated; sclerosis of the blood-vessels develops; hemorrhages from mucous membranes, into the skin, or into the internal organs including the brain may occur; the eye-grounds show choked disc and perhaps hemorrhage and thickening of the vessels and albuminuric retinitis; and uremic convulsions close the scene.

The symptoms and course which have been described vary somewhat, depending upon whether glomeruli, tubules, or interstitial tissue are preponderatingly involved. In some cases the term "subacute" or "subchronic" might better be applied, since the total duration of the disease may be only a few months or a year or two. In more chronic forms the kidney gradually reaches a stage when there is marked involvement of all its structures, with overgrowth of interstitial tissue and subsequent contraction leading to great shrinkage. To this the terms chronic interstitial nephritis, atrophic kidney, contracted kidney, and granular kidney have been applied. Apparently this may rarely occur as a primary condition in children, Greene[61] having been able to collect but 19 certain cases.

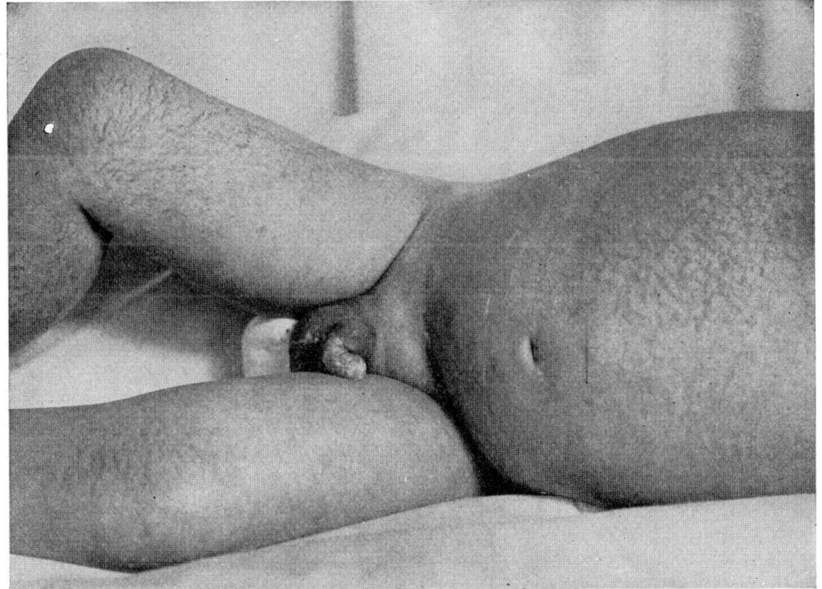

Fig. 192.—Chronic nephritis. Patient in the Children's Ward of the Hospital of the University of Penna. Exhibits widespread ascites, a yellowish-white tint to the skin, and a white mottling produced by the stretching.

Oftener it is a final development of a nephritis involving the parenchyma; but even with this there are seldom found in early life cases exhibiting the clinical features of contracted kidney as seen in adults. The designation *nephrosclerosis* best expresses the pathologic condition. When this marked renal insufficiency has come about in very early life there are, in addition to the symptoms already described, decided effects on the growing organism, which result from the disturbances of metabolism (Mitchell and Guest[62]). These consist in retardation of growth (*renal dwarfism*), lack of sexual development (*renal infantilism*), and, in some cases, lack of mental development. Of great interest are the osseous changes, which are often designated *renal rickets*. There may be enlargement of the epiphyses of the wrist and of the costochondral junctions, pigeon-shaped chest, bossing of the frontal and parietal bones, and deformities of the extremities. The sudden or gradual onset of genu valgum is an especially pronounced symptom. By roentgenologic and histologic study the changes in the bone have been found to be somewhat different from those of infantile rickets, in that the shafts of the long bones and the flat bones have greater translucence and a more spongy appearance. The cause of the changes is of great interest. With increasing lack of ability of the kidney to excrete waste products, the inorganic phosphates of the blood rise to the upper limits of normal or over, and the calcium diminishes below normal. We[62] have offered the hypothesis that in renal rickets a shift of the excretion of endogenous phosphorus to the intestine occurs, and that the concentration of phosphorus in the intestine by the formation of insoluble calcium phosphate blocks the absorption of calcium from the food, and the child suffers a true calcium starvation. Cases of renal infantilism and renal rickets have been reported by Lucas,[63] Fletcher,[64] Parsons,[65] Miller,[66] Barber,[67] and many others. We[29] have been able to collect about 80 such cases.

Prognosis.—The course and prognosis of chronic nephritis have been alluded to in the discussion of symptoms. In a group of cases collected by us[29] the average age at death was about nine to ten years in those who had contracted the disease early.

In many cases in children the disease differs considerably from the usual type, and there is assumed early a subacute or latent form, which either is consecutive to a mild attack of acute nephritis or often comes on without discoverable cause. The child develops irritability, moderate loss of strength, and a variable degree of anemia with perhaps headache and digestive disturbance, but usually no edema. This group of symptoms is present only at times, and during these the urine may exhibit a small amount of albumin and a few casts. To this group Heubner[68] has well applied the term *paedo-nephritis* and considers the prognosis comparatively favorable, reporting apparently complete recovery in 9 out of 16 cases followed during several years. Nevertheless, the longer this type of the disease continues the more liability there is of the functions of the kidney becoming dangerously involved, and the ultimate prognosis is consequently uncertain. The general tendency is toward a fatal ending. In a series of about 300 cases of nephritis in children which we have collected the large majority finally died of the disease. Among unfavorable symptoms of chronic nephritis are high blood-pressure; uremia; and marked renal insufficiency, as manifested by a fixation of the specific gravity, decided and continued azotemia, and elevation of the blood-phosphorus. (For renal function tests see p. 813.)

Complications and Sequels.—Those of uremia, hemorrhages, infantilism, and rickets have been mentioned. Acidosis may occur, due, among other factors, to the retention of acid phosphate. Tetany is rare in spite of the tendency to low blood-calcium, probably because acidosis makes the calcium more utilizable.

Diagnosis.—The early stage of chronic nephritis must be differentiated from *orthostatic albuminuria* by the entire lack of any other symptom of nephritis in this condition, and the transitory character of the albuminuria with its absence in the morning. The diagnosis from the *chronic passive congestion* of heart-disease is made by the disappearance of symptoms when the heart-condition improves. The headache, vomiting, and convulsions of nephritis have sometimes led to the diagnosis of *brain-tumor*, but evidences of localizing neurologic signs on the one hand, and the presence of symptoms of renal insufficiency on the other, should serve to differentiate. Pallor is sometimes one of the first noticeable symptoms of nephritis, and this may or may not be accompanied by anemia. At any rate a persistent secondary *anemia*, not otherwise explicable, should lead to the suspicion of chronic nephritis. The hematuria of a chronic nephritis, while intermittent, is accompanied by cylinduria and other signs of renal disease, which are absent in *hematuria* due to other cause (p. 809). From *nephrosis* the diagnosis of chronic nephritis is made by the absence in the former of hematuria, azotemia, uremia, and increased blood-pressure. It must be remembered, however, that the change in the albumin-globulin ratio in the blood, lipemia, and doubly refractile lipoid bodies in the urine, may all occur in chronic diffuse nephritis with considerable involvement of the tubules. It should also be mentioned that all the results and symptoms of chronic diffuse nephritis may come about from congenital or acquired obstructive *malformations of the genito-urinary tract.*

(7) NEPHROSIS

(Tubular Degenerative Nephritis)

The term "nephrosis," first used by Müller,[69] and since then by Munk,[70] Volhard and Fahr,[71] Epstein,[72] Elwyn,[49] Fishberg,[50] and many others, has been applied to the degenerative lesions of the kidney affecting chiefly the tubules. Epstein and others conceive of this condition as a general metabolic disturbance of some sort, in which the kidneys as well as other body

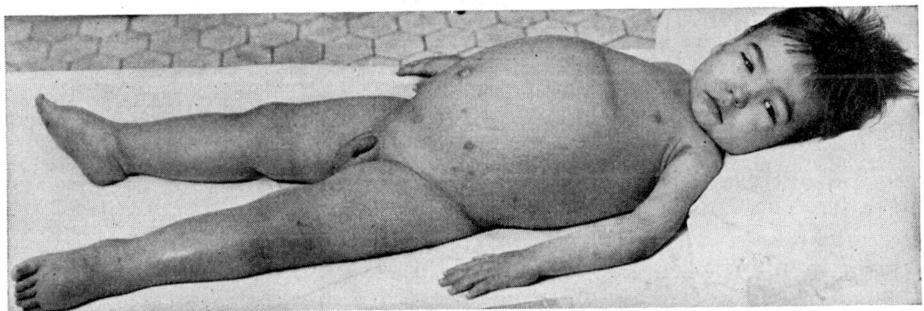

Fig. 193.—Nephrosis. Child of four years of age in The Children's Hospital, Cincinnati. Edema of insidious origin started several months before admission without any preceding infection, and varied from time to time. Urine contained large amounts of albumin and some hyaline casts, but never blood. No increase in blood-pressure and no azotemia. Total blood protein 3.86 per cent; albumin 1.79 per cent and globulin 2.07 per cent; cholesterol 300 mg. per 100 cc.

tissues are affected, *i. e.*, it is a perversion of protein metabolism with albuminuria, analogous to the perversion of carbohydrate metabolism in diabetes with its glycosuria. Amberg[73] well reviews other theories of causation of nephrosis and its symptoms. Diphtheria, typhoid fever, sepsis, influenza, cholera, syphilis and tuberculosis are rarely the apparent cause of forms of nephritis in which the tubules are primarily involved, and which are sometimes classified as nephrosis. The majority of cases of nephrosis, however, are without any known etiology. By many writers the term degenerative nephritis and tubular nephritis are avoided, and the title nephrosis preferred, both on the etiologic basis and because pathologically the lesions do not appear to be inflammatory in origin. It should, however, be said on the other hand that other investigators, among these Christian,[74] Bell,[75] Davison and Salinger,[76] and Lyttle and Rosenberg,[46] do not regard nephrosis as other than a variety of chronic nephritis. Some authors insist upon reserving the designation nephrosis for the lipoid form, and consider other types as tubular nephritis. It is evident, then, that it is still uncertain as to the actual position of the syndrome to which the title nephrosis has been applied; but, assuming provisionally the term "lipoid nephrosis" as expressing an entity, the following description may be given:

Lipoid Nephrosis.—This is apparently a rare condition, some clinicians of wide experience claiming to have seen only a few cases. It is, however, more common in children than in adults. **Etiologically** Marriott,[77] Clawsen,[78] and Aldrich[79] emphasize the importance of infection of the paranasal sinuses, but this must certainly seldom be operative. **Pathologically** there is a large, smooth, pale kidney with a widened cortex, which microscopically shows fatty degeneration, chiefly of the cells of the proximal convoluted tubules and the presence in them of doubly refractile lipoids, but the collecting tubules are comparatively or entirely normal, and there is little or no change in the glomeruli, especially in the early stage. Bell,[75] and Bell and Clawsen[80] have, however, found slight alterations in the glomeruli by special staining methods. The interstitial tissue contains lipoid material and perhaps leukocytes, and the arteries are normal. The **symptoms** are extensive edema (Fig. 193), pallor, anorexia, gastro-intestinal disturbances, urine of a high or normal specific gravity with large amounts of albumin and often casts, but never blood. Uremia does not occur. There is absence of high blood-pressure and azotemia, unless for some reason the urinary output is temporarily diminished. Tests for renal function are normal. The blood-fat and the cholesterol are increased above normal (see p. 41), especially during the period of edema. A characteristic feature is a reduction of the total blood-protein below normal and a relative increase of globulin as compared with albumin. (See p. 41.) When the total blood-protein falls below 5.5 per cent or the albumin below 2.5 per cent, edema is usually present (Moore and Van Slyke[81]). Edema, while paralleling these findings, changes more rapidly than do the alterations in the blood-protein (Calvin and Goldberg[82]). Probably the plasma-proteins, by their osmotic attraction for water, assist in preventing the hydraulic pressure from forcing fluid from the capillaries into the tissue-spaces. The increase in blood-fat so often present also helps in maintaining the osmotic pressure (Fishberg[83]). The blood-chlorides are increased during periods of edema. Doubly refractile lipoid bodies are found in the urine by means of the polarizing microscope, as first described by Munk.[70] There is a decrease in basal metabolism, probably due largely to the decrease of functioning body-tissue as compared with the large amount of fluid. The **course** of lipoid nephrosis is essentially chronic, lasting over a period of years with longer or shorter intervals of complete disappearance of edema and decrease of albuminuria. The **prognosis** for ultimate recovery is by no means hopeless. Of 20 children apparently belonging in this group whom Davison and Salinger[76] were able to follow, 6 were well, and 5 of these had been so for more than seven years; 6 died; and in 8 the disease continued active. Death is usually the result of an intercurrent disease; but it is an interesting observation that sometimes after an acute febrile disease edema is lost and the patient seems remarkably improved. Streptococcic infection may occur, but not infrequently the pneumococcus is responsible for infections, particularly in causing a peritonitis. This fact, and the occasional discovery of the pneumococcus in blood-cultures, have led to the thought that this germ may be in some way causative. The pneumococcic peritonitis is not necessarily fatal. The **diagnosis** of nephrosis must be made from diffuse nephritis. In the latter condition there may be a large "nephrotic" element. The confusion is increased by the fact that in diffuse nephritis there may be, as in nephrosis, sometimes low blood-protein, change in the albumin-globulin ratio, lipemia, and the presence of doubly refractile bodies in the urine. Continued observation, however, will usually disclose that in chronic diffuse nephritis there eventually develops increasing blood-pressure and azotemia, that occasionally there is hematuria, and that the history may show that the edema and other nephrotic symptoms followed an acute glomerular nephritis or began after a streptoccic-infection of some sort. The ingestion of bichloride of mercury or other heavy metals, as bismuth, causes a degenerative necrotizing form of renal disease often classified among the nephroses, or termed the "bichloride kidney." In this condition oliguria or anuria quickly follows, edema seldom occurs or is not marked, and there is increase in blood-pressure, azotemia, acidosis, and diminished blood-chloride; none of these belonging to the picture of true nephrosis.

TREATMENT OF NEPHRITIS

Prophylaxis.—During any acute febrile disorder, and especially those of a streptococcic nature, the kidney should be spared as much as possible. No drugs should be administered which would be irritating to these organs, and rest in bed is essential. The bowels should be kept open by laxatives if necessary; and the skin active by warm sponging or warm baths, and the avoidance of chilling. No measures should be employed which will result in concentration of the urine, and fluids should be taken freely. The diet may be largely of milk, itself an excellent diuretic, and amylaceous foods. There is no good evidence that a high protein or salt content of the diet incites acute nephritis, but these elements may be kept at a minimum during acute fevers. Mild alkaline diuretics, such as potassium citrate, are often given during fevers, but are hardly necessary if fluid is ingested freely. The prevention of recurrence of acute nephritis, in addition to measures which make for good general health, consists in the avoidance of chilling and infections, the treatment of foci of infection in the upper respiratory tract or elsewhere, and the removal to a warm, dry climate if possible.

Treatment.—In *acute nephritis* this consists essentially in the measures outlined above. Rest in bed must be continued until all symptoms, including hematuria, have ceased for ten days or more, and exercise allowed with caution for some time after this. Any resulting anemia should be treated. Sometimes when all symptoms have disappeared except albuminuria, exercise or a change of environment to a warm, dry climate may prove beneficial. Contrary to the usual practice, Basch[84] allows children with acute nephritis to be out of bed and to exercise, claiming that thereby diuresis is produced and albuminuria and hematuria favorably influenced.

Further than the measures outlined, the management of both *acute* and *chronic nephritis* resolves itself largely into certain dietary considerations and the treatment of symptoms.

Diet.—The amount of liquid must not be too much reduced, especially when toxic symptoms and azotemia are present; and even with edema little if any good, and often much suffering, results from water-restriction. During the acute symptoms a bland diet, consisting largely of milk, fruit-juices and starches, is indicated. In chronic nephritis a balanced diet must be supplied and protein not too greatly or too continuously reduced. Especially in growing children must a negative nitrogen balance be prevented. In nephrosis a high protein diet has been recommended, because of the low blood-protein and the large amounts of protein lost in the urine, and this sometimes appears to have a good effect in removing edema, although frequently disappointing in this respect. Since sodium chloride and water-storage in the body are related, a salt-poor diet may be employed during periods of edema, but must not be continued indefinitely. The comparatively low salt-content of milk constitutes one of its good properties. Bratke[85] and others have used successfully in producing diuresis a diet purely of sugar, giving for a few days 125 to 250 Gm. (4.4 to 8.8 oz.) of it with moderate amounts of water. Smith, Gibson and Ross[86] recommend high caloric diets, largely carbohydrate and reinforced with sugar. The Karell[87] diet is used for renal as well as cardiac dropsy (p. 796). An abnormally balanced diet of any sort should not be too long continued.

Edema.—The dietetic measures used for this have been described. Alkalies of various sorts, as sodium bicarbonate and potassium citrate, may exert a diuretic action in some cases. Osman[88] has found that in chronic nephritis there may be a decrease in plasma-bicarbonate, and that in decided renal insufficiency an actual acidosis may develop. However, since vomiting or some other factor may cause an alkalosis, it is advisable to determine the alkali reserve, if possible, when large doses of alkali are being given. Fischer[89] claims that edema depends on an acidosis and hydration of tissue-colloids, and recommends that a solution consisting of sodium chloride 14 Gm. (0.45 oz.) and sodium carbonate 10 Gm. (0.32 oz.) in 1000 cc. (33.8 fl. oz.) of water be given rectally or intravenously. This is undoubtedly effective in some cases, but fails entirely in others. Such acid substances as calcium chloride, ammonium chloride, and potassium chloride, given to an older child in doses of 5 or 6 Gm. (77 to 92 grains) daily, may have a diuretic action. In our own experience alkalies seem to be effective in some cases and acids in others, and clinical trial may be necessary in the individual case to determine which to use. Calcium lactate, recommended by Schultz,[90] and by Blum, Aubel and Hausknecht,[91] as well as other calcium preparations, may remove edema or prevent it, perhaps by rendering the capillaries less permeable. Calcium gluconate in doses of 1 Gm. (15.4 grains) in 10 cc. (0.34 fl. oz.) of distilled water may be given daily under the skin, intramuscularly, or intravenously. Certain salts of mercury (Novasurol, Salyrgan), given intramuscularly every three or four days in doses of 0.5 to 1 cc. (8.1 to 16.23 minims) of a 10 per cent solution are used for edematous conditions, but must not be employed in acute nephritis or when there is marked azotemia. Their mode of action is not yet fully understood. Instead of sugar by the mouth, urinary output may be stimulated by intravenous injections of glucose in 40 per cent solution. Magnesium sulphate in 1 to 2 per cent solution has also been used (Blackfan and Mills[92]), not more than 15 cc. per kilogram (0.23 fl. oz. per pound) of body-weight being administered slowly, and stopping when the systolic blood-pressure is 10 to 20 points above normal. If respiratory paralysis should result 5 cc. (0.17 fl. oz.) of a 5 per cent solution of calcium chloride is injected intramuscularly. A 25 per cent solution of magnesium sulphate intramuscularly (0.2 to 0.4 cc. per kilogram) (0.003 to 0.006 fl. oz. per pound) has the same effect (Blackfan and McKhann[93]). Large doses of magnesium sulphate, *i. e.*, from 1 to 5 or more ounces of a 50 per cent solution, when given by mouth may cause improvement in edema and exert surprisingly little cathartic action (Aldrich[94]). Caffeine and the purine derivatives, theobromine sodio-salicylate (diuretin), and theophylline (theocine), are useful diuretics on occasion. Urea is also a diuretic. It should not be used if the blood-urea is high. It must always be remembered that in acute inflammatory renal lesions, vigorous attempts at diuresis by drugs may do no good or may even be harmful; and that a chronic nephritis may have proceeded to a stage when stimulation of renal function by any diuretic is no longer possible.

In nephrosis, in addition to the measures outlined, Eppinger,[95] Epstein[72] and others have employed thyroid extract. Because of the low basal metabolism large doses of this may be given, but the results in removing edema are often disappointing. Grossmann[96] reports success by giving a salt-free liver-diet. Transfusion, by increasing the blood-proteins, may be followed by diuresis. However, this is often of only temporary benefit, since the transfused protein is quickly lost. Hartmann and Senn[97] have had good results in raising the colloidal pressure of the blood and producing diuresis by the injection of a 30 per cent solution of acacia intravenously, employing about 1 Gm. of acacia per kilogram (3.4 grains per pound) of *ideal* body weight (*i. e.*, allowing for the edema present).

Uremia.—When uremia has developed or when there are such threatening symptoms as increase in blood-pressure and marked azotemia, the necessity for treatment becomes urgent. The diuretic measures already mentioned are indicated, particularly those which have a dehydrating effect, as magnesium sulphate employed in various ways. Bleeding is also helpful, with subsequent transfusions of blood or injections of 5 per cent glucose solution in an amount smaller than that removed by bleeding. Nitroglycerin may be indicated; lumbar puncture may give relief; and sedative treatment with morphine, chloral and the like is needed if convulsions are present. Hot-packs, hot-air baths, and vapor-baths are an important part of the treatment, and it can be shown that large amounts of water, urea, and creatinin can thus be eliminated through the skin. Free purgation is helpful, but this and other measures must not be pushed to the point of weakening the patient. Hot poultices or dry cups over the region of the kidneys have been used when the amount of urine was greatly diminished.

Acidosis.—If this has been proven by laboratory examination to be present therapy with alkalies is indicated (p. 490), in addition to attempts to provoke diuresis.

Renal Rickets.—This according to most observers is not amenable to the usual antirachitic measures, such as ultraviolet light and the administration of cod liver oil and viosterol; although these may be tried. Diuresis and eliminative procedures are indicated, but the presence of osseous changes usually denotes such an advanced renal insufficiency that therapy is of little avail.

Decapsulation of the Kidney.—Incision to relieve tension of the capsule was first recommended by Harrison,[98] and decapsulation has been practiced by Edebohls[99] and others. It has given relief at times in chronic nephritis, but this is usually only temporary.

AMYLOID KIDNEY

This is uncommon in early life, and is oftenest the result of a long-continued suppurative process in the bones; but may occur also in tuberculous, suppurative, or syphilitic conditions in other parts of the body, and sometimes in chronic malnutrition from any source. **Pathologically** the kidneys are firm, pale, peculiarly translucent; on section stain red with iodine; and the glomeruli, and finally the other vessels and the epithelium of the tubules exhibit a thickened, waxy appearance. The renal condition is only a part of a general amyloid alteration of the organs of the body. The **symptoms** are much like those of chronic nephritis. Edema is frequent, and the skin exhibits a peculiar waxy pallor. The liver and spleen are enlarged. Hypertrophy of the heart is uncommon. The urine is generally abundant and contains albumin in large amount and waxy casts. According to Elwyn[49] amyloid disease of the kidney causes no symptoms except albuminuria unless there is a complicating lipoid nephrosis, in which case the symptoms characteristic of this disorder develop. The prognosis is unfavorable, death occurring often after a prolonged course from uremia, increasing debility, or a complicating illness. The **treatment** is that of the primary cause combined with measures appropriate for chronic nephritis.

TUBERCULOSIS OF THE KIDNEY

Etiology and Pathologic Anatomy.—Tuberculosis of the kidney is uncommon in early life except as a manifestation of a general tuberculosis.

It is rarely a primary lesion. It may manifest itself by the presence of small tubercles developing on the surface and in the parenchyma of the kidney, the tubercle bacilli having reached the organ through the blood (*excretory* or *hematogenous tuberculosis*). In other cases it may be combined with tuberculous disease elsewhere in the genito-urinary tract, the process being either an ascending or, more often, a descending one with the kidney the first part attacked. The disease may develop by contiguity from a tuberculous pleuritis or peritonitis. The caseous form of renal tuberculosis is more common in males and rare in early life. The process is often unilateral at first, but finally bilateral.

Symptoms.—No special symptoms occur with acute miliary tuberculosis of the kidney. Those of the caseous form are often masked by the existence of tuberculosis elsewhere in the body. In addition to the general symptoms of fever, emaciation, and the like, there may be pain, tenderness, and enlargement in the renal region, and frequent and painful urination. The urine is acid and shows the presence of blood, pus, and tubercle bacilli.

Course and Prognosis.—The course of miliary tuberculosis of the kidney is short, the patient soon dying from the general infection. The duration of caseous renal tuberculosis depends often upon the tuberculous condition elsewhere in the body. Occurring primarily it may last months or years, but the final prognosis is usually unfavorable.

Diagnosis.—The disease is to be distinguished from *pyelitis* by the continuance of symptoms, and by the discovery of tubercle bacilli in the urine. *Renal calculus* produces the more typical pain of renal colic; exhibits little pus in the urine; and is not accompanied by fever unless there is a complicating inflammation. Roentgenograms may reveal the stone. *Tuberculosis of the bladder* can be differentiated by cystoscopic examination, and its presence suggests involvement of the kidney also. The function of the individual kidney may be tested by the elimination of dye through ureteral catheters, but remembering that the excretion of this may be good, even with partial failure of the renal function. In examining the urine for tubercle bacilli care must be taken to differentiate these from the smegma bacillus, and for this inoculation of guinea-pigs with the urine may be required. Even this procedure is not entirely diagnostic, Morse-Braasch,[100] for example, finding 8 negative guinea-pig tests in 45 cases of proven renal tuberculosis.

Treatment.—All possible means must be employed to sustain the general health. Operative treatment may be adopted at times in unilateral cases, when it has been proven that the other kidney is functioning normally.

SUPPURATIVE NEPHRITIS

(Abscess of the Kidney)

Although even the new-born may exhibit this lesion, it is uncommon in early life, and almost never primary. In most cases the infection is hematogenous in origin, but in other instances may be an ascending process, or may reach the kidney by contiguity to other suppuration lesions, or may result from the presence of a calculus or from trauma. Micro-organisms of many different sorts may be present, but commonly the streptococcus, staphylococcus, colon bacillus, or typhoid bacillus. **Pathologically** the lesions vary somewhat with the cause. In those of hematogenous origin both kidneys are involved, with numerous abscesses of varying size. The **symptoms** in the variety resulting from sepsis are overshadowed by those of the general infection. Only when tenderness is discovered in the renal region, and blood and pus in the urine, is diagnosis possible. The same difficulty in diagnosis and similarity of local symptoms occur in abscess from other causes. In cases of abscess secondary to pyelonephritis the urinary findings are inconclusive. The general symptoms of suppurative nephritis, however, are more severe. In walled-off abscesses the urine may be normal. The **prognosis** is unfavorable in the metastatic cases, and the course short. In other forms the outlook is grave, being best when there is free communication with the urinary tubules and ready discharge of pus. A perinephritic abscess may develop, or the pus burrow its way beyond the perinephritic region. The **treatment** for abscess of the kidney which is part of a general septicemia is primarily that of the general infection. Operation in other cases may be indicated when it is suspected that there is localization, and it is known that the other kidney is functionally active.

HEMORRHAGIC INFARCTION OF THE KIDNEY

This has been described by Rayer,[101] Bednar,[102] Pollak,[103] Oppenheim,[104] and others. It occurs in marantic infants in the early weeks of life. The symptoms develop acutely and there are a yellowish tint to the skin, hematuria, and anemia. Death occurs after a few days.

RENAL CALCULUS

Etiology.—Uric-acid infarction of the kidney in the new-born has been referred to (p. 41). Reports by Civiale,[105] Collins,[106] Bugbee and Wollstein,[107] Thomas and Tanner,[108] Lignac,[109] Campbell,[110] Borman,[111] and others indicate that renal calculi are not uncommon in children and occur with about the same frequency as in adults. They have been discovered even in the new-born. Calculi are found much more frequently in some geographical regions than in others, and an inherited tendency is observed at times. Suppuration of bone and prolonged recumbent posture are supposed to predispose to their formation (Borman[111]).

Pathologic Anatomy.—The calculi consist oftenest of uric-acid or its salts, although oxalates, phosphates, carbonates, cystin, or xanthin occasionally compose them. Of over 500 calculi removed from children, according to Bókay[112] seven-twelfths were of uric acid or urates and four-twelfths of phosphate of lime. The stones may be many or few, and vary in size from that of gravel up to calculi which fill the entire pelvis of the kidney. In about 20 per cent of cases both kidneys are involved. There may be inflammation of the tissue surrounding stones in the renal parenchyma. Stones in the pelvis of the kidney produce irritation and dilatation.

Symptoms.—Characteristic symptoms are tenderness in the renal region; pyuria and hematuria; and attacks of renal colic with pain radiating to the lower part of the abdomen, the testicle, penis and thigh; and a constant desire to urinate. Vomiting may occur with the renal colic, and in some cases convulsions and collapse. The attack lasts for a few hours or sometimes, with remissions, for several days. The calculus may return to the pelvis of the kidney, or advance and be passed into the bladder and later voided, or perhaps only gravel found. The description given applies to typical cases, but in infancy symptoms may be absent or indefinite, and the pain of renal colic supposed to be intestinal in origin. In other patients there is hematuria without colic, particularly when the calculi are in the substance of the kidney. The **prognosis** is on the whole good in children, although the course may be much prolonged and repeated attacks of colic occur before the stone is passed. There is a decided tendency for new calculi to form. With impacted stone pyonephritis, hydronephrosis, or renal abscess may develop.

Diagnosis.—With the typical symptoms described the diagnosis is easy. In chronic pyelitis one of the causative factors to be looked for is calculus. The appearance of uric-acid crystals in the urine does not necessarily mean that they have been passed from the kidney, but perhaps that they have been precipitated after the urine has been evacuated. Roentgenograms and pyelograms may be of value, except that uric-acid stones cast no shadow.

Treatment.—During attacks of colic the patient should be immersed in a warm bath, and morphine and atropine given. In the case of impacted stone ureteral catheterization may be necessary to cause dislodgment. After the attack any remaining pyelitis should be treated, and the attempt made to discover whether other stones are present. To aid in preventing recurrence water should be taken freely, and any disorder of digestion corrected. If the stone passed has been of uric acid, it may be advisable to keep the urine somewhat alkaline for a while, and to avoid the excessive ingestion of meat. In phosphatic calculi the urine should not be alkalinized. It should be remembered that such foods as rhubarb, egg-plant, spinach, and asparagus increase the excretion of oxalates.

MORBID GROWTHS OF THE KIDNEY

These are more frequent in early life than later, and, according to the studies of Taylor,[113] Steffen,[114] and others, are encountered especially in the first five years. Warner[115] found that 20.4 per cent of all tumors in children were in the kidney. They may sometimes be congenital in origin (Walker,[116] Deming[117]).

Pathologic Anatomy.—One of the most common growths is a mixed tumor, sometimes called embryonal adenosarcoma (Doderlein and Birch-Hirschfeld[118]), Wilms's[119] tumor, or embryoma (Gage and Adams[120]). (For review of literature, see Dean and Pack.[121]) Epithelioma is reported. Renal hypernephroma, which may be of the type of a neuroblastoma, is a frequent variety, in which the tumor originates in misplaced adrenal tissue situated in the kidney. Malignant tumors of the kidney are usually primary, although occasionally secondary, and as a rule unilateral. Benign tumors, such as fibroma, lipoma, myoma and adenoma are rare.

Symptoms.—The tumor often reaches great size, more or less filling the abdominal cavity on one side, and growing rapidly (Fig. 194). It appears to project forward from the flank, and the anterior portion can be lifted by palpation with the hand in the lumbar region. It is more often soft than hard, and sometimes seems almost fluctuating. The surface may be smooth or lobulated. The urine contains blood and sometimes casts, but this is not always the case. Pain in the renal region is usually absent. As the tumor grows debility, emaciation and anemia develop; digestive disturbances may be observed; and symptoms due to pressure and metastasis may occur. Among such symptoms are vomiting, diarrhea, edema, cough, and paralysis.

Course and Prognosis.—The course is rapid, particularly in cases of sarcoma. According to the studies of Walker,[116] Schippers,[122] Lyman,[123] Wollstein,[124] Warner,[115] and Dean and Pack,[121] the average duration of life may be said to be from twelve to eighteen months from the time that diagnosis is obvious, operation prolonging life for several months or longer and radiologic treatment still longer. Hypernephroma often runs a longer course. Warner[115] gives the ultimate mortality for sarcoma as about 90 per cent.

Diagnosis.—This rests upon the presence of cachexia and hematuria, and sometimes solely upon the discovery of the renal tumor. The majority of abdominal tumors in childhood are renal or suprarenal. The growth appears to be largest in the renal region, and projects forward. There may be tympany over the tumor due to the presence of the colon there. The roentgenogram may be of value in differentiating renal tumor from other abdominal masses, and the latter are usually less movable. Splenic enlargements seem to take origin beneath the costal border, have a sharp edge and often a splenic notch, and move with respiration. Perinephritic abscess is accompanied by septic symptoms. A hypernephroma may exhibit fever, and peculiar somatic changes may accompany it (p. 1082). Suprarenal and renal tumors can hardly be differentiated by palpation. A tumor arising in the liver is directly continuous with it and moves with respiration. Fecal accumulations seldom extend to the flanks and generally disappear after purgation.

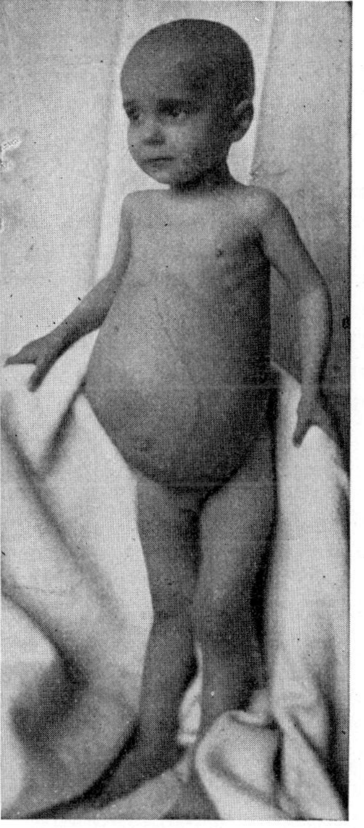

Fig. 194.—Tumor of the kidney. Ida D., aged two and one-half years. Had a swelling of the abdomen for some time, which had gradually grown larger. Entered the Children's Hospital of Philadelphia. Emaciation, diarrhea, no pain, leukocytes 9000, hemoglobin 70 per cent. Large tumor of the right kidney, weighing 2½ pounds (1134) removed. Pronounced to be sarcoma. Operational recovery. Discharged. Further history unknown. Faint outline in the photograph shows the margin of the growth.

Treatment.—Nephrectomy should be performed as early as possible and in malignant cases radiologic treatment given. It is sometimes advised to employ this before operation as well as after.

PERINEPHRITIS

(Perinephritic Abscess)

This is not a frequent disease in early life, but we have seen a number of instances, and there are reports of it in children by Gibney,[125] Nieden,[126] and others. Schatz[127] collected over 171 instances in children including cases of his own. It seems most often to follow an infection of the skin, which may be of minor character. It is apparently often a primary affection, the causative germs being carried by the blood-stream and lodging in the arteries which supply the renal cortex and the perirenal fat (Brunn and Rhodes[128]). Less often it may be secondary to suppurative nephritis, trauma, disease of the spine, pleurisy, septicemia, and the infectious fevers, and sometimes appears to follow exposure to cold without other discoverable cause. **Pathologically** the inflammation is usually unilateral, and almost always advances to suppuration. The pus accumulates chiefly below the kidney and may extend in different directions, rupturing into the ileo-costal space or above Poupart's ligament, or into the peritoneum, intestines, kidney, bladder or pleura. The **symptoms** may come on suddenly or more slowly, with fever and other manifestations of infection. There is pain in the lumbar region or referred to the groin, hip, thigh, or knee. Movement of the spine or walking causes pain, the patient bends toward the involved side, and later, when confined to bed, keeps the thigh flexed. Locally there is tenderness on palpation and increased resistance, and finally an indefinitely outlined tumor, perhaps fluctuating and not moving with respiration. Local edema and redness may develop on the cutaneous surface. The urine is not often altered in character nor are there usually urinary symptoms. The **course** in acute cases is generally several weeks; in chronic cases sometimes months or years if the cause persists and the pus finds an exit. Without operative interference the abscess finally ruptures in some of the directions mentioned. In secondary abscesses the prognosis is influenced by the nature of the primary disease. The **diagnosis** may be difficult, especially in the chronic cases. *Disease of the hip-joint,* which is to be distinguished, is more chronic in onset; lameness and deformity are slower in developing; there is tenderness over the hip-joint; and passive movement is restricted in all directions instead of in extension only. *Caries of the spine* may produce symptoms resembling perinephritis, but there should be found a prominence of some of the vertebrae and a roentgenogram may settle the matter. When perinephritic abscess ruptures into the pleura, the origin of the pus may not be suspected. Roentgenograms of perinephritic abscess may show changes in the psoas shadow and the fluoroscope reveal delayed excursion of the diaphragm. The **treatment** consists in local application of cold or heat over the renal region; but as soon as the presence of pus is proven, by an exploratory puncture if necessary, the abscess should be drained.

PYELITIS

This condition is variously denominated pyelitis, pyelonephritis, and pyelocystitis, indicating the combinations of lesions which may exist. (See also Cystitis, p. 838.)

Etiology.—Pyelitis is twice as common in children under two years as after that age. Its frequency is shown by the study of Fromm,[129] who found urinary infection in 4.4 per cent of an unselected group of 225 sick children, and of Hurt,[130] who observed pyelitis in 1.4 per cent of 773 infants. While uncommon under three months of age it has been seen even in the first week (Smith,[131] Sauer[132]). In very young infants as many boys as girls are affected, but after this period it occurs from three to four times as frequently in females. It may depend upon the presence of a renal calculus, renal tumors, inflammation of the bladder, and tuberculous or suppurative processes in the kidney. It may follow acute respiratory infections, the infectious fevers, or gastro-intestinal disturbances, especially of a diarrheal nature, or be part of a septicemia. The frequency and importance of kinking or stricture of the ureter, or of pressure upon it, in chronic and recurrent pyelitis is emphasized by Beer,[133] Mixter,[134] Smith,[135] Helmholz,[136] Hunner,[137] McKhann,[10] Campbell and Lyttle,[15] and others. Helmholz[138] believes that these anomalies do not predispose to infection, so much as prevent proper drainage when infection is present. An important cause in some cases seems to be stricture of the urethral meatus (Boyd[139]). Sometimes there appears to be an atony of the ureters, perhaps dependent upon a neuromuscular fault (Eisendrath et al.[140]), or a "neurogenic dysfunction" of the bladder (Campbell[141]). In recurrent cases diseased tonsils and teeth may occasionally be suspected of acting as foci of infection. In many cases, however, especially in young infants, pyelitis appears suddenly, without any preceding infection or known causative factor.

Whatever the cause, the active agents are bacteria which have penetrated to the pelvis of the kidney. There is much discussion whether the infection is ascending from the urethra, by way of the blood, or by the anastomosing lymphatics of the intestine and urinary organs; but probably all three routes are possible. In favor of the first is the presence of the colon bacillus, and the frequency in females with their shorter urethra, and in favor of the second is the frequency with which pyelitis follows acute infections. The colon bacillus is found alone or in combination in probably from about 60 to 80 or more per cent of the cases. The question has been raised whether this is the primary infecting germ or a later secondary invader. Other germs discovered are the streptococcus, staphylococcus, typhoid bacillus, bacillus pyocyaneus, bacillus lactis aerogenes, bacillus proteus, tubercle bacillus, and diphtheria bacillus. In spite of the frequency of vulvovaginitis, the gonococcus seldom infects the pelvis of the kidney.

Pathologic Anatomy.—Cases due to obstruction, calculus, and the like may be unilateral; otherwise both kidneys are affected. In acute cases there is a catarrhal inflammation of the mucous membrane of the pelvis. In more chronic cases the mucous membrane may become thickened. Other lesions, such as the malformations described, may be found. In severe cases the pathologic condition is in reality a pyelonephritis, and Wilson and Schloss[142] among others present strong evidence that focal inflammatory lesions in the interstitial tissue constitute the initial pathologic process in so-called "pyelitis." Yet these studies were made on fatal cases, and it seems probable that in the majority of instances of acute pyelitis, any such lesions which may develop must be temporary and leave no residual damage.

Symptoms.—In typical cases of the acute form there is sudden rise of temperature, reaching 103 to 105 F. (39.4 to 40.5 C.), preceded by chilliness, and continuing steadily elevated or oftener remittent. There is dull pain in the renal region; sometimes tenderness over the kidney; frequent micturition; debility; and anorexia. Leukocytosis is present. The urine is acid, of a normal specific gravity, and the quantity may be decreased. There is a small amount of albumin, and microscopically are found pus-cells and sometimes red blood-cells, epithelial cells, and perhaps a few hyaline casts. Bacteria may be present in varying number. The amount of pus varies from time to time in the same patient. When the fever and other constitutional disturbances are marked, the pus may be less in quantity on account of being retained. The condition as detailed is characteristic especially of cases dependent upon renal calculus. In the large majority of instances, however, especially in infants, the symptoms are uncharacteristic, and the disease is readily unrecognized unless an examination of urine is made. The fever may be only moderate, and is apt to show decided variation (Fig. 195), the child possibly being afebrile at times for a day or two. Pain, tenderness, and disturbance of micturition are oftener absent than present. There may be very few general symptoms, or those suggestive of a digestive disturbance may develop. Cases of chronic pyelitis exhibit often merely pyuria; fever and other symptoms developing only during the acute exacerbations which are liable to occur. In chronic cases, or in those which have had a large number of relapses, epithelial or granular casts may appear at times in the urine, indicating that the process has extended beyond the pelvis and that a pyelonephritis is present.

Course and Prognosis.—The condition is liable to be more severe and the mortality higher in infants under two years of age, but the average simple case of pyelitis seldom ends fatally. The acute attack lasts from two to four weeks, although the fever and general symptoms may disappear in less than this time. Recurrences are strikingly common, and liable to extend over a period of months or years, these later attacks often being less severe than the primary one. In other cases dependent upon strictures, tuberculosis, calculus, or the like, the pyuria is persistent. Occasionally cases are severe from the onset and run a rapidly fatal course, the condition then being a pyelonephritis.

Complications.—The most frequent is cystitis and some degree of pyelonephritis. Associated with pyelitis as causes or sequels, are perinephritis, pyonephrosis, malformations of the kidney, tumors, calculus, and tuberculosis. Severe anemia may develop.

Diagnosis.—This rests upon pyuria with an acid urine and the symptoms described. The pus-cells are often found in small clumps. The estimation of the number indicating pyuria has been discussed elsewhere (p. 808). Pyelitis should be suspected in every child with fever of an obscure nature. The urine should be examined frequently in febrile disorders of any kind, since pyelitis may complicate so many diseases. Recurrent or persistent pyuria should always lead to a search for a condition other than pyelitis, of which it may be a symptom. In *cystitis* there is pain over and

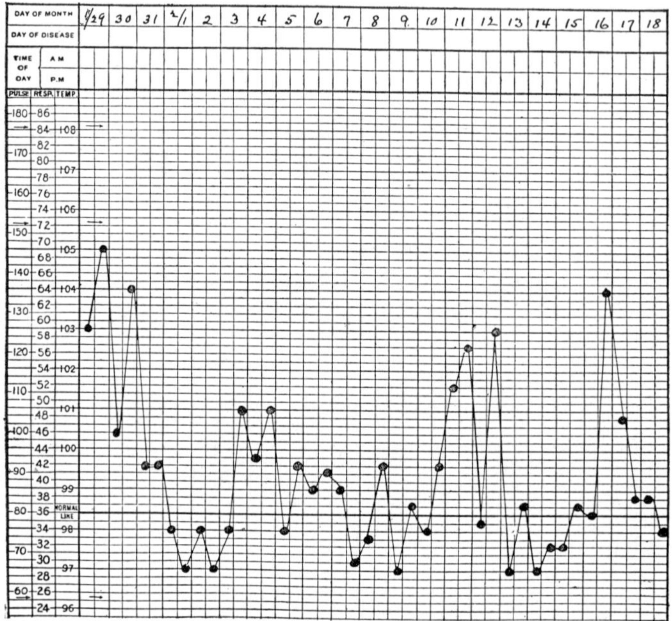

Fig. 195.—Pyelitis, characteristically vague symptoms as usually present, exacerbations of fever. Jeanette F., aged two years. Sudden onset Dec. 25, with vomiting and fever. Latter persisted, with fretfulness, malaise and cough. About Jan. 1, dysuria. Improved, but about Jan. 20 grew worse, with irregular fever, lost much weight, was anemic, restless, fretful, and very weak. Entered Children's Ward of the University Hospital, Philadelphia, Jan. 28. In hospital same symptoms continued, then gradually improved. Physical examination negative, except that urine was acid and contained pus, and on culture colon bacilli, and there was tenderness in the left renal region.

more irritability of the bladder than in pyelitis, and no pain or tenderness in the renal region; nor are fever and constitutional symptoms marked. The urine may be alkaline and contain mucus and many epithelial cells. Cystitis and pyelitis may, of course, be combined. Acute glomerular *nephritis* gives casts and more blood and less pus in the urine than usually found in pyelitis, and generally more albumin; and it may be accompanied by edema, increase in blood-pressure, and the like. *Renal calculus* produces colic and hematuria, and may often be discovered by roentgenograms. *Tuberculosis* of the kidney generally exhibits tuberculous lesions elsewhere in the body, and tubercle bacilli may be found in the urine. In *appendicitis* the localization of the tenderness over the right lower quadrant of the abdomen rather than over the renal region is the chief distinguishing characteristic from pyelitis, in addition to the examination of the urine. An inflamed retrocecal appendix may, however, give pain posteriorly and, by its proximity to the ureter irritate this and cause some increase of pus-cells in the urine. Furthermore, appendicitis and pyelitis may coexist. In the differential diagnosis of these several conditions from pyelitis and in the study of pyelitis itself roentgenograms of the urinary tract, with or without the injection of opaque substances, may be useful. (See p. 814.) The germs present should be searched for and cultures of the urine made.

Treatment.—In prophylaxis the external genitals should be kept as clean as possible. In chronic or recurrent pyuria study should be made to determine the presence of calculus or anomalies of the genito-urinary tract of the type already discussed, and these should receive appropriate treatment. In some cases it may be indicated to remove diseased teeth or tonsils. Great care should be used whenever catheterization is necessary in infancy. At all times, and especially during acute febrile illnesses, an abundant fluid intake should be insisted upon.

When the colon bacillus is the infecting organism it has been recommended that potassium citrate or sodium bicarbonate be given in doses sufficient to render the urine alkaline, since this organism prefers an acid medium for its growth. Clinically this seems to be of undoubted benefit, although Helmholz and Millikin,[143] and Helmholz,[144] could not find that any change in reaction of the urine had appreciable effect on the growth of colon bacilli. When the urine is already alkaline and the colon bacillus is not present, it may be rendered strongly acid by benzoic acid, acid sodium phosphate, calcium chloride or ammonium chloride, giving to a child five or six years of age from 1 to 3 Gm. (15 to 46 grains) three or four times a day. Even in colon bacillus infection it may be advisable to alternate the acid with the alkaline treatment every week or ten days. Hexamethylenamine will effectively render the urine antiseptic if given in full doses when the urine is acid. Infants of one year require from 1 to 3 grains (0.065 to 0.194 Gm.) several times daily, but much larger doses are necessary for older children. Renal irritation and even the passage of bloody urine may be caused by this drug, and repeated examinations should be made for the presence of red blood-cells and casts. Among other drugs used are acriflavine in doses of 0.025 to 0.05 Gm. (0.39 to 0.77 grain) by mouth two or three times a day (Davis and Beck[145]), mercurochrome 3 mg. per kilogram (0.02 grain per pound) of body-weight given intravenously in a 1 per cent solution (Young, Hill and Scott[146]), hexylresorcinol 0.3 Gm. (4.6 grains) three times a day by mouth (Leonard[147]), and pyridium 0.1 Gm. (1.54 grains) by mouth four times a day (Ostromislensky[148]). Draper, Darley and Harvey[149] have had success with the intramuscular injection of pituitary extract and pitressin. The doses of these various drugs as mentioned are those for older children. Somewhat smaller amounts should be given to younger children and infants.

Autogenous vaccines are sometimes of value and may be tried in persistent pyuria. Bacteriophage therapy has been used with variable results. (For review see Krueger, Faber and Schultz.[150]) Lavage of the pelvis of the kidney with 0.5 per cent solution of silver nitrate has been employed by Kretschmer and Helmholz,[151] and others. During the febrile period the patient should be kept at rest and a nonirritating diet employed. Aron and Hirsch[152] recommend high carbohydrate, low protein, and low salt diet. Complications naturally require treatment, and also, as mentioned, anomalies of the urinary tract. Helmholz[153] has had success with ketogenic diets.

Of all the measures outlined the most important during the acute febrile stage is the administration of large amounts of fluid, which it may be sometimes necessary to give parenterally. It is doubtful whether urinary antiseptics have much effect in shortening the course; their value is greatest in the chronic cases. We have not infrequently found autogenous vaccines to be helpful in continued pyuria. In other cases they have been entirely without result. Occasionally the removal of tonsils or infected teeth has been useful. Our experience with lavage of the pelvis of the kidney has been favorable.

References

1. J. Pharmacol. and Exp. Therap., 1909–10, **1,** 579. 2. Gittings and Mitchell, Am. J. Dis. Child., 1917, **14,** 174. 3. Deutsch. Arch. f. klin. Med., 1914, **114,** 120. 4. J.A.M.A., 1920, **75,** 596. 5. Arch. Int. Med., 1915, **16,** 733. 6. J.A.M.A., 1928, **90,** 1092. 7. J. Clin. Invest., 1929–30, **8,** 357; Medicine, 1930, **9,** 257. 8. J.A.M.A., 1931, **97,** 913. 9. J.A.M.A., 1924, **82,** 1425. 10. Am. J. Dis. Child., 1928, **36,** 315. 11. Am. J. Dis. Child., 1930, **39,** 386. 12. Brit. J. Child. Dis., 1916, **13,** 80. 13. Am. J. Dis. Child., 1929, **38,** 960. 14. Am. J. Dis. Child., 1929, **38,** 1202. 15. J.A.M.A., 1929, **92,** 544. 16. Quart. J. Med., 1929, **22,** 567. 17. Brit. M. J., 1902, **2,** 678. 18. Rev. mens. d. mal. de l'enf., 1893, **11,** 441. 19. Pediatrics, 1898, **6,** 439; Traité d. mal. de l'enf., 1904, **2,** 712. 20. Thèse de Paris, 1902. 21. Lancet, 1903, **1,** 731. 22. Beitr. z. path. Anat. u. z. allg. Path., 1890, **8,** 21. 23. New York M. J., 1896, **63,** 65. 24. La semaine méd., 1918, **25,** 58. 25. Rep. Soc. Study Dis. Child., 1901, **1,** 129. 26. Riv. di clin. pediat., 1903, **1,** 505. 27. Arch. Pediat., 1889, **4,** 1, 103. 28. Rev. mens. d. mal. de l'enf., 1900, **18,** 308. 29. Mitchell, Am. J. Dis. Child., 1930, **40,** 101; 345. 30. Prag. Vtljschr., 1870, **105,** 79; 1870, **106,** 60; Ref. Schmidt's Jahrb., 1871, **149,** 180. 31. J.A.M.A., 1919, **73,** 1747. 32. J.A.M.A., 1921, **76,** 505. 33. Am. J. Dis. Child., 1922, **23,** 375. 34. Practitioner, 1925, **114,** 222. 35. Atlantic M. J., 1926, **29,** 201. 36. Bull. Johns Hopkins Hosp., 1926, **39,** 60. 37. J. Clin. Invest., 1927, **5,** 7. 38. J. Path. and Bact., 1928, **31,** 191. 39. Griffith, Penna. M. J., 1918, **11,** 971. 40. Vorlesungen ü. Kinderkrankh., 1895, 697. 41. Jahrb. f. Kinderh., 1909, **69,** 652. 42. Nord. Med. Ark., Sec. 2, Innere Medicin, 1911, Pt. 2, No. 5, 1. 43. Jahrb. f. Kinderh., 1913, **77,** 1. 44. Surg., Gynec. and Obstet., 1916, **23,** 495. 45. Am. J. Path., 1931, **7,** 57. 46. Am. J. Dis. Child., 1929, **38,** 1052. 47. Jahrb. f. Kinderh., 1931, **130,** 215. 48. Bull. Johns Hopkins Hosp., 1931, **48,** 193. 49. Nephritis, 1929. 50. Hypertension and Nephritis 1930. 51. J. Exper. Med., 1898, **3,** 393. 52. Arch. Int. Med., 1919, **24,** 359; 1921, **28,** 1; 1928, **42,** 801; J. Clin. Invest., 1931, **10,** 153. 53. Bull. Johns Hopkins Hosp., 1923, **34,** 168. 54. Ann. Int. Med., 1931, **5,** 579. 55. Birmingham Med. Rev., 1903, **53–54,** 511. 56. Lehrb. d. Kinderkr., 1902, 992. 57. Am. J. Dis. Child., 1927, **34,** 218. 58. Arch. Int. Med., 1922, **30,** 817. 59. München. med. Wchnschr., 1930, **77,** 1657. 60. München. med. Wchnschr., 1930, **77,** 1922. 61. Am. J. Dis. Child., 1922, **23,** 183. 62. Mitchell and Guest, J.A.M.A., 1931, **97,** 1045. 63. Lancet, 1883, **1,** 993. 64. Proc. Roy. Soc. Med. Sec. Study Dis. Child., 1910–11, **4,** 95. 65. Brit. M. J., 1911, **2,** 481. 66. Brit. J. Child. Dis., 1912, **9,** 22. 67. Quart. J. Med., 1921, **14,** 205. 68. Kinderheilk., 1911, **2,** 502. 69. Verhandl. d. deutsch. path. Gesellsch., 1905, **9,** 64. 70. Ztschr. f. klin. Med., 1913, **78,** 1; Pathol. und Klinik der Nephrosen, Nephritiden, und Schrumpfnieren 1918. 71. Die Brightsche Nierenkrankheit 1914. 72. Am. J. M. Sc., 1917, **154,** 638; 1922, **163,** 167; M. Clin. N. Amer., 1922, **5,** 1067. 73. J.A.M.A., 1931, **97,** 1048. 74. J.A.M.A., 1929, **93,** 23. 75. Am. J. Path., 1929, **5,** 587. 76. Bull. Johns Hopkins Hosp., 1927, **41,** 329. 77. M. Clin. N. Amer., 1924, **7,** 1413. 78. Am. J. Dis. Child., 1925, **29,** 587. 79. Am. J. Dis. Child., 1926, **32,** 163. 80. Am. J. Path., 1929, **5,** 587; 1931, **7,** 57. 81. J. Clin. Invest., 1930, **8,** 337. 82. Am. J. Dis. Child., 1931, **42,** 314. 83. J. Biol. Chem., 1929, **81,** 205. 84. Ztschr. f. Kinderh., 1926, **42,** 589. 85. Jahrb. f. Kinderh., 1918, **88,** 268. 86. J.A.M.A., 1927, **88,** 1943. 87. Arch. gén. d. méd., 1866, **8,** 513. 88. Lancet, 1930, **2,** 945. 89. Edema and Nephritis, 1921. 90. Ztschr. f. klin. Med., 1918, **86,** 111. 91. Bull. et mém. soc. méd. d. hôp. de Paris, 1922, **46,** 206. 92. Trans. Am. Pediat. Soc., 1923, **35,** 197. 93. J.A.M.A., 1931, **97,** 1052. 94. Am. J. Dis. Child., 1931, **41,** 1265. 95. Zur Path. u. Ther. d. menschlichen Oedema, 1917. 96. Wien. klin. Wchnschr., 1928, **41,** 450. 97. Trans. Am. Pediat. Soc.; Am. J. Dis. Child., 1932, **44,** 673. 98. Lancet, 1896, **1,** 18. 99. New York Med. Rec., 1901, **60,** 961. 100. J. Urol., 1927, **17,** 287. 101. Traité d. mal. d. reins., 1837, **3,** 428. 102. Krankh. d. Neugeb. u. Säugl., 1850, **3,** 188. 103. Wien. med. Presse, 1871, **12,** 456. 104. Ztschr. f. Kinderh., 1920, **26,** 192. 105. Traité de l'affection calculeuse, Paris, 1838, 646. 106. Am. J. Dis. Child., 1913, **6,** 245. 107. J.A.M.A., 1924, **83,** 1887. 108. J. Urol., 1922, **8,** 171. 109. Nederl. Tijdschr. v. Geneesk., 1929, **1,** 3008. 110. J.A.M.A., 1930, **94,** 1753. 111. Am. J. Dis. Child., 1930, **40,** 804. 112. Traité d. mal. de l'enf. (Grancher) 1904, **2,** 753. 113. Am. J. M. Sc., 1887, **94,** 461. 114. Die malig. Geschwülste im Kindersalter 1905, 30. 115. Arch. f. klin. Chir., 1927, **145,** 347. 116. Ann. Surg., 1897, **26,** 529. 117. J.A.M.A., 1923, **80,** 902. 118. Zentralbl. f. d. Krank., d. Harn.-u. Sex.-Org., 1894, **5,** 3; 88. 119. Die Mischgeschwülste der Niere, 1899, **1,** 1. 120. Ann. Surg., 1923, **78,** 226. 121. J.A.M.A., 1932, **98,** 10. 122. Nederl. Maandschr. v. Geneesk., 1924, **12,** 400. 123. Arch. Pediat., 1925, **42,** 96. 124. Arch. Path. and Lab. Med., 1927, **3,** 1. 125. Chicago M. J., 1880, **45,** 61. 126.

Deutsch. Arch. f. klin. Med., 1878, **22,** 492. 127. Jahrb. f. Kinderh., 1927, **116,** 99. 128. J.A.M.A., 1930, **94,** 618. 129. Centralbl. f. Kinderh., 1904, **9,** 367. 130. Am. J. Dis. Child., 1930, **40,** 137. 131. M. Clin. N. Amer., 1918, **1,** 165. 132. J.A.M.A., 1925, **85,** 327. 133. Internat. Clin., 1923, **3,** 272. 134. Ann. Surg., 1926, **84,** 533. 135. Am. J. Dis. Child., 1924, **28,** 678. 136. J.A.M.A., 1927, **89,** 1932. 137. Am. J. Dis. Child., 1928, **34,** 603. 138. Tr. Northwest. Ped. Soc.; Am. J. Dis. Child., 1930, **40,** 1374. 139. J.A.M.A., 1929, **92,** 2154. 140. Am. J. Dis. Child., 1929, **38,** 1006. 141. J.A.M.A., 1929, **93,** 183. 142. Am. J. Dis. Child., 1929, **38,** 227. 143. Am. J. Dis. Child., 1924, **28,** 700. 144. Brit. J. Child. Dis., 1929, **26,** 247. 145. J. Urol., 1921, **5,** 215. 146. Arch. Surg., 1925, **10,** 813. 147. J.A.M.A., 1924, **83,** 2005. 148. Scientific Basis of Chemotherapy. 149. J. Urol., 1931, **26,** 1. 150. J. Urol., 1930, **23,** 397. 151. J.A.M.A., 1920, **75,** 1303. 152. Monatschr. f. Kinderh., 1929, **43,** 385. 153. Proc. Staff Meet. Mayo Clinic, 1932, **7,** 260.

CHAPTER III

DISEASES OF THE BLADDER

MALFORMATIONS

A FEW instances of **absence of the bladder,** and of two or more **rudimentary bladders** have been reported. **Congenital diverticula** are uncommon. **Congenital dilatation of the bladder** may occur (Fig. 196), being due to a complete or partial obstruction in the course of the urethra, to a **congenital valve-like deformity** of the posterior urethra (see p. 846), or to **congenital fibrosis** of the neck of the bladder (Campbell[1]). There may be **entero-urethral fusion** (Baldwin[2]), or the intestine may communicate with the bladder. In **persistent urachus** (*umbilical fistula*) the urine is discharged through the navel, and there may be an associated occlusion or stenosis of the urethra. The condition has been studied especially by Herrman.[3] All these are of very unusual occurrence.

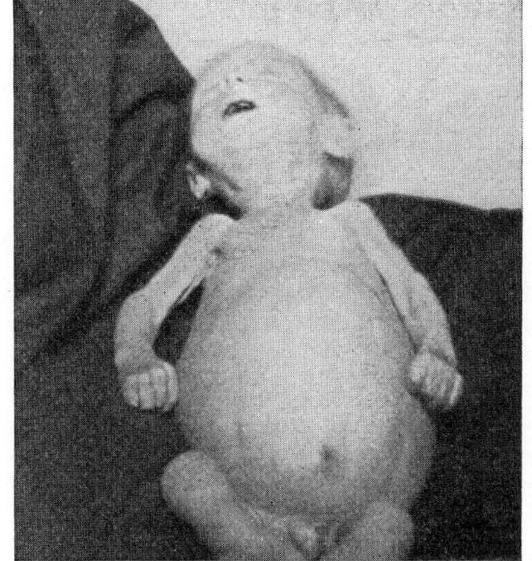

Fig. 196.—Congenital dilatation of the bladder. Child, aged three months, with partial hypospadias. The abdominal distention was noted at birth, and steadily increased. The necropsy revealed a distended bladder extending to the diaphragm, and containing over a quart (946 cc.) of urine. (*Courtesy of Dr. J. Madison Taylor.*)

EXSTROPHY OF THE BLADDER.—This comparatively uncommon malformation is seen, with few exceptions, only in boys. There is a defect in the anterior wall of the bladder and of the abdominal parietes over it. In complete cases there is fissure of the pubic bone and of the penis or the clitoris, and other anomalies of development are often combined. The posterior wall of the bladder is seen as a red, roughened area with the orifices of the ureters visible. In females the vagina may be absent or be replaced by a cloaca including vagina and rectum. The chief danger is the development of pyelonephritis. The treatment is surgical, with perhaps the possibility of replacing the anterior wall of the bladder by tissue from the abdominal wall or, in other cases, transplantation of the ureters into the intestine.

PROLAPSE OF THE BLADDER

This is occasionally seen in female children, and may be congenital or acquired. Part or all of the bladder-wall projects through the urethra, sometimes as the result of trauma, or of straining caused by dysentery or cystitis. The prolapse should be reduced and recurrence prevented by compresses and bandages. Occasionally a plastic operation on the dilated urethra may be necessary.

VESICAL CALCULUS

This condition is probably as frequent in children as in adults. The incidence in childhood appears to be less in the United States than in other countries; as England, India, Russia and Hungary. Among reports on vesical calculi in children are those of Bókai,[4] Borobio,[5] Cahill,[6] Crenshaw,[7] Thomas and Tanner,[8] Rocher and Blanc,[9] Campbell,[10] and Borman.[11] Vesical calculi are most common during childhood from the age of two to seven years, and occur much oftener in boys; the short, wide female urethra allowing stones to be passed while they are still small. The calculus usually is formed in the kidney, but in the bladder increases in size by repeated deposits on it. Occasionally a foreign body introduced into the bladder forms the nucleus for a stone. The usual composition is of urates, but in alkaline urine phosphates may form the bulk of the stone. The **symptoms** are vesical irritability, enuresis; and often attacks of pain, especially at the close of micturition, felt in the neck of the bladder or at the end of the penis, or in the vagina, rectum or perineum. Tenesmus is frequent both on urination and defecation, and may produce prolapse of the rectum. There may be a sudden arrest of micturition, accompanied by severe pain and straining. Priapism is common, and incontinence may occur and be continuous. As cystitis develops the symptoms grow worse, and the urine exhibits mucus, pus, and red blood-cells in small numbers. Large stones may perhaps be discovered by bimanual palpation with one finger in the rectum. The **prognosis** is uncertain. The only positive **diagnosis** is by cystoscopic or roentgenographic examination, or by exploration with a sound. The **treatment** for large stones is surgical.

FOREIGN BODIES IN THE BLADDER

Occasionally boys and girls, especially at the age of puberty, introduce foreign bodies into the urethra, and these may pass into the bladder. The nature of the bodies is varied, among them being hair-pins, pencils, shot, beads, etc. They may give rise to inflammation or form the basis of a calculus. Treatment usually consists in removal through the operating cystoscope, or operation may be necessary.

CYSTITIS

This affection is not common in older children, but in infants and young children may be combined with pyelitis. The majority of cases of pyelitis, however, exhibit no vesical symptoms. The preponderance of cases of cystitis is in girls. Among causes are vesical calculi, foreign bodies, tumors, rupture of an abscess into the bladder, an ascending spread of the gonococcus or the colon bacillus, or the action of other germs, sometimes transmitted by way of the blood-stream. Cystitis may accompany infectious or intestinal disorders. Chilling of the body appears to be a predisposing cause in some instances. Tuberculous cystitis is uncommon, and is associated with other tuberculous lesions. It is discussed elsewhere (p. 843). The organism oftenest found is the colon bacillus (*colicystitis*). A very rare form is *cystitis emphysematosa*, in which there are gas-containing vesicles in the wall of the bladder (Ravich and Katzen[12]). The constitutional **symptoms** include fever, restlessness, and anorexia. The local disturbance varies in intensity, being greater in older children. In these there are pain and tenderness in the region of the bladder, and painful and frequent urination. The straining may produce prolapse of the rectum, and there may be constant dribbling of urine. In infants the painful urination may be evidenced only by crying. In acute cases the urine is cloudy; usually acid; and contains pus and red blood-cells, mucus, vesical epithelium, bacteria, and albumin in small amounts. In chronic cases pus and mucus are present in larger quantity; the reaction is often alkaline; and crystals of triple phosphate and ammonium urate may be found. The **prognosis** is good when there is a removable cause and the attack is acute. Cases due to the colon bacillus are more favorable than when other germs are present. The disease tends to be prolonged and relapses readily occur, and in chronic cases with thickening of the mucous membrane of the bladder is difficult to cure. The **diagnosis** is usually easily made by study of the symptoms and the examination of the urine. Cystoscopic and roentgenographic examinations assist in discovering the cause and determining the local condition of the wall of the bladder. Pyelitis produces more severe constitutional reactions, less marked local symptoms; and the urine, while containing pus, does not exhibit much mucus or many epithelial cells. The **treatment** consists in search for the cause and its removal if possible. In acute cases rest in bed is needed, with a nonirritating diet and large amounts of water. Urinary antiseptics have been discussed elsewhere (p. 835). Pain and straining may be relieved by hot or cold applications over the bladder, or the administration of opiates or other analgesics if required. In severe and obstinate acute cases, and especially in chronic ones, lavage is indicated, employing boric acid solution (2 to 3 per cent); and later weak solutions of permanganate of potash (1:8000), bichloride of mercury (1:10,000), nitrate of silver (1:6000), or argyrol or silvol (5 per cent). The stronger injections should be left in the bladder for a short time and then washed out with sterile water.

SPASM OF THE BLADDER

This is more frequent in early childhood than later. Among causes are sudden chilling of the body; excitability of the nervous system; vesical calculus; and secretion of highly concentrated urine. It may also be a reflex symptom of renal calculus or of lesions of the rectum, vulva, urethra, hip-joint, appendix, or other neighboring structures. The chief **symptom** in the less frequent form is a spasm of the sphincter, making the child unable to void. More commonly there is irritation of the detrusor apparatus, resulting in frequent emptying of the bladder. The former condition is attended by pain and straining without the passage of urine. In the latter the urine is passed frequently, sometimes only in drops, and there may or may not be pain. There is no alteration in the character of the urine other perhaps than concentration. When dependent upon temporary irritability of the bladder the attack is of short duration. If produced by reflex disturbance, vesical calculus, or the like, the course is variable with a tendency to recurrence. **Treatment** consists in elimination of the cause if possible. When the urine is highly acid alkalies may be given, water should be ingested freely, and atropine or the bromides administered. During spasm of the sphincter hot compresses may be applied over the bladder or a warm bath given, and catheterization done if necessary.

ENURESIS

Incontinence of urine due to organic or similar causes has been considered elsewhere (p. 806). Here will be discussed the lack of control which is dependent, at least in part, upon a neurosis. It is a common disorder occurring, in our experience, in about 5 per cent of children.

Etiology.—By the end of at most the second year every normal child should have learned while awake to void into a vessel, and lapses during sleep should not occur often. If after the age of two years there is frequent bed-wetting, enuresis exists. The age, therefore, at which the disease can begin is two years, and it remains common until about puberty. Sex and race exert little influence. Many cases show the influence of heredity (Grover[13]). Most cases are a persistence of the condition normal to infancy, which period is characterized by a powerful detrusor apparatus and insufficient sphincter control of the bladder. A smaller number begin after normal control has been acquired (20 per cent; Anderson[14]).

In considering the influencing factors it is important to remember that urination is a reflex act, in which are concerned the wall of the bladder, the efferent and afferent nerves connecting this with the spinal centers, and these centers themselves. This reflex arc may be disturbed by irritation in other parts of the body. Finally there is the inhibition exerted by the brain, which is active even during sleep. Disorder of any part of this apparatus may produce enuresis. Among reflex disturbances outside of the direct reflex arc are phimosis; balanitis; a narrow meatus; vulvovaginitis; adherent clitoris; local irritation from masturbation; renal calculus; irritability of the rectum caused by fissures, parasites, inflammation, or the presence of a mass of feces; irritation of any portion of the intestinal canal; adenoids; foreign bodies in the nose, etc. These agencies appear to stimulate the detrusor urinae to contract or the sphincter vesicae to relax. Reflex irritation may arise in the bladder from calculus, cystitis, highly acid urine or overdistention. Another group of causes consists in disturbance of the nerves connecting the bladder with the spinal centers, and of the centers themselves; here belonging the not infrequent cases of occult spina bifida. The fact that enuresis may respond to psychic treatment would appear to justify the belief that some cases are psychogenic. Any agent producing nervous excitability or general debility may be operative, among such being febrile diseases, malnutrition, anemia, chorea, epilepsy, organic central nervous lesions, emotional instability, masturbation, fright or other nervous stress, and various other conditions such as the influence of habit and of thyroid insufficiency. Yet no reflex cause within or without the bladder is sufficient alone to produce enuresis, there apparently being necessary for its action undue excitability of the muscular walls or pathologic weakness of the sphincter.

There remains to be considered the control of the brain. During sleep the complete removal of this may be favored by a number of causes which make the sleep unusually profound, as the ingestion of a hearty evening meal, sleeping on the back, fatigue, or too heavy bed-covers.

Symptoms.—In *enuresis nocturna* the condition exists only during sleep. Patients with *enuresis diurna* are unable to control the bladder during the waking hours. The latter is much less frequent occurring alone, but is often combined to a varying degree with the nocturnal form. From the mild cases with occasional lapses there are all grades up to the inveterate bed-wetters, where scarcely a night passes without the accident occurring from one to several times. Sometimes children dream that they are passing urine, and may then perhaps be awakened by the accident; but as a rule the patient is not roused by the involuntary micturition. Perhaps oftenest the bed-wetting occurs during the first sound sleep before midnight; in others it is toward morning; in others at variable hours.

Diurnal enuresis often develops after nocturnal enuresis has continued for some time. In this form there is a too frequent desire to evacuate the bladder, perhaps coming on so suddenly that the clothing is wet before the child can retire. In bad cases the patient is constantly wet with offensive, decomposing urine. In some children play, exercise, sudden laughing, fright, or other emotion is followed immediately by evacuation of the bladder. Often the patient is of a decidedly neurotic temperament or exhibits some evidence of malnutrition; in other cases some other nervous condition is associated; but in the majority the general health is excellent. Not infrequently the psychic state is affected by the mortification which the disease produces or by the frequently repeated punishment.

Course and Prognosis.—If following an acute illness the disease lasts usually but a short time. If it is the persistence of the infantile condition, the longer it has lasted the more resistant is it to treatment. It is seldom absolutely continuous. Periods of days, weeks or months, especially during the summer, may occur when there is little if any incontinence. Infrequently the disease may appear to be cured, and then redevelop with the establishment of puberty. The majority of cases which come under treatment in early childhood can be cured, although it may require months to accomplish this result. The disorder usually disappears of itself as puberty is approached, and may, indeed, cease at any time before this even without treatment. Occasionally in girls it does not disappear at puberty, and then offers an unfavorable prognosis.

Diagnosis.—Cases of incontinence of urine due to malformations or to paralysis of the bladder suffer from dribbling of the urine. In enuresis in the narrower sense the urine is always passed in a stream. The cause can often be discovered by careful study. Nocturnal enuresis occurring at long intervals is sometimes merely a symptom of nocturnal epilepsy, as pointed out by Pfister,[15] and is not to be classed with the ordinary enuresis of childhood. Persistent enuresis occurring both by day and night may be due to spina bifida occulta.

Treatment.—It must be emphasized that the causes are so diverse and so often combined that therapy should be varied and suited to the individual case. First to be sought for and treated is any possible cause or influencing factor. It must be admitted, however, that the treatment of such supposed agents as enlarged tonsils and adenoids, phimosis, eye-strain, malnutrition and the like seldom influence the enuresis.

The *general hygiene* and *method of life* are to be carefully supervised. The child should pass much time in exercise in the open. Sometimes a temporary change of residence benefits promptly. All mental overwork and all undue excitement must be avoided. The child with diurnal enuresis should not be sent to school, since his trouble makes him the object of ridicule, and this reacts upon his psychic state; and children with nocturnal enuresis must avoid school also, if it is found to be too much of a strain upon the general health. Punishments only exceptionally do good but usually have the opposite effect. The child must be encouraged in every way, and assured that he can and will recover; and perhaps be rewarded when he has been successful. In this connection the value of suggestion, hypnotic or of other nature, may be referred to. We have even known the suggestion that he shall not wet the bed, whispered to the child in a state of natural sleep, to be of service; and Dunham[16] reports a series of cases benefited by having the child repeat several times daily such sentences as "I am not going to wet the bed," and the like. The *diet* should be of a nonirritating nature, with the absence of food liable to produce indigestion, constipation, or a highly acid urine. Liquid of any sort should be restricted after about 4 P.M. The child should *sleep* in a well-ventilated room and retire early, but too profound sleep is to be avoided. The bed-covering should therefore be rather too light than too heavy, the bed too hard rather than too comfortably soft, and fatigue before retiring should be avoided. Attention to *general health* is necessary. Cool morning baths have a stimulating effect. A cold douche to the spine before retiring is sometimes serviceable. All possible causative factors, such as malnutrition, anemia, disordered state of the nervous system, and the like, must receive appropriate treatment.

Local treatment may be important. Adhesions of the prepuce or clitoris may need to be broken up; phimosis may require correction; vulvovaginitis should be treated; the local irritation from masturbation prevented. An evacuation of the bowels before the child goes to bed should be procured if possible, and the presence of seat-worms excluded. Examination of the urine may show that pyelitis, cystitis, or calculus demands treatment. If the urine is highly acid, alkalies may be administered and the amount of meat ingested restricted; with water given in large amounts rather than curtailed. In most cases, however, the urine is secreted in large quantity and the fluid intake should be diminished. In nocturnal enuresis the child should be taken from bed several times in the night; if possible before unconscious urination occurs, the habit of continence thus being established. To avoid urinary pressure on the neck of the bladder there should be no pillows beneath the head; the foot of the bed should be elevated; and the patient prevented from sleeping on the back by tying a large spool over the spinal column. In the daytime the child should be taught to retain the urine as long as possible. The sphincter may be strengthened by having the child stop and start the stream several times during the act of urination.

Various sorts of local treatment of the bladder have been recommended to increase the tone of the sphincter or to diminish the hypersensitiveness of the nervous apparatus. Many of these act by their psychic effect. The passage of sounds of large size is one procedure, and has proven effective in obstinate cases. The employment of the faradic current has also been strongly recommended, one pole being placed over the bladder and the other in the rectum or vagina, or sometimes in the urethra itself. Cauterization of the neck of the bladder, or, in girls, of the meatus has also been advised, as has massage of the neck of the bladder through the rectum or by deep pressure over the lower abdomen. Circumcision has been recommended even when no phimosis exists. Finally is to be mentioned the epidural injection of normal salt-solution, as used by Cathelin,[17] Hintze[18] and others, with which success has repeatedly been obtained. For girls past puberty and with enuresis persisting, the bladder may have become unusually small and unable to retain a normal amount of urine. In such cases dilatation by the injection of increasing amounts of a boric acid solution may be tried, as used successfully by Thompson.[19] None of these more radical methods mentioned are to be employed except in obstinate cases which have resisted other forms of treatment.

Treatment with drugs is often very effective; often of no value whatever. That remedy should be chosen which counteracts the action of the cause. Thus strychnine is useful when there is a lack of tone in the sphincter; atropine when there is excessive irritability of the detrusor apparatus; iron or arsenic if there is anemia; alkalies when the urine is highly acid. As, however, it is often impossible to determine the exact cause or causes at work, the drug-treatment of the disease is to a large extent empirical, and a number of remedies have been advocated. Of all of them atropine is one of the most successful, since it lowers the pressure in the bladder and influences the amplitude and frequency of contractions (Amberg and Grob[20]). A useful method is to prepare an aqueous solution of which each minim (0.062) contains $\frac{1}{2000}$ grain (0.00003) of atropine. The initial dose at five or six years of age may be 4 minims, or even less owing to the idiosyncrasy to atropine sometimes encountered. This dose should be rapidly increased day by day, remembering that a large drop, from the edge of the bottle, equals approximately 1 minim. Children generally tolerate atropine in relatively large dosage, and enough must be given either to control the enuresis or to produce the physiologic effect, especially the flushing of the forehead. Pushing the remedy beyond this amount is not advisable. It may be administered three times a day, or better, in cases of nocturnal enuresis, the first dose late in the afternoon and a second just before getting into bed. It is important to hold the dosage at a maximum for a number of weeks, even if the result is good, and after that to diminish it very gradually. Sodium bromide, antipyrine, phenobarbital, and the like may be given in combination with the atropine. In other cases where the trouble appears to depend upon the sphincter alone, or in combination with the detrusor, strychnine may be given, perhaps combined with atropine.

Among other remedies recommended and of service in some instances are tincture of rhus aromatica, humulus, ergot, valerian, zinc, chloral, hyoscine, phenacetin, and sulphonal. Thyroid extract has been given, but should be used with caution unless the basal metabolic rate is known. Pituitary extract (posterior lobe) given hypodermically has been claimed by Jacobs[21] and others to cause improvement.

TUBERCULOSIS OF THE BLADDER

This affection may infrequently be found in childhood in combination with or secondary to tuberculosis of other parts of the genito-urinary apparatus, especially the kidney; or may be associated with tuberculosis in some more distant region. It is rarely primary. It appears in the form of scattered, small grayish, or larger caseous nodules, and of ulcers in the mucous membrane. The clinical manifestations are those of chronic cystitis with hematuria. The diagnosis can be made by the discovery of tubercle bacilli in the urine or by cystoscopic examination.

MORBID GROWTHS OF THE BLADDER

These are uncommon in early life and may be primary or oftener secondary. Steinmetz[22] could collect but 32 reports of primary cases. The most frequent growths are sarcoma and myxoma, and papilloma has also been observed. As the growth develops the symptoms of cystitis are liable to appear, hematuria being common. Palpation per rectum may aid in the diagnosis if the tumor is of considerable size; or a cystoscopic examination may be made. The growth may spread to the prostate or the vagina, or may give rise to pyelonephritis, hydronephrosis, or peritonitis. Removal offers the only hope of cure.

References

1. J.A.M.A., 1930, **94,** 1373. 2. Bull. Johns Hopkins Hosp., 1922, **33,** 440. 3. Inaug. Dissert. Berl., 1885. Ref. Baginsky, Lehrb. d. Kinderkr., 1902, 1020. 4. Gerhardt's Handb. d. Kinderkr. **4,** 3, 580; Jahrb. f. Kinderh., 1895, **40,** 32. 5. Arch. espanoles de pediat., 1918, Feb. Ref. Arch. de méd. d. enf., 1918, **21,** 657. 6. Internat.

J. Surg., 1920, **33**, 389. 7. J.A.M.A., 1921, **77**, 1071. 8. J. Urology, 1922, **8**, 171. 9. Gaz. hébdom. d. sc. méd. de Bordeaux, 1928, **49**, 203. 10. J.A.M.A., 1930, **94**, 1753. 11. Am. J. Dis. Child. 1930, **40**, 804. 12. J.A.M.A., 1932, **98**, 1256. 13. J.A.M.A., 1918, **71**, 626. 14. Am. J. Dis. Child., 1930, **40**, 591, 818. 15. Monatschr. f. Psychiat. u. Neurol., 1905, **15**, 113. 16. Am. J. Dis. Child., 1916, **12**, 618. 17. Thèse de Paris, 1902. 18. Mitt. aus. d. Grenzgeb. d. Med. u. Chir., **35**, 484. Ref. Jahrb. f. Kinderh., 1923, **101**, 356. 19. Brit. J. Child. Dis., 1922, **19**, 10. 20. Am. J. Dis. Child., 1931, **41**, 507. 21. Pennsylvania M. J., 1922, **25**, 867. 22. Deutsche Ztschr. f. Chir., 1894, **39**, 313.

CHAPTER IV

DISEASES OF THE GENITAL ORGANS

ADHERENT PREPUCE

In the majority of new-born male infants there is more or less adherence between the inner lining of the prepuce and the glans. When this persists it may be considered pathologic. The adhesions may be complete, or involve only the posterior portion of the glans. The smegma collects behind the corona and may be the cause of irritation, producing priapism, painful urination, or balanitis. The condition should be treated in the new-born by forcible retraction of the foreskin, followed by cleansing and the application of a bland ointment, and the drawing of the foreskin forward. After this the prepuce should be retracted daily sufficiently to expose the sulcus behind the corona, always pulling the foreskin forward again. (See Paraphimosis, p. 845.) If the adhesions are allowed to become firm, separation with a blunt probe is required.

PHIMOSIS

This consists in a narrowing of the prepucial opening sufficient to prevent retraction. In rare cases there is no opening whatever. Adhesions may be combined with phimosis. The prepuce may be of normal length, or much elongated and hypertrophied (*redundant prepuce*), the latter not necessarily accompanied by phimosis. When the opening of the prepuce is very small urination can be accomplished only by straining; the urine flows in drops or a very small stream; and if adhesions are not present, the foreskin during micturition is ballooned by the urine beneath it. Hernia or prolapse of the rectum may be produced by the straining, and there may develop inflammation of the urethra, pyelitis, or, rarely, hydronephrosis or pyonephrosis. Ramaroni[1] reports a case of phimosis with 45 calcareous concretions distending the prepuce. In the majority of cases urination is not difficult, but the inability to keep the mucous membrane clean commonly leads to posthitis or balanitis, with consequent dysuria from the swelling. The persistence of a constant degree of irritation readily leads to masturbation. Among conditions attributed to phimosis are enuresis, insomnia, night-terrors, digestive disturbances, convulsions, epilepsy, and various neuroses. The influence of phimosis in many of these is certainly over-rated. Even a decided degree of phimosis may be present and produce no symptoms at all, or at the most those of slight local irritation. In many cases **treatment** by forcible retraction or stretching with dressing forceps is sufficient, or the preputial orifice may be widened by incision, or preferably circumcision performed. A redundant prepuce without phimosis does not necessitate circumcision. Although circumcision removes the necessity of constant care for cleanliness, it is much disputed whether it is a procedure without subsequent disadvantages. The operation by no means prevents the habit of masturbation.

PARAPHIMOSIS AND STRANGULATION OF THE PENIS

In this condition the prepuce, which has been retracted beyond the corona, cannot readily be replaced. The circulation in the glans is interfered with by the constriction, and edema and bluish discoloration and even gangrene develop. There are the attending symptoms of pain and dysuria. The accident follows usually the retraction of the prepuce by the patient himself, or by the mother or nurse when cleansing the organ. Cold compresses should be applied to reduce the swelling, and an effort made to draw the foreskin forward into the normal position. To aid in this the glans should be well oiled, steadily compressed, and a smooth instrument such as a grooved director or, in emergency, the curved end of a sterilized metal hairpin, slipped under the constricting skin. This serves as a starting-point for the replacement. If this procedure does not succeed, incision of the constricting ring of skin at the rear of the swelling may be required. If the foreskin is unduly narrow, circumcision should follow. A condition similar to that of paraphimosis or involving a larger portion of the penis may be produced by the patient tying a string around the organ, or slipping a ring or other object over it. The treatment consists in division of the constricting body.

ABNORMAL SIZE OF THE PENIS

The size of the penis varies greatly. Sometimes in infancy the organ appears to be unusually small, due to a large deposit of fat in the mons and scrotum, which partially buries the penis from view. In other cases there is a decided retardation in the development of the organ, which as puberty approaches may assume its normal size. In infantilism (p. 1085) the penis may remain small, or, on the contrary, become greatly hypertrophied, as in certain cases of physical precocity (p. 1091), and tumors of the suprarenal gland (p. 1082) or pineal gland (p. 1079).

BALANOPOSTHITIS

Inflammation of the prepuce (posthitis) and glans (balanitis) is oftenest produced by phimosis, resulting in retention of smegma. It may follow injury caused by masturbation, or occur as a complication of urethritis. A diphtheritic balanoposthitis is sometimes seen. The prepuce becomes red, edematous, and itching, with the orifice narrowed and the mucous membrane producing a purulent secretion. There is dysuria, and cystitis or hydronephrosis may result in severe cases. In ordinary cases the inflammation lasts but a few days. **Treatment** consists in the injection of a solution of boric acid or one of potassium permanganate, 1:8000, under the foreskin; after which a little boric acid ointment or zinc ointment may be worked in with a probe. In severer cases cold compresses should be applied to reduce the swelling. In the worst instances splitting the foreskin or circumcision is necessary.

MALFORMATIONS OF THE URETHRA

Hypospadias.—In this congenital malformation the urethra opens on the lower surface of the penis behind the glans, or in the body of the organ; while in the worst cases it is in the perineum, sometimes as a fissure, the scrotum being split into halves. As the penis is usually rudimentary in such cases and the testicles undescended, the appearance of the external genitals strongly suggests that of the female (*pseudohermaphroditism*).

Treatment is surgical, and in many cases a plastic operation is successful. Rarely an analogous condition is seen in girls, the opening of the urethra being within the vagina just behind the hymen, or still farther inside.

Epispadias.—In this uncommon congenital anomaly the opening of the urethra is upon the dorsal surface of the penis. It may be small and just behind the glans in the less severe cases; or in the form of a fissure the entire length of the penis, and is then combined with exstrophy of the bladder. Treatment is surgical.

Other Anomalies.—A congenital **atresia of the urethra** may range in degree from mere closure of the meatus by adhesions to complete obliteration. Patulous urachus or exstrophy of the bladder may accompany the latter. There may be a congenitally **narrow urethra,** perhaps only at the meatus; or a cylindrical narrowing of some portion of the canal. Boyd[2] claims that congenital stricture of the meatus in the female is quite common. **Acquired stricture** may be the result of a gonorrheal urethritis, or rarely of cicatricial contraction from other causes. **Urethral diverticulum** or a **valve-like obstruction** is not uncommon. (Bókay;[3] Frontz;[4] Bigler;[5] Addison;[6] Kretschmer and Pierson;[7] Campbell.[8]) The end result of urethral obstruction of any sort, if continued, is dilatation of the bladder and ureters, and hydronephrosis. **Fusion of the urethra and intestine** may occur (p. 1037). **Urethral fistula** is rare, and may be congenital or be due to injury by a calculus or foreign body in the urethra, or to trauma. The external opening of the fistula may be in the penis, in the perineum, or elsewhere.

URETHRITIS

This is not common in early life. Simple urethritis may be due to extension of inflammation from balanoposthitis; to irritation by highly acid urine; or to introduction of foreign bodies into the urethra or other onanistic acts. Specific urethritis is due to the gonococcus. The latter, like the simple form, is seen oftener in females, in whom it is secondary to gonorrheal vaginitis, although by no means occurring in every case of this. We[9] saw one instance in a boy of three months, and collected 132 instances of gonorrheal urethritis in male infants, and others have since been reported. The **symptoms** are dysuria, swelling and redness of the urethral orifice, and discharge of pus from it. In the simple form the **course** is usually short; in the gonorrheal cases much longer and there are liable to develop balanitis, sometimes proctitis, and rarely epididymitis, arthritis, and conjunctivitis. Stricture may be a sequel. The **diagnosis** between the two forms is made by bacteriological examination. **Treatment** consists in the administration of alkalies, in keeping the parts clean, and, in gonorrheal cases, the same therapy as for adults. A protective dressing should be worn to prevent extension and the carrying of the infection to the eyes.

INFLAMMATION OF THE EXTERNAL URETHRAL ORIFICE

This condition, probably due to ammoniacal urine, is quite common, and apparently confined to circumcised infants. It causes dysuria and a tendency to retention of urine. Even superficial ulceration of the orifice may be produced (Brennemann,[10] Bokay[11]). In the line of **treatment** the reaction of the urine should be altered. If the diet is high in fat, this should be reduced and the carbohydrate increased. A thick layer of bland ointment should be applied locally and the diaper should not be tight-fitting.

FOREIGN BODIES IN THE URETHRA; URETHRAL CALCULUS

Not infrequently a stone, after its passage from the kidney and bladder, becomes impacted in the urethra, oftenest in the membranous portion of the penis. Englisch[12] analyzes the reports of 405 such cases. Foreign bodies may be introduced into the urethra, oftenest by boys during later childhood, and become impacted there. The **symptoms** depend somewhat upon the size and character of the stone or foreign body. There is dysuria and obstruction to the flow of urine. Urethritis may develop, perhaps with periurethritis and infiltration of urine into surrounding tissues, and the flow of urine may then be entirely cut off. The detrusor force of the bladder may finally succeed in expelling smooth calculi and foreign bodies, but frequently surgical interference is necessary.

INFLAMMATION OF THE SCROTUM

The most common cause of this is irritation from uncleanliness in the case of infants, but the scrotum may also be attacked by eczema or erysipelas, or become diseased by contiguity with inflammations of neighboring structures. The scrotum becomes intensely red, and, owing to the laxness of the tissues, much swollen. The inflammation may be of an erythematous nature, as when due to eczema, or may become phlegmonous and abscess develop. **Treatment** consists chiefly in cleanliness and in keeping the scrotum dry with mild antiseptic powders and leaving the parts exposed to the air. In severe inflammation wet dressings may be indicated. Eczematous and erysipelatous processes require treatment appropriate for these diseases. Surgical procedures are necessary if abscess develops.

GENITAL EDEMA

The cause of this unusual condition is not understood. It was first described by Zappert[13] and has been discussed by Friedjung,[14] Ylppö,[15] Petényi,[16] and Woringer.[17] It occurs especially in premature infants, and consists in noninflammatory edema of the entire genital region, perhaps extending over the abdomen and thighs, and appearing at any time in the first month or two of life. It usually disappears in a few days, but may last a month or more. The disorder is differentiated from sclerema by the limitation and the good general condition; from erysipelas by the lack of inflammation and the good prognosis. No particular treatment is indicated.

UNDESCENDED TESTICLE

The testis should descend into the scrotum in the 8th month of fetal life, but in about 0.1 to 0.7 per cent of males (Willard,[18] Southam and Cooper[19]), arrest in the advance of one or both testes takes place and the organ may remain within the abdomen (*cryptorchidism*) or, more frequently, in the inguinal canal (*retentio inguinalis*). Infrequently it may wander into some abnormal position (*ectopia testis*), oftenest the perineum. The subject of undescended testicle is reviewed exhaustively by Wangensteen.[20] A testis retained in the inguinal canal may descend into the scrotum in the course of some weeks or months, but if this has not taken place by the third year, it is unlikely to do so later. When in the inguinal canal the organ is a small, movable body, and may be mistaken for hernia, by which, in fact, it is accompanied in one-half or more of the cases. It may be complicated also by hydrocele or torsion of the spermatic cord (p. 848). Its exposed position subjects it to trauma, and renders it more subject than a normally placed testicle to malignant degeneration. A testicle remaining persistently out of place finally becomes atrophic and functionally useless, and does not secrete semen. In continued double cryptochidism the patient will probably be sterile, but only occasionally is the development of masculine characteristics interfered with. **Treatment** is not required in infancy, since the testis may descend of itself. By the end of the third year, or certainly before puberty, operation should be performed in bilateral cases, with the attempt to transplant the organ into its normal position. In unilateral cases operation is not so imperative, but is indicated if there is hernia or persistent pain. Ordinarily the testis should not be removed, but replaced in the abdominal cavity when it cannot be transplanted to the scrotum.

HYPERORCHIDISM

In this rare condition more than the normal number of testicles is present. Haas[21] reports an instance of a third testicle and collects 6 other cases confirmed by necropsy.

ORCHITIS. EPIDIDYMITIS

An **acute orchitis** is occasionally seen in children, the result of trauma, rheumatism, and infectious fevers, especially mumps. Gonorrhea is more liable to produce **epididymitis** than orchitis (Mitchell and Quinn,[9] Weisner[22]). Epididymitis may also be due to the staphylococcus, streptococcus, and other organisms (Campbell[23]). The prognosis of both orchitis and epididymitis is favorable unless suppuration occurs. Atrophy and subsequent sterility of the involved side may result. The testicle should be elevated and cold wet dressings applied. **Syphilitic orchitis** runs a more chronic course, is painless and does not suppurate, and is not infrequent in cases of hereditary syphilis.

TORSION OF THE SPERMATIC CORD

This is more common in incompletely descended testes. Sloughing and infection and subsequent atrophy may occur. It must be differentiated from epididymo-orchitis, strangulated hernia, and inguinal adenitis. It has been described particularly by Mouchet,[24] Feldstein,[25] and Donovan.[26]

MORBID GROWTHS OF THE TESTIS AND PROSTATE GLAND

Neoplasms of the **testis** are infrequent in early life, but may even be congenital (Steffen;[27] Kutzmann and Gibson[28]). The majority are malignant (13 collected cases; Steffen[27]), carcinoma being more common than sarcoma. Usually only one testis is affected, and those undescended somewhat more frequently than others. The scrotum becomes involved and the growth becomes nodular and ulcerated, and metastasis may occur. Early operation and radiologic treatment are indicated, but recurrence is frequent. Malignant tumors of the **prostate gland,** usually carcinomatous, are rare, Steffen[27] having collected reports of but 6 cases.

HYDROCELE

This common disorder consists in an accumulation of fluid around the testis or the spermatic cord. It may be congenital or acquired; the latter, less frequent in children than the former, being produced by pressure, inflammation, or injury. Several varieties are encountered:

1. Communicating Congenital Hydrocele.—In this common form the extension of the serous membrane from the peritoneal cavity has never become closed above and a communication exists, either freely or through a very small opening.

2. Communicating Hydrocele of the Cord (*Communicating Funicular Hydrocele*).—In this comparatively uncommon variety, also of congenital origin, the pouch containing the fluid is shut off from the testis below, but communicates with the peritoneal cavity above.

3. Infantile Hydrocele (*Hydrocele of the Tunica Vaginalis Testis*).—This title is applied to a collection of fluid in the tunica vaginalis, the communication with the peritoneal cavity having been cut off, making it irreducible. It is one of the commonest varieties.

4. Encysted Hydrocele of the Cord.—Here the funicular process of the peritoneum is closed both above and below, forming a sac containing liquid in the course of the cord, with the testis below it.

5. Hydrocele of the Canal of Nuck.—This is a variety occasionally seen in females. It develops in the peritoneal process, which, in the fetus, surrounds the round ligament.

Symptoms and Diagnosis.—**Communicating congenital hydrocele** forms a swelling extending throughout the whole length of the cord to the lower part of the scrotum. The testis is at the posterior part of this and rather high. The fluid may be present at birth or may not be discoverable until later. It is readily reducible, either spontaneously, by gravity, or by pressure. This makes the condition readily mistaken for hernia, with which it is, indeed, often combined. In contrast with hernia, however, the swelling is dull on percussion, more fluctuating, translucent, and does not under manipulation slip back suddenly into the peritoneal cavity with a gurgling sound.

Communicating hydrocele of the cord forms a small, elastic, fluctuating, elongated swelling above the scrotum. It is reducible like hernia, but is distinguished in the same way as in the form just described. After reduction the cavity soon refills. The testicle is in the normal position near the bottom of the scrotum. Hernia may complicate the condition.

Infantile hydrocele presents an accumulation of fluid filling the scrotum and forming an oval, elastic, fluctuating, tense, translucent sac. The spermatic cord and ring can be distinctly felt above it. The testis is posterior and rather high in position. The swelling is irreducible and not affected by cough or position, and is in other respects distinguished from hernia by the characteristics described for the first variety of hydrocele.

Encysted hydrocele of the cord forms a small cyst, spindle-shaped or globular, suggesting often an undescended testis, small hernia, lymphatic gland, or a tumor of some sort. From the testis it is distinguished by its translucency and by the finding of this organ in its normal position in the scrotum; from a lymphatic gland or tumor by its elasticity and translucency; and from hernia by the same qualities together with its irreducibility and dulness on percussion.

It may happen, however, that in hernia the intestine may sometimes be distended by gas and be somewhat translucent, thus, perhaps, making repeated examinations necessary to establish a diagnosis. Further, two forms of hydrocele may be combined, or the sac of a congenital hydrocele with a large opening into the peritoneal cavity may contain fluid at one time and intestine at another.

The **prognosis** in early life is good, the majority of cases, especially of the communicating forms, recovering of themselves in a few weeks or months. If not, treatment, which consists in applying a truss, will usually effect a cure by producing a mild obliterating inflammation. Irritating local solutions should not be applied. It is not often that aspiration or operation of any sort is necessary in early life.

TUBERCULOSIS OF THE MALE GENITAL ORGANS

Tuberculosis of the prepuce may be acquired through ritual circumcision (Holt,[29] Reuben,[30] Wolff[31]). General tuberculosis is very likely to follow. **Tuberculosis of the testis** has been reported by Dreschfeld;[32] Jullien;[33] Kantorowicz;[34] and Poissonier.[35] The disease may even be congenital, is seen in childhood oftenest in the first two years of life, but is generally less common in early life than in adults. It is usually unilateral, may be primary or secondary, and trauma may be a predisposing cause. The testis with the epididymis becomes enlarged and hard and the scrotum discolored. The process later may undergo absorption or, especially in infants, break down. The course is protracted and tuberculosis of other parts of the body may develop. Treatment is constitutional as well as local; a suppurating testis being removed only if other means fail.

DISORDERS OF THE BREASTS

The frequent presence of milk in the breasts soon after birth, and the common development of **mastitis** at this age, has already been described (p. 241). Later mastitis may occasionally result from trauma or infection. **Absence of the breasts** is extremely uncommon, and is usually combined with other malformations such as would affect ectodermal tissues. **Supernumerary breasts** are more frequently seen. They occur in either sex, oftenest on the trunk and just below the normal breast or sometimes in the axilla or elsewhere. Four breasts is the most frequent number reported. The condition may be hereditary. **Early enlargement of the breasts,** apart from the temporary condition in the new-born alluded to, is seen oftenest as an accompaniment of precocious menstruation (p. 854). However, it occasionally occurs independently of this, either in the female or male. **Tumors of the breast** in early life are rare. Those reported comprise angioma, fibroadenoma, carcinoma, sarcoma, and cysts. (See Jopson and Speese.[36])

MALFORMATIONS OF THE VULVA, VAGINA AND CLITORIS

Atresia of the vulva is rare. There may be only epithelial adhesions of the greater or lesser labia, or there may be a firmer union, which, if not complete, will cause a retention of mucous secretion, and later of the menstrual discharge; and if complete will also interfere with the passage of urine. A similar result in the retaining of menstrual discharge is produced by an **imperforate hymen.** Sometimes there is an **absence of the vagina** through a considerable part of its extent. In any of these conditions operative measures are required. Adhesions between the labia often need only to be broken up by the employment of a probe, if they do not become detached spontaneously. Malformations of the vulva or vagina are often associated with those of the rectum, anus and bladder, and communication may exist between the vagina and the rectum or bladder. There is frequently **adherence between the labia and the clitoris** sometimes causing irritation from the retained smegma, with a consequent reflex nervous condition or masturbation. With a probe the adhesions can be readily broken up. In pseudohermaphroditism there is decided **hypertrophy of the clitoris. Congenital fissure of the clitoris** is a rare condition usually seen in combination with fissure of the urethra.

VULVOVAGINITIS

This disease is one of the most common affections of girls. It occurs in two forms: (1) Simple, and (2) Gonorrheal, the latter by far the most frequent. A dissenting opinion is that of Stein, Leventhal and Sered,[37] who could prove as gonorrheal only 20 per cent of 296 cases of vaginitis.

1. Simple Vulvovaginitis (Nongonorrheal).—This, while occurring even in the newborn as the result of the normal desquamative process, is more frequent after infancy has passed. It is then caused by uncleanliness;

traumatism; masturbation; eczema; thread-worms, trichomonas or other parasites in the vaginal canal; anemia and other debilitating influences; and the various infectious fevers. The vesicles of varicella may appear upon the mucous membrane of the vagina, and in measles a catarrhal inflammation may develop. Germs of various sorts other than the gonococcus are the active agents, and at times the thrush fungus (Plass, Hesseltine and Borts[38]). We have seen Döderlein's bacillus in pure culture and apparently pathogenic. The **symptoms** are redness and swelling of the internal and external genitalia. There is a vaginal discharge which is scanty or abundant, thin or purulent, and often offensive in odor. If the cause can be removed, the **prognosis** is good; but in debilitated subjects the discharge continues for a long time in spite of treatment. The **diagnosis** of the simple form from the gonococcic lies in the greater involvement of the vulva; the slight degree of contagiousness; and the absence of complications and of the gonococcus in the discharge (p. 852). The **treatment** consists primarily in the search for and removal of the cause. Cases associated with debility demand tonic remedies, and possibly change of air. Locally the treatment is much the same as for the gonorrheal form (p. 852). A 1 per cent aqueous solution of gentian violet may be used locally for infection by the thrush fungus, combined with alkaline douches. In trichomonas infection lactic acid (0.5 per cent) douches are employed.

2. Gonorrheal Vulvovaginitis.—This disease is especially common in infancy and in the first five years of life. It is impossible to estimate its incidence, but from figures gathered by Yesko[39] it would seem that from 2 to 10 per cent of young girls in institutions suffer from it. Blum[40] claims that there is a seasonal incidence, with the peak in winter and spring. In infants the disease may be acquired during the process of birth, or later from a mother with a gonorrheal discharge; or may spread in other ways, as by the hands or garments of the attendant, or by infected bath-tubs, diapers, bed clothing, wash cloths, or thermometers. It is commoner among the poor on account of lesser cleanliness, but is not infrequent among those in apparently good hygienic surroundings. In girls past the period of infancy it may be acquired by sleeping with a mother or sister who has gonorrhea, or by contaminated water-closet seats or baths. The contracting of the disorder by any sort of sexual act is uncommon in children.

The acting organism is one which has the characteristics of the gonococcus as seen in adults. Yet the lesser intensity of the inflammation in children as compared with adults, the infrequency of complications, and the failure of attendants to contract the disease from patients, suggest either that the virulence of the germ as it occurs in early life is greatly modified, or that it is a different strain of gonococcus from that which infects the adult. Pearce[41] by studies of agglutination and complement-fixation tests found a difference between the adult and infantile type of gonococcus. The two types were found active in early life; the adult, capable, for instance, of producing ophthalmia as a complication; the other, much the most frequent at this period, never doing this.

Symptoms.—In milder cases there may be only a small amount of thin discharge, but in others this is abundant, yellow, and purulent. The mucous membrane of the vulva and vagina is inflamed, and there may be involvement of the urethra and of the rectum. Ordinarily there is little or no discomfort, but in severe cases there may be fever, dysuria, and excoriation of the skin of the vulva and thighs.

Course and Prognosis.—Although seldom serious, the disease is tedious and a source of great anxiety and often of unwarranted mortification to the parents. It appears to recover of itself as time passes, and apparently leaves no permanent after-effects. There is considerable evidence (Frank,[42]

Dooley[43]) that the disease seldom if ever is carried over the age of puberty or causes sterility. Recovery as puberty is approached may depend upon the development of more mature squamous epithelium (Norris and Mikelberg[44]). From six to ten weeks is required for the cure of the acute stage, but months or even years may elapse before complete recovery takes place. Relapses are common, and between them the disease is latent, but may be infectious. It is such cases that spread the disease in institutions.

Complications.—Serious complications are much less frequent than in adult life, and occur chiefly in later childhood. In a series of 188 collected cases, we[45] found the percentage of complications of all sorts to be 13.3 per cent. Among the more common are inguinal adenitis, urethritis, and proctitis (Flugel,[46] Stumpke[47]). Much less common are cystitis, pyelonephritis, endometritis, salpingitis, peritonitis, arthritis (see p. 1008), gonorrheal septicemia, and gonorrheal rhinitis (Miller[48]). Gonorrheal ophthalmia is observed with surprising infrequency, and chiefly in new-born infants, where there is a possibility that the condition had been acquired during birth.

Diagnosis.—All leukorrheal discharges, particularly in infancy and early childhood, should be considered as gonorrheal until proven otherwise. A smear negative for the gonococcus, especially one carelessly taken, does not rule out gonorrheal vaginitis. The material for examination should be secured from the vagina itself, or the cervix of the uterus, preferably through a speculum or a small vaginoscope (Levy[49]). Another procedure is to fill a syringe or a medicine dropper with normal salt solution, insert this into the vagina, after several flushings centrifuge the fluid, and examine the stained sediment.

Treatment. *Prophylaxis.*—Before any female patient is admitted to a hospital ward, and perhaps to other institutions, the vaginal secretion should be examined for gonococci. Every child who is in a hospital and develops leukorrheal discharge should be examined in the same way and, in order to diagnose cases which have been latent on admission, it would be well to repeat such examinations every week or two. It is necessary to remember that occasionally urethritis in the male or, more frequently proctitis in either sex, may be the focus from which infection spreads. Rarely a gonorrheal conjunctivitis or rhinitis may act in the same way.

In hospitals individual service for every patient should be established, in so far as possible, in the matter of thermometers and other toilet articles. A single-service diaper made of cotton, absorbent gauze, or paper, which can be destroyed after use, should be employed instead of the ordinary textile one; or the latter, if used, be disinfected before going to the general laundry. The U-shaped toilet-seat should be recommended, and individual paper protectors used. Spray-baths are preferable to tub-baths. All of these precautions should be applied, if possible, as routine hospital practice.

A patient with vaginitis or other gonorrheal discharge must be treated in a separate ward or institution, since apparently even the greatest precautions will not otherwise prevent spread of the disease. When a case develops in a home, or institution other than a hospital, the same principles should be followed. School authorities should be familiar with the disease and its implications; and, while too radical measures cannot be adopted, U-shaped toilet-seats and, if possible, paper protectors should be provided, and the sanitation of the washroom carefully supervised.

Treatment of the Attack.—Locally scrupulous cleanliness should be observed. The vulva and, with a small catheter, the vagina, should be douched daily, employing a saturated solution of boric acid; potassium permanganate (1:8000); corrosive sublimate (1:10,000); acriflavine (1:1000); or mercurochrome (1 per cent). Following this a 25 per cent solution of argyrol or other silver preparation should be instilled; elevating the hips in order to keep the solution retained as long as possible. Suppositories of 25 per cent argyrol or 1 to 2 per cent mercurochrome may be used. Norris and Mikelberg[44] employed a 1 per cent Dakin's solution in olive oil, of which about 3 drams were introduced night and morning. Schauffler[50] recommends instilling to the point of distention a 1 per cent solution of silver nitrate in anhydrous wool-fat. In cases with infection of the cervix and the urethra, local applications should be given through a small vaginoscope. Any treatment must be continued for two or three months, although not as frequently as in the beginning. Following an apparent cure vaginal smears should be taken every two or three months for at least a year because of the tendency to relapse. It should be emphasized that too vigorous and often repeated treatment may have a bad psychic effect and is not always necessary. In fact, we have frequently noted improvement with little local treatment when attention was given to the general health of the patient.

Among other treatments is that recommended by Weiss[51] which consists in subjecting the patient to baths at a temperature of 41 C. (105.8 F.), this being based upon the principle that the growth of the gonococcus is retarded at this temperature. The secondary effects of this treatment have often been found too severe to justify it (Kaiser;[52] Schultz[53]). Courtin[54] uses malarial treatment to induce fever. *Vaccine treatment* has been extensively employed. While it seems of value in some cases, its success is not sufficient to warrant its routine use.

3. Herpetic Vulvitis (*Aphthous Vulvitis*).—This disease consists in the development of numerous small vesicles, soon becoming placques and in a few days superficial ulcers, situated on the cutaneous and mucous vulvar surfaces, and often upon neighboring parts. It is most frequent in infancy or early childhood, in unhealthy or neglected subjects, and after infectious diseases, especially measles. It is sometimes seen in nephritis. The ulcers may coalesce and cause pain and itching and a vaginal discharge. Under treatment the disease disappears in a few days, although rarely gangrene develops. The **treatment** consists in keeping the parts clean, and in the application of iodoform or of zinc oxide and starch in powder or ointment form.

4. Phlegmonous Vulvitis (*Abscess of the Vulva*).—This is the result of trauma, erysipelas, or the extension of inflammation from a vaginitis. The external labium on one or both sides becomes red, tender, swollen, and usually develops pus. The general constitutional symptoms of inflammation are present. **Treatment** consists in the application of cold compresses, or in incision if necessary.

5. Gangrenous Vulvitis (*Noma pudendi*).—By this title is designated a gangrenous condition analogous to noma seen in the mouth. It occurs in conditions of malnutrition, especially after infectious diseases as measles or erysipelas, or it may follow aphthous inflammation. Spirochetes and fusiform bacilli may sometimes be found. A swollen, tense, dark-red area which proceeds to gangrene appears on one of the external labia. In severe cases the process spreads with great rapidity. There are pain, fever, and great prostration, followed by death. In mild cases the process is limited to a small area which heals with cicatricial deformity. **Treatment** consists in supportive measures and in prompt excision followed by cauterization.

6. Diphtheritic Vulvovaginitis.—Occasionally diphtheria involves the female external genitals either as a primary disease or as a complication of nasopharyngeal diphtheria. The typical pseudomembrane develops on an inflammatory base. In addition to local **treatment** antitoxin should be administered.

MORBID GROWTHS OF THE VULVA AND VAGINA

These are exceptional, but may occur very early in life or even congenitally. Of malignant growths sarcoma is that oftenest seen (Steffen;[27] Mergelsberg;[55] Morse[56]). Among benign growths are to be mentioned the vaginal polyp and benign acuminated warty growths of the vulva.

DISEASES OF THE UTERUS AND TUBES

The uterus may be absent, rudimentary, doubled, or divided in varying degrees. One or both Fallopian tubes may be absent or rudimentary. Rarely there is extension to the uterus and tubes from a gonorrheal vaginitis. In cases of imperforate hymen the vagina and uterus may become dilated by mucous or watery secretion, and after puberty a hematocolpos or hematometra may develop. Uterine prolapse is often combined with spina bifida. Complete prolapse has been reported in the new-born (Qvisling[57]). Malignant tumors are rare, but have been recorded (Steffer;[27] McLean;[58] Kehrer and Neumann;[59] Morse[56]).

DISEASES OF THE OVARIES

One or both ovaries may be absent, or there may be accessory ovaries. **Ovarian hernia** is not rare. It may be congenital or acquired, and the ovary on one or both sides be found in the inguinal canal, less often beneath the femoral ring, and occasionally elsewhere (Peuch[60]). In inguinal prolapse the pedicle of the ovary may become twisted and the organ strangulated. Sometimes the ovary can be restored to the abdomen by manipulation, and then a truss be applied. If this is not possible it should be protected against injury. Among **morbid growths** are sarcoma, carcinoma, teratoma, adenoma and cysts. Cases have been reported by Mergelsberg;[55] Hunt and Simon;[61] Lanman;[62] Frank;[63] and others. Dermoid cysts and sarcoma are among the most frequent varieties. They may be congenital, but are oftener observed in later childhood. Some of them may be associated with sexual precocity and early menstruation. The pedicle of a cyst may undergo torsion. The diagnosis from tumors of other organs is of great difficulty. Growths of the spleen appear to start under the left costal border, and those of the kidney are nearer the flank and often have the tympany of the intestine in front. Frequently, however, the diagnosis can be made certain only by exploratory laparotomy. Removal is the only treatment, followed by energetic postoperative roentgenotherapy.

TUBERCULOSIS OF THE FEMALE GENITAL ORGANS

This is uncommon, and generally secondary to disease in the peritoneum or intestine, or perhaps other parts of the body (Brüning,[64] Gräfe[65]). The external genitals may be involved, but the internal genital tract more frequently. The condition is of pathologic rather than clinical interest.

GENITAL HEMORRHAGE; PRECOCIOUS MENSTRUATION

Discharge of blood from the vagina may result from inflammation, injury, the presence of tumors, or asphyxia at birth; be an evidence of the hemorrhagic diatheses; or attend in hemorrhagic forms of infectious diseases, including sepsis. It may occur in the new-born (Schukowski,[66] Zacharias[67]). The blood may arise from the vulva, vagina or uterus. **Precocious menstruation** (p. 1092), in which the flow takes place at more or less regular intervals, is often accompanied by other evidences of sexual and somatic precocity, and is of great infrequency, although a number of cases have been reported (Hennig;[68] Dodd;[69] Gautier;[70] Morse;[71] Lenz;[72] Reuben and

Manning[73]). Some of the children menstruate for a time and then cease, others continue regularly to and through adult menstrual life. Some age rapidly or become debilitated and die early; in more no influence on the general health is apparent. A number have early become mothers. Precocious menstruation may also be a symptom of tumors of the ovary, pineal body, or suprarenals; and, according to Craven,[74] of hypersecretion of the anterior lobe of the pituitary. Treatment of genital hemorrhage itself is seldom needed, although the underlying cause may demand appropriate therapy.

References

1. Nourrisson, 1917, **5,** 270. 2. J.A.M.A., 1929, **92,** 2154. 3. Jahrb. f. Kinderh., 1900, **52,** 181. 4. South. M. J., 1922, **15,** 570. 5. Am. J. Dis. Child., 1929, **38,** 960. 6. Arch. Dis. Childhood., 1929, **4,** 255. 7. Am. J. Dis. Child., 1929, **38,** 804. 8. J.A.M.A., 1931, **96,** 592. 9. Arch. Pediat., 1915, **32,** 846. 10. Trans. Am. Pediat. Soc. 1920, **32,** 52; Am. J. Dis. Child., 1921, **21,** 38. 11. Jahrb. f. Kinderh., 1922, **99,** 303. 12. Arch. f. klin. Chir., 1904, **72,** 487. 13. Wien. klin. Wchnschr., 1904, **17,** 1247. 14. Wien. klin. Wchnschr., 1906, **19,** 732. 15. Ztschr. f. Kinderh., Orig., 1916, **14,** 243. 16. Monatschr. f. Kinderh., 1921, **19,** 461. 17. Rév. franç. de pédiat., 1926, **2,** 63. 18. Surgery of Childh., 1910, 213. 19. Lancet, 1927, **1,** 805. 20. Arch. Surg., 1927, **14,** 663. 21. Deutsche Ztschr. f. Chir., 1922, **168,** 1. 22. Jahrb. f. Kinderh., 1920, **48,** 305. 23. Am. J. Dis. Child., 1929, **38,** 794. 24. Presse méd., 1923, **31,** 485. 25. Am. J. Dis. Child., 1928, **36,** 1231. 26. Ann. Surg., 1930, **92,** 405. 27. Die maligne Geschwülste im Kindersalter 1905. 28. Ann. Surg., 1923, **78,** 761. 29. J.A.M.A., 1913, **61,** 99. 30. Arch. Pediat., 1917, **34,** 186. 31. Berl. klin. Wchnschr., 1921, **58,** 1531. 32. Brit. M. J., 1884, **1,** 860. 33. Arch. gén. de méd., 1890, **165,** 1, 420. 34. Dissert. Berlin 1893. 35. Gaz. d. hôp., 1907, 375. 36. Ann. Surg., 1908, **48,** 662. 37. Am. J. Dis. Child., 1929, **37,** 1203. 38. Am. J. Obst. and Gynec., 1931, **21,** 320. 39. Am. J. Dis. Child., 1927, **33,** 630. 40. Arch. Pediat., 1928, **45,** 357. 41. J. Exper. Med., 1915, **21,** 289. 42. Monatschr. f. Kinderh., 1927, **36,** 483. 43. Am. J. Dis. Child., 1931, **42,** 1086. 44. Arch. Pediat., 1922, **39,** 281. 45. Gittings and Mitchell, Am. J. Dis. Child., 1917, **13,** 448. 46. Berl. klin. Wchnschr., 1905, **42,** 325. 47. München. med. Wchnschr., 1916, **49,** 1720. 48. Am. J. Dis. Child., 1930, **40,** 588. 49. J.A.M.A., 1929, **93,** 1379. 50. Am. J. Dis. Child., 1932, **43,** 305. 51. Arch. f. Kinderh., 1919, **67,** 429. 52. Monatschr. f. Kinderh., Ref., 1919, **15,** 413. 53. Ref. No. 51. 54. Arch. f. Kinderh., 1928, **86,** 28. 55. Inaug. Dissert. Berlin, 1913. 56. Am. J. Obst. and Gynec., 1930, **19,** 520. 57. Arch. f. Kinderh., 1890, **12,** 81. 58. Med. Rec., 1922, **101,** 170. 59. Monatschr. f. Geburtsh. u. Gynäk., 1929, **81,** 68. 60. Gaz. obstet. de Paris, 1876, 129; Ref. Hennig in Gerhardt's Handb. der Kinderkr., 1878, **4,** 3; 24. 61. Ann. Surg., 1928, **87,** 84. 62. New England J. Med., 1929, **201,** 555. 63. Am. J. Dis. Child., 1932, **43,** 942. 64. Monatschr. f. Geburtsh. u. Gynäk., 1902, **16,** 144. 65. Monatschr. f. Geburtsh. u. Gynäk., 1914, **40,** 448. 66. Spareda Vop., 1902, H. 3; Ref. Jahrb. f. Kinderh., 1903, **57,** 105. 67. Med. Klin., 1914, **10,** 1643. 68. Gerhardt's Handb. d. Kinderkr., 1878, **4,** 3, 18. 69. Lancet, 1881, **1,** 601. 70. Rev. méd. de la Suisse romande, 1884, **4,** 501. 71. Arch. Pediat., 1897, **14,** 241. 72. Arch. f. Gynäk., 1913, **99,** 67. 73. Arch. Pediat., 1922, **39,** 769. 74. Am. J. Dis. Child., 1932, **43,** 936.

SECTION VIII

DISEASES OF THE NERVOUS SYSTEM

CHAPTER I

INDICATIONS OF SYMPTOMS

Anatomical and physiologic peculiarities consequent upon incomplete development of the nervous system in early life (p. 45) are the necessary causes of certain characteristics of nervous disease at this period. There is a resulting instability and excitability which renders the nervous system much more susceptible to pathologic influences. Convulsions, delirium, and coma are produced with great readiness; this depending upon the feeble inhibitory power of the nerve-cells, due to incomplete development. There is imperfect functioning of those centers which control temperature, and children consequently readily develop high fever from slight cause. The influence of inheritance is also decided, as seen in numerous nervous disorders, and the great frequency in childhood of infectious diseases of many kinds renders nervous disturbances common. The prevalence and indication of some of the nervous symptoms seen in early life can receive attention here only to a limited extent. For fuller discussion such books as those of Sachs,[1] and of Bruns, Cramer and Ziehen[2] may be consulted.

Atrophy.—Lack of use produces atrophy of the muscles to a certain degree, as in cerebral palsies, in which the paralyzed limb is smaller and shorter than normal; but the condition is more marked when either the anterior horns are involved, as in poliomyelitis and some other affections, or the nerves themselves. Here, in addition to the muscular wasting, there are trophic disturbances as glossiness, pallor, blueness and coldness of the skin, and bed-sores readily develop. Atrophy of the muscles is seen also to a high degree in the later stages of the various muscular dystrophies.

Paralysis.—Rickets, syphilis, scurvy and congenital dislocation of the hip may produce a condition of muscular weakness or of pain which simulates paralysis closely, and a similar pseudoparalysis may also be seen in hysterical conditions. True paralysis is dependent upon a number of causes, the lesions being located in the brain, spinal cord, nerves, or muscles. Paralysis of both arms is oftenest due to poliomyelitis, less frequently to some form of muscular dystrophy; that of one arm alone may be dependent upon the former affection or upon injury to the brachial plexus, as in obstetrical paralysis, or upon a very limited lesion in the brain. In the last condition the paralysis is of a spastic nature, while in the others it is flaccid. Hemiplegic paralysis is oftenest cerebral, and consequently of a spastic type; that of both lower extremities, if spastic, is usually dependent upon spinal caries, cerebral spastic diplegia, or upon diseases involving primarily the lateral tracts of the cord. Flaccid paralysis of one or both lower extremities occurs in neuritis, poliomyelitis, and muscular dystrophies.

Ataxic movements are normally present in young infants. Later they are often symptomatic of hereditary ataxia, cerebellar disease and neuritis, or may sometimes be seen after epidemic encephalitis.

Choreiform movements are witnessed most typically, of course, in chorea. Some of the habit-tics have a certain resemblance; but movements most suggesting those of chorea are found among the postparalytic symptoms of the cerebral palsies and after encephalitis.

Athetoid movements, although irregular, are slow and without jerking, in contradistinction to choreiform movements. They occur chiefly in the hands; sometimes in the feet or the face. They are usually residual symptoms of the cerebral palsies.

Tremor may be general or limited. It may be dependent upon a cerebral lesion, but we[3] have seen unilateral tremor of hemiplegic distribution apparently a purely functional disturbance. Encephalitis is an important cause. Tremor may sometimes follow enteritis, pneumonia or measles, and then subside in a few weeks. It may be an evidence of hyperthyroidism. In other cases it is hereditary or familial (Schippers[4]).

Nystagmus may be vertical, horizontal, or rotatory. It may be an inherited condition, and it is seen in a variety of nervous disorders, among them diseases of the brain, as encephalitis, meningitis, cerebellar tumor; Friedreich's ataxia; gyrospasm; hydrocephalus; disseminated sclerosis; labyrinthine disease; and diseases of the eye. Dizziness usually accompanies nystagmus of central origin. Vertical nystagmus occurs only in central nervous disturbance, and points to disease in the posterior fossae of the skull. Generally it indicates some organic disorder, but sometimes is dependent upon reflex causes or a greatly weakened state.

Hiccup is in nature a spasmodic action of the respiratory muscles, especially the diaphragm. Although occurring at any time of life, it is probably commonest in young healthy infants in the first three months, developing oftenest when the stomach is full of food or of gas. It may, however, be associated with indigestion or with more serious conditions, as intestinal obstruction, peritonitis, or some nervous disorder; or it may occur in an epidemic form. (See p. 402.) By some it is considered to be due to irritation of the esophagus from regurgitated food, and it can be demonstrated experimentally that irritation of this organ will produce hiccup (Pendleton[5]).

Reflexes.—(See also pp. 46, 150.) *The knee-jerk* is abolished or diminished in poliomyelitis, neuritis, Friedreich's ataxia, late in the course of muscular dystrophy, and often in severe acute and chronic disorders not of a nervous nature. In some individuals it may be absent or diminished when no disease is present. It is exaggerated in cerebral and meningeal diseases, and in involvement of the lateral tracts of the cord. The *Achilles jerk* carries the same implications as the knee-jerk. Since both these reflexes may be disturbed in functional disorders, the coexistence of *ankle clonus* is evidence, although not actual proof, of organic disease. The *Babinski*[6] *reflex, i. e.*, dorsal flexion of the great toe on stroking the sole, has the same indications as the knee-jerk. This is true, however, only after the age of two years. At one year 50 per cent of infants will show dorsal flexion (Engstler[7]). *Kernig's*[8] *sign* consists in the inability to extend the leg by passive movement when the thigh is at right angles with the trunk. It is frequently present in meningitis, but by no means always so; and the indisposition of many children to permit the test under any circumstances renders it of limited value. *Brudzinski's*[9] *sign* called also the "neck phenomenon" or the "identical" reflex consists in the involuntary flexion of the thighs on the trunk, when the head is forcibly bent forward. It is a symptom of meningitis, and of increased intracranial tension. Under the same conditions will be present the *contralateral reflex* (Brudzinski[10]) in which flexion of the leg on one side causes the other leg to flex. An early sign of basilar involvement, as described by Gingold,[11] consists in the development of unilateral or bilateral strabismus, perhaps accompanied by retraction of the upper eyelid, when the head is flexed on the chest. The

Moro *embrace reflex* (p. 46) is normally present up to about the fourth month of life. Absence of it indicates motor paralysis or injury, as in brachial paralysis or fractured clavicle; diminished intensity occurs in cerebral injury and great general weakness; and persistence of it over the age of six months signifies injury of the brain or the pyramidal tracts (Gordon;[12] Sanford[13]).

Tache Cérébrale (Tache meningitique).—This consists of a broad, slowly appearing and long-continuing red line developing where the finger-nail has been drawn over the skin (Fig. 197). It indicates meningeal irritation, but, although corroborative, it is not conclusive, since it appears in other conditions accompanied by vasomotor instability.

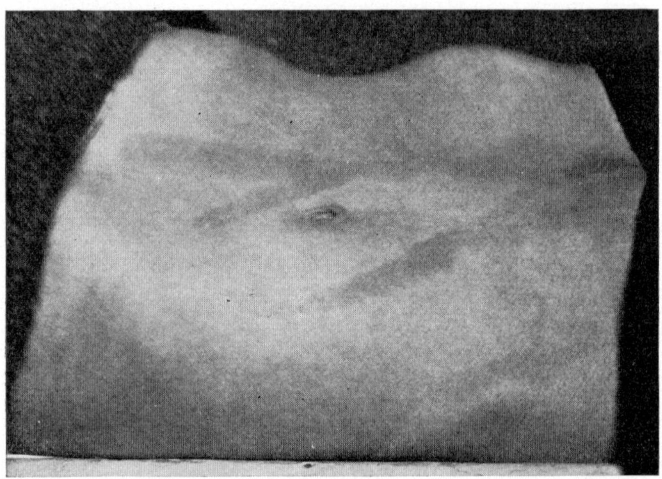

Fig. 197.—Tache meningitique. From a patient, aged four years, suffering from cerebrospinal fever, in the Children's Ward of the Hospital of the University of Pennsylvania. The broad red lines are shown black in the photograph.

Muscular Rigidity.—In the neck-muscles this may be due to rheumatism (torticollis), disease of the cervical spine, meningeal irritation, and increased intracranial pressure; and it is also observed in tetanus, cervical adenitis, and retropharyngeal abscess. Retraction of the head with some rigidity of the muscles may accompany extreme malnutrition in infants. Elsewhere in the body it may be produced similarly, or may depend upon cerebral paralysis, tetanus, or tetany.

Electrical Reactions.—Normal electrical reactions are seen in cerebral diseases, except those of the cranial nerve-nuclei; in disease of the lateral and posterior columns; in functional disorders; and in some muscular dystrophies. There is reaction of degeneration in poliomyelitis; neuritis; to some extent in Pott's disease; and, in general, in affections of the anterior horns. Amyotonia congenita and some of the muscular dystrophies show loss or diminution of both faradic and galvanic response, without the reaction of degeneration. Spasmophilia gives a distinctive electrical response (p. 870). The *reaction of degeneration* may be summarized as follows: There is no longer response to faradic stimulation, but there is contraction with a galvanic stimulus, even with a weaker current than normal, although the response is more sluggish. The minimum stimulus which will cause a contraction is obtained when the current is made and the anode (positive pole) is on the affected muscle (anodal closing contraction), while a stronger current is necessary if the cathode is on the muscle (cathodal closing contraction). This is the reverse of normal, in which the cathodal closing contraction is the greater.

Sensation is diminished or lost in neuritis, or there may be paresthesia. There is anesthesia in involvement of the posterior nerve-roots or the gray matter of the posterior horns, as in transverse myelitis. Hyperesthesia is encountered in irritability or inflammation of the nervous system, as in poliomyelitis, meningitis, sometimes early in neuritis, in hysteria, and the like.

Cerebrospinal Fluid.—In normal children this is clear, and contains a few leukocytes, but certainly not more than 8 to 10 to the cubic millimeter; a substance (sugar) which reduces copper solutions; and traces of albumin, but no globulin in response to the usual clinical tests. It contains approximately 28 mg. of protein per 100 cc.; 10 of urea-nitrogen; 70 of sugar; 700 of chlorides; 5 of calcium; 1.5 of inorganic phosphorus. The amount of spinal fluid and its pressure are less in young infants and children than in adults, but the former may be said to be approximately 100 cc. and the latter about 3 to 5 mm. of mercury, and more when the child is sitting up, crying, or struggling. Under normal conditions when the child is quiet the fluid will drop from the average sized needle, rather than flow in a stream. In meningitis and sometimes also in meningeal irritation globulin is present, the cell-count and the pressure are above normal, sugar may be diminished, and bacteria are found. The extent of these deviations from normal will be discussed under appropriate headings. In *xanthochromia* there is a yellowish tint dependent upon effusion of blood, with subsequent release of pigment from it. This occurs in meningitis, tumor, and trauma, and is usually associated with obstruction of some sort. In the so-called "Nonne's[14] syndrome" there is in addition to xanthochromia a marked globulin-reaction, and in "Froin's[15] syndrome," which is a later stage of this, there is massive spontaneous coagulation of the fluid after its removal; this appearing particularly with tumors of the spinal cord. The Wassermann reaction is positive in the spinal fluid in many cases of syphilis.

References

1. Nerv. Dis. of Children. 2. Handb. d. Nervenkr. im Kindersalter. 3. Griffith, Trans. Am. Pediat. Soc., 1897, **9**, 158. 4. Nederl. Tijdschr. v. Geneesk., 1920, **2**, 983. 5. Am. J. Dis. Child., 1927, **34**, 207. 6. La Semaine méd., 1898, **18**, 286; 321. 7. Wien. klin. Wchnschr., 1905, **10**, 567. 8. Berl. klin. Wchnschr., 1884, **21**, 829. 9. Arch. de méd. d. enf., 1909, **12**, 745. 10. Wien. klin. Wchnschr., 1908, **21**, 255. 11. Arch. Pediat., 1920, **37**, 19. 12. Am. J. Dis. Child., 1929, **38**, 26. 13. Am. J. Dis. Child., 1931, **41**, 1304. 14. Deutsch. Ztschr. f. Nervenheilk., 1910, **40**, 161. 15. Gaz. d. hôp., 1903, **76**, 1005.

CHAPTER II

FUNCTIONAL NERVOUS DISEASES

ECLAMPSIA

(Convulsions)

THE title is applied here to the attacks of more or less general convulsions with loss of consciousness, occurring in early life, and chiefly of functional origin. The condition is a symptom rather than an independent disorder.

Pathogenesis.—An eclamptic convulsion consists of an involuntary irregular discharge of motor impulses from the cells in the brain, resulting in muscular contractions. The predisposition depends on the imperfect inhibitory control by the cerebral nerve-cells, and the increased reflex irritability of the lower centers seen in early life. It is evident, however, that the lack of nervous stability is not of itself sufficient to occasion eclampsia; otherwise every infant would suffer. The tendency is magnified by any condition which increases the irritability or decreases inhibition. With such existing, any slight stimulus applied to the motor area of the brain, or reflexly from elsewhere in the body, may be a sufficient causative agent; and consequently many organic central nervous disturbances, or toxic or reflex causes, may act as excitants.

Etiology.—The incidence is great and the disease stands well towards the head of the list among the assigned causes of death under two years of age. (See Prognosis p. 861.) The majority of cases occur at this period, and especially in the first year. After early childhood convulsions are seen much less often, except as evidence of some organic disease of the brain. Inheritance and familial influence seem to exist at times, several children in a family perhaps showing a tendency to the disorder, or the parents being of a distinctly neurotic type. Rachitic subjects are especially prone to it. Other nutritional disturbances likewise predispose, such as anemia, syphilis, lymphatism, malnutrition, and spasmophilia; the subjects of the last condition having a peculiar tendency to convulsions, often combined with laryngospasm or tetany. (See p. 869.)

The **exciting causes** may be divided into several classes, which, however overlap:

(1) The *acute infectious diseases* are frequently ushered in by a convulsion, instead of the chill seen in older subjects. The exciting cause here is probably the direct first influence of the poison peculiar to the disease. Later in the course of infectious disorders convulsions depend upon various causes, as hyperpyrexia, toxic influences, uremia, asphyxia, cerebral hemorrhage, encephalitis, and anoxemia. (2) *Acute* and *chronic gastro-intestinal disorders* constitute frequent causes, perhaps from toxins elaborated in the intestinal tract or elsewhere. (3) *Toxemic* convulsions of other origin are seen in asphyxia, especially in the new-born; acidosis; alkalosis; hyperglycemia; hypoglycemia; anoxemia; uremia; and occasionally as a result of some of the metallic or vegetable poisons such as lead, opium, and strychnine. (4) *Hyperpyrexia* is an occasional cause, although children, as a rule, bear a moderately high temperature well. (5) *Reflex irritation* may be of the most varied sort. The presence of undigested food in the stomach or intestines may act by mechanical irritation before toxic material could have been produced. Among other reflex causes are colic; earache; phimosis; trauma of any sort; retention of urine; burns; violent crying; fright; etc. Yet although the influence of many reflex irritations is of moment, it is only so if the susceptibility and predisposition are great, and especially in

spasmophilic subjects. Many other assigned conditions, as worms, dentition and the like, probably possess little, if any, reflex influence. (6) *Disease or injury of the brain* is frequently accompanied by eclampsia. This is seen in meningitis; encephalitis; poliomyelitis; hydrocephalus; tumors; hemorrhage; embolism; and thrombosis. The sudden anemia following severe loss of blood, and the venous stasis accompanying diseases of the heart and lungs, may become factors. The majority of instances of convulsions in the new-born and up to the age of three or four months probably depend upon hemorrhage or other intracranial lesion. (7) *Hereditary syphilis* is liable to be attended by fatal convulsions in the new-born, without any causative organic lesion being discoverable at necropsy. (8) *Terminal convulsions* are of frequent occurrence in infants dying from many different disorders.

Symptoms.—In a typical convulsion there may be such premonitory symptoms as twitching of the mouth or extremities; flexing of the thumbs; rolling upward or crossing of the eyes; and restlessness, fretfulness or peevishness. Oftener the onset is sudden. There is sometimes an initial cry; the body stiffens; the elbows flex; the face pales; the eyes have a staring expression, or may be rolled upward; the pupils are contracted; respiration is momentarily arrested; consciousness lost; and there is more or less general rigidity. In a moment the tonic spasm is succeeded by violent rhythmical clonic movements of the extremities; the face being distorted, cyanotic, and covered with sweat; the mouth often foaming; the lips cyanosed; the eyes congested; the pupils dilated; the head retracted or turned in various directions; the back arched; the abdomen flattened; respiration irregular and shallow. There is rattling in the throat; the pulse is irregular, rapid and weak; the hands made into fists with the thumb in the palm; the rectum and bladder may be emptied. The jerking movements continue; sometimes equally everywhere, sometimes now worse in one region and then in another. After a variable time,—usually several minutes, sometimes longer,—the convulsive movements grow less violent and frequent, respiration becomes regular, and cyanosis disappears; but a stuporous condition and often some rigidity persist for a short time. Then complete relaxation follows, often with decided prostration if the convulsion has been severe, and the child passes into natural sleep or begins to cry.

Not infrequently, either after complete or partial relaxation, another paroxysm follows after some minutes or hours. Repeated convulsions may occur in this way during several days, with only short intervals of complete freedom; or with the partial rigidity and stuporous state continuing during the intervals.

Not all the symptoms described are witnessed in every case. Often the convulsion is merely partial. It may be of only momentary duration and limited to a slight twitching of the extremities with brief cessation of respiration, crossing or rolling of the eyes, transitory distortion of the face, and unconsciousness. To this condition the laity often apply the term "inward-spasms" or "internal convulsions." In other cases the spasm begins upon one side, and either is confined here or spreads to the rest of the body, while in others there is little more than temporary loss of consciousness and the symptoms simulate syncope. In still other cases the convulsion is so severe that cyanosis becomes extreme, respiration greatly interfered with, the extremities cold, the body covered with cold sweat, and the pulse too rapid and weak to be counted.

Prognosis.—The immediate and subsequent prognosis is so intimately linked to the numerous disorders of which the convulsion is but a symptom, that it is better discussed under the headings of the acute infectious diseases, meningitis, encephalitis, and the like. Convulsions are so often a terminal process that statistics regarding mortality are misleading. When due to reflex irritation, or to the onset of acute infectious or digestive disturbance, they are rarely dangerous. The actual danger from the convulsive attack itself is from asphyxia or from exhaustion.

Sequels.—Sometimes after severe attacks there is a temporary paralysis, the result of the exhausted nervous condition or of cerebral edema; or there may be aphasia, or a stuporous state. These are all functional and temporary disturbances. Any sequels of a permanent nature depend usually upon the condition of which the convulsion was a symptom. An exception, however, is the possibility of a convulsion being severe enough to produce intracranial hemorrhage, with resulting permanent damage. (See also Epilepsy, p. 864.)

Diagnosis.—Most important is the diagnosis of the cause of the convulsion, and for this a careful study of the history and of all the symptoms is required.

Convulsions in the first three or four months of life are most frequently dependent upon an organic cause. After this through the remainder of the first two years they are oftenest spasmophilic. In the first few days of life they are oftenest due to traumatic hemorrhage, or to asphyxia from atelectasis. In the latter case they are attended by cyanosis and feeble respiration, and in the former are liable to be frequently repeated during, perhaps, several days. It is possible, too, for asphyxia to produce eclampsia after this period, as in bad cases of pneumonia, pertussis, cardiac disease, and diphtheritic laryngitis. Convulsions dependent upon cerebral abscess or tumor are often localized at the start, and then become general. It is possible, however, for limited convulsions to occur not dependent upon cerebral lesions. Imperfect cerebral development is a cause of repeated attacks covering a long period. General convulsions with high fever point to some acute infectious disorder, acute digestive disturbance, or meningitis. In most of these cases the attack is prone to be single, except meningitis where there is liable to be frequent recurrence with the development of other evidences of this malady. Convulsions from reflex irritation may or may not be attended by fever. Uremia may be a cause, and the urine should always be examined; but on the other hand, albuminuria does not necessarily indicate uremia. Spasmophilic convulsions exhibit low blood-calcium and characteristic electrical and mechanical reactions (p. 870), and often carpopedal spasm. Attacks occurring in the morning may be hypoglycemic from faulty carbohydrate metabolism. We[1] have seen a number of such cases, and the condition has been described by Josephs.[2] In some such instances pancreatic disease may exist (Howland;[3] Nielson and Eggleston[4]). The diagnosis of eclampsia from epilepsy will be discussed in considering the latter disease.

Treatment.—The **preventive treatment** of convulsions is often dependent upon the cause, and is better considered under the appropriate headings. Judicious sedative treatment may sometimes prevent a convulsion, and should be employed whenever convulsive seizures are likely to be symptoms. If the attacks are hypoglycemic, a heavy carbohydrate evening meal should be given, and perhaps orange juice or glucose in the late evening or early morning. In infancy the possible existence of spasmophilia must always be investigated (p. 869).

In the **treatment of the attack** immediate relief is indicated, and treatment for the cause likewise employed. The child is placed in a warm tub bath of 98 to 100 F. (36.7 to 37.8 C.), and a cold compress, frequently changed, or an ice-bag applied to the head, if there is fever. For great hyperpyrexia a cool bath may be given if the reaction is satisfactory. If the bowel contains undigested food a large enema may be administered. In obstinate attacks inhalation of ether or chloroform is indicated. Chloral, bromides, or phenobarbital may be given by the mouth, or in a small enema, or morphine hypodermically. The last is especially serviceable where convulsions are rapidly repeated. Amyl nitrite, compression of the carotids, inhalation of oxygen, and lumbar puncture are also used; the last if there is an increased amount of cerebrospinal fluid, provided no brain-tumor is present. If there is an indication an emetic, or a purgative or enema, may be given, but not if the procedure distresses or excites the child, since quiet and rest are imperative. Sedatives should be continued for several days, the child kept quiet, and the diet light.

EPILEPSY

The title *idiopathic epilepsy* is applied to a chronic convulsive disorder with loss or disturbance of consciousness, not dependent upon a demonstrable pathologic lesion. *Symptomatic, secondary,* or *organic* epilepsy designates the convulsions associated with organic intracranial lesion. More properly this form should be described under Organic Diseases of the Nervous System; but the symptoms are often so similar that, for the sake of convenience, the two forms will be considered together here.

Pathologic Anatomy.—It is usually considered that there are no causative lesions in idiopathic epilepsy. In patients dying during attacks there are sometimes found edema and hemorrhages in the pia and the brain-tissue, but these may well be the result rather than the cause. Areas of degeneration in the brain have been found at operation and by ventriculography, and Dandy[5] reported dilated subarachnoid spaces and ventricles; these changes not being present at necropsy. In symptomatic epilepsy various gross or microscopic lesions of the brain may be present.

Pathogenesis.—There exists some disturbance of the brain which allows the irregular discharge of impulses from the motor cells of the cortex. These disturbances differ from those initiating eclampsia in early life, in that they first manifest themselves at a time when the normal lack of inhibitory control of early life has diminished, and in that they are chronic and persistent. The nature of the disturbances is unknown. Among the theories advanced are changes in oxidation, in the acid-base balance of the tissues, and in their fluid content or permeability. There have been reported a slight shift of the blood to the alkaline side before the attack, and to the acid side after it; water retention during the attack and diuresis and increased excretion of sodium and chlorine afterwards; and edema of the central nervous tissue. The value in some cases of dehydrating measures point to an influence of hydration of the tissues as an important factor. (See studies and reviews by Fay;[6] Gamble and Hamilton;[7] Lennox and Cobb;[8] McQuarrie and Keith;[9] McQuarrie;[10] Gamble;[11] Fay and Winkelman;[12] McQuarrie and Peeler.[13]) Even in secondary epilepsy it seems that there must be something other than the lesion which precipitates a convulsive attack at one time rather than another.

Etiology.—The *incidence* of epilepsy is great, Davenport[14] estimating that there are about 500,000 epileptics in the United States. Undoubtedly *heredity* has an influence, since, according to Gowers,[15] Green,[16] Peterman,[17] and others, there is found in about 40 to 50 per cent of epileptics a family history of some such nervous disorder as convulsions, feeble-mindedness, insanity, alcoholism, migraine, fainting spells, and the like. The frequency of epilepsy itself in the families of epileptics is variously estimated, Thom[18] for example, finding it in only about 6 per cent of epileptics; others, as Green[18] and Brain[19] in almost 30 per cent. It is usually believed that the offspring of known epileptics frequently develop the disorder, Echeverria,[20] for example finding this in 14.6 per cent of 533 such children. Both *sexes* are attacked, with perhaps slight preponderance in the male (Talbot[21]). The *age* at which most cases of idiopathic epilepsy begin is from ten to twenty years, although a good many develop it at a younger age. The statistics concerning this are, however, at considerable variance. The first-born child is more susceptible to epilepsy. The relation of *eclampsia* in early life to epilepsy developing later is disputed. It is certain that the ordinary infantile convulsion seldom in itself predisposes to epilepsy. The *direct* cause of an epileptic seizure generally cannot be traced. Among the possible initiating factors assigned are infectious diseases, trauma, fright, other reflex and toxic influences, masturbation, and especially digestive disturbances.

Symptoms. **Major Epilepsy** (*Grand Mal*).—In typical attacks there are in many cases prodromal symptoms, *i. e.*, an *aura*. There may be a sensory disturbance such as pain, numbness, or tingling in the pharynx, the region of the heart, the stomach, or some other part of the body. Motor aurae may be represented by slight localized twitching and paresis, as sometimes of the tongue producing temporary inability to speak; and vasomotor aurae by flushing or pallor. There may be psychic aurae, such as a sudden feeling of dread or anxiety, restlessness, excitability, or other psychic conditions of varied nature; or disturbances connected with the auditory or optic apparatus, such as flashes of light, momentary blindness, vertigo, sounds as of whistles, bells, and the like. In the rare cases of *procursive epilepsy* there is a tendency to run rapidly and without purpose for some moments before falling in the ordinary fit. The aura is a warning that an attack is about to begin. Its duration varies, but it is generally only a few seconds. Frequently there is no aura, and the onset is entirely sudden. The attack then begins with an abrupt loss of consciousness, pallor of the face, dilated pupils, and often a cry; and the child falls if in a position to do so. Immediately a more or less widely spread tonic spasm develops. The head is retracted or drawn to one side; the jaws tightly shut; the face cyanotic; the extremities rigid; the forearms flexed; the hands clenched; respiration is interfered with by the contraction of the muscles of the chest. This tonic spasm lasts a few seconds up to half a minute, and is then followed by the clonic stage with movements and symptoms similar to those of eclampsia. During this period the tongue is often bitten as a result of the spasmodic movements of the jaws; foam, often bloody, comes from the mouth; the face is distorted; the eyes roll in different directions; cyanosis persists, but to a less degree; there are irregular rhythmical spasmodic movements of the trunk and extremities; respiration is jerking and irregular; the bowels and bladder are often emptied involuntarily. This stage lasts usually only two or three minutes, sometimes longer; the symptoms gradually moderating, then disappearing, and the patient, relaxed, passing into coma with snoring respiration from which he cannot be wakened. This in turn lasts from a few minutes up to a quarter of an hour, and the patient can then be roused, or perhaps awakes of himself bewildered; yet oftener, if not disturbed, passes into a natural sleep. From the beginning of the attack there is complete loss of consciousness and insensibility to pain. A moderate elevation of temperature is frequent during the attack. Some headache, fatigue, or general pain may be experienced when the child wakens from sleep. Changes in the chemical composition of the blood and the spinal fluid as occurring during the attack have been described by different investigators (see Pathogenesis p. 863), but their relationship to it is not clear. (See Patterson;[22] Lennox;[23] Robinson et al.;[24] Kulkow;[25] Lennox and Allen.[26])

Not every instance of major attacks shows the completely developed syndrome. Occasionally, even without a focal organic lesion, convulsive movements begin in some region, and consciousness is fully lost only as the spasm spreads to the remainder of the body.

Minor Epilepsy (*Petit Mal*). This is more frequent than the major form. It exhibits many diverse modifications and degrees of intensity, but there is always the characteristic complete or partial loss of consciousness, although often momentary. The child may suddenly stop talking; have a far-away expression of face, with pallor; and then in a moment continue his conversation at the point of interruption without knowledge that anything has happened. Any object in the hand will probably have been dropped. Such attacks may be supposed by the parents to be dizziness, absent-mindedness, faintness, and the like; and their true nature never suspected. The patient may in some cases actually experience a sensation of dizziness or faintness, but there is seldom a distinct aura. Sometimes there is confusion of mind for a moment after the attack, and automatic acts of very varied sorts may be performed, such as partially undressing; and occasionally these acts may be violent. In other instances there may be a few slight twitching movements of the face or a trembling of the body accompanying the seizure. Still other cases are more severe in that the loss of consciousness is attended by falling, although this loss is of such brief duration that consciousness immediately returns, and crying begins on account of the pain from the fall. Some of the cases of procursive epilepsy (p. 864) belong in the present category, since consciousness is not entirely lost, and no general convulsion follows.

Symptomatic Epilepsy.—This form may be either general, or localized and perhaps hemiplegic; or may remain localized over a long period of the disease and then become general. The first movements in any attack are liable to be seen in the region presided over by the portion of the brain affected, but may be widespread from the beginning and distinguished in no way from those of the idiopathic form. Any aura occurring is prone to be motor in character and may indicate the seat of the organic lesion. There is, as a rule, loss of consciousness; but in one form this is preserved either throughout or until late in the attack (Jacksonian epilepsy) (Jackson[27]).

Course of the Disease.—Sometimes the attacks occur only during the night (*nocturnal epilepsy, epilepsia larvata*), and it is solely from bed-wetting on certain occasions, combined with injury to the tongue, exhaustion, or headache in the morning, that the disease is suspected. Generally the early attacks of idiopathic epilepsy come at first at long intervals, perhaps one or two in a year; and then become more frequent. Sometimes the disease begins with well-marked attacks of grand mal; in other cases with petit mal, which tends to change gradually to the major form; or there may be an alternation of an occasional major attack with a number of minor ones. The attacks of petit mal are usually more frequent than those of the major form, and sometimes reach as many as 20 or 30 up to occasionally nearly 100 in a day. In some severe cases of major epilepsy the seizure is rapidly succeeded by others without recovery of consciousness (*status epilepticus*). In general, symptomatic epilepsy exhibits a more rapid increase in the frequency of the attacks than does idiopathic epilepsy; the attacks are longer and status epilepticus is oftener seen; and psychic degeneration is more frequently present and is greater. The general health of epileptics suffers but little unless the attacks are severe and frequent and the course prolonged. However, especially in repeated petit mal and in symptomatic epilepsy, there may be such psychic disturbances as alteration of personality, irritability, attacks of temper, and the like; or mental backwardness in all degrees up to that of idiocy. While many epileptics remain entirely normal mentally, or are even precocious, Dawson and Conn[28] found that the intelligence of a group of epileptic children was below the average.

Prognosis.—Epilepsy is seldom fatal during an attack, except as a result of some accident, or of exhaustion in status epilepticus. The prognosis as regards final recovery is, on the whole, poor. Unfavorable factors and symptoms are distinct inheritance; cases beginning in late childhood or after this, and also those developing earlier but not responding to treatment; great frequency of attacks; psychic or mental disturbance; and association with organic cerebral lesions, unless these are amenable to operative interference. Even when children cease to have attacks for a time, caution in prognosis is necessary, since there may be recurrence at puberty. In the few cases apparently depending on syphilis, treatment of this may benefit little, if organic change in the brain is already present. If a factor which initiates attacks can be eliminated early in the course and before the "epileptic habit" has been established, or if the patient responds readily to dietetic treatment, the outlook is brighter. Acute febrile disease may cause increase in number or severity of the attacks, or may sometimes result in temporary improvement. The duration of life is variable and depends largely upon the severity and frequency of attacks. Status epilepticus is a serious condition.

Diagnosis.—It is only by its chronic character and the repetition of convulsions that epilepsy can be diagnosed. Unless the seizures occurring solely at night are witnessed, the diagnosis in these cases must rest on the conditions described (p. 865) found present in the morning. The varied manifestations of minor epilepsy need continued study before their nature can be determined. The convulsion of *eclampsia* may be similar to that of idiopathic epilepsy, but it is likely to be secondary to some discoverable toxic or other cause, is not preceded by aura, and is more liable to occur in the first three years of life. When spasmophilic it is usually seen between the sixth month and the end of the second year, and the mechanical and electrical nervous changes and the low blood-calcium will be found. (See p. 870.) There is usually in eclampsia, no sudden cry or fall; often fever; and less tendency to stuporous sleep following. However, a differential diagnosis is often difficult, and frequently only time can solve the question. Eclampsia in early life dependent upon organic lesion is in reality symptomatic epilepsy. *Syncope* may be recognized by the entire lack of convulsive movements, although these are not always present in petit mal; by the slower development of unconsciousness; the absence of tongue-biting or relaxation of the sphincters; and the infrequency of attacks. In older children there may be difficulty in distinguishing *hysteria* from epilepsy, but in the former the convulsive movements may be obviously voluntary, the tongue is not bitten nor the sphincters relaxed, the apparent unconsciousness is not accompanied by analgesia, and the patient remembers the details of the attack. *Pyknolepsy* (p. 868) differs from petit mal chiefly in its good prognosis and in its failure to respond to sedative treatment. *Hypoglycemic* convulsions occur usually in the morning or after a long fast (p. 862) or following the injection of insulin; are associated with low blood-sugar; and respond favorably to the administration of carbohydrates. The diagnosis of *symptomatic* from *idiopathic* epilepsy is based on the history; the localization of the convulsive movements or their onset in a given region; and sometimes by the aid of ventriculography (p. 154). However, localization of symptoms is not a necessary proof that circumscribed lesions exist.

Treatment.—During the seizure the patient should be placed in a position to avoid injury, the clothes loosened, and a piece of wood, cork or rubber inserted between the teeth to prevent biting of the tongue. The subsequent sleep should be undisturbed. If there is an aura, inhalation of amyl nitrite will sometimes prevent or shorten the seizure. On the theory that hyperpnea tends to initiate attacks, it has been recommended that the patient exhale and maintain exhalation as long as possible. Lennox[29] found that the inhalation of pure oxygen or of air containing a high percentage of CO_2 tends to inhibit seizures. In severe and prolonged attacks morphine may be given, or sometimes inhalations of ether or chloroform. In cases of status epilepticus phenobarbital sodium in doses of 2 to 10 grains (0.13 to 0.65) may be given intravenously and spinal puncture performed.

Treatment of the disease involves a careful study of the patient and his environment. The amount of rest required, the association with older children, and the necessity for institutional treatment depend upon the circumstances in the home and the severity of the disease. Any factor which might initiate attacks should be removed or avoided if possible. In a few cases correction of faulty posture is helpful (Talbot[21]). The food should be simple and digestible; tea, coffee and alcohol eliminated; and constipation avoided. There is no physiologic objection to the giving of protein in the amount required for the age. A salt-poor diet has been recommended on the basis that chlorides increase nerve-irritability, and in large quantities favors water-retention. (See p. 863.) At least excessive amounts of salt should be avoided.

In cases in which convulsions are frequent and severe, some form of sedative medication must be employed. The effort should be to prevent the seizures, yet without producing constant mental sluggishness by the drugs. The usual remedies selected are the bromides and phenobarbital or some similar preparation, the dose of these varying with the age and condition of the patient. It is well to alternate these drugs, using one type for several weeks and then the other. Phenobarbital seems to be the least disturbing of the two. When bromides are employed, the possibility of a bromide rash developing should be borne in mind (p. 1098). Among the numerous other drugs recommended are chloral, antipyrine, acetanilid, arsenic, belladonna, borax, silver nitrate, and opium. Calcium has also been given, although there is no calcium deficiency in the usual case. Ammonium chloride, calcium chloride, and other acid substances have been tried on the basis that alkalosis is a factor (p. 863).

On the ground that the cause is some disturbance of metabolism Guelpa and Marie,[30] Geyelin,[31] and others recommended starvation for from one to three weeks, and reported benefit from this, giving only water or perhaps thin broth and orange juice. Yet Lennox and Cobb[32] obtained permanent results in only 1 of 27 patients; and this form of treatment has been largely supplanted by the ketogenic diet proposed by Wilder,[33] and used by many clinicians (Peterman;[34] Helmholz;[35] Helmholz and Keith;[36] McQuarrie and Keith;[37] Talbot[21]). The action of this is probably a dehydrating one, as pointed out by McQuarrie[37] and others. (See also p. 863.) We have had some success with this treatment, which appears more successful when started before attacks have become severe and frequent. When effective the relief may continue only so long as the diet is in force, yet in some cases appears to be permanent. Sedative drugs may be employed, if needed, in combination with the dietary treatment. Helmholz and Keith[36] found that of 141 patients receiving the ketogenic diet 43 had remained free from attacks for from one to seven years; 32 had shown improvement; and 66 were not benefited. The method of procedure, as outlined by Peterman,[34] consists in giving only broth, bran wafers, and orange juice for a week, and then gradually increasing to a larger intake of not more than 20 Gm. of carbohydrate and 1 Gm. of protein per kilogram of body-weight daily, *i. e.*, 3.2 oz. carbohydrate and 0.16 oz. protein per pound, with the remainder of the caloric needs derived from fat. (For further details see Diabetes, pp.

496, 500, and Talbot.[21]) For a growing child this amount of protein is low, and we prefer, as does McQuarrie[38] to give at least 1.75 Gm. per kilogram (.28 oz. per pound). Another objection to the diet is that ketosis produces a negative calcium and phosphorus balance (Nelson[39]). The diet should be continued for several months before deciding on its therapeutic value, and for at least three months more if the attacks have been controlled, after which the return to a normal diet may be made gradually. Acetone bodies should be excreted in the urine during the period of the diet. The type of food which must be offered often becomes distasteful.

In view of the possible factor of hydration of tissues in epilepsy (p. 863) McQuarrie[10] recommends the combination of a mild ketogenic diet with a restriction of fluid intake. This restriction should at first be decided, but later the amount increased to from 15 to 30 cc. per kilogram (0.3 to 0.6 fl. oz. per pound) of body-weight per day, this including the amount in the food.

Operative treatment, consisting of decompression and, in the case of symptomatic epilepsy, the excision or destruction of the so-called "epileptic area," has been practised, and in some instances with apparent success. The cases for this form of treatment must be carefully selected. Injections of air (p. 154) have sometimes made the condition worse, but a few authors have reported at least temporarily cessation of convulsions. Fay,[6] for example, combines injections of air with limitation of fluid, and drainage of the spinal canal. Among other operative procedures is excision of the cervical sympathetics, but the results of this are inconclusive.

NARCOLEPSY

This condition, considered by some to be a form of epilepsy, may be "idiopathic," or occur in syphilis, multiple sclerosis, some tumors of the brain, or encephalitis. It is characterized by an overwhelming desire to sleep. The sleep is apparently normal and the patient easily aroused. The attacks last a few seconds to several minutes and as many as 20 may occur in the course of a day. The return to consciousness after an attack is not followed by a confused mental state. The resemblance to petit mal is only slight, and, furthermore, narcolepsy is not succeeded by the later development of grand mal. We have not seen in children the so-called "idiopathic form" of the disease, nor has it been observed in our experience in syphilis of the nervous system in early life. Idiopathic narcolepsy apparently, however, can occur in childhood (Redlich;[40] Weech[41]), and as a secondary affection may be seen as a sequel of epidemic encephalitis. Doyle and Daniels[42] had good results with ephedrine sulphate in doses of 25 mg. (.375 grain) two or three times a day; and thyroid extract, caffeine, and strychnine also have been used.

PYKNOLEPSY

(Absences. "Crowded Little Attacks")

This has been considered an independent affection by Friedmann;[43] Schroeder,[44] who first suggested the term "pyknolepsy"; Sauer;[45] Meyer;[46] Stier;[47] and Kochmann.[48] Some place it in the category of epilepsy or of hysteria. It develops oftenest between the ages of four and ten years, apparently independently of any nervous disorder or inheritance. The attacks begin with a staring expression of the eyes; the head may be turned in some direction, but there is never any actual convulsion; the limbs are relaxed, but there is never falling; consciousness may be impaired but is never entirely lost; and any evidence of vasomotor disturbance is absent. With the onset of the seizure, the child ceases speaking or whatever he is doing, and resumes it immediately after it. The attacks begin without warning, last ten to thirty seconds, and occur five or six or perhaps one hundred times daily. The general health is not affected, nor do nervous and psychic disturbances develop. The **course** is prolonged and the disease may last for months or years, but always ceases, usually abruptly, as puberty is approached and without leaving sequels. The **diagnosis** is made from minor epilepsy by the absence of falling, deep unconsciousness and convulsions; by the good prognosis; and by the failure to respond to treatment with bromides or other sedatives. Often the diagnosis can be made only after years have passed, and the outcome seen. The **treatment** consists merely in attention to the general health.

SPASMOPHILIA

(Spasmophilic Diathesis)

Nature.—Under the title Spasmophilia, as first used by Thiemich,[49] is designated that condition seen in children in which there is a peculiar tendency to convulsive disorders of various sorts, notably laryngospasm and tetany, as well as many instances of eclampsia. It is probable that most cases of eclampsia in the first two years of life, after the period of the first few months, are spasmophilic in nature. The chief characteristic, apart from the actual spasmodic attack, is the increased mechanical and electrical excitability of the nerves, which may be latent in children who never suffer from active manifestations of the disease. The disturbance is based upon no known pathologic lesion, and apparently is not connected with the imperfect development of the nervous system characteristic of early life. The condition in its latent form is frequent; the development of visible manifestations is less common.

Etiology.—Although it is sometimes claimed that there is a familial influence (Pincherle and Pollidori[50]), environmental factors are the more important. Spasmophilic manifestations are most frequent from the age of six months to two years, but may sometimes be observed in the third and fourth years, although rarely later. That the disorder may occur in the first six months of life, and even in the first weeks, is shown by the reports of Wolff;[51] Klose;[52] Nassau;[53] Powers;[54] and Shannon.[55] We[56] also have observed it in very young infants. Tetany appearing in the first few days of life may sometimes accompany hyperpyrexia and vomiting (Bass and Karelitz[57]). Spasmophilic manifestations are seen oftenest in winter and spring (Escherich;[58] Hochwart;[59] Moro[60]). Males are more frequently affected than females, in the proportion of 2:1, according to Bakwin and Bakwin.[61] The disease is closely associated with rickets, from 50 per cent (Kirchgässer[62]) to 95 per cent (Escherich[58]) of cases of spasmophilia being in rachitic subjects. It is more common in artificially fed infants than in the breast-fed. There sometimes appears to be an association, but without an obvious etiologic connection, with the lymphatic diathesis (p. 482).

Pathogenesis.—Since the studies of Howland and Marriott[63] practically all observers have found, that when there are active manifestations of spasmophilia, the blood-calcium is usually below 8 mg. per 100 cc. (normal 10 to 12 mg.). It may be as low as 5 to 6 mg. and occasionally 3 to 4 mg. The calcium in the spinal fluid is also below the normal level of 4.3 mg. per 100 cc. (Ingvar[64]). The lowering of the blood-calcium is not, however, an invariable rule, and we[56] have seen well marked cases in which it was over 8 mg. Still, any measure which raises the blood-calcium above 8 mg. usually results in the cessation of symptoms. At times there is an increase in the blood-phosphorus, although this may be simply a secondary matter, since anything which tends to raise the level of one of these elements tends to lower the other. The lowered calcium in the blood, and, therefore, presumably also in the tissues, in some way brings about an increased irritability. The action of such factors as season, diets poor in vitamins and minerals, artificial feeding as opposed to breast feeding, and gastro-intestinal disorders, are all related to the poor absorption of calcium from the intestinal tract, probably dependent upon increased alkalinity there. (See p. 444, chapter on Rickets.)

The studies of Gerstenberger[65] and his coworkers, and of Rominger, Meyer and Bomskov[66] would indicate that tetany develops when there is healing in the first stage of rickets, since at that time calcium may be withdrawn from the tissues to be deposited in the bones; and Shipley[67] and his coworkers state that it is in the cases of rickets with less severe bony deformity that spasmophilia is prone to occur, since the blood-calcium is liable to be low in these cases. The increased incidence of spasmophilia in the spring months may be related to this factor of healing of rickets, because of increased exposure to sunshine at that time and a consequent lowering of blood-calcium. Spasmophilia has also been described as associated with over-dosage from ultraviolet light (Karger[68]), and with hemorrhage into or hyperplasia of the parathyroid and other glands of internal secretion. The connections are, however, not clear.

It should be remembered that carpopedal spasm (tetany) while a symptom of infantile spasmophilia, also occurs in a number of other conditions. Thus it may follow extirpation of the parathyroid glands or deficiency of them (p. 1073), marked vomiting, forced respiration, hypochloremia, administration of sodium bicarbonate, and injection of phosphates or of guanidine. In some of these conditions the calcium of the blood is normal, in others reduced; and even when not reduced there may be an action on the diffusibility of the calcium or on its ionization, *i. e.*, the effectiveness of calcium is diminished. In some of the conditions mentioned the pH and the bicarbonate of the blood are normal; in others there is an alkalosis. This last diminishes the ionization of calcium. In infantile tetany there does not usually appear to be an alkalosis (Calvin and Borovsky;[69] Ockel;[70] Drucker and Faber;[71] Rohmer and Woringer[72]).

Symptoms.—Apart from active manifestations, as eclampsia, tetany and laryngospasm, there are the electrical and mechanical characteristics and the chemical alteration in the blood already referred to. The *altered electrical reaction* described by Erb[73] is satisfactorily determined over the course of the median or the peroneal nerve. Contractions of the muscles supplied by these nerves occur with less current than in the normal infant. There is much variance of opinion regarding the significance of the reaction, especially after infancy. The following conclusions of Holmes[74] may be taken as representing the preponderance of views:—A cathodal opening contraction under 5 milliamperes is pathognomonic of spasmophilia in children under five years of age. An anodal opening contraction obtained with less current than for the anodal closing contraction, and with less than 5 milliamperes during the first six months of life, and of 2 milliamperes from the age of four to five years, is probably characteristic of spasmophilia, but is of little value after this age. It would appear that in older children no certain conclusions can be drawn from the altered reactions.

Mechanical irritability of the nerves is well seen in the *facialis* symptom, or *Chvostek's*[75] *sign.* A slight tapping or stroking in front of the auditory canal, or over the malar bone, or farther along the branches of the seventh nerve, causes sudden clonic contraction of the muscles of that side of the face. The patient should be quiet and preferably sleeping. There is much discussion of the value of this sign. (Hochsinger;[76] Raudnitz;[77] Graham and Anderson;[78] Veronese;[79] Schultze;[80] Lombardi.[81]) The conclusion may be fairly drawn that occurring after the period of infancy it cannot be considered a proof of the presence of spasmophilia; but when appearing in infancy it points strongly to this disease, although its absence is no proof that spasmophilia is not present. Found in the first few weeks of life it is without significance, since, as we[82] have shown, it may be obtained almost routinely at this age on sleeping infants with normal blood-calcium. Another evidence of the same mechanical excitability is *Trousseau's symptom.* If firm circular pressure by the fingers or the band of a blood-pressure apparatus be made over the nerves and arteries of the upper arm in a spasmophilic subject, the tetanoid position of the hands will be increased if already present, or sometimes brought on even if evidences of tetany have been absent. The *chemical alteration of the blood,* consisting in a diminution of the calcium content, has already been discussed (p. 869).

Eclampsia.—Generalized convulsions may or may not be associated with carpopedal spasm. If not, they differ in no way from the usual convulsive attack due to any other cause. Whether they are, in fact, spasmophilic in origin can be determined only by the study of other features, as described.

Tetany.—This term was first applied to the condition by Corvisart.[83] "*Arthrogryposis,*" or carpopedal spasm, is a term employed when only the hands and feet are involved. Although tetany is a symptom of diverse conditions (p. 870) yet, as far as children are concerned, it is practically always a manifestation of spasmophilia, and as such is discussed here. Tetany may be *intermittent* or *persistent.* The onset is usually sudden. There is a tonic spasm of the hands as a result of which the thumb is drawn into the palm, the fingers adducted and flexed at the metacarpo-phalangeal articulations, but extended at the more distal joints, and the wrists flexed ("accoucheur's hand") (Fig. 198). This typical position may be replaced by a tight flexing of the fingers over the thumb. Often the forearms are flexed and the upper arm drawn to the body. Usually the spasm soon extends to the lower limbs, the foot being extended in the position of talipes equinus, or equino-varus, the toes flexed, and the sole hollowed. (Fig. 199.) Less often the knee-joints are rigidly flexed, and the thighs flexed and adducted. In most cases the contraction is limited to the extremities, especially the hands and feet, and occasionally occurs in the feet only. Sometimes there is a widespread tonic spasm throughout the body, including the muscles of the trunk and face and interference with respiration and swallowing, but this is uncommon in infantile tetany. There is never any loss of consciousness. In the intermittent type the condition may last a few minutes or an hour, be frequently repeated, and pain and often paresthesia are present. In the more persistent form, which is the most frequent in infancy, the spasm is oftenest limited to the hands and feet, and may continue for hours or for weeks, but may lessen or cease for some hours and then be renewed. There is no pain unless the parts are disturbed. Edema may develop in the parts affected. The cutaneous- and tendon-reflexes are exaggerated.

Laryngismus Stridulus.—This title may conveniently be limited to that form of laryngospasm which is a manifestation of spasmophilia. It is closely allied to tetany, and is seen nearly always only in rachitic subjects and in the first two years of life, (90 per cent of 443 cases, Kirchgässer[62]). Among causes precipitating an attack are sudden fright, anger, hard attacks of crying, and the like; but very frequently no cause is discoverable. There is absence of fever and of evidences of laryngitis. In the milder cases the child suddenly stops breathing, the head is thrown back, and the face is pale. This condition lasts only a few seconds, and the attack ceases with a loud crowing inspiration. In severe cases the closure of the glottis is more complete and long-continued, and suffocation seems imminent. Generally these cases terminate like the milder in a crowing inspiration, which may be repeated several times. In still more threatening cases there may be unconsciousness, with a few clonic spasmodic movements, or even general eclamptic convulsions; and carpopedal spasm may attend. There are severe cases in which, without convulsions, tonic spasm of the thoracic muscles of respiration suddenly develops, accompanying the spasm of the larynx and producing entire apnea and complete asphyxia, and an appearance of death (*expiratory apnea* of Kassowitz[84]). Should recovery take place, respiration is re-estab-

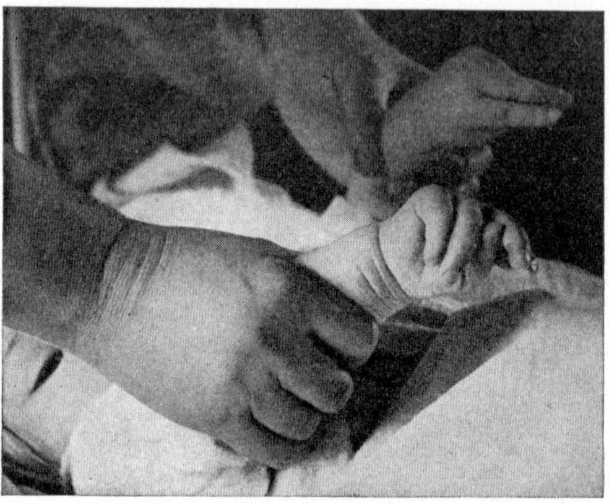

Fig. 198.—Tetany. Male infant of one and one-half years, in the Children's Hospital of Philadelphia. Somewhat rachitic. Illustration shows the flexion of the fingers and the position of the thumb often seen.

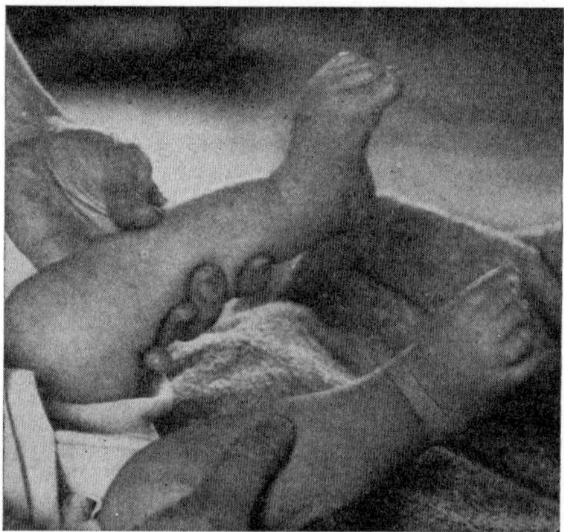

Fig. 199.—Same case as in Fig. 198. Well-marked plantar flexion of the toes.

lished with a crowing inspiration, or quietly if the spasm has passed off completely.

Other Symptoms of Spasmophilia.—There has been described by Czerny and Moser;[85] Klose;[86] Gregor,[87] and others a condition of general persistent **muscular hypertonia** (Fig. 200). It occurs usually in the early weeks of life and is associated with severe nutritional disturbances. The flexors of the extremities are especially involved, and in some cases the head is retracted and there is some degree of opisthotonos. Certainly not all of the cases are spasmophilic; yet there exist intermediate forms which indicate a close affiliation. A form has been described by Haas[88] and

Lemaire and Olivier[89] in which, associated with the hypertonia, there are irritability and vomiting. The relationships of these two forms are not clear. Lederer[90] gave the title **bronchotetany** to a syndrome occurring in spasmophilic subjects, and described as consisting of spasmodic contraction of the bronchioles, obstruction of the alveoli, and atelectasis. The **spurious whooping cough** of Wernstedt[91] consists of a spasmodic pertussis-like cough occurring in spasmophilic children. Escherich[58] designated as **pseudotetanus** a condition characterized by generalized rigidity and extreme hardness of the muscles, with paroxysmal increase of the spasm accompanied by pain, and lasting three or four weeks. All of these symptom-complexes in some instances appear to be associated with and to be due to spasmophilia. On the other hand they may have no etiological connection whatever, and investigation must always be made for other symptoms present, and for the mechanical, electrical, and chemical findings characteristic of spasmophilia.

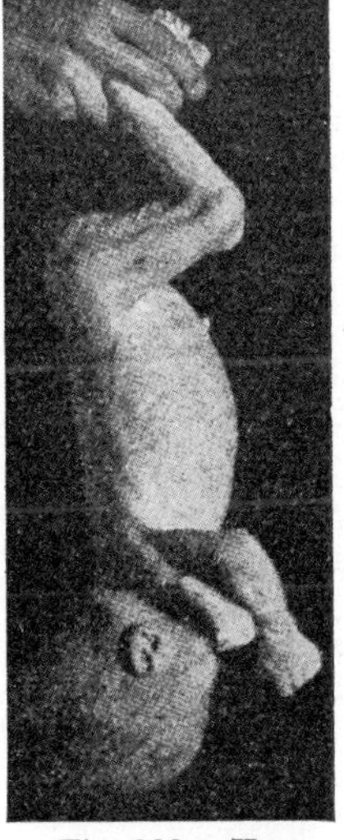

Fig. 200.—Hypertonia in an infant of eleven weeks. Had been fed on rice-water and condensed milk. The illustration shows the persistence of flexion at the knees in spite of the suspension of the child. (*Klose, Jahrb, f. Kinderh.*, 1915, **82**, 362.)

Course and Prognosis of Spasmophilia.—Spasmophilia may be *latent* without active signs of the disease, but examination will reveal the increased mechanical and electrical excitability and the lowered blood-calcium. The prognosis of latent spasmophilia appears entirely favorable, although some claims to the contrary have been made (see Hendriksen[92] and Hjärne[93]). The altered nervous and hemic conditions disappear after infancy, or probably at longest by the end of the fifth year. As regards *active* spasmophilia, eclampsia dependent upon it is seldom fatal; the duration of tetany is very uncertain (p. 871), but the prognosis is good; the outcome of muscular hypertonia depends on the associated conditions; that of bronchotetany is uncertain; and cases of pseudotetanus recover. The majority of cases of laryngismus recover, but sometimes death occurs in an attack.

Diagnosis.—Latent spasmophilia is characterized by the altered condition of the blood and of the electrical and mechanical reactions as already described (p. 870). The most characteristic manifestation of active spasmophilia is carpopedal spasm. When this is present in an infant the diagnosis is practically certain, although other conditions may produce this symptom (see p. 491). A generalized eclamptic convulsion cannot be regarded as certainly spasmophilic unless accompanied by carpopedal spasm or by the characteristic evidences of latent spasmophilia referred to. The combination of these symptoms with active spasmophilic manifestations is diagnostic especially within the age-period of six months to two or three years. In addition to such aids in diagnosis, there are clinical distinctions from certain other diseases. In *tetanus*, which is a much rarer condition than tetany, the hands and feet do not assume the typical position of carpopedal spasm and trismus is present. In *meningitis* the hands may occasionally contract somewhat as in carpopedal spasm, and the feet likewise, but there are other distinguishing characteristics of this disease. The tonic contractions of *cerebral diplegia* may be mistaken for tetany, but the persistence over long periods of time, the much exaggerated reflexes, and the history of the case should remove doubt. *Laryngospasm* other than the spasmophilic form may be an attendant upon certain diseases of the brain, but there are usually other medullary or bulbar symptoms. *Pertussis* occurring in an infant, especially when there is absence of the whoop, might cause confusion with laryngismus, but there is always an accompanying cough, and lymphocytosis soon develops. *Spasmodic laryngitis* and *diphtheritic laryngitis* are attended by fever, hoarseness, and cough; and the attack of stenosis, although apparently sudden in onset, is slower in passing in the former, while in the latter it is persistent. *Congenital laryngeal stridor* occurs earlier in life, and the difficulty in respiration is more continuous, but the symptoms are not threatening. Cases of sudden death in *status lymphaticus* may be improperly attributed to laryngospasm (see p. 483). Attacks of *holding the breath* may in some instances be in reality spasmophilic in nature (see p. 893).

Treatment.—The **prevention** of spasmophilia is similar to that of rickets. Breast-milk is the ideal food. Especially to be avoided are diets which are high in carbohydrate and low in minerals and fat. Proper exposure to the sun should be practised; and cod liver oil, and probably also viosterol, recommended as routine measures in the temperate zone in winter. When **active** symptoms are present more urgent procedures are required. These consist chiefly in the administration of viosterol and cod liver oil; and the exposure to ultraviolet irradiation, preferably from a mercury-vapor-quartz lamp. Bakwin, Bakwin, and Gottschall[94] found that viosterol in average dose for the spasmophilic subjects raised the blood-calcium to normal in about seven days; ultraviolet irradiation in about fourteen days; and that cod liver oil acted slowly and inconstantly. Excessive ultraviolet irradiation is not necessary in treating active symptoms, and may even be harmful. A total of four to six minutes exposure daily with a mercury-vapor-quartz lamp at 50 cm. (19.5 in.) is sufficient (Bakwin and Bakwin[95]). When urgent symptoms are present it is often well to administer some form of calcium, although ordinarily the intake of this in the food is sufficient. Calcium chloride is more efficient than the lactate and may be given in doses of 15 to 30 grains (0.97 to 1.195) four to six times a day. If necessary calcium gluconate may be administered subcutaneously, intramuscularly, or intraspinally, in 7.5 per cent solution in doses of 3 to 4 cc. (0.1 to 0.13 fl. oz.) to young infants. Hydrochloric acid milk for prophylaxis and treatment has been recommended by Sheer[96] and others, and ammonium chloride by Freudenberg and György.[97] It is probable that these acid substances increase the ionization and consequent effectiveness of calcium, even if the total blood-calcium is not increased thereby. They also tend to cause a better intestinal absorption of it.

Although seldom necessary, parathyroid extract may also be employed to raise the blood-calcium rapidly (see Hoag and Rivkin[98]). During attacks of laryngismus efforts should be made to relieve the spasm. Immersion in a warm bath, or slapping the face with a cold wet towel may incite an inspiration, although sometimes these procedures seem to make matters worse. Inhalation of an anesthetic is serviceable if the attack is prolonged and some degree of respiration is present.

CHOREA

(Chorea Minor, St. Vitus's Dance, Sydenham's Chorea)

According to Hecker[99] pilgrimages were made to various shrines, including that of St. Vitus, in the effort to obtain relief from the dancing manias which were so prevalent from the fourteenth to the sixteenth century. From this fact the title "St. Vitus's Dance" has been derived. There would appear to be no actual relationship between these conditions and the disease now under consideration, which was first clearly described by Sydenham.[100] It is one of the commonest of the disorders of childhood and adolescence.

Pathogenesis.—There is close clinical association of chorea with other rheumatic manifestations; many studies showing that from 30 to even 75 per cent of the cases exhibit, either before or after the chorea, evidences of rheumatism in some form. Micro-organisms of the streptococcus group have been recovered from the blood or central nervous tissue of cases of chorea, but this has been exceptional. It would appear that the disease is one of the brain, perhaps due to some functional or toxic disturbance in the basal ganglia, or more widespread throughout the central nervous system. Pathologic changes which have been found, such as multiple emboli or round-celled infiltration, may be only of a secondary nature. Cases which recover are not left with any residual intracranial damage. There probably exists an instability of the nerve-cells in those suffering from chorea. The sudden development of the condition after fright and similar mental disturbances is difficult to explain, although in some cases the disorder was probably present but unnoticed before the psychic insult. It is likewise difficult to understand an association of such cases with rheumatism, and probably these are not to be included as instances of that disease.

Etiology.—The disease is especially one of the *age* of later childhood and puberty. It has, however, been seen in infancy, and even congenital chorea is reported; St. Florent[101] having collected 29 instances in which this diagnosis had been made. The identity of these with true chorea is, however, doubtful. In Starr's[102] 1400 cases 5 per cent were in the first five years and 83 per cent from five to fifteen years. In the matter of *sex* females are more frequently attacked than males, in the proportion of about 2:1 (Starr[102]). *Heredity* operates only indirectly, the children of parents of a nervous disposition or with nervous diseases being those most likely to suffer from chorea. We have repeatedly seen it in more than one child of a family. As regards *season* the general experience is that the larger number of cases are seen in the spring, as pointed out by Lewis,[103] and as most authorities agree. Nordgen[104] and Abt and Levinson[105] publish views dissenting from this. *Climate* and *race* have some influence. Chorea is distinctly less common in hot climates, and infrequent in the negroes of the U. S. and in the North American Indians. Although not truly *epidemic* there is no doubt, as we have seen, that in certain localities it is much more common in some years than in others. Local epidemics in homes for children may occasionally occur, in this case the influence of imitation being apparently decided. The relationship of chorea to *rheumatism* is very intimate, as pointed out under Pathogenesis. (See also Rheumatism, p. 473.) There is a decided association with tonsillitis, such cases being clearly of a rheumatic nature. The direct effect of *psychic* causes is in our experience very positive. A neuropathic, excitable disposition predisposes, and frequently chorea develops promptly after fright, sudden grief, fear, and the like. We have seen the nervous influence of school-life an evident cause. It is more likely to occur in the mentally alert and more intelligent than in the phlegmatic child. Imitation is an occasional psychic factor to which reference has already been made. The *acute infectious fevers*, especially scarlatina, are sometimes followed by chorea. Syphilis probably possesses no etiologic relationship. *Reflex influences* of various sorts have been mentioned as predisposing causes, but are not prominent factors.

Symptoms.—All degrees exist, from mild to more severe and sometimes fatal cases. The onset is usually gradual, the child seeming merely awkward, nervous, restless or emotionally disturbed, and perhaps being reproached by the parents for spilling its food, dropping objects, stumbling when walking, crying without reason, making grimaces, and the like. Soon in average cases jerking movements become evident; frequently, however, first discovered by the physician before the parents had suspected their presence. They begin oftenest on the right side, and are most marked in the upper extremities. In about one-third of the cases they are largely limited to one side of the body (*hemichorea*), with only some slight jerking being observed elsewhere. More often the movements soon involve to some degree all the extremities and the face. They are then characteristic, taking place without any symmetry or regularity, both when the patient is at rest and during attempted action; frequently being accentuated by excitement, fatigue, or effort to control them. As a rule they cease during sleep. In cases of slight severity, the jerking does not interfere greatly with the patient's acts, and he may sometimes be able to control it for a short time during examination. In such cases we have found that the grasping of the wrist as though the pulse were being felt, or requesting the patient to put out the tongue or button the clothing, may reveal the condition by distracting the patient from the effort at control. At the wrist there are felt slight twitching of the muscles, while the tongue is often suddenly jerked back into the oral cavity before the order is given to close the mouth. In the early stages there may occur the Czerny[105] phenomenon, in which, when the child takes a deep breath, the abdominal wall does not swell out during inspiration as in normal cases, but is drawn in and the diaphragm drawn upward into the thorax. Stephens[107] describes a characteristic hypersensitiveness on both sides of the spine from the third dorsal level down to the buttocks. Some degree of psychic disturbance is present and sleep is generally poor and restless, with dreaming.

In many instances the jerking and grimacing are nearly constant, and the patient is unable to feed himself or dress, or even to walk. The respiration is jerking and irregular from the involvement of the diaphragm. Speech is hurried, interrupted, and stumbling, or the patient may not be able to articulate at all. In mild cases the affection of speech may be elicited by having the child count rapidly up to ten, and then backward to one. Part of this interference of speech in the severer cases appears to be of psychic origin. There is often loss of power in the limbs, simulating paralysis, and sometimes this paresis is much in excess of the choreic movements (*paralytic chorea; chorea mollis*).

The majority of cases do not pass beyond the conditions described. Occasionally, however, a choreic state of frightful intensity is observed (*chorea insaniens*). In this the movements are so severe and persistent that the child is tossed violently about the bed and becomes covered with bruises, and forcible restraint is required. The jerking continues during the night and there is almost no sleep. Speech is almost or quite impossible, swallowing is difficult, the sphincters are relaxed, the expression of the face is that of a maniacal person.

Tactile sensibility in chorea is usually not disturbed. There may be headache; pain in the limbs is frequent; paresthesia is exceptional. The reflexes are sometimes exaggerated, sometimes diminished. Loss of adipose tissue occurs; there is diminution of muscular power, especially in the limbs most affected; the patient is easily fatigued; and anorexia and anemia may develop. The action of the heart is often accelerated and murmurs may be present; often soft, blowing, and dependent upon anemia, or, according to some views, on chorea of the muscles of the heart, and therefore functional and temporary. Still oftener the murmurs are the result of a developing endocarditis. Fever of moderate degree is sometimes observed, usually dependent upon a complicating endocarditis or some other condition. The urine may exhibit albumin in severe cases, and glycosuria has been recorded. Urohematoporphyrin was found by Garrod[108] and guanidine by Fanton.[109] The spinal fluid has shown lymphocytosis in some instances (Richardière, Lemaire and Sourdel[110]). Leopold,[111] Fanton[108] and others believe that eosinophilia occurs in the majority of cases. We have noted its presence, but not constantly. A slight lowering of the serum-calcium was found by Warner.[112]

The psychic disturbance alluded to may show itself only in fretfulness, wilfulness, sudden causeless attacks of crying or laughing, and lessened memory and mental concentration. In the severer attacks the condition suggests imbecility, or there may be violent maniacal excitement.

Course and Prognosis.—The disorder reaches its height in one or two weeks, remains stationary for a time, and then gradually grows less and disappears after from eight to ten weeks, or sometimes several months, from the onset. The prognosis, as regards the chorea itself, is good in the majority of cases. The psychic disturbances disappear with the choreic movements, and all traces of paresis are lost. The severest cases may die from a complicating endocarditis or cerebral lesion, or worn out by the violence of the movements. The general mortality may be placed at 2 or 3 per cent, most of the fatal cases occurring after puberty. The prognosis for perfect recovery must be guarded, on account of the danger of the occurrence of permanent cardiac lesions. These, usually endocardial, develop in approximately 30 to 50 per cent of the cases (pp. 473, 786).

Relapse and Recurrence.—Relapse is not very often seen, but the tendency to recurrence, especially in the spring, is well known. It is more frequent for a second attack to occur than otherwise.

Diagnosis.—The jerking, arrhythmical movements of chorea are quite characteristic, yet mistakes in diagnosis sometimes occur. The movements of *postparalytic chorea* are generally unilateral and chronic in their course; the intelligence is often not normal; and the affected limbs are spastic. The paralysis of *poliomyelitis* results in atrophy and the reaction of degeneration. We have seen *Friedreich's* ataxia mistaken for chorea, but here the ataxic movements are not quick and jerking; and there are present characteristic slowness of speech, nystagmus, and a peculiar habitus. (See p. 967.) *Post-encephalitic choreiform movements* resemble closely those of chorea, but the course is more chronic and there is the history of preceding encephalitis. *Hysteria* seldom causes confusion in early life; the movements are usually more rhythmic; and there are other evidences of that disease. *Huntington's chorea* is not a disease of childhood. *Habit spasm* may resemble mild instances of chorea very closely, and repeated observations and a careful history of the case may be needed to differentiate. However, the course is chronic, the movements are limited to certain regions, and they can be restrained for a time by the efforts of the child. *Chorea electrica* is like chorea minor in name only, the movements being peculiarly sudden and speech unaffected (see p. 880).

Treatment.—To **prevent** chorea in those predisposed careful regulation should be made of the general life, avoiding over-study, undue excitement, exposure to cold and damp, and any deterioration of the general health. While foci of infection, such as diseased tonsils, should be removed if this seems indicated, little can be promised in the prevention by this of the occurrence or recurrence of chorea, and in our experience operation is inadvisable during the attack (see p. 542).

In the **treatment of the attack** itself, association with other children should be avoided, a digestible diet given with the omission of stimulants, and punishment or scolding guarded against. Rest in bed but in the open air, if possible, is important, although in mild cases and during convalescence this may be for only a part of the day. Mental rest is as vital as physical rest, but judgement should be used in recommending strict isolation, since this may produce unhappiness and fretting. Mental occupation which is not disturbing will busy the child's mind; and there is no objection, unless the choreic movements are excessive, to playing with puzzles, blocks, and the like, and to a limited amount of reading. Daily warm tub-baths or warm packs, and general massage are often beneficial. The worst cases demand, necessarily, forcible restraint or other protection against injury. Throughout the entire course of the attack the heart must be carefully watched. The rest in bed may sometimes be allowed to cease before the movements have entirely disappeared, provided, of course, there is no cardiac complication.

Drugs hold a minor therapeutical place. Arsenic has long enjoyed repute, being given as Fowler's solution; intramuscularly as sodium cacodylate; or as arsphenamine, neoarsphenamine, or sulpharsphenamine (Talent;[113] Bókay;[114] Moffett and Smith[115]). There is considerable doubt as to the real value of arsenic in the treatment of chorea. If used at all it should be in fairly full doses, and the possibility of detrimental effects remembered. Among sedative remedies are antipyrine, phenobarbital, and the bromides. Apomorphine has been employed. Because of the association with rheumatic manifestations, salicylates have been given, although it is questionable whether they are helpful. In bad cases it may be necessary to administer morphine or hyoscine hypodermically. In very severe cases with evidence of increased intracranial pressure treatment with magnesium sulphate has also been employed, giving intraspinally 0.5 to 1 cc. (0.017 to 0.03 fl. oz.) of a 25 per cent solution for each 20 lb. (9072) of body-weight. Its use is not without danger. For the relief of intracranial pressure simple lumbar puncture is to be recommended. Intraspinal injection of autoserum, proposed by Goodman,[116] is little used at present, and the same is true of intrathecal injection of horse-serum (Porter[117]). Among other therapeutical measures which have been recommended are the subcutaneous injection of the patient's cerebrospinal fluid (Block[118]); foreign protein therapy for the production of fever (Sutton[119]); streptococcic serum perpared from steptococci derived from the throat and nose of patients with chorea (Rosenow[120]); and the employment of a ketogenic diet. One of the latest drug-treatments for chorea is with phenylethylhydantoin (nirvanol) first used by Roeder.[121] This is given orally once a day for seven to ten days, a safe daily dose being 0.2 Gm. (3 grains) in the second year, increasing to 0.5 Gm. (8 grains) in older children. After about one to two weeks a morbilliform or scarlatiniform rash appears, together with leukopenia or eosinophilia, and the treatment should be discontinued, if it is still being given. Toxic effects such as delirium, edema, nephritis, and agranulocytosis are sometimes seen.

The multiplicity of treatments recommended for chorea indicates that none of them are particularly efficacious. The average case should be treated hygienically as described, and sedative treatment and drugs employed as symptomatically indicated. Our experience with the various recommended therapies has been for the most part disappointing, little benefit having been obtained with most of them. Apparently the course of chorea can be shortened by foreign protein therapy, as also by the use of nirvanol, but it would seem that the cure may sometimes be worse than the disease. There is no convincing evidence that any form of treatment lowers the incidence of cardiac complications.

After recovery from chorea a period of several weeks should elapse before the child is permitted to resume school-life or be exposed to other exciting conditions. Anemia, malnutrition, and any other fault of general health must be treated. If a cardiac complication has developed, especial care is needed during convalescence.

SPASMUS NUTANS. GYROSPASM

(Nodding Spasm)

This not uncommon condition first described by Eberth[122] occurs chiefly between the ages of four and twelve months, although cases beginning in the second year or later are occasionally seen. It is somewhat more common in females. The causes are not clearly understood. Almost all the cases observed in infants are associated with rickets. About 70 to 75 per cent of the cases develop in the winter (Thomson,[123] Herrman[124]), this probably being due to the lesser amount of light at this time of year; since residence in dark houses and streets appears to be an important cause, the child having to turn its eyes obliquely or upward in order to see distinctly such objects as toys and the like. Yet there are many cases in which no history of such influence can be elicited. Debilitating disorders and sometimes trauma of the head aid in producing the symptoms. The **symptoms** consist in constant or intermittent involuntary nodding of the head, or a rotary movement of it. The range of movement is slight, and the rapidity about once a second. The movements increase with efforts to fix the eyes upon an object, and disappear during sleep or if the eyes are bandaged. They may sometimes be observed only when the light comes in a particular direction. The head may be held obliquely or bent a little backward. Nystagmus, either of one or both eyes, may occur at the same time with the movements of the head, or before or after them. The movements of the eyes are rapid, of slight extent, may take place in any direction, and are increased by forcible fixing of the head. There may be an attendant convergent strabismus. The intelligence is normal. The **duration** is several months, as a rule, and occasionally recurrence is observed. The **prognosis** is entirely good. In **diagnosis** the age of the patient and the absence of all other symptoms than those described serve to distinguish the disorder. *Congenital nystagmus* is accompanied by ocular defects, and is without movements of the head. *Eclampsia nutans*, to which the title "Salaam convulsion" is also properly applied, is a rare affection of older subjects, usually without nystagmus, and attended by psychic or hysterical manifestations. The *head-nodding* which occurs more as a habit (p. 893) is seen in older children, is without nystagmus, and has a much larger range of movement. The *rocking* of the head on the pillow observed in rachitic infants is slower in movement and attended by fretfulness and irritability. The **treatment** consists in remedying the insufficiency of light, and in treating rickets or other debilitating disorder present. Antispasmodics or sedatives are hardly required.

THE TICS

Here are included several affections, bearing in some respects a resemblance to chorea.

1. Habit-spasm (*Habit-tic; Simple Tic; Habit-chorea*).—This, the most frequent of the tics, is a common disorder, seen oftenest in early and later childhood, and especially in subjects of a neuropathic disposition, with the general health below normal, or when there is mental strain. There is frequently a local cause, such as chronic infection in the upper respiratory tract, adenoids, defective vision, or localized pain or discomfort in some region, which determines the localization of the movements. Occasionally imitation is the starting-point of the disease, or the movements of habit-spasm may develop with recovery from chorea. The **symptoms** consist in spasmodic and irregular movements oftenest connected with the face, such as twitching or distortion of the mouth, wrinkling of the forehead, elevating the eyebrows, forcible winking, and the like; or there may be sighing or sniffing, or jerking movements of the whole head. The movements are only occasional at first, but soon become frequent; are made worse by excitement; and are done unconsciously, although the child is able to restrain them by force of will. Sometimes the effort at control produces such a sensation of discomfort that the patient is unwilling to make it. Other cases have jerking movements of the body, especially of the hands, arms or shoulders, while others exhibit repeated forced efforts at coughing. There may be only one sort of movement, or a number of various kinds; or one sort may be replaced by another. The **duration** of the disease is uncertain. Sometimes it lasts but a few months, while in other cases it may continue for years or perhaps for a lifetime. Generally the much longer duration and the limitation of the movement to some one region serve to distinguish it from chorea. In **treatment** it is important to enlist the efforts of the child to control the movements. The parents should call the attention of the patient to the matter, but not so frequently that this degenerates to nagging, or makes the child over-conscious. A careful search is required for all possible exciting causes, especially nasal disease or defective vision, and the proper treatment instituted. Particular attention must be given to the general health, with insistence upon sufficient physical and mental rest. As far as drugs are concerned arsenic appears to be the most beneficial.

2. IMPULSIVE TIC (*Gilles de la Tourette's Disease*).—This condition, studied especially by Gilles de la Tourette[125] and often bearing his name, begins oftenest in later childhood or at puberty, is infrequent, and generally exhibits a marked neuropathic inheritance. It is more closely allied to hysteria and psychasthenia than to habit spasm. The **symptoms** consist in convulsive and often violent twitchings, especially of the muscles of the face and arms, but in some cases of other parts of the body. With the movements is associated the production of explosive sounds, such as a loud barking cough; or the enunciation of certain words. A frequent symptom accompanying the movements is the tendency to repeat several times a word just heard (*echolalia*) or the involuntary uttering of foul language (*coprolalia*). In many cases imperative conceptions are associated with the movements, resulting in the child performing certain acts, such as the touching of some object, sudden jumping, counting a certain number of times, the making of hissing sounds, the speaking of a number of words in sequence, and the like. The **course** is chronic, and the **prognosis** is not favorable, although the disease occasionally disappears. The **treatment** consists in efforts to improve the neuropathic disposition. Isolation, change of scene, hydrotherapy, gymnastic exercises, and the like may be instituted. Suggestion may be of value in cases possibly hysterical. Self-control should be taught; but not too much notice taken of the attacks.

3. CHOREA ELECTRICA.—There are several forms of this rare affection. It appears to belong to the tics, but in some instances may be of a hysterical or possibly epileptic nature. One form confined chiefly to Italy and described by Dubini[126] occurs in older children and adults, and exhibits a series of violent frequently repeated, convulsive movements of various parts of the body, especially the head. Epileptiform convulsions also occur, and paralysis finally develops, with wasting of the muscles. There is much pain. Coma is a terminal phenomenon. There may be a fatal ending in a few weeks, or sometimes not for months. The cause is unknown.

A second form described by Henoch[127] occurs in children from nine to fifteen years of age. There are sudden, shock-like contractions of the muscles of the head and neck, or less often of other parts of the body. The movements are of momentary duration and slight degree, may be repeated at intervals of seconds or minutes, and occur by day and occasionally during sleep at night. Speech is unaffected, and the muscular control undisturbed except during the jerking. The cause is unknown, the course chronic, and treatment without avail.

A third form was observed in children by Bergeron and described by Berland[128] in 1880. The onset is sudden, sometimes following a nervous shock, and the condition may be a hysterical one. The patients are generally debilitated or neurotic. The movements are similar to those of the second variety, but the prognosis is good.

A fourth form, so-called *lightning convulsions,* appears in most reported cases between four and six months of age. A sudden lightning-like convulsion of the entire body occurs, with the head bent forward on the chest and the legs drawn up. Soon there is arrest of physical and mental development, and idiocy appears (Moro and Asal;[129] Lederer;[130] Lehmkuhl[131]).

The true nature of these varieties of electric chorea is uncertain, as is their relationship to each other. The **diagnosis** of chorea electrica may be made from *chorea minor,* which exhibits more widespread and irregular movement, but less sudden and jerking. *Paramyoclonus multiplex* (p. 988) presents close similarity to the electric chorea of Henoch and is held by some authors to be identical with it. *Postencephalitic* movements occasionally resemble electric chorea. *Habit-spasm* is without the sudden shock-like movements, and *impulsive tic* exhibits echolalia.

NERVOUS CHILDREN

(Neuropathic Children; Nervousness; Neuropathic Diathesis)

In a broader sense this term includes children suffering from one or more of a number of different conditions, such as disturbances of sleep, headache, neurasthenia, anorexia, bad habits, psychasthenia, moral insanity, and hysteria. It does not follow, however, that all children with some of these manifestations are to be classed among the simply "nervous," and for this reason these individual topics referred to will receive independent consideration. (See Index.) No attempt will be made here to explain, or even to use, much of the newer terminology which has arisen in connection with the subject, and the reader is referred to such books as those of Watson,[132] Cameron,[133] Gesell,[134] Thom,[135] Arlitt,[136] and Morgan.[137]

Etiology.—In the narrower sense here employed there are many children who, without necessarily suffering from any distinct nervous disease of moment, are to be denominated *nervous.* Usually there is an *inherited tendency,* one or both of the parents or other members of the family distinctly possessing this character. There is this underlying neuropathic basis present in most cases, but sufficient to produce the symptoms only under the influence of *exciting causes.* Among these are the natural physiologic and anatomical peculiarities of early life. There is, in the first place, the incomplete development of the centers in the cerebral cortex, with consequent lack of control over reflex excitations. There is, further, the rapid growth of the intellect and the interest in the outside world, without a balancing experience and judgement. These conditions favor the development of nervous symptoms in those with or without inherited nervous disposition. There is also the very strong tendency to imitation seen in early life, which may readily give rise to pathologic nervous states. Further there is combined an amount of mental and of physical strain, undergone by children from infancy through the school-years, which is enormous, and the evil influence of this on many subjects is great; since a child will exert itself physically at play until absolutely tired out, or will be allowed to spend more hours at mental work in school than many of its seniors could well endure. This overstrain of body and of mind in the absence of proper control by the parents, or even abetted by them, is a very important cause of the development of nervousness. The constant association with nervous excitable relatives is another cause, as are the efforts to make an infant learn quickly, or to show, in general, evidences of precocity. One often sees, too, the development of nervousness in an only child who is pampered and over-guarded by the parents, mingles only with older persons, and is without that association with other children which is so important for proper mental development.

The influence of school-life has already been referred to. Undue mental labor; worry about unfinished lessons and imperfect recitations; the strain of keeping near the head of the class; the fear that he will fail to pass examinations, are all powerful influences for the development of nervousness in a child predisposed to it. Most teachers and, still more, the parents, are to blame, but often the fault lies in the school-system. There should be no method which forces all children to keep the same pace in the same studies. Finally may be mentioned shock, fright, trauma of any sort, or the influence of some debilitating disease. Fears may be established by improper training, injudicious punishment, the reading of unsuitable books, the hearing of gruesome stories, or the attendance at moving-pictures.

Symptoms.—The symptoms seen in the nervous child are very varied and differ with the individual. They may appear even in the first year of life, among them at this period being, for instance, vomiting produced by slight emotional excitement or a trifling alteration in the taste of the food; the refusal to take any new article of diet (see Anorexia Nervosa, p. 559); starting from sleep from very insignificant causes; precocious development in various directions; the early acquiring of unusual fear of or great shyness at the approach of strangers; thigh-friction; very active emotional facial expression; excitement without sufficient reason; and the like. Babies of this class are often subjects of imperfect nutrition.

Older children of the neurotic type frequently are delicately built, anemic, easily tired mentally and physically, suffer readily from digestive disturbances, and have capricious appetites. There may be a tendency to undue cardiac irregularity or rapid respiration. Nervous coughing or vomiting is sometimes seen following any excitement. Some of the stigmata of degeneration to be described later (p. 901) may be present, but are not constant accompaniments. These nervous children are very impressionable, emotional, and easily excited, and express this to a degree in excess of that seen in normal children. In some cases there is an unusual movement of the face during speech, with the production of grimaces. The power of imagination, always great in a child, is unusually developed, and may be the cause of terror at night from the images which the mind creates, and often of fear of remaining alone or without a light. Nervous children are disposed to worry; are timid; unduly anxious over minor matters; and in some instances have an uncontrollable fear of harmless animals and other objects. They are sensitive, and slight reproof becomes the cause of unhappiness and morbidity. This self-consciousness makes them shy with strangers and even with associates. Various idiosyncrasies are liable to develop. At school and at home the children may be conscious of the difference between themselves and others, and they may become self-repressed, reticent and silent; self-conscious and brooding. Headache is a common and troublesome symptom.

The intellectual power of the nervous child is often unusually great, and the mastering of the school-work is a matter of no difficulty. In other cases the vanity of the parent or child makes pre-eminence at studies attained only by undue effort. In very many the intellectual power becomes easily fatigued on slight mental exertion, and the child finds it difficult to keep up with classmates at school.

Course and Prognosis.—The state of nervousness may be of but temporary duration when the exciting cause was a rapidly acting one, such as trauma or acute illness. If not properly cared for the course may be prolonged, and the condition readily pass beyond the domain of mere nervousness into that of neurasthenia, psychasthenia, psychoses, or other nervous disorder. Yet the prognosis for nervous children is not unfavorable under proper management. The underlying neuropathic tendency, present in practically all cases, always remains, but may cease to give trouble if the life is properly regulated. The outcome often depends on the care and exactness with which the treatment can be carried out; and especially on how well the parents can be instructed in the proper management of the child. It is to be remembered that the strain thrown upon these children must continue always to be in accord with the diminished resisting power which is characteristic of them; otherwise at any time during life there may be a return of nervous symptoms.

Diagnosis.—Simple nervousness, neurasthenia, hysteria, and psychasthenia often appear to shade into each other, or to be variously combined, making differentiation difficult. The diagnosis of simple *nervousness* rests upon the congenital origin usually present; the absence of intellectual defect; the easily developed mental and bodily fatigue; the tendency to excitability and timidity; and the other symptoms as detailed. *Neurasthenia,* as it occurs in children, does not necessarily possess any congenital origin but may be acquired. In the stricter sense it is characterized by the excessive degree of weakness and excitability of mind and body. *Psychopathic children* may exhibit some of the characters of the neuropathic, but with the addition of a great prominence of psychic manifestations. The condition is congenital in origin. Some of the stigmata of degeneration are liable to be exhibited. The state of the intelligence is variable. *Hysteria* is characterized by defective will-power, emotional excitability, and the control of the body and mind by perverted notions and fixed ideas, which are not uncommonly produced by suggestion (Rachford[138]).

Treatment.—This lies most frequently and largely within the province of the physician; the psychiatrist, especially the nonmedical one, being when needed an aider in the study and direction of the individual case. The great frequency of some sort of maladjustment to environment must be recognized and the situation dealt with accordingly. Much can be done by proper training and securing correct environment. From early infancy the evidence of a neurotic disposition must be watched for and guarded against by proper education and control. Late hours, broken sleep, excitement of the young baby by visitors, and other disturbing causes are to be carefully shunned. Later in infancy great caution must be used against forcing the baby into precocity by strenuous efforts to teach it to talk or walk. Both at this period and after it there must be an abundance of mental and bodily rest and of sleep (see Hygiene, pp. 57–59). It is especially in the school-years that constant supervision and most careful judgment are required. A middle ground must be chosen between too much and too little study. The child must necessarily receive instruction, association with other children is very important; and too constantly keeping him at home from school makes him lazy or indifferent and gives him no occupation and no playmates. Most important is it that the parents cease to pamper a nervous child, yielding to his whims, supplying specially prepared food according to his fancies, and constantly exhibiting anxiety over his condition. This concentrates his thoughts upon himself. It is a common habit of parents to show their solicitude and to detail a child's symptoms and behavior to the physician in the presence of the patient. Little could be more harmful than this. Beginning early, with either nervous or normal infants, self restraint must be taught, and the knowledge inculcated in the child that there are things that he must or must not do, and that he can or cannot have. It is claimed by many psychologists that traits of character are largely formed by six years of age.

One of the most vital elements of treatment is, unfortunately, one which frequently cannot be fulfilled; viz., the removal entirely from the nervous influence of home-associations. So-called "nursery schools" or "mother's training centers" have value here when properly conducted. The sending of the older child to a boarding school is often greatly to be desired. In other instances the spending of the summer-vacation where there are new sights and associations is of very great benefit; always localities being selected where there are other children to be had as playmates. The direct influence of change of climate is in itself beneficial.

Naturally, every method possible must be employed to improve the general health; such as properly chosen gymnastic exercises; life and exercise in the open air; suitable diet; and the treatment of any disordered condition present. After any acute illness there should be no haste in returning the child to school; since the strength of nervous children often suffers decidedly during the attack. Throughout there must be encouragement given, and the symptoms openly made light of rather than dwelt upon. The unreasoning timidity which is usually present is to be managed carefully. Thus a nervous child who has developed, for instance, a fear of sleeping in the dark, should be allowed a light in the room, and that without question. Nothing can be accomplished by compulsion, scolding, or ridicule in such cases; but encouragement and reward will aid greatly. With older children a quiet and sympathetic discussion of their fears, and explanation of the groundlessness of them, may be helpful; while with infants pleasant sensations may be gradually associated with the cause of fear, if the source can not be removed. Disciplining nervous children is, of course, required on occasion, or they become self-willed and uncontrollable; but such forms must be varied from time to time, and those chosen which cannot awaken fright or other nervous shock, lest the nervous symptoms be made worse thereby.

NEURASTHENIA

In the condition of Nervousness, as just described, are included many of the cases designated by some writers as neurasthenia. While the symptoms are to some extent those seen in nervous children, neurasthenia is not common in early life, and is especially marked by a profound exhaustion of the mental and bodily powers, very often combined with severe and prolonged headache and attacks of fainting. There may or may not be an underlying congenital predisposition. The intellect is unaffected except for the mental asthenia, which renders long continuance of thought impossible. The **treatment** is quite similar to that for simple nervousness. Great physical and mental repose is required. Rest in bed may be needed for a time, with removal of all exciting surroundings. Change of air and scene are advisable, with massage and hydrotherapeutical measures. Constant encouragement of the patient is necessary. The malady is curable, but the course is prolonged.

HEADACHE

Etiology and Symptoms.—Headache, although but a symptom, may be dependent upon many and diverse conditions, some of which are as follows:

(1) **Organic diseases of the brain or meninges,** as in intracranial tumor, meningitis, poliomyelitis, encephalitis, brain-abscess, sinus thrombosis, and syphilis. Pain is more or less persistent, frequently severe, and localized. (2) **Infectious diseases,** in which headache is common as a prodromal symptom. There are accompanying fever and other symptoms. The headache is usually frontal, and the pain lasts over a few hours or days. (3) **Toxemia** dependent upon gastro-intestinal disorders ("bilious headache"); poisoning by lead, alcohol, opium, and the like; and metabolic disturbances such as hypoglycemia, ketonemia (Cameron[139]), uremia, and disturbed states of the acid-base balance. The headache is generally frontal or vertical. Perhaps here may be placed the headaches accompanying chronic infections and rheumatic disease. (4) **Disturbance of the cerebral circulation,** often observed in anemia. The headache is frontal or oftener vertical, dull, and most marked in the morning. *Congestive headache* may sometimes be seen in pertussis, cardiac disease, difficult or delayed menstruation in girls approaching puberty, sunstroke, and intense mental activity. This form is due to hyperemia of the brain, and may be attended by flushing of the face and injection of the eyes. (5) **Nervous causes** due to mental and bodily fatigue, or occurring in hysteria, neurasthenia, and epilepsy. This headache is liable to occur day after day and is often vertical. "School-headaches" are frequently of a nervous nature. Anemia and insomnia are often attendant symptoms. (6) **Disorders of the special senses,** of which eye-strain is the most frequent variety. This headache is frontal or occipital in position, and develops after the eyes have been used for study, or after prolonged exposure to bright light. Conjunctivitis or keratitis is present in some cases. Disorders of the nose, as adenoids, rhinitis and polypi, may be a reflex cause of headache. Otitis may produce an intense pain in the parietal or temporal region. (7) **Neuralgia,** which is produced by many of the causes mentioned, and is characteristically limited to the distribution of certain of the cranial nerves. The pain is sometimes supra-orbital; oftener is situated lower on the face and may then be dependent on carious teeth. (8) **Migraine (sick headache; hemicrania),** which has distinctive features. In our experience it is uncommon in infants, but seen with more frequency in older children. It is often distinctly hereditary, or may occur in those with an inherited neurotic tendency. Among assigned causes are toxemia of some sort, cerebral anemia, cerebral congestion, conditions of faulty metabolism, and allergy. It is more common in females. Slight causes, as fatigue, emotional disturbance, or dietary indiscretion may start an attack. The attacks occur at intervals of weeks or months, and usually begin with prodromal symptoms, especially derangements of vision or vertigo. The headache is intense and generally unilateral. It may be accompanied by photophobia, tinnitus, paresthesia, vertigo, or temporary difficulty in speech. After a few hours the pain is followed by nausea and vomiting, and then by deep sleep from which the patient wakens free from pain. In young children headache may be a minor feature, and nausea and vomiting marked. As pointed out by Rachford[140] attacks of recurrent vomiting may be later replaced by migraine.

Diagnosis of Headache.—In young infants headache may be shown by wrinkling of the forehead, rubbing of the head, restlessness, and crying. In older subjects localized persistent pain in the head depends oftenest upon organic disease of the brain; that in the course of a certain nerve is neuralgic in nature; temporary headache with fever is most frequently from gastro-intestinal disturbance, or the onset of some febrile disease; periodic headache may be due to migraine; frequently recurring headache may depend upon nervous conditions, anemia, or eye-strain. The position of the pain, too, is often to a certain extent a guide to the cause. Frontal headache is most frequently from eye-strain, acute infectious disorders, disease of the nose, anemia, or gastro-intestinal disturbances. Vertical headache is generally of a nervous nature, or the result of anemia. Occipital headache is often from eye-strain, otitis, or pharyngitis. Only careful study will serve to determine the cause in many instances.

Treatment.—The cause must be sought for and appropriate treatment instituted. Apart from this, direct relief of the headache may be obtained by rest, both bodily and mental; mustard plasters to the back of the neck; hot foot-baths; cold cloths or an ice-bag to the head; and the application of ointments or liquids containing menthol or alcohol. Analgesic drugs may be necessary. The ketogenic diet (p. 867) has been used with some success for migraine in adults (Barborka[141]).

Disorders of Sleep

The physiology of sleep is so imperfectly understood that discussion of it is not warranted here. Reviews and studies of the subject are given by Freeman,[142] Stephenson et al.,[143] and Kleitman.[144] The following conditions may receive attention.

INSOMNIA. DISTURBED SLEEP

Etiology.—The need for abundant sleep and the number of hours of it required have been discussed previously (p. 57). Among the many causes of disturbed sleep in infancy are hunger; pain of some degree; itching, as in eczema; local irritation, as from a wet diaper; an uncomfortable bed; and fever. Nervous infants may be wakeful, either crying during the night or sometimes lying awake but entirely happy. The nervousness is sometimes inherent; sometimes brought about by the nervous anxiety of the mother or nurse. Rickets is a frequent cause of nervous wakefulness, and in some cases lowered blood-calcium may possibly be a factor (Shannon[145]). Among other causes are too much light, poor ventilation, or too low or too high a temperature in the sleeping room; insufficient or too heavy bed-covering; unusual noises; undue excitement, as of play, before the sleeping hour; and over-fatigue. An important etiologic factor is improper training, such as walking with the child or rocking it, or giving the bottle or the breast as soon as it begins to cry.

In addition to the causes already mentioned, certain others are operative in older children. These are mental overwork; mental stimulation from hearing exciting stories, or emotional excitement of any sort, even pleasurable, shortly before going to bed; insistence upon sleep when there is no desire for it; abnormal fear of being alone at night; diseases of the heart or lungs, or obstruction of the upper respiratory tract, accompanied by dyspnea and cough; and any cause productive of pain. Epidemic encephalitis may have obstinate insomnia as a sequel.

Symptoms.—There may be actual insomnia, or only disturbance of sleep, and various degrees of these. Wakefulness may be present when the child first goes to bed, but the sleep later be sound; sleep may come early but the child waken later; or while asleep there may be excessive restlessness.

Treatment.—Any such condition as nervousness, anemia, debility, and the like should receive appropriate treatment, the diet and digestion being particularly studied. Sometimes a lighter evening meal is helpful; sometimes the increasing of the amount taken. In infancy the securing of an opening of the bowels before bedtime may be efficacious. The daily warm bath may often be given in the evening with good results. Careful inquiry into the hygienic methods and the general life and training of the child should be made, and all the possible disturbing factors removed. Sometimes a change of nurses gives excellent results. The room should be darkened, or a low light allowed, according to the case. Everything should be avoided which centers the child's mind on the existence of sleeplessness. Drugs should be resorted to only when really necessary, and their use should not be long continued. Sometimes the other members of the family need hypnotics more than the infant, who, in spite of a restless night, enters upon the next day in good condition. Of sleep-producing drugs a choice may be made between the bromides, chloral, and the barbital derivatives.

EXCESSIVE SLEEPINESS

In weakly new-born infants there is not infrequently seen a disposition to constant sleep, so great that nursing is interfered with. Either debility or a toxemia appears to be the active agent, some toxic substance in the mother's milk occasionally seeming to be the cause, since temporary withdrawal of this has good effect. Organic disease of the brain may also produce excessive sleepiness. Later in infancy and in childhood it may be seen at the onset or during the course of febrile diseases, especially measles; in uremia; as a result of exhaustion; in hypothyroidism; in organic cerebral diseases as tuberculous meningitis, thrombosis of the cerebral sinuses, epidemic encephalitis, or brain-tumor; after epileptic convulsions; and as a result of drugs. Narcolepsy has already been discussed (p. 868).

DREAMING; NIGHTMARE; SOMNAMBULISM

Even infants may dream, as shown by the sudden startled screaming or by evidently purposeful movements of the hands. Dreaming occurs particularly in nervous children; in the restless disturbed sleep of indigestion; in respiratory disturbances; with fever; and following some definite excitement or mental strain. Often dreams are repeated night after night. They can sometimes be traced to a decided mental impression associated with fear. When dreams of this sort reach an extreme degree, *nightmare* is spoken of. It seems hardly necessary to do more than mention in passing that the Freudian school believe that even in childhood dreams may have a sexual basis. In *somnambulism* the patient, oftenest an older child, performs various systematic acts during sleep, actual walking not being a necessary feature. Occurring alone or often combined with somnambulistic acts is *talking during sleep*. The **treatment** of these conditions consists in searching for and removing any exciting cause. Children with somnambulism may require tying in bed in order to prevent accidents. The temporary administration of hypnotics and sedatives may be helpful.

PAVOR NOCTURNUS

(Night-terrors)

Etiology.—This disorder occurs in children with a neurotic inheritance; or with anemia, adenoids, or other causes of general ill health. Exciting influences may be operative, such as are seen in ordinary dreaming; yet in many instances the terrors occur repeatedly without any exciting cause being discoverable. The subjects are of both sexes and oftenest between the ages of three and eight years, but may be older.

Symptoms.—Two classes of cases have been described. In the first, denominated *symptomatic night-terror*, the child wakens from sleep in terror and perhaps confused; but ultimately cognizant of the dream which disturbed him. On the evening before there may have been some warning, such as excessive malaise, visual disturbance, or the like. The dreams are not those resembling any actual experience and they are associated with great fear. There is no recurrence on the same night. The attack comes on oftenest soon after going to sleep. The condition is so closely allied to nightmare that it may be regarded as an unusually severe form of this. In *cerebral* or *idiopathic night-terror* the attack comes on usually after an hour or two of sleep and when it is deepest. Without previous warning the child suddenly sits upright in bed bathed in perspiration, screaming, and trembling with terror; or in some instances gets out of bed and is found sitting upon the floor. Sometimes he repeats words or points with his finger, indicating the imaginary object which has frightened him. Although he clutches at his mother or nurse he does not recognize her or know where he is. Considerable time is required before he can be quieted. Sometimes he sleeps again without returning to consciousness; or in other cases he becomes partially conscious, quiet, and then quickly falls asleep. In contradistinction to nightmare and symptomatic night-terror, the child is unable to describe the occurrence of any dream, does not attain complete consciousness, does not recognize his surroundings, and has no remembrance of the attack upon the following day.

Course and Prognosis.—The frequency of the attacks varies. They may occur nightly, or only at intervals of weeks or months. Only rarely is there more than one during a night. There are no after-effects seen upon the next day. It may be months before the recurrences cease, but there seems to be no certain evidence that pavor nocturnus predisposes to the development later of epilepsy or other nervous affection. Epilepsy, however, may sometimes exhibit symptoms which closely resemble night-terrors.

Treatment.—Search should be made for any exciting cause, and this treated as well as any disturbance of general health. Constipation should be corrected and usually the evening meal should be light. Excitement before bed-time must be avoided. Frequently a light may be allowed to burn in the bed-room, and someone should sleep in an adjoining room with the door open, if the child demands these things. Generally late hours should be avoided; but we have known attacks to cease after a later hour for retiring was chosen, this producing a tendency to a deeper sleep. Bromides, chloral, or phenobarbital may be administered at bed-time, although such treatment is not feasible if the attacks are at long intervals.

PAVOR DIURNUS

Very much less frequently attacks corresponding to pavor nocturnus occur in the day-time during the morning-sleep, or even when the child is awake. The child may be subject to night-terrors also. The prognosis of pavor diurnus is guarded on account of a more possible closer relationship with hysteria, epilepsy, insanity, or other nervous diseases. In quite young children pavor diurnus may be represented by fits of violent screaming without discoverable cause. The element of anger must be excluded in making the diagnosis.

DISORDERS OF SPEECH

Some of the disorders of speech depend upon organic defects, but most are functional in nature. They will be grouped together here as a matter of convenience. Speech defects of various sorts are common. In 18 large cities in the United States, the ratio of speech defectives to the total school-enrollment in a recent year was 1.8 per cent (Rogers[146]). While statistics vary, lisping appears to be the most common difficulty, and next in order comes either stammering or defective phonation ("baby-talk").

RETARDED ACQUIRING OF SPEECH

Children should normally begin to speak by two years of age (p. 48) and those who do not may perhaps be suffering from mental defect. Other causes are prolonged illness and retarded physical development; rarely deafness; and exceptionally disorders or malformations of the mouth, nose and throat. In many cases no cause can be discovered, the delay in talking being but an individual characteristic which time will improve; in these cases the child appearing to understand perfectly. Others chatter in a jargon unintelligible to all but the attendants. The only **treatment** consists in continued efforts to teach the child. Children indisposed to talk should not have their wants immediately gratified when they have signified them merely by pointing or other gesture.

APHASIA; DUMBNESS; MUTISM

In a strict sense the term "*aphasia*" is applied only to the loss, through the disease of the speech-centers or their connecting apparatus, of the power to talk previously acquired; those who never had the power of speech, or who have lost it through early developing deafness, being described as suffering from *dumbness* or *mutism*. Deaf-mutism may be either congenital in nature, due to defect of the auditory apparatus, or acquired through injury or disease of the middle or internal ear or of the auditory nerve occurring early in life, especially in the course of the infectious fevers. Dumbness of varying degree is present in imbecility. It is occasionally seen where the organs of articulation are defective, and temporarily when the acquisition of speech is retarded (p. 888). Aphasia may be either *functional* or *organic*. The first, of a temporary nature, is observed in such conditions as chorea, hysteria, migraine, shock, or following severe febrile diseases, especially typhoid. Organic aphasia results from trauma, hereditary syphilis, cerebral paralysis, brain-tumor, meningitis, encephalitis, etc. Aphasia may be complete, or the child can speak some syllables or words. The **prognosis** is good in the functional cases, and even in organic ones the regaining of the power of speech is sometimes surprising. The only **treatment** possible in any case of aphasia is that of education, combined with efforts to improve the general health.

Alexia (*Congenital Word-blindness*).—This is an inability or retardation in the learning to recognize written or printed words or letters; some patients recognizing them but being unable to put them into speech. Intelligence is normal, vision unaffected, and the understanding of spoken words and the ability to talk are unimpaired. There may be complete incapability of learning to read, or mere slowness in acquiring the power, which could wrongly be attributed to stupidity or defective eyesight.

STAMMERING; STUTTERING

Stuttering denotes a difficulty in beginning a word or syllable, often with frequent repetition of the first portion of it; while *stammering* consists in difficulty in uttering certain sounds at all, is not accompanied by repetition, and is in some cases associated with malformation of the organs of speech or with imperfect intellectual development. The two terms are often used interchangeably.

Etiology.—Grouping stuttering as a form of stammering the underlying cause seems to be a lack of nervous coordinating control over the respiratory and articulating mechanisms. Often the action of the brain appears to be too fast for the articulating apparatus. Heredity plays an important rôle, in over 25 per cent of the cases more than one member of the family being affected (Gutzmann[147]). Many of the cases apparently of inheritance are due to unconscious mimicry. The asserted relationship of left-handedness to stammering has not been proven (Quinan;[148] Tompkins;[149] Kistler[150]). Many subjects are of neuropathic disposition and may exhibit other nervous disturbances; but most of them are of normal intelligence (Lima[151]), although shy and sensitive, perhaps as an effect rather than a cause. Males are more predisposed (3:1). The condition is a common one especially in later childhood, although it may appear before the age of four years. It has been estimated as occurring in from 0.4 per cent (Priestly[152]) to 1 per cent (Gutzmann[147]) of school-children. Among possible exciting causes, or those which exaggerate the condition, are excitement; impairment of general health; digestive disorders; and disturbances of the respiratory tract, such as adenoids.

Symptoms.—The principal symptom is produced by a spasm of the articulating apparatus which prevents for a moment the word being spoken, or breaks in upon it during its utterance. In the milder cases the stammering is only moderate and at times entirely absent; but reappears when the patient is excited or hurried. Often only certain sounds cause the chief hesitation and difficulty, the words which immediately follow being spoken rapidly. There may be complete momentary stopping over the difficult word or syllable, with a final explosive enunciation of it; or the initial sound may be repeated a number of times in rapid succession before the rest of the syllable can be pronounced. In the severer cases various movements may accompany the effort at articulation; such as contortion of the face, or certain systematic motions of the arms and legs; while in some instances there is the interjection of grunting or other noises, or of words without bearing upon the sentence. It is a curious fact that many stammerers can whisper without stammering, some can read or recite poetry, and most of them can sing without difficulty.

Prognosis.—When stammering begins in children less than four years of age the condition is usually less severe and only temporary, and soon disappears permanently under treatment. In older children the prognosis is much more uncertain, and the longer the disease has continued untreated, the less likely it is to be cured even by intensive training. Relapses are very liable to occur unless treatment is persisted in.

Treatment.—Every means must be taken to diminish any nervous tendency and to improve the general health. Removal of a stammerer from school is advisable, both for his own sake and for that of other children; since it is during school-life that stammering develops or is liable to become worse if already present, and the association with a stammerer may induce the disease in other children. Attempts to talk with undue rapidity should be stopped and the child made to tell slowly, in a low voice, and in short sentences, what he has to say. The direct treatment of stammering already established requires much knowledge and experience of a specialized nature. There are given exercises to cause muscular relaxation and correct the breathing, together with instruction in phonetics and vocal gymnastics. The methods to be employed are described by Gutzmann,[147] Wylley,[153] Glassburg,[154] Twitmyer and Nathanson,[155] and others.

LISPING

(Lalling; Alalia; Idioglossia)

Lisping (sigmatismus) is an imperfect phonation in which certain letter-sounds are replaced by others, as "th" for "s," or, less often, other letters as "r," "k" and "g" being mispronounced. Such replacement is a normal attendant of the early efforts of a child to talk, but in some instances it continues to a greater or less extent and is then pathologic. In some of the severer cases of lisping or other forms of imperfect phonation there may be an organic defect present, such as hare-lip, cleft palate, paralysis of the lips or palate, adenoids, abnormalities of the uvula, tongue-tie, deformed teeth and dental arches. The worst form of lisping is **lalling**, which consists of persistence of infantile speech. It is observed oftenest in children with mental deficiency, but occurs sometimes because all the adults in contact with the child employ "baby-talk" to address it. The term **idioglossia** has been used to designate certain excessive degrees of lalling in which, although the child is mentally normal, speech is voluble but practically unintelligible. **Alalia** is entire inability to articulate. The **prognosis** of lisping is good under treatment in all functional cases, there being a natural tendency to spontaneous cessation. The **treatment** consists in education by mechanical measures and the like, as in the oral methods with deaf-mutes by aid of touch and sight. Organic defects require suitable operative measures.

Neurotic Habits

In many instances these are of little moment, while in others they appear to be manifestations of degeneration, or to be evidences of minor psychic disturbances or even of true psychoses. There has already been discussed certain aspects of the training of children (p. 60). The learning of habits begins soon after birth, the acquiring depending largely upon how often the acts are repeated and the pleasure derived. The habits of eating and sleeping are acquired automatically; with later ones imitation and suggestion are influential. Such qualities as honesty, self control, sociability, and the like, often considered "traits of character," are largely due to proper habit-formation (Thom[135]). The **treatment** of neurotic habits in general, and of the underlying nervous temperament so often present, is very similar to that for the management of nervous children (p. 883). Efforts should be made to replace a bad habit by a good substitute, the bad habit being condemned, and the child being made to associate it with unpleasant results, other than bodily punishment. With older children rewards are often valuable, and sympathetic discussion may secure their coöperation.

THUMB-SUCKING; TEETH-GRINDING; NAIL-BITING, ETC.

Thumb-sucking; Tongue-sucking.—Besides the thumb there may be sucking of the tongue, fingers, toes, lips, etc.; or such objects as a rubber nipple or "comforter," a blanket or sheet, or part of the clothing. Tongue-sucking is common in Mongolism and may occur in other mental defectives, and occasionally in normal infants. Sucking of the thumb, fingers, rubber nipple, or other objects is common in infancy, and usually a matter of little moment. Few pediatrists would be willing to accept the view sometimes advanced that it has any sexual basis. It arises from the natural disposition of the hungry infant to put something into his mouth. The sucking may be of the "combined" form, *i. e.*, accompanied by other acts, such as rubbing at the nose, pulling at the hair, and the like. Thumb-sucking is more liable to occur when the child is about to go to sleep, or when hungry, sleepless, or ill. In milder cases it is only occasional, and the child easily diverted from it. If it is continuous, there may be produced permanent deformity of the thumb or jaws, with malposition of the teeth. The **duration** of the habit is indefinite. Most infants cease of their own accord, but it may last well into childhood. The ultimate **prognosis** is usually good, but recovery is often tedious and relapses readily occur if the child's general health suffers. Final cure is uncertain only in cases of mental deficiency. **Treatment** should be commenced early if the habit is unduly frequent or of the combined type, and in all infants over one year of age. Occasionally, however, the sucking at a rubber nipple or "comforter" may be temporarily permitted in an ill or nervous child who has long had the habit. In the early stage of thumb-sucking mechanical restraint is most effective, an elbow-splint of pasteboard, or one made of wooden tongue-depressors and adhesive plaster, being put upon the elbows. Globular aluminum mitts or other coverings for the hand or thumb may be used. The application to the thumb of bitter substances, as aloes or quinine, is of service only in the mildest cases. Mechanical interference with tongue-sucking or lip-sucking is hardly practicable. In older children, addicts of thumb-sucking, similar restraint is necessary. Ridicule by school-mates sometimes effects a cure. Rewards may be helpful, but punishment is useless (see p. 891).

Among other neurotic habits may be mentioned **tongue-chewing** seen oftenest in the second year, in which one side of the tongue is subjected to a chewing movement between the molars. **Teeth-grinding** is observed chiefly during sleep, or in unconscious states dependent upon disease. It occurs with greatest frequency in neurotic children suffering from some reflex peripheral irritation, as in gastro-intestinal disorders. It may result from intracranial disease, and hence is a characteristic symptom of meningitis. It in no way especially indicates the presence of "worms." Occurring during the waking hours it is not infrequently observed in imbeciles, and in other cases seems to be simply a vicious habit. In bad cases the teeth become much worn. *Treatment* must be directed against the cause, including both the general condition and any peripheral irritation present. **Nail-biting** is observed only in decidedly nervous children. It is more significant of a disordered state of the nervous system than is thumb-sucking. It may be done only when the general nervous condition is worse, or when the patient is under some sort of excitement or worry. *Treatment* is the same as that for thumb-sucking. The nails should be kept cut very short, and the fingers protected by gloves. In addition measures should be employed for the relief of the inherent nervous condition. **Picking,** pulling, rubbing, or scratching at some portion of the body is seen in infants and children of nervous disposition, or those affected by some disorder of general nutrition, such as rickets. Fatigue and emotional stress may initiate or exaggerate the condition. To these factors is often added a localized irritation. Children suffering from illness of many sorts, such as typhoid fever, often pick at the lips so continuously that restraint is necessary. Fretful infants frequently pull at the hair, and large areas of the scalp may be almost denuded in some cases. Certain infants have a tendency to pull at the foreskin, the ear, the navel, or other parts of the body while sucking the thumb. The most frequent and annoying habit is that of picking at or boring into the nose, for which there is sometimes a distinct local irritating cause. In the way of *treatment* for picking of any sort, forcible restraint may be necessary in infancy; and admonition and restraining measures of other nature in older subjects. Of especial importance is it to improve the general nervous condition and to remove the local irritation.

RHYTHMICAL MOVEMENTS

(Head-banging; Swaying; Head-nodding; Head-rocking, etc.)

Certain rhythmical movements occur oftenest in those mentally defective, but others may be seen in subjects merely of a nervous disposition or even apparently normal. The movements may be always of one sort, or one form may alternate with another.

Head-banging, as it was named by Gee,[156] is encountered in extremely nervous children, usually from two to six years of age, who may be suffering from rickets, or in those mentally defective. The child rhythmically bangs his head against the pillow or the side of the crib, and may continue this for minutes or hours while awake, or sometimes in sleep. Occasionally there is evidence of anger; generally none. **Head-rolling** is not uncommon in nervous infants, especially with rickets. The child lying in bed rolls its head from side to side, and continues this day after day. As a result the hair is almost completely worn away from the back of the head. **Head-nodding** is another of the nervous movements sometimes seen. It is to be distinguished from the gyrospasm and nodding spasm previously described (p. 879) in that it is much more energetic and apparently intentional. It occurs while the child is sitting, and may be either a vigorous nodding or a lateral shaking movement. **Swaying,** or **body-rocking** to and fro is a common habit, especially, but not only, observed in mentally defective children. The child in a sitting position rocks rapidly forward and backward, and continues this for hours. Generally it is without the evidence of excitement seen in masturbation.

The **treatment** of these various conditions consists in improving the general health, in combating any nervous condition present, and in forcible restraint as far as possible.

PICA

Pica, or perverted appetite, is a common disorder observed oftenest in the first and second years of life, although sometimes developing later; and consisting in the desire to eat some of a large variety of unsuitable substances, according to the case, such as sand, earth, wool from blankets, broken glass, goat-droppings, hair from the head, paint from the furniture, coal, ashes, plaster from the wall, etc. Often there is an underlying digestive disturbance, while in other cases the presence of intestinal parasites, especially hook-worm, is a cause. In many instances the mental and general health is good; in others there is anemia, malnutrition, or a distinctly neurotic disposition. The habit is frequent in mentally defective subjects. There is a natural tendency for pica developing in infancy to cease of itself by the age of three or four years, and this renders the **prognosis** good; but the habit may sometimes continue much longer and be very intractable. The general health may finally be seriously affected by the harmful action of the various objects swallowed, and the anorexia which commonly attends. **Treatment** should be given promptly, and consists principally in preventing the eating of the unnatural articles and in general hygienic measures.

HOLDING THE BREATH

The attacks of holding the breath, as now under consideration, cannot strictly be called a bad habit, although sometimes seemingly voluntary, but are to be classified as the direct effect of yielding to violent anger or to other excitement. They are seen in highly neurotic, uncontrollable, or psychopathic children who show no effort at self-control of their emotions or impulses. A temporary spasm of the larynx is probably produced. The attacks occur at a somewhat later period of life than laryngismus stridulus, exhibit no evidences of spasmophilia, and appear to possess no relationship to epilepsy. There seems to be no good reason to consider them as related to any enlargement of the thymus. They begin oftenest in the second or third year of life, but generally disappear by the age of four or five years at latest. Although anger is the most frequent cause, in some cases sudden fright is operative.

Symptoms.—Under the influence of something which displeases or startles him, the child exhibits a sudden cessation of respiration, cyanosis, and rigidity of the body; and then in severe cases loss of consciousness, possibly convulsive twitching, pallor which is sometimes extreme, and general relaxation. In a few seconds the attack is over, and in a very brief time the patient seems as well as before. There may be recurrence several times a day or at longer intervals. In some cases the holding of the breath is the terminal stage of an attack of rage, in which the child throws himself on the floor and screams violently for a few moments; or the holding of the breath may be both preceded and followed by crying. The **prognosis** is good and, unlike laryngismus, the condition is rarely a fatal one.

Treatment.—This consists in measures to improve the nervous condition and the correction of any fault of general health. Especially important is the teaching of the child to exercise self-control. Rewards and encouragement may do much; and certainly the yielding by the parents on every occasion for fear of precipitating an attack can do only harm. The question of punishment depends upon the individual case, since the punishment itself is liable to cause an attack in some instances. Yet knowledge that punishment, not corporeal, will follow, may aid the child in learning control. Certainly nothing must be done to frighten the patient, and kindness will do more than harshness with the neurotic condition which these children possess. The attack itself may sometimes be curtailed by the sudden application of cold water or a cold cloth to the face; yet this is seldom required and is not well-tolerated in every instance.

MASTURBATION

Etiology.—A marked neurotic disposition is a powerful predisposing cause of this very common habit, and it is only in such cases that it becomes a matter of serious moment. In many imbeciles, or in those who later show themselves vicious in other respects, masturbation has often begun early and is practised to great excess. Anything which impairs the general health may predispose to masturbation or cause its renewal. Some local irritation is active in many instances, such as the presence of phimosis, the accumulation of smegma behind the corona, balanoposthitis, the irritation from tight diapers or drawers, vulvovaginitis, the itching produced by eczema or by the presence of thread-worms in the rectum or vagina, constipation, highly acid urine, preputial adhesions of the clitoris, and the like. Sometimes irresponsible nurses have habitually rubbed the penis of an infant for the purpose of soothing him. In older children masturbation may be initiated accidentally, as by sliding down a baluster rail, climbing trees, horseback riding, irritation of tight clothing, and the like; but oftenest at this age it is taught by companions. It is at this period much oftener practised by boys, although as puberty is approached or even much before this it is frequently encountered in girls as well. It is much more common in later than in early childhood.

Symptoms.—In infancy masturbation shows itself usually in the form of *thigh-friction* or associated movements. The infant, usually a female, sitting on the floor, or lying on its back with the lower extremities drawn upward, rubs the thighs vigorously together, thus catching and rubbing the clitoris between them. The face meanwhile becomes flushed and the eyes have a fixed, somewhat staring expression. Often the attention of the attendant will be drawn by the unusual absence of noise, or the uttering of a grunting sound on the part of the child. After a short time something suggesting an orgasm is produced, sweat breaking out on the forehead, the face growing paler, and the infant lying back relaxed from temporary exhaustion. The procedure is repeated possibly many times a day or even during sleep.

Various modifications or substitutions of this typical thigh-friction are seen. Some infants, lying on the back or sitting, rub the buttocks from side to side on the bed or floor; others rub the genital organs against some object, such as a pillow, the leg of a chair, or the like. Sometimes movements of other parts of the body are associated with or even appear to take the place of those which directly cause friction of the genitals.

Infants with thigh-friction may exhibit other signs of neurotic excitability or show evidences of retardation. Many such manifestations present are, however, less often the result than the cause of the habit. Many infants seem perfectly healthy. The examination of the genitals will frequently show redness of the entrance of the vagina, and probably some local source of irritation.

After the period of infancy, masturbation is more clearly associated with an early development of sexual excitability. The hand is generally used, thigh-friction being uncommon. As a result of reproof and consequent consciousness of wrongdoing, the habit soon becomes a secret one. Generally it is occasional only, but in bad cases in children of a very highly neurotic nature the child may lie awake at night masturbating, or do it many times in the day, and sometimes loses all sense of shame and power of self-control, and masturbates in public as well. The local manifestations are varied. The penis may be unusually turgid or enlarged, and with a tendency to ready erection, or the organ may seem relaxed. The prepuce may be swollen and slightly inflamed. In girls the clitoris and labia may be larger than normal and reddened, and there may be some degree of vaginitis. None of these signs, however, are positive, and all may be wanting. As regards the general symptoms there is much uncertainty. In many cases there are none discoverable. Excitability, nervousness, apathy, mental hebitude, depression, morbidness, shyness, reticence, pallor, loss of memory, debility, headache and many similar conditions have often been described as the result of masturbation; but it seems more probable that, in the majority of instances, these are manifestations of the neurotic state upon which the habit itself largely depends. Feeblemindedness or other psychic disturbance, for instance, is far oftener the cause of masturbation than its sequel; and the same is true of hysteria, epilepsy, nymphomania, insanity, sexual perversion, and the like. These conditions were developing, and excessive masturbation was but one of the early manifestations. On the other hand, frequent masturbation certainly has an exhausting effect upon the nervous system, and may make worse the symptoms of general nervous debility already present; and the consciousness of concealed wrongdoing is harmful to the child's moral nature.

Prognosis.—This is generally good in the case of infants with thigh-friction, and there is even a disposition for the habit to cease of itself as early childhood is approached. In early childhood there is a tendency to recover from the habit, as from any other habit-neurosis. An exception exists in those cases where the masturbation is very frequent and where there is a distinct pathologic psychic condition shown in other ways. In older children the habit readily becomes a fixed one, and as it is carried on without the knowledge of the parents, supervision and control become a matter of great difficulty. The prognosis, however, of the general condition of the patient is good, except in the cases where the masturbation is excessive. Here it is frequently an evidence of degeneration and but little can be done for it. It is remarkable how little damage seems to result in some instances, even in the case of masturbation in young children carried on to an extreme degree.

Treatment.—In cases of thigh-friction constant supervision is important, and the act must be interrupted as soon as it begins, by picking the child up and diverting its thoughts into other channels. In bad cases, and especially if the act occurs during sleep, some appliance must be employed which will mechanically make friction impossible. A small pillow may be placed between the thighs and a bandage applied around them; or the knees kept separate by a rod terminating at each end in a leather collar fastened around the thigh just above the knees. In infants or quite young children where the hands are employed, it may be necessary to confine these, as by elbow-splints or in other ways. In cases of any age, search must be made for local causes and these removed. Adhesions of the prepuce should be separated, and cleanliness of the penis insisted upon. Circumcision is of value if there is a narrow prepuce. It is also sometimes curative in older children through the soreness produced by the operation, and the consequent breaking in upon the habit. Adhesions of the preputial hood in females should be freed, and if necessary circumcision of the clitoris performed. Vulvovaginitis, if present, demands treatment, as do threadworms, constipation, and eczema. Guarding against tight clothing is important.

Further treatment in the case of older children is difficult and varied, must often be long-continued, and is frequently unsatisfactory. The general health must be looked after in most instances, and hygienic measures employed to control nervous excitability. A life in the open air with abundance of exercise is greatly to be desired; avoiding the climbing of trees, horseback riding, and the like, which might cause local stimulation. No reading should be permitted which excites the nervous system in any way. Sleeping in very warm soft beds under warm bed-clothing is to be avoided. Cool morning baths have a beneficial effect. The meals should not be too large or too stimulating, and constipation is to be prevented. The child must be kept from vicious companions, and, conversely, his associations must be so controlled that he cannot teach the practice to others. A constant supervision must be kept over the patient, making this as complete as possible, so that few opportunities are given to be alone. Punishments are of little value, and only make the patient more secretive. Dwelling upon the matter as a sin may breed in nervous children only despair and cessation of effort, if good resolutions are broken. Such warnings of the terrible results as appear in the quack-medicine advertisements have rather a bad than a good effect on neurotic subjects. The confidence of the child should be sought, and encouragement given; and the practice put before him as one which will make him inferior to other boys in the matter of strength of body, and of a less manly nature. Meanwhile, great caution is to be observed lest even such advice is too often given; and surveillance which is too apparent serves only to concentrate the mind of the patient upon his practices and to establish the habit more firmly.

References

1. Griffith, J.A.M.A., 1929, **93**, 1526. 2. Am. J. Dis. Child., 1926, **31**, 169. 3. J.A.M.A., 1929, **93**, 674. 4. J.A.M.A., 1930, **94**, 860. 5. Bull. Johns Hopkins Hosp., 1923, **34**, 245; Am. J. Psychiat., 1926, **6**, 519. 6. J.A.M.A., 1923, **80**, 1445; 1925, **82**, 1261; Am. J. Psychiat., 1929, **8**, 783; Arch. Neurol. and Psychiat., 1930, **23**, 920. 7. Bull. Johns Hopkins Hosp., 1927, **41**, 389. 8. Medicine, 1928, **7**, 105. 9. Am. J. Dis. Child., 1929, **37**, 261. 10. Am. J. Dis. Child., 1929, **38**, 451. 11. Arch. Neurol. and Psychiat., 1930, **23**, 915. 12. Am. J. Psychiat., 1930, **9**, 667. 13. J. Clin. Investig., 1931, **10**, 915. 14. Arch. Neurol. and Psychiat., 1923, **9**, 554. 15. Epilepsy and Other Chronic Convulsive Disorders, 1901, 5. 16. Michigan State M. S. J., 1929, **28**, 749. 17. Am. J. Dis. Child., 1916, **32**, 416. 18. Boston M. and S. J., 1916, **174**, 573. 19. Quart. J. Med., 1926, **19**, 299. 20. On Epilepsy, 1870; Ref. Binswanger, Nothnagel's Handb. d. spec. Path. u. Therap., 1904, **12**, 1; 1, 77. 21. Treatment of Epilepsy, 1930. 22. Psychiatric Quart., 1929, **3**, 82. 23. Arch. Neurol. and Psych., 1928, **20**, 345. 24. Lancet, 1927, **2**, 325. 25. Arch. f. Psychiat. u. Nervenheilk., 1929, **88**, 114. 26. Arch. Neurol. and Psychiat., 1930, **23**, 521; 525. 27. St. Andrew's Medical Graduates Assn., 1869, **3**, 162. 28. Arch. Dis. Childhood, 1929, **4**, 142. 29. J. Clin. Investig., 1928, **6**. 23. 30. Bull. gén. de thérap., 1910, **160**, 616. 31. Med. Rec., 1921, **99**, 1037. 32. Arch. Neurol. and Psychiat., 1928, **20**, 771. 33. Mayo Clin. Bull., 1921, 2, No. 307. 34. Am. J. Dis. Child., 1924, **28**, 28; Minnesota Med., 1924, **7**, 708; J.A.M.A., 1927, **88**, 1868; 1928, **90**, 1427. 35. J.A.M.A., 1927, **88**, 1427. 36. J.A.M.A., 1930, **95**, 707. 37. Am. J. Dis. Child., 1927, **34**, 1013. 38. J. Nutrition, 1929, **2**, 31. 39. Am. J. Dis. Child., 1928, **36**, 716. 40. Ztschr. f. d. ges. Neurol. u. Psychiat., 1925, **95**, 256. 41. Am. J. Dis. Child., 1926, **32**, 672. 42. J.A.M.A., 1932, **98**, 542. 43. Deutsche Ztschr. f. Nervenheilk., 1906, **30**, 462. 44. Allg. Ztschr. f. Psychiat., 1913, **70**, 631; Med. Klin., 1917, **17**, 467. 45. Monatschr. f. Psychiat. u. Neurol., 1916, **40**, 276. 46

Ztschr. f. Kinderh., Orig., 1920, **27**, 293. 47. Ztschr. f. d. ges. Psychiat. und Neurol., 1923, **80**, 143. 48. Arch. f. Kinderh., 1923, **73**, 163. 49. München. med. Wchnschr., 1899, **46**, 1449. 50. Riv. di clin. pediat., 1918, **16**, 169. 51. Arch. f. Kinderh., 1918, **66**, 385. 52. Arch. f. Kinderh., 1919, **67**, 439. 53. Ztschr. f. Kinderh., 1921, **28**, 310. 54. J.A.M.A., 1925, **84**, 1907. 55. Arch. Pediat., 1931, **48**, 153. 56. Griffith, J.A.M.A., 1926, **86**, 828. 57. J.A.M.A., 1931, **97**, 1372. 58. Traité d. mal. d. l'enf. Grancher, 1905, **4**, 404; 416; 420. 59. Nothnagel's Spec. Path. u. Therap., 1898, **11**, 2; 116. 60. München. med. Wchnschr., 1919, **66**, 1281. 61. Am. J. Dis. Child., 1928, **35**, 964. 62. Deutsche Ztschr. f. Nervenh., 1900, **16**, 356. 63. Quart. J. Med., 1918, **11**, 289. 64. Acta paediat., 1928, **8**, 198. 65. J.A.M.A., 1930, **94**, 523. 66. Ztschr. f. d. ges. exp. Med., 1930, **73**, 343. 67. Am. J. Dis. Child., 1922, **23**, 91. 68. Jahrb. f. Kinderh., 1925, **109**, 1. 69. Am. J. Dis. Child., 1922, **23**, 493. 70. Arch. f. Kinderh., 1923, **73**, 273. 71. J. Biol. Chem., 1926, **68**, 57. 72. Bull. de la soc. pédiat., 1926, No. 6–7, 245. 73. Ziemssen's Handb. d. spec. Path. u. Therap. 12; 2; 1; 335. 74. Am. J. Dis. Child., 1916, **12**, 1. 75. Wien. med. Presse, 1878, **19**, 822. 76. Wien. klin. Wchnschr., 1911, **24**, 1487. 77. Verhandl. der Gesellsch. f. Kinderh., 1913, **30**, 62. 78. Lancet, 1924, **1**, 1307. 79. Il Policlinico, 1921, **28**, 1465. 80. Monatschr. f. Kinderh., 1922, **22**, 484. 81. Riv. di clin. pediat., 1925, **23**, 744; 1926, **24**, 649. 82. Stevenson and Mitchell, Am. J. Dis. Child., 1927, **34**, 425. 83. De la contracture d. extremit., ou tétanie chez l'adulte, 1852. Ref. Soltmann, Gerhardt's Handb. d. Kinderh., 1880, **5**, 1; 1; 141. 84. Praktische Kinderh., 1910, 266. 85. Jahrb. f. Kinderh., 1894, **38**, 449. 86. Jahrb. f. Kinderh., 1915, **82**, 347. 87. Monatschr. f. Psychiat. u. Neurol., 1901, **10**, 81. 88. Am. J. Dis. Child., 1918, **15**, 323. 89. Nourrisson, 1922, **10**, 305. 90. Ztschr. f. Kinderh., 1913, **7**, 1. 91. Hygeia, 1920, **82**, 559. 92. Spasmofili og. epilepsi, Thesis, Copenhagen, 1920. 93. Acta paediat., 1931, **10**, 281. 94. Am. J. Dis. Child., 1929, **37**, 311. 95. J.A.M.A., 1930, **95**, 396. 96. Jahrb. f. Kinderh., 1922, **97**, 130. 97. Klin. Wchnschr., 1922, **1**, 140. 98. J.A.M.A., 1926, **86**, 1343. 99. Epidemics of the Middle Ages, Sydenham Soc. Trans., 1884, 87. 100. Sydenham's Works, 1850, **2**, 198; 257. 101. Thèse de Paris, 1895. 102. Jacobi Festschrift, 1900, 5. 103. Trans. Assoc. Am. Phys., 1892, **7**, 249. 104. Acta paediat., 1922, **2**, 159. 105. J.A.M.A., 1916, **67**, 1342. 106. Monatschr. f. Kinderh., 1916–18, **14**, 1. 107. Brit. M. J., 1931, **1**, 303. 108. Lancet, 1892, **1**, 793. 109. Clin. pediat., 1928, **10**, 137. 110. Ann. de méd. et de chir. inf., 1911, **15**, 276. 111. New York M. J., 1914, **100**, 225. 112. Lancet, 1930, **1**, 339. 113. Thèse de Paris, 1913. 114. Deutsche med. Wchnschr., 1911, **37**, 111; Med. Klin., 1929, **25**, 1060. 115. Arch. Pediat., 1924, **41**, 657. 116. Arch. Pediat., 1916, **33**, 649. 117. Am. J. Dis. Child., 1918, **16**, 109. 118. New York M. J., 1920, **111**, 949. 119. J.A.M.A., 1931, **97**, 299. 120. Am. J. Dis. Child., 1923, **26**, 223. 121. Therap. Monatsh., 1919, **38**, 54. 122. Charité Ann., 1850, **1**, 752. 123. Traité d. mal. de l'enf. Grancher, 1905, **4**, 278. 124. Am. J. Dis. Child., 1918, **16**, 180. 125. Arch. d. Neurol., 1885, **9**, 19. 126. Giorni di Milano e gaz. med., 1840; Ref. Bruns, Berl. klin. Wchnschr., 1902, **39**, 1185. 127. Vorlesungen ü. Kinderkr., 1895, 193. 128. Ref. Bézy in Grancher, Traité d. mal. d. l'enf., 1905, **4**, 377. 129. Jahrb. f. Kinderh., 1925, **107**, 1. 130. Jahrb. f. Kinderh., 1926, **113**, 275. 131. Monatschr. f. Kinderh., 1927, **36**, 138. 132. Behaviorism, 1924. 133. The Nervous Child., 1919. 134. Human Growth, 1928; The Guidance of Mental Growth in Infant and Child, 1930. 135. Everyday Problems of the Everyday Child, 1929. 136. Psychology of Infancy and Childhood, 1930. 137. Psychology of the Unadjusted Child, 1930. 138. Neurotic Disorders of Childhood, 1905, 328. 139. Brit. M. J., 1930, **2**, 717. 140. Diseases of Children, 1912, 259. 141. J.A.M.A., 1930, **95**, 1825. 142. J.A.M.A., 1928, **91**, 67. 143. Am. J. M. Sc., 1929, **178**, 663. 144. Am. J. Physiol., 1928, **84**, 386. 145. Arch. Pediat., 1929, **46**, 679. 146. U. S. Dept. Interior, 1931, Bull. No. 7; The Speech-defective School-child. 147. Grancher and Comby, Traité d. mal. de l'enf., 1905, **4**, 209. 148. Arch. Int. Med., 1921, **27**, 255. 149. Med. Rec., 1921, **100**, 941. 150. Schweiz. med. Wchnschr., 1930, **60**, 32. 151. Mental Hygiene, 1927, **2**, 795. 152. Brit. J. Child. Dis., 1916, **13**, 104. 153. The Diseases of Speech, 1894. 154. J.A.M.A., 1929, **92**, 958. 155. Correction of Defective Speech, 1932. 156. St. Bartholomew's Hosp. Rep., 1886, **22**, 97.

CHAPTER III

PSYCHIC DISORDERS. PSYCHOSES

The psychic disorders are in a way a connecting link between the functional and the organic nervous diseases. Some are functional; some, at least, rest upon a distinct anatomic basis, and are often associated with the stigmata of degeneration described later (p. 901). The range of subjects included varies according to the classification of different writers. The following may be considered:

HYSTERIA

Although the symptoms of hysteria are manifold and many shade imperceptibly into those of neurasthenia, various neuroses and psychoses, and organic diseases, the malady in itself is entirely distinct from other affections. Its underlying character is a lack of will-power, with emotional and reflex excitability; combined with the production of a great variety of symptoms apparently due to corporeal affections, but in reality simulative and of a psychic nature. There exist fixed or perverted ideas which are often produced by suggestion or autosuggestion. There are an exalted egoism, and a desire to attract attention and gain the sympathy of others; and the power of self-control is enormously decreased.

Etiology.—The occurrence of hysteria in childhood is more common than often supposed, and it may be observed even in infancy. Heredity is a prominent *predisposing factor*, and children born of neurotic parents are particularly liable to develop hysterical symptoms. The more nearly puberty is approached, the more frequent the disease, and the greater proportion of females attacked. That all cases of hysteria in children are the result of earlier forgotten repressed emotions of a sexual character, as claimed by Freud and his followers, is unproved. The neurotic disposition upon which hysteria rests is congenital, and the tendency has been lying dormant. The actual production of symptoms depends upon a variety of influences.

Among the *direct causes* of the development of hysteria are malnutrition of any sort; surroundings favorable to emotional excitement; the strain of school-life; imitation from association with hysterical or other nervous individuals; faulty training by parents; the incurring of fright, fear, or trauma; the impairment of health following acute diseases; and sometimes masturbation or other genital irritation.

Symptoms.—These may come on suddenly and disappear rapidly, or may be persistent, and may simulate diseases of any part of the body. Commonly there is in early life only a single symptom prominently manifest (monosymptomatic); and stigmata of hysteria are more often absent until puberty is approached, when suggestion may develop some of these, especially during examinations. Among the stigmata may be mentioned anesthesia and hyperesthesia of different sorts, the globus hystericus, contraction of the visual fields, ovarian and spinal tenderness, and various convulsive conditions. The general health of patients with hysteria is usually not perfect. Disorders of digestion, disturbances of appetite, anemia, insomnia, and intellectual derangements are common.

Sensory Symptoms.—Prominent here are neuralgic pain; pain with contracture about the joints, and widespread or localized hyperesthesia, paresthesia or anesthesia, although these are not as frequent as in adults.

Motor Symptoms.—These may consist in *spasm* of some sort, either tonic or clonic; hysterical convulsions, seen usually in older children; and catalepsy.

The limited tonic and clonic spasms are not infrequently of a choreiform nature. In others the spasm is represented by contortions of the face, irregular action of the diaphragm and other muscles of respiration, torticollis or hysterical contraction elsewhere. Some of the cases of tic and of chorea electrica are probably hysterical. *Paralysis* may develop, with or without contracture. This may be flaccid or spastic; paraplegic, hemiplegic, or monoplegic; or affect only one portion of a limb. It is less common in children than are the evidences of spasm. Astasia abasia is one of the commonest forms of hysterical paralysis in children; the child being able to make all or many of the normal movements with the limbs, yet unable to stand or walk, or doing it with difficulty. Aphonia may occur from hysterical paralysis of the muscles of the larynx. The tendon-*reflexes* in hysteria are usually active; never absent. The cutaneous reflexes are variable; those of the cornea and pharynx perhaps being absent. Ankle-clonus does not occur. *Tremor* is an uncommon symptom.

Psychical Symptoms.—Here are to be classed attacks of laughing or crying without sufficient cause; violent paroxysms of anger; great excitability of the nervous system; disturbed sleep with night-terrors or somnambulism; capriciousness of disposition; unreasonableness; impulsiveness; hysterical aphasia; a stuporous condition; mental depression; delirious states sometimes of a maniacal nature; hallucinations. Not all of these, of course, are necessarily hysterical. An extreme power of imagination, excitability, egoism, and a remarkable tendency to deception without reason, are characteristic psychic alterations. Noteworthy, too, is the extreme interest of the patient in his symptoms, and the disposition to imitate the symptoms of others.

Symptoms Connected with the Special Senses.—In this category are such manifestations as blindness; contraction of the visual fields; asthenopia; blepharospasm with closure of both eyes; paralysis of some of the ocular muscles; deafness.

Symptoms Connected with Other Organs.—*Respiratory symptoms* may be represented by sighing or rapid respiration; yawning; hysterical cough; attacks of dyspnea; rapid respiration; aphasia from the paralysis of the laryngeal muscles, as already mentioned; hiccup from spasmodic action of the diaphragm. Among *circulatory symptoms* are palpitation, tachycardia, pallor, flushing and edema. The disturbances connected with the *digestive organs* are hysterical dysphagia; gastralgia; umbilical colic; and vomiting, often of a very persistent nature, the last occurring even in infants. Anorexia nervosa (p. 559) is a characteristic hysterical disturbance. Among other symptoms connected with the alimentary tract, which may sometimes be of a hysterical nature, are meteorism, long-continued diarrhea, constipation, incontinence of feces, and recurring anal prolapse. Of *genito-urinary* manifestations are frequent urination, polyuria, ischuria, and paralysis of the bladder. That enuresis nocturna is sometimes amenable to treatment by suggestion places such instances among urinary manifestations of hysteria.

Prognosis.—The prognosis is, as a rule, good if treatment is instituted early; yet this statement applies only to the cure of the visible conditions present. When the disease appears in a child of a distinctly neurotic tendency or inheritance, return of hysterical manifestations is liable to occur in later years. The suddenly developing attacks offer the best prognosis, especially where imitation has been an active cause.

Diagnosis.—Although organic disorders of all sorts are closely simulated, certain features will aid in distinguishing the hysterical condition. Primarily there is to be noticed the lack of proportion between the assigned cause and the symptoms produced, and a tendency for all symptoms to become worse when much attention is paid to them. There is also a grouping of symptoms which it is impossible to attribute to any known lesion or series of lesions. One of the chief difficulties in diagnosis is that the explanation of symptoms on the basis of hysteria does not occur to the physician encountering them in subjects of so early age. It is possible, too, to have a combination of hysteria with the evidences of an actual organic lesion.

The major hysterical convulsive attack suggests epilepsy, but is distinguished by the absence of biting of the tongue or injuries by falling, of real unconsciousness, of relaxation of the sphincters, and of terminal sleep; while the movements of the body are suggestive more of purpose, and the patient may later recall and speak of what took place. As regards other motor symptoms, hysterical contractures are marked by the greater rigidity on passive movement, as compared with those of organic nature. Hysterical paralytic conditions and contractures may disappear completely during sleep or under anesthesia. There is also no atrophy of moment or absence of the tendon-reflexes, such as should accompany some of the paralytic conditions of organic origin; and there is often a distribution and an association with other symptoms which it is impossible to explain except on a hysterical basis. Hysterical chorea often exhibits more violent and systematic movements than does true chorea, and there is a tenseness of the limbs rather than the hypotonia of the latter disease.

Sensory symptoms exhibit similar suggestive characteristics. It is an important observation that through the diverting of the mind of the child, or during sleep, tender regions may entirely cease to be tender. Areas of hyperesthesia, too, do not show the distribution which organic lesions would necessarily produce. Hysterical involvement of the joints comes on more suddenly than one of an organic nature, often with more sensitiveness, with an absence of evidences of inflammation, and a greater variation in the symptoms. In hysterical headache no cause for the condition can be found, and the attack is liable to develop at a time when it may be of service to the child, or when suggestion is given by too much attention; and it disappears when something happens to entertain the patient or to divert the attention in other ways. The aphasia of hysteria is rather a dumbness. It comes on suddenly and there is no effort whatever to speak; such as would occur in many cases of true aphasia. In some instances, too, the patient can sing, whisper or cough, although he cannot speak in the ordinary manner. Severe barking cough, or attacks of dyspnea occurring without sufficient discoverable cause, may frequently be determined to be hysterical from autosuggestion, if the child at an earlier period has suffered from such symptoms depending upon actual organic cause. The repeated vomiting of hysteria is in many cases only partial, and not followed by the emaciation and loss of strength which one would naturally expect. Also suggestive are the ease with which the vomiting occurs, and the frequent apparently direct intention of the child. Hysterical anorexia may be traced to the earlier administration of some food distasteful to the patient, or may be found to have been started by some actual dyspeptic disturbance and kept going by suggestion, often through the great urgency of the parents that the child should eat. Meteorism of hysterical nature disappears under anesthesia.

Treatment.—**Prophylactic treatment** of a child with nervous inheritance or one who has shown nervous or hysterical symptoms is of the utmost moment. All those factors and the management of them discussed under the subject of nervous children (p. 883) demand attention. Of especial importance in **direct treatment** of the disease already developed is the removal from the parents' care or from association with any nervous individuals. A nurse should be found who will win the affection of the patient, but who will show no sympathy whatever, and take as little notice of the symptoms as possible. The principle of suggestive treatment is of the greatest value in hysteria. Sometimes it is well to do nothing to entertain the child; sometimes better to fill its mind with matters which will divert it from a consideration of itself. A very careful study of the individual case is necessary, and no general rules can be formulated. Changes from time to time in the surroundings and in the things done for the patient are an important part of the mental cure. Hydrotherapy, electrical treatment, massage, may follow one another, and do good partly through the improvement in tone, largely through the impression made. In some cases the rest-treatment is of service.

In certain selected cases the discomfort caused by the use of the cold douche, counterirritation of the spine, application of a strong faradic current, or the like, may be employed to cause symptoms to disappear. Sometimes symptomatic cure results from sudden, sharp insistence by the physician that a paralyzed child get up at once; or the command to speak given to one with dumbness, at the same time that a painful stimulant, such as an electric current, is applied over the larynx. The danger of failure by these methods is great, and then the malady is harder to relieve. The ignoring of symptoms is more certain, although more tedious.

STIGMATA OF DEGENERATION

These consist of bodily or mental characteristics which are prone to be present in children with diminished power of resistance in the nervous system; in nervous children; and in those with neurasthenia and especially with mental deficiency. They are not, however, necessarily present, nor when observed are they by any means positive indications of a nervous or mental weakness. They can be looked upon merely as corroborative signs. They are referred to here because at times associated with functional or psychic disturbances.

The *head* may be brachycephalic; dolichocephalic; macrocephalic; hydrocephalic; microcephalic; asymmetrical; or deformed in other ways. The face may be asymmetrical; the lower jaw very prominent or markedly receding; the forehead abnormally narrow. An unusually high arching of the palate has been claimed to be a suggestive stigma, but Channing's[1] observations confirm the opinion that it possesses no real significance. Among other deformities connected with the head are bifid uvula, harelip, and cleft palate; enlargement of the tongue; malposition or imperfect development of the teeth; and deformity of the nasal bones. The eyes may show irregular coloring of the iris; congenital coloboma; albinism; opacities; congenital cataract; strabismus; irregular form or position of the pupils; oblique inclination or narrowness of the palpebral fissure; hypertelorism; pigmentary retinitis. The ears may exhibit irregularity in shape; adhesion of the lobule; crumpling of the helix; or be unusually large or prominent. In the region of the *trunk* are to be noted spina bifida; hernia; polymastia; deformities of the breasts. In the *genital organs* are epispadias; hypospadias; rudimentary penis; cryptorchidism; early development of genital hair; atresia of the vagina; and double vagina or uterus. The *limbs* may show such lesions as webbing or alteration in the number or formation of the fingers or toes; very long or very short arms, and the like. The *development* as a whole may be altered; the child seeming prematurely old or having retarded puberty; or there may be evidences of feminism; masculinism; infantilism; gigantism; albinism; etc. *Functions*, too, may show degenerative signs; to be mentioned here being delay in learning to sit or walk; defective speech; congenital deaf-mutism; stammering; enuresis; poor circulation of the blood; abnormalities of appetite; and diminished resistance to disease. Among *psychical stigmata* are, in milder cases, the manifestations of nervousness, debility, and excitability mentioned in discussing nervous children;

and in the severer cases the evidences of mental deficiency, moral insanity, sexual perversion, precocity in a limited direction, fixed ideas, phobias, truancy, etc.

MENTAL PRECOCITY

In itself not a disease, the condition is often attended by distinct pathologic conditions. A child who is precocious within normal limits shows merely an unusual and rapid development of his intellectual powers as compared with his age. This may take place in all directions equally, or only, perhaps, along one or two lines; the mental condition being average in other respects. Precocious children may be born so, and advance without effort on the part of the parents, or even in spite of restraint. In many other instances there is at first little more than the normal degree of intellectual power; but over-prompt beginning of teaching of a forcing character, or association only with those older than themselves, develops in them an early acquisition of knowledge, and a precocity which is more apparent then real. Precocity of this sort is to be guarded against, as the premature stimulation of the intellect is liable to result in the development of some of the various characteristics of the nervous child. True precocity in all directions needs no checking except so far as is necessary to keep the bodily health in good condition. In the case of children precocious in certain directions only, great care should be taken that in the training along these lines others are not neglected. It is often better to make an effort to retard development on the precocious side. (See also Idiots savants p. 909.)

PSYCHASTHENIA. BEHAVIOR DISORDERS

(Conduct Disorders; Delinquency; Antisocial Acts)

While Behavior Disorders, strictly speaking are not necessarily a part of Psychasthenia they may be referred to here for convenience of discussion.

Etiology.—Some of the conditions discussed in this connection are allied to Nervousness (p. 881), but with predominance of psychic manifestations; the severer forms closely approaching insanity. There is also a relationship to some of the tics with imperative ideas. The psychasthenic tendency appears to be an inborn one, with a dormant existence until awakened by some exciting cause. Some of the antisocial acts, however, seem to depend entirely upon improper training, or lack of training of any sort. Operative, too, are physical defects, as undersize or oversize, perhaps related to dysfunction of the endocrine glands; faults of the special senses; cleft palate or some other deformity which puts the child at a handicap with his fellows; malnutrition; chronic infections; and the like. Disease of the central nervous system, particularly encephalitis, may be followed by behavior disorders of a psychasthenic appearance, which are in reality dependent upon organic lesions.

While some of the patients may be normal intellectually or even possess special mental power, as a class they have a lower mentality than an average group (Wile[2]). In regard to environmental influence, already referred to, there may be mentioned poor discipline and training both at home and in school; the expectation that the child should do more than his innate ability will permit; and too great restriction of normal activities. Antisocial acts may be caused by a desire for adventure and power; by imitation; or serve as an outlet for emotions when normal and less harmful activities have been denied. All such factors are more likely to act in children with an inherited tendency to psychasthenia and nervousness than in those with a stable nervous disposition.

Symptoms.—*Psychasthenia* in its strict sense, denoting an inborn tendency, and referring to that group of symptoms frequently designated the *inferiority complex*, is found in nervous, impressionable, imaginative children, who often have the so-called "shut-in" personality; and who wish to be by themselves or prefer the society of adults rather than of children. While the symptoms may develop earlier, they appear oftenest about puberty. One of the most important is the feeling of doubt, and, closely associated with this, phobias of all sorts; and with these is combined an over-conscientiousness, which finally leads to obsessions and to imperative ideas. These result in hesitation in action and in reaching conclusions; lack of will-power and of concentration; restlessness; repetition of acts for fear they have not been properly performed; melancholic states from the consciousness of personal imperfection; hallucinations; fear of certain objects, places, and conditions; the fear of personal contamination, leading to frequently repeated washing of the hands and the like; impulses to spring into the water or out of a high window, etc. The disease may advance still further, and the obsessions and imperative ideas become so uncontrollable that criminal acts may be performed, such as theft or murder; or they may lead to self-mutilation or suicidal attempts. Truancy from school or the running away from home is, in many instances, a symptom of psychasthenia; as is sexual perversion of various sorts. In fact some of these children appear to be moral degenerates (p. 904).

Behavior disorders are committed from willfulness, rather than from lack of will-power or morbid fears. While true psychasthenics may also perpetrate antisocial acts, those of lying, stealing, thievery, jealousy, eroticism, destructiveness, truancy and the like are often due to bad environmental factors and training, without any innate viciousness as a background.

Prognosis.—This is uncertain, yet even in psychasthenia with its underlying tendency the symptoms can often be made to disappear under proper treatment. Behavior disorders without the inherited neurotic predisposition offer a still better prognosis, if treated early. In both, relapses are prone to occur, especially when the environment continues bad, or when health deteriorates for any reason.

Diagnosis.—Psychasthenia is distinguished from simple nervousness (p. 883) by the predominance of psychic disturbance; from insanity and imbecility by the fact that the patient recognizes that the idea and the acts which follow are wrong, even though he lacks the ability to control them. Behavior disorders not associated with poor inheritance are less likely to be found in children with a retiring, melancholic, self-doubting disposition; and the history and subsequent course show that the antisocial acts committed depend solely upon bad environment. In behavior disorders caused by organic disease of the central nervous system there can usually be demonstrated other symptoms suggestive of the latter, as well as definite mental deterioration.

Treatment.—Measures are to be sought which improve the general health and quiet nervous excitability. (See Treatment of Nervous Children, p. 883, and Neurotic Habits, p. 891.) Physical defects should be remedied if possible. All mental over-strain is to be avoided, and yet the child's mind must be kept filled with healthy ideas and diverted by occupations. Of special importance is the removal of the patient from unsuitable surroundings. Without this but little can be accomplished. The confidence of the child is to be obtained without fail, and then every effort put forth to increase the will-power. The attempt must be made to discover the nature and origin of the obsession which possesses the child, to remove the cause which occasions this, and to produce a conviction of the unreasonableness of the doubt, fear, or antisocial act. Gymnastic exercises are useful both in improving the general condition, and in awakening the concentration upon healthy thoughts. In spite of lack of prompt results, treatment must be persevered with.

INSANITY

The distinction between insanity and idiocy is that the former is disease of a mind previously sound, coming on after mental power has been fairly well attained; while the latter is mental feebleness, depending on disease or defect of the brain, congenital or acquired during its development, which has arrested the growth of the mental powers (Peterson[3]).

Etiology.—While insanity is comparatively uncommon in childhood, cases in very early life have been reported. It is only in later childhood that its occurrence becomes significant. There is an inherited tendency, the parents being neurotic, or suffering from some nervous affection. Insanity may result from lesions of the brain, as in trauma, meningitis, encephalitis or syphilis; or may follow epilepsy, chorea, acute infectious fevers, shock, or undue mental work. Excessive masturbation, sometimes given as a cause, more often depends upon a diseased nervous state which finally terminates in insanity.

Symptoms.—One of the most frequent forms is an *acute delirious state*, reaching even *mania*. This is encountered oftenest in connection with acute infectious fevers. Mania may also develop independently of infections; may be a symptom of severe chorea; be witnessed in some cases of hysteria; and be temporarily present in epilepsy. *Dementia* often occurs in long-continued and severe epilepsy; and may also depend upon the cerebral lesions of hereditary syphilis, being then seen in early childhood. *Melancholia* is found in later childhood, especially after mental over-work. In *moral insanity* there is an entire absence of moral sense. All the tendencies are vicious; sexual impulses may be dominant and perverted; cruelty is a prominent feature; the intelligence is usually defective; and, as the child grows older, he is liable to commit criminal acts. Strictly speaking the majority of these cases are *moral imbecility*, since the disease is a congenital one, and the moral nature has been arrested in its development. There are, however, instances in which the moral perversion is the result of accident or disease occurring in those who have previously shown no abnormality in this respect, and to those the title moral insanity is properly applied. These are usually dependent upon undue mental strain or bodily exhaustion; or may follow trauma of the head, or encephalitis.

Many of the perverted tendencies and feelings seen in neurotic children and in psychasthenia are present in increased degree in insanity; differing in the latter, however, in that the patient does not recognize their unreality and groundlessness. Often in early childhood, or even later, there is seen a great degree of perverted behavior and maliciousness, which is not in reality a moral insanity, but depends upon an unusually exaggerated ego, and the desire to attract attention. Stigmata of degeneration (p. 901) are prone to occur in the insane.

Prognosis.—This varies according to the cause and the form of insanity exhibited. In melancholia and hypochondriasis recovery generally takes place, as also in acute delirious insanities and those accompanying hysteria or chorea. The prognosis of dementia following syphilis, epilepsy or encephalitis is unfavorable. Forms of insanity with fixed delusions are unfavorable, and the well-marked cases of moral insanity even more so. Always to be remembered in any form of insanity is the liability to recurrence.

Treatment.—Details cannot be discussed here, but there should be mentioned the maintenance of general health; the removal of any discoverable cause or exciting factor; the separation of the patient from unfavorable surroundings; and the careful guarding against injury by the patient to himself or others. The whole question of marriage, contraception, and sterilization may arise in connection with individual cases, and advice concerning these becomes part of the function of the physician.

MENTAL DEFICIENCY

(Idiocy; Imbecility; Feeble-mindedness)

The distinction from insanity has already been defined (p. 904); deficiency being regarded as mental feebleness due to organic cerebral defect or disease at birth, or arising in the brain while the mental powers are in a developing state. Cretinism (p. 1067) is an exception, the mental arrest being due to deficiency of thyroid secretion.

Idiocy, imbecility, and feeble-mindedness can all be included under the title "idiocy"; yet this and the term "imbecility" suggest opprobrium to the laity, and should be avoided by the physician in speaking to parents. The three varieties mentioned constitute merely degrees of the same clinical condition; the typical "idiot" never reaching the mental age above that normal for two years; the "imbecile" never above that normal for about seven years; and the moron, the subject of slight feeble-mindedness, being but little separated from the normal. There is further a moral imbecility (p. 904).

The term "*backwardness*" is often applied to children who have not attained the stage of mental development average for their age. In some instances this depends upon an attendant slowness of physical development, perhaps the result of debilitating diseases, lack of training, defective eyesight or hearing, the presence of adenoid growths, and the like. Such cases are not properly included among the mentally deficient. Allied to this are cases of *idiocy by deprivation*, in which mental defect of mild degree results from physical disorders, as illustrated by congenital deaf-mutism.

Etiology.—The condition is a common one. In 1927 there were in State schools in the United States, 49,791 feeble minded and subnormal children; in City day-schools 51,814, and in private schools 2416.[4] Of 52,514 public school children in several States, 3.4 per cent were classified as superior mentally, and 62.7 per cent as normal (Haines[5]). Ferguson[6] found 16 imbeciles per 10,000 children attending school, 98 feeble minded, and 24 with gross mental instability. *Inheritance* is a factor in from one-fourth to one-half of all the cases according to various statistics. The parents may themselves have been degenerates, or only neurotic, or the subjects of nervous disease of some sort. Alcoholism and tuberculosis in the parents are possible factors. *Syphilis* seems operative in some instances, but there are great differences in the statistics, the percentage of positive Wassermann reactions in idiots ranging from 1.15 per cent to 43 per cent (Atwood;[7] Weiss and Izgur;[8] Dayton;[9] Hall;[10] Masten;[11] Woodall[12]). In general, statistics often show no greater incidence of idiocy in groups of syphilitic children than in nonsyphilitic groups. On the other hand, 15 to 20 per cent of syphilitics have mental retardation (White and Veeder,[13] Woodall[12]). *Debility of the mother* during pregnancy possesses no proved influence. *Consanguinity* is operative only if both parents are neurotic, when the tendency to all nervous conditions in the offspring is increased. *Irradiation of the pelvic region* by the roentgen-ray or radium during pregnancy may affect the fetus, especially by producing microcephalus (Murphy[14]). In most cases the symptoms of idiocy appear at an early *age*. *Sex* is a factor, male defectives being perhaps somewhat more common, approximately in the ratio of 6:5 (Tredgold,[15] Bridgman[16]). *Trauma* at birth and meningeal hemorrhage at that period are important factors. It is to be noted here that the employment of forceps is an element of less importance than prolonged labor, and that a sufficiently early use of them will probably prevent the development of many cases of cerebral paralysis and mental defect. Cases of *premature birth* are liable to exhibit mental deficiency, either from the imperfect development of the brain or, more often, because of the tendency to intracranial hemorrhage.

Mental deficiency arising from causes after birth may be the result of eclamptic convulsions; trauma; central nervous disease as meningitis or encephalitis. Mental shock or mental overwork is liable to be operative only upon the basis of an underlying neurotic predisposition. Prolonged calcium disturbance during the period of active growth of nervous tissue is supposed to be a factor in some cases.

In regard to the frequency of the various causes, Barr and Whitney[17] found in 5000 cases that 6 per cent were due to trauma or injury at birth; 28 per cent to illness or injury in infancy or early childhood; and 25 per cent were on a hereditary basis.

Pathologic Anatomy.—Organic lesions of the brain of some kind are often found, among them being alteration in size and shape, hydrocephalus, porencephalus, general atrophy, absence of a hemisphere, cysts, and improper development of the subarachnoid space (Winkelman[18]). The changes may be only microscopical. (See also p. 913.) Here may be mentioned the condition described as agenesis corticalis (Sachs[19]) in which there has been an arrest of development of the cortex. In another class there is sclerosis of some sort (p. 949) or lesions following encephalitis, meningitis, hemorrhage, thrombosis, embolism and tumors. In the mongolian type of the disease there is usually present lack of proper development of the brain, which is oval, small, and with poorly formed convolutions; and microscopically there is exhibited diminution in the number of cortical cells, with perhaps diffuse sclerotic changes. In amaurotic family idiocy the lesion in the brain consists in degenerative changes, especially in the cortex, but the gray matter of the entire cerebrospinal axis may be involved. Lipoid degeneration has also been found, and Sachs,[20] Schmitz and Thoenes,[21] Goldstein and Wexler,[22] and others view the disease as a disturbance of lipoid metabolism allied to Gaucher's disease, lipoid histiocytosis, and the like.

Symptoms.—There is first to be noted in all classes the predominant feature of enfeeblement of mind, inability to fix the attention, and diminution in the power of receiving impressions and forming concepts or reaching conclusions. This appears early in well-marked cases. The patients are commonly extremely restless and uncontrollable and often destructive, and without awe of strangers or of strange surroundings. With these symptoms are frequently combined lack of proper physical development and some of the stigmata of degeneration (p. 901). Some alteration in the expression of the face or shape of the head is nearly always present.

In the typical *idiot* the mental faculties are more or less completely impaired. There is inability to say more than a few words or to understand anything said; and no note is taken of anything put before the child. It is much after the normal age for doing this that he is able to sit up or even to hold the head erect. Saliva dribbles from the mouth; and the ability to walk comes very late or not at all. The *imbecile* is slow in learning to walk. The power of fixing the attention is poor. He may learn to talk fairly well, but only late and after continued teaching. He understands to a degree, and can obey orders if so disposed; but the behavior in many cases is unreasonable and mischievous, and there may be attacks of maniacal excitement or rage. Some imbeciles, however, are good-natured and industrious. Imbeciles are able to feed and dress themselves. Automatic or rhythmical movements are common. Some imbeciles exhibit remarkable mental talents in certain directions (*Idiots savants* p. 909). In others the intellectual defect is combined with moral imbecility (p. 904). The practice of masturbation is frequent and often excessive. Typical idiocy and imbecility shade into each other, and there are many gradations between them. Children with only slight *feeblemindedness* or *deficiency* (*morons*) speak usually without difficulty, but are slow in acquiring ideas and never become able to reason quite normally. Even in the mildest cases they are behind in their classes. They may, under favorable conditions, later become self-supporting; but they drift readily into crime, the women often becoming prostitutes.

Varieties.—A few of the many clinical varieties of idiocy may be mentioned in more detail.

1. Paralytic Idiocy.—This depends upon lesions producing infantile cerebral paralysis. While the degree of mental defect, which varies from idiocy to slight deficiency, is not always proportionate to the extent of the paralysis, it is prone to be greatest in diplegia. It dates usually from meningeal hemorrhage occurring during birth; less often from this or other lesions developing later (p. 916). Lack of development of the brain, porencephalus, and the like are also causes. What appears to be but a variety of paralytic idiocy is described by Garbiso and Marotta[23] and others under the title "Congenital regressive rigidity."

2. Mongolian Idiocy.—This is a frequent form, constituting about 20 per cent of all cases of mental deficiency. Its cause is obscure. Both *sexes* are about equally affected. It is observed chiefly in the white race. We[24] have seen 4 cases in negroes and collected reports of 11 others. Demuth[25] describes a case in a Chinese infant. We[26] have seen it in one of twins, and others have reported it in one or both of them, Macklin[27] collecting a total of 47 such cases. In no instance has it been shown that it can occur in one of twins the result of a single-ovum pregnancy. Usually only one child in a family is affected, although a number of exceptions to this are reported (Van der Scheer;[28] Scott;[29] Pardee;[30] Glassburg;[31] Babonneix and Villette;[32] Orel;[33] Borovsky[34]). Steinen[35] noted an increase in the number of mongols during and after the World War. While often born of mothers of nearly forty years of age or over, or as the last of a large family, there are numerous exceptions to this. We have often seen mongolism in the first child of young mothers, and Macklin[27] in 788 collected cases found that 20 per cent were first-born. There does not, in fact, seem to be any proven influence of the age of the mother or the number of pregnancies. Among other causative factors sponsored by various authors, none of which has satisfying proof, are marked differences in the age of the parents; alcoholism; tuberculosis; neuropathic tendency of the parents; disease of the mother or mental strain during pregnancy; fetal hyperthyroidism or hypothyroidism; and immaturity or senility of the ovum. Interesting reviews are those by Macklin[27] and Brousseau.[36]

There are peculiar somatic conditions in mongolism (Fig. 201) some, but not all, of which are present in every case. The skull is small and brachycephalic, the occiput flattened, the mouth usually small and open, the nose flat and broad, the nostrils narrow, and adenoid growths are common. The tongue may be enlarged and is prone to protrude, even although of normal size, and later is characteristically fissured (*scrotal tongue*). Sucking of the tongue is a common symptom. The palpebral fissures are narrow and slope upward outwardly, with an unusual development of the inner epicanthic fold, suggesting the Mongolian type of face. Nystagmus is not uncommon. Some degree of opacity of the crystalline lens is frequent, Koby[37] finding it in 22 of 36 patients; and Van der Scheer[38] in all of 100 who had reached an age of eight years or over. The hands are often broad and square, with the fourth finger and the thumb abnormally short, the former being incurved. This stigma is not infrequently absent, and sometimes occurs also in normal persons. The feet are broad and flat, the limbs are short, and roentgenograms show delay in ossification. The muscles and ligaments are flaccid, often allowing unusual passive movement. There is a tendency to congenital heart-disease as a complication, the incidence of this varying with the age at which the patient is studied, since the patients with more severe cardiac disease die early. Malformation of other parts of the body is not infrequent. Growth and development are slow, and normal size never attained. After puberty there is a tendency to fatness. Mongolian imbeciles are generally good-natured and lively.

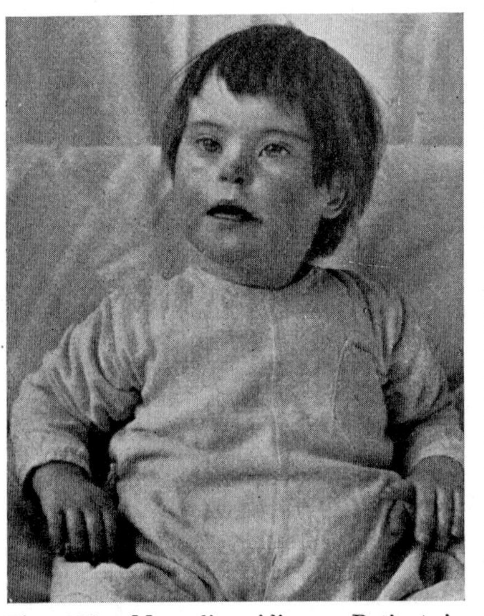

Fig. 201.—Mongolian idiocy. Patient in the Children's Hospital of Philadelphia.

3. Microcephalic Idiocy (*Aztec Type*).—(See also p. 913.) In these patients, who constitute about 10 per cent of all forms of idiocy, there is a small cranium, the forehead is narrow, the vertex pointed, and the occiput flat (Fig. 202). The sutures are often prematurely ossified, and the fontanelles close early. In other respects the infants are usually well-formed and well-nourished. The mental power is very defective, and little improvement in it can be expected. A marked degree of muscular rigidity is often present; convulsions are frequently observed; walking is delayed, and speech, if acquired, is limited. Less severe cases are seen without spasticity, and in these there is more possibility of mental development. The cranium is small because the brain does not grow, rather than the reverse of this; consequently craniotomy can be of no benefit.

4. Hydrocephalic Idiocy.—Children with hydrocephalus may have a remarkable preservation of intellectual power as compared with the amount of brain-substance present. Sooner or later, however, with the increase of intracranial pressure, there occurs mental impairment of varying degree (p. 947).

5. Epileptic Idiocy.—Here a gradual mental deterioration may take place, with the symptoms of dementia. The condition may be consecutive to epileptic mental disturbances of a more active form.

6. Amaurotic Family Idiocy.—This title was given to the disease by Sachs,[39] although alterations in the macula had been previously observed by Tay.[40] (See also Disturbances of the Reticulo-endothelial System p. 1050.) Numerous cases have been reported. It is seen usually in Hebrew infants, and often several members in the family are subject to it. Cases in other races are reported by Lebbetter;[41] Scotti;[42] Cordes and Horner;[43] and Greear.[44] The ordinary evidences of idiocy become apparent generally in the latter half of the first year, up to which time the child has seemed entirely normal. Now it grows weak, apathetic, lies quietly in bed and loses muscular power, and the condition of stupidity gradually increases. Study of the eyes shows that the child cannot see, and there is found a reddish spot surrounded by a bluish-white halo in the region of the macula lutea, with more or less atrophy of the optic nerve. Rarely there is no change in the macula lutea. The muscular flaccidity at first seen is replaced by spasticity and increased reflexes. Convulsions may occur, and death generally takes place about the age of two years.

There occurs also a *familial maculo-cerebral degeneration* which develops in later childhood, exhibits a decided familial occurrence, and has generally been considered as much similar to amaurotic family idiocy, or a juvenile form of it. There are the macular changes, but not complete blindness. Gradual mental deterioration takes place, but life may continue for years.

7. Idiots Savants.—In this group there are special mental powers in certain limited directions, yet the individual is not above a condition of feeblemindedness in all other respects. There may be remarkable aptitude for music, painting, mathematical calculations, mimicry, games, or other accomplishments.

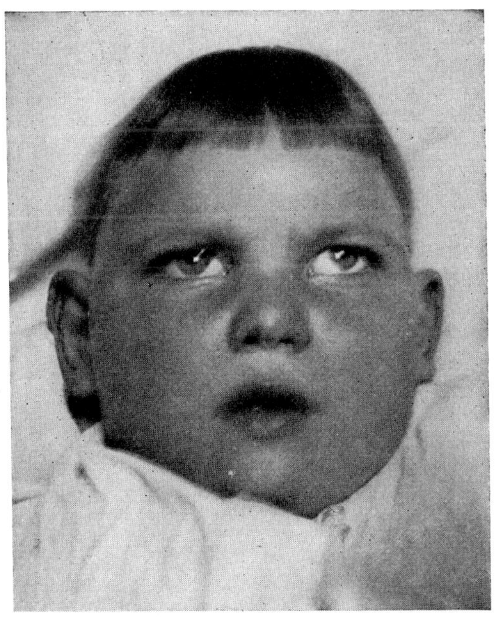

Fig. 202.—Microcephalus. Robert S., two and one-half years old. Children's Medical Ward of the Hospital of the University of Pennsylvania. Labor was slow but without instruments. Infant had convulsions after the first three days. Never made any effort to talk, walk or play. Constant dribbling of saliva. Muscles slightly spastic, and tendon-reflexes somewhat increased. No control over bladder or bowels.

About 50 per cent of idiots cannot be classified in any of the types described, and a number of other uncommon forms are mentioned in the literature. De Sanctis[45] described under the title of *Dementia precocissima catatonica* a form of idiocy of which Jancke[46] collected 13 cases and added 2. Typical cases begin in the third or fourth year, with disturbance of speech, restlessness, increasing mental deterioration proceeding to complete dementia, and arrest of bodily development. The cause is unknown. A familial variety of it is described by Higier.[47]

Idiocy also occurs in the various types of atrophy and sclerosis of the brain (p. 949).

Prognosis.—Complete recovery in those whose minds are actually defective can hardly occur; but the possibility of errors in diagnosis is not to be forgotten. From all points of view the prognosis should be made guardedly. That as to improvement depends upon the nature of the cause, the variety of deficiency and its degree and time of development, and the treatment. The lower grade idiot can improve but little. Subjects of imbecility of not too great a degree can be taught personal cleanliness; to talk to some extent; and, in the case of slight feeblemindedness, even to learn some occupation. As to the prognosis of some of the specific forms, the microcephalic idiot usually shows little if any improvement, and generally does not survive infancy. The improvement in mongolian imbeciles is often steady and decided for a time, and then ceases. They learn to talk to a certain extent and even exceptionally to write and read a little. The general strength is subnormal, and they have little resistance to disease and may die from various infectious disorders, including tuberculosis and pneumonia. Many statistical studies show that only about 10 or 15 per cent live beyond puberty (Orel,[48] Steinen,[35] Spühler[49]). Brousseau[36] found the average age at death fourteen years. Idiots savants are liable early to suffer from increasing mental degeneration. Epileptic and paralytic idiots of low grade seldom improve. In general patients with severe mental defect die in childhood or adolescence, those with mere feeblemindedness may improve remarkably with good training. The earlier in life mental defect becomes apparent, the worse the prognosis. An interesting study of mortality among mental defectives is that by Dayton.[50]

Diagnosis.—The diagnosis is easy in well-marked cases past the age of infancy. Often there are features which clearly proclaim the type. In milder cases, especially in very early life, the diagnosis often presents difficulty. One should know the ages at which the normal child begins to notice, sit, stand, walk, talk, and to exhibit other signs of intelligence. (See pp. 45–48.) The application of the Binet-Simon tests and their numerous modifications are of service as aids for determining the degree of backwardness. (See Dana,[51] Knox,[52] Goddard,[53] Terman,[54] Kuhlmann,[55] Tredgold,[15] Gesell[56].) The following is an outline of certain of the mental and motor characteristics of average normal development. Those up to the age of two years are selected from one of Gesell's[57] publications; those from three to fifteen years follow Goddard:[53]

Twelve Months.—Shows a preference for one hand in reaching; scribbles imitatively with a crayon; comprehends simple verbal commissions; says two words besides "Mama" and "Dada"; can wave "bye-bye" and often say it; places a cube in a cup on command; recovers a cube concealed by a cup; retains a cube in either hand and takes a third; plays with or reaches for his mirror-image; co-operates while he is being dressed; inhibits simple acts on command; imitates simple acts like scribbling and rattling a spoon.

Eighteen Months.—Says five or more words; comprehends simple questions; points to nose, eyes, or hair; builds blocks in tower, imitatively; uses spoon without much spilling; shows dramatic mimicry in play; habitually inhibits certain acts; tries, definitely, to put on shoes.

Two Years.—Plays catch and toss with a ball; uses simple sentences and phrases; names familiar objects like key, penny, watch; builds a tower of three or more blocks; folds paper once imitatively; listens to stories with pictures; tells experiences; asks for things at table by name.

Three Years.—Points out nose, eyes, and mouth; repeats two numbers; enumerates the objects in a picture; knows name; repeats a sentence of six syllables—*e. g.*, "It is cold and snowing." (An average child of three can repeat six, but not ten, syllables.)

Four Years.—Tells whether a little boy or a little girl; names familiar objects—*e. g.*, key, knife, penny; repeats three numbers; points out the longer of two lines.

Five Years.—Tells which is the heavier of two weights; copies a square; repeats a sentence of ten syllables—*e. g.*, "His name is John. He is a very good boy."; counts four pennies; reconstructs an oblong card which has been cut diagonally into two pieces.

Six Years.—Knows whether it is morning or afternoon; says what common objects are used for—*e. g.*, fork, chair, table, horse, mother; obeys triple commands;—*e. g.*, puts key on chair, brings box, shuts door; shows right hand and left ear; says which is pretty and which ugly of a series of drawings of faces.

Seven Years.—Counts 13 pennies; describes pictures (the same pictures as for three years are used, but the child is now required to describe them, not merely enumerate objects); notices that certain parts are missing from drawings of incomplete figures; can copy diamond; names four colors,—*e. g.*, red, blue, green, yellow.

Eight Years.—Compares two things from memory, such as fly and butterfly, wood and glass, paper and cloth; counts backwards from 20 to 1; repeats the days of the week; repeats 5 figures, 4, 7, 3, 9, 5.

Nine Years.—Gives change out of quarter; describes common objects in detail, not merely their use; knows date; repeats the months in order; arranges five weights in order of heaviness.

Ten Years.—Knows money, $1.00, 0.50, 0.25, 0.10, 0.05, and 0.01; copies two simple designs from memory, having seen them for ten seconds (a prism and a Greek moulding); repeats 6 figures, as 8, 5, 4, 7, 2, 6;—2, 7, 4, 6, 8, 1;—9, 4, 1, 7, 3, 8; comprehends easy questions; uses three given words in two sentences.

Eleven Years.—Sees absurdity in statements,—*e. g.* "An unfortunate bicycle-rider broke his head and died instantly; he was picked up and carried to a hospital, and they do not think he will recover,"—"I have 3 brothers, Paul, Ernest, and myself,"—"We met a man who was finely dressed, he was walking along the street with his hands in his pockets, and twirling his cane;" uses 3 given words in a single sentence; gives 60 words in three minutes; gives simple rhymes; rearranges a simple sentence of words which have been put out of order.

Twelve Years.—Repeats 7 figures, as 2, 9, 6, 4, 3, 7, 5;—9, 2, 8, 5, 1, 6, 4;—1, 6, 9, 7, 2, 3, 8; defines charity, justice, goodness; repeats a sentence of 23 syllables,—*e. g.*, "I saw in the street a pretty little dog. It had curly brown hair, short legs, and a long tail"; resists suggestion made by lines of different lengths (the child is confronted by a series of pairs of unequal lines, and this is then followed by a series in which the lines are equal, and he is asked which are the longer. The test is passed if he recognized the equality of the second series); explains an incomplete account of some incident,—*e. g.*, "My neighbor has been having strange visitors. He has received one after the other a physician, a lawyer, and a clergyman. What has happened in his house?"

Fifteen Years.—Tells the impression produced by a picture; interchanges hands of clock—*e. g.*, if 6:20, what would the time be if hour and minute hands were interchanged; writes a simple code which has previously been explained to him; gives the opposite to a list of words supplied.

Intelligence tests should be performed by specially trained persons unless the pediatrist is himself proficient in their use. The results of the tests are aids to a study of the situation, and must be interpreted in conjunction with other facts ascertained about the physical and mental status of the patient and his environment. The reaction of the child while being tested is important, and it should be remembered that the tests in some particulars represent the degree to which the child has been instructed, as well as his innate intellectual capacity. Before reaching a diagnosis of mental deficiency the possibility should be entertained that some other condition may be present, which would cause slowness of mental development. Among such factors are blindness, deafness, marked malnutrition, prolonged illness, and lack of proper instruction. In general a child who has not learned to talk at all by the age of two and one-half years probably is suffering from actual mental defect, particularly if the understanding of words is not normal. (See p. 888.) The presence of any of the stigmata of degeneration is a corroborative diagnostic symptom of idiocy. In certain forms of idiocy help may be had in ascertaining the extent of cerebral injury, cerebral atrophy, dilated ventricles and the like by air-injections (p. 154).

Treatment.—For low-grade idiots little more can be done than to care for cleanliness and to guard the general health and prevent injury. It is usually better to remove the subject from the household. For those less seriously affected constant attention and training may do an astonishing amount of good. The underlying principles consist in the effort to arouse and increase the interest and power of attention; to awaken the association of objects with the names for them; to encourage the child's affections; to inculcate self-control; and to develop mechanical skill. These efforts should not be employed to a degree sufficient to fatigue or worry the patient. Glandular therapy does little good unless specially indicated. Thyroid extract is of some value in mongolian idiots, but only in those whose basal metabolism is low (Talbot[58]).

References

1. J. Ment. Sc., 1897, **43,** 72. 2. Am. J. Dis. Child., 1930, **40,** 1076. 3. Church and Peterson, Nerv. and Ment. Dis., 1911, 851. 4. Biennial Survey of Educat., 1927–28; U. S. Bureau of Educat., 1930. 5. Proc. Am. Assoc. Study of the Feeble Minded, 1931, **55,** 31. 6. Edinburgh M. J., 1929, **36,** 526. 7. J.A.M.A., 1910, **55,** 464. 8. J.A.M.A., 1924, **82,** 12. 9. Boston M. and S. J., 1925, **193,** 671. 10. Am. J. Syph., 1926, **10,** 563. 11. J. Nerv. and Ment. Dis., 1929, **70,** 379. 12. Am. J. Psychiat., 1930, **9,** 1065. 13. Am. J. Syph., 1922, **6,** 353. 14. Surg., Gynec. and Obstet., 1928, **47,** 201. 15. Tredgold, Mental Deficiency 1914, 4th edit. 16. Mental Hygiene, 1929, **13,** 62. 17. New England J. Med., 1930, **203,** 872. 18. Am. J. Psychiat., 1931, **10,** 611. 19. J. Nerv. and Ment. Dis., 1887, **14,** 541. 20. Arch. Neurol. and Psychiat., 1929, **21,** 247. 21. Monatschr. f. Kinderh., 1929, **43,** 341. 22. Arch. Ophth., 1931, **5,** 704. 23. Arch. de méd. d. enf., 1928, **31,** 197; 276. 24. Mitchell and Cook, J.A.M.A., 1932, **99,** 2105. 25. Ztschr. f. Kinderh., 1922, **33,** 110. 26. Mitchell and Downing, Am. J. M. Sc., 1926, **172,** 866. 27. Am. J. M. Sc., 1929, **178,** 315. 28. Nederl. Tidjschr. v. Geneesk., 1919, **1,** 328; Nederl. Maandschr. v. Geneesk., 1926, **13,** 407. 29. Atlantic M. J., 1924, **27,** 841. 30. J.A.M.A., 1920, **74,** 94. 31. J.A.M.A., 1924, **82,** 1196. 32. Arch. de méd. d. enf., 1916, **19,** 478. 33. Ztschr. f. Kinderh., 1926, **42,** 440. 34. J.A.M.A., 1928, **90,** 459. 35. Monatschr. f. Kinderh., 1927, **35,** 495. 36. Mongolism, 1928. 37. Rev. gén. d. ophth., 1924, **38,** 365. 38. Nederl. Maandschr. v. Verlosk. en Vrouvenz. en Kindergeneesk., 1919, **8,** 217. 39. New York M. J., 1896, **63,** 697. 40. Tr. Ophth. Soc. of the United Kingdom, 1881, **1,** 55. 41. Canad. M. A. J., 1925, **15,** 367. 42. Ann. di ottal. e clin. ocul., 1928, **56,** 333; Am. J. Dis. Child., 1929, **37,** 648. 43. Am. J. Ophth., 1929, **12,** 558. 44. South. M. J., 1930, **23,** 324. 45. Folio neuro-biol., 1908, **2,** 9. 46. Arch. f. Kinderh., 1929, **88,** 114. 47. Ref. Monatschr. f. Kinderh., 1927, **36,** 452. 48. Ztschr. f. Kinderh., 1927, **44,** 449. 49. Rev. méd. de la Suisse Romain, 1929, **49,** 258. 50. Proc. Am. A. Study of Feebleminded, 1931, **55,** 127. 51. Med. Rec., 1913, **83,** 1. 52. New York M. J., 1914, **99,** 527. 53. The Training School, 1910, Jan. 54. The Measurement of Intelligence, 1916. 55. J. Psycho-Asthenics 1913, **17,** 132; Handbook Ment. Tests, 1922. 56. J.A.M.A., 1926, **86,** 1277; Infancy and Human Growth 1928; The Guidance of Mental Growth in Infant and Child, 1930. 57. The Mental Growth of the Pre-School Child, 1925. 58. Arch. Pediat., 1922, **39,** 419.

CHAPTER IV

DISEASES OF THE BRAIN AND ITS MENINGES

HERE are included, for the most part, those affections in which there is organic disease chiefly marked in or limited to the brain and its membranes.

MALFORMATIONS

ANENCEPHALUS.—In this condition there are absence of the cerebral hemispheres and of the vault of the cranium, and atrophy of the cerebellum. It is combined with other malformations, especially of the spinal cord. There is sometimes seen a familial tendency to it. It is incompatible with life for more than a few days. It has been variously attributed to hypoplasia of the suprarenals, dysthyroidism in the mother, or to other endocrine faults. A useful review is given by Marcus and Nickman.[1]

CYCLOPIA.—Here the vault of the cranium is present, but the hemispheres imperfectly formed, united anteriorly, and perhaps cystic. There is in typical cases but a single eye in a median position. It is possible for life to continue throughout childhood, if the malformation is only partially developed.

MICROCEPHALUS.—This malformation has already been referred to (p. 908 and Fig. 202). As shown by Zappert,[2] Murphy,[3] and others, roentgenologic or radium irradiation of the ovary before and during pregnancy may produce microcephalus, anencephalus, and other malformations; this, of course, accounting for only a very small number of the cases. The head is small and oftenest brachycephalic, or it may be dome-shaped, or the forehead sloping and narrow. The fontanelles are closed and the sutures united. The brain is correspondingly small, and imperfectly formed in portions, or degenerated. In some cases the circumference of the head may be normal, but the brain microcephalic.

PORENCEPHALUS.—In this there is absence of some of the cerebral tissue, producing a depression in the surface of the brain. The interior of the affected region may be cyst-like and contain serous fluid, or no cavity may be present. It is congenital, or may be acquired from a degenerative process following inflammation, thrombosis, embolism, or hemorrhage. One or both hemispheres may be involved. There may be an associated deformity of the skull. The **symptoms** vary with the position of the lesion. With large cerebral defect there are mental deficiency and spastic cerebral palsy, and death usually occurs in infancy.

HYDROCEPHALUS.—Although some cases are acquired, the greater number are congenital even when there is no evidence of the condition at birth. (See p. 945.)

MACROCEPHALUS.—In this rare congenital affection the size of the brain is increased. The skull may be enlarged; the convolutions flattened; the ventricles compressed. The symptoms are chiefly those of hydrocephalus. A different condition termed "*Megacephalus*" will be considered later (p. 951).

NUCLEAR APLASIA.—This lesion consists in defective development of the cranial nerve-nuclei. It affects oftenest those governing ocular movements, but in some cases the expression of the face and the movements of the tongue are involved. (See p. 950.)

AGENESIS CORTICALIS.—There is here one of the causes of infantile cerebral paralysis and idiocy. There is congenital failure of development of the cortical cells, especially of the pyramidal cells (Sachs[4]). All parts of the cortex of both hemispheres are involved.

ENCEPHALOCELE; HYDRENCEPHALOCELE; MENINGOCELE

Etiology.—These malformations depend in some way not understood upon defect in fetal development.

Symptoms.—In all three of these conditions there is an opening in the skull and dura mater through which a portion of the brain or of its membranes protrudes. The opening is oftenest between two of the bones rather than in the substance of one. There results a tense, smooth tumor, globular or pyriform in shape, generally with a narrow pedicle, and varying from perhaps 1 in. (2.54 cm.) in diameter to a size equaling that of the infant's head. It is oftenest in or near the median line in the occipital region, and sometimes almost as far posteriorly as the foramen magnum. The fronto-nasal region, slightly to one side of the median line, is another favorite position, perhaps involving the root of the nose. Sometimes it projects into

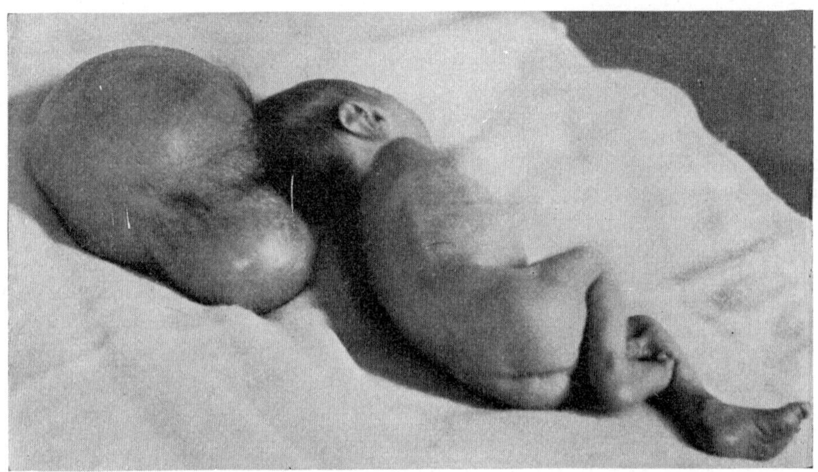

Fig. 203.—Hydrencephalocele of unusual size. Infant aged four months. Children's Medical Ward of the Hospital of the University of Pennsylvania. Large globular mass attached to occipital region, present at birth. At first about size of infant's head, but has grown rapidly. Feels cyst-like; no solid masses discoverable, and is largely of cerebral spinal fluid, but probably contains brain-tissue as well.

the pharynx or the mouth. When external, it is covered by skin, which is often thin, shining and without hair, and sometimes exhibiting cicatricial markings. Deformities of other sorts are often associated with any of the forms; among them spina bifida, cleft palate, harelip and club-foot.

In **encephalocele** (*hernia cerebri*), an uncommon variety, the tumor contains brain-substance and membrane, is usually small, without pedicle, opaque, pulsates but does not fluctuate, and is often reducible. In **meningocele,** also uncommon, the opening in the skull is usually smaller, the tumor contains only meninges distended by cerebrospinal fluid, and, with occasional exceptions, communicates with the arachnoid cavity. It is fluctuating, pediculated, does not pulsate, becomes more tense on crying, and is translucent and reducible. In **hydrencephalocele,** the most common variety, the tumor contains brain-substance with cerebrospinal fluid within it which communicates with the ventricle. It is generally of large size and provided with a pedicle, is only partially translucent, fluctuates, is partly reducible, and often pulsates (Fig. 203).

The general symptoms depend upon the size, position, and nature of the tumor. Meningocele is without nervous manifestations, except that efforts at reduction may produce increased intracranial pressure. Encephalocele may also be free from symptoms, except those of pressure. Hydrencephalocele is liable to be attended by hydrocephalus, optic atrophy, idiocy, nystagmus and strabismus.

Prognosis.—In meningocele the tumor grows larger and there is always danger of rupture and secondary infection. Yet a chance exists that the communication with the arachnoid cavity may become closed. Encephalocele offers the most favorable prognosis, since it increases but little in size. Hydrencephalocele is liable to secondary infection or rupture, and the prognosis is entirely unfavorable.

Treatment.—A meningocele should be protected from injury. A small quantity of fluid may be aspirated if rupture threatens, or a plastic operation may be performed. Encephalocele should merely receive protection. Hydrencephalocele may be subjected to plastic operation if rupture threatens. The results of plastic operation on any of the forms are not encouraging, and even if immediately successful hydrocephalus is liable to develop later.

Spurious Meningocele.—This is the result of trauma, producing fracture of the skull and rupture of the dura mater; union of the opposing fractured edges having failed to take place. Sailer[5] collected 37 such reported cases. Operation may be successful in curing the condition.

DISEASES OF THE MENINGES OF THE BRAIN

PACHYMENINGITIS EXTERNA

Inflammation of the dura is uncommon in children, but may be seen as a *chronic form* secondary to tuberculosis or syphilis of the skull, or as represented by fibrous adhesions to the skull accompanying chronic leptomeningitis. An *acute form* is represented by the serous or purulent external pachymeningitis which may follow purulent processes elsewhere, oftenest infection of the mastoid or of the nasal sinuses. The abscess which develops may remain small or may become extensive and involve secondarily the inner surface of the dura and even the piarachnoid. The **symptoms** of the acute form are sometimes slight and often concealed by those of the primary suppuration elsewhere. In other cases there are evidences of cerebral compression, such as headache, vomiting, slow and irregular pulse and respiration, somnolence and optic neuritis. There are less often localizing symptoms than in cerebral abscess. In circumscribed forms following otitis, which may be more of a serous than a purulent nature, it will be found that drainage of the middle ear and mastoid results in cure. In other cases where an epidural abscess has formed, drainage of this is necessary.

PACHYMENINGITIS INTERNA HEMORRHAGICA; SUBDURAL HEMORRHAGE; CHRONIC SUBDURAL HEMATOMA

There is reason to believe that this condition occurs oftener than has been supposed. Among **causes** are traumatism, as at birth; syphilis; severe infectious diseases; rickets; cachexia; hemorrhagic disorders; scurvy; pertussis; and venous congestion from cardiac and pulmonary disease. It is more common in infancy than in later life. Reviews on the subject are those of Herter,[6] Hunt,[7] and Sherwood.[8]

It is sometimes maintained that the primary lesion is a subdural hemorrhage, this being followed by inflammation. Virchow[9] designated the pachymeningitis as primary, the hemorrhage being secondary, and this view is more generally accepted. There appear to be cases of primary subdural hemorrhage without inflammation, as there are certainly others of pachymeningitis with the presence of a false membrane on the inner surface of the dura mater, but with little effusion of blood; and there are mixed forms. Hemorrhages are usually punctate and scattered, combined with some of larger size, and with perhaps an effusion of blood covering portions of one or both hemispheres. Later the effused blood clots and organizes, and still later is absorbed and leaves cysts; or in the cases where the false membrane predominates this thickens and becomes adherent to the dura, and perhaps to the pia. The **symptoms** are often uncharacteristic, especially in marantic infants or those otherwise severely ill. There may, however, be vomiting; headache; cyanosis; convulsions; unconsciousness; and later, bulging of the fontanelle, slowness of the pulse and respiration, hypertonicity of the muscles, increased reflexes, choked disc, retinal hemorrhages, stupor and convulsions. Lumbar puncture gives a fluid in small amount, which may be clear, xanthochromic, or even distinctly blood-stained. The presence of blood and its quantity depend upon the stage of the disease. Puncture of the ventricles may show a clear fluid, but puncture of the fontanelle and merely through the dura gives a bloody fluid in the acute stages. Fever may or may not be present. In cases of long duration with cystic formation the head becomes decidedly enlarged, and evidences of paralysis and rigidity appear. The **prognosis** is unfavorable, and death may take place within a week, or the condition may become chronic and last for some weeks or months, with characteristic remissions and exacerbations. Recovery, complete or with paralytic symptoms, may occur, but chiefly in older children. In **diagnosis** the retinal hemorrhages, the alterations in the spinal fluid, and the bulging fontanelle are the most important symptoms. In *epidural hemorrhage* the effusion of blood tends to be slower, but not sufficiently so to give much aid in differentiation. *Meningitis* is slower of onset and has a higher fever with less tendency to localizing symptoms. The **treatment** is symptomatic, combined with measures to relieve intracranial pressure, such as purgation, the administration of hypertonic solutions (p. 198), and lumbar and cranial puncture.

EPIDURAL HEMORRHAGE

This rare condition results from trauma with rupture of the meningeal vessels, occurring oftenest during birth. Blood is effused between the dura mater and the skull, producing an internal cephalhaematoma (p. 221). The symptoms are those of gradually increasing intracranial pressure. They develop more slowly than in other forms of meningeal hemorrhage, but the diagnosis is difficult or impossible. Death usually occurs soon.

LEPTOMENINGEAL HEMORRHAGE

Etiology and Pathologic Anatomy.—Intracranial hemorrhage, which in the large majority of cases is meningeal, is common in the new-born if we include here the scattered punctiform hemorrhages, or even some of larger size, which produce no symptoms. (See also p. 935.) Discarding these, studies on the frequency of intracranial hemorrhage give varying figures, but it would appear that about one-half of the still-births and of deaths promptly after birth are due to it, and necropsy studies show that perhaps two-thirds of new-born infants coming to necropsy have some degree of it (Wilson,[10] Wehye,[11] Hedren,[12] Vischer,[13] Irving,[14] Cruickshank,[15] Yagi,[16] Greene,[17] Burpee,[18] Ehrenfest,[19] Fleming and Morton[20]). One of the most common causes is trauma. Consequently the condition is especially frequent in the new-born as a result of the continued pressure of a difficult and prolonged labor, with the accompanying asphyxia; and much less often produced by the employment of forceps, and probably sometimes resulting from a too rapid delivery with the consequent alteration of intracranial pressure and the accompanying intense congestion. It would appear from recent studies, as those of Ford,[21] Ehrenfest,[19] Fleming and Morton,[20] Crothers,[22] and others, that the mechanical injury of labor is the most important factor, and that asphyxia is relatively unimportant. Intracranial hemorrhage occurs oftenest in first-born children. It is more frequent in premature infants according to some studies, although others, such as those of Cruickshank,[15] do not show this. That hemorrhage happens so readily in the new-born may depend, too, upon the delicate structure of the pial vessels at this period. The existence of the hemorrhagic disease of the new-born may be a factor in some cases (Warwick,[23] Foote,[24] Munro and Eustis[25]). There may possibly be operative, too, the physiologic delay in coagulation-time sometimes found in new-born infants (p. 40).

Much less often meningeal hemorrhage is produced by trauma later in childhood, or occurs as the result of some infectious disease, including occasionally syphilis; or may develop during a hemorrhagic disorder. It may be a secondary lesion to the congestion attending a convulsion or a paroxysm of pertussis; or sometimes to embolism or thrombosis of the cerebral vessels or sinuses. In 10,150 children who died at birth or before twelve years of age Sheldon[26] found intracranial hemorrhage in 0.5 per cent. He included only those cases with actual extravasation of blood.

The hemorrhage is often confined to the region below the arachnoid, but it may burst through this and produce a complicating subdural hemorrhage. It may be only punctiform, or much larger and occupy the arachnoid space. It may be either superficial and cover a considerable area over the convexity of the brain, usually on both sides; or it may be at the base, in the latter situation being beneath the tentorium, and caused by a rupture of this. There may be lacerations of other dural folds. Hemorrhage does not constantly accompany laceration of the dura. There may be blood in the ventricles in cases of subarachnoid hemorrhage. Basal hemorrhage is oftenest seen in head-presentations, and hemorrhage over the convexity in breech- or foot-presentations. Hemorrhages in other viscera are not infrequent complications. Later secondary changes consist in softening of the brain-tissue, cysts, meningo-encephalitis, sclerosis, atrophy, and degeneration in the lateral tracts of the spinal cord.

Symptoms.—With hemorrhages of very small size occurring at birth there are generally no immediate or later symptoms. Such hemorrhages are probably frequent. Larger ones, too, may produce at the time no characteristic symptoms, and the infant promptly, or a day or two after birth, merely becomes constantly or intermittently cyanotic, atelectatic, apathetic or drowsy, and nurses poorly. Sometimes these symptoms do not appear until three or four weeks after birth; an explanation advanced for this being that at that time contraction of a subtentorial clot presses on the vital centers (Glaser[27]). In other cases there are at birth, or shortly after, distinct signs of increased intracranial pressure, with unconsciousness, slow pulse, irregular respiration, and bulging of the anterior fontanelle. Evidences of irritation, as represented by convulsions, rigidity, and increased reflexes, are of very frequent occurrence and usually bilateral. Convulsions occur more frequently when the hemorrhage is over the cortex; less when it is basal. Paralysis is less common among the early manifestations. Strabismus and nystagmus may be both early and late symptoms. Retinal hemorrhages are common early, as is jaundice. In some instances manifestations of a residual nature are not observed until the latter part of the first year. There is no characteristic alteration of temperature. Lumbar puncture may give a bloody or reddish fluid with degenerated red blood-cells, but this by no means always occurs.

Course and Prognosis.—Punctiform hemorrhages are of little importance, and are absorbed without residue. Small effusions may give rise to no immediate symptoms, but may in later years show evidence of the damage done. Hemorrhages of decidedly large amount may produce death in a few hours or days. Sometimes a lesion becomes infected and suppuration follows. Grouping all forms of intracranial birth-injury together, the large majority being meningeal hemorrhage, Munro[28] gave as the results in 177 cases, 56 as fatal, and of 48 living 39 were known to have recovered; and Fleming and Morton[20] found that of 33 infants who survived what was believed to be intracranial hemorrhage, only 5 had persistent mental and physical defects.

Diagnosis.—This is based on the symptoms of increased intracranial pressure and the results of lumbar or cisternal puncture. It should be remembered that blood may not be present in the fluid, and, further, that about 10 per cent of all new-born infants may have red blood-cells in the spinal fluid when there are no clinical symptoms at the time nor residual effects later. In addition, symptoms such as nystagmus and retinal hemorrhages may occur when the lesion seems to be simply edema or when, at least, hemorrhage is a minor lesion. Xanthochromia of the spinal fluid is not a necessary sign of intracranial hemorrhage, inasmuch as it may occur from icterus; in which case, however, it will not give the benzidine reaction for blood. Paralytic symptoms are of more aid than general convulsions in forming a diagnosis, since the latter occur in so many conditions. Localized convulsions are of greater import, although often not present even with circumscribed lesions. From *subdural hemorrhage* leptomeningeal hemorrhage is distinguished by the usually wide spread of the effusion, and the consequent less marked localization. From *epidural hemorrhage* leptomeningeal hemorrhage is difficult to differentiate, although in the former the symptoms may be slight, unless the effusion is large.

Treatment.—If there is increased intracranial pressure, as shown by the lumbar puncture, this or cisternal puncture may be performed and repeated until the condition is relieved. Increased pressure seems to be the proper criterion for the performance of puncture, although some clinicians advise against its use except for diagnosis. Even when hemorrhagic disease is not suspected, intramuscular injections of blood may be given for their hemostatic effect. Sedatives should be used for restlessness and convulsions. When there is a depressed fracture, operative interference is indicated. Preventive treatment consists in proper obstetrical practice.

MENINGISMUS

This title was first used by Dupré,[29] and refers to a syndrome resembling meningitis symptomatically, but without any evidence of pathologic lesions or abnormality in the spinal fluid except, perhaps, increase in pressure. It occurs especially with acute infectious fevers, pneumonia, and marantic states in infancy. Most writers are disposed to abandon the term, and to consider the condition as serous meningitis. The prognosis, apart from that of the causative disease, is favorable. No special treatment is required, unless increased intracranial pressure indicates lumbar puncture.

LEPTOMENINGITIS

Among the several forms of this are (1) Serous meningitis; (2) Acute purulent meningitis; and (3) Tuberculous meningitis.

SEROUS MENINGITIS

(Serofibrinous Meningitis; Ependymitis; Serous Apoplexy; Acute Acquired Hydrocephalus)

The title, first used by Quincke, applies properly to cases with acute meningeal symptoms in which the cerebrospinal fluid is increased in amount and shows evidences of inflammation, but exhibits a normal or but a slight increase in the number of leukocytes; while no micro-organisms, or only a few, are discoverable in it. (Fig. 204.)

Etiology.—The disease is liable to develop especially in the first two years of life, although not confined to this period. It is almost always secondary; not infrequently to otitis media or other neighboring purulent processes, the effusion resulting from irritation rather than transmitted infection. Other causes are trauma of the head; syphilis; lead poisoning; and acute diseases, as typhoid fever, gastro-enteritis, measles, pertussis, and particularly pneumonia.

Pathologic Anatomy.—Early in the attack there is a circumscribed and often edematous swelling of the meninges involving various regions, with effusion of fluid. Later there may be dilatation of the ventricles and flattening of the convolutions, and, in some instances, evidences of circumscribed meningitis.

Symptoms.—These vary depending upon the severity of the attack, the portion of the meninges chiefly involved, and the disorder to which the condition may be secondary. In the most acute cases (*serous apoplexy*) the condition begins with high fever, severe repeated convulsions, contracted pupils, possibly slight stiffness of the neck, and coma. Much more frequently the development is more gradual and the course less intense. There is then moderate fever, headache, stiff neck, muscular rigidity, sometimes vomiting, often delirium, grinding of the teeth, convulsions or stupor, and evidences of intracranial pressure. The convulsions may be general or localized. Especially in ventricular involvement (*acute acquired internal hydrocephalus*) will symptoms of intracranial pressure develop, as choked discs; slow irregular pulse; either convulsions or coma; and, in infancy, bulging of the anterior fontanelle. In some forms the onset is so gradual that tuberculous meningitis is simulated.

Course and Prognosis.—The violent, acute cases may end in death in a few hours up to a few days, the fatal ending being influenced largely by the primary disease. In the less violent form the symptoms often disappear rapidly, either with the subsidence of an acute infectious disease, or as a result of operation on some neighboring purulent focus, or spontaneously without this. Other cases go on to a fatal ending after days or weeks; and still others pass into the condition of chronic acquired internal hydrocephalus, with optic atrophy, paralysis of cranial nerves and spasticity. In

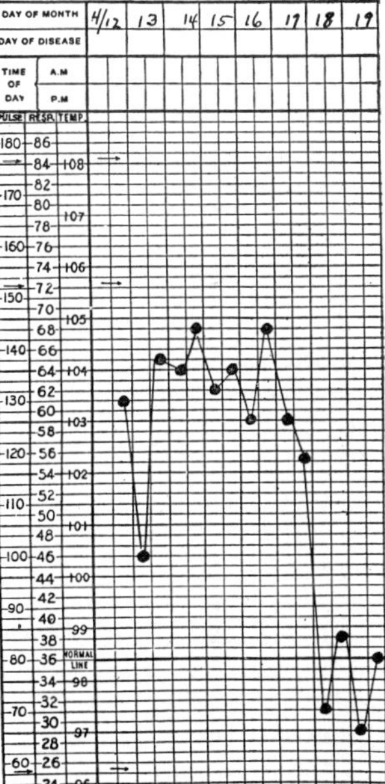

Fig. 204.—Serous meningitis with cell-count not abnormal but pressure increased. Antonio DeM., aged twenty-eight months. Admitted to Children's Hospital of Philadelphia, Apr. 12. Said to have developed pneumonia eight days before. Rigidity of body began three days ago, first in legs, and followed by opisthotonos. Diarrhea last few days. While in hospital respiration from 30 to 60+, pulse 110 to 160, restless, coughing, lesions of pneumonia found in lungs, body and limbs very rigid, general symptoms those of meningitis; Apr. 13, spinal puncture gave 12 cc. (0.41 fl. oz.) of clear, watery fluid under increased pressure, no organisms, 7 leukocytes to the c.mm.; Apr. 14, stiffness still marked, knee-jerks exaggerated, tache very marked, lesions of pneumonia still well-developed; Apr. 15, condition poor, pulse rapid, comatose, vasomotor flushing and paling as in meningitis; Apr. 18, critical fall of temperature; Apr. 19, rigidity has disappeared, lungs clear, knee-jerks normal, examination of lungs practically negative. Recovery.

recovered cases a tendency to recurrence later is noted; and certain instances of epilepsy, slight mental defect, or psychic disturbance may have had their origin in earlier serous meningitis. On the whole, however, the prognosis is favorable and the majority of cases recover completely.

Diagnosis.—This rests upon the presence of meningeal symptoms combined with the results of lumbar puncture. The spinal fluid is clear, under slight pressure, contains an increased amount of protein, globulin is present, there are but few or no germs, and only a moderate increase of the cells, these being of a mononuclear type. Sugar is usually present, and a delicate fibrin-clot may sometimes form on standing. The fluid of *tuberculous meningitis* may be much like that of serous meningitis, and the differential diagnosis may rest upon the finding of tubercle bacilli or the inoculation of a guinea-pig, and clinically upon the slower onset and more prolonged course of tuberculous meningitis. *Purulent meningitis* is readily differentiated by the cloudy fluid with polymorphonuclear cells and, generally, bacteria. Exceptionally in the early stages of cerebrospinal fever the fluid may be quite clear, and also in the later stages when adhesions prevent the free drainage of exudate. Occasionally, too, in serous meningitis, there may be an unusual increase in the cell-count. *Encephalitis* and the meningitic form of *poliomyelitis* may have a spinal fluid much like serous meningitis, but other symptoms, especially paralysis, should serve to differentiate these conditions from it. The diagnosis from *cerebral abscess* will be considered under that heading. If there is a distinction from *meningismus* it is that this condition is not accompanied by any evidence of meningeal inflammation in the spinal fluid.

Treatment.—Prompt and repeated lumbar puncture often gives decided aid, and hypertonic solutions and magnesium sulphate may be employed (p. 198). The causative disease should be treated and its symptoms relieved by appropriate remedies.

Lymphocytic Meningitis. (*Acute Aseptic Meningitis, Benign Acute Idiopathic Serous Meningitis, Epidemic Meningitis Serosa.*)—This condition, of which we have seen a number of instances, possesses features which distinguish it from ordinary serous meningitis. Cases of it have been reported by Wallgren,[31] Krabbe,[32] Viets and Watts,[33] Andersen and Wulff,[34] Gibbens,[35] Eckstein,[36] Roch,[37] and others. Its cause is unknown, but the cases are evidently not tuberculous or syphilitic in nature. It has been suggested that the disease is an abortive form of poliomyelitis, but there is no proof of this. An epidemic influence is sometimes observed. Headache and vomiting are initial symptoms, but the evidences of meningitis are usually mild, and the patient more or less alert. The spinal fluid is under increased pressure; globulin is present; the amount of sugar is normal; cultures, guinea-pig inoculation and Wassermann reaction are all negative; and the cells, which are practically all lymphocytes, may be increased to as many as 500 or more per c.mm. Recovery almost invariably occurs.

ACUTE PURULENT LEPTOMENINGITIS

That variety of purulent leptomeningitis due to the meningococcus has already been described (p. 319.) To the remaining forms the title *meningitis simplex* is sometimes applied.

Etiology.—A large variety of germs are capable of producing the disease. Among them being the pneumococcus, streptococcus, staphylococcus, influenza bacillus, Friedländer bacillus, typhoid bacillus, bacillus pyocyaneus, bacillus proteus, bacillus lactis aërogenes, bacillus acidi lactici, colon bacillus, micrococcus catarrhalis, diphtheria bacillus, diphtheroids, Koch-Weeks bacillus and gonococcus. Frequently the infection is a mixed one. Acute meningitis has repeatedly been observed with mumps; many

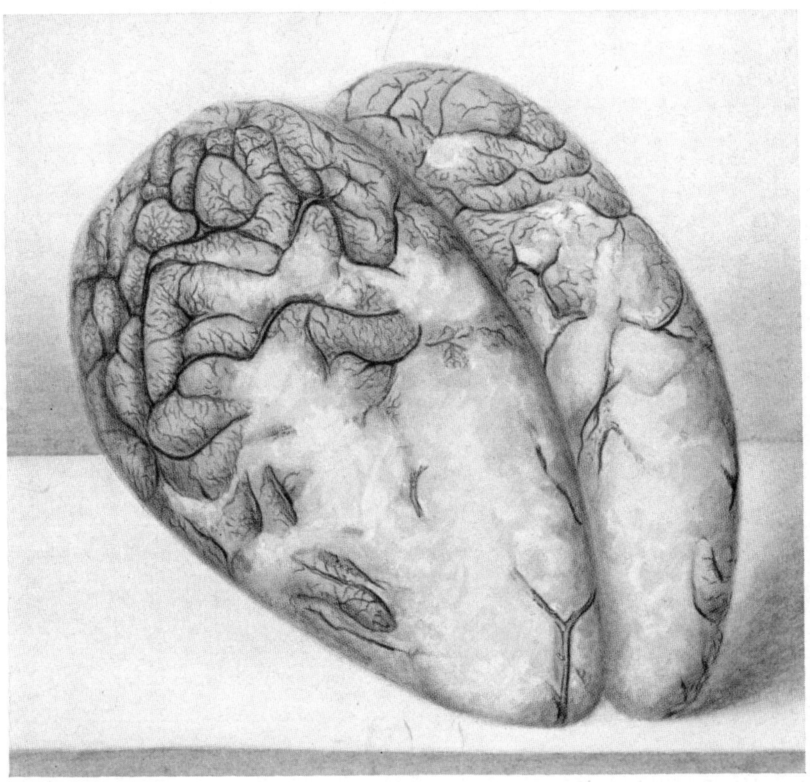

Fig. 205.—Pneumococcic meningitis. Infant of seven months in the Children's Medical Ward of the Hospital of the University of Pennsylvania. Vague nervous manifestations followed by symptoms of pneumonia, otitis media, and mastoiditis. Necropsy showed a thin layer of lymph over a portion of the cortex and at the base. Pneumococci found, with staphylococci and streptococci probably as secondary development.

of these cases, however, being of the serous rather than the purulent variety (p. 371). It may occur in the course of other infectious fevers, without necessarily being dependent upon the germ causing these diseases. Syphilitic meningitis, while generally chronic, may rarely be acute. Meningitis has been reported due to the streptothrix, blastomyces, and torula histolytica (Massee and Rooney[38]). The majority of instances of meningitis occur in infancy, although the first three months of life are relatively immune, except for the cases of septic meningitis seen in the new-born.

Clinical Forms.—A few of the clinical forms dependent upon different germs require brief description:

PNEUMOCOCCIC MENINGITIS.—This is perhaps the most common variety next to those due to the tubercle bacillus or the meningococcus. Sometimes the affection is primary, the pneumococci having penetrated to the meninges through the ethmoid bone; while in other instances there is a pneumococcic inflammatory focus primary elsewhere in the body, although undiscovered during life. So far as our own experience goes, in most cases of pneumococcic meningitis encountered either an otitis media was present or no primary focus could be discovered. The number of occasions on which a pneumococcic meningitis develops in connection with pneumonia is relatively very small.

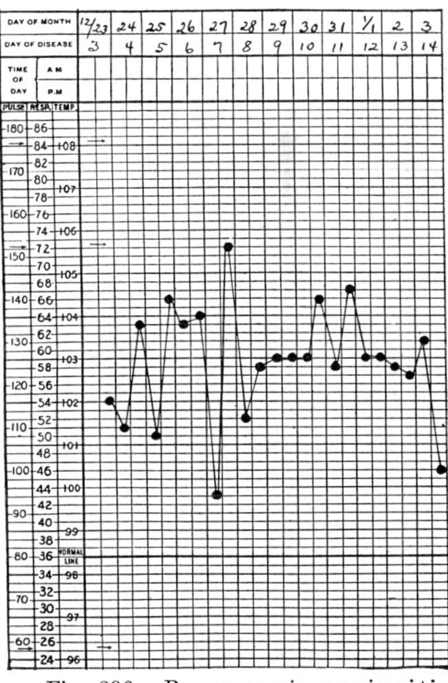

Fig. 206.—Pneumococcic meningitis, high fever. Lillian S., ten months old. Admitted to Children's Hospital of Philadelphia, Dec. 23. Taken ill Dec. 22 with convulsions. These continued more or less. No positive symptoms of pneumonia were found, but respiration was from fifty to seventy per minute, and lumbar puncture showed slightly cloudy fluid, with numerous polymorphonuclear cells, globulin ++, pneumococci found. Died Jan. 3.

Pathologically there is often a greater development of fibrino-purulent exudate than in cerebrospinal fever, especially on the convexity of the brain; and the base is involved to a lesser degree and sometimes not at all (Fig. 205). The ventricles may occasionally be more effected than the surface. Involvement of the spinal cord is usually slight or absent. The **symptoms** and physical findings are largely those characteristic of cerebrospinal fever and have already been described (p. 319). (See also Indications of Symptoms p. 856.) In the cases developing in children previously entirely well, or at least not severely ill with other affections, there is an abrupt onset with high fever, headache, vomiting, frequently convulsions, delirium, and stupor (Fig. 206). Stiffness of the neck, retraction of the head, opisthotonos and hyperesthesia are not as common as in cerebrospinal fever or tuberculous meningitis. This is dependent upon the lesser frequency and degree of involvement of the base as compared with the convexity of the brain. In subjects seriously ill with other disease, pneumococcic meningitis may run a latent course, the diagnosis being made at necropsy. The **course** is short and usually severe, the attack lasting seldom more than three or four days. While nearly always fatal, exceptionally recovery has occurred. In a review of the literature in 1927 Goldstein and Goldstein[39] estimated that there are about 150 such instances. Other reported recoveries are noted by Sala,[40] Harkavy,[41] and Globus and Kasanin.[42] The apparently primary cases cannot be certainly **diagnosed** from other forms of acute leptomeningitis except by lumbar puncture, which gives a turbid fluid in which pneumococci can be found, together with numerous polymorphonuclear cells. The existence of the disease should be suspected when, during the course of pneumonia, empyema, pericarditis, peritonitis or otitis, the symptoms of meningitis suddenly develop; although much more frequently under these conditions the manifestations are produced by a serous meningitis or are perhaps toxic in nature. The diagnosis of pneumococcic from tuberculous meningitis will be considered elsewhere (p. 929).

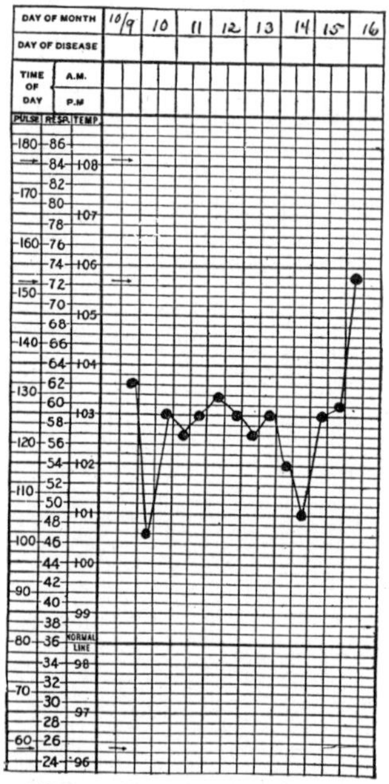

Fig. 207.—Septic (staphylococcic) meningitis. Thomas W., aged twelve years. Entered Children's Ward of University of Pennsylvania Hospital, Oct. 9. About two weeks previously developed diffuse pain in left leg, with fever; then on Oct. 7 in the left arm, and became delirious. Examination showed no positive localization in the limbs, slight dry cough, condition supposed to be typhoid fever with neuritis, grew steadily worse, very hypersensitiveall over, rigidity of neck, evident signs of meningitis. Lumbar puncture on Oct. 13 gave fluid under pressure, containing staphylococcus pyogenes citreus; Oct. 14, delirious, unconscious, papulovesicular eruption over the body, some places in the form of blebs. Fluid obtained today was turbid, under high pressure, cell-content 98 per cent polymorphonuclears and 2 per cent lymphocytes. Died Oct. 16.

Septic Meningitis (Fig. 207).—Here are included the cases depending upon the action of such pyogenic germs as the streptococcus and the staphylococcus. In the newborn the disease is oftenest associated with umbilical infection; in older subjects with otitis, sore throat, empyema, erysipelas, scarlet fever, measles, pertussis, diphtheria, and suppuration of the joints. In some cases no preceding infection can be discovered. The **lesions** are quite similar to those of pneumococcic meningitis, although with the production of a smaller amount of fibrin, and the **clinical features,** too, are like those of this variety. The **course** is short, and the **prognosis** almost entirely unfavorable. According to Appelbaum[43] writing in 1932, and reviewing the literature, there are only 56 reported recoveries from streptococcic meningitis in patients of all ages. In staphylococcic meningitis a chronic meningitis may follow the acute form. We have three times seen it lead to a chronic hydrocephalus, one of these cases being reported by Lamb.[44] Cases of staphylococcic meningitis may recover. We have seen this, and an instance is reported by Ballenger[45] who gives a short review of the literature. The **diagnosis** of septic meningitis is confirmed by spinal puncture, which shows a turbid fluid containing many polymorphonuclear cells and the causative micro-organism. A localized septic meningitis is diagnosed from abscess of the brain chiefly by the fact that in the latter the spinal fluid is generally clear and contains relatively few cells, unless the abscess has ruptured. In abscess there is more headache and a greater degree of optic neuritis.

Influenzal Meningitis.—This seems to be more common than formerly. Of 124 cases of purulent meningitis, Ward and Fothergill[46] found that 20 per cent were influenzal. It has been studied especially by

Adams,[47] Wollstein,[48] Torrey,[49] and Rivers.[50] In our own experience it ranks in frequency with pneumococcic and streptococcic forms. In the majority of instances it seems to be primary and not preceded by manifestations of influenza elsewhere in the body. Most cases occur in infancy. The **lesions** and the **symptoms** are similar to those of other forms of purulent meningitis (Fig. 208). Lumbar puncture gives a turbid or purulent fluid with numerous polymorphonuclear cells and with influenza bacilli, often pleomorphic and both extra- and intracellular. On culture the strains are found to differ from the ordinary respiratory strains (Rivers[50]). Bacteremia with influenza bacillus is not infrequently present. A nitrate reaction in the spinal fluid, described by Greenthal[51] is said to be specific. The **prognosis** is unfavorable,

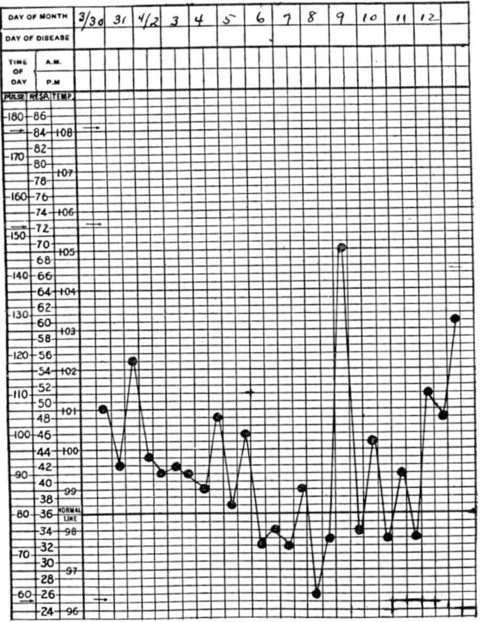

Fig. 208.—Fatal influenzal meningitis. Samuel M., aged two years. Entered the Children's Hospital of Philadelphia, Mar. 30. Earache two weeks previously, ear been discharging for two days. Promptly developed signs of meningitis with restlessness and deviation of the eyes; Apr. 3, lumbar puncture gave cloudy spinal fluid which yielded a pure culture of the influenza-bacillus, 70 leukocytes to the c.mm.; Apr. 7, condition unimproved, intraspinal injection of influenza-serum given yesterday and again on this date; Apr. 8, lumbar puncture showed very cloudy fluid. Died Apr. 12.

the mortality being, according to most reports, almost 100 per cent, only a few cases of recovery having been observed.

Treatment of Simple Purulent Leptomeningitis.—Symptomatic treatment consists in keeping the child quiet in a somewhat darkened room; the administration of suitable nourishment; and medication for pain, convulsions and the like. Repeated lumbar or cisternal punctures should be used to reduce intracranial pressure and for drainage. In the pneumococcic type antipneumococcic serum has been given intravenously and intraspinously, employing, if possible, the serum specific for the type of pneumococcus present. Kolmer,[52] Harkavy[41] and others have used Felton's concentrated antipneumococcus serum intrathecally, intravenously, and intramuscularly (see p. 742); Kolmer reinforcing each 10 cc. of the serum with 0.5 cc. of a 1:100 solution of optochin hydrochloride (ethylhydrocupreine), and injecting this into each common carotid artery as well as by other routes. Optochin hydrochloride has been used intraspinously in pneumococcic meningitis by a number of other clinicians, some employing 2 or 3 injections of as much as 15 cc. of a 1:1000 solution. Huntoon's pneumococcus antibody has also been employed intravenously and intramuscularly, and iodine solution (Pregel's) intraspinously (Apfel[53]). In streptococcic meningitis, antistreptococcic serum may be given intravenously and intrathecally, some authors recommending, even in cases not accompanying scarlet fever, the use of antiscarlatinal serum. In staphylococcic meningitis we have tried the effect of intravenous and intraspinal injections of blood-serum from an individual receiving staphylococcus vaccine, but cure did not result. Wollstein,[54] Ward and Fothergill,[46] and others have produced sera to be used intraspinously in influenzal meningitis, but these have not given the results hoped for. It should be remembered that in some of the reported cures of any of the forms of purulent meningitis there has been employed only simple drainage by lumbar puncture. Dandy[55] and others have cured a few cases of pneumococcic and streptococcic meningitis by operation, removing part of the occipital bone and securing continuous drainage. A method first proposed by Reiche[56] has been used by Gardner[57] and others, in which spinal fluid is withdrawn and air injected until all the spinal fluid has been replaced; then salt solution, perhaps with the indicated serum, is injected. Intrathecal injection of dyes such as gentian violet, 5 to 10 cc. of a 1 per cent solution, may be employed for gram-positive organisms, or the same amount of a 1:1000 solution of neutral acriflavine for gram-negative ones. Mercurochrome also has been given intraspinously in pneumococcic meningitis in doses of from 2 to 4 cc. of a 0.5 per cent solution (Stoessinger[58]).

TUBERCULOUS MENINGITIS

Although a disease long existing and mentioned by other writers before Whytt,[59] this author was the first to give a clear description of it. It is the most frequent form of leptomeningitis occurring in children, equaling more than all the others combined if the epidemic outbreaks of cerebrospinal fever be disregarded. Of 239 cases of meningitis occurring in the Children's Hospital of Philadelphia during a period of years, during some of which cerebrospinal fever in an epidemic form was present in the city, 121 were diagnosed as tuberculous. The influence of the disease upon the mortality in early life is decided.

Etiology.—Inheritance and family relationship play the *predisposing* part seen in all tuberculous affections. The age of the child is a matter of moment. It is generally maintained that the period from the second to the sixth year inclusive exhibits the greatest number of cases; the majority of these being in the second and third years. Yet a large number occur in the second six months of life, and cases are reported earlier than this (Rilliet and Barthez,[60] Reich,[61] Herter,[62] Holt,[63] and others). Sex appears to have no certain influence. The largest number of cases are observed in the spring, apparently because the winter's confinement to the house and the frequency of respiratory infections have led to the acquiring or awakening to activity of a tuberculous focus in the body. Acting in the same way many other diseases, and particularly measles, pertussis and typhoid fever, are liable to be followed by tuberculous meningitis. Trauma, especially of the head, seems to be a predisposing cause in some cases. The *direct cause* is, of course, infection by the tubercle bacillus, which, while it may appear from a clinical point of view to have attacked the meninges primarily, is always transported to the brain by way of the lymph-vessels or often by the blood from some small unrecognized focus, very frequently in the lungs or especially in the tracheobronchial lymphatic nodes. Quite commonly meningitis is the terminal process of a general tuberculosis, the symptoms of which had been of the usual vague nature, and the diagnosis often questionable or wrongly made. In older children it is not uncommon to see tuberculous meningitis develop as a sequel to an active or a healed tuberculous process in the bones or joints. The method by which the primary infection has taken place has already been discussed. (See p. 410.)

Pathologic Anatomy.—The process in brief consists of the formation of miliary tubercles together with an inflammatory exudate. The dura is tense, the convolutions flattened, and the cavity of the arachnoid and the ventricles more or less filled with serofibrinous or fibrinopurulent exudate; the presence of pus perhaps depending upon a mixed infection. The amount of fibrin and of pus is usually small as compared with other forms of meningitis, and the fluid is clear or slightly cloudy. Tubercle bacilli are found in the fluid, and perhaps other germs in addition.

The degree of pathologic change varies with the case. Miliary tubercles may be numerous, and be found on the convexity as well as at the base; or they may be so few that they easily escape notice. The membranes at the base may be only slightly turbid, or in long-continued cases much thickened, gelatinous, and matted; the ventricles contain only a normal amount of fluid, or be much distended; the exudate clear or seropurulent, watery or gelatinous; the brain-substance firm or show the superficial congestion and softening of a meningo-encephalitis. Tuberculous lesions of other parts of the body are, as stated, always present; sometimes small, often extensive.

Symptoms.—In the typical form the symptoms may be divided into three stages: (1) *irritation*, or the prodromal stage; (2) *pressure*, or the transitional stage; (3) *paralysis* or coma, the terminal stage. These are never sharply demarcated, and, in general, the disease is subject to many variations.

The onset is usually slow, but not infrequently in infants, acute. There develop irritability; fretfulness; malaise; sometimes drowsiness; disinclination to play; perhaps headache, discovered if the children are old enough to complain of it; loss of appetite; constipation; vomiting without discoverable cause; restless sleep with dreaming or grinding of the teeth. Sometimes the mental state and the disposition are strangely altered. The temperature is often slightly and irregularly elevated; sometimes high, but oftener moderate. It is impossible at this time to come to an accurate or even a provisional diagnosis, and the children are supposed to have some one of a large range of maladies other than the true one.

The second stage, that of pressure, then begins with a sudden or gradual increase in the severity of the symptoms, and distinct cerebral manifestations appear. Most marked here is the development of unusual drowsiness, perhaps ushered in by a convulsion. The child lies still, with the eyes half-open and apparently fixed on some distant object; and when roused with difficulty from this drowsy state cries out or may become delirious. With the stupor are rigidity of the neck and often of much of the body; slowness or irregularity of the pulse; irregular or sighing respiration; and a tendency to assume the "gun-hammer" position; *i. e.*, with the head thrown backward, the back arched, the thighs flexed on the abdomen, and the arms flexed at the elbows and drawn to the sides of the thorax. In other instances the position assumed is on the back with the arms extended along the sides of the trunk, and perhaps with the head turned to one side. There is headache; sometimes photophobia; moderate hyperesthesia; a disposition to sudden screaming, particularly at night, *i. e.*, the so-called "hydrencephalic cry"; exaggerated reflexes; scaphoid abdomen; bulging of the fontanelle in infancy; and often repeated general convulsions, or mere twitching of some of the muscles. The eyes frequently are turned to one side or rolled in different directions, or there may be nystagmus; the pupils are contracted or normal; vomiting may occur at intervals. Fever is present, but not often high and occasionally is absent. During this stage there is a well-marked *tache cérébrale,* with which is frequently associated an irregular flushing of the body, as of the trunk, following the exposure of the surface to the air; or seen as a suffusion of the face, the flush coming and going slowly and without discoverable reason.

The symptoms gradually grow worse, and after a variable and uncertain time the evidences of irritation from pressure give way largely to those of the paralysis of the final, or third, stage of the disease. Convulsions and rigidity of the neck, however, often persist. There is now complete coma; the patient rapidly loses strength; the pulse becomes more accelerated and irregular; paralysis is widespread; voluntary movements cease; the reflexes are abolished; the pupils respond little if at all to light and are dilated; the

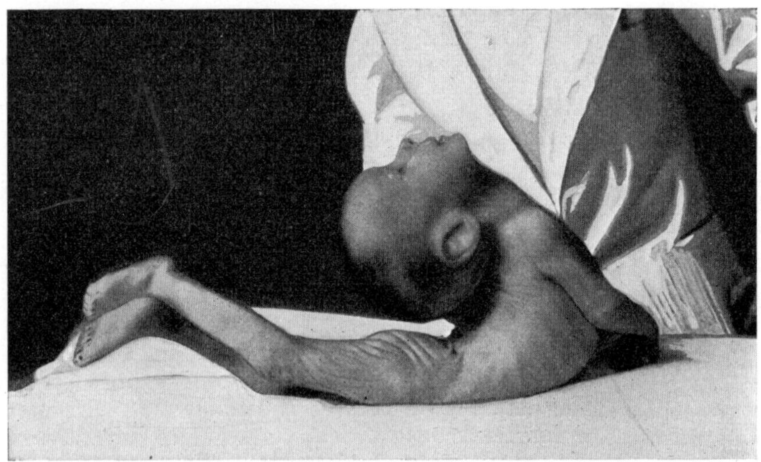

Fig. 209.—Tuberculous meningitis with an unusual degree of opisthotonos. From a patient aged six months in the Children's Hospital of Philadelphia. Had had opisthotonos for three weeks. The occiput was almost against the shoulders, and the heels sometimes touched the head; tubercle bacilli in the spinal fluid.

cornea is insensitive to touch; the respiration is irregular, sometimes rapid, and sometimes approaching the Cheyne-Stokes type. The temperature may often rise to 104 or higher, or may be normal or even subnormal; there is incontinence of urine and feces, or the urine may be retained; swallowing is difficult or impossible; glycosuria may occur. Death takes place in coma with or without convulsions.

Certain of the symptoms referred to, and others not mentioned in detail, require a fuller elaboration.

Clonic convulsions, may occur at any period of the disease, being sometimes initial, sometimes observed just before death. They may be general, or limited to certain localities. They may, for instance, be in the form of a constant rhythmic twitching of a hemiplegic distribution lasting for hours, and then disappearing or being replaced by convulsive movements in other parts of the body. Not infrequently widespread convulsions do not occur at all; and they are as a rule less frequently seen than in other forms of meningitis, and oftenest in the first year.

Rigidity of various distribution is a prominent symptom. That of the neck occurs early among the manifestations of pressure. It may persist throughout the attack, although it often is absent for a time and then returns. There is usually less retraction of the head and opisthotonos (Fig. 209) than in cerebrospinal fever. One or more limbs may develop a tetanic rigidity. Distention of the abdomen may take the place of retraction, especially in infants.

The tendon-*reflexes* are increased until coma is well established, when they may be abolished. The spastic condition of the limbs often makes the examination unsatisfactory. Kernig's sign (p. 857) may or may not be present, and we have not found it of any special diagnostic value in tuberculous meningitis. The Babinski reflex (p. 857) is frequently observed, but is without certain significance in infancy. Brudzinski's reflexes, identical and contralateral (p. 857) are usually seen as in other forms of meningitis.

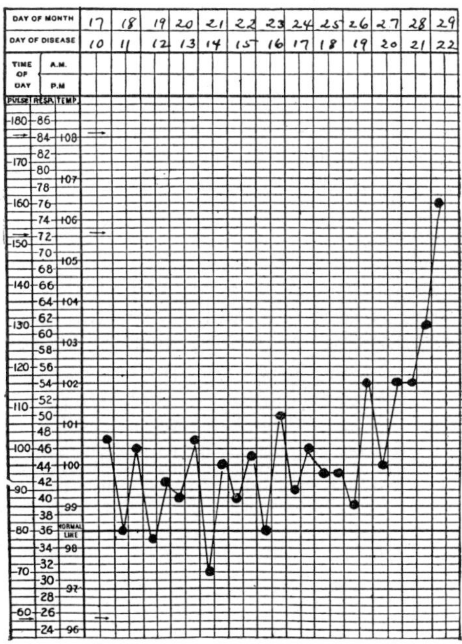

Fig. 210.—Tuberculous meningitis with low degree of fever until hyperpyrexia on the last day. Catherine McC., eight months old. Admitted to the Children's Hospital of Philadelphia, Dec. 17. Ten days previously began to vomit, apparently result of bad feeding; was constipated; Dec. 19, examination negative except for rapid cardiac action; Dec. 20, drowsy, abdomen distended, Cheyne-Stokes respiration, neck-reflex marked. Lumbar puncture revealed tubercle bacilli with polymorphonuclear cells 83 per cent and lymphocytes 17 per cent.

Ocular symptoms are of interest. The pupils are often contracted in the earlier stages, dilated in the last. Hippus may be present. Moderate swelling of the disc is frequently seen early; choked discs not so often. Tubercles may be present in the choroid, oftenest in the cases where tuberculous meningitis is but one of the manifestations of general miliary tuberculosis, but even then only rarely in our experience. Paralysis of the movements of the eyeballs is common, either of the oculomotor or the abducens nerve. It is usually unilateral. As the disease advances the eyes are not shut completely, and the cornea loses its sensitiveness to touch and becomes injected and cloudy.

Paralysis may be widespread in the parts supplied by other cranial nerves, or may involve other regions of the body. It is often hemiplegic in type, but may be paraplegic or monoplegic, or may change from time to time. On the whole, paralyses are less frequent than convulsive symptoms.

The *bowel-movements* are usually constipated, but diarrhea may occur, especially in infancy. *Vomiting* not attended by nausea or by retching is one of the most characteristic of the early symptoms, and, as the disease advances, it sometimes grows more projectile.

The *temperature* is variable and uncharacteristic. It may never rise to over 100 F. (37.8 C.), but as a rule there is slight irregular fever throughout the prodromal period, becoming somewhat higher in the stage of pressure, but still tending to be moderate and generally not reaching over 102 F. (38.9 C.); while shortly before death the temperature often reaches 104 F. (40 C.) or more (Fig. 210), or sometimes becomes subnormal.

An early rapidity and irregularity of the *pulse* is of no diagnostic value; but the slowness and irregularity which are symptoms of the fully developed second stage are of great importance when present. These are, however, not infrequently absent in infancy. During the final stage the pulse becomes rapid because the period of vagal stimulation is past.

While the *tache cérébrale* is not a pathognomonic sign, yet in association with other symptoms it is extremely suggestive (p. 858, Fig. 197). Although seen at its best in the stage of pressure, it may occur well-marked among the prodromes. We have seen well-developed tache, without evidence or suspicion of meningitis, soon followed by characteristic symptoms of the disease.

The *tuberculin-reaction* is of limited diagnostic importance owing to the large number of children without active tuberculosis who react. It is usually discoverable in the earlier stages, and is of corroborative value if suspicious symptoms are present; but in the terminal stage it may be absent.

The *blood* often exhibits little, if any, increase in the number of white corpuscles early in the course of the disease, but as the attack advances there is generally some degree of leukocytosis, chiefly of the polymorphonuclear cells, equaling about 20,000 or less per c.mm. The leukocytosis is, therefore, less marked, as a rule, than in cerebrospinal fever.

Examination of the *spinal fluid* obtained by lumbar puncture (see p. 151) is of great importance. The fluid generally flows under increased pressure, reaching about 50 mm. or more of mercury, and is either limpid, or shows only a faint haziness with minute floating particles. The specific gravity is 1.010 to 1.011. A chloride content as low as 500 to 600 mg. per 100 cc. is common (normal 720 to 750), but this may occur in other forms of meningitis. Noguchi's globulin-test is positive, as in all forms of meningitis, and the sugar-content is diminished. Later sugar may disappear, but this is by no means constant. When examined microscopically a few cells are obtained, perhaps from 100 to 200 or more to the c.mm. Although they are usually nearly all mononuclear, yet a predominance of polymorphonuclear cells does not exclude tuberculous meningitis (Fig. 210). To discover tubercle bacilli the last portion of the fluid obtained should be placed in a sterilized test-tube, corked with raw sterilized cotton, and allowed to stand for twelve to twenty-four hours. Generally a delicate fibrin-coagulum forms by this time, and this is further proof of the inflammatory nature of the exudate. In the coagulum are enmeshed most of the tubercle bacilli. It should be drawn out carefully upon a cover-slip, dried, and stained. The bacilli are usually but few in number, and prolonged search may be required to detect them. They may, however, be found in the majority of cases, in our experience, particularly as the disease progresses. These are almost invariably of the human strain, the bovine type being rarely found. If no coagulum forms, the fluid should be centrifuged, and successive drops, taken from the bottom of the centrifuging tube, placed upon a cover-slip, evaporated, and examined.

Course and Duration.—The duration of the disease is generally from two to three weeks after definite symptoms appear; sometimes four weeks or even longer; and sometimes apparently lasting only a week or less. The prodromal symptoms last perhaps about a week, but varying from a few days to two or three weeks. The duration of the second stage can hardly be computed, as it begins and ends in so indefinite a manner. An average of a week would probably cover this also. From the time coma fully sets in, life is generally of but short duration; usually under or slightly over a week; but not infrequently the terminal stage is prolonged remarkably. Death takes place usually quietly in coma. Much less often there are terminal convulsions.

The course is subject to many variations. Thus the prodromal stage may be absent; the onset may be sudden and the course short; hemiplegia or some other localizing symptom may first occur and later give place to the ordinary prodromal symptoms; the usual stages of pressure and paralysis may be practically absent, and after the prodromal symptoms death may occur suddenly in convulsions; there may be psychic symptoms of a violent nature. Temporary improvement for even as long as two weeks may occur in the stage of pressure, this being especially true of patients past infancy. Even remission for months may be witnessed; in this case, perhaps, there actually being temporary recovery followed by recurrence. (See collected instances by Martin.[64]) As a rule the course in infancy is more abrupt in onset than in childhood, general convulsions are more frequent, the symptoms are less characteristic, diarrhea is more common, and the course is shorter.

Prognosis.—This is practically always unfavorable. Among reports of recovered cases and collected series are those by Pitfield,[65] Bókay,[66] Hollis and Pardee,[67] Harbitz,[68] Bickel,[69] Koch,[70] Niedhardt,[71] Wiese,[72] deLuca,[73] and Selter.[74] The last author states that of 250 reported cases of recovery, only 64 will stand critical examination. Recovery has been more common in patients past infancy. Before recovery can be accepted as a fact, the patient must be observed for months to make sure that there is not simply a remission; and there should have been tubercle bacilli in the spinal fluid demonstrated by cultural and inoculation tests.

Diagnosis.—This is not always easy in the early stages. The most suggestive prodromal symptoms are vomiting without evidence of indigestion, drowsiness, and a well marked tache cérébrale. The persistence of these symptoms without relief by treatment should lead to lumbar puncture. In the later stages the diagnosis of intracranial lesion becomes more obvious, its nature again being ascertained by examination of the spinal fluid. Among other signs of increased intracranial pressure is that of Macewen[75] in which the percussion-note over the cranium is clearer than normal. To determine the presence of tuberculosis elsewhere in the body roentgenograms are of great value, not only of the chest but also to ascertain whether there are calcified tuberculous nodes in the neck or in the abdomen. Tuberculous meningitis may resemble *typhoid fever*, since there are in both continued fever and lack of marked leukocytosis, and sometimes there are meningeal symptoms in the latter disease. The Widal reaction and the results of lumbar puncture will settle the matter. *Pneumonia* beginning with meningeal symptoms may be differentiated by the development of signs of acute consolidation in the chest and by the results of lumbar puncture. From *poliomyelitis* and *encephalitis* the diagnosis at first is sometimes impossible. The spinal fluid in these diseases is practically identical with that of tuberculous meningitis, except in the matter of the tubercle bacilli. There may, however, be an increase in the sugar in encephalitis (p. 403) and a decrease of it in tuberculous meningitis. The onset of tuberculous meningitis is usually more insidious than that of these other diseases, and the meningitic symptoms more persistent. From *other forms of meningitis* the tuberculous variety may be differentiated by the more gradual onset, the longer continuance and lower grade of fever, the absence of marked leukocytosis, and the results of lumbar puncture. It should be remembered that meningitis other than tuberculous may occur in tuberculous subjects. *Chronic basilar meningitis*, while having a fluid which may be clear and without organisms, is an essentially chronic disorder and probably in all cases a sequel of cerebrospinal fever. *Serous meningitis* usually exhibits a spinal fluid which has fewer cells than in tuberculous meningitis, with no tubercle bacilli present; its onset is more rapid and its outcome favorable.

Aiello[76] and Lichtenberg[77] describe a test with tryptophan which was positive only in tuberculous meningitis.

Treatment.—The most important is that of *prevention*, following out the procedures already discussed (p. 423). The *treatment of the disease* consists in supportive measures; the administration of nutriment, if necessary by gavage; and the relief of intracranial pressure by repeated lumbar puncture or the administration of hypertonic solutions (pp. 151, 198). Tuberculous meningitis is in many cases a terminal stage of generalized tuberculosis, but in others it is in itself the cause of death in a patient who has minor tuberculous disease elsewhere. In view of this latter consideration, and since recovery may occasionally take place, it is worth while to persist with the therapeutic measures outlined. In a few cases we have tried intraspinous injections of blood-serum obtained from adults in a healed or quiescent stage of pulmonary tuberculosis. Cure did not result, but there appeared to be amelioration of the symptoms and a prolongation of the course. Intraspinal injections of tuberculin (0.25 to 1 mg. in 10 cc. of salt solution) have been used by Neidhardt,[71] Weise,[72] and Selter,[74] their patients recovering.

CHRONIC MENINGITIS

(Syphilitic Meningitis)

Chronic meningitis subsequent to meningococcic infection has already been described (p. 326). There remains to be discussed the chronic leptomeningitis occasionally seen as a result of hereditary syphilis. The pathologic changes consist in thickening, opacity and adhesion of the piarachnoid over the vertex or the base of the brain, with some shrinking of the convolutions, and often hydrocephalus. The **symptoms** in infancy consist in idiocy and diminished muscular power, perhaps with rigidity. When the base of the brain is involved the clinical manifestations may be quite similar to those of chronic basilar meningitis (p. 326). The **diagnosis** rests upon the presence of other manifestations of syphilis; the positive Wassermann reaction in the blood and spinal fluid, and in the latter a positive globulin reaction, increased cell-count, and a characteristic "meningitic curve" in the colloidal gold test (p. 325). The **prognosis** is unfavorable, but vigorous antisyphilitic treatment should be employed, perhaps with the intraspinal Swift-Ellis method (p. 440). We have found it advisable to treat these patients continuously and without the period of rest which is allowable in other forms of syphilis. Cessation of treatment for a few months may result in great increase of severity of symptoms.

References

1. Arch. Pediat., 1930, **47,** 739. 2. Arch. f. Kinderh., 1926, **80,** 34. 3. Surg., Gynec. and Obstet., 1929, **48,** 766. 4. J. Nerv. and Ment. Dis., 1887, **14,** 541. 5. Univ. of Pennsylvania Med. Magaz., 1900, **13,** 515. 6. Am. J. M. Sc., 1898, **116,** 202. 7. Am. J. Dis. Child., 1930, **39,** 84. 8. Am. J. Dis. Child., 1930, **39,** 980. 9. Verhandl. phys.-med. Ges. in Würzburg, 1857, **7,** 134. 10. Philadelphia M. J., 1901, **7,** 226. 11. Ref. Sloan, Cleveland M. J., 1915, **14,** 808. 12. Socuska Läkaresällskapets Handlinger, 1918, **44,** 53; Ref. J.A.M.A., 1918, **70,** 1988. 13. Correspondbl. f. Schweiz. Aerzte, 1919, **49,**

230; Ref. J.A.M.A., 1919, **72**, 1194. 14. Boston M. and S. J., 1921, **184**, 539. 15. Lancet, 1923, **1**, 836. 16. Jap. J. Obst. and Gynec., 1927, **10**, 30. 17. Boston M. and S. J., 1928, **197**, 1302. 18. Boston M. and S. J., 1928, **197**, 1449. 19. Am. J. Dis. Child., 1923, **26**, 503; J.A.M.A., 1929, **92**, 97. 20. Arch. Dis. Childhood, 1930, **5**, 361. 21. Bull. Johns Hopkins Hosp., 1928, **42**, 70. 22. J.A.M.A., 1929, **92**, 99. 23. Am. J. M. Sc., 1919, **158**, 95. 24. Am. J. Dis. Child., 1920, **20**, 18. 25. Am. J. Dis. Child., 1922, **24**, 273. 26. Quart. J. Med., 1927, **20**, 353. 27. Am. J. Dis. Child., 1929, **37**, 807. 28. Surg., Gynec. and Obstet., 1928, **47**, 662. 29. Congress de Lyon, 1895; Traité d. mal. de l'enf., Grancher, etc., 1905, **4**, 27. 30. Volkmann's Sammlung klin. Vorträge, 1893, Inner. Med. No. 23. 31. Acta paediat., 1925, **4**, 158; Acta med. Scandinav., 1927, **65**, 722. 32. Bibliot. f. laeger, 1929, **121**, 511. 33. J.A.M.A., 1929, **93**, 1553. 34. Ugesk. f. Laeger, 1930, **92**, 572. 35. Lancet, 1931, **2**, 12. 36. Ztschr. f. Kinderh., 1931, **50**, 564. 37. Rev. méd. de la Suisse rom., 1931, **51**, 1. 38. J.A.M.A., 1930, **94**, 1650. 39. Internat. Clin., 1927, **3**, 155. 40. Pediatria, 1927, **35**, 492. 41. J.A.M.A., 1928, **90**, 597. 42. J.A.M.A., 1928, **90**, 599. 43. J.A.M.A., 1932, **98**, 1253. 44. Arch. Pediat., 1928, **45**, 306. 45. J.A.M.A., 1930, **94**, 1040. 46. Am. J. Dis. Child., 1932, **43**, 873. 47. Arch. Pediat., 1907, **24**, 721. 48. Am. J. Dis. Child., 1911, **1**, 42. 49. Am. J. M. Sc., 1916, **152**, 403. 50. Am. J. Dis. Child., 1922, **24**, 102. 51. Am. J. Dis. Child., 1930, **40**, 569. 52. J.A.M.A., 1931, **96**, 1358. 53. Arch. Pediat., 1929, **46**, 516. 54. J. Exper. Med., 1911, **14**, 73. 55. Surg., Gynec. and Obstet., 1924, **39**, 760. 56. Monatschr. f. Kinderh., 1925–26, **31**, 295. 57. Kentucky M. J., 1930, **28**, 326. 58. Brit. J. Child. Dis., 1930, **27**, 35. 59. Observations on the Dropsy in the Brain, Edinburgh, 1768. 60. Sanné, Mal. d. enf. 1891, **3**, 1027. 61. Berl. klin. Wchnschr., 1878, **15**, 551. 62. New York M. J., 1901, **73**, 42. 63. Am. J. Dis. Child., 1911, **1**, 26. 64. Brain, 1909, **32**, 216. 65. Am. J. M. Sc., 1913, **146**, 37. 66. Jahrb. f. Kinderh., 1914, **80**, 133. 67. Arch. Int. Med., 1920, **24**, 49. 68. Am. J. M. Sc., 1921, **161**, 212. 69. Ann. de méd., 1922, **12**, 226. 70. München. med. Wchnschr., 1925, **72**, 793. 71. München. med. Wchnschr., 1926, **73**, 823. 72. München. med. Wchnschr., 1926, **73**, 1937. 73. Riv. di clin. pediat., 1930, **28**, 663. 74. Ztschr. f. Kinderh., 1930, **49**, 437. 75. Pyogenic Dis. of the Brain and Spinal Cord, 1893, 148. 76. Riforma med., 1927, **43**, 35. 77. Am. J. Dis. Child., 1932, **43**, 32.

CHAPTER V

DISEASES OF THE BRAIN-SUBSTANCE AND VESSELS

CEREBRAL HYPEREMIA

THE *active* form of this condition may result from over-eating, exposure to the sun, the use of alcohol, undue mental work or excitement, and the existence of the acute infectious diseases or disorders of the kidneys. There occurs an over-filling of the brain with arterial blood. The condition plays a very slight rôle in the production of symptoms in early life. *Passive* hyperemia, a congestion of the brain with venous blood, may be seen in chronic diseases of the heart with dilatation of the right side of the organ; or in any disorder which interferes with respiration and induces distention of the right cardiac chambers, as general convulsions, laryngospasm, pseudomembranous laryngitis, straining at stool, severe coughing, and the like. Pressure of any growth upon the jugular vein or the descending cava constitutes other cause. The **symptoms** may be of a temporary or of a more persistent character. They consist in distention of the veins of the head and neck, vertigo, headache, sleeplessness, and sparks before the eyes. The condition may be so severe that convulsions occur; or stupor or, finally, coma may develop. The **prognosis** depends upon the nature of the cause, and the **treatment** is directed chiefly to this. In addition cold compresses applied to the head and the keeping of the head in an elevated position may be beneficial.

CEREBRAL ANEMIA

Among the **causes** of this condition is sudden hemorrhage, or the development of general anemia in other ways. Other agents are passive hyperemia and cerebral edema, either of which may finally diminish the blood-supply to the brain by pressure upon the small vessels. Sudden fright or other shock, the sight of blood, etc., may produce a sudden anemia by a weakening of the heart's action, or through other vasomotor disturbance. The **symptoms** in the *acute* form are ringing in the ears, bright or dark spots before the eyes, dizziness, drowsiness, yawning, pallor, sweating, nausea, rapid respiration and pulse, and often loss of consciousness; the symptoms, in fact, of syncope. Convulsive movements may sometimes develop. In the more *chronic* cases there are mental exhaustion with inability for mental work, noises in the ears, flashing of light before the eyes, great excitability from slight causes, headache, insomnia, and in severe cases delirious states or coma. In marantic infants, especially after prolonged diarrhea, the symptoms of meningismus (p. 918) or of the hydrocephaloid disease of Marshall Hall[1] may develop. There are then observed restlessness; jactitation; rolling or crossing of the eyes; retraction of the head; depression of the fontanelle; feeble and rapid pulse; rapid and often irregular respiration; narrowed and, later, dilated pupils; convulsions; and finally coma. The **prognosis** in the acute cases is generally favorable if the cause can be removed. The **diagnosis** is sometimes one of difficulty. In the acute severer cases the syncope may suggest the existence of epilepsy, especially if convulsive movements occur; and in the absence of such movements petit mal or pyknolepsy may be suspected. The presence of some cause for anemia, the longer duration of the attack, and the absence of repetition of this serve to eliminate these conditions. In the more chronic forms the evidences of anemia elsewhere in the body render the diagnosis easy. **Treatment** is primarily that of the cause. During an attack the patient should be placed in a horizontal position or with the head lowered, the temperature of the body maintained, and the circulation favored by the use of friction of the extremities and the application of heat. Internally aromatic spirits of ammonia, or whiskey or other liquor may be given. In the worst cases hypodermoclysis or transfusion may be required.

CEREBRAL EDEMA

In this disorder there is a saturation of the brain-substance with fluid transfused from the vessels. It may be general; or be a localized condition dependent oftenest upon some focal disease, such as abscess, tumor, hemorrhage, or embolism or thrombosis of the vessels. It may occur, too, as a result of trauma or of a serous meningitis, or may be caused by the passive hyperemia of cardiac disease or by nephritis. The symptoms may appear rapidly, or after some days of illness. They are to an extent those produced by the original focal lesion; but, as the edema increases, drowsiness and finally coma develop. The diagnosis, especially from cerebral anemia, cannot be made with certainty during life. The prognosis and treatment are those of the original cause. The employment of intravenous dehydrating solutions may be tried (p. 198), perhaps combined with lumbar puncture.

EMBOLISM

This is oftenest the result of endocarditis, but it occurs also with the acute infectious diseases. The plugging of the arteries may be by a vegetation whipped off from a cardiac valve, or by a portion of a thrombus from the cavity of the heart or elsewhere. The disorder is uncommon and is oftener seen after the age of ten years than earlier.

Much most frequently embolism occurs somewhere in the course of the middle cerebral artery, one or more branches being affected, oftener in the cortex than in the central region. The first alteration following the plugging is anemia in the tissues supplied by the vessel. The area involved is softened, and at first red from hyperemia and the presence of small hemorrhages. Inflammatory changes then occur; and if the embolism is of a septic nature, suppuration may follow. The final condition is localized sclerosis or the formation of a cyst. The **symptoms** are sudden in onset, often with convulsions; followed by headache, moderate fever, vomiting, delirium, or coma. With these general symptoms are the focal ones, their nature and distribution depending upon the position of the embolism. The **prognosis** is serious, more than $\frac{1}{2}$ of the patients dying in coma and with increasing cardiac weakness. Those who recover exhibit permanent localized sequels, unless the original lesion is very small. The **diagnosis** must be based chiefly upon the sudden onset, combined with the existence of chronic disorders known to favor the production of embolism. The disease is especially apt to be confounded with *cerebral hemorrhage.* The chief distinction is the more rapid disappearance of the general cerebral symptoms in the cases of embolism which recover. Cerebral *thrombosis* is slower in its onset; otherwise the symptoms are much the same. *Acute hemorrhagic encephalitis* (p. 936) may be distinguished with difficulty, except for its greater early elevation of temperature and the less rapid onset of paralytic symptoms. *Epidemic encephalitis* may also begin with hemiplegic shock. *Tumors of the brain* in which there is sudden onset of symptoms may be difficult to differentiate from embolism, although they lead to more permanent increase in intracranial pressure and may also exhibit choked disc. In a few instances we have seen *tuberculous meningitis,* which began with unilateral symptoms, cause confusion in diagnosis until the examination of the spinal fluid was made. The **treatment** is entirely symptomatic in the early stage of the disease. The management of paralytic sequels will be discussed elsewhere (p. 956).

THROMBOSIS

Thrombosis of the cerebral veins and especially of the arteries is uncommon in early life. It is at this period nearly always the result of an endarteritis or endophlebitis dependent upon hereditary syphilis. It may also occasionally be produced by extreme feebleness of the circulation, or of the extension of the process from a sinus-thrombosis. The disease occurs much less frequently after the age of ten years. The pathologic processes which develop after the thrombosis has formed are identical with those seen in embolism. The **symptoms** are slower in onset than in that condition; in general less striking; and the production of paralysis is slower, requiring sometimes even several days to develop fully. Defective intelligence is a frequent sequel. In other respects the symptoms are the same as attend embolism. The **prognosis** is unfavorable for complete recovery. There is also the danger of recurrence, although there is a good hope of the prevention of this by appropriate treatment. The **diagnosis** rests especially upon the slowness of the onset, and the history of syphilis or the presence of its manifestations. Syphilis should be vigorously treated if present.

SINUS-THROMBOSIS

(Thrombosis of the Cerebral Sinuses)

Etiology.—The disease falls naturally into two classes: the first the marantic or primary; the second the inflammatory or secondary. As the name implies, *marantic sinus-thrombosis* occurs in connection with greatly debilitated states accompanied by feebleness of the circulation or alteration of the character of the blood, such as may be seen in the course of severe, long-continued gastrointestinal disease, prolonged suppurating processes, tuberculosis, syphilis, and the acute infectious diseases. Sometimes the shock of an operation will be followed by a thrombosis of the sinuses. The more frequent *inflammatory* form is an extension of inflammation from neighboring regions, such as disease of the ear, orbit, nose or bones of the cranium; traumatism; inflammatory process within the skull; suppuration situated on the face or scalp; facial erysipelas; and septic conditions in the mouth or pharynx, as in diphtheria or scarlet fever. Of the causes in this form the most frequent in early life is inflammation of the ear. In cases of inflammatory nature germs of some sort, especially streptococci, are always present; as in those, too, of the marantic form which depend upon suppurative processes in distant parts of the body. There is, in fact, a tendency for every thrombosis, however produced, finally to exhibit bacteria and consequently to be septic. Marantic thrombosis occurs oftenest in early childhood and especially in infancy. Inflammatory cases may develop at any age, but are less frequent in the first ten years of life.

Pathologic Anatomy.—In the *marantic* cases the wall of the sinus is entirely unaffected and there is found only a fairly firm clot, more or less adherent to the vessel-wall, and of a color varying from dark-red to a more yellowish-red tint depending upon the age of the lesion. The surface of the brain and of the meninges in the vicinity of the thrombus may sometimes be deeply congested and covered with effused blood. The most frequent seats of marantic thrombosis are the superior longitudinal and the lateral sinuses, and the process may extend secondarily into most of the sinuses of the brain.

In the *inflammatory* variety there is a phlebitis present in addition to the thrombus. The clot in this form may show purulent softening. The meninges may be locally or generally inflamed, and the brain-substance exhibits congestion or hemorrhage, perhaps with areas of softening or even abscess. Pyemic abscesses may be discovered also in other organs of the body. The seat of the primary thrombosis in the inflammatory form depends upon the location of the primary process. As this is in the ear in most instances, thrombosis is most frequently found in the lateral sinus. Involvement of the cavernous sinus follows oftenest disease of the nasal cavity, sometimes that of the mouth, orbit, or base of the skull; that of the longitudinal sinus is a sequel to disease of the vault of the cranium or of the skin covering it.

Symptoms.—Especially in the *marantic* form the symptoms, if any, are overshadowed by those of the primary disease, and as a rule the condition is unrecognized during life. However, prodromes may be present, as vomiting and headache; followed by delirium, hyperesthesia, rigidity, convulsions, paralysis, and coma. In some cases there are external evidences of interference with cerebral circulation, as nose-bleed and dilatation of the veins of the scalp and face. The symptoms of the *inflammatory* form are more characteristic, and evidences of decided sepsis are generally present; pyogenic germs may be discovered in the blood; and abscesses develop in other parts of the body. Local manifestations depend upon the sinus involved. Thrombosis of the lateral sinus secondary to otitic disease produces dilatation of the superficial veins, with swelling and tenderness in the mastoid region. Sometimes the jugular vein is involved, becoming tender and cord-like, and the head may be bent toward the affected side. Thrombosis of the longitudinal sinus may give rise to fulness of the veins and edema of the forehead, temples, and top of the head; cyanosis of the face; nose-bleed; and papillitis. Thrombosis of the cavernous sinus occasions edema of the eyelids, usually on one side, and of the root of the nose; exophthalmos; dilatation of the veins of the forehead; paralysis of the ocular muscles; and sometimes optic neuritis and choked discs.

Course and Prognosis.—The prognosis is unfavorable. Marantic cases generally last only a few days, pulmonary embolism being a frequent cause of death. In the inflammatory cases death takes place in from a few days up to three weeks through pyemia, meningitis, or encephalitis; the prognosis being entirely unfavorable except in those instances, as in involvement of the lateral sinus, where operative interference is possible.

Diagnosis.—That of marantic thrombosis may be impossible during life. It rests principally upon the existence of a disease which is liable to be followed by this condition, and upon symptoms pointing to an intracranial affection. Yet meningitis and encephalitis may produce symptoms similar to those of thrombosis. The diagnosis of the inflammatory form varies with the primary lesion, and the symptoms have already been sufficiently described. In either variety there may be a brown-red or green-red discoloration of the spinal fluid.

Treatment.—That of the marantic form is of little avail, since the primary disease is liable in itself to be fatal. Surgical treatment of the inflammatory form is especially applicable to cases of thrombosis of the lateral sinus. Prompt operation is often successful in the course of otitic disease where the beginning of thrombosis is feared. The internal jugular on the affected side may be tied or excised, and the lateral sinus opened and drained.

INTRACEREBRAL HEMORRHAGE

Hemorrhage connected with the meninges has already been described (p. 915). Here only is to be considered the effusion of blood from the vessels into the brain-substance itself in an amount capable of producing symptoms. Most of the studies referred to in connection with meningeal hemorrhage show that intracerebral hemorrhage of any degree is much less frequent than the former, especially in very young infants.

Etiology.—The most frequent cause is trauma, which acts in a manner described for leptomeningeal hemorrhage (p. 917). In addition diseases of the heart or kidneys may, in rare instances, increase intracranial pressure and produce hemorrhage in early life. Operative also may be the endarteritis of hereditary syphilis; hemorrhagic diseases, as leukemia and the like; encephalitis; tumors; and embolism, thrombosis and sinus-thrombosis. Probably in some cases convulsions may give rise to hemorrhage instead of being the result of it.

Pathologic Anatomy.—The bleeding may be either arterial or venous; oftener the former. There occurs a rupture of small arteries, generally branches of the middle cerebral; or of the veins, most frequently those emptying into the longitudinal sinus. When the hemorrhage is large the surrounding brain tissue is torn, and softening and edema occur. Small capillary hemorrhages may be entirely absorbed without leaving any change. The larger ones later, after encapsulation of the effused blood, either are finally absorbed or the damaged brain-substance is replaced by sclerotic tissue, or by the formation of a cyst or perhaps the development of pus.

Symptoms.—Sudden loss of consciousness develops with or immediately following the hemorrhage, or occasionally not for several days. There is relaxation of the body with abolition of reflexes, and sometimes general convulsions. Unconsciousness may last for a few minutes up to several days, coma perhaps continuing until death. In more favorable cases these early symptoms diminish, focal manifestations develop, and the general paralytic condition disappears, with evidences of paralysis being confined to certain regions only. As a rule in arterial hemorrhage the focal symptoms are hemiplegic in type, and after improvement perhaps monoplegic only: Venous hemorrhage, occurring as it does oftenest near the sagittal suture and as a result of birth-trauma, is more liable to exhibit paralysis of a paraplegic type. (See p. 954.)

Course and Prognosis.—The prognosis is always serious, both as regards death shortly after hemorrhage and with respect to final complete recovery without residual symptoms. Minute arterial hemorrhages may disappear without even having shown any symptoms. Large effusions may be followed by death in a few days. Following injuries to the head in older children, there may be such sequels as headache, vertigo, insomnia, and behavior disorders (Strecker and Ebaugh[2]).

Diagnosis.—This rests upon the sudden onset of the symptoms, combined with the existence of conditions liable to produce intracerebral hemorrhage. Arterial hemorrhage differs from the venous form chiefly in its tendency to produce hemiplegia, and in the fact that venous hemorrhage is limited practically to cases occurring at birth. The distinction from *embolism* is chiefly that the general cerebral symptoms disappear in favorable cases of this more rapidly than in hemorrhage. *Leptomeningeal hemorrhage*, while difficult to distinguish, usually gives fewer focal symptoms and more irritative ones, and especially in infancy is more common than intracerebral hemorrhage.

Treatment.—Prevention consists in good obstetrical practice, with avoidance of too prolonged a delivery, and in the prompt relief of asphyxia. Treatment of the hemorrhage itself is similar to that described for leptomeningeal hemorrhage (p. 918).

NONSUPPURATIVE ENCEPHALITIS

(Acute Toxic Encephalitis)

The form of acute encephalitis occurring in poliomyelitis has been described (p. 392), as also that of epidemic encephalitis (p. 398). Special forms of encephalitis, such as Schilder's disease and the like, are considered under Atrophy and Sclerosis of the Brain (p. 959), and the variety due to vaccination, referred to under that heading (p. 300). There remain to be reviewed cases of encephalitis depending upon other causes.

Etiology.—The disease may follow any of the acute exanthemata, pneumonia, pertussis, mumps, sepsis, diphtheria, grippe, and otitis. Other causes are trauma, tuberculosis, and gastro-intestinal intoxication. Superficial secondary encephalitis accompanies severe meningitis. Another variety is caused by syphilis (p. 950). Poisons such as lead and arsenic may produce encephalitis; when caused by the latter drug being of hemorrhagic form. A special variety of congenital interstitial encephalitis described by Virchow[3] has been reviewed by Berkholz,[4] who points out a possible familial tendency. Nonsuppurative encephalitis would appear not to be a common disease, occurring oftener in early life than later. It is possible, however, that with acute infections some mild degree of encephalitis may be more frequent than supposed; and, while exhibiting few symptoms at the time, may later result in mental and psychic disturbances.

Pathologic Anatomy.—In the congenital form there are small, scattered foci, chiefly in the white matter, containing round-cells and other cells filled with fatty granules, and evidences of hyperplasia of the glia. In early infancy the process is generally a *diffuse encephalitis* with widespread softening, disappearance of ganglion cells, atrophy of white matter, and perhaps followed later by a sclerosing process. There is less destruction of ganglion cells and perivascular cellular infiltration is less marked than in poliomyelitis or epidemic encephalitis. In older children the process may be more circumscribed, and is oftenest that of *acute hemorrhagic encephalitis*, the hemispheres being usually predominantly involved. There may be foci of softening with effusion of blood, combined with capillary hemorrhage and cellular infiltration into the surrounding tissue. Bacteria may be present. The lesions are similar to those of the polio-encephalitic type of poliomyelitis. *Multiple disseminated myelo-encephalitis* is another variety with scattered foci in both brain and spinal cord, and in still another form there is *hyperplastic encephalitis* (p. 951).

Symptoms.—These are variable and uncharacteristic and depend upon the position of the lesion and the age of the patient. In the diffuse form, the most serious, as seen oftenest in infants, the symptoms in typical cases consist in rapid development of high fever, unconsciousness, and convulsions. The pulse is weak and the respiration irregular, perhaps with asphyxia; there is rigidity of the neck and extremities. Focal symptoms may be absent or only slightly marked.

In the form with more circumscribed lesions, the usual one in children past infancy, there are in severe cases sudden onset, high fever, rigidity, convulsions, vomiting, delirium or coma, and perhaps optic neuritis. Soon evidences of localization are found. In the more frequent hemiplegic cases there may be rolling of the eyes always in one direction; convulsions limited to, or severer on, one side of the body or one limb; hemiplegia, or paralysis limited to one extremity or to the face; tremor on one side of the body (Griffith[5]), or localized diminution of sensibility. These symptoms last for a week or more, although after a few days fever generally disappears and tendon-reflexes begin to increase on one side. After this period gradual improvement begins and continues for months; there usually being left, however, some degree of paralysis or other evidence of cerebral disorder. The symptoms detailed may affect both sides of the body. In many cases the fever is less high and the general cerebral symptoms less marked as compared with the paralytic manifestations. Sometimes the course is more chronic, the onset insidious, and symptoms suggest those of brain tumor; yet the patient finally recovers entirely or with evidence of cerebral disorder persisting. Involvement of the cerebellum may predominate, producing the uncommon condition of *acute cerebellar ataxia* (p. 966). Here the initial symptoms are those of encephalitis in general, but with the later development of staggering gait, ataxia, vertigo, nystagmus, disturbance of speech, and tremor. We[6] have seen 4 such instances and collected a number of others. Encephalitis affecting the *pons* and *medulla* is observed oftenest in connection with poliomyelitis (p. 392) or in epidemic encephalitis (p. 402), but may occur independently of these. Here, after subsidence of the early manifestations, there is discovered involvement of some of the cranial nerves. In *multiple disseminated myelo-encephalitis* the final symptoms may be those of multiple sclerosis with disturbances of speech, idiocy, convulsions, and tremor.

Course and Prognosis.—Most patients affected by the diffuse form in the first year of life die after a few weeks or less. In less typical cases, with lesions not so diffuse, recovery may occur. Berkholtz[4] reports several instances of recovery in cases diagnosed as the congenital interstitial form. Older subjects suffering from more circumscribed lesions may die in a few days; yet many milder cases recover, some showing no evidence later that the disease has occurred but others having residual symptoms. The prospect for complete recovery, however, is better than in epidemic encephalitis. In fact, it is remarkable how complete the recovery may be in patients who have had the most severe symptoms during the acute stage.

Diagnosis.—The principal diagnostic characteristics are the acute febrile onset with general cerebral manifestations, followed soon by distinct localizing symptoms. In early infancy the frequent failure of localizing symptoms to develop makes the diagnosis from *meningitis* uncertain. In encephalitis the spinal fluid is normal or the only changes consist in slight increase in pressure, a faint globulin-reaction, and a moderate increase of cells. In meningitis, on the other hand, there are usually marked evidences of irritation and inflammation, the globulin reaction is distinct, sugar is absent or the amount of it diminished, and the causative organism may be discovered. In severe encephalitis death may occur before diagnosis is possible. Disseminated myelo-encephalitis is distinguished from *multiple sclerosis* chiefly by the sudden febrile onset following some infectious disease in the former as well as the failure of symptoms to show persistent increase. Disseminated encephalitis may also be confused with some of the other forms of sclerosis of the brain (p. 949). *Cerebral embolism, sinus-thrombosis,* and *cerebral hemorrhage* are difficult to differentiate from encephalitis, but in them the fever is not apt to be so high, the history and associated conditions are different, and in some of them the spinal fluid findings may be of value. (See pp. 932, 933, 935.) *Abscess of the brain* is of slower onset, the fever is not so uniformly high, and distinct stages are exhibited (see below). *Intracranial tumor* lacks the sudden febrile onset.

Treatment.—At the onset there may be employed such measures as free purgation, ice-bags to the head, hot mustard foot-baths and the like. Rest and quiet are imperative; the fever should be combated; and sufficient nourishment should be given, by gavage if necessary. Nervous and convulsive symptoms require sedative drugs and hydrotherapy. Dehydrating substances may be given intravenously, orally, or rectally (pp. 185 and 198); and lumbar puncture may be repeated if there is increased intracranial pressure.

ABSCESS OF THE BRAIN

(Suppurative Encephalitis)

Etiology.—The condition is not common in early life according to statistics collected by Gowers,[7] Holt,[8] Holmes[9] and others. It is rare in infancy, Sanford[10] finding only 17 cases in patients under twelve months of age and adding 2 more. The most frequent cause is extension from disease of the ear, usually chronic, or of the petrous bone or less frequently of other cranial bones. A prominent factor is trauma of the head with or without fracture. Among less frequent causes are infectious emboli from pyemia, cutaneous infections, or local infection from spina bifida or meningocele. Various germs may be found in the abscess, particularly staphylococci and streptococci. Rarely the thrush-fungus has been reported present (Ribbert[11]). In a number of cases no cause whatever can be discovered.

Pathologic Anatomy.—When the result of distant causes, the lesions are usually multiple. In most cases, however, abscess depends upon nearby local conditions and is single. It may then occupy different parts of the brain, oftenest the temperosphenoidal lobe, or less frequently, the frontal lobe or the cerebellum. Traumatic abscess is generally in the cerebrum; otitic abscess here or in the cerebellum; that depending upon disease of the orbit or the nose in the frontal lobe. The final size of the abscess ranges from that of a pea up to an accumulation filling a large part of the hemisphere. Many abscesses remain always without a capsule; others begin to form one in the second or third week and develop this completely by the end of the second month. The surrounding tissue is edematous. An abscess may cause death through local pressure; may produce a purulent meningitis; may rupture in various directions, as into a ventricle, on the surface of the brain, or occasionally through the ear or nose.

Symptoms.—These are often obscure. They are both general and focal in nature; the latter often absent. Ordinarily they are classified in three stages, which, however, are not always sharply distinct from each other or present in every case. The **initial stage** often commences insidiously, but may have an abrupt and stormy onset. When well-marked it is characterized by headache, perhaps localized; vomiting; prostration; chills; and fever of a continuous type and of moderate severity. There are sometimes general or local convulsions. In acute abscess the advance from this stage is directly to a terminal fatal one. In chronic abscess, however, the initial period lasts for a few days or weeks and is often followed by the **latent stage,** which is characterized by a disappearance of symptoms; or there may remain occasional headache and rises of temperature, chills at irregular intervals, some degree of somnolence or mental disturbance and, in some cases, convulsions. Focal symptoms which have appeared during the first stage persist. The duration of latency is extremely variable. It may be a few weeks or shorter and occasionally may last for several years. The **terminal stage** begins gradually or suddenly, and marks the rupture of the abscess, or inflammatory extension to contiguous regions. When the initial stage has been mild, the symptoms of the third stage may be the first to attract notice. It is characterized by return of early symptoms in increased force. Fever is high and continuous; headache often severe and persistent; symptoms of meningitis develop; the pulse is irregular and either slow or rapid; respiration may be Cheyne-Stokes in type; vomiting and vertigo may occur; there are often delirium, convulsions, paralysis and optic neuritis; and finally the patient passes into coma. The duration of this stage is usually not more than a few days.

In addition to these general symptoms, there are not infrequently *localizing* ones. These are, however, much less often observed than with tumor. Even large abscesses may present no localizing symptoms, since the regions oftenest affected are not those which produce them. Headache when localized is most frequently on the same side of the head as the abscess. If occipital, it indicates cerebellar lesion, with which, too, may occur inco-ordination and nystagmus. If the abscess is in the motor area, paralyses of various sorts or localized convulsions may result, corresponding to the regions involved. Vomiting and giddiness, while often seen in cerebellar abscess, are frequent in cerebral cases also. Slow and difficult speech, ptosis, and disturbance of the ocular movements point to pressure upon the pons. Severe headache, vomiting, drowsiness, choked disc, and slow pulse indicate obstruction of the ventricles. In involvement of the left temporal lobe in right-handed persons there may be aphasia. Local tenderness of the scalp may indicate the position of a superficial abscess. (For localization see also Symptoms of Brain-tumor, p. 942.)

Prognosis.—This is always grave, especially in infants; nearly all cases dying unless operation gives relief. In half of the cases collected by Gowers,[7] the duration did not exceed two weeks. Exceptionally the wall of the capsule may become calcified and the contents dry and harmless.

Diagnosis.—This is generally difficult and sometimes impossible. The principal diagnostic symptoms are slow onset with gradual increase of headache, the presence of fever, the development later of convulsions and coma, and focal symptoms. These, combined with such possible causes as otitis or trauma, may make diagnosis possible. The occurrence of symptoms in stages is of diagnostic assistance when the stages can be recognized. If lumbar puncture is performed for diagnostic purposes, only a small amount of fluid should be withdrawn, since diminution of intracranial pressure is dangerous. The fluid in the acute stage, even without generalized meningeal inflammation, almost invariably contains 100 or more polymorphonuclear cells to the cubic millimeter. In chronic walled-off abscess the spinal fluid may be normal.

Meningitis is more rapid in onset and shorter in course; the pulse oftener accelerated than in abscess; initial fever is higher; there is a greater tendency to rigidity and convulsions, although the latter are less often localized; and focal symptoms are not common. To all this, however, there are numerous exceptions. Lumbar puncture reveals more cells in the purulent forms of meningitis than in abscess, unless the latter has ruptured. *Serous meningitis* depending upon otitis or trauma is distinguished with difficulty, since the primary cause may produce either affection, and optic neuritis may occur in either. The principal clinical differences consist in the more sudden onset and often rapid disappearance of symptoms of meningitis. The examination of spinal fluid obtained by lumbar puncture does not certainly aid, although the procedure often gives relief to the symptoms in meningitis but not in abscess. *Intracranial tumor* has no febrile stage; choked discs are more uniformly present; and focal symptoms more constantly seen. *Sinus-thrombosis* shows more rapid production of high and irregular fever; rigors are more common, with the evidence in general of sepsis; and focal symptoms are absent. The diagnosis of many of the conditions which simulate abscess is rendered still more difficult by the fact that this condition may be combined with them as a sequel or a cause.

Treatment.—The only palliative treatment consists in rest, ice to the head, purgatives, and remedies to quiet nervous excitation. The curative treatment is surgical, and this should be employed when the lesion can be localized, and is often followed by recovery (60 in 134 cases; Oppenheim[12]). In chronic abscess, Dandy[13] has had success by simple aspiration without subsequent drainage.

TUMORS OF THE BRAIN

Etiology.—With the exception of those of a tuberculous or syphilitic nature, the causes are entirely unknown. Some of the tumors are formed of primitive embryonal tissue or fetal rests. The growth may be primary, or secondary to similar formations elsewhere. There is no statistical evidence that trauma of the head has any etiologic connection (Parker[14]). The ratio of tumors in children as compared with adults is given as 1:7 by Cushing[15] and as 1:17 by Leavitt.[16] Other good reviews and studies on this subject are those by Gowers,[7] Critchley,[17] Starr,[18] Horrax,[19] Cutler et al.,[20] and McIntyre.[21]

TABLE 70.—BRAIN-TUMORS IN PERSONS UNDER FIFTEEN YEARS OF AGE

Diagnosis.	Age in years.			
	One to five.	Five to ten.	Ten to fifteen.	Total.
Gliomas (varia)	15	48	53	116
Pituitary adenomas	..	..	2	2
Meningiomas	..	1	1	2
Neurinomas (acoustic)	..	..	1	1
Congenital tumors	4	4	13	21
Invasive and metastatic	..	..	1	1
Blood-vessel tumors	2	..	..	2
Tuberculomas	2	4	..	6
Papillomas	1	..	..	1
Miscellaneous	..	..	2	2
Totals	24	57	73	154

Nature and Position.—The growths found in early life are not of numerous sorts. The preponderance of subtentorial tumors in childhood is shown by the studies of Starr,[18] Taylor,[22] and Cushing;[15] the last author giving the proportion of cerebellar to cerebral tumors in children as 2:1, whereas in adults it is 1:5. The table on p. 940 is after Cushing.

Glioma is the most common tumor. It is always primary; usually single; and of various sizes, sometimes miliary, sometimes very large. It is not sharply defined. It may be of several pathologic types, as medulloblastoma, spongioblastoma, neuroblastoma, astrocytoma, etc., some being more malignant than others. It is situated oftenest in the pons or cerebellum. The so-called "congenital tumors" arise from Rathke's pouch; are usually situated above the level of the sella turcica; are liable to become calcified; and may interfere with the function of the pituitary gland. While they have existed since birth, they may not cause symptoms until much later. *Tuberculous tumors,* while, according to older statistics, very frequent, are shown by the studies of Cushing,[15] Leavitt,[16] Van Wagenen[23] and others to constitute approximately only 2 to 4 per cent of all brain tumors. In some cases they are very numerous and small, but are oftener single, vary in size from that of a pea to a walnut or larger, and are usually cerebellar. *Meningioma* or meningeal fibroblastoma is a benign tumor which arises from the mesoderm and occurs chiefly in the anterior fossa of the skull. This may cause pressure-symptoms, but does not infiltrate the brain. *Sarcoma* is either primary or secondary, generally single, of varying size and growth and oftenest found in the cerebellum. *Carcinoma* is rare but may attack even young infants, as in the case of Fuhrmann.[24] Among other uncommon tumors are *gummas, papillomas* and *neurinomas. Cysts* may be encountered. Lindau[25] in a monographic review collects 275 cases of cerebellar cysts. He states that these constitute 10 per cent of all cerebellar tumors and divides them into dermoids; those due to softening and following hemorrhages; parasitic cysts as from cysticercus; cysts with tumors; simple cysts; and those with direct connection with the fourth ventricle. Cysts and cystic degeneration may, of course, occur in other situations than the cerebellum. Not infrequently they may become calcified.

With tumors may be associated *secondary changes* in contiguous parts of the brain; such as hemorrhage, localized meningitis, and conditions arising from pressure. This last includes flattening of the convolutions, hydrocephalus, and erosion of cranial bones.

Symptoms. General Symptoms.—These may appear gradually, but quite often suddenly. Headache is a frequent early one, and may be paroxysmal or continuous; diffuse or localized; severe or slight; and later may improve if the head enlarges, as it often does provided the sutures have not become ossified. Localized tenderness of the skull may accompany it. Vomiting is seen in well over half the cases, although perhaps not until late. It is more frequent with cerebellar tumors than with those in the posterior fossa. It is forceful and usually independent of any evidence of indigestion or nausea. Convulsions occur during some part of the course in about 30 per cent of the cases. They are attended by unconsciousness, and may be general or sometimes local; severe or slight; and be seen only at long intervals or be of frequent occurrence or increasing severity. They occur particularly with tumors near the motor areas. In some cases of nonmalignant and slow-growing tumors they may be for years the only marked symptom present; and, since an aura is sometimes witnessed, may readily be mistaken for epilepsy. *Choked disc* is not as common in children as in adults; especially in young children in whom increased intracranial pressure can more readily be accommodated by expansion of imperfectly ossified cranial sutures. It is uncommon or occurs late in frontal tumors, pituitary adenomas, congenital cysts and meningiomas above the level of the sella turcica (Van Wagenen[26]). It develops early in cerebellar tumors and in those at the base of the brain or in the crus. Vertigo is nearly always present in subtentorial tumors. The pulse may be slow and the respiration irregular or slow when there is increased intracranial pressure. Particularly in tumors of the frontal lobe or corpus callosum there may be psychic disturbances. These are varied and consist of irritability, altered disposition, apathy or somnolence, insomnia, increasing mental deficiency, hallucinations, delusions, etc. The *spinal fluid* is normal or at most may show a slight increase in the number of cells and perhaps globulin.

Local Symptoms.—These are not always present and are necessarily varied depending upon the situation of the tumor, the rapidity of its growth, the presence of a complicating meningitis, or the results of irritation or pressure. Not infrequently they come on suddenly due to hemorrhage within or around the tumor. Careful neurologic examination should localize the tumor in about 75 per cent of the cases before operation.

Growths of the motor area produce hemiplegic or monoplegic symptoms on the contralateral side, their extent depending upon the convolutions involved and the size of the growth. There may be localized anesthesia, convulsive movements in the paralyzed part, or generalized and epileptiform convulsions. There may be conjugate deviation of the eyes to the side opposite the tumor; or toward the side of the tumor in destructive lesions of the pyramidal tract. If the meninges are involved there will be the usual symptoms of this. If the growth is in the *frontal lobe*, of rare occurrence in children, there may be few or no symptoms. On the other hand, the psychic disturbances already noted may occur; and from extension of irritation there may be convulsions, but generally without paralysis. Motor aphasia is produced by growth in the 3d frontal convolution on the left side, and ataxia is occasionally witnessed on the contralateral side; sometimes exophthalmos on the affected side; and so-called "reflex-grasping" in the contralateral hand in irritative lesions of the pyramidal tract (Freeman[27]). *Tumors of the temporosphenoidal lobe*, uncommon in early life, give rise to sensory aphasia and disturbances of hearing, and sometimes of the senses of smell and taste. Those of the *Island of Reil* cause aphasia in right-handed individuals, if the lesion is on the left side. Growths of the *parietal lobe* are rare in childhood and usually produce no localizing symptoms, unless secondarily by pressure upon the motor region there may develop hemiparesis and Jacksonian convulsions. There may, too, be sensory disturbances as of the sense of touch and of muscle sense, ataxia, word-blindness, impaired joint-sensation, astereognosis on the opposite side, and apraxia. Tumors of the *hypothalamic region* or the *floor of the 4th ventricle* may occasion glycosuria; of the *floor of the 3d ventricle*, polyuria; of the *pituitary region*, Fröhlich's syndrome (p. 1088); of the *pineal region*, precocious puberty (p. 1092). In addition there may be with pineal tumors, symptoms of increased intracranial pressure, as headache, failing vision and vomiting; and perhaps bilateral difficulty in hearing. Pressure on the motor and sensory pathways is uncommon (Horrax[19]). Involvement of the *occipital lobe* is rare but produces homonymous hemianopsia, or sometimes other disturbance of vision. Tumors of the *centrum ovale*, uncommon in children, are liable to cause symptoms similar to those of the corresponding cortical region, except that convulsions are infrequent. In deeper lesions the basal ganglia may be pressed upon. Growths involving the *basal ganglia* are of comparatively common occurrence in childhood and are difficult to localize. Convulsions are not frequent. The nature of the symptoms depends upon the conducting paths involved. If the internal capsule is pressed upon, hemiplegia follows. With tumors of the optic thalamus there is hemianesthesia, hemiathetosis or hemichorea. There is frequently involvement, too, of the functions of the cranial nerves, and speech may be affected. Tumors of the *corpora quadrigemina* cause paralysis of the ocular muscles, affections of hearing, tremor, ataxia, nystagmus, and, from compression of the aqueduct of Sylvius, internal hydrocephalus. Lesions of the *crura cerebri* occasion paralysis of the oculomotor nerve on the side of the lesion; hemiplegic paralysis, including the face, on the contralateral side; and sometimes tremor, ataxia, hemianesthesia, and convulsions. In tumors of the pons, comparatively common in early life, there is produced a crossed paralysis, including the cranial nerves on the side of the tumor and the extremities on the contralateral side, sometimes with loss of sensation. If the lesion is high in the pons, the cranial nerves escape; if somewhat lower, the more usual situation, the 3d and 5th nerves are involved, with paralysis of the ocular muscles in the former, and facial neuralgia and sometimes ulceration of the cornea in the latter; if lower in the pons, the 6th, 7th and 8th nerves are affected, producing internal strabismus, facial paralysis and disturbance of hearing. With pontine tumors the general symptoms are usually not marked; convulsions are infrequent; drowsiness is an early symptom; and there is often rigidity of the extremities, which may be diplegic if the tumor occupies both sides of the pons. *Tumors of the medulla*, not common, affect the last four of the cranial nerves, and often by extension some of the other cranial nerve-nuclei as well. The principal symptoms are dysphagia, deafness, difficult articulation, and involvement of the tongue. There are often disturbance of cardiac and respiratory action, flushing, and sweating. Polyuria and glycosuria have been reported. There is frequently a unilateral and later a bilateral involvement of the pyramidal tracts, with rigidity and increased reflexes; or the sensory tracts may be affected, with consequent ataxia and anesthesia. Tumors of the *cerebellum* cause symptoms when the middle lobe is involved, and large tumors in one hemisphere affect the middle lobe by pressure. The most characteristic indications are cerebellar ataxia, often so great that walking is impossible; vertigo; and nystagmus; these being combined with the early development of marked general symptoms as headache, vomiting, choked disc with blindness, and rigidity of the neck. Drowsiness occurs very late. Late pressure-symptoms of a cerebellar growth are those characteristic of the cranial nerves or the pyramidal tracts. Pyramidal signs, if present, usually involve the contralateral side. Tumors of the cerebellar-pontine angle, which are of the type of acoustic neurinomas, are very uncommon in children. Subtentorial tumors frequently cause hydrocephalus.

Course and Prognosis.—In general the course is slowly progressive, although periods of intermission may sometimes occur with stationary symptoms, these being followed by exacerbations. In other cases there may be a rapid increase in symptoms. Sudden death may take place without any preceding symptoms, especially in the case of cysts, the condition being diagnosed only at necropsy. Certain of the gliomata grow more rapidly than others. Tuberculous growths are liable to be of long duration. Frontal tumors usually produce fewer symptoms than those involving the pons or the medulla. The duration may be said to vary from about six months to two years. Brain-tumors usually result fatally, although certain of them, which are favorably located, are accessible to operation and sometimes can be removed with restoration of normal cerebral function. Tuberculous growths may become encapsulated and uncommonly the condition arrested, and gummatous tumors may disappear under antisyphilitic treatment.

Diagnosis.—The course and various general and localizing symptoms have already been described. When lumbar puncture is employed for diagnosis, only a small amount of fluid should be withdrawn, since diminishing the intracranial pressure too greatly is dangerous, especially in subtentorial tumors and those of the posterior fossa. Roentgenograms may demonstrate convolutional markings on the skull, spreading of sutures, and sometimes increased density in the region of the tumor or calcification of it. In pituitary tumors enlargement of the sella turcica may be demonstrable. Encephalography (p. 154), although not without danger, may in some cases reveal the location of the lesion. Roentgenograms taken after air has been injected into the subarachnoid space may show the lateral ventricle to be compressed on the side of the tumor when this is above the tentorium; while in tumors in the posterior fossa, no air may enter the ventricles, or there may be an internal hydrocephalus. A study of the visual fields may be helpful in diagnosis.

Intracranial abscess differs from tumor in the existence of a definite primary cause; a more rapid and irregular course, often with characteristic stages; less frequent and later development of choked disc; less intense headache; the presence of fever and chills or of a definitely subnormal temperature; less common involvement of the cranial nerves; and lesser frequency of the localizing symptoms. *Tuberculous meningitis* can be confounded with tumor only when it runs an exceptionally slow course. In this disease optic neuritis is less common and less marked; rigidity of the neck more frequent; there is some fever; localizing symptoms less often appear; and the spinal fluid shows abnormalities not present in brain-tumor. *Poliomyelitis of the cerebral type* or *encephalitis* may suggest brain-tumor with hemiplegic paralysis. There is, however, a sudden febrile onset and the course of the case eventually differentiates.

Treatment.—In the case of gummata, antisyphilitic treatment should be employed. In all other cases surgical intervention is indicated if the situation and type of tumor permit of this. It is surprising how large a tumor of certain regions, such as one in the frontal lobes, can be removed without leaving residual symptoms. Simple decompression may relieve the symptoms for a time, delay the loss of sight, and prolong life. Radiotherapy of certain pituitary tumors and of gliomas may alleviate symptoms, and is indicated in inoperable tumors and also, at times, following operation. Tuberculomas should not be removed, but decompression performed if necessary.

HYDROCEPHALUS

It is customary to divide the disease into *external hydrocephalus* and *internal hydrocephalus*, the latter being again subdivided into the *acute* and the *chronic* forms. The condition in all these consists in an accumulation of serous fluid within the cranium.

1. External Hydrocephalus

In this uncommon chronic form there is an excess of fluid in the subdural space. It occurs as a sequel to pachymeningitis, is seen in chronic meningoencephalitis and serous meningitis, or encountered where there has been either wasting or lack of development of a portion of the brain (*hydrocephalus e vacuo*). The fluid is clear or sometimes blood-tinged, and the amount generally small; but sometimes it is large and the skull grows progressively more distended. There is no evidence of inflammation of the membranes found at necropsy. Sometimes an external hydrocephalus is combined with one of the internal variety, or may possibly be produced by the rupture of one of the latter form into the subdural space. The **symptoms** are at first those of the primary causative disorder. Later the amount of fluid may be not large enough to produce any characteristic manifestations; but in the cases with progressive increase of the quantity the symptoms are those seen in chronic internal hydrocephalus.

2. Acute Internal Hydrocephalus

The title is applied synonymously both to tuberculous meningitis and to the cases of serous meningitis in which the ventricles are especially involved. The course is not prolonged and the amount of fluid in the ventricles is not large.

3. Chronic Internal Hydrocephalus

This variety is the one oftenest seen. It may be divided into *congenital* and *acquired*, the former, however, not necessarily being noticeable at birth.

Etiology.—*Congenital* cases may be due to some abnormality of development, and are not infrequently associated with other malformations, such as spina bifida, harelip and club-foot (Fig. 211). They are probably oftenest the result of an earlier intra-uterine meningitis. In about 50 per cent there is a cicatricial stenosis of the aqueduct of Sylvius (Dandy[28]). Maclaire[29] believes some cases are due to the organization of adhesions

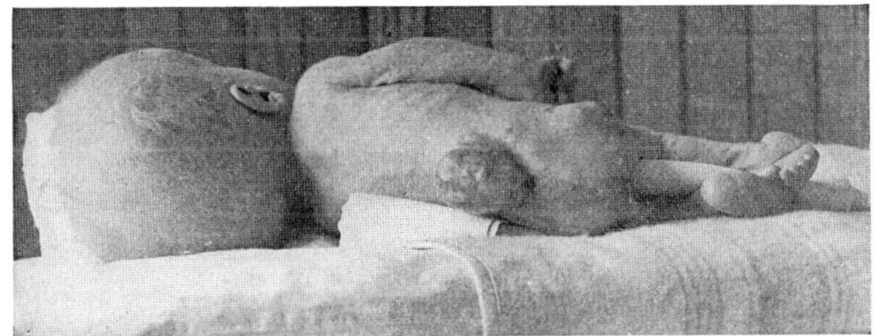

Fig. 211.—Hydrocephalus, spina bifida and club-foot. From a patient in the Children's Hospital of Philadelphia.

following intracranial hemorrhage at birth. A familial tendency is sometimes observed. Among the causes of chronic *acquired* hydrocephalus may be mentioned cerebrospinal fever, and occasionally other forms of purulent meningitis, as from staphylococcus or streptococcus; abscess or tumor of the brain; and trauma. Syphilis would appear to have a causative influence in some instances. In many rachitic heads there seems to be a tendency to an unusual accumulation of fluid. This, however, is but temporary. In the domain of trauma may be included the effect of operation upon spina bifida, which not infrequently is followed by hydrocephalus, or by an increase in the symptoms in cases where this is already present.

There is general agreement with the results of the investigations of Dandy and Blackfan[30] and of Frazier and Peet.[31] According to these the cerebrospinal fluid is secreted by the choroid plexuses in the different ventricles. It finds its exit through the aqueduct of Sylvius into the 4th ventricle and thence through the foramina of Magendie and of Luschka into the subarachnoid space. It is absorbed from the entire subarachnoid space but more particularly from the cerebral portion. Hydrocephalus may be produced in several ways; from a hypersecretion from the choroid plexuses or due to the products of inflammation; or diminished absorption from the subarachnoid spaces. There may be, in one form, an *obstructive hydrocephalus* in which absorption is absent because the fluid cannot find egress from the ventricles to the subarachnoid space. The second form is the *communicating type*, in which there is sufficient communication between the ventricles and the spinal subarachnoid space, but the cerebral subarachnoid, the chief seat of the absorption, is cut off by adhesions involving the various cisternae, and absorption is thus prevented. Hydrocephalus due to hypersecretion is of rare occurrence. A view differing from the usually accepted one is that of Hassin[32] who claims that hydrocephalus may sometimes occur even when the choroid plexuses are destroyed, and when, in addition, obstruction exists; this indicating that the cerebrospinal fluid does not come from the choroid plexuses.

Pathologic Anatomy.—The characteristic lesion is a dilatation of the lateral ventricles with a corresponding thinning of the cortex of the hemispheres. The 3d and 4th ventricles also may be distended, as well as the passages connecting the ventricles, this depending upon the nature of the

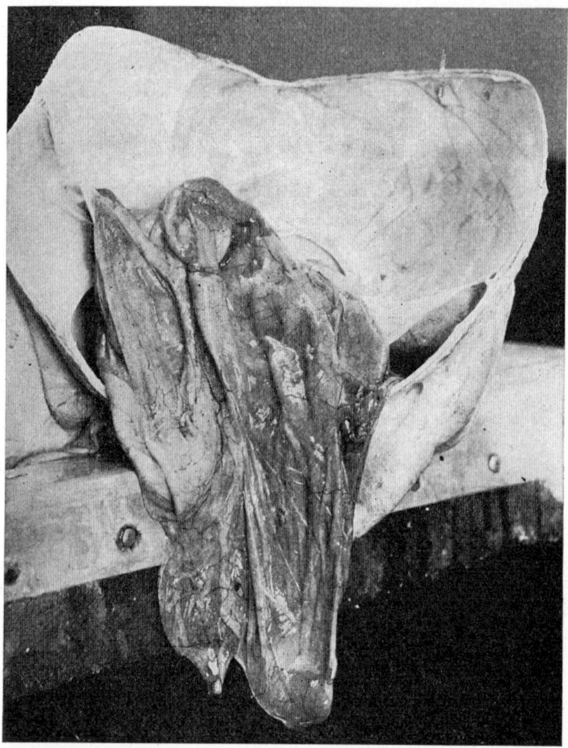

Fig. 212.—Opened skull in hydrocephalus. Same case as in Fig. 213. On removing the calvarium a gush of liquid occurred and a collapsed sac of thin membrane remained, all cerebral tissue above the basal ganglia seeming to have disappeared.

cause. The amount of fluid varies from a few ounces up to ½ pint (237) and exceptionally a quart (946) or more. In the noninflammatory cases the fluid is usually normal. When active inflammation is the cause of the disease, it may be turbid and perhaps purulent, and is richer in albumin. When fluid is in large amount, as characteristic chiefly of congenital hydrocephalus, the convolutions are much flattened and thinned; and in such cases the brain-substance of the hemispheres may even appear macroscopically to be entirely destroyed (Fig. 212). The choroid plexus may be of natural appearance, or thickened, enlarged, firm and unduly vascular. The walls of the ventricles and the meninges may show evidence of inflammation in acquired hydrocephalus. The aqueduct of Sylvius and the foramina of Luschka and of Majendie may be closed, and the capacity of the cisterna magna much diminished. The bones of the cranium are greatly altered in cases beginning early. They become much thinned and translucent and show convolutional markings; the sutures are very wide; the fontanelles much enlarged; the roof of the orbit depressed. Naturally all the changes described vary in degree, depending upon the amount of fluid. If hydrocephalus is acquired after the bones of the skull have become ossified, the skull may exhibit a slowly developing and moderate increase in size.

Symptoms.—In the most common variety, the *congenital form*, the head may be so much enlarged before birth that labor is interfered with, and perforation of the skull may be required. More often, however, the head is but little, if any, larger than normal at birth, and no change is noticed for a period varying from days or weeks often up to two or three months. Then the growth of the cranium in all directions is abnormally rapid. In well-developed cases the head has a shape approaching the globular; the parietal regions may project beyond the ears, and the forehead is overhanging with prominent frontal eminences (Fig. 213). The fontanelles are widely open and bulging; the sutures wide and often with wormian bones situated in them. The veins of the scalp are prominent and the hair scanty. The cranium may be translucent and fluctuate readily in severe cases, and there may be a somewhat tympanitic note on percussion. The face by comparison appears unusually small. The depression of the roof of the orbit causes a corresponding downward displacement of the eyeballs, the sclera showing above the iris, and the lower part of this latter or even a portion of the pupil being covered by the lower lid. There is sometimes nystagmus, strabismus, sluggishness of the pupils or optic atrophy. The external ear is somewhat depressed. The degree of distention of the head is very variable. A circumference of from 50 to 70 cm. (19.7 to 27.6 in.) is not uncommon, and one of even 100 cm. (39.4 in.) has been reported.

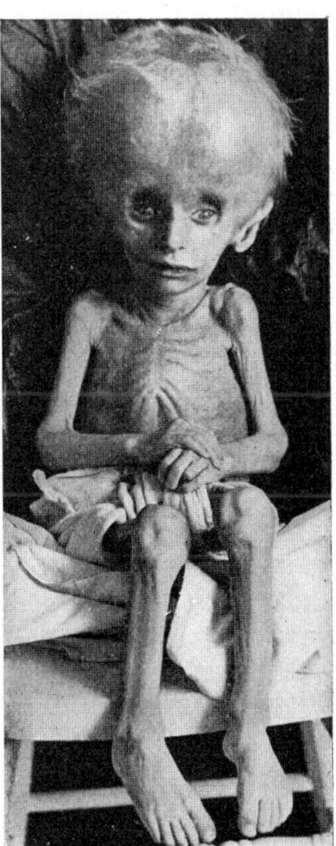

Fig. 213.—Hydrocephalus. From a patient admitted to the Children's Hospital of Philadelphia, Nov. 17, aged thirteen months. Head large at birth, and continued to increase in size. Examination showed the circumference 22½ inches (57 cm.), veins dilated, sclera visible above iris, arms and legs usually rigid and with tremor, no optic neuritis. Died Jan. 3.

In addition to these alterations of the head there appear sooner or later failure of satisfactory development of the body, with general weakness; inability to hold the head erect; slowness in learning to sit up or to walk; and either paresis of a flaccid type, or a tendency to spasticity with marked increase of the reflexes and clenching of the hands. Convulsions are not uncommon. The digestion may be disturbed, and much emaciation develops as the case advances. The intelligence may long be normal, but oftener there is some degree of apathy, dulness, irritability, imperfect speech, and finally often idiocy. It is remarkable, however, in cases in which the advance has been slow, how little the intellect may be affected for a long period.

In the *acquired cases* the symptoms are usually less marked, if ossification has not yet occurred, and the head may increase in size but little, owing to the small amount of fluid which accumulates in the ventricles. After ossification has taken place, a small quantity of fluid may produce by its pressure as severe general symptoms of intracranial pressure as are observed in advanced congenital cases with a large amount present.

Course and Prognosis.—The course is extremely variable. Some cases end fatally within a few weeks after birth. Others advance slowly for a time, and then the head ceases to grow in size and no increase in general symptoms develops, or improvements may even take place. Such cases, not numerous, may reach adult life. Others exhibit periods of temporary cessation of advance alternating with exacerbations. The prognosis is on the whole unfavorable. The cases due to syphilis are to a degree susceptible of benefit by antisyphilitic treatment. Acquired hydrocephalus dependent upon cerebrospinal fever presents usually an unfavorable prognosis. The large majority of cases of congenital hydrocephalus die in the early years of life, and most of them in the first year. The cause of death is either progressive wasting and exhaustion, or some intercurrent complication. In general the duration of life is dependent upon the rapidity of the accumulation of the fluid and the degree of yielding of the bones of the skull.

Diagnosis.—Rachitis is the disease causing most confusion, especially as it is not uncommon for temporary hydrocephalic accumulation to be associated with it. Rickets, however, is distinguished by the peculiarly square shape of the head; the deposition of bone on the frontal and parietal eminences and about the fontanelles; the failure of the head to increase rapidly in size; and the evidences of the disease elsewhere in the body. The suspicion of hydrocephalus is sometimes aroused, too, in the case of children in the first year who have abnormally large heads with prominent foreheads, but in whom this is merely an individual peculiarity. The absence of widely distended sutures and fontanelles and of abnormally rapid growth of the head will soon remove all doubt. (See p. 447.) In acquired cases in older children, with well-advanced ossification of the bones of the cranium, hydrocephalus often closely resembles tumor. Encephalography (p. 154) has proved of diagnostic value in many cases. The interior of the ventricles has been examined through a small endoscope (ventriculoscopy) by Dandy,[33] Fay and Grant[34] and others.

The diagnosis of the type of hydrocephalus is a matter of interest. As shown by Dandy and Blackfan, if a solution of *neutral* phenolsulphonephthalein is injected into one of the ventricles, the dye appears within three minutes in the fluid obtained by lumbar puncture or cisternal puncture, provided no obstruction is offered to the flow of fluid from the ventricles. Under normal conditions, if a known amount of phenolsulphonephthalein is injected into the spinal canal or into the ventricles and its excretion in the urine estimated, the presence and degree of *communicating* hydrocephalus can be determined. After ventricular injection it should normally appear in the urine in from ten to twelve minutes, and during two hours from 12 to 20 per cent of it should be eliminated. After injection into the spinal subarachnoid space it should appear in the urine in from six to eight minutes; from 35 to 60 per cent being excreted in two hours. In cases of the communicating type of hydrocephalus, the difficulty being one of absorption, the dye, injected into the ventricle or into the spinal subarachnoid space, is absorbed from the latter very slowly and elimination by the kidneys is much retarded. When the patient is suffering from the *obstructive* type of hydrocephalus the solution injected into the ventricle does not enter the spinal subarachnoid space before from thirty to fifty minutes if at all. Febrile reactions may follow the injection of dye, and occasionally such temporary disturbances as weakness of the lower extremities. Even without injections some information can be gained by lumbar puncture, inasmuch as a large amount of spinal fluid under normal or increased pressure would suggest that there was no obstruction to the flow from the ventricles into the basal cisterna. We[35] have proposed a method by which after injection of dye the total amount of fluid in the subarachnoid space can be estimated during life.

Treatment.—None of the various methods of treatment by drugs proposed in the past have proven of any value, except the employment of mercury and of the iodides in cases the result of syphilis. The administration of thyroid extract has been urged by Frazier[36] in cases dependent upon hypersecretion, on the ground that this substance has a distinctly inhibitory effect upon the secretion from the choroid plexus. Marriott[37] was able to increase the absorption of cerebrospinal fluid in a few instances of the communicating type by the administration of about 0.2 Gm. (3 grains) of theobromine sodiosalicylate (diuretin) three times a day. External pressure of the head, as by bandages, does not seem to be a logical procedure. Various operative measures have been proposed. Among them lumbar puncture is employed to relieve the intracranial pressure. This it will sometimes do, if there is no mechanical obstruction existing in the passages from the ventricles to the spinal subarachnoid space; and by its frequent repetition undoubted relief is sometimes given, but this is almost invariably only temporary. The same is true of puncture of the ventricles when lumbar puncture does not avail. Various efforts have been put forth to establish permanent drainage of the ventricular fluid into the subarachnoid space, the subcutaneous tissue, the jugular vein and elsewhere. There have been a few remarkable cases of improvement, but the operations are serious ones, and the mortality is high. Puncture of the corpus callosum is probably one of the simplest procedures, but any benefit obtained is but temporary. Dandy[38] has proposed removal of the choroid plexus in cases of communicating hydrocephalus, and has performed the operation with success. Ligature of the common carotids is another procedure which is designed to decrease secretion, and which has resulted in some benefit (Fraser and Dott[39]). In cases due to closure of the aqueduct of Sylvius, Dandy[28] has attempted reconstruction of this passage. All other treatment is supportive and symptomatic. Radiotherapy has apparently been successful in some cases, perhaps by inhibiting secretion from the choroid plexuses (Francioni[40]). (See also Treatment of Cerebrospinal Fever, p. 331.)

ATROPHY AND SCLEROSIS OF THE BRAIN

1. General or Local Atrophy of the Hemispheres.—This may be seen in porencephalus (p. 913) and agenesis corticalis (p. 913) occurring as congenital affections, or may result later from compression in hydrocephalus. As a local process it may be due to the pressure exerted by tumors, to meningo-encephalitis, or be the result of hemorrhage. It is observed, too, as a sequel to conditions of long-continued or extreme exhaustion, such as marantic states. Atrophy is commonly combined with a certain degree of sclerosis, exhibited in increase of connective tissue. The affection may involve only a few convolutions, a larger portion of one or both hemispheres, the basal ganglia, or the cerebellum. Secondary degeneration may follow in the pyramidal tracts of the cord. The primary **symptoms** are those of the original disease; later manifestations are those of infantile cerebral paralysis (p. 954).

2. Calcification of the Brain.—There may be calcification of tuberculomas, or calcareous deposits in other tumors. Independently of these there occur rarely scattered patches of calcification seen on the roentgenogram, which pathologically appear to be due to a calcifying endarteritis.

A symptomatic epilepsy may result. Cases of this sort of calcification in children are reported by Geyelin and Penfield[41] and Sauer.[42]

3. Tuberous Sclerosis.—This uncommon affection was described under this title by Bourneville.[43] Sherlock[44] used for it the term *epiloia*. The cause is unknown. There develop pea-sized or larger nodular masses of hypertrophied glial tissue, scattered upon the cortex, and extending into the gray matter beneath. The **symptoms** are observed soon after birth in most instances; the most marked being idiocy. Convulsions appear in the early months of life; and paralysis, with or without contractures, may develop. There is tumor-formation in the heart; kidneys; retina (Hoeve[45]); and the skin, especially of the face, where adenoma sebaceum is found. The prognosis is unfavorable, although the patient may not die until early adult life. The subject has been reviewed by Freeman,[46] and Brushfield and Wyatt.[47]

4. Diffuse Cerebral Sclerosis.—This rare acquired form begins oftenest in infancy. Assigned as **causes** are syphilis, fetal meningitis, and trauma of the head. There is a diffuse sclerosis of the base of the brain, the medulla, and the spinal cord; the white matter being affected more than the cortex. The **symptoms** consist in a progressive decrease of intelligence, difficulty in speech, slowness in movement, ocular paralysis, and finally extensive rigidity with contractures. There may be nystagmus, tremor, ataxia, and convulsions. The course is short and the termination fatal.

5. Lobar Sclerosis.—This unusual affection may be congenital or develop in early life. It is probably secondary to various causes, as thrombosis or meningo-encephalitis. It affects one or both hemispheres. There is a decided increase of the glial tissue, with degeneration of the ganglion-cells and nerve-fibers. The **symptoms** vary with the region involved, but are oftenest motor in nature, consisting of those seen in infantile cerebral paralysis (p. 953). There are various degrees of mental impairment.

6. Nuclear Atrophy.—In one variety of atrophy, uncommon in early life, a degenerative process is limited to the cranial nerve-nuclei (*nuclear ophthalmoplegia, nuclear bulbar palsy*). Some of the cases are merely instances of nuclear localization of poliomyelitis. Others depend upon syphilis or the acute infectious diseases, and in some there is a familial tendency. There occurs also a *nuclear aplasia* (p. 913), which differs pathologically in that it consists in congenital failure of development of the nuclei. The **symptoms** in cases due to poliomyelitis or to an aplasia do not exhibit a progressive course. In the more typical cases of nuclear atrophy due to other causes, the course is progressive to a fatal ending, although often with remissions, and rarely with a permanent cessation of advance. In *progressive nuclear ophthalmoplegia* the external ocular movements are involved, ptosis being an early symptom. In *progressive bulbar palsy* various nuclei in the pons and medulla are affected. There are increasing difficulty in articulation, swallowing, and retention of saliva; disappearance of facial expression; tremor of the tongue; palatal paralysis; hoarseness; and interference with respiratory and cardiac action.

7. Disseminated Sclerosis of the Brain and Spinal Cord.—This is an affection of adolescence and early adult life, but it may exceptionally occur in late childhood (8 in 260 cases, Frankl-Hochwart[48]). The disease appears to be a primary degenerative one, but in some cases is apparently inflammatory in origin and secondary to acute infectious diseases. The **lesions** involve the brain and spinal cord in scattered patches, and consist of a sclerosis or, in primary cases, a gliosis. The meninges and blood-vessels exhibit no characteristic alteration. The **symptoms** vary greatly, depending upon the seat of the lesions. The most characteristic are scanning speech, intention-tremor, nystagmus, bilateral or unilateral spastic

paresis, and increase of the tendon-reflexes. There may be disturbances in the regions supplied by any of the cranial nerves, anesthesia or paresthesia in various localities, and some degree of mental deficiency. The onset is insidious and the course chronic, with remissions and acute exacerbations. The **prognosis** is unfavorable.

8. ENCEPHALITIS PERIAXIALIS DIFFUSA (Progressive Degenerative Subcortical Encephalopathy; Schilder's Disease).—Schilder[49] described what he believed to be a special form of cerebral sclerosis. This has been studied also by Globus and Strauss;[50] Shelden, Doyle and Kernohan;[51] Gesul,[52] and others. Pathologically the condition is limited to symmetrical subcortical involvement of the white matter. Cerebral blindness (eye-grounds normal) is an early symptom. There occur also spastic quadriplegia, mental apathy, gradual failure of hearing and speech, increasing spastic paralysis, and sensory manifestations. It is seen mostly in males, and is more common in older children than in adults. The onset is either acute or gradual and the course steadily progressive to a fatal termination within a few days or years.

HYPERTROPHY OF THE BRAIN

As a true hypertrophy it is doubtful whether this affection exists. Uncommonly, however, there is found a hypertrophic encephalitis in children. This occurs especially in connection with rickets, but also with disorders of the thymus gland or the suprarenals; or the condition may be congenital. The **lesions** consist in hyperplasia of the neuroglia, although the nervous tissues may be involved to some extent in a degenerative process. The total weight of the brain may be decidedly above normal. The convolutions are flattened and the cerebral fluid greatly diminished. The earliest **symptoms** consist in disturbance of sleep, headache, and other signs of cerebral irritation; much as in chronic hydrocephalus, which is likewise suggested by the gradual enlargement of the head. The **prognosis** is entirely unfavorable. As the disease advances symptoms of increasing intracranial pressure are observed.

MEGACEPHALUS.—In addition to the form of hypertrophy just described there exists in many premature infants an abnormally large head and brain. It is encountered especially in the smallest subjects, but is present in the large majority of premature infants of low body-weight. It appears about the second month of life and the maximum growth is observed at from the sixth to the eighth month, after which normal relative proportions are gradually attained. The fontanelles are unduly wide and the size and shape of the head suggest hydrocephalus, no evidence of which, however, is found at necropsy. The affection appears to be merely an early increase in the growth of the brain, without corresponding development of the body. (See Ylppö,[53] Hess,[54] and Rosenstern.[55])

JUVENILE GENERAL PARALYSIS

(Paralytic Dementia; General Paresis; Progressive Dementia)

This syphilitic disorder is not often seen before the age of twelve years, but has been reported as early as three. Cases are recorded by Thiry,[56] Zappert,[57] Leonard,[58] Krapelin,[59] Bunker,[60] Ferguson and Critchley,[61] and others. Menninger[62] states that over 500 cases are reported and adds 40 more. Leavitt[63] reports a case in a third generation of a syphilitic family. The proportion of males to females is 1:1.6 (Menninger[62]). The **lesions** consist in an atrophic condition of the entire brain, but especially of the convolutions; the result, apparently, of a diffuse chronic meningo-encephalitis. The **symptoms** may be divided into somatic and psychic. The former consist in a gradual increase of hesitation and indistinctness in speech; Argyll Robertson pupil; inequality of the pupils; ataxia; tremor of the lips and tongue; unsteadiness of gait; exaggeration of the tendon-reflexes and other symptoms suggesting spastic diplegia; increasing weakness of the limbs; and often a stunting of growth which may amount to infantilism. Peculiar chewing or sucking movements constitute a common symptom in early life. There are also sudden paralytic attacks with vertigo, loss of speech, headache, local paralyses, or epileptic seizures. The psychic disturbances comprise a progressive diminution of intelligence, listlessness, depression, and inability to perform many acts formerly done with ease. Hallucinations and delusions are less common than in adult life. In the later stages the mental condition is that of dementia; while the body wastes, rigidity develops, and there is paralysis of the sphincters. The **prognosis** is entirely unfavorable, treatment having little effect. The **duration** is variable, death taking place in from a few months to several years. Before the end is reached, symptoms of tabes may become associated (p. 968). The **diagnosis** rests upon the symptoms as described. In addition there may be other evidences of syphilis, while a Wassermann reaction may be obtained on the blood, and the cerebrospinal fluid show a lymphocytosis, increased globulin, a colloidal gold test positive in the syphilitic zone, and a positive Wassermann reaction. Vigorous antisyphilitic treatment is indicated, including perhaps intraspinal injections of arsphenaminized serum (p. 440), although without the expectation of any marked benefit. Malarial treatment and foreign protein therapy, so often beneficial in adults, have, in our experience, little effect on the disease in childhood.

INFANTILE CEREBRAL PARALYSIS

This is not a primary disease, but a terminal condition secondary to a number of intracranial affections. The paralyses produced by hydrocephalus, tumor, abscess, and polio-encephalitis have been discussed in other sections. Infantile cerebral paralysis may be subdivided in various ways. Based upon the nature of the paralysis, the disease resolves itself into (1) *Spastic hemiplegia*, and (2) *Spastic diplegia* and *paraplegia;* while, following the classification of Sachs,[64] according to the time of development, one may speak of (1) *Paralysis of intra-uterine origin;* (2) *Birth or natal palsy;* (3) *Acute acquired paralysis*, or *postnatal palsy*.

The antenatal is the least common of these, and those produced at birth are generally considered the most frequent. Ford,[65] however, believes that cerebral paralysis due to birth-injury is rare. The antenatal and birth-injury cases are oftenest diplegic or paraplegic; the acquired much oftener hemiplegic.

Etiology and Pathologic Anatomy.—The lesions and causes are as follows:

1. Paralysis of Intra-uterine Origin.—It is possible that injuries received by the mother, such as blows upon the abdomen, may produce damage to the brain of the fetus. Among the lesions of large size are cysts, microcephalus, and porencephalus (p. 913). Imperfect formation of the cells of the cortex (Agenesis Corticalis, p. 913) is an occasional cause, and of the same nature is the undeveloped structure of the brain present in prematurely born children.

2. Birth-palsies.—The primary factor in nearly all such cases is meningeal hemorrhage incurred during birth (p. 916). Only rarely is intracerebral hemorrhage the cause (p. 935).

3. Postnatal Palsies (*Acquired Palsies*).—A large number of pathologic lesions have been found, many of which are only terminal processes. The large majority of cases develop in infancy or early childhood. The primary lesions are most frequently hemorrhage, thrombosis, embolism, and encephalitis. The method of production in these cases has been discussed in the chapters treating of them. Strümpell[66] thought that most of the encephalitic cases were due to the virus of poliomyelitis attacking the cerebrum. While this may sometimes be the case, the pathologic changes are usually quite different from those found in poliomyelitis, and consist of hemorrhage and cerebral softening (Peabody, Draper and Dochez[67]). Hemorrhage is the lesion most frequently encountered, but it is not always clear that this is primary; and it may, perhaps, be part of an encephalitic process. Intracerebral hemorrhage is rare. Embolism is an exceptional etiologic factor, but thrombosis of the vessels and sinuses is more frequent. Diffuse sclerosis of the brain is an unusual cause (p. 950). Hereditary syphilis may be an agent through the production of chronic meningo-encephalitis.

Symptoms.—The cases may be divided into (*A*) *hemiplegia;* (*B*) *diplegia* and *paraplegia*. The very rare cerebral monoplegia may be disregarded in this connection. (See p. 955.) The decided majority of cases of infantile cerebral paralysis are of the hemiplegic type; but inasmuch as most of the diplegic cases are short-lived, it is possible that the greater number of cases in early infancy are diplegic, and statistics must be accepted with caution. Comparatively few cases of hemiplegia are natal or prenatal in time of development.

(*A*) Infantile Hemiplegia.—The term infantile as used here includes infancy and childhood, and is applicable because of the greater incidence during the first of these periods. Usually the condition is acquired, and seen oftenest from a few months up to three years of age. The onset is usually sudden, the first symptom in about 50 per cent of the cases being a prolonged convulsive attack, most marked on, or confined to, one side of the body. This may sometimes last, with interruptions, for several days. The spinal fluid is usually normal. The temperature may be elevated, and consciousness is lost between the convulsive seizures if the case is severe. Paralysis of a hemiplegic nature, including the face on the affected side, appears early. In infancy and early childhood speech is frequently lost at first, if it has previously existed, no matter which side of the brain is involved. It may, too, be rendered difficult or indistinct by the facial paralysis. In later childhood in right-handed subjects, speech is affected only when the lesion is in the left hemisphere. As time passes spasticity, rigidity, and exaggeration of the reflexes develop in the affected side, these perhaps varying in intensity from time to time. Occasionally flaccidity is present instead of rigidity. As improvement takes place the lower extremity and the face recover usually more quickly and to a greater extent than the arm. Sometimes one limb, generally the leg, recovers so completely that the condition appears to be a monoplegia. Often, however, some involvement of the leg remains, and there may be a typical spastic paralysis of it, with equinovarus, stiff dragging with outward swinging of the extremity, and a gait upon the ball of the toe; or the limb may be too weak to permit of standing. In some cases, contrary to the rule, the leg remains decidedly affected and the arm very little so. Sometimes paresis predominates; in other cases rigidity. Involvement of the cranial nerves other than the facial is occasionally observed.

Later there persists a moderate degree of atrophy with shortening of the limb; scoliosis; and asymmetry of the pelvis, the shoulder-girdle, and sometimes of the face resulting in a facial hemiatrophy. The general bodily development is often much below normal. Contractures may appear after one or two years, or occasionally sooner. Sensory disturbances are usually absent. There is no alteration of the electrical reactions, other than a moderate quantitative diminution of response. Among later disturbances of a post-paralytic nature, coming on from a year or two after the onset, are athetosis and choreiform movements, unilateral tremor of the paralyzed limbs, and epilepsy. The last may be of the Jacksonian type, but later become general in character. Mental defect is not so often witnessed as in diplegia, many subjects remaining entirely normal mentally. The mental defect is the result of a diffuse sclerosis which has spread from the original focal lesion. It is seen oftenest when the frontal lobes are involved.

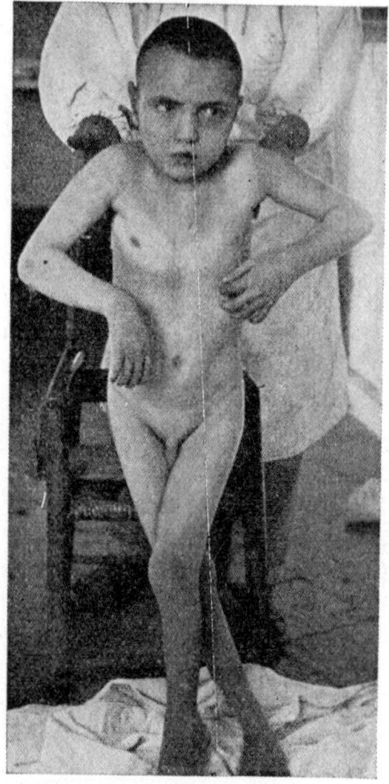

Fig. 214.—Spastic diplegia. Illustrating cross-legged progression. (*Concetti, Arch. f. Kinderh.*, 1913, **60–61**, 175.)

(*B*) Spastic Diplegia and Paraplegia. Little's Disease. (See also Paralytic Idiots, p. 907, and Hereditary Paraplegia, p. 968.)—Diplegia and paraplegia, both dependent upon a bilateral intracranial lesion, differ from each other in the limitation of the paralysis in the latter to the legs. Most cases are diplegic at the beginning, although the paralysis in the arms may later recover and only paraplegia remain. Most cases, too, are prenatal in origin or occur at birth. Only rarely are they acquired later. In diplegia, paralysis is a much less prominent symptom than certain others. The lower extremities are often more involved than the upper. The face is frequently attacked at first, but later appears to be normal. The two sides of the body are seldom affected equally. Generally rigidity is a prominent manifestation, either present at birth or developing soon after it, although no symptoms may have been observed until the time comes for sitting or walking. Contractures soon appear in most cases. The degree of stiffness of the whole body is often remarkable; and, as the child grows older, voluntary efforts may be impossible on account of the incoordination. He may be unable for years to sit unsupported or to hold up his head. Walking is impossible, or, if accomplished, exhibits a typical cross-legged progression (scissor-gait) due to the adductor spasm (Fig. 214). Increase of the tendon-reflexes is marked, ankle-clonus is present, and bilateral athetosis or choreiform movements are frequent. In other instances inability or slowness in muscular power may be dependent rather upon general physical and mental debility.

In the occasional instances of the "atonic astasic" type of diplegia, as denominated by Förster,[68] the spastic state is replaced by general muscular hypotonia and inability to stand, sit, or hold the head erect; although the child while lying in bed can make ordinary movements with the limbs, and the muscular strength appears to be preserved. The tendon-reflexes and electrical reactions are normal. There is decided mental defect. The lesion is supposedly situated in the frontal lobe. The condition has been further described by Clark,[69] Batten and von Wyss,[70] Orrico[71] and others.

Batten[72] described a cerebral type of diplegia in which speech, walking and standing are involved (p. 966), and Hunt[73] reported a condition which he called the ataxic type of cerebral birth paralysis, in which coordination is especially disturbed; without paralysis, spasticity, convulsions, or mental defect. The symptoms suggest cerebellar ataxia, but the condition is distinct.

The incoordination often present in cerebral diplegia makes speech difficult or impossible; or the lack of speech or the slow acquisition of it may depend upon the mental defect, which ranges from slight impairment up to complete idiocy. We have seen cases in which the intelligence was apparently unaffected, but talking was entirely impossible because of the lack of muscular control. Involvement of the intracranial nerves may be present, especially that producing optic atrophy, and there may occasionally be an *infantile pseudobulbar palsy* suggesting bulbar paralysis, yet dependent upon lesions of the cortex, not of the pons and medulla. The symptoms here are difficulty in swallowing, interference with speech, dribbling of saliva, hanging of the jaw, immobility of the tongue, and inability to chew. Epileptiform convulsions are observed in fully 50 per cent of the cases of diplegia. They may appear early, or sometimes at frequent intervals later. The head may be variously malformed or unduly small, the nature and degree depending upon the extent of the involvement of the brain. The paralyzed limbs are smaller than normal.

Not all cases show such marked symptoms, and the milder ones may not become apparent until several months after birth.

Little's Disease.—This term has been applied broadly to all forms of cerebral spastic diplegia. In his first publication Little[74] expressed the view that the symptoms depended upon defective formation of the pyramidal tracts of the brain and cord of premature and imperfectly developed infants. Later, however, Little[75] recognized that some of the cases he had described were instances of intracranial hemorrhage. The characteristic features of Little's Disease are a spastic rigidity, chiefly of the lower extremities, dating from birth, with some degree of loss of power. The speech is not necessarily affected; convulsions are not common; intelligence may be entirely normal or slightly defective. Obviously these symptoms might occur with intracranial hemorrhage as well as from lack of development of the pyramidal tract.

Cerebral Monoplegia.—This very uncommon condition might be confounded, in some cases, with the brachial injury resulting from obstetrical paralysis (p. 981).

Course and Prognosis.—The prognosis of infantile *hemiplegia* is good as regards life, but unfavorable for complete recovery. The degree of improvement depends upon the severity, nature and extent of the lesion, and the age of the patient at the time of onset. The older the child when the disease occurs the less liability is there of serious damage to the brain. The more marked and extensive the early symptoms, the more uncertain the final outcome. Yet it is impossible to determine at the beginning of the attack how complete recovery will be, especially in regard to the final mental condition. Most children will have remaining some traces of paralysis, spasticity, deformity, and some psychic disturbance. The paralytic symptoms are less liable to persist than the spastic. Decided permanent paralysis may be accompanied by perfect mental power; or, on the other hand, mental deficiency or epilepsy or both may remain the prominent final symptoms. According to several studies, (Gowers,[76] König,[77] Fuchs,[77] Sachs and Peterson[78]) 40 to 75 per cent of cases of cerebral paralysis develop epilepsy, and at least 50 per cent show permanent mental impairment (Ziehen[79]). Diplegias and paraplegias exhibit a greater percentage of persistent mental defect than do hemiplegias. Persistent aphasia and facial paralysis are seen each in about 15 per cent or more of cases.

Prognosis can be made only after several weeks from the onset. By this time it may be evident that no improvement will occur; or in favorable cases recovery then commences, first and most marked in the leg in many instances, while the power of speech begins to return, unless the mind has been affected. Repeated convulsions, as improvement in other respects goes on, suggest that symptomatic epilepsy is developing. However, epilepsy may not appear for a year or more after the original lesion.

The prognosis in *diplegic* cases—nearly all of which are natal or prenatal in origin—is uncertain even as regards life (p. 954). Repeated convulsions in the early weeks indicate a severe lesion. Many die during the acute symptoms in the first few weeks of life; but a surprisingly large number who have survived that period recover without residual symptoms. In true cases of the so-called *Little's disease*, dependent upon prematurity, there is a tendency to more or less recovery of mental power and improvement in muscular control. In cases of infantile cerebral paralysis Hempelmann[80] found that the following symptoms in the order given were unfavorable prognostically: Mental deficiency, progression of symptoms, athetosis, ataxia.

Diagnosis.—Well-marked cases of infantile cerebral paralysis offer no difficulty in diagnosis, and the symptoms have already been detailed. Among the conditions which may be confounded with it, is the paralysis due to *poliomyelitis.* The atrophy in this affection is, however, much greater; the reflexes diminished or absent; there are altered electrical reactions; the paralysis is flaccid; the distribution of this is not hemiplegic or diplegic, but greater in certain limbs than others. There are, further, characteristic prodromal symptoms and less likelihood of an initial stupor and coma. The spinal fluid in cerebral paralysis is usually entirely normal, whereas some change is found in the early stage of poliomyelitis. The paralysis of *Pott's disease,* although spastic in type, has a history entirely different from that of cerebral paralysis. *Obstetrical paralysis* of one arm exhibits a flaccid paralysis with atrophy. The pseudoparalysis of some cases of *rickets* suggests rather a poliomyelitis than a cerebral paralysis. We have seen the spastic condition in diplegia supposed to be *tetany* of the persistent type. *Pontine tumors* may produce spastic symptoms suggesting cerebral diplegia, but the presence of other evidences of intracranial tumor, combined with paralysis of the cranial nerves, should serve to distinguish. The form of infantile cerebral paralysis called *pseudobulbar palsy* (p. 955) in which, with lesions in the cortex, the symptoms are apparently bulbar ones, is distinguished from the paralysis due to atrophy of the cranial nerve-nuclei in the medulla and pons by the fact that in the latter there are progression of symptoms, tremor of the tongue, and interference with respiratory and cardiac action. Cases of *congenital nuclear aplasia* (p. 913) might perhaps be considered as a form of congenital infantile diplegia. *Postparalytic epilepsy* and *postparalytic chorea* are recognized by the history of the case and the existence of other evidences of cerebral paralysis.

Treatment.—The treatment of leptomeningeal hemorrhage, the most frequent cause, has been discussed elsewhere (p. 918). After the quiescent stage of cerebral palsy is reached and when residual symptoms are present, the only treatment is symptomatic. Deformity should be prevented; massage and physiotherapy used to strengthen the muscles and lessen the rigidity; and the mental condition dealt with by special training. Orthopedic apparatus may assist in correction of contractions. Operative procedures such as tenotomy, tendon- and nerve-transplantation, nerve-stretching, division of the posterior nerve-roots, resection of the sympathetic nerves and the like, have been attempted and are successful in many cases. Decompression operations in the late stages after the cerebral damage has already been done have been of no avail in our experience.

DISORDERS OF THE CORPORA STRIATA

Disorders occurring in children and showing such symptoms as choreiform movements, tremor, athetosis, juvenile paralysis agitans and the like strongly suggest some involvement of the striated body. The subject has been reviewed by Förster,[81] Crothers,[82] and others. Here will be given descriptions of two conditions seen especially in childhood.

1. Progressive Lenticular Degeneration

(Wilson's Disease)

The title was given by Wilson[83] to a rare disorder earlier described by several other authors. Monographs on the subject are those by Hall,[84] who collected 68 cases, and by Rauh,[85] who published abstracts of 62 cases. More than one member of the family is usually affected, but the disease may occur singly. The proportion of males to females is over 2:1. It develops usually toward the end of childhood or in adolescence, although cases beginning as early as three years are recorded. **Pathologically** there is found a bilateral, symmetrical degeneration of the lenticular nucleus, especially the putamen, and to a less extent of the globus pallidus. The liver is cirrhotic; yet there are seen none of the symptoms ordinarily associated with this condition. Wilson regarded the lenticular degeneration as probably the result of a selective toxin which possibly arose in the liver. Yakovlov and Cobb[86] suggest that metallic poisoning of some sort might possibly produce the disorder. The **symptoms** consist of rhythmical, bilateral tremor, increasing with effort; and a rigidity and spasticity of the muscles producing a stiff, open-mouthed smile, distorted attitudes of the limbs, a fan-shaped position of the toes; and convulsive laughter. Later there are contractures, inability to sit or stand, dysarthria, and dysphagia. The reflexes are normal and there is no real paralysis. Mentality is normal at first, but eventually becomes defective. There is cirrhosis of the liver. The duration of acute cases is a few months, and in those of slower course four or five years may elapse before the fatal ending.

2. Dystonia Musculorum Deformans

(Progressive Torsion Spasm)

This unusual condition was first described by Ziehen[87] and called by him "*torsion spasm.*" The title employed here was first applied by Oppenheim.[88] Reports and reviews are those by Thomalla,[89] Hunt,[90] Mendel,[91] Flater,[92] Home,[93] Wechsler and Brock,[94] Navarro and Marotta,[95] Urechia and Groza,[96] Ibrahim,[97] and others. It is described as a torsion spasm of the trunk and extremities, seen almost exclusively in Russian and Polish Jews; incurable; progressive; but finally becoming stationary. Occasionally there is evidence of familial tendency. The cause is unknown, although some cases clinically resembling the condition appear to be post-encephalitic (Kaufman[98]). It begins usually in late childhood; males are more frequently attacked than females. The **lesions** would appear to be in the corpora striata, but not limited to this. In a few cases there has been found an hepatic cirrhosis similar to that of Wilson's Disease. The **symptoms** consist in peculiar twisting movements of the whole trunk, with curious alterations of position in standing, and a rocking of the hips and pelvis in walking. These usually disappear during sleep or when the patient ceases to make voluntary efforts. Hypotonia is commonly associated when the patient is at rest, but marked stiffness develops with effort at movement. There is no paralysis. The lower extremities are usually more involved than the arms. The face and speech are not affected except terminally;

the knee-jerks are diminished; clonic movements are sometimes observed. The course is slow and progressive, and no treatment is of avail.

References

1. Diseases and Derangements of the Nervous System, 1841, **5**, 153; see also Medical Essays, 1825. 2. Arch. Neurol. and Psychiat., 1924, **12**, 443. 3. Virchow's Archiv., 1867, **38**, 129; 1868, **44**, 472. 4. Monatschr. f. Kinderh., 1929, **42**, 12. 5. Arch. Pediat., 1897, **14**, 809. 6. Griffith, Am. J. M. Sc., 1916, **151**, 24; 1921, **162**, 787; Am. J. Dis. Child., 1920, **20**, 82. 7. Diseases of the Nervous System, Amer. Edit. 1888, 852. 8. Arch. Pediat., 1898, **15**, 81. 9. Arch. Int. Med., 1916, **17**, 591. 10. Am. J. Dis. Child., 1928, **35**, 256. 11. Berl. klin. Wchnschr., 1879, **16**, 617. 12. Nothnagel, Handbuch d. spec. Path. u. Therap., 1896, **9**, 1, 3, 253. 13. J.A.M.A., 1927, **87**, 1477. 14. J.A.M.A., 1931, **97**, 535. 15. Am. J. Dis. Child., 1927, **33**, 551. 16. Am. J. M. Sc., 1929, **178**, 229. 17. Brit. J. Child. Dis., 1926, **23**, 165. 18. Brain Surgery, 1893, 202. 19. Arch. Neurol. and Psychiat., 1927, **17**, 179. 20. Ohio State M. J., 1929, **25**, 269. 21. Ohio State M. J., 1930, **26**, 1011. 22. Nervous Diseases in Children, 1905. 23. Arch. Neurol. and Psychiat., 1927, **17**, 57. 24. Ztschr. f. Kinderh., 1928, **45**, 725. 25. Acta path. et microbiol. Scandinav., 1926, Supp. 1, 1. 26. Am. J. M. Sc., 1928, **176**, 346. 27. J.A.M.A., 1929, **93**, 7. 28. Surg. Gynec. and Obstet., 1920, **31**, 340. 29. J. Nerv. and Ment. Dis., 1925, **62**, 498. 30. Am. J. Dis. Child., 1914, **8**, 406; 1917, **14**, 424; 1919, **19**, 525; Ann. Surg., 1918, **68**, 569. 31. Am. J. Physiol., 1914, **35**, 268. 32. Arch. Neurol. and Psychiat., 1932, **27**, 406. 33. Bull. Johns Hopkins Hosp., 1922, **33**, 189. 34. J.A.M.A., 1923, **80**, 461. 35. Mitchell and Zeligs, Am. J. Dis. Child., 1925, **30**, 189. 36. Am. J. Dis. Child., 1916, **11**, 95. 37. Am. J. Dis. Child., 1924, **28**, 479. 38. Ann. Surg., 1918, **68**, 569. 39. Brit. J. Surg., 1922, **10**, 165. 40. Riv. di clin. pediat., 1929, 1. 41. Arch. Neurol and Psychiat., 1929, **21**, 1020. 42. Ztschr. f. Kinderh., 1928, **46**, 457. 43. Arch. de neurol., 1880, **1**, 81. 44. The Feebleminded, 1911. 45. Graefe's Arch. f. Ophthalmol., 1921, **105**, 880. 46. Arch. Neurol. and Psychiat, 1922, **8**, 614. 47. Brit. J. Child. Dis., 1926, **23**, 178. 48. Arb. aus dem neurol. Inst. an der Wien. Univ., 1903, **10**, 19. 49. Ztschr. f. d. ges. Neurol. u. Psychiat., 1912, **10**, 1; 1913, **15**, 359. 50. Arch. Neurol. and Psychiat., 1928, **20**, 1190. 51. Arch. Neurol. and Psychiat., 1929, **21**, 1270. 52. Am. J. Dis. Child., 1930, **39**, 595. 53. Ztschr. f. Kinderh., Orig., 1919, **20**, 202. 54. Premature and Congenitally Diseased Infants, 1922, 307. 55. Ztschr. f. Kinderh., 1922, **32**, 129. 56. Thèse de Nancy, 1898. 57. Pfaundler und Schlossmann, Handb. der Kinderh., 1906, **2b**, 661. 58. Illinois M. J., 1915, **27**, 443. 59. Ueber die juvenile Paralyse, 1920; Ref. Pollock, Am. J. Dis. Child., 1921, **22**, 320. 60. Am. J. Syph., 1926, **10**, 553. 61. Brit. J. Child. Dis., 1929, **26**, 163. 62. J.A.M.A., 1930, **95**, 1499. 63. Arch. Neurol. and Psychiat., 1931, **26**, 665. 64. Nerv. Dis. of Childh., 1905, 447. 65. Medicine, 1926, **5**, 121. 66. Jahrb. f. Kinderh., 1885, **22**, 173. 67. Monograph, Rockefeller Institute of Medical Research, 1912. 68. Deutsch. Arch. f. klin. Med., 1909, **98**, 216. 69. Am. J. Dis. Child., 1913, **5**, 425. 70. Brit. J. Child. Dis., 1915, **12**, 65. 71. Arch. latino-am. de pediat., 1927, **21**, 675; Ref. Am. J. Dis. Child., 1928, **35**, 922. 72. Brain, 1905, **28**, 484. 73. Am. J. M. Sc., 1918, **155**, 503. 74. Lancet, 1843–44, **1**, 318. 75. Trans. Obst. Soc. London, 1862–63, 293. 76. Dis. of the Nerv. Syst., 1888, Amer. Ed., 843. 77. Ref. Bruns, Cramer u. Ziehen, Handb. d. Nervenkr. im Kindesalter, 1912, 636. 78. J. Nerv. and Ment. Dis., 1890, **17**, 295. 79. Handb. d. Nervenkr. im Kindersalter, 1912, 635. 80. Am. J. Dis. Child., 1927, **33**, 296. 81. Ztschr. f. d. ges. Neurol. u. Psychiat., 1921, **73**, 1, 169; Ref. Am. J. Dis. Child., 1924, **27**, 90. 82. Am. J. Dis. Child., 1921, **22**, 145. 83. Brain, 1912, **34**, 295. 84. La dégénérescence hépato-lenticulaire, 1921. 85. Arch. f. Kinderh., 1931, **95**, 17. 86. New England J. Med., 1932, **206**, 207. 87. Neurolog. Centralbl., 1911, **30**, 109; Allg. Ztschr. f. Psychiat., 1911, **68**, 281. 88. Neurolog. Centralbl., 1911, **30**, 1090. 89. Ztschr. f. d. ges. Neurol. u. Psychiat., Orig., 1918, **41**, 311. 90. J.A.M.A., 1916, **67**, 1431. 91. Monatschr. f. Psychiat. u. Neurol., 1919, **46**, 309. 92. Ztschr. f. Neurol. u. Psychiat., 1921, **69**, 27. 93. Neurol. Bull., 1921, **3**, 253. 94. Arch. Neurol. u. Psychiat., 1922, **8**, 538. 95. Arch. de méd. d. enf., 1927, **30**, 29. 96. Bull. et mém. soc. méd. d. hôp. de Paris, 1931, **47**, 650. 97. Pfaundler u. Schlossmann, Handb. der Kinderh. 3, 1924, **4**, 390. 98. Arch. Neurol. u. Psychiat., 1928, **20**, 824.

CHAPTER VI

DISEASES OF THE SPINAL CORD AND ITS MEMBRANES

In this chapter will be described conditions in which the cord alone or its membranes are affected, or the most marked symptoms are referable to disease there. Other disorders of the cord may arise secondary to disease in the brain, such as tumor; or be part of a process which involves both brain and cord or their membranes, as poliomyelitis, encephalitis, meningitis, and disseminated sclerosis. Some of the muscular atrophies and dystrophies, although probably of primary muscular or neural origin, are included in this chapter as a matter of convenience.

MALFORMATIONS

Most of these are of infrequent occurrence. They may be found alone, or in combination with malformations of the brain or of other parts of the body. Much the most common is spina bifida.

Spina Bifida

Etiology and Pathologic Anatomy.—This is analogous to cerebral meningocele and encephalocele, but is more frequent, being encountered in about 0.1 to 1.15 per cent of births (Chaussier,[1] Demme[2]). A familial tendency is sometimes observed. It is often associated with other deformities, as hydrocephalus, club-foot, hare-lip, encephalocele or meningocele, ectopia of the bladder, etc. (Fig. 215). There has been a failure of the bony arches of the spinal canal to close completely. The opening may be small and no effusion of spinal fluid or projection of membranes takes place (*spina bifida occulta*), such a lesion being usually in the lumbar region. In typical cases there is perforation of the dura, and a globular, tense, fluctuating tumor is produced, which may be several inches in diameter. In the simplest and least common form only the membranes protrude (*meningocele*), the fluid which distends them being either in the arachnoid cavity or the posterior subarachnoid space. The opening connecting the sac with the spinal canal is small or may be closed. This variety, situated oftenest in the cervical or sacral region (Fig. 216), is globular, translucent, often pedunculated and covered with normal skin. The commonest and most serious form of spina bifida is *meningomyelocele,* with the spinal cord and meninges contained in the sac. The tumor is generally smaller than in the previous variety, oval, soft, fluctuating, usually sessile with a broad base; the skin over it is thin, reddish, vascular, and usually depressed in the center, and often ulcerated (Fig. 215). It is situated oftenest in the sacrolumbar region, and the fluid accumulates in the anterior subarachnoid space or the anterior arachnoid cavity. In some instances the tumor may be pedunculated and present its greatest swelling lateral to the spine or in the buttocks. *Myelocystocele* (*syringomyelocele; hydromyelocele*) is uncommon. The central canal of the cord dilates and pushes its posterior portion with its covering through the opening in the spinal canal. This produces a sessile tumor, oftenest in the dorsolumbar or sacral region. On palpation it is found to contain solid contents as well as fluid. The skin covering it is at first normal, but may later become ulcerated.

Symptoms.—These vary with the form and situation. In *spina bifida occulta* there may be visible at most a slight depression in the skin, often covered by a hairy mole. The bony defect may be palpable. Adhesions of the cord to the skin may produce interference with the growth of the former, resulting in incontinence of urine, paralysis, and neuralgias, perhaps not evident until puberty. Club-foot developing in later life may be due to occult spina bifida (deVries[3]). *Meningocele* is unattended by any symptoms of paralysis, and this is often true of *myelocystocele*. *Meningomyelocele* often exhibits flaccid paralysis and atrophy of the legs. There may also be paralysis of the bladder and rectum; prolapse of the rectum and of the uterus; flexion of the thighs at the hip-joint; anesthesia; and trophic disturbances, as ulceration of the buttocks, genitalia, and inner surface of the thighs. Less severe cases, particularly those in the sacral region, may present only incomplete paralysis of the legs and feet, and perhaps of the sphincters.

Course and Prognosis.—The occult form may sometimes develop a visible tumor when adolescence is reached. In other varieties the lesion tends to become larger. The ulcerated skin in *meningomyelocele* may finally be covered with epithelium, but septic infection is very liable to occur and involve the spinal and cerebral meninges. Rarely a local infection obliterates the sac. There is always danger of rupture, with a rapidly fatal ending. Even with operative interference, the mortality is 50 per cent or more, and

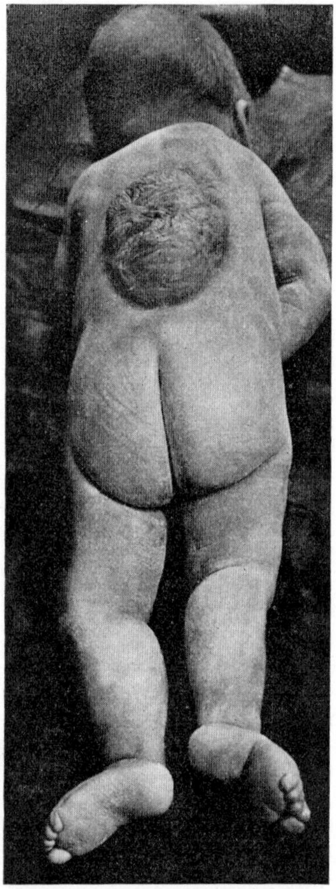

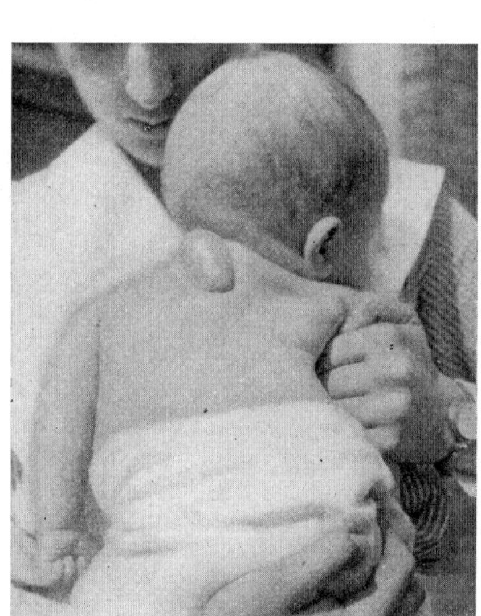

Fig. 215. Fig. 216.

Fig. 215.—Spina bifida and club-foot. Male infant of six months in the Children's Hospital of Philadelphia. Large spinal bifida with talipes cavus.

Fig. 216.—Cervical spina bifida. Female infant of three months in Children's Hospital of Philadelphia. Swelling increasing from birth; some degree of hydrocephalus present. Radical operation on spina bifida followed by recovery, but hydrocephalus unchanged.

hydrocephalus is liable to develop in those who survive. Without operation the prognosis is worse. *Meningocele* grows to large size, seldom ruptures or becomes infected, and is the least serious variety and more amenable to operative treatment, although here, too, hydrocephalus may later occur.

Diagnosis.—Lumbosacral tumors, as lipoma and teratoma, should be diagnosed from spina bifida by lack of fluctuation and absence of symptoms. The different varieties of spina bifida are to be differentiated from each other by the characteristics already described. In spina bifida occulta the roentgenogram may reveal the vertebral defect.

Treatment.—Such methods as injection into the sac, ligation, compression, and the like have largely given place to plastic operations. Surgical intervention is, however, contraindicated when hydrocephalus is also present, when flaps cannot be formed, or when there are severe paralytic symptoms. The operation is in itself dangerous, and after surgical recovery symptoms may continue, or hydrocephalus develop later. Meningocele offers the best hope, and operation may also be justified in myelocystocele, or in other cases when rupture is threatening. The occult cases may frequently be successfully operated upon with relief of symptoms.

Other Malformations of the Spinal Cord

These are of rare occurrence. There may be complete absence of the spinal cord (**amyelia**), or entire failure of closure of the spinal canal posteriorly (**rachischisis**), with splitting open of the cord,—conditions incompatible with life. In other cases there is partial deficiency of the cord (**atelomyelia**); **heterotopia** of small areas of grey matter into the white matter; partial **degeneration** of the pyramidal tracts; a congenital dilatation of the central canal (**hydromyelia**); or a doubling of the cord (**diplomyelia**) or of the central spinal canal (**diastematomyelia**) through a portion of its extent. With all of these conditions malformations of other regions of the body are very prone to be associated. To hydromyelia there may be later joined a **syringomyelia,** dependent upon a diffuse gliosis of the cord with the formation of cavities. It seems doubtful whether syringomyelia ever occurs alone in early life.

SPINAL MENINGITIS

1. Serous Spinal Meningitis, circumscribed in nature, may occur after trauma or be due to syphilis. Adhesions may form between the pia and arachnoid and cyst-like accumulations of fluid result. The **symptoms** are usually those of spasticity of the legs and disturbances of sensation (Hassin and Andrews[4]).

2. Pachymeningitis may occur secondarily to spinal caries, tumor or trauma, or suppuration outside of the spine, as in retropharyngeal abscess. The inflammation is usually limited to the external surface of the dura, and is semipurulent in character, terminating in abscess. The early **symptoms** are those of compression-myelitis (p. 965), except that in pachymeningitis they are slower in onset, and show a preponderance of pain and muscular spasm, and an absence of paralysis. *Pachymeningitis cervicalis hypertrophica* is a rare affection with firm deposit of fibrous tissue on the inner layer of the dura. The symptoms result from compression-myelitis of the cervical region, with involvement of the nerve roots; the most prominent being pain in the upper extremities, shoulder, and neck; hyperesthesia; and atrophy, partial paralysis, and contractions of the hands. The onset is gradual and the course may last for years. The prognosis is serious, but arrest of the process or complete recovery may occur.

3. Spinal Leptomeningitis may be acute or chronic and occurs rarely except in combination with analogous inflammation of the brain. With cerebrospinal fever the lesions may be widespread; in tuberculous meningitis often confined to the cervical region of the cord. A gummatous meningitis may involve the membranes of the cord. As a localized process, spinal meningitis may also depend on spinal caries, tumor, and trauma. Inflammation may readily extend to the cord, or, conversely, from a myelitis to the meninges. The principal **symptoms** are usually those occurring in connection with the associated cerebral meningitis. In cases with solely or

predominantly spinal involvement there is more or less paroxysmal, severe pain in the back or limbs, worse on movement. This is accompanied by moderate fever. There may be paresthesia or hyperalgesia; and rigidity, contractures, increased reflexes, stiffness of the neck, or opisthotonos may appear. Later there develop paralysis, perhaps also of the sphincters, and loss of sensation. If the lumbar cord is affected these symptoms are in the lower extremities; if the dorsal, there is also involvement of the trunk; if the cervical, there may be difficulty in respiration and disturbance of arm-movements. In the circumscribed spinal form there may be spastic paraplegia without other central nervous symptoms. The **prognosis** is uncertain. Disregarding meningococcic and tuberculous meningitis of the brain and cord, it can be said that the probability of recovery depends upon the extent and severity of the inflammation, its cause, its nearness to the medulla, and the degree to which the cord itself is involved. In some cases death occurs in a few days; others are liable to terminate fatally after long-continued exhaustion, attended by muscular atrophy. Adhesions may form and shut off circulation of spinal fluid, producing symptoms suggesting those of cord-tumor (p. 963), but differing from these in having a history of some acute condition, in their slow progress, in the greater chance of complete block, and in the absence of xanthochromia. Spinal meningitis caused by trauma gives a better prognosis than that due to other causes. The **diagnosis** must be made from myelitis, which gives little pain; from rheumatism, which causes pain only on movement; and from tetanus, which produces rigidity and usually shows the presence of a wound and other distinguishing symptoms. The **treatment** is that of the cause. Syphilitic cases require the usual remedies for this; spinal caries the appropriate treatment; traumatic cases sometimes surgical treatment if fracture is present. In circumscribed spinal meningitis with cyst-formation, laminectomy and emptying of the cyst may be curative.

INJURY TO THE SPINAL CORD. HEMATORACHIS. HEMATOMYELIA

Injury to the spinal cord, nearly always consecutive to or accompanied by hemorrhage, is usually the result of application of traction during labor, most commonly in breech-deliveries. Crothers and Putnam[5] saw 26 cases of cord-injuries and during the same period 260 instances of cerebral palsy due to birth-injury. With partial or complete tears of the cord there may occur hemorrhage into the spinal meninges (*hematorachis*), or into the substance of the cord (*hematomyelia*). Hemorrhages may take place even when relatively little injury has been done to the cord itself, and are then liable to be associated with bleeding into other parts of the body, oftenest within the cranium. Exceptional causes are trauma other than birth-injury, rupture of vessels during pertussis, and hemorrhagic diseases. Among other reports of cord-injury and hemorrhage are those of Spencer,[6] Burr,[7] Kohlbry,[8] and Ford.[9] We have seen 4 cases in infants who survived the birth-period.

The **symptoms** of damage to the cord depend upon whether it is partial or complete, and on its location. Complete destruction of the lower part of the cord results in flaccid paraplegia and absent reflexes, and there may be incontinence of urine and feces and severe trophic ulcers. In partial transection feeble voluntary movement may persist with unaltered reflex activity. Symptoms due to intracranial injury may complicate the picture. *Meningeal hemorrhage* produces radiating pain, hyperesthesia or paresthesia, and muscular rigidity; while later there are paralyses of the limbs or sphincters and diminished sensation in the parts below the seat of the hemorrhage. The symptoms are similar to those of spinal meningitis, but of more sudden onset. In hemorrhage into the substance of the cord, unless of the slowly infiltrating form, the onset is sudden, and paralysis is the most prominent early symptom and pain less characteristic. There are also varying focal symptoms depending upon the position of the hemorrhage. In flaccid paralysis associated with hemorrhage, Gött[10] believed that there was injury to the nerve-roots through secondary meningitic thickening. The **prognosis** is always serious. In injury from hemorrhage or other cause high in the cord death may occur shortly. If paralytic symptoms continue there may develop infection of the urinary apparatus and intractable trophic ulcers of the skin. Absorption of hemorrhage may occur, and partial or complete recovery follow after several weeks, this being less likely in hematomyelia than in hematorachis. In the former secondary myelitis is liable to develop. The **treatment** is entirely symptomatic.

TUMORS OF THE SPINAL CORD

About 5 to 10 per cent of tumors of the spinal cord occur in children (Mills and Lloyd,[11] Schlesinger,[12] Stookey[13]). They may be primary or secondary, and may involve the meninges or the cord itself. In the former situation they are oftenest sarcoma or gliosarcoma; in the latter, tubercle or sometimes glioma. Gumma is uncommon; lipoma may occur. The **symptoms** vary greatly. There may be pain in some of the extremities; sometimes hyperesthesia, or spastic rigidity and contractures; and later loss of sensation, motion, or control of the sphincters. The character and location of the symptoms depend upon the extent and position of the lesion. When the meninges are chiefly involved, evidences of irritation predominate; when the cord itself, loss of motion or of sensation. A growth of one side of the cord may produce a Brown-Séquard paralysis; while if the entire transverse section is involved the symptoms are those of transverse myelitis. The pressure of the spinal fluid above the tumor is greater than that below. Characteristic is an exaggeration of symptoms following lumbar puncture (Elsberg and Stookey[14]). Dye, such as phenolsulphonephthalein, when injected below the tumor may not appear in the fluid obtained by puncture made above it. If iodized oil is injected intraspinally and roentgenograms taken, a diagnosis of obstruction may be made; but the liquid may lead to chronic irritation unless removed later at operation. The fluid below the tumor may approximate blood-serum in some of its characteristics and xanthochromia and the syndromes of Nonne and of Froin be present (p. 859). These changes are not, however, entirely diagnostic, since they may occur in any condition causing complete block, as, for example, an adhesion produced by spinal meningitis (p. 962). The slow onset and course of the disease may suggest spinal caries. The **prognosis** is unfavorable unless the tumor can be removed by operation without leaving residual destruction of the cord.

SYRINGOMYELIA

This has rarely been reported in early life (di Giorgio,[15] Bruns[16]). It is in most instances a gliomatous infiltration of the spinal cord, with the production later of cavities, and may be combined with dilatation of the central canal (p. 961). There are usually no symptoms during childhood, but any seen are similar to those in adult life.

MYELITIS

This term may be applied broadly to all affections in which inflammation of the spinal cord is present. Among these are poliomyelitis, amyotrophic lateral sclerosis, and certain other disorders considered elsewhere.

1. Acute Myelitis

In childhood the process is nearly always diffuse, affecting especially the gray matter, and is identical in lesions and symptoms with poliomyelitis (p. 387). Among the causes are an intoxication or an acute infectious disease, as diphtheria (Powers[17]), extension from a meningitis, or trauma. The influence of syphilis is uncertain. The whole of the transverse section of the cord may be affected throughout a considerable extent of its length (*diffuse myelitis*), and the process less often involve the brain as well (*encephalomyelitis*); or the inflammation may be in scattered foci (*disseminated myelitis*), or may affect the transverse section of the cord in a limited region only, and rarely completely (*transverse myelitis*). In rare instances a transverse myelitis may be in reality due to an abscess (*purulent myelitis*), following trauma or oftener as a result of septic metastasis or purulent meningitis. The **symptoms** vary greatly, depending upon the locality, the amount of the cord involved, or on whether the lesion remains localized or undergoes a rapid extension. As seen in transverse myelitis of the dorsal region, for example, there may early be moderate pain in the limbs or back, numbness in the limbs, a girdle-sensation, and muscular twitching. Paralysis of the lower limbs develops rapidly and may be marked in a few hours or days. It is paraplegic and combined with increase of reflexes, and later spastic symptoms, anesthesia, paralysis of the sphincters, and the production of bed-sores. High fever, loss of appetite, debility, headache, and similar constitutional disturbances are usually present. The occurrence of spastic symptoms and the like depends upon the situation of the lesion. In the parts of the body receiving their nerve-supply from the cord *below* the seat of the lesion, the tendon-reflexes are increased and there are rigidity and anesthesia, but no excessive atrophy or degenerative reaction. On the other hand atrophy is marked, degenerative reaction present, tendon-reflexes absent, and the paralysis is of the flaccid type in the parts supplied by the diseased portion of the cord, provided that the anterior horns are involved. Thus, when the lumbar cord is affected the paralyzed legs are flaccid, anesthetic and atrophic, and exhibit reaction of degeneration but no increase of the knee-jerks; but when the dorsal cord is diseased the knee-jerks are exaggerated, the paralysis is spastic, there is anesthesia, atrophy of the lower extremities is little marked, and the reaction of degeneration is absent. When the lesion is situated in the cervical region the arms exhibit paralysis and anesthesia; the paralysis finally becoming spastic and with increased reflexes if the lesion is above the origin of the brachial nerves, but flaccid and with atrophy and reaction of degeneration if the gray matter of the cord from which these nerves arise is involved. The **course** may be rapid, ending in death from exhaustion or some complication, as nephritis or pneumonia. In other cases the symptoms may remain stationary or show slight increase; and then improvement may begin after a few weeks. Final recovery may be complete, but is oftener only partial. The **diagnosis** is to be made from compression-myelitis by the more rapid onset and the absence of the earlier root-symptoms of that disease. In spinal hemorrhage the onset is sudden rather than rapid. In Landry's paralysis the sensation is not affected, and the paralysis is ascending in type. Meningitis has more severe pain, hyperesthesia, and earlier rigidity. The only **treatment** possible is absolute rest, with the patient preferably on the face; and dry cupping to the spine or the application of an ice-bag, if the case is seen early. Other treatment is symptomatic. Paralysis of the bladder may necessitate catheterization. When improvement begins gentle massage may be employed.

2. Compression-Myelitis

This condition is sometimes a result of trauma, pachymeningitis, or pressure by tumor, but the most frequent cause is caries of the spine (p. 1010). As a result of this last disease a pachymeningitis is set up (p. 961), often with an accumulation of pus; and this, together with, on the one hand, the narrowing of the spinal canal by curvature resulting from the destruction of the vertebrae and, on the other, the development of granulation tissue within the canal, exerts a gradually increasing pressure upon the cord (generally exercised from in front, sometimes from one side) and produces decided flattening. In most instances the cord is not affected for more than 2 in., although some minor degree of inflammation reaches both above and below the position of greatest involvement. In addition there is degeneration in certain tracts; a descending degeneration in the motor, an ascending one in the sensory. The nerve-roots coming from the region of compression are earlier and more extensively diseased than the cord itself, with corresponding degenerative changes in the nerves and the muscles supplied by them. The **symptoms** vary with the stage of the disease and with the position of the lesion. Only exceptionally is the process acute; as in cases due to trauma or to a sudden giving-way of carious vertebrae. Among the earliest symptoms is constant or intermittent pain, developing in the course of the involved nerves. Hyperesthesia is frequent, and later often localized anesthesia; together with muscular weakness, atrophy and the electrical reactions of degeneration, all of these occurring in the same region as the pain. These are "root-symptoms," and are dependent upon the complicating neuritis, not upon the lesion of the cord itself. "Cord-symptoms" are seen chiefly in regions of the body the nervous supply of which arises from the cord *below* the lesion. They consist first of all in paralysis coming on rapidly or much oftener slowly. This is bilateral and of the spastic type, with increase of deep and superficial reflexes, pain, paresthesia, and often anesthesia. There is no reaction of degeneration. There may sometimes be loss of sphincter control. **Course** and **prognosis** vary greatly. When the principal lesion has been edema, there may be entire recovery after a few weeks under appropriate treatment. Even when there has been more or less destruction of the nervous tissue, regeneration may take place and the cord resume its power of conduction. In older cases, when the paralysis has been long-continued and the sclerosing process has become well-established, there is less hope of improvement. It is surprising, however, to what degree recovery may follow even after the disease has persisted for several years. (See p. 1011.) The **diagnosis** depends largely upon the earlier development of sensory disturbance, followed later by paraplegia. Acute transverse myelitis exhibits a rapid development of paralysis. Tumors of the cord are less likely to produce pain on movement of the body than is caries of the vertebrae, and in the latter there may be deformity of the spine. **Treatment** is chiefly that of the cause. Operation is indicated for tumor and for trauma. The treatment for spinal caries will be described later.

LANDRY'S PARALYSIS

(Acute Ascending Paralysis)

The majority of cases described as occurring in early life and called by this name were in reality but one of the forms of poliomyelitis (p. 392). Others probably were neuritis; others forms of myelitis. There are, however, still other cases rarely encountered which, for the most part, correspond clinically with the account first given by Landry,[18] and which seem to warrant a separate description. The disease appears to be an acute toxic or infectious process. A condition suggesting it has been observed in some cases of botulism and of rabies, and the ascending paralysis reported by McCornack[19] may be of a similar nature. We have twice seen it follow chicken-pox. The anatomical condition is a varying one. In some instances there are no lesions whatever; in others there is the early evidence of myelitis, in others involvement of the nerve-roots; and in still others micro-organisms of different sorts are found. The enlargement of the spleen usually observed indicates the toxic-infectious nature of the malady. The **symptoms** consist often of an initial stage with malaise and fever, followed by a progressive, ascending paralysis. This begins in the legs, is of the flaccid type, without electrical changes or trophic symptoms; and sensory disturbances are absent or little marked. The paralysis extends rapidly, attacking the trunk and upper extremities, and, as the medulla becomes involved, the respiration, speech and swallowing. The action of the sphincters is usually normal. Moderate fever may continue. Occasionally the upper extremities are first attacked, or the bulbar symptoms may even appear first and the advance be a descending one. The disorder reaches its full development in from one to two days, or sometimes longer. Death takes place in one or two weeks or a shorter time, often from asphyxia; yet cases of recovery are reported. The **diagnosis** is not difficult, except that no clinical distinction exists betwen this Landry's paralysis and the ascending form of poliomyelitis. An ascending multiple neuritis is recognized by the presence of decided pain and tenderness in the nerve-trunks, the atrophy, altered electrical reactions, longer course, and more favorable termination. **Treatment** can be symptomatic only, and consists in absolute rest and the employment of supporting measures.

THE ATAXIAS

Ataxia may exist as a symptom of various conditions, in some of which, as after infectious diseases, or in chorea, infantile cerebral paralysis, certain cases of tumor of the cerebellum or mid-brain, multiple neuritis, and hydrocephalus, it is but one of other manifestations. In other diseases it constitutes the most striking symptom, and it is to these affections that some special attention must now be given. The different forms are grouped here as a matter of convenience.

One of the most important is *Friedreich's ataxia*. Intermediate forms doubtless exist between this and certain other ataxic disorders, such as the *hereditary cerebellar ataxia* to be described. Mention should be made in passing of the forms of *cerebellar ataxia* as classified by Batten.[20] The first of these is congenital cerebellar ataxia, depending upon imperfect development of the cerebellum or upon lesions analogous to those producing infantile cerebral paralysis. The second is acute cerebellar ataxia, which has already been mentioned (p. 937) under the topic of acute encephalitis. The third is chronic progressive cerebellar ataxia, which is certainly closely allied to, or perhaps a form of, hereditary cerebellar ataxia.

1. Friedreich's Ataxia

This disorder was first described by Friedreich[21] in 1861. In 1889 we[22] published an analysis of 143 collected cases including 3 of our own, but some of these reports, however, later studies would probably show perhaps belong in the category of other ataxic diseases. We have since seen a number of other cases, and many have been reported by other physicians.

Etiology.—The direct cause is unknown. Hereditary or familial influence is a striking feature, a number of brothers or sisters being attacked, and sometimes the disease being directly inherited through several generations. In other instances nervous diseases of some other sort have been present in the ancestors or in other children of the family. The malady makes its appearance in early childhood, sometimes after puberty, and occasionally in infancy. The influence of acute, and usually infectious, disorders in precipitating the onset of the symptoms of Friedreich's ataxia is very decided.

Pathologic Anatomy.—The process is a degenerative one with sclerosis, and attacks especially the posterior columns of the cord, the lateral tracts, the direct cerebellar tracts, and the posterior nerve-roots, and sometimes extends to the medulla.

Symptoms.—The first symptom seen is ataxia, beginning in the lower extremities, and shown by uncertainty or staggering in the gait. When standing the patient may sway from side to side (*static ataxia*), and when the eyes are closed the swaying increases in some cases (*Romberg's*[23] *symptom*). The sphincters are unaffected. The knee-jerks are absent. Trembling or oscillating movements of the legs when in certain positions are common. The feet often exhibit a characteristic deformity, consisting of high arching of the instep, shortening of the foot, and hyperextension of the great toe, sometimes with flexion of the last phalanx. This may be an early or a late symptom. Gradually, sometimes only after several years, the process extends to the trunk and the upper extremities, and finally to the head. The patient now sways while sitting and scoliosis is common. The hands exhibit marked ataxic movements on voluntary effort, the attempt at grasping being often peculiarly claw-like and over-reaching; and even while lying passive in the lap there may be choreiform or athetoid movements of the fingers. There is an irregular nodding or jerking movement of the head. The face develops a peculiar expressionless appearance. Nystagmus is common; optic atrophy rare; the pupillary reflexes are generally unaffected. The speech is jerking and peculiar, with alternation of pauses and of rapid enunciation of several words together. When the symptoms are well-developed the difficulty in walking increases to an entire disability, and in advanced cases there may be actual paralysis, both in the lower and upper extremities. There is no loss of control of the bladder and rectum. Sensory symptoms are of little prominence in Friedreich's ataxia. There are no trophic symptoms of moment, and muscular atrophy is usually not great even in well-developed cases. Vertigo is not infrequent. Salivation, disturbance of respiration, palpitation, and uncontrollable laughing are among rare symptoms. The intelligence is usually normal, although the vacuous expression and the difficulty in enunciation suggest the opposite of this.

Course and Prognosis.—The course is slowly onward, often with stationary periods. Occasionally the upper and lower limbs are affected almost simultaneously, and sometimes the speech as well. Generally, however, the upper extremities do not show involvement until from one to five years after the lower, and the speech about one and one-half years later still. To all this there are, however, many exceptions. In one of our cases seventeen years elapsed between the involvement of the lower and that of the upper limbs. The patient often reaches at last a state of comparative helplessness, and death may occur from asthenia or from some intercurrent disorder.

Diagnosis.—From *tabes dorsalis* the disease is distinguished by the characteristic uncertain gait, nystagmus, the early age of onset, and the family history; and by the absence of severe pain and of other sensory manifestations, pupillary symptoms, optic atrophy, and visceral disturbances. Friedreich's ataxia is frequently supposed to be *chorea*. The latter, however, is an acute disease of more sudden onset, which generally involves the arms first and most decidedly, and is lacking the club-foot, scoliosis and nystagmus of Friedreich's ataxia. *Disseminated sclerosis* usually develops later in life, the speech is scanning rather than irregular and jerking, the knee-jerks are increased, there is intention-tremor, the nystagmus is more extreme, spastic paralysis may develop, and the intellect is often affected. *Cerebellar tumor* gives a more typically drunken gait, and there are headache, decided vertigo and optic atrophy; while the tendon-reflexes are not abolished. The distinction from *hereditary cerebellar ataxia* will be considered below.

Treatment.—This is entirely unavailing and can be only symptomatic.

2. Hereditary Cerebellar Ataxia

Until the publication by Marie[24] in 1893, cases of this nature were generally classified under Friedreich's ataxia. It would appear that the two may be regarded as different types of the same disorder, and the clinical distinctions cannot be sharply drawn. In the one the spinal symptoms predominate (Friedreich's ataxia); in the other the cerebellar (cerebellar ataxia). In the type described by Marie there is a strong family tendency; the disease begins usually after the period of childhood; and the anatomical lesions are seen chiefly in the cerebellum. There are cases reported, however, in which both cord and cerebellum were involved. The **symptoms** are much the same as in Friedreich's ataxia (p. 967), except that the knee-jerks are increased; the gait is more drunken; oculomotor involvement is not uncommon; optic atrophy is frequent; derangements of sensation are more common, although still not frequent, and deterioration of the intellect is liable to occur. **Treatment** is unavailing.

3. Tabes Dorsalis

(Locomotor Ataxia)

This condition rarely appears in early life, but collected cases have been reported by Marburg,[25] Cantonnet,[26] Ferguson and Critchley,[27] and others. The majority of these have developed after puberty (*juvenile tabes*), yet cases have been seen as early as five years of age. Females are as frequently affected as males. Oftenest the syphilis upon which the disease depends is hereditary in origin, but sometimes it may have been acquired early in life. The **symptoms** are similar to those seen in adults, except that the onset is more indefinite, the characteristic ataxic gait is less marked, sensory manifestations are less prominent, reflexes may not be absent, and paralysis of the ocular muscles and loss of sphincter-control are somewhat less often seen. On the other hand, optic atrophy is unusually frequent and often the earliest symptom. Disturbances in urination are among early manifestations. Tabes and general paresis may be combined. The blood and spinal fluid will usually give a positive Wassermann reaction; and in the spinal fluid there is increase in globulin and cells, and the colloidal gold test may show a "syphilitic" curve. The **course** and **prognosis** are as in adults. The **diagnosis** is to be made from Freidreich's ataxia, this being a familial disorder, exhibiting nystagmus, disturbed speech, a prominence of ataxic symptoms and an absence of optic atrophy. The ataxia of hereditary cerebellar ataxia is more marked than in tabes, and the knee-jerks are normal or increased. Vigorous antisyphilitic **treatment** should be tried, including intraspinal injections of arsphenaminized serum (p. 440).

HEREDITARY SPASTIC PARAPLEGIA

Spastic paraplegia arises from numerous causes, as cerebral diseases, birth-injuries, spinal caries, tumors, spinal meningitis, etc. There exists, however, a distinct form in which the familial tendency is marked, as pointed out by Strumpell,[28] Newmark,[29] Erb,[30] Bayley,[31] Spiller,[32] Powdermaker,[33] and others. The disease usually begins early in life. The **lesions** consist in degeneration of the crossed pyramidal tracts; and sometimes to a slight extent of the direct cerebellar tracts and of the columns of Goll. It has been suggested that the **cause** may be an unknown intra-uterine condition; or that there may be a defect of the germ-plasma. The **symptoms** come on gradually, the first being increased reflexes and a spasticity of the lower extremities causing the foot to be pushed stiffly along the floor in walking. There is no loss of sensation, and the sphincters are not involved. A final inability to walk is not the rule. The arms are only exceptionally affected. Bulbar symptoms are absent and the intellect is normal. The **course** is prolonged, and although symptoms may reach their height comparatively rapidly they may then remain unchanged. The **diagnosis** from other conditions which produce paraplegia is made chiefly by the evidence of familial occurrence. The existence of intellectual defect points to spastic paraplegia of cerebral origin, and of bulbar symptoms to disseminated sclerosis. Systematic exercises may possibly be of benefit in overcoming the spasticity.

THE MUSCULAR ATROPHIES AND DYSTROPHIES

Although some of these appear to be primarily muscular diseases, others are spinal in origin, and others perhaps neural. The interrelationship of all seems so close that they may well be studied together.

The different types are conveniently divided into (*A*) *Spinal muscular atrophy* or *amyotrophy*, which may be subdivided into: (1) Amyotrophic lateral sclerosis; (2) Progressive muscular atrophy of the hand-type; and (3) the Werdnig-Hoffman type. (*B*) *Neural muscular atrophy.* (*C*) The *primary myopathies* or *muscular dystrophies*, consisting of a number of types presently to be considered. Intermediate forms undoubtedly occur, and no classification can be absolute. Many of the varieties have certain features in common, such as a distinct familial tendency and a slowly progressive course. Some of them are peculiarly characteristic of early life; others are seen principally or only in adult life.

A. Progressive Spinal Muscular Atrophy

1. Amyotrophic Lateral Sclerosis (*Charcot's*[34] *Type of Muscular Atrophy*).—Only a few cases of this beginning in childhood have been reported. In some of these there has been shown a decided familial tendency, several sisters or brothers having been attacked. In some cases the syndrome may be due to syphilis (Ostheimer, Wilson and Winkelman[35]). The pathologic **lesion** is a degeneration of the pyramidal tracts and of the anterior horns of the spinal cord. The **symptoms** in brief consist in an atrophic paralysis, yet with a spastic condition; the atrophy being seen especially in the arms, and the spastic manifestations in the legs. The loss of power and the spastic symptoms appear before any atrophy shows itself, this being in sharp contrast with the relations obtaining in the hand type of progressive muscular atrophy, in which the atrophy precedes the paralysis. Contractures develop, with pain on movement, increase of the tendon-reflexes, and fibrillary twitchings. The patient at last becomes helpless. Bulbar symptoms finally appear, with interference with speech and swallowing. The **course** of the disease is slow, lasting over several years, and the **prognosis** is unfavorable and uninfluenced by treatment.

2. Progressive Muscular Atrophy; Hand-type (*Duchenne-Aran Type*).—This malady was brought into prominence through the writings especially of Duchenne[36] and of Aran.[37] It is not common at any time of life, and is rare before puberty (Seidel[38]). Males are much more frequently attacked than females. A familial tendency is sometimes seen. The **lesions** consist in degeneration of the anterior horns of the spinal cord, with

secondary involvement of the nerve-roots and the muscles. The **symptoms** are characteristic. Atrophy appears first in the thenar eminences, then the hypothenar and the interossei, and extends thence to the forearms. Here it may cease; or may spread to the arms, shoulders, neck, back, and finally, late in the disease, to the lower extremities. The claw-like appearance of the hand is characteristic (*main en griffe*). Exceptionally the disease attacks other localities before the hands and arms. The fibrillary twitchings which the muscles exhibit, sometimes before atrophy is seen, constitute a very striking symptom. The faradic contractility disappears gradually in proportion to the amount of atrophy present; and in well-advanced cases there may be a reaction of degeneration. The tendon-reflexes are diminished or absent. The **course** is progressive, the wasting being only gradual, and perhaps some years passing before the lower extremities become involved. Finally the patient grows powerless and wasted to an excessive degree. The **diagnosis** from amyotrophic lateral sclerosis is made by the absence of spastic symptoms, and, still more important, by the fact that the atrophy precedes the paralysis, the latter being in proportion to the degree of the former. The differences between the two diseases are not always sharply defined, and some writers class them together. **Treatment** is without avail, but the malady is fatal only through complications; except in certain instances where the paralysis involves the tongue and the muscles of respiration.

3. The Werdnig-Hoffman Infantile Type of Progressive Muscular Atrophy.—This very unusual disorder, described by Werdnig,[39] Hoffmann,[40] and others, exhibits lesions similar to those seen in the Duchenne-Aran type just described, but has certain definite distinguishing clinical features. Parsons and Stanley[41] found but 21 well-authenticated cases in medical literature, and Ziehen[42] places the number at over 30. Lyon[43] reports 1 case. Foremost among the characteristics is the striking familial history. It begins usually in the 1st or sometimes the 2d year. The **lesions** consist especially in degeneration of the cells of the anterior horns throughout the whole of the cord. The anterior nerve-roots are also involved. There is no change in the lateral tract. The muscles and the motor nerves show extensive atrophy also. The **symptoms** develop first in the pelvic region or the trunk, and consist in progressive weakness and atrophy; and this spreads to the neck, shoulders, thighs, and last to the arms, hands and feet. The order is almost the reverse of that seen in the Duchenne-Aran type. The tendon-reflexes are abolished, the limbs are flaccid, and fibrillary twitchings are sometimes seen. The cranial nerves are not affected or but slightly so, the sensation and sphincters are not disturbed, the electrical contractility is much diminished or abolished, and the reaction of degeneration may sometimes be present. The extension and increase of the paralysis is rather rapid, and the patient soon becomes helpless, greatly wasted, and variously deformed; and death takes place usually in from one to five years through involvement of the respiratory muscles and consequent disease of the lungs, or through some other complication. The **diagnosis** is to be made from the Duchenne-Aran type especially by the familial occurrence, early age, and the sequence of symptoms. The two types are, however, very closely allied. From some forms of hereditary muscular dystrophy unattended by hypertrophy the diagnosis is difficult, but the course in the Werdnig-Hoffmann type is much more rapid and the onset earlier. Amyotonia congenita is distinguished especially by the still earlier age of onset, the much less degree of atrophy, the slower course, and the tendency to improvement sometimes seen. In progressive neural muscular atrophy the disease begins with distal rather than with proximal groups of muscles.

B. Progressive Neural Muscular Atrophy

(Peroneal Type)

To this form the title "Type of Charcot-Marie[44]-Tooth"[45] is often applied. It is an infrequent variety, of a very positive familial and hereditary nature, occurring sometimes through several generations (Herringham[46]). It is rather more common in males, and develops oftenest in early childhood, but may first appear in later childhood or even after puberty. It seems to occupy a midway position between the spinal muscular atrophies and the muscular dystrophies. The **lesions** are not certainly established, and those described have varied with the case. The most frequent are degeneration of certain of the nerves, with interstitial changes; simple atrophy of the muscles; and sclerosis of the posterior columns, and to a slight extent of the lateral tracts and the anterior horns. Not all of these changes have been present in every case examined; and which of them may be primary is not yet determined (Potts and Wilson[47]). The title "neural" is not, therefore, strictly speaking, applicable. The first **symptoms** in typical cases consist in wasting and loss of power in the peroneal muscle-group and the extensors of the toes of both legs; with consequent walking upon the outer side of the foot, foot-drop, high-stepping gait, and later club-foot in the equinus or equino-varus position. The atrophy spreads to the rest of the muscles below the knee, and the ankle-jerks are diminished; but the knee-jerks are unaffected unless the muscles of the thigh become involved. Fibrillary twitchings are common. The electrical response is diminished, and there may be a partial reaction of degeneration. In some cases there are such sensory disturbances as pain, hyperesthesia, or anesthesia. Sometimes antedating or simultaneously with the involvement of the legs, but oftener from one to four years later, the disease may appear in the hands,—with the production of the claw-hand,—and perhaps in the forearms also. The power of walking is retained, since the muscles of the thigh are involved only late if at all. The trunk, shoulders, arms, neck and face usually escape entirely. An Argyll Robertson pupil may be present. Mental deterioration occurs in some cases. The course of the disease is very slow and often with long intermissions; and the prognosis for recovery is unfavorable, although little change may take place for years. The **diagnosis** is to be made from progressive muscular atrophy of the hand-type by the commencement in, and limitation early to, the lower extremities, and the marked familial tendency. The Werdnig-Hoffmann type begins earlier, attacks the legs and pelvis first instead of the feet, and runs a more rapid course. The muscular dystrophies oftenest commence in the muscles of the trunk or shoulder-girdle, not in the muscles below the knee, and disturbances of sensation do not occur. Multiple neuritis produces much greater sensory disorder; has no familial history; if beginning in the feet soon shows itself elsewhere as well; is of much more rapid development and course, and offers a more favorable prognosis. **Treatment** is of no avail in restoring damage once done; but much may often be accomplished in preserving muscles as yet unaffected and maintaining the ability to walk, by the employment of massage and electricity and of suitable orthopedic apparatus, tenotomy and the like.

C. The Muscular Dystrophies

The remaining forms of muscular atrophy are to be classed together under the title "Muscular Dystrophies," or "Primary Myopathies." The different varieties have many points in common distinguishing them from the atrophies already described. All begin before adult life, and a familial or hereditary tendency is often observed. Atrophy is decided in all, although a pseudohypertrophy or actual hypertrophy is an early and prominent symptom in one variety. The disease is first manifested in other regions of the body than the distal portion of the extremities; fibrillary twitching, qualitative electrical changes, and disturbances of sensation are absent; and in typical cases the nervous system does not exhibit lesions. The principal forms are (1) the pseudohypertrophic, (2) the simple atrophic, (3) the facio-scapulo-humeral, and (4) the juvenile type. All these forms are practically one disease with variations of localization.

1. Pseudohypertrophic Type of Muscular Dystrophy (*Pseudohypertrophic Paralysis*). **Etiology.**—This is one of the more frequent varieties. Hough[48] estimates the incidence of the condition in the New England States to be 6 per 100,000 of the total population. Although isolated cases may be met with, the hereditary and familial tendency is very marked, the inheritance coming through the mother, herself often not a sufferer from the disease. Males are more often affected. The majority of cases begin in early childhood; seldom after puberty; sometimes apparently in infancy.

Pathologic Anatomy.—The lesions consist at first of hypertrophy of the individual muscle-fibers, at least in certain muscles. This is followed by atrophy, with loss of striation, vacuole-formation, increase of muscle-nuclei, and fatty degeneration. The increase of size in some of the muscles at first is due in part to actual hypertrophy, but later depends upon increase of connective tissue and infiltration by fat. This description of the lesions applies to all the muscular dystrophies, with the exception that in those of types other than the one now under consideration the lipomatosis and connective-tissue hypertrophy are not so great, and no visible macroscopic pseudohypertrophy is produced. It is ordinarily stated that the muscular dystrophies exhibit no lesion of the spinal cord or the nerves, although in some advanced cases changes in the anterior horns have been found which are perhaps of a secondary nature. Kuré[49] presents some evidence that the muscular dystrophies in general are caused by lesions of the various parts of the autonomic nervous system, these being in the brain, along the course of the nerves, or in their endings.

Symptoms.—The onset is insidious. Sometimes the gait has always been unsteady; but generally there develops slowly increasing weakness in the legs in children previously normal. The gait is waddling, and while standing there is lordosis, with the trunk very rigid or inclined backward. The characteristic manner of rising from the floor is shown in the accompanying illustrations (Fig. 217). With the weakness there is a symmetrical increase in the size of certain of the muscles, usually especially well seen in the calves (Fig. 218). The glutei, too, are often large, and occasionally also other muscle-groups of the legs. In the upper extremities an enlargement of the infraspinati is frequent, and often also of the supraspinati, deltoids, and triceps. On the other hand, atrophy is commonly observed in other muscles, notably the flexors of the thigh, latissimi dorsi, serrati, biceps, and the lower part of the major pectorals. A hypermobility of the shoulder develops on passive movement, shown especially by the manner in which the arms and shoulders slip upward and through the examiner's hands placed in the armpits in the attempt to lift the child. The distribution of atrophy and of hypertrophy detailed represents the general rule, but other muscle-groups may be involved. Sometimes even the tongue may be hypertrophied, but, as a rule, the face is not involved. We[50] had under our care a patient dying in adolescence where extreme wasting was almost universal (Fig. 219), except that the tongue was phenomenally large.

The large muscles, although appearing powerful, are in reality weak. The tendon-reflexes are normal at first, but grow less active and finally disappear. Superficial reflexes are disturbed; fibrillary contractions are absent; electrical response gradually diminishes, but there is no reaction of degeneration; sensation is normal; and the sphincters are unaffected. The intellect is usually normal. Several authors have reported hypoglycemia, and Magee[51] found that in a case of extreme muscular dystrophy there was inability to convert creatine into creatinine.

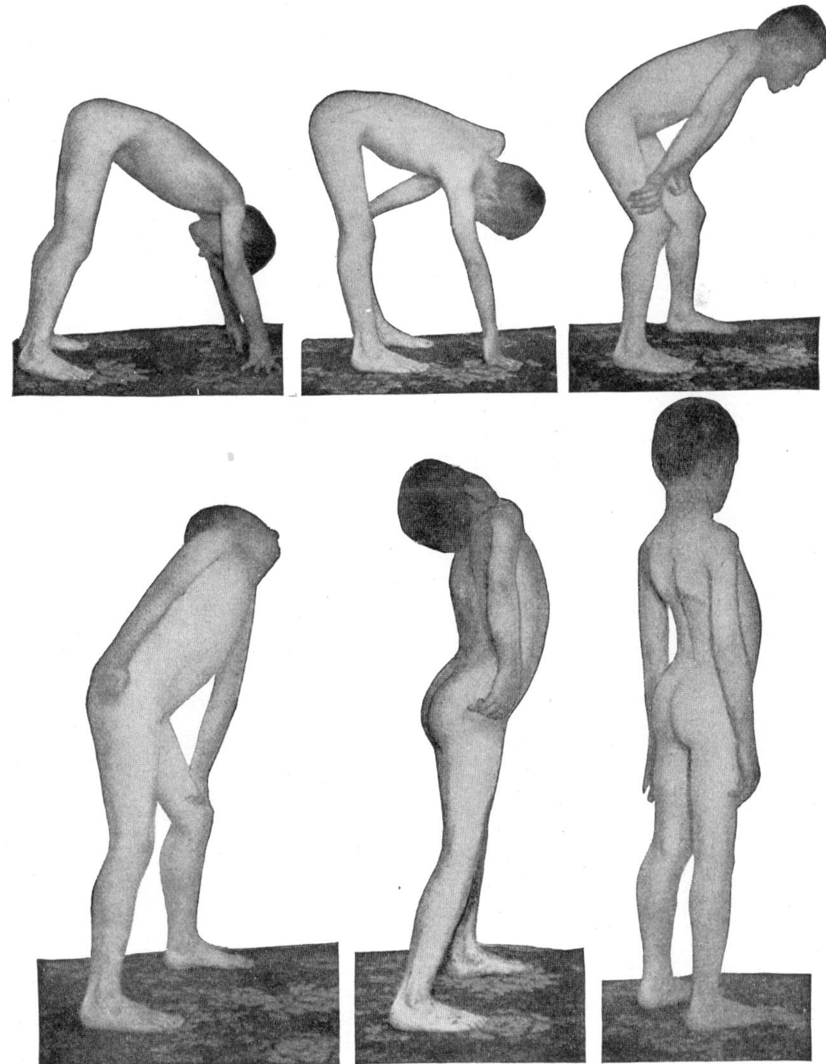

Fig. 217.—Method of rising from the floor in pseudohypertrophic muscular dystrophy. (*Church and Peterson, Nervous and Mental Diseases*, 1914, 421.)

Course and Prognosis.—The course is slow, often with periods of intermission. It is more rapid in cases developing early, and generally advances more slowly after puberty. There is gradual loss of power, and in long-continued cases great wasting of the muscles of the limbs; all signs of pseudohypertrophy disappear; and various deformities result. Death is liable to occur from some complicating affection before adult life is reached.

Diagnosis.—In far-advanced cases the diagnosis of this type of dystrophy must be made from the earlier history. In the early stage the awkwardness shown in rising from the floor is suggestive, but this can occur in other diseases, as spinal caries, or in other forms of muscular dystrophy.

2. Simple Hereditary Atrophic Type (*Hereditary Muscular Atrophy, Leyden*[52]*-Möbius*[53]).—This less common form has a remarkable familial and hereditary tendency. It begins usually at from eight to ten years of age. The earliest symptoms are atrophy and weakness in the muscles of the back and lower extremities. There are lordosis and difficulty in walking. Evidences of pseudohypertrophy are never seen, but in other respects the symptoms are very similar to those present in the pseudohypertrophic form.

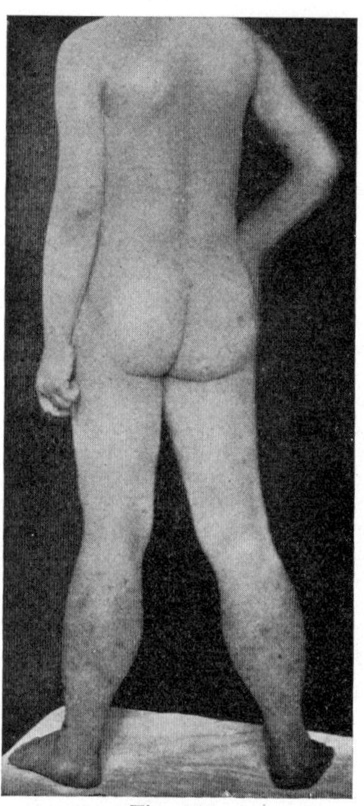

Fig. 218.

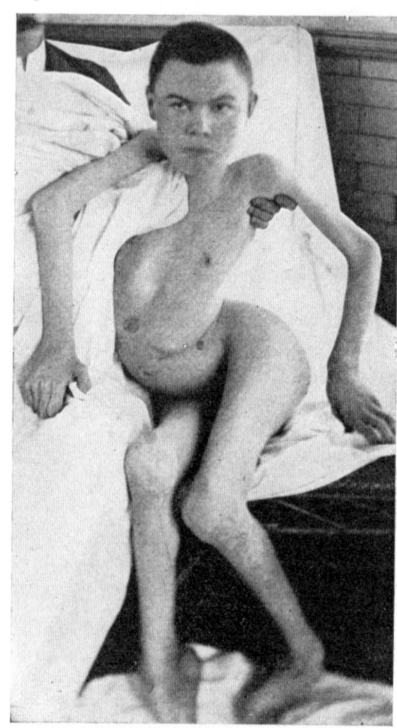

Fig. 219.

Fig. 218.—Pseudohypertrophic muscular dystrophy. Showing enlargement of the calves. (*Courtesy of Dr. Howard C. Carpenter.*)

Fig. 219.—Pseudohypertrophic muscular dystrophy, advanced case. Boy of fifteen and one-half years, in whom the disease began at about the age of seven years. (*Griffith, Univ. Med. Magaz.*, 1889, I, 310.)

The disease advances slowly, involving finally the muscles of the upper extremities, as in the case of the pseudohypertrophic type. It is questionable, indeed, whether the two should not be classed together, cases of Leyden's type being merely those in which the pseudohypertrophy has been transitory and overlooked.

3. Facio-scapulo-humeral Type (*Type of Landouzy and Déjérine*).—Although previously described by Duchenne,[54] this infrequent form of myopathy generally bears the names of Landouzy and Déjérine.[55] The familial and hereditary characteristics are usually prominent. The disease begins oftenest in childhood; sometimes as early as two years of age, or possibly even before this. The changes are seen first in the facial muscles, and earliest here in the orbicularis oris and orbicularis palpebrarum. As the disease develops the face becomes peculiarly impassive and expressionless, the eyelids cannot be tightly closed, the eyebrows lifted, or the forehead

wrinkled. There may be difficulty in sucking, but not in chewing or swallowing; while older children cannot whistle, and speech may be indistinct. The muscles undergo marked atrophy, although the lips do not suffer from this but are prominent and thickened, the upper extending beyond the lower (*tapir-mouth*). The progress of the disease may stop here for a while, generally for from five to fifteen years or longer but sometimes for a short time only, before it advances to the muscles of the shoulder-girdle and the upper arms. It spares for the most part the infraspinati, supraspinati, and the muscles of the forearm. Later those of the pelvis and lower extremities may become involved. The atrophy of the shoulder-girdle causes the scapulae to stand out in wing-form; but other deformities, as of the hands and feet, are seen only in very long-continued and advanced cases. Fibrillary contractions are absent. There is diminished electrical contractility but no reaction of degeneration. The **course** is one of the slowest seen in the muscular dystrophies, and as a result, little, if any difficulty in walking or in rising from the floor is usually observed.

4. Juvenile Type of Muscular Atrophy (*Erb's Type; Scapulohumeral Type*).—Under this title are included cases as first described by Erb,[56] in which the paralysis, usually symmetrical, begins in the shoulder-girdle, leaving the face unaffected. It is probably the least frequent variety. Hereditary and familial relationships are present as in other forms. It begins oftenest at, or soon after, puberty or early in adult life. The scapulae become markedly winged from the affection of the serrati magni and trapezii, and there is difficulty in raising the arms above the head. Other muscles involved are the pectorals, latissimi dorsi, rhomboids, and later the muscles of the upper arm. All the affected muscles are not only paralyzed but atrophic; while the deltoids, infraspinati and supraspinati are not affected until very late if at all, and are even hypertrophic. The muscles of the forearms and hands escape. Disturbances of sensation, fibrillary contractions, and reaction of degeneration are absent. The tendon-reflexes are at first unaltered; later diminished. Occasionally the pelvis and thighs are attacked simultaneously with, or before, the upper portion of the body, the muscles affected being especially the quadriceps extensors, the adductors, and the iliac and psoas groups. As a result the patient is unable to flex the thigh easily upon the abdomen. The **course** of the disease is slow, often with periods of long intermissions which perhaps last several years. The **diagnosis** rests upon the age of development and the muscular regions first attacked. The disease is closely allied to the facio-scapulo-humeral type, differing from it in the later age at which it appears and in the freedom from atrophy of the face.

Treatment of Muscular Dystrophy.—This is sustaining and orthopedic in nature. Apparatus should be used when necessary to prevent deformity. Electricity is of some slight value. Among various therapies which have been recommended are the employment of thyroid, pineal, and pituitary products; calcium lactate; high vitamin-containing diets; and epinephrine and pilocarpine. None of these has been proven to be of actual curative value, although the combined use of adrenaline and pilocarpine has seemed to be of temporary benefit in some instances (Kuré and Okinaka,[57] Hough,[48] Lewin[58]).

AMYOTONIA CONGENITA

(Myatonia Congenita)

The close affinity of this disease, first described by Oppenheim,[59] to the muscular dystrophies and possibly to diseases of the spinal cord makes it advisable to consider it here. Its exact relationships are not yet understood. The condition should not be confused with myotonia congenita (p. 988).

In 1910 and 1911, we[60,61] collected 60 cases including 1 of our own, and instances have since been reported and collected by Reuben,[62] Faber,[63] Reh,[64] Haushalter,[65] Katz,[66] Nielsen,[67] Bielschowsky,[68] Moe,[69] Gurdjian,[70] Tuthill and Levy,[71] and others.

Etiology and Pathologic Anatomy.—Hereditary influence appears to be absent, although familial cases are reported by Pearce,[72] Allaban,[73] Katz,[66] Gurdjian,[70] and others. Nearly always the disease is a congenital

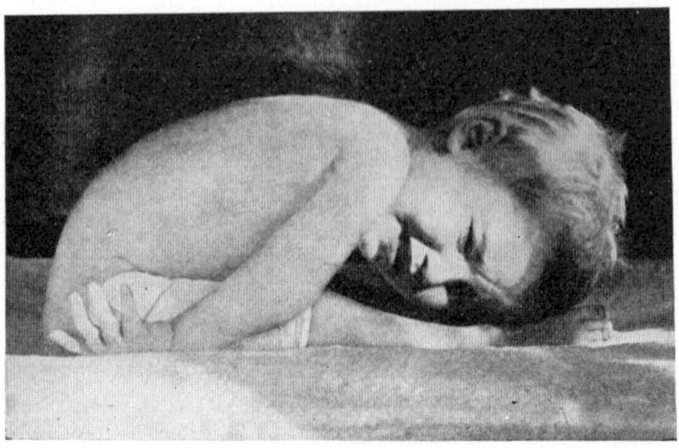

Fig. 220.—Amyotonia congenita. Boy of fifteen months, in the Children's Ward of the Hospital of the University of Pennsylvania. Admitted Dec. 8. Never able to sit up or hold the head erect. Voluntary movement of the limbs very slight, moderate passive hypermobility. Improved decidedly under treatment, but developed pneumonia and died the following October.

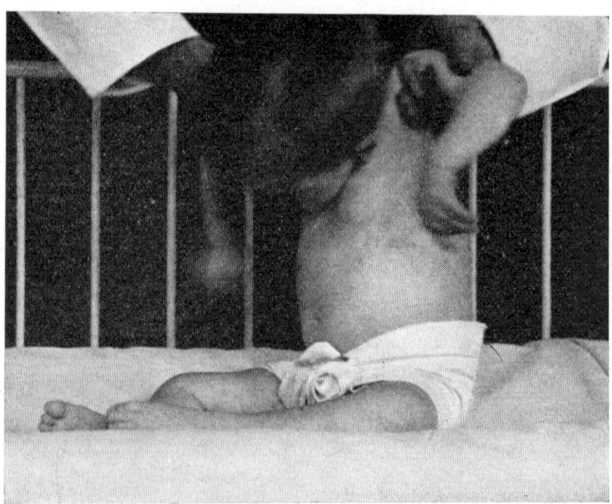

Fig. 221.—Amyotonia congenita. Same case as in Fig. 220. Shows hypermobility at the shoulder-joint.

one. The lesions vary considerably. It is maintained by Krabbe,[74] Slauk,[75] Leenhardt and Sentis,[76] Tuthill and Levy,[71] and others that there is no difference pathologically between amyotonia and the Werdnig-Hoffmann type of muscular dystrophy (p. 970). Batten[77] placed amyotonia among the dystrophies. The changes in the muscles are usually slight, although there have been reported lipomatosis, sclerosis, diminution of muscle-fibers, and absence of the motor plate endings. In some cases there have been found changes in the anterior horn cells of the cord, chromatolysis of ganglion cells, and atrophy of the anterior nerve-roots.

Grinker[78] claims that in the Werdnig-Hoffmann type of dystrophy there is actual degeneration of the ganglion-cells and neuronophagia, whereas in amyotonia congenita there is paucity of cells in the anterior horn; and Holmes[79] and others favor the theory of retarded embryological development in certain muscle-cells and in the anterior horns. There has been observed in amyotonia a lowered excretion of creatinine, a normal one of uric acid and phosphorus, and a normal retention of calcium (Spriggs,[80] Gittings and Pemberton,[81] Ziegler and Pearce[82]).

Symptoms.—These consist of remarkable flaccidity and loss of power, mostly in the lower extremities, but extending more or less over the body. The weakness may be so great that the limbs are powerless except for slight movements of the fingers and toes. Few patients retain the ability to stand. Any movements possible are made with peculiar slowness, yet without any ataxia; there is often seen a great degree of passive hypermobility of the joints (Figs. 220 and 221); sensation is not disturbed; electrical contractility is much diminished or absent, but without reaction of degeneration; the sphincters are not involved; the patellar and other reflexes are usually diminished or absent; the face is rarely attacked; intelligence is normal; there are no fibrillary contractions; the muscles do not appear to be atrophied, although they are flaccid and soft; general nutrition is well-preserved; and contractures of some of the muscles are not infrequent. This description applies to typical cases. Mild degrees of amyotonia are not infrequent, but it is doubtful whether many of these are instances of the disease. On the other hand, probably to be classed as mild instances of amyotonia congenita are certain cases in which walking or holding the head erect is greatly delayed, but in which there is not the widespread lack of muscular power described.

Course and Prognosis.—There is no tendency for the condition to grow worse, and in a number of instances decided improvement has been seen. Since cases are extremely rare in adult life, the patients must either have recovered or, much more probably, died in childhood.

Diagnosis.—The disease is to be distinguished from the Werdnig-Hoffman type of dystrophy by the absence of progressive advance or of marked familial disposition, and the remarkable atony of the muscles without visible atrophy. Milder cases of amyotonia might be confounded with mental defect or with rickets, although the progress of the case should remove doubt. It should be remembered that many asthenic conditions show marked secondary myatonia, and it is present also in the ataxias, paralytic conditions, and the like.

Treatment.—This consists in the employment of electricity and massage; although these are of little avail. Thyroid extract has been recommended.

References

1. Fürst, Gerhardt's Handb. d. Kinderkr., 1880, **5**, 1, 1, 347. 2. Wien. med. Blätter, 1884, **7**, 804. 3. Am. J. M. Sc., 1928, **175**, 365. 4. J.A.M.A., 1929, **92**, 877. 5. Medicine, 1927, **6**, 41. 6. Trans. Obst. Soc. London, 1892, **33**, 203. 7. Am. J. Dis. Child., 1920, **19**, 473. 8. Am. J. Dis. Child., 1923,**26**, 242. 9. Arch. Neurol. and Psychiat., 1926, **14**, 742. 10. Jahrb. f. Kinderh., 1909, **69**, 422. 11. Pepper's Syst. of Med., 1886, **5**, 1090. 12. Beitr. z. Klin. der Rüchenmarks-und Wirbeltumoren, 1898, 99. 13. Am. J. Dis. Child., 1928, **36**, 1184. 14. Arch. Neurol. and Psychiat., 1922, **8**, 502. 15. Pediatria, 1920, **28**, 226. 16. Bruns, Cramer and Ziehen, Handb. der Nervenkrank. im Kindersalter, 1912, 456. 17. Boston M. and S. J., 1922, **186**, 45. 18. Gaz. hebdom., 1859, **6**, 472. 19. J.A.M.A., 1921, **76**, 260. 20. Brain, 1905, **28**, 484. 21. Virchow's Archiv., 1863, **26**, 391; 443; **27**, 1; 1876, **68**, 145; 1877, **70**, 140. 22. Griffith, Tr. Coll. Physicians, Philadelphia, 1888, **10**, 196. 23. Lehrb. d. Nervenkrankh., 1st Ed., 1840, 795. 24. La sem. méd., 1893, **13**, 444. 25. Wien. klin. Wchnschr., 1903, **16**, 1295. 26. Arch. d'opht., 1907, **27**, 708. 27. Brit. J. Child. Dis., 1930, **27**, 1. 28. Arch. f. Psychiat., 1880, **10**, 711; Deutsch. Ztschr. f. Nervenheilk, 1893, **3**, 495. 29. Am. J. M.

Sc., 1893, **105**, 432. 30. Deutsch. Ztschr. f. Nervenheilk., 1895, **6**, 137. 31. J. Nerv. and Ment. Dis., 1897, **24**, 697. 32. Philadelphia M. J., 1902, **9**, 1129. 33. Am. J. Dis. Child., 1930, **39**, 148. 34. Charcot and Joffroy, Arch. de physiol. norm. et path., 1869, **2**, 344. 35. Am. J. M. Sc., 1924, **167**, 835. 36. Atrophie musculaire avec transformation graisseuse, 1849. Ref. Duchenne L'electrisation localisée, 1855, 814. 37. Arch. gén. de méd., 1850, **24**, 5. 38. Gerhardt's Handb. d. Kinderkr., 1889, **5**, 2, 9; 10. 39. Arch. f. Psychiat., 1890, **22**, 437. 40. Deutsch. Ztschr. f. Nervenheilk., 1893, **3**, 427. 41. Brain, 1912, **35**, 50. 42. Bruns, Cramer and Ziehen, Handb. der Nervenkrank. im Kindersalter, 1912, 415. 43. South. M. J., 1929, **22**, 839. 44. Rev. de méd., 1886, **6**, 97. 45. The Peroneal Type of Progressive Muscular Atrophy, Thesis, Cambridge, 1886. 46. Brain, 1888, **11**, 230. 47. Arch. Neurol. and Psychiat., 1923, **9**, 431. 48. J. Bone and Joint Surg., 1931, **13**, 825. 49. Lancet, 1928, **1**, 441. 50. Griffith, Univ. Med. Mag., 1889, **1**, 310. 51. Am. J. Dis. Child., 1932, **43**, 19. 52. Rückensmark's Krankheiten, 1876, **2**, 2, 525. 53. Volkmann's Sammlung, 1879, Intern. Med., No. 171. 54. L'électrisation localisée, 1855, 328; 833; Arch. gén. de méd., 1868, **11**, 421. 55. Rev. de méd., 1885, **5**, 81. 56. Ziemssen's Handb. d. allg. Therap., 1882, **3**, 389; Deutsch. Arch. f. klin. Med., 1884, **34**, 467. 57. Klin. Wchnschr., 1930, **9**, 1168. 58. J.A.M.A., 1926, **87**, 399. 59. Monatschr. f. Psychiat. u. Neurol., 1900, **8**, 232. 60. Griffith, Arch. f. Kinderh., 1910, **54**, 241. 61. Griffith and Spiller, Am. J. M. Sc., 1911, **142**, 165. 62. Arch. Int. Med., 1917, **20**, 657. 63. Am. J. Dis. Child., 1917, **13**, 305. 64. Rev. méd. de la Suisse rom., 1920, **40**, 247. 65. Arch. de méd d. enf., 1920, **23**, 133. 66. Monatschr. f. Kinderh., 1927, **35**, 517; Arch. f. Kinderh., 1928, **85**, 161. 67. Am. J. Dis. Child., 1928, **35**, 82. 68. J. f. Psychol. u. Neurol., 1929, **38**, 199. 69. Norsk. Mag. f. Laegevidensk., 1930, **91**, 1392. 70. Arch. Neurol. and Psychiat., 1930, **24**, 52. 71. Am. J. Dis. Child., 1931, **41**, 591. 72. Am. J. Dis. Child., 1920, **20**, 393. 73. J.A.M.A., 1924, **83**, 842. 74. Brain, 1920, **43**, 166. 75. Deutsch. Ztschr. f. Nervenheilk., 1920, **68**, 1. 76. Arch. de méd d. enf., 1921, **24**, 137. 77. Quart. J. Med., 1910, **3**, 313. 78. Arch. Neurol. and Psychiat., 1927, **18**, 982. 79. Am. J. Dis. Child., 1920, **20**, 405. 80. Quart. J. Med., 1907, **1**, 63. 81. Am. J. M. Sc., 1912, **144**, 732. 82. J. Biol. Chem., 1920, **42**, 581.

CHAPTER VII

DISEASES OF THE PERIPHERAL NERVES

In this connection will be considered certain disturbances of the nerves themselves, omitting those in which the primary cause is some disorder of the brain or spinal cord.

A. Polyneuritis

(Multiple Neuritis; Toxic Neuritis)

Etiology.—With the exception of the neuritis following diphtheria (p. 343), this is a decidedly uncommon disease in early life. We have not seen over a dozen cases in children. It may, however, occur even in infancy. No reference is made here to the neural form of muscular atrophy (p. 971) or to the neuritic type of poliomyelitis (p. 392). Factors of various sorts may be operative. (1) *Primary causes* include such agents as over-exertion and exposure to cold. Some cases are classed as "rheumatic," although it is questionable whether rheumatism has any influence. In some instances no cause can be discovered. (2) *Toxic causes* include arsenic, lead, and alcohol. Arsenical neuritis may follow the continued administration of this drug in the treatment of syphilis or chorea; or may rarely occur in childhood through chronic intoxication by arsenic from wallpaper, carpets, and the like. Plumbic neuritis occurs less frequently in early life than later, but the poison may be ingested by children when present in cakes, candies, medicines, drinking-water, and paint on cribs or toys. Alcohol is a rare cause in childhood. Neuritis occurring in cachectic conditions and that following injections of foreign protein can be classed as toxic. (3) *Post-infectious* neuritis may develop after any of the infectious diseases, especially diphtheria. Epidemics of multiple neuritis are probably in many instances due to poliomyelitis, and in others to a group-exposure to one of the several toxic factors mentioned above.

Pathologic Anatomy.—The lesions are both inflammatory and degenerative. Many cases stop short of serious destructive change, and complete restitution occurs. The changes in localized neuritis are often greater than in the multiple form. The degree of regeneration varies with the severity of the lesion and its duration. Accompanying the neuritis there is in some cases slight degeneration in the anterior horns of the spinal cord, apparently secondary or appearing simultaneously. Atrophic changes develop in the muscles supplied by the affected nerves.

Symptoms.—These vary largely with the cause and the regions affected.

1. Acute Primary Polyneuritis.—The onset is sometimes rapid but oftener gradual; two to four weeks being required for full development. The earliest manifestations are a symmetrical weakness and possibly pain in the extremities, especially below the knee. Constitutional symptoms may be present or absent. There is foot-drop, with a characteristic high-steppage gait. The forearms may be attacked simultaneously with the legs, or oftener later, and wrist-drop develop. The muscles atrophy; the tendon-reflexes, and generally the cutaneous also, are weakened or abolished; electrical contractility is diminished; reaction of degeneration is often present; the sphincters are not affected; contractures may develop; and ataxia and tremor may occur. In some instances ataxia is more prominent than paralysis. Paralysis is of the flaccid type, and may advance to a flail-like condition of the joints. In severe cases it may be widespread and even involve the muscles of respiration or the cranial nerves. Sensory disturbances consist of pain, hyperesthesia, paresthesia, or less often anesthesia. These are usually most marked early in the attack and may be largely absent. The disturbance involves the cutaneous sensibility to pain, the temperature-sense and the muscle-sense. Trophic conditions, as edema, glossy skin, and sweating are sometimes seen. The **course** is often several months, and sometimes much shorter or longer. The **prognosis** is usually entirely favorable, except in cases dependent upon diphtheria. Persistence of atrophy and paralysis is uncommon. There is a tendency for an attack of neuritis to recur, perhaps several times. This is, however, especially rare in children (Sereni[1]).

2. Toxic Neuritis.—In *arsenical cases* paralysis and pain are oftenest limited to the extremities, especially the lower; ataxia is usually prominent; and trophic disturbances are frequent. *Plumbic neuritis* in children attacks the legs first, and then the forearms. The supernator longus and abductors of the thumb usually escape. In *alcoholic neuritis* the paralysis spreads over the body, and ataxia and sensory manifestations are prominent. The **prognosis** in toxic neuritis is generally favorable. Permanent paralysis seldom remains. Death may occur from other effects of the poison.

3. Post-infectious Neuritis.—Post-diphtheritic paralysis has been considered elsewhere (p. 343), but here may be mentioned the tendency of this form to involve the muscles of the throat, especially the palate; the muscles of the eye; the extremities; the heart; and the respiration. The patellar reflex is almost invariably lost; atrophy occurs; but pain in the nerve trunks is absent. Neuritis after other infectious diseases is uncommon. Malaria occasionally produces it. The **prognosis** of post-infectious neuritis is usually good, except in the event of severe cardiac or respiratory paralysis, in which a fatal ending is frequent.

Diagnosis of Polyneuritis.—The principal diagnostic indications are the combination of sensory and motor symptoms in the same region;

muscular atrophy; and altered electrical conditions, especially the reaction of degeneration. The disease might be confounded with *poliomyelitis.* The onset in the latter is, however, usually more sudden; the general nervous symptoms more severe; the distribution is not so widespread nor so symmetrical; the affection does not begin in the terminal portions of the limbs; and there is less localized tenderness and pain along the nerve-trunks. Cases occur, however, in which the diagnosis is difficult; and it is probable that some of the epidemics of multiple neuritis should be classed as poliomyelitis. *Landry's paralysis* shows a progressive ascending advance, while polyneuritis involves parts far removed from each other, as, for instance, the upper and lower extremities with the trunk still unaffected. *Compression-myelitis* gives pain and paralysis, but the tendon-reflexes are increased. The *muscular dystrophies* are of slower onset and sensory disturbances are not common. *Neural muscular atrophy* exhibits foot-drop, as does often multiple neuritis; but there is less marked sensory disturbance in the former and the extension of the process is slow. *Infantile scurvy* has occasioned confusion on account of the pseudoparalysis and the pain which are present (p. 458). The distinguishing of the different forms of polyneuritis from each other has been sufficiently indicated.

Treatment.—The cause of the condition must be removed if possible. Apart from this the treatment is entirely symptomatic. The pain is to be relieved by the application of heat, or, when required, by the internal administration of analgesics. Heat must be applied cautiously in order not to produce burns in a skin perhaps partly anesthetic. Counterirritation is not advisable. Quinine should be employed in malarial cases. Later in the disease, galvanic or faradic electricity and massage are advisable. Contractures are to be guarded against by splints or bandages. In diphtheritic paralysis the element of cardiac weakness must receive first consideration, and any sudden movement of the body avoided. Full doses of strychnine, considered a favorite remedy in diphtheritic neuritis, may be of service in other forms.

B. Localized Peripheral Neuritis

Only those forms of localized neuritis will be considered which are of importance in early life.

1. Facial Paralysis (*Bell's Palsy*). **Etiology and Pathology.**—This is one of the commonest varieties. The cause may be trauma of the facial nerve incurred during birth from the pressure by forceps, or there may have been intra-uterine compression of the nerve if the head of the fetus has been held against its shoulder or against some maternal bony prominence. Surgical operations, as the removal of cervical glands, may injure the nerve; or the pressure of an inflamed parotid or lymphatic gland may produce a neuritis. An important cause is exposure to chilling, instances of this sort being often called "rheumatic." Some cases appear to depend upon foci of infection in the tonsils, nasal sinuses, or elsewhere. With all these causes the injury is peripheral to the stylomastoid foramen. Within the aqueduct of Fallopius the nerve may be compressed by caries of the petrous bone as a result of disease of the middle ear. Within the cranium the nerve may be injured by pressure of tumors, a basilar meningitis, or other disease of the base of the brain. In some congenital cases there has been found agenesis of the nucleus of the seventh nerve or of its root or trunk (Bonar and Owens[2]). The **lesions** are those of neuritis of any sort. (See Polyneuritis, p. 979.)

Symptoms.—These vary with the position of the lesion. The degree of paralysis due to compression by obstetrical forceps depends upon the point where the nerve was pressed upon. Operations for removal of cervical glands affect only the lower branches of the nerve. Rheumatic neuritis and that the result of disease of the middle-ear involve, partially or completely, the whole nerve-trunk before branching occurs. In well-marked cases the forehead on the affected side cannot be wrinkled, nor can the eye be closed, the mouth put in position for whistling, or the edge of the nostril raised. The cheek on this side is flabby and smooth; and on efforts at smiling or at showing the teeth the mouth is drawn to the healthy side while the other side remains unmoved. The facial nerve being purely motor, there is no disturbance of sensation. In lesions up to and including the nucleus in the pons there is great or complete loss of faradic contractility, and soon of galvanic response as well. Later both may return, the latter then showing the reaction of degeneration. Lesions above the nucleus are not productive of these changes. In cases due to intra-uterine pressure other local deformities or atrophies may be present. In some cases the paralysis may be bilateral.

Course and Prognosis.—In paralysis dependent upon birth-lesions recovery generally is complete in from one to two weeks; although more serious cases may continue longer or persist permanently. In instances due to exposure to cold, recovery is the rule after a few weeks or months. Neuritis following middle-ear disease has a longer course with periods of temporary improvement, and the ultimate recovery is more uncertain. Prognosis is unfavorable when the condition depends upon intracranial lesions. Recovery is slow after injury by operations, but generally is finally complete.

Diagnosis.—Paralysis in all the branches of the facial nerve indicates a peripheral lesion; while only the lower branches may be peripherally affected by operation on the neck, or centrally by a lesion above the pontine nucleus. In the latter case there is no reaction of degeneration, and, if the lesion is at the base of the brain, other cranial nerves, especially the auditory, may be affected. When the lesion is in the pons, paralysis of the face is usually complete and hemiplegia generally present also. Lesions below the stylomastoid foramen have no attending disturbances of taste, hearing, or of salivary secretion. This is true also when the nerve is diseased within the canal below the departure of the chorda tympani; but where, in addition, the posterior auricular branch of the nerve is involved. If the lesion is in the region of the chorda tympani there are disturbance of taste and diminution of salivary secretion. If the portion above this, but below the geniculate ganglion, is affected there is also abnormal acuteness of hearing. A lesion of the geniculate ganglion shows, besides these symptoms, disturbance of lacrimation and perhaps paralysis of the palate.

A facial palsy which is part of poliomyelitis usually shows paralysis elsewhere, but we have seen it practically the only symptom remaining after poliomyelitis.

Treatment.—When the cause is entirely cerebral, little can be done. When disease of the ear is at fault, prompt treatment for this condition is indicated. In cases depending upon exposure to cold the iodides may be given, although most cases recover in any event. Later a weak galvanic current may be applied, if needed.

2. Obstetrical Paralysis (*Neuritis of the Brachial Plexus; Erb's Paralysis*). **Etiology.**—This is oftenest associated with difficult and prolonged labors (most frequently in primiparae) which have been manually assisted. The majority are vertex-presentations, although some are breech- and foot-presentations (Stransky,[3] Sever[4]). It has been claimed that, allowing for the greater frequency of vertex-presentations, relatively the larger number of cases occur in breech-presentations, but Sever's figures do not support this. The **lesions** may be produced by pressure of the forceps on the nerves in the neck; by a finger or traction hook pulling

in the axilla; or, in breech presentation, by pressure above the clavicles, or efforts at bringing the arms down.

Symptoms.—The paralysis is flaccid and usually unilateral. Oftenest the upper portion of the brachial plexus upon one side is involved (*Erb's*[5] *paralysis*), especially the fifth and sixth cervical nerves. There results paralysis especially of the deltoid, biceps, brachialis anticus, and supinator longus, and often also the supraspinatus, infraspinatus, supinator brevis, and teres minor. All the muscles may be affected, or only some of them. In milder instances the condition may not be discovered for some weeks. The arm, oftener the right, is rotated inward, the forearm pronated, and the palm of the hand directed outward (Fig. 222). The forearm cannot be voluntarily flexed at the elbow, but if passively flexed can be extended by the patient. The movements of the muscles of the forearm and of the fingers are unaffected. Sensory disturbances, if present, are limited to moderate anesthesia of the shoulder and outer side of the upper arm. The extremity is colder than normal. The Moro embrace reflex is absent (p. 46). Atrophy of the muscles develops in a few weeks. The electrical contractility is diminished, and the reaction of degeneration obtained in severe cases.

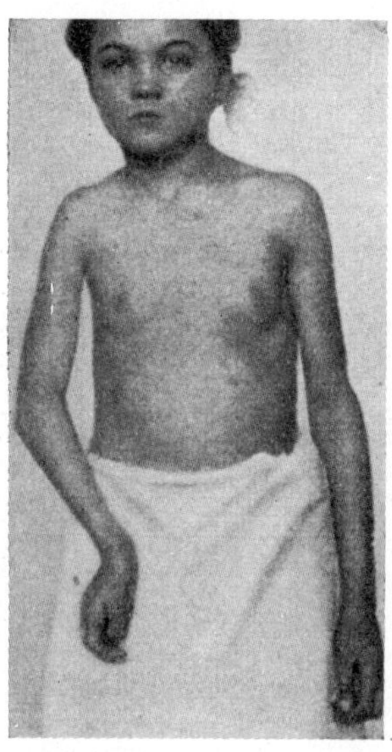

Fig. 222.—Obstetrical paralysis, upper arm type. Characteristic position of the paralyzed right arm. (*Bullard, Am. J. M. Sc.*, 1907, **134**, 99.)

In the much less frequent instances where only the seventh and eighth cervical and first dorsal nerves are affected, the upper arm is normal, but the hand and forearm are paralyzed (*Klumpke's paralysis*[6]). When the whole plexus is involved—a still less frequent condition—the forearm, hand, and upper arm are paralyzed. All degrees of paralysis are present in lesions of the plexus, from slight weakness to complete helplessness. Fracture of the clavicle or of the humerus, separation of the epiphysis, or dislocation of the shoulder-joint may be complications. The phrenic nerve may be injured in these obstetrical paralyses and paralysis of the diaphragm result (p. 625).

Course and Prognosis.—The prognosis in general is favorable. Approximately $\frac{2}{3}$ of the cases recover completely after two or three months or sooner (Meyer[7]). In others the progress is slow, and yet recovery is finally complete. When faradic contractility has never been entirely lost, recovery is rapid; but if both it and galvanic contractility disappear, or the reaction of degeneration is present, the recovery is slow and uncertain. In severe cases growth of the limb may finally be interfered with and there may develop atrophy of the bone and contractures.

Diagnosis.—Brachial monoplegia dependent upon an intracranial lesion is rare, the paralysis is spastic, and there is no diminution of faradic contractility. Syphilitic epiphysitis and infantile scurvy are later in development than obstetrical paralysis, and there is no true paralysis present. Fractures occurring at birth are painful.

Treatment.—For a few weeks after birth there should be no treatment except perhaps supporting the arm with a splint. After this time, if rapid improvement is not beginning, there should be employed massage, passive movement, and electricity; using the faradic current if contractions are obtained with it, otherwise the galvanic. At this time a splint should not be employed, but the arm allowed free, and use of it encouraged by limiting movement of the normal arm. Dislocation of the shoulder should be reduced if present. The advisability of operation and the time at which it is performed are difficult to decide. A steady improvement under conservative treatment, even though slow, warrants delay. In cases showing no improvement after three months, it is probably advisable to attempt to suture the ends of the ruptured nerves.

3. Other Peripheral Paralyses.—Peripheral neuritis may occur in almost any nerve. Exceptionally there may be a paralysis of the lumbar and sacral plexus, due to injury occurring at birth. This must be distinguished from injury to the spinal cord (p. 962), the latter condition inducing complete anesthesia. Later in life the peroneal nerve may suffer through injury to the legs, or the crural nerve be affected by pressure from a psoas abscess or appendicitis. Nerves in the forearm may be paralyzed by trauma; those of the upper arm damaged by dislocations and fractures. Various cranial nerves may suffer from neuritis, depending upon nuclear lesions or the result of pressure by tumor, meningitis, or encephalitis.

4. Facial Hemiatrophy.—(See also p. 1091.) This rare condition often begins in childhood, and sometimes in the first six months of life. It is more common in girls. It has been supposed to depend upon inflammation of the trigeminal nerve and Gasserian ganglion, or on disease of the sympathetic nervous system. In some cases it is associated with congenital facial paralysis (p. 980). It has been known to develop after trauma of the face, extraction of a tooth, cervical adenitis, or infectious diseases. The **symptoms** consist in progressive wasting of the tissues of one side of the face, including the skin, subcutaneous tissue, muscles, and bone. Electrical reactions and muscular movements are normal. Neuralgic pain may occur early in the disease. The pupil on the affected side may be somewhat dilated. In some cases facial hemiatrophy is associated with congenital torticollis (p. 986).

MORBID GROWTHS OF THE PERIPHERAL NERVES

Both primary and secondary neoplasms of the nerves are rare in early life. **General neurofibromatosis**, or von Recklinghausen's[8] Disease, is sometimes hereditary or familial and has been observed at this period. The symptoms consist in development of numerous cutaneous tumors; small pigmented spots in the skin; and tumors of any of the cranial, spinal, or sympathetic nerve-trunks, or of the spinal nerve-roots. When the tumors are on the cranial nerves or spinal nerve-roots varied symptoms suggesting morbid growths of the central nervous system are produced.

References

1. Il Policlinico, 1903, **10**, sez. med., 357. 2. Am. J. Dis. Child., 1929, **38**, 1256. 3. Centralbl. f. d. Grenzgeb. d. Med. u. Chir., 1902, **5**, 669. 4. J.A.M.A., 1925, **85**, 1862. 5. Ziemsson's Handb. d. spec. Path. u. Therap., 1874, **12**, 1, 492. 6. Rev. de méd., 1885, **5**, 591. 7. Monatschr. f. Neurol. u. Psych., 1917, **41**, 250. 8. Ueber multiplen Fibrome der Haut und ihre Beziehung zu den multiplen Neuromen, Berlin, 1882.

SECTION IX

DISEASES OF THE MUSCLES, BONES AND JOINTS

CHAPTER I

DISEASES OF THE MUSCLES

THE most important of these have already been described under Diseases of the Nervous System for reasons there explained.

MALFORMATION OF THE MUSCLES

These have been carefully studied by Bing.[1] The most common is partial or total congenital **absence of the pectoralis muscles.** Less frequently there may be a **defect** in the trapezius, serratus, quadriceps femoris, or other muscles including the diaphragm, the last producing diaphragmatic hernia or eventration. Other deformities are frequently combined with the pectoralis defect, such as imperfect development of the breast; abnormally high position of the shoulders (*Sprengel's deformity*); defective formation of the hand, etc. Sometimes a number of different malformations of the muscles are encountered in the same individual. Congenital **absence of the abdominal muscles** is a rare anomaly (Garrod and Davis,[2] Taillen[3]). A small localized **defect in the abdominal muscular wall** may give rise to ventral or lumbar hernia.

MYOSITIS

A *suppurating myositis* in one or more muscles may occur as a result of trauma or through pyogenic infection acquired in other ways. A *non-suppurating localized myositis* is represented by muscular rheumatism, as in some cases of torticollis; or may be the result of trauma, or follow some of the infectious diseases. A *multiple suppurating myositis* may occur as an unusual manifestation of general sepsis, or we have seen it apparently independent of this.

To be considered here are (1) Simple polymyositis, (2) Trichinous myositis, (3) Progressive myositis ossificans.

1. PRIMARY SIMPLE POLYMYOSITIS

This is a rare affection, perhaps more common in childhood than later, of which there are several subvarieties. The cause is often obscure, although cases may occur apparently as complications of acute infections. Streptococci and staphylococci have sometimes been found in the muscles. The muscles are stiff and firm and show edema and small-celled infiltration, increase of interstitial connective tissue, and secondary degeneration of the muscle-fibers. Inflammatory edema of the skin may also be present (*dermatomyositis*). Hemorrhage into the skin or mucous membranes may occur (*hemorrhagic polymyositis*); or there may be foci of hyperplasia of the interstitial connective tissue (*myositis fibrosa*). The **symptoms** begin acutely in *dermatomyositis*, with fever, loss of appetite, malaise, headache, enlargement of the spleen, and gastro-intestinal disturbances. Then, with other symptoms persistent, the extremities, usually first the lower, become painful on touch and movement, and the muscles swollen and hard; and later other muscles of the body including those of the face are affected. The patient finally loses the power to move, and is confined, helpless and stiff, to bed. Contemporaneously, or sometimes later, there develops a wide-spread, tense, inflammatory cutaneous edema, not readily pitted, with the surface suggesting an erythema of different sorts, and involving the whole body including the face. This edema may obscure the underlying condition of the muscles. Occasionally endocarditis develops. (For bibliography see Friedman[4] and Lehmkuhl.[5]) The *fibrous form* is without acute general symptoms and the cutaneous edema is absent. This form is more chronic than the type previously described, there is less pain, and the condition less often becomes so widespread. The final deformity, however, may be very great. The **course** in the severer cases is rapid; the functions of the larynx, swallowing, respiration, and cardiac action are interfered with, and death occurs in from one to eight weeks. In other instances the acute symptoms are absent; or they subside and the condition passes into a subacute or chronic form, lasting three to six months or even several years. Periods of remission are often seen, followed by exacerbations; favorable cases finally recovering, although with the muscles perhaps atrophied. The **prognosis** is always serious, more than half the cases ending fatally. The outlook is more favorable when the onset occurs in childhood, and decidedly so in the fibrous variety. The **treatment** is entirely symptomatic and consists in complete rest in the acute stages, with measures to relieve pain. Later gentle massage and electricity can be tried.

2. Trichinous Myositis

This is a special form of myositis due to the invasion of the muscles by the larvae of a nematode worm, the trichinella spiralis, acquired through the eating of infected pork. It involves among other muscles those of the arms and legs, the larynx, the intercostal muscles, and the diaphragm. We have seen several cases in children. The parasites can be found by biopsy of the muscles. The general symptoms consist in fever; perspiration; prostration; pain, tenderness and stiffness of the muscles; and diarrhea. Characteristic symptoms are edema of the eyelids and decided eosinophilia. The **prognosis** is uncertain.

3. Myositis Ossificans

Of this uncommon affection reports or statistical collections have been made by Lorenz,[6] Johannessen[7] and Mair;[8] Johannessen putting the number at 78 and Mair at over 66. The disease is one of early life and is seen oftener in males. The cause is probably a congenital constitutional disturbance, although a local trauma undoubtedly may precipitate the development in the region injured. The lesions consist at first of cellular infiltration, and later of connective-tissue overgrowth; these advancing to the production of nodules of true bone, situated primarily in the muscles, but later attaching themselves to some extent to the bones of the body, or sometimes developing originally there also. The **symptoms** show themselves first in the muscles of the neck and back, but eventually spread to a less extent to other regions. With fever and pain there develops a localized and sometimes tender swelling in the muscles, with edema in the surrounding parts. In a few days the symptoms, including the swelling, disappear completely, the latter becoming permanent only after several recurrences in the same locality. In other cases the primary swelling does not disappear, but remains as a hard nodule, and gradually, perhaps with recurrent attacks of inflammation, becomes actually bony. There occur repeated attacks of this nature, often after some slight localized trauma, with development of fresh nodules; until in advanced cases a large majority of the muscles are involved, including finally the masseters and the temporals. The muscles of the hands and feet, the sphincters, and some other muscles escape, as do all those with unstriped fiber. The bony masses once formed are not tender; are at first of pea-size; but gradually enlarge and many of them coalesce into irregular masses. They are at the beginning movable, but are finally fixed through attachment to the bones. At first there are no subjective symptoms produced by the bony masses; but eventually there is interference with muscular activity, and the joints become stiff and the patient rigid and helpless. Microdactylia is a very common attendant, the thumb and big toe being congenitally smaller than normal. The **course** is prolonged, although generally with long intermissions, the disease lasting over many years. Sometimes the course is more rapid. The **prognosis** is entirely unfavorable. The **diagnosis** is easy after the formation of bone has taken place. Multiple exostoses are attached to the bone from the very beginning, and cause no widespread interference with the movements of the body. **Treatment** is entirely unavailing, although in a few cases the process seemed to have been arrested by radiologic therapy. Even slight traumata should be guarded against.

CALCINOSIS

This condition is closely allied to myositis and sometimes accompanies it. In calcinosis, however, the calcareous deposits are usually located in the skin or subcutaneous tissues, but may occasionally be elsewhere. They consist of small chalky nodules, movable or fixed, few in number or numerous, and scattered over most of the body. They are much harder than are rheumatic nodules. Cases have been reported by Morse,[9] Lowenburg,[10] Langmead,[11] Tisdall and Erb,[12] and Wilens and Derby.[13]

TORTICOLLIS

(Wry Neck)

This condition is common at any time of life. Much the most frequent cause is muscular rheumatism. Less often torticollis may be brought about by caries of the cervical vertebrae; or be caused by pressure of an inflamed cervical gland or of an abscess or tumor in the neck upon the spinal accessory nerve; or be the result of some primary affection of the nerve itself. Cases dating from birth or seen soon after it may be dependent upon a congenital anomaly, such as a shortening of the muscles or malformation of the cervical spine; or may be the sequel to a hematoma or a rupture of the sternocleido-mastoid muscle the result of trauma received during birth (p. 222). Spasmodic wry neck dependent upon a primary spinal-accessory affection is of very uncommon occurrence in early life. Exceptionally a torticollis may be the result of paralysis of the nerve of the healthy side, allowing the head to be gradually drawn to the other.

Symptoms.—The congenital cases, or those dependent upon trauma at birth, both of them uncommon, are chronic in their course; the rheumatic cases are oftener acute; those due to other causes persist while the acting cause remains. The *congenital* condition is not infrequently combined with other deformities, among them facial asymmetry. The alteration in the position of the head is generally not discovered for some time after birth. In typical *acquired* cases the disease is situated chiefly in the sternocleido-mastoid muscle upon one side, as a result of which this stands out as a rigid, prominent cord, and the head is drawn to the affected side and downward toward the thorax, with the chin tilted upward and toward the sound side

(Fig. 223). Frequently the trapezius is also involved on the same side, in this event the head being also drawn somewhat backward. Sometimes the posterior muscle-groups on both sides are the seat of the disease, in which event the head is pulled backward, the chin slightly elevated, and turning the head to either side is interfered with. In such a condition cervical caries must always be suspected. The amount of pain and tenderness existent also varies with the case. Pain may be constantly present and severe, or develop only when efforts are made to move the head. Pain and tenderness are especially marked in the acute rheumatic cases. The **course** in the acute cases is generally short and recovery takes place in a few days or weeks, although rheumatic cases may sometimes be much prolonged. Recurrence in torticollis is not uncommon and there is a tendency for it to become chronic. When torticollis is due to some involvement of the spinal-accessory nerve the duration and **prognosis** will depend upon the possibility of the removal of the lesion. When the cause is a cervical caries the prognosis is unfavorable, unless the treatment of the primary disorder is successful. The congenital cases continue indefinitely, although the milder ones may be relieved by appropriate treatment. Any case which has lasted a considerable time has the prognosis made more unfavorable by the probability of some permanent alteration of the muscle developing. The **treatment** consists in the attempt to remove the cause. In the acute rheumatic form relief is obtained by the administration of the salicylates, often advantageously combined with phenacetin; the protection of the neck from cold; the employment of a hot-water bag, and the application of such counterirritants as mustard or capsicum. Congenital cases, and others which have lasted some weeks, require efforts at correction and support by orthopedic apparatus. Massage and electricity may also be tried, but after the condition has continued a few months surgical procedures are to be considered.

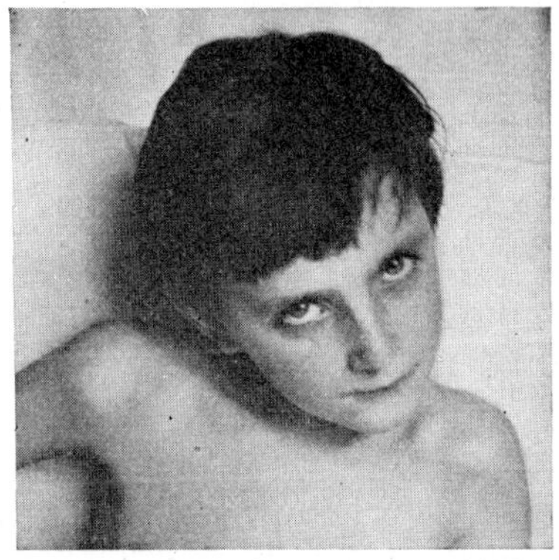

Fig. 223.—Rheumatic torticollis. From a patient in the Children's Ward of the Hospital of the University of Pennsylvania.

MYASTHENIA GRAVIS

(Asthenic Bulbar Paralysis)

This is a very rare affection in childhood, although a few cases are on record (Palmer,[14] Thomson,[15] Adie[16]). The cause is unknown, and the only lesions which have been observed consist in the occurrence of masses of small round-cells in the muscles. An enlargement of the thymus gland has sometimes been noticed. Nothing has been found wrong with the nervous system. The **symptoms** consist in excessive fatigue and ready exhaustion, seen first and especially in the muscles controlling the movements of the eyes, swallowing, speech, and mastication; and extending to those of the neck, trunk, and the extremities. There are ptosis, indistinct speech, and altered expression of face. Movements of the muscles are possible only for a few minutes at a time; then after a short rest the power returns for a similarly brief period. There is no muscular atrophy and sensation is undisturbed. The electrical excitability is normal but soon exhausted; to reappear after a short rest. The onset is rather slow; the course chronic, often with periods of temporary improvement. Death may occur after some months or years of illness; often from respiratory involvement, interference with swallowing, or inanition. Recovery, however, may take place. Good effects have followed the administration of glycine (Boothby[17]), and of ephedrine (Edgeworth[18]).

MYOTONIA CONGENITA

(Thomsen's Disease)

Although cases had been reported previously, this rare condition was brought into prominence by the writings of Thomsen[19] in 1876. It should not be confused with amyotonia congenita (p. 975). It is usually congenital, but oftenest not recognized until late childhood or adolescence; and is typically familial and hereditary. Males are more frequently affected. There are no characteristic pathologic **lesions.** The **symptoms** of the well-developed cases consist in a temporary rigidity of the muscles when efforts are first made to put them into action. This is oftenest experienced in the legs or arms. The patient on starting to walk is able to do so only stiffly and slowly, but after a few steps the stiffness disappears and he can walk entirely normally. If grasping any object, he is unable to let go of it for several seconds. Less often the muscles of other parts of the body are involved. Thus sucking, crying, masticating, talking, or opening the eyes may be rendered difficult by the slow, stiff action of the muscles. The obstruction to all these movements disappears promptly if effort is persisted in, and does not return until a renewed attempt at movement is made after a period of rest. The distribution of the malady is symmetrical, although it may perhaps be more marked on one side. The condition is made worse by exposure to cold or by excitement or the consciousness of being observed. There are no sensory disturbances, and the muscles are well-developed or abnormally large. Tapping a muscle reveals an increase of mechanical excitability, shown by a slow contraction and increased prominence of the muscle, with a central depression which disappears slowly after some seconds. The muscles also exhibit an unduly active but slow response to both the faradic and the galvanic current of weak strength (Myotonic reaction of Erb[20]), while strong currents produce a series of small wave-like contractions. The disease lasts through life, although sometimes with periods of temporary improvement. It does not affect the duration of life. Persistent employment of massage and of active and passive muscular movements has been recommended.

Paramyoclonus Congenita.—Eulenberg[21] has described a condition which he called paramyoclonus congenita. The symptoms resemble those of Thomsen's disease in most particulars, but there is absence of the altered mechanical and electrical reactions. The muscular contractions appear to be brought on by the action of cold rather than by attempted movement. The disease was observed in seven generations of one family. Similar cases have been reported by others, but it is questionable whether the condition is not merely a variant of myotonia congenita (Rosett[22]).

PARAMYOCLONUS MULTIPLEX

(Myoclonia)

This uncommon condition, described by Friedreich[23], is rare in childhood. It occurs principally in males and is sometimes hereditary or familial. Over-excitement or over-exertion operates as a direct cause. The disease resembles somewhat, but is distinct from electric chorea, convulsive tic, and hysteria. The **symptoms** consist in very rapidly repeated, irregular, clonic contractions in many different muscles of the body, as a rule symmetrical in distribution. The extremities are oftenest involved, while the face usually escapes. The excursion of the movements is generally slight, but the action may be violent. They come on in paroxysmal attacks and are entirely beyond the control of the patient, or may be constantly present except during sleep. Tremor may occur between the attacks. There are no sensory, psychic, or electrical disturbances. The **prognosis** as to recovery is very uncertain; although some cases of cessation of the disease have been reported. **Treatment** is without effect.

PERIODICAL PARALYSIS

This uncommon malady exhibits distinct hereditary and familial occurrence. Cases have been reported and collected by Taylor,[24] Buzzard,[25] Oddo and Audibert,[26] and Adie.[16] The condition may begin even in early childhood, but usually develops at puberty or later. Over-exertion, unusual rest, or a too hearty meal would appear to bring on individual attacks, but generally no cause is discoverable. Sections of muscle have shown no changes sufficient to explain the condition. The **symptoms** consist in attacks of flaccid paralysis of varying degree, developing often during sleep, and affecting generally first the lower limbs, but in the course of a few hours or less extending to the upper extremities and the trunk. The muscles supplied by the cranial nerves usually escape, although ptosis and dysphagia have been observed. Sensation and the mental condition are unaffected; the reflexes are abolished; the electrical response is greatly diminished or even entirely absent. Excretion of urine is often interfered with by the paralysis of the abdominal muscles. Profuse perspiration may occur, and sometimes signs of cardiac dilatation. The duration of an attack is variable, the symptoms gradually disappearing and recovery being complete in from a few hours up to two or three days. The frequency of the recurrence varies from daily up to every few weeks, although sometimes there may be intervals of months. The disease generally ceases after the age of fifty years, but has occasionally been directly fatal. On the theory that a toxic state is present, alkaline diuretics have been recommended in **treatment,** with apparent benefit. In the way of prevention over-excitement is to be avoided.

References

1. Virchow's Archiv., 1902, **170,** 175. 2. Med.-Chir. Trans., 1905, **88,** 363. 3. Nourrisson, 1928, **16,** 291. 4. Med. J. and Rec., 1926, **123,** 382. 5. Arch. f. Kinderh., 1929, **86,** 179. 6. Nothnagel's Handb. d. spec. Path. u. Therap., 1904, **11,** 3, 1, 273. 7. Jahrb. f. Kinderh., 1917, **86,** 442. 8. Edinburgh. M. J., 1932, **39,** 13; 69. 9. Trans. Am. Pediat. Soc., 1921, **33,** 332. 10. Pennsylvania M. J., 1922, **26,** 21. 11. Arch. Pediat., 1923, **40,** 112. 12. Am. J. Dis. Child., 1924, **27,** 28. 13. Am. J. Dis. Child., 1926, **31,** 34. 14. Guy's Hosp. Rep., 1908, **62,** 64. 15. Brit. J. Child. Dis., 1919, **16,** 92. 16. Brit. J. Child. Dis., 1928, **25,** 128. 17. Proc. Staff Meetings Mayo Clinic, 1932, **7,** 557. 18. J.A.M.A., 1930, **94,** 1136. 19. Arch. f. Psychiat. u. Nervenkr., 1876, **6,** 702. 20. Die Thomsensche Krankheit, 1886. 21. Neurol. Zentralbl., 1886, No. 12, Ref. Med. Klinik., 1916, **12,** 505. 22. Brain, 1922, **45,** 25. 23. Virchow's Archiv., 1881, **86,** 421. 24. J. Nerv. and Ment. Dis., 1898, **25,** 637. 25. Lancet, 1901, **2,** 1564. 26. Arch. gén. de méd., 1902, **189,** 290.

CHAPTER II

DISEASES OF THE BONES, JOINTS AND EXTREMITIES

ALTHOUGH a subject largely surgical, certain topics require discussion here.

MALFORMATIONS AND OTHER DEFORMITIES OF THE BONES AND JOINTS

These are varied and numerous. Some are described with the primary diseases of which the deformities constitute but a part, and others receive independent consideration.

There may be congenital or acquired deformities of the head. Some, as those dependent upon rachitis, hydrocephalus, idiocy, chloroma, suprarenal sarcoma (neuroblastoma), syphilis, and cleidocranial dysostosis are referred

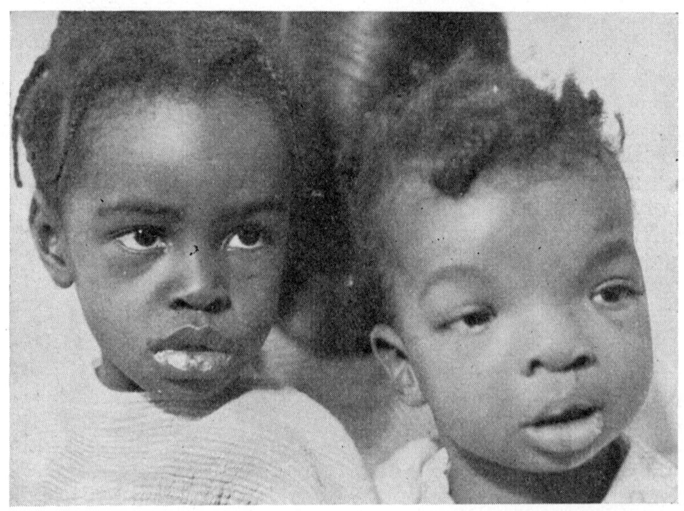

Fig. 224.—Hypertelorism. Patient seventeen months old in Cincinnati General Hospital. Also had cleft palate and harelip, and an incomplete accessory auditory canal. The fontanelle was closed and there was no bony deficiency of the forehead. Mother also had hypertelorism and father had harelip. Picture shows contrast with normal child of about the same age.

to elsewhere. **Asymmetry of the skull,** later disappearing, is frequent in new-born infants and due to pressure within the uterus or to molding during labor. (See p. 17.) There may be a **nonrachitic softening of the skull,** often accompanied by softening of the ribs (Hess;[1] Greene[2]), which may lead to flattening of the occiput, asymmetry of the face, or deformity of the dental arches. **Ocular hypertelorism** (Fig. 224), first described by Greig[3] is probably more common than reports would indicate. Reilly[4] found only 17 cases noted in the American literature. It is due to excessive growth of the lesser wings of the sphenoid bone, causing the orbits to be widely separated. Mental deficiency may be associated, and there is often a familial tendency. Hypertelorism may be unilateral. A form of hypertelorism termed **hereditary craniofacial dysostosis** was described by Crouzon[5] and by Roubinovitch et al.[6] Dzierzysky[7] published a remarkable family history of what he designated **"dystrophia periostalis hyperplastica familiaris"** in which the affected members exhibited from early life acrocephalic heads, combined with thickening of the long and short bones and the clavicles. In **oxycephaly** (*acrocephaly, tower-skull*) (Fig. 225), first described by Virchow,[8] there is a malformation, sometimes hereditary, in which the cranial vault is dome-shaped and brachycephalic, with a high, pointed vertex. Of the same nature is **scaphocephaly** in which the skull is long and narrow, with arching of the vault. With these deformities are liable to be associated others, among them webbing of the fingers, to which combination Apert[9] gave the title **acrocephalosyndactylism,** and of which Toni[10] states that there are not over 40 cases reported, and Nørvig[11] makes the number 40. With scaphocephaly there may be a combination of cloudy cornea, ankylosis of joints, claw-like hands and feet, lumbar kyphosis, and mental retardation, as in the cases described by Helmholz and Harrington.[12] With oxycephaly are often associated exophthalmos, nystagmus, paralysis of the ocular muscles, optic atrophy, and mental deficiency. It is usually believed that oxycephaly is produced by premature ossification (*synostosis*) of the coronary and sagittal sutures, the other changes in the skull being secondary to this, and any defect of the brain resulting from the pressure. (For recent studies on oxycephaly and allied conditions, see Jacobsen,[13] Helmholz and Harrington,[12] Bronfenbrenner.[14]) Faber and Towne[15] among others recommend the prevention of pressure-symptoms by the operative removal of strips of the calvarium.

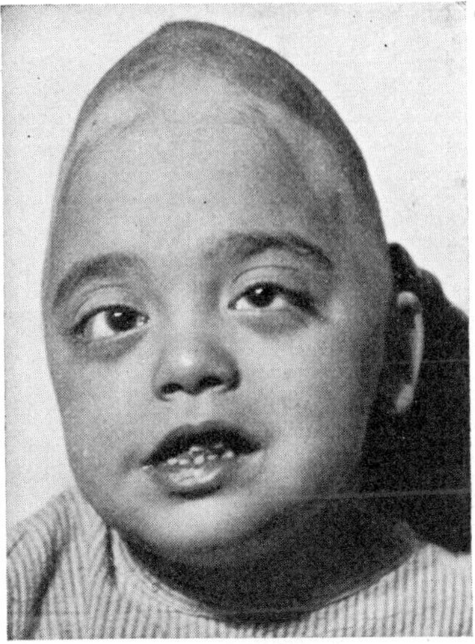

Fig. 225.—Oxycephaly. Patient in the Cincinnati General Hospital. Paralysis of ocular muscles and mental deficiency.

The bones of the extremities, together with the accompanying soft parts, may be absent or imperfectly developed. Mall[16] in a summary of 81,000 births found 0.14 per cent of defective extremities. There may be **ectromelia** (absence of a limb), which is usually not complete; **micromelia** (shortening); **hemimelia** (distal portion absent); **phocomelia** (proximal part missing and the remaining portion arising directly from the trunk). (See Fig. 226.) Barkman[17] reports absence of the leg and of the corresponding acetabulum, and states that there are only 4 similar cases recorded. The deformities described have in some instances followed radiologic treatment of the pregnant mother (Murphy and Goldstein[18]). Club-hand may occur (Fig. 227). **Congenital absence of bones** with little deformity of the soft parts has been reported, as has also **congenital fusion of the ulna and radius.** Especially to be mentioned are **polydactylism** (Fig. 228) and **syndactylism** (Fig. 229). These conditions are often hereditary and combined with other malformations. Syndactylism may vary from simple webbing of some of the fingers to much more complete fusion. **Ectrodactylism** (absence of digits) (Fig. 226) may in some instances be hereditary (Klein[19]), as may also **symphallangism** (absence or fusion of joints of the finger). In **amyoplasia congenita** (*arthrogyrosposis multiplex congenita, multiple congenital articular rigidity*), of which Sheldon[20] collected 49 cases, there is immobility of one or more joints, generally symmetrically distributed; the fixation being in a straight or flexed

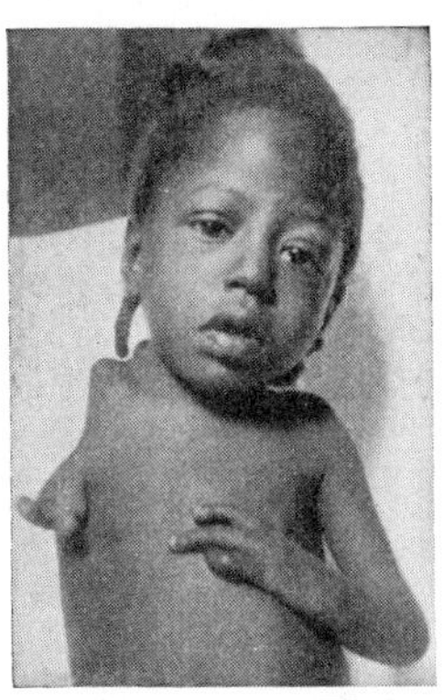

Fig. 226.—Phocomelia and ectrodactylia. Patient three and one-half years old in Cincinnati General Hospital.

position. **Supernumerary foot** has been reported (Mayer and Sashin[21]). **Congenital hypertrophy of the fingers and toes** is occasionally observed (Annandale[22]). **Arachnodactylia** is the title applied by Achard[23] to a rare malformation in which there is abnormal length of the hands and feet and of

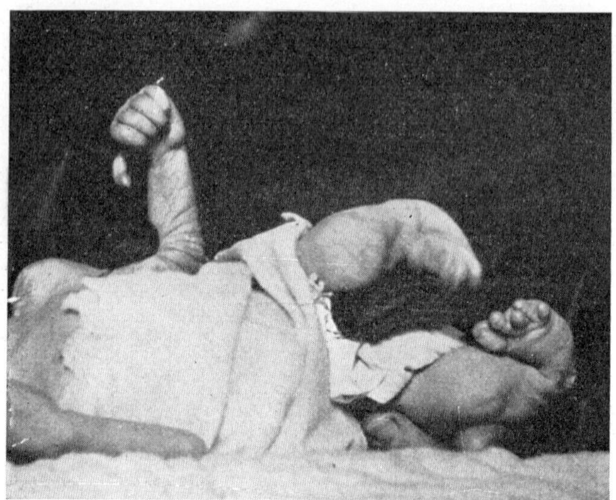

Fig. 227.—New-born infant showing club-hand and club-foot. (*Courtesy of Dr. John D. Target.*)

the entire extremities, with undue slenderness of the bone (Fig 230). Marfan[24] described this under the term *dolichostenomelie*. It may be associated with other defects, as congenital heart-disease and pathologic conditions of the eyes (luxation of lens, megalocornea). The subject is reviewed by Börger,[25] Nieresheimer,[26] Piper and Irvine-Jones,[27] Zuber,[28] Thaden,[29] and by Young,[30] who states that there are only 22 cases on record. **Congenital shortness of the neck** is in some cases due to absence or fusion of the cervical vertebrae. In addition to these faults of development there are such deformities as **amputation** or other injury of a limb by amniotic bands or through strangulation by the umbilical cord.

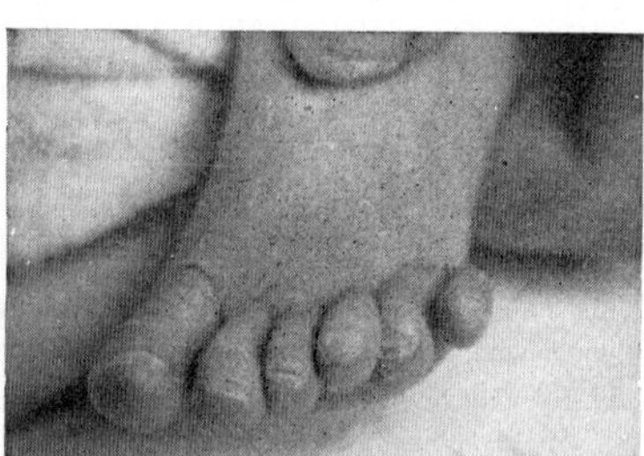

Fig. 228.—Polydactylism. Infant of five weeks in the Children's Hospital of Philadelphia. Six fingers on each hand, and six toes on each foot. Nystagmus.

The **nails** may be deformed and aplastic, this often being associated with other ectodermal defects (p. 518). A familial dystrophy of the nails has been reported by Walter and Bradford,[31] Jacobsen,[32] Thompson[33] and others. Grooving, thinning, and thickening of the nails may accompany or follow severe illnesses and malnutrition.

Acrocyanosis, described in children by Comby,[34] begins usually about puberty. There are lividity and hyperhidrosis of the hands and feet. Suggested causes are disorders of the sympathetic nervous system and endocrine disturbances. Delay in development of **epiphyses** accompanies such states as hypothyroidism and severe diabetes or extreme malnutrition, and early union of epiphysis with diaphysis is usual in conditions associated with precocious sexual development.

Congenital elevation of the scapula (*Sprengel's*[35] *deformity*) is an unusual condition in which the scapula, oftenest on one side, is displaced upward and rotated, with the lower angle too near the spine. Sometimes a bridge of bone unites the spine to the scapula. The arm on the affected side cannot be raised above a right angle with the body, the head is inclined toward this side, scoliosis is present, and other deformities may be combined. Massage and exercises may do good, but operation is sometimes required.

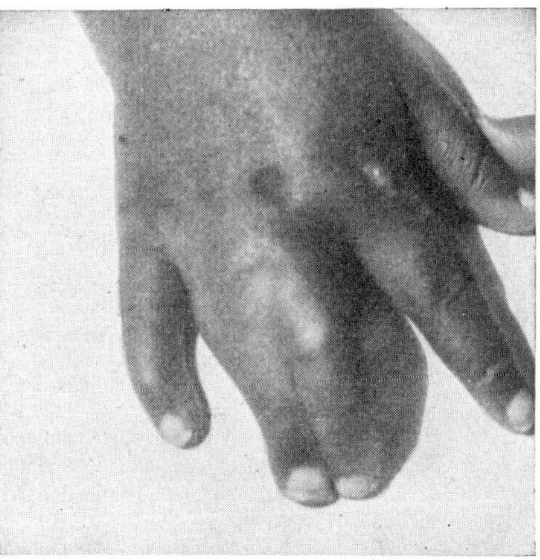

Fig. 229.—Syndactylism. Patient in the Cincinnati General Hospital.

Winged scapulae (*Scapulae alatae*) may result from displacement of the latissimi dorsi, lateral curvature, muscular debility or wasting, paralysis of the serrati magni, or pseudohypertrophic muscular dystrophy. The angles of the scapulae are tilted outward, causing the characteristic winged appearance.

Pigeon-breast (*Pectus carinatum; Chicken-breast; Keel-shaped Chest*) is a prominence of the sternum and cartilages, with a depression of the sides of the thorax. It is a symptom in rickets; but also results from prolonged interference with respiration, as from the presence of adenoids, and occurs in well-marked kyphosis from dorsal caries. Treatment in all but the last is satisfactory, and consists in removing the cause, and in practising deep inspiration and forced expiration, and such gymnastic exercises as swinging from a horizontal bar and the like, which tend to pull out the sides

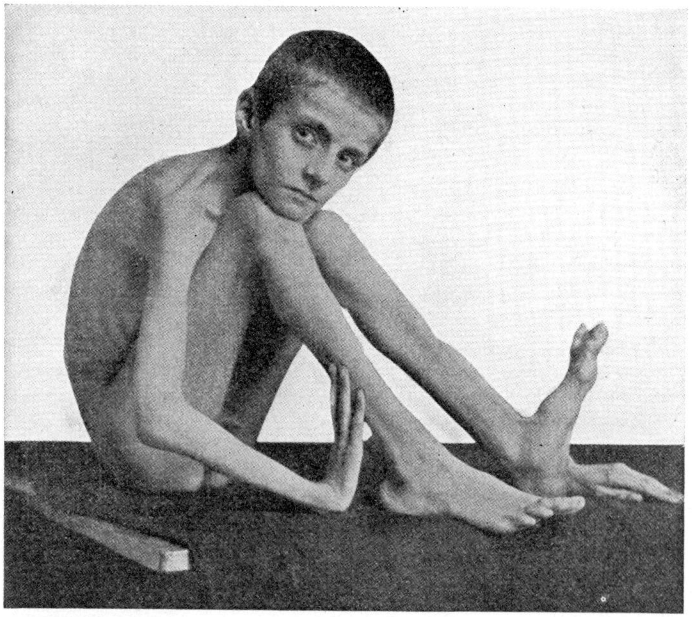

Fig. 230.—Arachnodactylia. Child of nine years. Shows the extreme slenderness and length of the limbs, especially of the hands and feet. (*Börger, Ztsch. f. Kinderh. Orig.*, 1914, **12**, 161.)

of the chest and expand the lungs. Systematic pressure at intervals upon the sternum is also recommended.

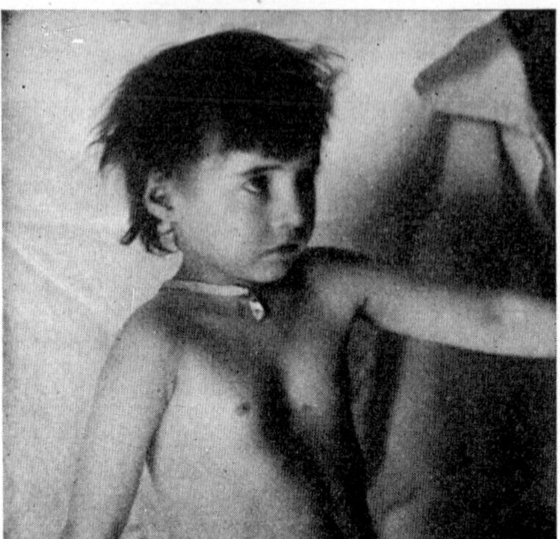

Fig. 231.—Funnel-chest. From a patient in the Children's Hospital of Philadelphia.

Funnel-chest is a depression of a funnel-like form in the sternum. It may be either of considerable extent along the course of the sternum (Fig. 127, p. 544) or much smaller and more abrupt (Fig. 231). In some cases it depends upon rickets or obstruction to respiration, and in others appears to be a congenital anomaly. Treatment for rickets or nasal obstruction, and the employment of suitable gymnastic exercises and of forcible expiration against resistance may be of avail.

CONGENITAL DISLOCATION OF THE HIP-JOINT

This is encountered in less than 0.5 per cent of births (Willard[36]); oftenest in females in the proportion of about 7:1; and is bilateral in about 40 per cent of the cases. The characteristic **symptoms** are generally first observed when the child begins to walk. In unilateral dislocation there then develops a limp; the trochanter can be found above Nélaton's line; there is moderate lordosis; the thigh is shorter than normal and the nato-femoral fold higher; the head of the bone is absent from the normal position in the groin to the outer side of the femoral vessels and rests finally on the dorsum of the ilium; and when the child is standing upon the dislocated leg and elevating the other the pelvis is inclined toward the healthy side (Trendelenburg's symptom). In double dislocation, in addition to the features mentioned, the gait is waddling; the lordosis decided (Fig. 232); and the perineum and the distance between the thighs widened. Apart from these symptoms there are sometimes pain in the joints and fatigue on walking, and in some cases inability to walk at all, except with crutches. The **diagnosis** is made from coxitis by the freedom of movement of the joint; and from coxa vara by earlier development, absence of rickets, absence of a right-angled inclination of the neck of the femur, and the presence of lordosis. Roentgenography will establish the diagnosis in doubtful cases. Various methods have been employed in **treatment.** Whether this should consist in operation with open incision or be manipulative is a matter of discussion, and is influenced to some extent by the age of the patient.

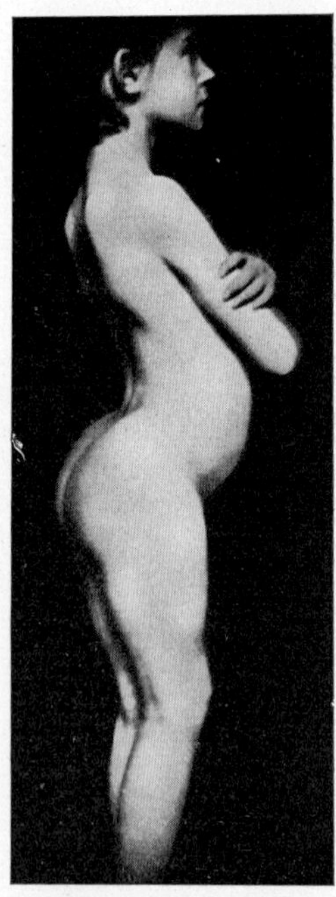

Fig. 232.—Bilateral congenital dislocation of the hip showing lordosis. (*Courtesy of Dr. H. R. Wharton.*)

CURVATURE OF THE SPINE

This is usually not congenital and is due to many causes. **Lordosis** (exaggeration of the normal anterior curve in the lumbar region) is observed in congenital dislocation of the hip (Fig. 232), coxitis, paralysis of the muscles of the back, and sometimes in spinal caries. A moderate degree of it is frequent with general lack of muscular tone, as from chronic indigestion, rickets, and other causes. **Kyphosis** (abnormal posterior curvature) occurs oftenest in the dorsolumbar region and is especially well seen in rickets (Fig. 105, p. 450). In childhood it is common in stooping, round-shouldered children. An angular kyphosis, which finally may become very decided and is chiefly in the dorsal region, results from spondylitis (Fig. 245, p. 1011). **Scoliosis** (lateral curvature) (Fig. 233) is common. Rarely it is congenital, and then due to malformations of ribs or vertebrae. It is very frequent as an acquired deformity. Early cases are oftenest seen in rachitic children. Other causes are poliomyelitis; faulty habits in standing, sitting, or lying; unequal length of the legs; contraction of the chest following empyema; poor musculature from malnutrition or other cause, etc. The curvature may be situated in any portion of the spine; may be single to either side, although as a rule there are other compensating curves present; and always there is also rotation of the vertebrae. The degree of scoliosis is usually slight and attracts little attention, but it may be decided. With the curvature there are unavoidable alterations in the position of the pelvis, the hip on the side of the convexity being more prominent and the shoulder higher; and there may be deformity of the chest.

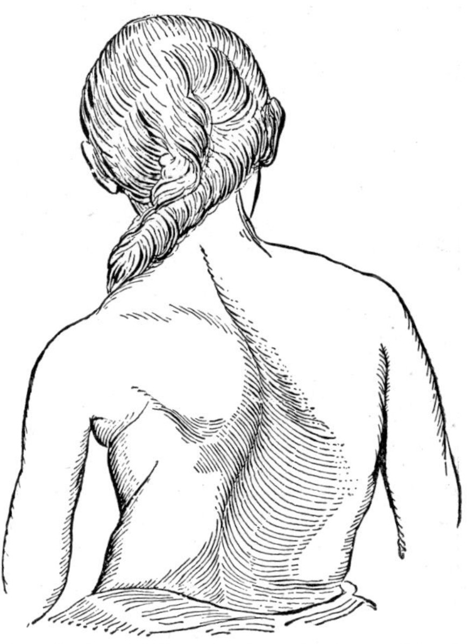

Fig. 233.—Well-marked scoliosis. (*Griffith, The Care of the Baby*, 1923, *7th Ed.*, p. 310.)

All forms of curvature require energetic **treatment.** Where the deformity is liable to occur, this should be anticipated by the employment of prophylactic measures. With curvature already present, the causes must be removed when possible. In many instances gymnastic exercises, massage, and the application of a suitable apparatus are indicated. For details reference must be made to works on orthopedic surgery.

CLUB-FOOT

Talipes may be congenital and is often hereditary. It is one of the most common of the deformities of the extremities, and occurs about once in every 1000 births (Willard[36]). Other deformities are frequently present. It is more common in boys, and is oftener than not bilateral. Congenital cases are probably produced by abnormal intra-uterine pressure. Acquired cases are more numerous and result from trauma or disease in the region of the ankle, cerebral paralysis, and poliomyelitis. Talipes may develop in adult life in cases of spina bifida occulta (deVries[37]). In *talipes varus* the foot is adducted and inverted, and the child walks on the outer border; in *talipes valgus*, the reverse of this, walking takes place on the inner border; in *talipes equinus* the heel is turned up and the child walks on tip-toe; in *talipes calcaneus* walking is on the heel with dorsal flexion of the foot. There may be various combinations of these. When the child begins to walk the deformity grows progressively greater. Treatment may be manipulative, mechanical, or operative, depending upon the case, and is within the province of the orthopedist.

FLAT-FOOT

Pes valgus is a common deformity. It may be congenital; develop early as a result of rickets; or be acquired by walking too soon. Later it may be produced by tight shoes and high heels, general muscular weakness, too much continuous standing, or poliomyelitis. It is often associated with knock-knee. The arch, generally of both feet, is lowered or entirely destroyed as a result of weakness of muscles and ligaments, and the inner aspect of the ankle is too prominent (Fig. 232). The child walks with the toes turned out too much; and seems to have weak ankles. The shoes wear out chiefly upon the inner side of the sole and over the internal malleolus. Fatigue occurs readily, and there is often pain in the feet and sometimes in the back. In severe cases pain may continue even when the patient is off his feet. Except in young children, where the fatty tissue normally present may be misleading, the examination of the foot will reveal the depression of the arch. Standing on a blotter or paper after the sole has been inked or wet, or on a glass stand below which a mirror has been placed, will give the outline of the foot. **Treatment** is satisfactory except in severe, long-continued cases. Prophylaxis is important. Early walking should be discouraged, particularly if the child is rachitic or abnormally heavy. Shoes should have a fairly stiff sole, a broad toe, sufficient length so that there is not pressure against the ends of the toes, and sufficient height across the toe and the vamp. Should evidence of flattening appear, the sole and heel of the shoe should be thickened upon the inner side, in order to throw the weight of the body toward the outer border of the foot, and to keep the toes from turning outward when walking. Perhaps a slight curved elevation of leather may be inserted as an insole to support the weakened arch. The muscles of the foot should be strengthened by massage, frequent forcible adduction of the foot by passive movement practised, and exercises prescribed, as walking without shoes on tip-toe with the feet turned inward. (See Brahdy.[38])

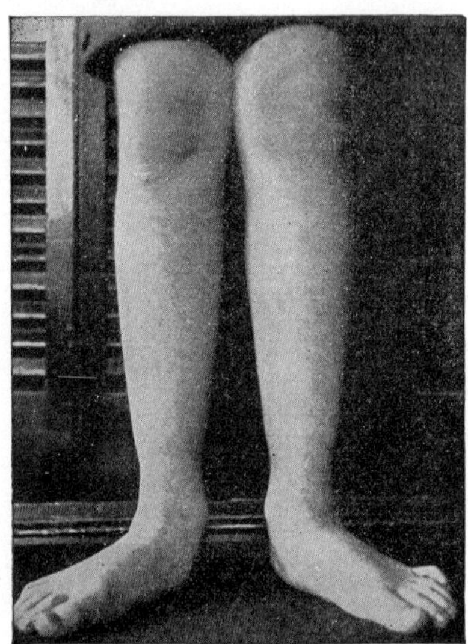

Fig. 234.—Pronated feet (flat-foot). (*Willard, Surgery of Childhood,* 697, *Fig.* 640.)

PIGEON-TOES

When first walking the normal child tends to keep the feet parallel or even to turn the toes in, and this should not be discouraged in infancy, since it will correct itself in due course. Too early turning out of the toes is liable to favor the production of flat-foot and knock-knee. The condition may, however, depend upon knock-knee, a certain degree of club-foot, or an inward rotation of the hips, and these may need orthopedic aid.

KNOCK-KNEE

Genu valgum is a common deformity, usually resulting from rickets, general debility, poliomyelitis, or from the child having been carried in a faulty manner. Relaxation of muscles and ligaments results, with deformity of the adjacent extremities of the femur and tibia. The internal condyles are always enlarged. Either one or both legs may be affected, usually one more than the other. When both legs are involved the child stands with the knees close together and the ankles apart (Fig. 235). In early cases the feet are turned in in walking. In more pronounced instances there is some degree of talipes valgus and flat-foot. The gait is somewhat waddling or, in unilateral knock-knee, limping. The child suffers readily from fatigue and sometimes from pain. Frequently children are temporarily knock-kneed up to the age of three or four years. In contradistinction to the pathologic knock-knee, such children consistently turn their toes in, and this is in no way to be interfered with. The deformity of the knee in such cases will soon disappear. In the way of prophylactic **treatment** rickets should be attended to if present, and standing and walking be delayed. When knock-knee begins to appear, the inner border of the sole and heel of the shoe should be thickened, as in flat-foot, in order to throw the knees out and turn the toes in; and if necessary the arch of the foot supported. Garters which suspend the stockings from the outer side of the leg should not be worn. If the patient is still quite young much can be accomplished by forcible bending of the knees outward while the leg is extended at the knee-joint. This should be done several times a day, using considerable pressure. Walking barefoot and on tip-toe is of benefit. The child should be taught to stand with the heels close together, and to walk with the toes turned in. In older children bicycle-riding and horseback riding are of service. Should such measures not avail, mechanical treatment must be employed.

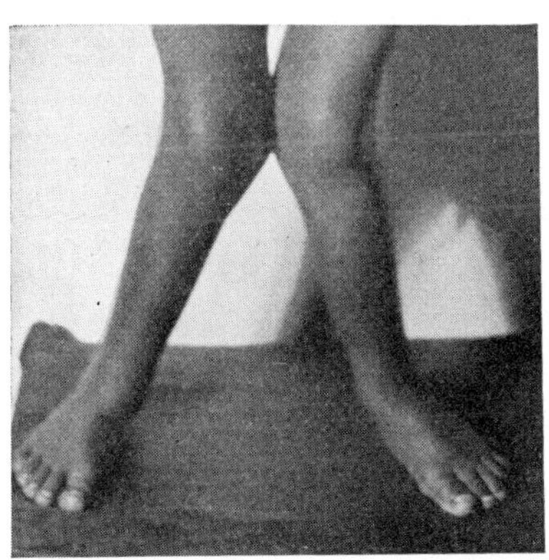

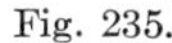

Fig. 235.

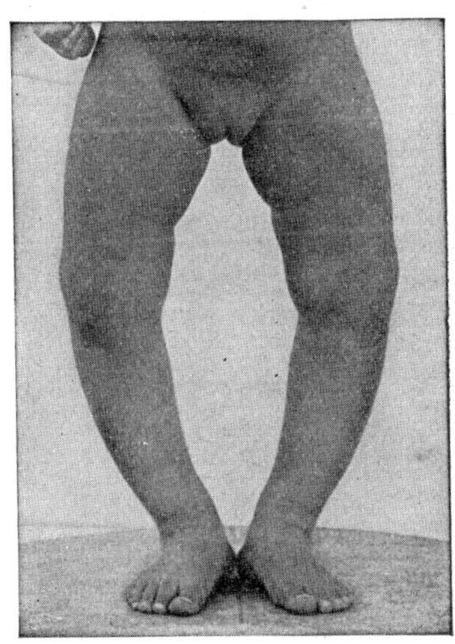

Fig. 236.

Fig. 235.—Knock-knee. Child three years of age in Cincinnati General Hospital.

Fig. 236.—Out-knee and bow-legs. Resulting from too early walking while rickety bones were soft. (*Willard, Surgery of Childhood*, 301, *Fig.* 252.)

BOW-LEGS

Genu varum is very common. All infants in the earliest months of life exhibit a certain degree of normal bowing (p. 20). The usual cause of pathologic bow-legs is rickets, especially when early standing or walking is permitted. It may result, too, even without rickets from wearing thick diapers. The soft bones of the legs and thighs of both sides become curved outward. When standing the knees are widely separated, and the feet tend to assume the position of talipes varus (Fig. 236). Sometimes one leg is bowed and the other exhibits knock-knee; this resulting from pressure of the arm of the nurse carrying a rachitic child always upon her one side. Sometimes the bones of the legs may be bowed, yet without the knees being bent outwardly. In severe rachitic cases there may be anterior bending as well as bowing, produced by the habit of sitting with the legs crossed, or the too early bearing of weight upon them. **Prognosis** is good except in advanced cases, many children recovering spontaneously. **Treatment** should be prophylactic, especially the prevention of too early standing in the case of rachitic children. In children with bow-legs whose bones are still soft, firm pressure should be made against the curvature several times a day and massage given. It may be necessary to resort to mechanical or even operative treatment, the latter being delayed until danger of recurrence of rickets is past.

COXA VARA

In this disorder the neck of the femur is at a right angle or even an acute angle with the shaft of the bone. The condition may be either bilateral or unilateral; is rarely congenital; often is the result of rachitic softening or of epiphyseal separation; still oftener (*coxa vara statica*) develops in later childhood or adolescence, and is dependent upon a yielding of the neck of the femur from such causes as poliomyelitis, epiphyseal disease, or fracture. In the unilateral cases the **symptoms** consist in pain in the affected hip, often extending to the knee; limping gait; shortening of the limb and of the abductors of the thigh; limited power of abduction; inward rotation of the hip; upward tilting of the pelvis on the affected side; and displacement of the trochanter above Nélaton's line. In bilateral cases the gait is waddling as in congenital dislocation, and the knees often pass each other with difficulty (*scissors-gait*). **Diagnosis** is made from congenital dislocation of the hip by the later period of development; the firmer gait; the decided knock-knee; the absence of lordosis; and the presence of the head of the femur in normal position (see also p. 994). Hip-joint disease exhibits a general fixation of the hip, while in coxa vara there is limitation only in abduction. Roentgenograms should always be made. The **treatment** is entirely surgical.

HYPERTROPHIC PULMONARY OSTEO-ARTHROPATHY

This disorder, so named by Marie,[39] is the result of prolonged suppuration, as in empyema, bronchiectasis, and chronic phthisis; but it may occur also in congenital heart-disease and sometimes with syphilis. There is no satisfactory explanation for its production. The lesions consist in an ossifying periostitis, effusion into the joint, erosion of the cartilages, and hypertrophy of the soft tissues. The condition is manifested in milder instances chiefly by clubbing of the ends of the fingers, the nails being broad and curved in form transversely and longitudinally (Fig. 237). (See also Fig. 184 p. 772.) In well-developed cases there is enlargement also of the ends of the long bones and of the hands and feet, with pain and swelling of the joints. Probably no distinction should be made between the condition limited to clubbing of the fingers and toes (*Hippocratic fingers*), in which there are said to be no changes in the bones, and the more severe condition in which the terminations of the long bones are involved. Roentgenograms show that in cases apparently of simple clubbing there is also involvement of the long bones (Locke[40]). Clubbing of the fingers does not appear until several weeks to a year or longer after development of the primary disease. In cases of congenital heart-disease clubbing of the fingers is not present until after several months, and only in cases of decided cyanosis.

CRANIOTABES

This term, first applied by Elsässer,[41] designates a condition of thinning of the cranium in spots. In 600 infants in the first 6 months of life we[42] found 32 with craniotabes. It is seen oftenest at from three to four months of age. Rickets and syphilis are considered causes, but, while both of these can produce it, it occurs in many infants who do not have these diseases. There appears to be a physiologic form of craniotabes without any particular significance. In a type of the condition present at birth or soon thereafter the thinning of the bone may be due to pressure in utero of the maternal pelvis (Abels and Karplus,[43] Abels[44]). This view is supported by the fact that it is rare in the skull of infants born by breech-labor, and that no defect

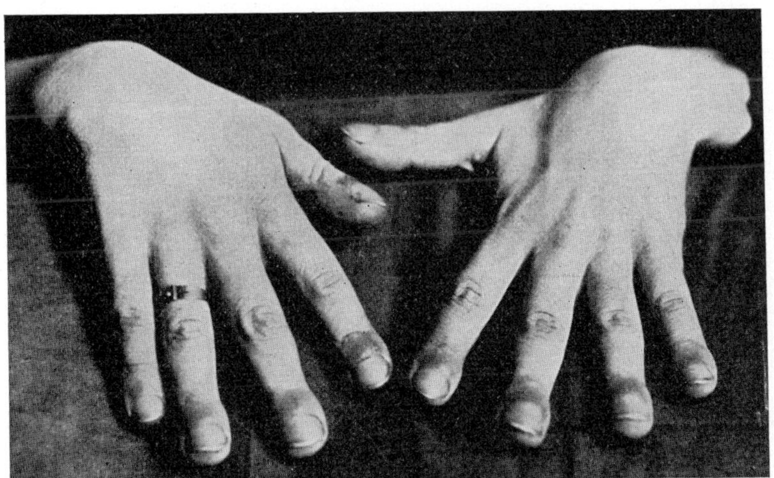

Fig. 237.—Pulmonary osteo-arthropathy. From a patient in the Children's Hospital of Philadelphia, with abscess of the lung.

in bones is found elsewhere; this indicating the absence of any general constitutional deficiency. The spots are situated oftenest in the parietal bones, less often in the occipital. The bone may be so thin that it yields readily to pressure by the fingers and gives a crackling sensation. Craniotabes located along the suture-lines is usually the type found in the first few months of life. When not so near the edge of the bone and developing after three months, a rachitic basis may be suspected. The condition disappears as the infant grows older.

ACHONDROPLASIA

(Chondrodystrophia Foetalis)

Achondroplasia is the title applied by Parrot,[45] and chondrodystrophia foetalis by Kaufmann,[46] to this particular type of dwarfism. There is reason to believe from sculpture that it had been recognized in ancient Egypt; and many of the dwarfs pictured in art were achondroplastics (Regnault[47]).

Etiology.—The cause is unknown. It has been supposed by some observers that the disease depends upon disordered internal secretion of some of the endocrine glands, while others place it among maladies of the nervous system. It has also been believed to have been produced by pressure of an abnormally small amnion (Jansen[48] and others). Heredity has played a part in many instances through the father; a woman with achondroplasia being seldom able to propagate.

Pathologic Anatomy.—The process begins in early fetal life as a failure of proper development of the ossifying process in the cartilaginous tissue. There occurs finally a premature ossification of the cartilage, and the long bones are shorter than normal but not thinner, since the production of bone beneath the periosteum is not interfered with. In the majority of cases the epiphysis is normal in size, and the increase in size at the ends of the bones is due to a cup-shaped enlargement of the diaphysis around the epiphysis (Fig. 238). The cartilaginous bones of the base of the skull are involved, and there is an early ossification of these and a failure to reach a

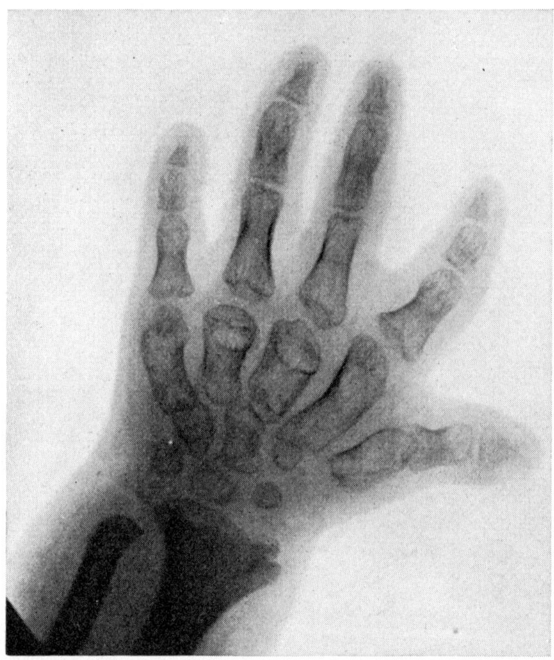

Fig. 238.—Roentgenogram of the hand in achondroplasia. Same case as Fig. 239, showing the expansion of the radius, and the stunting and increased breadth of phalanges and metacarpals.

fully developed size. This produces a distortion of the position of the remaining membrane-bones of the skull.

Symptoms.—These are visible at birth. The chief characteristic is the stunted growth of the extremities, while the trunk is normal in length (Fig. 239). The shortness in the thighs and arms is greater than in the legs and forearms. The hands may not reach below the hips, and are short and broad, with a separation between the second and third fingers (*trident hand*) (Fig. 240). The long bones of the body are not only short and thick, but often sharply curved at the epiphyseal junction. There is enlargement of these junctions, and the ribs are beaded. The skin of the limbs, especially on the extensor surfaces of the legs, shows folds and deep furrows, as though it were too abundant (Fig. 241). These furrows disappear as the patient grows older. There is generally a large amount of subcutaneous fat. The abdomen is prominent. The head appears large and brachycephalic, with prominent forehead, flattening of the bridge of the nose, and a forward projection of the lower jaw. The largeness of the head is due in part to the pushing upward of the brain as a result of the smallness of the base of the skull; in part often to the presence of a slight degree of hydrocephalus.

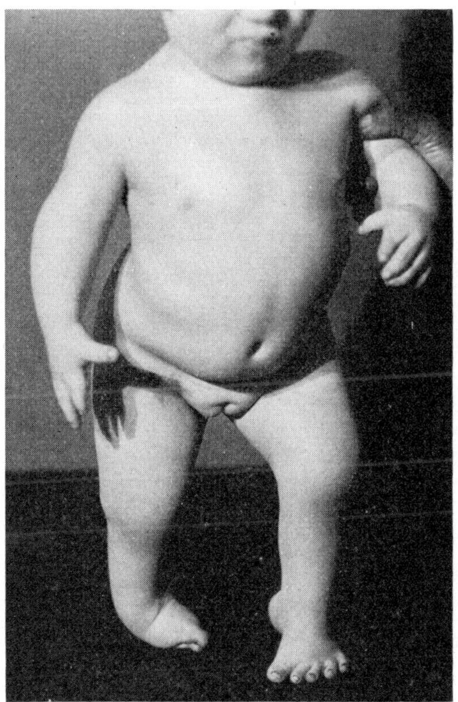

Fig. 239.—Achondroplasia. Patient aged four years in Cincinnati General Hospital.

The lips are thick. The fontanelle may not close for several years. Complicating defects, as polydactylism and inguinal hernia, are not infrequent.

Course and Prognosis.—The majority of achondroplasics are stillborn or die soon after birth. Many of the rest die during the first year;

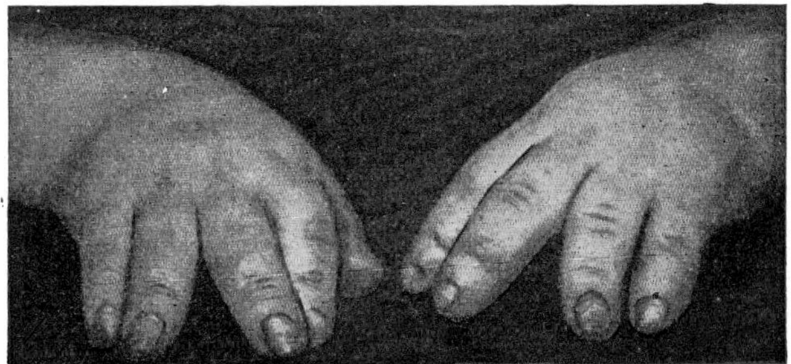

Fig. 240.—The "trident hand" in achondroplasia. (*Fussell, McCombs, deSchweinitz and Pancoast, Jour. Amer. Med. Assoc.*, 1909, **53,** 1615.)

but after this the duration of life is not affected by the disease. Dentition occurs at the usual time, but walking is often delayed until the third or fourth year. Growth is slow and the final height is seldom over $4\frac{1}{2}$ ft. After childhood the subjects often become very muscular. The gait is frequently waddling, the legs bowed, and there is lordosis. The pelvis is contracted, the second dentition unaffected, and the sexual functions are normal. The mental faculties are somewhat slow in developing, but the intellectual power may finally be normal.

Diagnosis.—At first achondroplasia strongly resembles *cretinism*. In this, however, there are at the beginning no lack of proportion between the limbs and the trunk and no characteristic alterations in the shape of the face and head, while fat pads are present in the region of the clavicles. The depression at the bridge of the nose in cretinism develops later. Achondroplasics exhibit a mental power which is either normal or, at the worst, far in excess of that of cretins. *Rickets* has often been confounded with achondroplasia. In fact, the disease was earlier known by the title "fetal rickets." In rickets there are delayed dentition, no early deformity of the face and head, and no disproportion between the extremities and the trunk. It is possible for an achondroplastic to be rachitic as well. *Infantilism*, or dwarfing from other cause, does not exhibit the peculiar disproportions seen in achondroplasia. The lesions in *osteogenesis imperfecta* are not in the cartilage at the epiphyseal junction, but in the shafts of the long bones or in the membrane-bones; there is a tendency to multiple fractures; and any shortness of the limbs is dependent upon fractures with union in malposition. Leri, Layani and Weill[49] describe under the term *dyschondrosteosis* 2 cases with marked shortness of the extremities but no other features of achondroplasia. The **treatment** is without benefit.

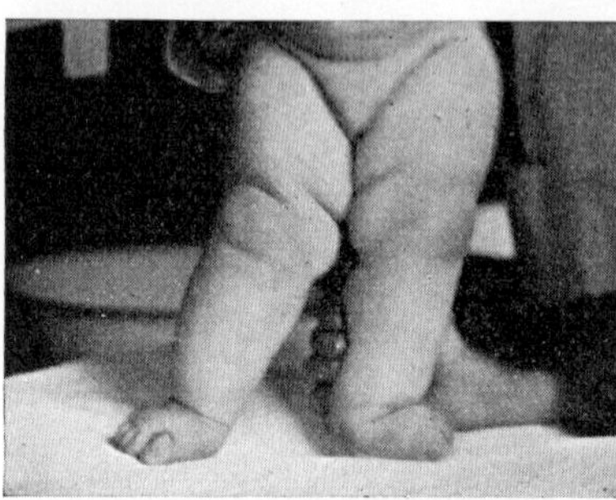

Fig. 241.—Achondroplasia, showing folds of the skin on the lower extremities. From a patient in the Children's Hospital of Philadelphia.

IDIOPATHIC OSTEOPSATHYROSIS

(Fragilitas Ossium)

Fragility of the bones in early life may occur secondarily to such conditions as scurvy, rickets, and syphilis. Under consideration here is only the tendency to multiple fractures without sufficient discoverable cause. Osteogenesis imperfecta with multiple intra-uterine fractures is discussed elsewhere (p. 1003). The two conditions are clearly allied. Writing in 1897 we[50] collected 67 cases of osteopsathyrosis (some of which should more properly be considered osteogenesis imperfecta) and we have since seen several instances of it. Additional cases have been collected and reported, among others by Porak and Durante,[51] Stewart,[52] Stobie,[53] Rosenblatt,[54] Apert, Bach and Odinet,[55] Gorter,[56] Harpøth,[57] Gleich,[58] and Bowcock and Lewis.[59] The **cause** is unknown, except that hereditary and familial influences play a part in many cases. A deficient absorption of phosphorus and calcium has been reported, but the amount of these minerals in the blood is usually normal. The **pathologic lesions** appear to vary, but there are usually slenderness of the shafts and thinness of the cortex of the bones. Lesions in various endocrine glands have been reported. The descriptions of chemical changes in the bones are contradictory, and the actual condition uncertain. The **symptoms** consist of fractures which may occur previous to or during normal labor. After birth inconsiderable movements may occasion them, such as the mere lifting of the child from bed. Fractures are oftenest situated in the long bones, ribs, and clavicles; may be complete or green-stick; occasion less pain than usual with this lesion; and unite readily in normal time with abundant callous, but often with malposition of all sorts. By no means all cases exhibit a marked degree of fragility, and it not infrequently happens that no fracture occurs until the child is several years old. It seems probable that fragilitas may be combined with osteogenesis imperfecta (see below). Frequently observed is dark-blueness of the sclerae, the association of which with fragility was first mentioned by Eddowes.[60] Sometimes there is deafness or benign glycosuria associated with brittle bones. The **prognosis** is unfavorable, although the brittleness of the bones may diminish. The **diagnosis** is readily made. *Rickets* produces bending of the bones without complete multiple fracture, and there are other characteristic manifestations. Inherited *syphilis* occasionally brings about a separation of several epiphyses which at first suggests fracture. *Achondroplasia* has shortening, but without fracture. *Osteogenesis imperfecta* exhibits distinct evidences of imperfect bone-formation, especially of the membranous bones; and the fractures are more numerous. Yet a sharp distinction cannot always be made, particularly in instances where fractures occur at or soon after birth. **Treatment** consists in the employment of extreme care in the handling of the patient. Fractures are managed as usual. Treatment with ultraviolet irradiation, cod liver oil and irradiated ergosterol, and the administration of calcium and phosphorus should be tried, but these have little effect. Feeding with thymus gland is claimed to do good. Radiologic treatment of the parathyroid gland has been tried, but hardly seems logical since hypercalcemia is not present.

OSTEOGENESIS IMPERFECTA

(Periosteal Aplasia; Periosteal Dysplasia)

Although it could be used in a broad sense to include achondroplasia, osteopsathyrosis, and certain other affections, it seems best to limit the term osteogenesis imperfecta to cases with defective osseous development of intra-uterine origin, most marked in the membrane-bones, but observed also in other regions. Cases have been reported and collected by Ostheimer,[61] Puech,[62] Bauer,[63] Klercker,[64] Sindler,[65] Fahr,[66] Welz and Lieberman,[67] Tauber,[68] Weber,[69] Wyatt and McEachern[70] and others. The **cause** is unknown. The blood usually shows normal calcium and phosphorus values, and normal retention of these minerals has been found. Several authors have reported abnormality of the parathyroid or of other endocrine glands. The disorder is encountered oftenest in fetuses or in still-born infants, but may be present in those who survive. The basis of the **lesions** is defective development of bony tissue both endochondral and periosteal, but especially the latter. Other mesodermal tissues, as blood vessels, dentine, and connective tissue, may show pathologic changes. As a result of this defective osseous development the vault of the cranium may suggest on examination a soft-shelled egg, and palpation produce a crackling sensation. The long bones, ribs, and clavicles may be soft and fragile, bending and breaking under slight pressure. Many deformities result, often producing a decided shortening of the extremities (Fig. 242). The **prognosis** is entirely unfavorable, death as a rule taking place early, but occasionally not until the second or third year. The **diagnosis** from osteopsathyrosis lies chiefly in the thinness of the vault of the skull combined with the deformities of the long bones; and the fact that osteopsathyrosis may not show itself until early infancy or later. Many cases of so-called "fetal rickets" are really instances of osteogenesis imperfecta. In achondroplasia the process is at the epiphyseal junctions, not in the shafts, and there are no fractures. **Treatment** is of no avail, but calcium, phosphorus, cod liver oil and ergosterol may be administered, and ultraviolet irradiation given.

CLEIDOCRANIAL DYSOSTOSIS

This rare affection appears to have been first described by Stahmann,[71] and was brought into prominence by Marie and Sainton.[72] Villaret and Francoz[73] collected 45 cases and Fitzwilliams[74] 60 more. An excellent review of the literature is given by Fitchet.[75] The cause is unknown, except that the condition is hereditary and familial. (Compare Langmead.[76]) There is delay in ossification of the cranial bones, with persistence to adult life of open anterior and posterior fontanelles. Large bosses develop on the frontal, parietal and occipital regions; the skull is brachycephalic and glob-

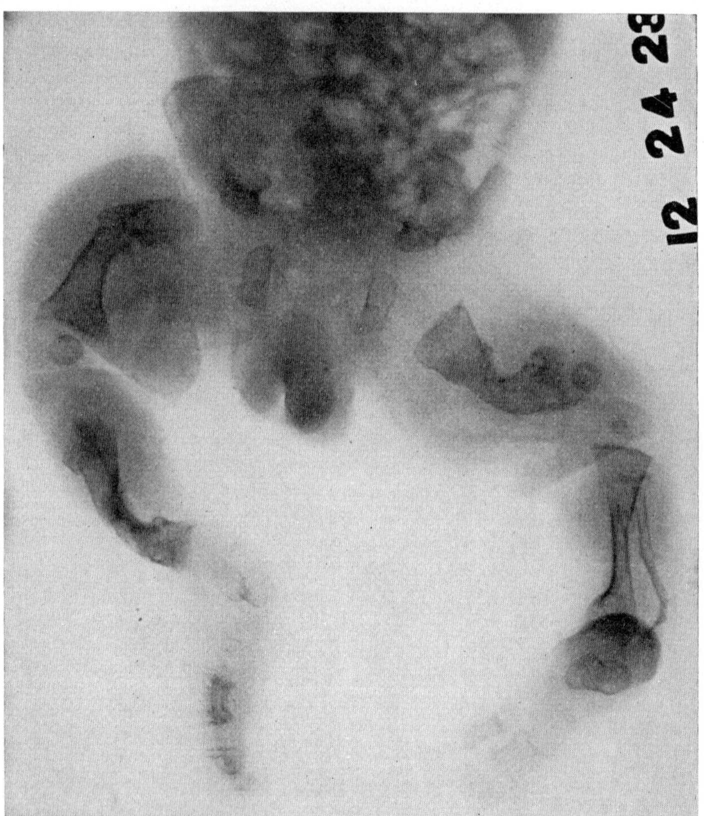

Fig. 242.—Roentgenogram of osteogenesis imperfecta. Infant of less five months. Bones of skull very soft. Fractures of all the long bones of the extremities. Blood-calcium 11.2 to 13.2. Blood-phosphorus 3.8 to 4.3. Illustration shows the numerous fractures involving the long bones of the legs.

ular; the forehead protruding; the facial bones small; the palatal arch high and perhaps cleft; the dentition irregular. The clavicles may be absent, or entirely cartilaginous; or the sternal ends present and the remainder absent; or the distal portions not united to intermediate parts. The shoulders can be drawn together in front to a remarkable degree (Fig. 243). The patients are generally shorter than normal, but with intellectual power and general health unaffected.

OSTEOMALACIA

Mollities ossium is rarely observed in children; and although described in infants (Rehn[77]) it is doubtful whether it ever occurs in them as an independent affection. Blank and Graves[78] report 3 cases in children in which there seemed to be roentgenographic evidence of bony changes characteristic both of rickets and osteomalacia. In older children it has been said to follow attacks of the infectious diseases, and, very possibly, some cases which have been called "late rickets" (p. 452) were, in fact, osteomalacia. In the same category probably belong most of the cases of so-called famine- or hunger-osteomalacia or war-rickets. Mollities has also been attributed to disorders of the internal secretion of the ovaries, the suprarenals, or the parathyroids. Lowered retention of calcium, phosphorus and magnesium has been reported. It may occur as a complication of osteopsathyrosis and osteogenesis imperfecta. The **lesions** comprise thickening of the perios-

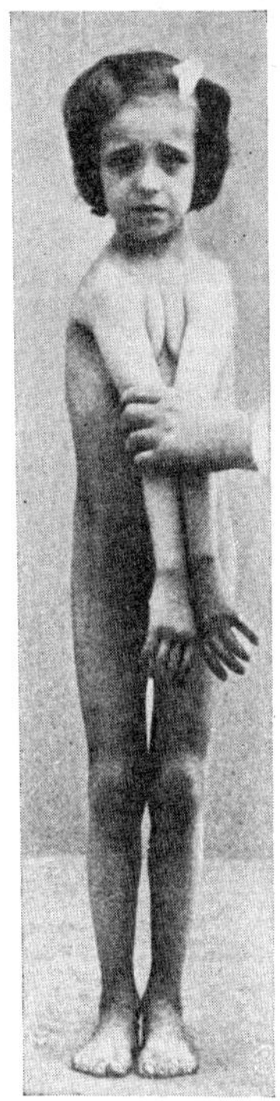

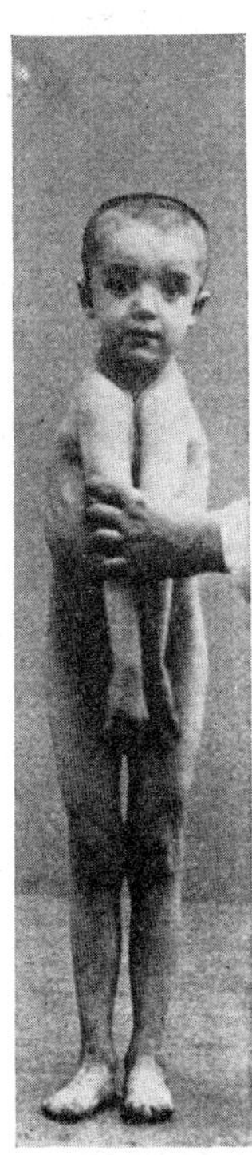

Fig. 243.—Cleidocranial dysostosis. Sister and brother aged nine and six years respectively. Illustrates broadness of the head and extreme mobility of the shoulder-joints, the result of imperfect development of the clavicles. A younger sister and the mother exhibited the same symptoms to a lesser degree. (*Villaret and Francoz, Nouv. iconogr. de la Saltpêtrière,* 1905, **18,** 302.)

teum, with softening of the bone beneath through the absorption of calcium salts and the occurrence of osteitis. The early **symptoms** consist in gradual development of pain in the bones, especially those of the legs. Bending then occurs, and fractures may later take place. The **course** is often long and progressive, although periods of remission may occur. The **prognosis** is unfavorable, except in famine-osteomalacia. White[79] distinguished this type by the ability to absorb and retain calcium and phosphorus; this power being lost in other forms. The **diagnosis** from rickets is made by the later period at which the softening takes place, and from osteopsathyrosis by the absence of early fracture or actual brittleness. In **treatment** bending and fractures are to be prevented as far as possible. Adrenaline is said to be of some value. The administration of calcium, phosphorus, cod liver oil, and irradiated ergosterol, and treatment by ultraviolet irradiation have curative value in famine-osteomalacia, but little if any effect in other types.

INFLAMMATION OF THE BONES AND JOINTS

Acute Infectious Osteomyelitis

(Acute Epiphysitis; Acute Septic Diaphysitis; Acute Periostitis)

This disease, which consists in an acute septic infection of the bone, occurs oftenest in males in later childhood, although it is seen even in infancy. It develops only during the period in which the bone is quite vascular and is growing. Under the influence of trauma, of some neighboring local source of infection, of some debilitating of infectious disease, or even without apparent predisposing cause septic germs lodge in the metaphyseal capillary loops among the cartilage cells. The species oftenest present are staphylococci, streptococci and pneumococci. An abscess later forms, the infection spreading by way of the Haversian canals to the periosteum (*acute periostitis*); or the pus extending to the shaft (*osteomyelitis*). The inflammation may involve the epiphysis (*acute epiphysitis*); and pus may penetrate into the joint (*septic arthritis*). Exceptionally inflammation starts beneath the periosteum. In severe cases of osteomyelitis the advance may be so rapid that in a few hours the periosteum has been lifted from the bone. Later, in more chronic cases, a sequestrum may be separated from the healthy bone which remains. Pus may penetrate the soft tissues, producing sinuses. In favorable cases the sequestra are finally softened or discharged, or can be removed by operation; although the medullary canal may be obliterated, and the destruction of epiphyseal cartilage may interfere with further growth of the limb. The favorite situations of the lesions are the terminal portions of the long bones, especially about the knee; less often about the shoulders, ankles, elbows, and in the ribs. Exceptionally the short bones are affected. The ilium is sometimes attacked and the disease supposed to be in the hip-joint. Osteomyelitis may attack the superior or inferior maxilla in young infants. Roehm[80] and Wilensky[81] review the literature on this subject. Pericarditis, pleuritis, or multiple abscesses may be present in some cases.

The **symptoms** at the onset develop suddenly, perhaps with a convulsion or chilliness, followed by high fever, delirium, and severe localized pain and tenderness, with slight redness and swelling. In rapidly fatal cases the child may promptly develop general sepsis; pericarditis often being an attendant complication. If the progress is slower, pain, swelling and redness extend over the whole section of the limb, and symptoms of arthritis may be added. This extension is especially liable to occur at the hip. Sometimes a metastatic multiple osteomyelitis is produced. In more chronic cases sinuses leading to the necrosed bone are formed; the acute manifestations subside; and the patient exhibits symptoms due to prolonged suppuration, as anemia, loss of weight, and possibly amyloid disease. In some cases there may be a chronic abscess involving most of the medullary cavity; in others, multiple localized abscesses develop, often in the vicinity of the epiphysis of the tibia, femur, or humerus, and surrounded by eburnated bone (*Brodie's*[82] *abscess*). In another chronic form there are thickening of cancellous bone and sclerosis of the medulla. In the chronic stage roentgenograms may reveal the softened area surrounded by thicker bone. A mild form of epiphysitis, occurring especially in the hip, which does not advance to actual pus formation, may follow trauma or infectious diseases. A nonsuppurative aseptic form of osteomyelitis affecting the epiphyses of the long bones may occur in smallpox. The **prognosis** is serious. Cases with severe septic symptoms may die after three or four days, perhaps before a diagnosis is made. Prompt incision and evacuation of pus may cause septic symptoms to disappear rapidly, but there is always the danger of complicating pyemic conditions. Later death may occur after prolonged suppuration. In cases which survive the limb is liable to be shortened. The **diagnosis** is not always easy. Roentgenography is of limited value, since it reveals no changes in acute cases before ten days or longer. Especially in infancy the local symptoms may not be evident when the condition is in the region of a deeply seated joint. In older subjects *acute rheumatism* must be differentiated. As a rule in this disease the inflammation is in the joint rather than the shaft of the bone; there is pain on movement of the joint itself; more than one articulation is affected; and constitutional symptoms are less severe. Tenderness on pressure over the bone below or above the joint aids in the exclusion of rheumatism. In infancy rheumatism is extremely rare. *Erysipelas* gives rise to redness and swelling, but there is no great tenderness or pain on movement. *Scurvy* produces painful and tender swelling in the shaft of the bone, with great pain on movement, pallor, and some fever, but does not exhibit the severe constitutional symptoms of osteomyelitis, and roentgenograms should be diagnostic (p. 461). **Treatment** must be instituted early. It consists in incision of such sort that pus shall be freely evacuated. In later stages vaccines may have some value, and various operative procedures may be required to remove sequestra. Reference may be made here to the treatment of chronic osteomyelitis by the implantation of maggots in the suppurating lesion (Baer[83]).

Tarsal Scaphoiditis

This was first described by Köhler.[84] It occurs in children between the ages of four and six years, affecting more boys than girls. It appears to be caused by repeated slight trauma to a delayed ossifying center in the scaphoid bone. There are pain, tenderness, swelling, and redness over the instep, associated with limping. The roentgenogram reveals a small scaphoid bone, irregular in outline, and increased in density. Prognosis is good and the treatment consists in immobilization.

Arthritis

This condition is often intimately associated with disease of the bones; in some varieties being secondary to it, in others followed by an extension of the process to the bones from the joint. Acute rheumatism, tuberculous arthritis, rheumatoid arthritis, and arthritis deformans are described elsewhere.

Acute Infectious Arthritis of Infancy (*Acute Infectious Epiphysitis*). This in cause and nature is similar to the osteomyelitis just described. Any of the ordinary pyogenic bacteria, as the streptococcus and staphylococcus, may be active; the gonococcus and the pneumococcus frequently so. Occasionally found are the meningococcus, colon bacillus, and typhoid or paratyphoid bacillus. The germs may enter the blood from various regions, not infrequently in young infants through the umbilicus or through trauma sustained at birth. The disease occurs chiefly in the first year of life, oftenest in the first six months. It may be monoarticular or polyarticular. The joints oftenest involved are the hip and shoulder; the small joints less frequently. Onset is sudden and the **symptoms** are indicative of sepsis. The swelling comes on rapidly, with pain, redness, and rigidity followed promptly by suppuration. Death may occur in a few days, usually from some visceral septic complication. In less severe cases suppuration develops more slowly, an abscess appearing in two to three weeks and discharging near the joint, or burrowing widely unless relieved by operation. In **diagnosis** rheumatism is excluded by the age of the patient. The **prognosis** is somewhat more favorable than in osteomyelitis, and the **treatment** similar to that for this disease.

Inasmuch as the symptoms in acute arthritis depend somewhat upon the nature of the germ, separate descriptions of the types of inflammation are desirable:—

Gonococcic Arthritis.—This occurs consecutively to gonorrheal ophthalmia, as first pointed out by Lucas,[85] gonorrheal vulvovaginitis, gonorrheal proctitis (Cooperman[86]), or gonorrheal coryza (Canino[87]). It is a relatively infrequent complication and we[88] found it but three times in 188 complications of gonorrheal vulvovaginitis reported by different observers. It begins acutely, often several weeks after the primary infection, or even after recovery from the symptoms of this; and may be monoarticular, but is frequently polyarticular, especially in infants. The **symptoms** are those of infectious arthritis as described, and the effusion may be purulent, but the process is usually limited to the synovial membrane. The wrist, knees, ankles, and especially the small joints of the fingers and toes are those oftenest involved. Recovery takes place after a number of weeks, with or without residual interference with motility. **Treatment** consists in the employment of measures to relieve pain and to put the part at rest, in evacuating pus if this is present, and perhaps the use of vaccines. Non-specific protein-therapy has been of benefit in this as in other forms of arthritis.

Pneumococcic Arthritis.—This occurs as frequently in early as in adult life, and probably more often in infancy. It is not necessarily associated with pneumonia, but may develop after empyema, otitis, or grippe, or apparently be primary. Probably a large proportion of cases of suppurative arthritis in the first five years of life are pneumococcic. The **lesions** are oftenest monoarticular, the joint involved being the knee, shoulder, hip, elbow or ankle in the order named. A widespread suppurative polyarthritis is generally dependent upon other germs than the pneumococcus. The effusion may be serous, but is oftener purulent. The **symptoms** are similar to those produced by other forms of arthritis, but the constitutional manifestations are often less marked. **Prognosis** is dubious. Half or more of the cases die, usually from pneumococcic complications in other parts of the body, although the outlook is better in children than in adults, and the destructive changes in the joint are usually not great as compared with other forms of suppurative arthritis. Cases in which the pus is thick and greenish-yellow are more favorable than those with a dark, watery fluid. Pneumococcic arthritis is to be **diagnosed** from the gonococcic by the absence of gonorrhea elsewhere, and by a lesser tendency to involvement of the small joints. In acute articular rheumatism the involvement is generally multiple, shifts from joint to joint, and is not purulent. Staphylococcic arthritis produces more decided local and constitutional symptoms. However, a positive diagnosis is to be made only by exploratory puncture and bacteriological examination. **Treatment** is entirely surgical.

Arthritis Depending upon Other Causes.—Arthritis may be due to other causes than those mentioned. In some cases the process may perhaps be toxic, as in the nonsuppurative arthritis seen after some of the infectious diseases, especially scarlatina, and rarely typhoid fever, measles, mumps, and other disorders. A frequent form is a mild arthritis limited to the synovial membrane (*synovitis*) caused by trauma, such as a sprain or a contusion, or which may follow injections of foreign protein as a symptom of serum-sickness. In arthritis due to such causes there are pain, tenderness, and swelling of the joints, but without decided constitutional involvement except in severe cases. Syphilitic and tuberculous arthritis are described elsewhere.

TUBERCULOSIS OF THE BONES AND JOINTS

Etiology.—Tuberculosis of these regions is of frequent occurrence in early life, but usually not until after infancy. That of the bones is dependent upon some primary, often distant, and generally unrecognized focus elsewhere in the body, as in the bronchial glands. Tuberculous arthritis is usually secondary to disease of the neighboring bones, but may occasionally be primary in the synovial membrane, especially in the knee. The occurrence of some infectious or debilitating condition, as measles or pertussis, or of a trauma, even slight, is a powerful inciting cause. Either variety of the tubercle bacillus may be active, but according to most investigators, it is more frequently the human type (p. 409).

Pathologic Anatomy.—The principal parts affected are the spinal vertebrae and the hip-joint, about a third of the cases occurring in each region. Other regions are attacked less frequently, among these being the knee, tarsus, carpus, ribs, wrists, shoulder-joints, and the bones of the skull. The upper extremities are much less often involved than the lower. In the former the elbow is the most frequent seat of the disease. The process in the bones is an osteitis beginning in the cancellous tissue of the bodies of the vertebrae; the bones of the carpus and tarsus; the central portion of the short tubular bones, such as the metacarpal bones and the phalanges, or the epiphyses of the long bones and extending thence to the joints; or the lesions may appear in the form of scattered nodules, as in the bones of the cranium. Small cavities may form which are shut in and encapsulated and the disease arrested; or the process may continue and extend to the periosteum or into the joint and an abscess form, burrow in various directions, and finally rupture spontaneously or be relieved by operation. Suppuration then continues until all the diseased bone has been softened and discharged. Meanwhile a reparative action goes on, new bone being formed. Occasionally in the more chronic lesions a cystic condition develops (*osteitis tuberculosa multiplex cystica*) (Schwentker[89]).

Tuberculosis involving a joint produces miliary tubercles and granulation-tissue upon the synovial membrane, which is finally separated from the cartilage leaving the bone exposed. A more or less purulent fluid accumulates and may discharge externally, or the process may be arrested earlier and heal without this. After recovery in the suppurative cases ankylosis or deformity of the joints may remain. Recovery from tuberculous lesions of the bones or joints is a matter of months or much oftener years. In many cases there is never any external evidence of suppuration, although a joint may be severely affected and finally recover ankylosed. Generally only one joint is involved. In the vertebral column one or several adjacent vertebrae suffer. Secondary tuberculous processes may appear, among the most frequent being meningitis. Amyloid degeneration of the liver, spleen, and kidneys is a frequent development after prolonged suppuration. The onset of tuberculous disease of the joints or bones is insidious, and the **symptoms** often misleading. There is in general but little pain early in the case. The formation of abscess is slow, without much fever, and with little constitutional disturbances. The early employment of roentgenography will often be of diagnostic aid. Further symptomatology is best discussed under the individual localizations of the tuberculous involvement.

1. Tuberculous Dactylitis

This disease, often called "spina ventosa," is the chief representative of tuberculosis of the short tubular bones, other bones of this class being rarely affected. It occurs most frequently in early childhood, and involves one or more of the phalanges and the metacarpal bones of the hands and feet, oftenest the index-finger. The center of the bone undergoes destruction and the periphery is thinned and expanded, while the periosteum thickens. The entire finger develops a spindle-shaped, hard and, later, red swelling, the soft tissues sharing in the inflammation (Fig. 244). An abscess generally develops. The course is comparatively painless, but long-continued, the process often ceasing only after many months, and with much deformity or even loss of the finger. The diagnosis is to be made chiefly from syphilitic dactylitis. This occurs in younger subjects, and is oftener multiple and symmetrical, while other evidences of syphilis are present. Treatment consists in measures suitable for the management of tuberculosis in general (p. 424). The part should be at rest with a splint or a plaster dressing applied. Operation should be performed only if abscess forms.

2. Tuberculous Spondylitis

(Caries of the Spine; Pott's Disease)

This is one of the most frequent tuberculous manifestations in early life. The greatest incidence is between the ages of three and fourteen years. It consists of a tuberculous osteitis beginning in the bodies of the vertebrae, producing caseous material, destroying the bone, and spreading to all the tissues of the articulation. The spinous process and arches are unaffected. Kyphosis (Fig. 245) gradually develops, with some degree of scoliosis if the vertebrae soften more upon one side. One or often several vertebrae are involved, and the extent and form of the kyphosis depend upon the number. The dorsal spine, especially the lower part, is the portion oftenest attacked in early life; the lumbar much less frequently, and the cervical still less often. The **symptoms** are insidious in onset and vary with the region of the spine affected. The earliest manifestations consist of fretfulness and disturbed sleep; and persistent or intermittent pain occurring in the course of the spinal nerves which arise from the affected part. There is muscular rigidity of the back, and pain there increased by pressure on the head or by jumping, but not by pressure applied over the seat of the lesion. The child assumes a position which will best take the weight from the diseased region and prevent jarring. Thus he may avoid bending to reach an object on the floor; walk stiffly or carefully upon the toes; prefer to lie on the abdomen; rest frequently across a chair, or over the mother's lap, or with the hands on the thighs. In cervical cases the child may hold the head stiffly or support it with the hands. Evidences of paralysis or other nervous disturbances often appear. These have been described under Compression Myelitis (p. 965). Paraplegia occurs in from 10 to 20 per cent of all cases. It is seen in about half of the cases of caries of the upper dorsal or cervical region, but is rare in involvement below the mid-dorsal spine. The average duration of the disease is three years before paralysis appears; but the symptoms may develop even after a few months. Abscess is most frequent in involvement of the lumbar vertebrae but may not occur at all, or may not appear for three or four months, or oftener not until the second year of the disease. It is prone to develop insidiously and without acute symptoms (*cold abscess*). Abscess in cases of cervical caries often opens in the pharynx (*retropharyngeal abscess*), or above the clavicle. In tuberculosis of the lower cervical and upper dorsal vertebrae it may burst into the pleura or make its way to the scapula, but

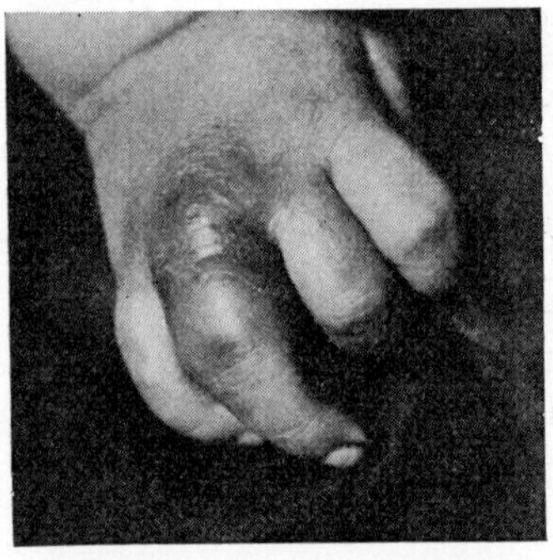

Fig. 244.—Tuberculous Dactylitis. Infant eleven months old in Cincinnati General Hospital. Process of five months' duration.

often it gravitates to the lower part of the trunk and is discharged above Poupart's ligament. Lower dorsal and lumbar abscesses may open above Poupart's ligament, in the loin, or in the upper portion of the thigh. Kyphosis also is a late symptom of spondylitis. It begins as a slight curved projection over one vertebra (Fig. 245), but increases in extent. It is most visible in the mid-dorsal region, and the worst curvatures are found here. It may fail to develop in the lumbar and cervical regions. With kyphosis of the dorsal region, if well-marked, there are flattening of the sides of the thorax and prominence of the sternum. The **course** may last from two to five years, unless the disease is recognized and treated early, in which case the duration is considerably shorter, and after two or three years the reparative process begins and recovery with ankylosis results with but slight deformity. Even many cases untreated until after paraplegia develops may finally regain the entire use of the limbs. There is always, however, great danger of relapse of a spondylitis, brought about by trauma or other cause. The **prognosis** in childhood is on the whole good, if treatment is begun promptly and systematically followed. Yet the disease is a serious one, with a mortality of 10 to 25 per cent, death occurring from the result of prolonged suppuration, myelitis, or general tuberculosis. The **diagnosis** should be made early and before curvature develops. When any of the symptoms mentioned are present, there must be studied the mobility of the spine; the position assumed; the gait; the distribution of pain; and the knee-jerks and other evidences of involvement of the spinal cord. Roentgenographic examination is of value only later in the disease. Certain other pathologic conditions are especially to be distinguished. *Rachitis* produces kyphosis; but it is of much greater length and uniformity, is unaccompanied by rigidity, and usually largely disappears when traction is applied to the legs or the child suspended from the armpits or placed face downward and the legs elevated. *Scoliosis* from rachitis or faulty position might suggest the lateral curvature sometimes produced by caries. It is, however, of considerable length, while that of caries is short, and the former is not accompanied by rigidity or pain. *Hip-joint disease* may be supposed to be present in cases where the lameness is in reality the result of caries of the lumbar spine. The latter disease is without the limitation of movement at the joint, except in the direction of extension if a concealed psoas abscess be present; and under these circumstances the thigh is kept more or less flexed. The paralysis and other symptoms attendant upon spinal caries are to be distinguished from *nervous symptoms due to other causes.* This has been considered under Compression Myelitis (p. 965). **Treatment** is principally medical and mechanical rather than operative, the last two being orthopedic in nature. The details will be found in works upon orthopedic and general surgery. In general it consists in rest of the diseased spine. Equally

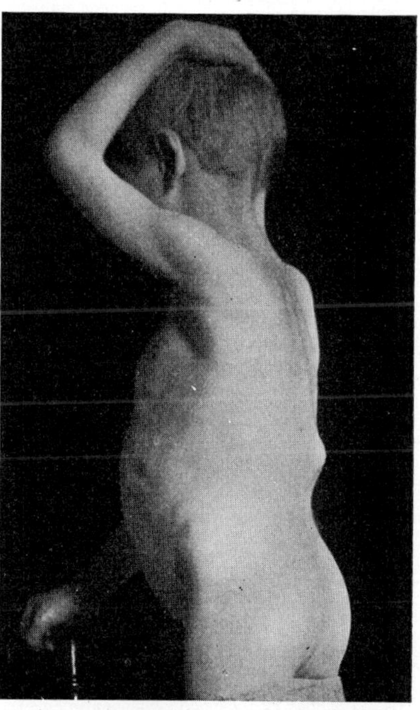

Fig. 245.—Caries of the vertebrae. Early deformity. (*Courtesy of Dr. I. Valentine Levi.*)

important is the maintaining and improving of the general health in every possible way, as in tuberculosis in any part of the body (p. 424).

3. Hip-joint Disease

Coxitis is the most common tuberculous disease of the joints in children, and 85 per cent of the cases occur before the tenth year. In the large majority of instances only one hip is involved, and if both, then not simultaneously. Sometimes the disease begins in the synovial membrane, but as a rule an osteitis of the epiphysis of the femur is the first process, followed later by arthritis in which all parts of the joint share, and still later by the formation of abscess and destruction of the head of the femur, displacement, and deformity. A reparative process may begin at any time.

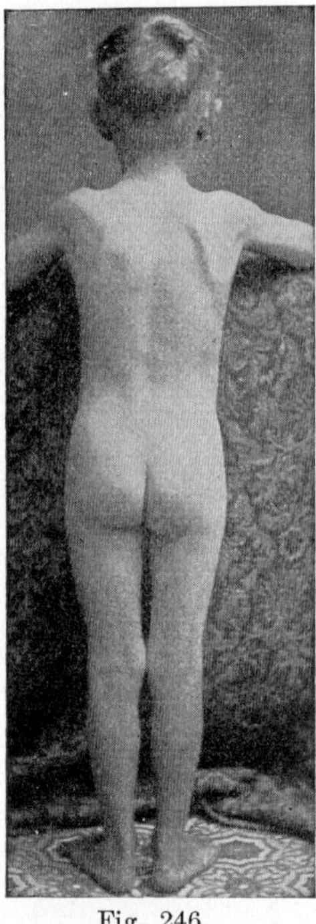

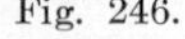

Fig. 246.

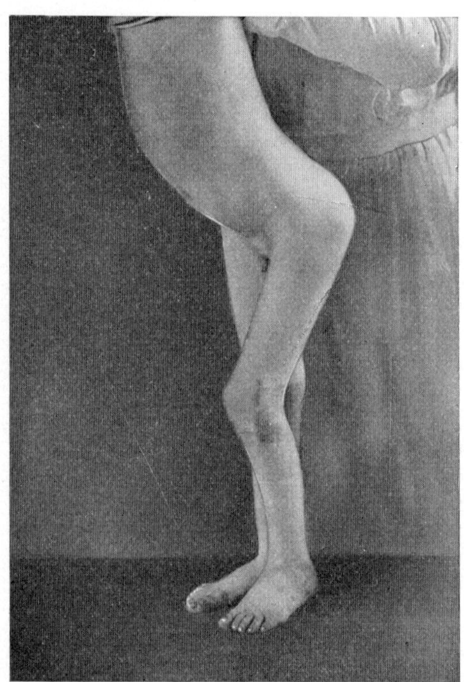

Fig. 247.

Fig. 246.—Disease of right hip-joint. Internatal crease inclined toward left thigh. Right buttock narrower, gluteofemoral crease shortened and less distinct, buttock fading away into thigh. (*Willard, Surgery of Childhood*, 462, *Fig.* 406.)

Fig. 247.—Hip-joint disease. Shows flexion at hip and knee and outward rotation. (*Courtesy of Dr. H. R. Wharton.*)

Symptoms.—The onset is usually gradual, the first symptom being slight lameness, which is generally intermittent and seen oftenest on first rising in the morning or after exercise. Days or weeks may then pass without lameness being again discoverable. Some degree of pain may be present, now or developing later, usually referred to the front of the knee or the inner side of the thigh. There is a disposition to stand with the weight of the body thrown upon the sound leg, the other being abducted and rotated outward. When standing with the feet close together, there is a flattening of the gluteofemoral fold on the diseased side, and a deviation of the internatal crease toward the healthy side (Fig. 246); and when placed on the back on a table with the legs together, the diseased side appears longer. Distinct muscular rigidity is shown if efforts are made by the examiner to move the diseased hip. At first this is found only during backward extension with the child on the abdomen or side, but later motion in any direction is restricted, and, with the patient on his back, the pelvis may be found to move with the leg if the fingers are placed upon the anterior superior spinous process of the ilium. Swelling and tenderness about the joint may be detected even early in the course by feeling for the head of the femur under Poupart's ligament close to the femoral artery. Atrophy of the thigh begins early.

As the disease advances there is an increase of the limp, with pain on walking; and there are startings and "night cries" from the occurrence of pain as the result of involuntary movement during sleep. Walking may become impossible, or accomplished only with a marked limp; and even when at rest the pain is often constant and intense. The thigh is now held partially flexed and rotated outwardly, and the knee flexed (Fig. 247). When the child is on his back upon a table, with the legs extended and parallel, the diseased leg now exhibits an apparent shortening, owing to tilting of the pelvis upward; and the back is arched. The atrophy of the thigh and leg become decided.

Destruction of the joint proceeds, with the production of pus; the thigh is flexed, adducted, and now rotated inward; the knee is flexed; the swelling about the hip increases, and an abscess may form with final discharge. This evacuation is oftenest immediately in front of the joint, but burrowing in other directions may occur before an opening forms. However, absorption of the head and neck of the femur may take place without any visible evidence of suppuration. Statistics upon the frequency of abscess vary from 23 to over 60 per cent (Young[90]), depending largely upon the time at which appropriate treatment is started. Actual shortening of the limb, often of several inches, is now present, resulting from destruction of the head of the bone, erosion of the acetabulum, and diminished growth of the femur. Marked lordosis of the spine develops.

Course and Prognosis.—It is usually three or four months, although sometimes less, before the osteitis extends to actual involvement of the joint and severe symptoms begin; and from two to four years, and still longer in cases with abscess, before the whole process is over and the symptoms of inflammation have disappeared. It is possible when treatment is begun in the first few weeks for the process to cease entirely before the joint itself is attacked, and for recovery to be complete without stiffness or any alteration of the gait. In the large majority of cases, however, more or less permanent lameness persists. If proper treatment has not been employed, many children recover with the hip-joint ankylosed in a faulty position. Even years after recovery recurrences may take place from slight trauma or over-use of the limb. The disease may end fatally from prolonged suppuration, or from the development of tuberculosis elsewhere, especially general tuberculosis or meningitis.

The prognosis on the whole is good, both for life and for the possessing of a fairly useful limb, especially in children and when the diagnosis is made early and the general health is not impaired. Probably from 10 per cent in patients treated early, to 60 per cent in neglected cases already suppurating, would fairly express the final mortality (Willard[36]).

Diagnosis.—This should be made as early as possible, and is based upon a consideration of the symptoms described, the child having been undressed and carefully examined throughout. Roentgenograms are of great aid, the joint early appearing indistinctly outlined, and in advanced cases showing undoubted evidences of destruction of the bone and of faulty position. *Rheumatism* is seldom confined to the one joint, and is of acute onset with fever and with localized swelling and pain. *Spinal caries* may produce flexion of the thigh from the production of a psoas abscess. The restriction of movement is generally, however, limited to extension. *Trauma* of the hip causes acute local pain, swelling, lameness, and even suppuration; but the onset is acute after injury and there is no muscular rigidity. In overweight children trauma may produce a partial separation of the epiphysis of the femur and cause pain and limping, and a mild transient coxitis, not tuberculous, may sometimes occur. An *infectious arthritis* is acute in nature and rapid in its course. The referred pain of hip-joint disease may suggest the existence of *tuberculous arthritis of the knee-joint*, but examination will readily show that there is no inflammation there. *Juvenile osteochondritis deformans* (Perthes'[91] disease) is a rare condition producing symptoms very similar to those of tuberculous coxitis. It is distinguished to a certain degree by the lack of pain and spasm; the limitation of motion chiefly on adduction; the absence of evidences of rarefaction of the bone on roentgenographic examination; and the negative tuberculin-reaction. Yet often the diagnosis cannot be made early in the case. The difficulty in diagnosis of hip-joint disease even in the early stages depends chiefly on lack of care on the part of the examiner.

Treatment.—The treatment consists in putting the part entirely at rest and removing the influence of muscular spasm by means of traction. The manner of accomplishing this is in the province of the orthopedist. The same remark is true of the treatment of abscesses which may occur. The medical management is similar to that for tuberculosis in general. Open-air life, preferably at the sea-shore and with heliotherapy, is a great desideratum.

4. Tuberculous Arthritis of Other Joints

Less frequently tuberculosis may affect other joints than the hip, most frequently the knee, next the ankle, and after this in childhood the elbow. In the elbow the lesions are oftenest first situated in the end of the humerus, and only exceptionally in the radius alone. In the ankle the disease appears usually first in the bones of the tarsus, less frequently in the end of the tibia. In the knee it begins in one of the condyles of the femur, and less often in the head of the tibia, or may develop first of all in the synovial membrane. One or more joints may be involved. The **symptoms** are analogous to those of hip-joint disease. The onset is slow. Pain may be severe, or often slight or absent early in the case; but it is later constant. Rigidity of the muscles is characteristic, and the joint is swollen and held in a flexed position. Redness is not an early symptom. Atrophy of the muscles develops, and high fever is present if suppuration occurs. The symptoms vary naturally with the location. In tuberculous arthritis of the knee (*white swelling*) the first manifestations are the swelling and an occasional slight limp, with a tendency to keep the knee flexed. The child walks on the toes, and the leg is adducted and rotated outward. If the ankle is affected there is likewise a limping gait, with abduction of the leg and eversion and outward rotation of the foot. In disease of the elbow-joint there is pronation of the arm with slight flexion of the elbow.

The course is quite similar to that of hip-joint disease, but the prognosis for life is better, although death may occur from the development of tuberculosis elsewhere, or from prolonged suppuration. The diagnostic distinctions from other diseases are in general similar to those discussed under Hip-joint Disease (p. 1012), and the same principles of treatment prevail, except that for some reason heliotherapy appears to be ineffective in tuberculosis of the knee-joint.

SYPHILITIC DISEASE OF THE BONES

(See also Syphilis, P. 432–434)

Although a syphilitic arthritis is occasionally seen (p. 432, Fig. 94), syphilis usually shows itself in the bony system as epiphysitis, dactylitis, and chronic osteoperiostitis. Excellent studies emphasizing the roentgenographic changes in congenital syphilis are those by Bromer[92] and McLean.[93]

1. Syphilitic Epiphysitis

Although recognized earlier this is often called "Parrot's[94] Disease," from his description of it in 1872. It generally appears within the first three months of life, and is found even in still-born infants. It is the most common early osseous manifestation of hereditary syphilis. The epiphyses of the large joints are oftenest affected, especially those of the humerus, and usually on both sides; but several of the long bones may be attacked simultaneously. The **symptoms** develop acutely and are those suggestive of flaccid paralysis, with swelling and tenderness in the neighborhood of the epiphysis involved (*syphilitic pseudoparalysis*). The affected limb is not moved voluntarily and passive movement causes pain. The swelling is generally moderate and sometimes scarcely visible. Occasionally crepitus can be elicited. There is little or no fever. Roentgenograms may show epiphyseal separation. The **prognosis** is favorable if treatment is prompt and thorough, the normal condition of movement often being regained in two or three weeks, or longer in severe cases. Spontaneous recovery may occur even without treatment. Occasionally there is suppuration, perhaps involving the neighboring joint, or osteomyelitis may develop and the prognosis is then unfavorable. The **diagnosis** rests upon the symptoms as described, evidences of syphilis elsewhere, the early age, and the Wassermann reaction. Examination shows no alteration in electrical response, while the presence of swelling and pain on movement exclude *obstetrical paralysis* of the upper arm type. *Scurvy* rarely occurs so early in life, is not limited to the epiphysis, is promptly cured by antiscorbutic treatment, and the roentgenographic appearances are different. *Infectious arthritis* is attended by severe septic symptoms. *Rickets* develops later and does not have marked pain. The **treatment** is that for syphilis in general (p. 438). In addition the part must be kept at rest and, if suppuration develops, surgical aid is needed.

2. Syphilitic Dactylitis

This is not common and is seen usually from the first four or five months to the second year of life, may be single or multiple, and is often symmetrical. It affects the phalanges more frequently than the metacarpal and metatarsal bones, and oftenest the proximal phalanx of the index finger. There is seldom suppuration, and the joint is not involved. It differs from tuberculous dactylitis (p. 1009) in being more often multiple; less liable to attack metacarpal and metatarsal bones; and of less frequent occurrence. Especially in its early stages it responds to antisyphilitic treatment.

3. Chronic Syphilitic Osteoperiostitis

This is a manifestation of late hereditary syphilis, seen oftenest in later childhood, although it may occasionally occur in infancy. There is a characteristic hypertrophic osteoperiostitis involving several bones, generally symmetrically, and oftenest the shaft of the tibiae, the bones of the arm, and the cranium. There may be great increase in the thickness of the long bones, as well as to some extent in their length; or the enlargement is nodular and chiefly near the epiphyses. Gummata may develop beneath the periosteum or within the bone, and undergo necrosis and softening, with suppuration and the formation of sinuses. The **symptoms** develop slowly. There is a variable degree of pain, especially at night, with tenderness and gradually increasing deformity. In characteristic cases the tibia of each leg is much thickened, often exhibits irregular nodules, and is bowed anteriorly (*saber tibia*) (Fig. 248 and p. 433, Fig. 96). If the cranium is involved there are irregular hyperostoses, especially of the frontal and parietal regions, making the forehead square (Fig. 248). The **course** is chronic, and the condition resistant to treatment unless this is commenced early. Any production of pus is of slow development and attended by little pain or constitutional disturbance. Sinuses are long in healing, and keep open until any necrotic bone has been discharged. Acute symptoms may be relieved by antisyphilitic treatment, but bony thickening changes little. The **diagnosis** need only be made from *rickets* which, however, shows a bowing of the legs, generally nearer the lower epiphyses, little if any pain in the bones, and an occurrence much earlier in life. *Tuberculosis*, if it produces necrosis and sinuses, affects more often the ends of the bones rather than the shaft. The periosteal elevation occurring in *scurvy*, *leukemia*, and *osseous tumors* should occasion little difficulty in diagnosis.

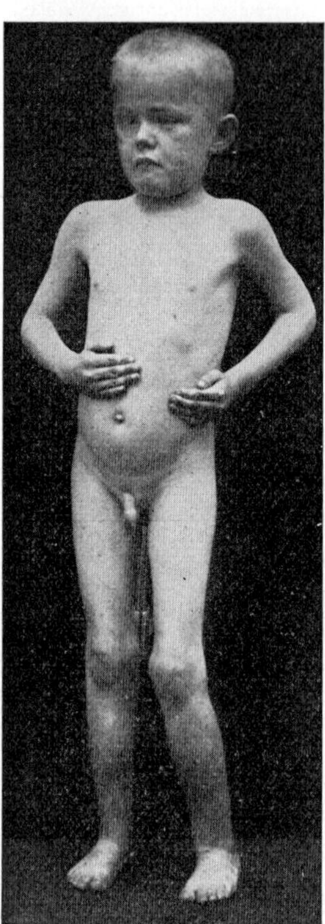

Fig. 248.—Chronic syphilitic osteoperiostitis. Child of eleven years in the Children's Ward of the Hospital of the University of Pennsylvania. Head brachycephalic, occipital region almost perpendicular, frontal tuberosities, flattening of the bridge of the nose and typical saber-tibiae, spleen enlarged.

MISCELLANEOUS DISEASES OF THE BONES

Multiple Exostoses.—These are not uncommon. They may be single or more often multiple and more or less symmetrically situated; affect males more frequently than females; and often are hereditary in nature. While still growing the exostoses are covered externally by cartilage. Under this is compact bone with a medullary cavity communicating with that of the bone from which the growth arises. The growths are benign and vary in size and form, and are situated chiefly in the long bones of the limbs, oftenest on the shaft near the epiphysis, and especially in the neighborhood of the knee, shoulder, and wrist. They may be present at birth, but usually appear during childhood and increase in number until early adult life, when they may diminish in size. They may be few or numerous; as a rule are painless except through pressure upon nerves; and may interfere with motion to a limited extent. There are no bony deposits in the muscles as in myositis ossificans (p. 985). The administration of iodides may be tried, and the growths removed if decided local symptoms develop.

Chondrodysplasia (*Multiple Cartilaginous Exostoses; Multiple Enchondromata; Diaphysial Aclasis; Chondro-osteoma; Ollier's*[95] *Disease; Hereditary Deforming Chondrodysplasia*).—According to Ray,[96] 157 cases of this have been reported in the American literature alone, and Leucutia and Price[97] place the total of those recorded at about 700 cases. The condition is frequently hereditary and familial. The growths are composed of cartilage and situated oftenest upon the hands, fingers, feet, and toes. They may produce thinning of the bone and cysts may form. In one variety of chondrodysplasia there are softening and bending of the bones but without outgrowths (Stocks,[98] Blount[99]).

Osseous Dystrophy.—Morquio[100] and Meyer and Brennemann[101] describe a rare form of familial osseous dystrophy, with rarefaction and absences of bony tissue and retardation of bony development. There is decided deficiency of osseous tissue involving practically the whole skeleton with the exception of the skull. This condition might possibly be classified with the chondrodysplasia just discussed.

Osteitis Fibrosa Cystica (*Von Recklinghausen's*[102] *Disease*).—This rarely occurs in children. There is painless enlargement of the bones, oftenest near the joints, which occurs because of resorption and atrophy of osseous material, with the subsequent formation of cysts. The first sign is often fracture. Roentgenograms show a honeycombed appearance in the long bones and occasionally in the flat bones. The cause of the condition is unknown, but hypertrophy of the parathyroid glands has sometimes been associated. Calcium and phosphorus may be administered, although they do little good; radiologic treatment may be of assistance; occasionally some of the cysts may be operated on. Ask-Upmark[103] found improvement following removal of the parathyroids. Good reviews on cystic disease of the bones are given by Morton[104] and Stoloff.[105] A *congenital form* of *osteodystrophy fibrosa* is described by Frangenheim.[106] *Leontiasis ossea*, in which hyperosteitic formations occur symmetrically on the tibiae and skull, is probably to be classified with osteitis fibrosa. A case in a child is reported by Capon.[107]

Cysts of Bone.—Cysts of the bone may be found in certain malignant conditions as well as in chondrodysplasia and osteitis fibrosa cystica. Nonmalignant solitary osseous cysts are found in children (Phemister and Gordon[108]).

Malignant Growths.—*Primary* new growths of the bone are not common in infancy, but are not infrequent in later childhood. The usual one is sarcoma. A type of this known as *Ewing's endothelioma* may occur in childhood (Reuben and Peskin[109]). *Secondary* neoplasms may be of various sorts, as those metastatic from suprarenal tumors. Xanthomatosis involves the bones. (See pp. 1051, 1052.)

Chloroma, so-called from the green color of the tumor on section, while rare, occurs as frequently in early as in later life. Mensi[110] reported 4 cases and collected 41, and Washburn[111] states that there are 162 reported cases. More males are affected than females. Chloroma develops in the bone-marrow especially of the skull, and metastases take place into the various lymphatic tissues of the body. The blood shows a condition similar to lymphocytic, or more frequently myelocytic, leukemia, and the disease has been considered a form of leukemia by some authors. Others believe that it is neoplastic in nature. There occur enlargement of lymph-glands and spleen, fever, emaciation, and hemorrhage from mucous membranes. Death occurs in a few months; occasionally not for twelve to eighteen months. Washburn's[111] patient, subjected to roentgenographic treatment, was apparently still well after two and one-half years.

Multiple Myeloma (*Kahler's Disease*[112]).—In this there is a circumscribed or diffuse myeloma of the bone-marrow, neoplastic in nature. Painful swelling of the bones, including the skull, occurs, and rarefactions are seen in the roentgenograms. Spontaneous fractures may take place. Bence-Jones protein is found in the urine (Lewis[113]).

References

1. Am. J. Dis. Child., 1931, **41,** 1309. 2. Am. J. Dis. Child., 1931, **41,** 1317. 3. Edinburgh M. J., 1924, **31,** 560; 1926, **33,** 189; 280; 357. 4. J.A.M.A., 1931, **96,** 1929.

5. Presse méd., 1912, **20,** 737. 6. Arch. d. méd. d. enf., 1927, **30,** 650. 7. Ztschr. f. d. ges. Neurol. u. Psychiat., Orig., 1913, **20,** 547. 8. Ges. Abhandl. z. wissenschaft. Med., Frankfurt, 1856. Ref. Am. J. Dis. Child., 1931, **41,** 793. 9. Bull. et mém. soc. méd. d. hôp., 1906, **23,** 1310. 10. Pediatria, 1926, **34,** 1305. 11. Hospitalstid., 1929, **72,** 153; 165. 12. Am. J. Dis. Child., 1931, **41,** 793. 13. Arch. Pediat., 1930, **47,** 556. 14. Am. J. Dis. Child., 1931, **42,** 837. 15. Am. J. M. Sc., 1927, **173,** 701. 16. J. Morphol., 1908, **29,** 1. 17. J.A.M.A., 1931, **96,** 441. 18. Surg. Gynec. and Obst., 1930, **50,** 79. 19. Am. J. Dis. Child., 1932, **43,** 136. 20. Arch. Dis. Childhood, 1932, **7,** 117. 21. J. Bone and Joint Surg., 1930, **12,** 649. 22. Malformations, Diseases, and Injuries of Fingers and Toes, 1866. 23. Bull. et mém. soc. méd. d. hôp., 1922, **19,** 834. 24. Bull. et mém. soc. méd. d. hôp., 1896, **13,** 220. 25. Ztschr. f. Kinderh., Orig., 1914, **12,** 161. 26. Arch. f. Kinderh., 1916, **56,** 391. 27. Am. J. Dis. Child., 1926, **31,** 832. 28. Nourrisson, 1927, **15,** 292. 29. Arch. f. Augenh., 1929, **100–101,** 278. 30. Arch. Dis. Childhood, 1929, **4,** 190. 31. J. Missouri M. A., 1928, **25,** 20. 32. J.A.M.A., 1928, **90,** 686. 33. J.A.M.A., 1928, **91,** 1547. 34. Arch. de méd. d. enf., 1928, **31,** 645. 35. Arch. f. klin. Chir., 1891, **42,** 545. 36. Surgery of Childhood, 1910, 721; 664. 37. Am. J. M. Sc., 1928, **175,** 365. 38. Arch. Pediat., 1927, **44,** 86. 39. Rev. de méd., 1890, **10,** 1. 40. Arch. Int. Med., 1915, **15,** 659. 41. Der weiche Hinterkopf, 1843. 42. Greenebaum, Selkirk, Mitchell and Bier, Ohio State M. J., 1929, **25,** 34. 43. Ztschr. f. Kinderh., 1927, **44,** 365. 44. Ztschr. f. Kinderh., 1930, **50,** 381. 45. Bull. soc. d'anthrop. de Paris, 1878; La syphilis héréd. et la rachitis, 1886, 280. 46. Untersuchungen ü. d. sogen. Rachitis foetalis, 1892. Ref. Centralbl. f. Gynäk., 1892, **16,** 358. 47. Arch. gén. de méd., 1902, **189,** 232. 48. Achondroplasia. Its Nature and Its Cause, 1912. 49. Presse méd., 1931, **39,** 262. 50. Griffith, Am. J. M. Sc., 1897, **113,** 426. 51. Nouv. icongr. de la Saltpêtrière, 1905, **18,** 481. 52. Brit. M. J., 1922, **2,** 498. 53. Quart. J. Med., 1924, **17,** 274. 54. J. Michigan M. Soc., 1927, **26,** 447. 55. Bull. de la soc. de pédiat. de Paris, 1928, **26,** 21. 56. Nederl. Tijdschr. v. Geneesk., 1929, **1,** 2022. 57. Ugesk. f. Laeger., 1930, **92,** 356. 58. New York State J. Med., 1930, **30,** 850. 59. Ann. Int. Med., 1930, **3,** 700. 60. Brit. M. J., 1900, **2,** 222. 61. J.A.M.A., 1914, **63,** 1996. 62. Ann. Paul. de med. e. chir., 1917, Nov., Ref. Arch. de méd. d. enf., 1918, **21,** 658. 63. Deutsch. Ztschr. f. Chir., 1920, **154,** 166; Berl. klin. Wchnschr., 1923, **2,** 624. 64. Monatschr. f. Kinderh., 1923, **25,** 338. 65. Ztschr. f. Kinderh., 1926, **42,** 85. 66. Virchow's Arch. f. path. Anat., 1926, **261,** 732. 67. Am. J. Obst. and Gynec., 1927, **14,** 49. 68. Monatschr. f. Kinderh., 1927, **36,** 12. 69. Arch. Path., 1930, **9,** 984. 70. Am. J. Dis. Child., 1932, **43,** 403. 71. Ztschr. f. Med. Chir. u. Geburtsh., 1857, **11,** 433. 72. Bull. et mém. soc. méd. d. hôp. de Paris, 1897, 3s, **14,** 706; 1898, **15,** 436. 73. Nouv. iconogr. de la Saltpêtrière, 1905, **18,** 302. 74. Lancet, 1910, **2,** 1466. 75. J. Bone and Joint Surg., 1929, **11,** 838. 76. Proc. Roy. Soc. Med., 1916, **10,** 1; Dis. Child., 1. 77. Jahrb. f. Kinderh., 1878, **12,** 100. 78. Am. J. Dis. Child., 1929, **38,** 84. 79. Arch. Int. Med., 1922, **30,** 620. 80. Am. J. Dis. Child., 1931, **42,** 1171. 81. Am. J. Dis. Child., 1932, **43,** 431. 82. London Med. Gaz., 1845, **36,** 1399. 83. J. Bone and Joint Surg., 1931, **13,** 438. 84. München. med. Wchnschr., 1908, **55,** 1923. 85. Brit. M. J., 1885, **1,** 429; **2,** 57. 86. Am. J. Dis. Child., 1926, **31,** 183; 1927, **33,** 932. 87. Pediatria, 1931, **39,** 264. 88. Gittings and Mitchell, Am. J. Dis. Child., 1917, **13,** 448. 89. Am. J. Dis. Child., 1931, **42,** 102. 90. Orthopedic Surgery, 1906. 91. Verhandl. d. Gesellsch. f. Chir., Berlin, 1913, **42,** Teil 2, 140. 92. New England J. Med., 1929, **200,** 524. 93. Am. J. Dis. Child., 1931, **40,** 131; 363; 607; 1129; 1411. 94. Arch. d. phys. norm. et path., 1871–2, **4,** 319. 95. Rev. de chir., 1900, **21,** 396. 96. Arch. Pediat., 1930, **47,** 152. 97. Am. J. Roentgenol., 1929, **22,** 338. 98. Hereditary Disorders of Bone Development, 1925. 99. Am. J. Dis. Child., 1930, **40,** 327. 100. Arch. de méd. d. enf., 1929, **32,** 129. 101. Am. J. Dis. Child., 1932, **43,** 123. 102. Festschr. Rudolf Virchow, 1891. 103. Hygeia, 1931, **93,** 704. 104. Arch. Surg., 1922, **4,** 534. 105. Am. J. Roentgenol., 1927, **18,** 26. 106. Deutsch. Ztschr. f. Chir., 1927, **200,** 484. 107. Arch. Dis. Childhood, 1928, **3,** 285. 108. J.A.M.A., 1927, **87,** 1429. 109. Arch. Pediat., 1928, **45,** 116. 110. Pediatria, 1920, **28,** 593. 111. Am. J. Dis. Child., 1930, **39,** 330. 112. Prag. med. Wchnschr., 1889, **14,** 33; 45. 113. Internat. Clin., 1927, 37th Series, **1,** 157.

SECTION X

DISEASES OF THE BLOOD, SPLEEN AND LYMPH-NODES

CHAPTER I

DISEASES OF THE BLOOD

Knowledge of blood-dyscrasias is constantly increasing because of newer studies, but the many unsolved problems make any classification a tentative one. The characteristics of the blood under normal conditions have been discussed elsewhere to some extent, and the approximate numbers of the cells noted (p. 39). Something has been stated, too, concerning the methods of examination (p. 149). In Fig. 249, prepared under the direction of Dr. Frank B. Lynch, Pathologist to the Germantown Hospital, Philadelphia, is shown the appearance of many of the blood-cells. In the following section will be considered chiefly certain pathologic considerations of these cells.

NORMAL AND PATHOLOGIC BLOOD-CORPUSCLES

Erythrocytes. **Microcytes** (3 to 5, in plate) are pathologic red cells which are smaller than the average normal erythrocyte, and often show crenation and poikilocytosis. They are seen in secondary anemias and chronic hemorrhagic conditions. **Macrocytes** (*megalocytes*) (6 to 10, in plate) are erythrocytes larger than the average, which often show granular degeneration and polychromatophilia. They are seen in pernicious anemia, sprue, dibothriocephalus latus infestation; to a lesser extent in syphilis, von Jaksch's anemia, aplastic anemia, malaria, sickle-cell anemia, exophthalmic goiter, marked secondary anemias, etc. **Anisocytosis** (variation in the size of the red cells) and **poikilocytosis** (irregular forms) (11 to 15, in plate) may occur in any anemia even if mild. **Polychromatophilia** (7 to 10, in plate) may be seen in any severe anemia, but especially in lead-poisoning, pernicious anemia, and leukemia. **Crenated cells** (16, 17, in plate) may be found to a slight extent in normal blood, or may indicate only poor preparation of the specimen. **Granular degeneration** (*basophilic degeneration*) (9, 10, 24, in plate) occurs in the new-born and in severe anemias; especially those accompanying lead-poisoning, pernicious anemia, and leukemia. **Reticulation** is found in normal blood in only 0.1 to 0.5 per cent of the red cells, but in anemias may appear in 1 to 2 per cent, and reaches 10 or 15 per cent or more in certain conditions, as hemolytic jaundice. **Howell-Jolly bodies** and **Cabot's rings** are presumably remnants of normoblasts, and found only in severe anemias. **Blood-platelets** (25, in plate) are constituents of normal blood and are decreased in certain hemorrhagic conditions particularly in thrombocytopenic purpura. For an excellent review on this subject see Mackay.[1]

Nucleated red cells (*erythroblasts*) (18 to 23, in plate) never occur in normal blood except in the first few days of life, and occasionally in the first year. They are found in any severe secondary anemia, in chlorosis, pernicious anemia, leukemia, sickle-cell anemia, and certain of the so-called "hemolytic anemias." There are three varieties: The normoblast (18, 19, in plate) of the same size, the microblast (20, in plate) smaller, and the megaloblast (21 to 23, in plate) larger than the normal erythrocyte; the last being characteristic of pernicious anemia.

Leukocytes (*granulocytes; microphages*).—In normal blood these consist of lymphocytes, large mononuclears, polymorphonuclear neutrophiles, eosinophiles, and basophiles. The figures given on p. 39 are for the normal percentages of the various forms found in a usual study of fixed preparations with Wright's stain or some similar method. With supravital staining lymphocytes are found to be approximately 10 per cent lower than these figures, and the polymorphonuclear cells approximately 10 per cent higher. There is considerable fluctuation in the total leukocyte-count and in the percentage of the different forms in a normal person during the course of a day. We[2] have studied this especially in children. (See also Leukocytosis, p. 1021.)

Lymphocytes (29 to 33, in plate) are increased in lymphocytic leukemia, pertussis, glandular fever and syphilis. A relative increase is seen in mumps, influenza, typhoid fever, tuberculosis, exophthalmic goiter, and during the invasion periods of rubeola and rubella. Occasionally there will be found in acute infections in childhood a lymphocytosis instead of an expected polymorphonuclear leukocytosis.

Large Mononuclears (*monocytes*) (26 to 28; 34 to 36, in plate) probably comprise two distinct groups. One of these, for which the title *monocyte* is often reserved, is supposed to develop like a blood-cell from a primitive form in the reticulo-endothelial system especially in the spleen, but also in the bone-marrow, liver, lungs etc. Monocytes include the so-called "transitional cell" formerly thought to be a forerunner of the polymorphonuclear neutrophile. The second variety, which under certain conditions may be found in the circulating blood, is variously termed *macrophage, histiocyte, endothelial leukocyte, polyblast, clasmatocyte,* and is supposed to arise from the endothelial lining of blood-sinuses and possibly of capillaries, and to be a normal constituent of connective tissue. Vital staining shows certain distinctions between the two types. An increase in large monomuclears may be found in leukemias, especially the so-called "monocytic form"; glandular fever; typhoid fever; variola; varicella; subacute bacterial endocarditis and rheumatic endocarditis; septicemia; malaria and other protozoal infections; agranulocytosis; Hodgkin's disease; and active tuberculosis, and has been described in other conditions also. It is generally believed that monocytic cells are more effective in defending the body against bacterial infections than are polymorphonuclear leukocytes (*microphages*).

Polymorphonuclear Neutrophiles (37 to 41, in plate) are actively phagocytic and play an important rôle in resistance to, and the combating of, many infections. (See also Leukocytosis, p. 1021.) **Polymorphonuclear Eosinophiles** (42 to 45, in plate) are increased with intestinal parasites, as the hookworm and the tapeworm; in trichinosis, hydatid cysts, and filariasis; in cutaneous disorders, as eczema, herpes zoster, pemphigus, psoriasis; in asthma and other allergic disorders; in certain diseases as gonorrhea, scarlet fever, and at times in tuberculosis; in Hodgkin's disease; and following injections of foreign serum. **Polymorphonuclear Basophiles** (*Mast-cells*) (46, 47, in plate) are increased in some cases of chronic cutaneous diseases, in bone-tumor, and in myelocytic leukemia.

Türk's irritation cells appear in stimulation of the bone-marrow, leukemia, marked anemia, and occasionally in leukocytosis from any cause or during recovery from infectious diseases.

Myelocytes (48 to 56, in plate) are not found in normal blood after the first few weeks of life, although throughout childhood they appear under

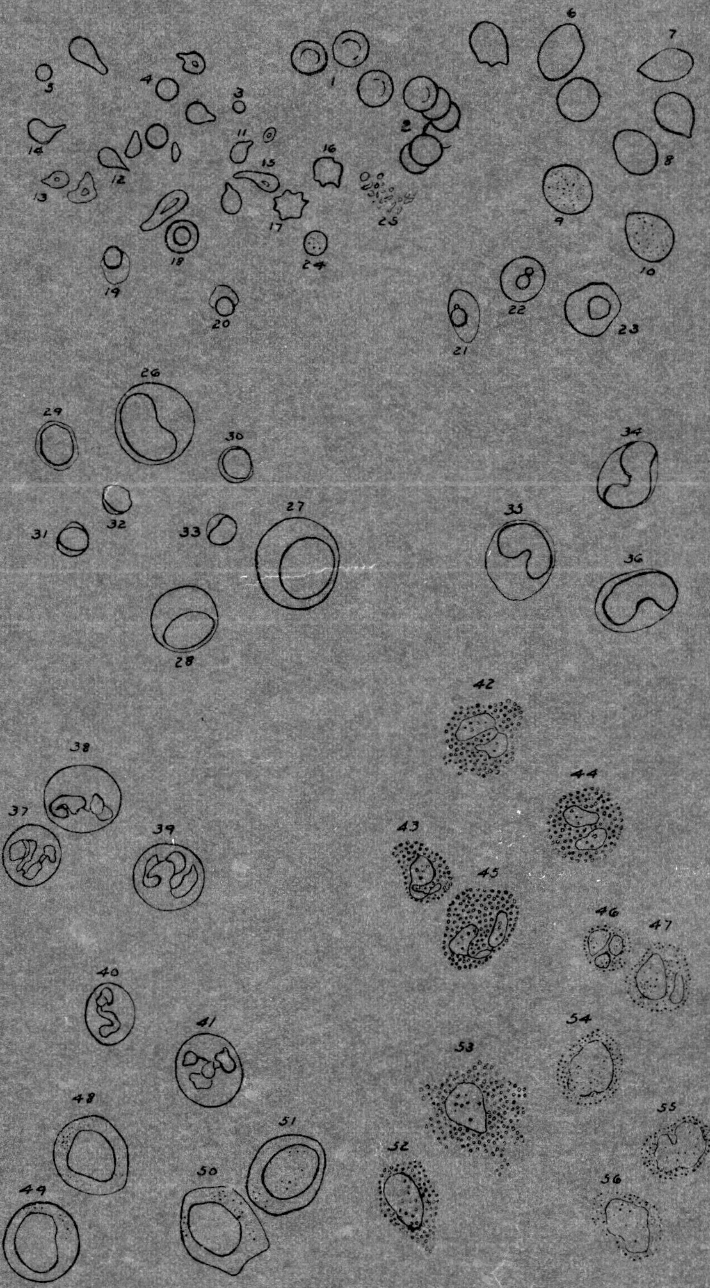

Erythrocytes: 1, Normal erythrocytes; 2, rouleaux of erythrocytes; 3, 4, 5, microcytes; 6, 7, 8, 9, 10, macrocytes; 7, 8, 9, 10, show polychromatophilia; 9, 10, granular degeneration; 11, 12, 13, 14, 15, poikilocytes; 16, 17, crenated red blood-cells; 18, normoblast; 19, normoblast extruding nucleus; 20, microblast; 21, 22, 23, megaloblasts; 24, granular degeneration (see also 9, 10); 25, blood-platelets.

Leukocytes: 26, 27, 28, Large mononuclear leukocytes; 29, intermediate type, classed as small lymphocytes; 30, 31, 32, 33, small lymphocytes; 34, 35, 36, transitionals; 37, 38, 39, 40, 41, polymorphonuclear neutrophiles; 42, 43, 44, 45, eosinophiles; 46, 47, basophiles (mast-cells); 48, 49, 50, 51, neutrophilic myelocytes; 52, 53, eosinophilic myelocytes; 54, 55, 56, basophilic myelocytes.

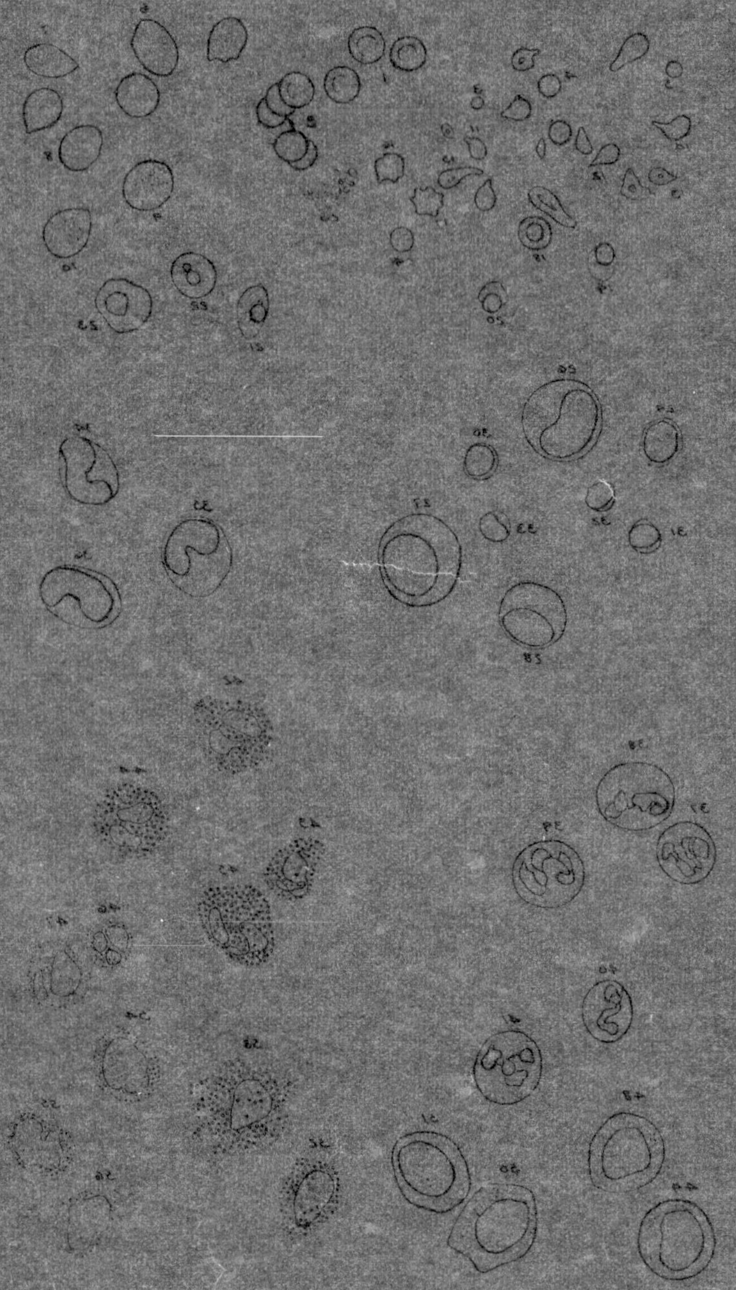

ERYTHROCYTES: 1, Normal erythrocytes; 2, rouleaux of erythrocytes; 3, 4, 5, microcytes; 6, 7, 8, 9, 10, macrocytes; 7, 8, 9, 10, show polychromatophilia, 9, 10, granular degeneration; 11, 12, 13, 14, 15, poikilocytes; 16, 17, crenated red blood-cells; 18, normoblast; 19, normoblast extruding nucleus; 20, microblast; 21, 22, 23, megaloblasts; 24, granular degeneration (see also 9, 10); 25, blood-platelets.

LEUKOCYTES: 26, 27, 28, large mononuclear leukocytes; 29, intermediate type, classed as small lymphocytes; 30, 31, 32, 33, small lymphocytes; 34, 35, 36, transitionals; 37, 38, 39, 40, 41, polymorphonuclear neutrophiles; 42, 43, 44, 45, eosinophiles; 46, 47, basophiles (mast-cells); 48, 49, 50, 51, neutrophilic myelocytes; 52, 53, eosinophilic myelocytes; 54, 55, 56, basophilic myelocytes.

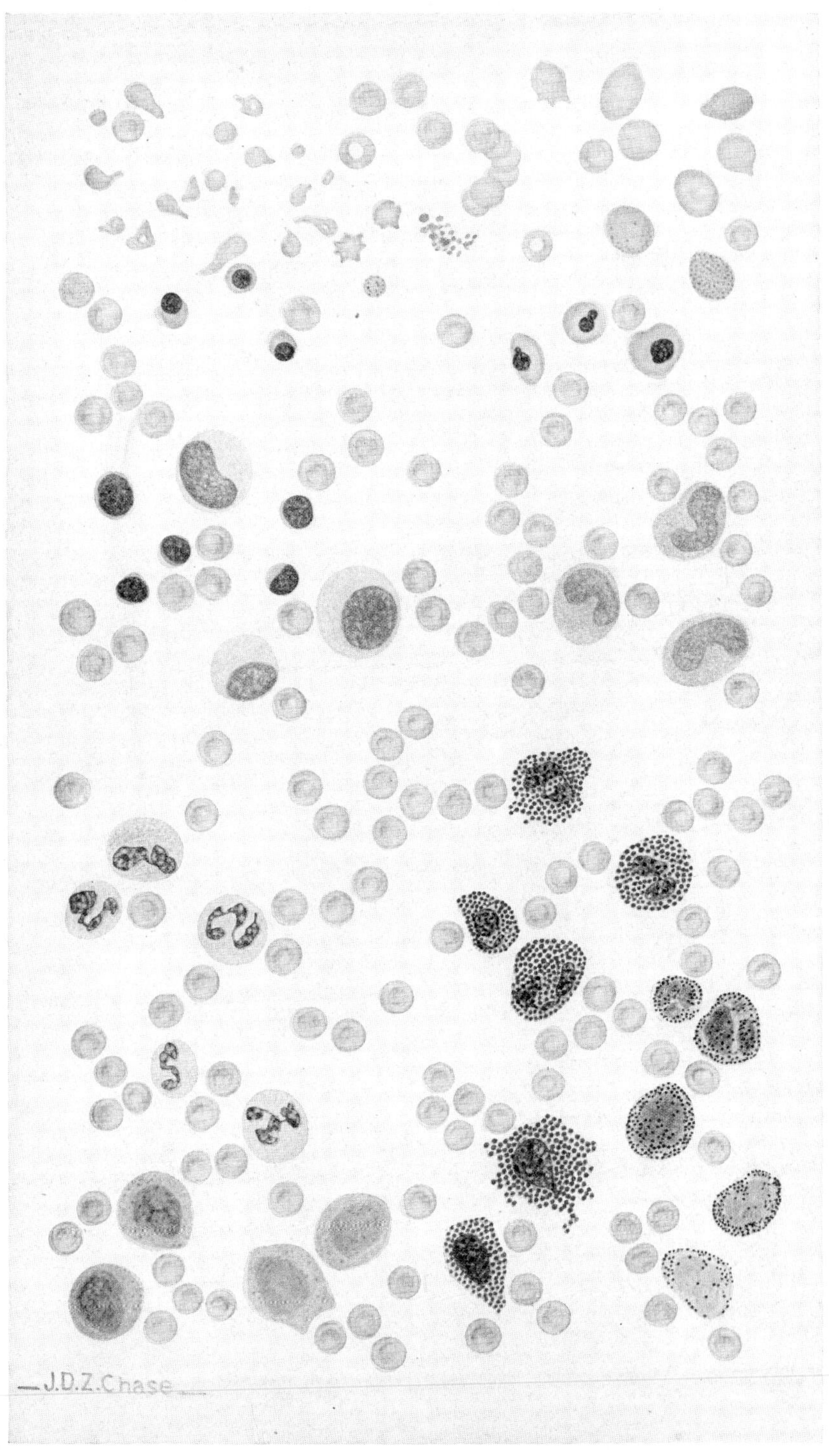

Fig. 249.—Varieties of erythrocytes and leukocytes in normal and pathologic conditions. (*Wright's stain.*)

lesser degrees of stimulation than in adults and, therefore, have less significance. They occur in myelocytic and lymphocytic leukemia, pernicious anemia, von Jaksch's anemia, variola, severe diphtheria, severe sepsis, and marked secondary anemias. There are several types of myelocytes. *Eosinophilic forms* (52, 53 in plate) are rare except in myelocytic leukemia, bone-tumor with involvement of the marrow, and von Jaksch's anemia. *Basophilic forms* (54 to 56, in plate) are rare even in myelocytic leukemia. Three other forms of myelocytes may appear in the blood in advanced states of the conditions mentioned. They are (1) *myeloblasts*, the parent-cells of myelocytes, (2) *promyelocytes*, which are earlier forms still, and (3) *metamyelocytes*, which are transitional forms between myelocytes and polymorphonuclear cells.

LEUKOPENIA

Diminution in the total number of leukocytes may occur, or there may be relative diminution of the polymorphonuclears or of the lymphocytes. Diseases associated with leukopenia are typhoid fever, malaria, rubeola, uncomplicated tuberculosis (excepting meningitis), and certain forms of influenza. Leukopenia may occur also in agranulocytosis; pernicious anemia; Kala-azar; aplastic anemia; Banti's disease; advanced cachectic states; certain stages of some of the leukemias; severe sepsis; and with certain poisons as benzol, arsenic, and some of the coal-tar products.

LEUKOCYTOSIS

This may be physiologic or pathologic. It has already been stated (p. 1020) that the leukocyte-count varies during the course of the day. Slight leukocytosis is normally present in the new-born, and after cold baths, emotional stress, exercise, and massage. Our[3] studies, which have since been confirmed by others, have shown that so-called "digestive leukocytosis" is uncommon in children. Pathologic leukocytosis is an evidence of inflammation, the increase usually being chiefly in the polymorphonuclear cells. It is seen in most acute febrile diseases with the exception of those mentioned under leukopenia. It is especially marked when there is suppuration, provided the patient has the power of reaction. Conditions showing increase of the monocytes and the lymphocytes have already been mentioned in the previous paragraph. In determining the presence and significance of leukocytosis the age of the child must always be considered (p. 39). Recently considerable stress has been put upon the maturity of the polymorphonuclear leukocyte in determining the severity and prognosis of disease. Severe infections so stimulate the bone-marrow that immature forms appear in the peripheral blood. Occasionally in infections cells as early in development as the myelocytes may be found in the stained smears. In the so-called "Arneth[4] count" the number of lobes of the polymorphonuclear cells is detailed. The greater the number of lobes the more mature the cell. Of the several modifications of this the one most widely used is the Schilling[5] index (*hemogram*) (Schilling-Gradwohl[6]). The count is made upon the smear stained in the usual way. Seven types of cells may be enumerated: Myelocytes; stab cells (*band-forms*) which contain a contracted, irregular nucleus with granules either deeply stained or replaced by vacuoles; juvenile cells with a sausage-, bean- or S-shaped nucleus, which is rather faintly stained; monocytes with a blue-staining irregular cytoplasm, and a polymorphic nucleus which may be segmented or sausage-shaped; the ordinary segmented polymorphonuclears with from two to five lobes in the nucleus connected by strands of filament; eosinophilic cells; basophilic cells. The adult has in his blood under normal conditions about 1 per cent basophiles; 2 to 4 per cent eosinophiles; no myelocytes; no juvenile cells; 3 to 5 per cent stab-forms; 58 to 65 per cent segmented forms; 21 to 25 per cent lymphocytes; and 4 to 8 per cent monocytes. These percentages differ somewhat in different periods of life, and in early life juvenile forms may occasionally be found under normal conditions. The term "*shift to the left*" means that there is an increase in juvenile and stab-forms, with which there is a decrease of lymphocytes and monocytes and a decrease or disappearance of eosinophiles. It occurs at the height of an infection and, if marked, indicates a severe infection and a guarded prognosis. A "*shift to the right*" implies that fewer juvenile forms are found and more segmented forms appear, at which time the lymphocytes and monocytes increase and the eosinophiles reappear. It occurs with improvement in infections. Rogatz[7] and Nussbaum[8] have studied the Schilling count especially in children. It has been found of value, when frequently repeated, and reflects the progress of an infection. Changes in the blood-picture may anticipate the appearance of a complication, or improvement of the disease, some hours before this actually occurs.

POLYCYTHEMIA

Cyanosis with red cells in the circulating blood much above normal in number is seen in congenital heart-disease; as a compensatory process at times in acquired cardiac or pulmonary disease; and in transition from a low to a high altitude. Increase of red cells may also occur in anhydremia; in acute hemorrhage; and in poisoning by carbon monoxide, phosphorus, and other substances. In idiopathic polycythemia (*polycythemia vera; Vaquez's*[9] *disease; erythraemia*), which is sometimes hereditary and familial, there are enlargement of the spleen, viscosity of the blood, and a red or bluish color of the skin; these symptoms being persistent and chronic. A few cases have been reported in children (Minot and Buckman,[10] Kretschmer[11]). The literature is reviewed by Weber[12] and Harrop.[13] Phenylhydrazine hydrochloride, as first used by Eppinger and Kloss,[14] may cause diminution in the number of erythrocytes, and radiologic treatment over the bones is said to be beneficial (Milani[15]). Splenectomy should not be performed.

BLOOD IN ANEMIA

For comparison, Table 71 (p. 1023) demonstrates the blood-picture in certain varieties of anemia and leukemia. For a more complete review see Osgood Haskins.[16]

SYMPTOMATIC ANEMIA

(Secondary Anemia; Simple Anemia)

Etiology.—The causes of symptomatic anemia may be divided into several groups.

1. *Hemorrhage.*—Any loss of blood whether from trauma or disease, visible or concealed, rapid or gradual, will cause anemia. In large acute hemorrhages there may be temporary concentration of blood with increase of hemoglobin and red cells.

2. *Debility.*—Under this term might be included a number of causes in which there would be deficiency of blood-formation, and in some of which there exists insufficient intake or assimilation of iron or other minerals. There may be such factors as congenital asthenia, prematurity, chronic nutritional disorders, or chronic diseases as syphilis and rickets. The anemia of premature infants is probably dependent in part upon poor development of the blood-forming organs, and in part upon the lesser iron-deposit in their tissues before birth. (See p. 212.) Operative in producing anemia may be poor hygienic conditions and lack of fresh air and sunlight. A frequent cause is a diet which is insufficient in iron or in other minerals concerned in blood-formation (see Treatment), such as would obtain when milk is given in too large quantities or too long continued. The severe

TABLE 71.—BLOOD IN ANEMIAS AND LEUKEMIAS

	R.B.C. millions per c.mm.	Hb.-Gm. per 100 cc.	Hb per cent normal (15 Gm. = 100 per cent).	Color index (Hb. count and ratio).	Volume index (Hb.-cell vol. and ratio).	W.B.C. per c.mm.	Myelocytes, per cent.	Lymphocytes, per cent.	Platelets No.	Fragility of R.B.C.	Nucleated red cells.
Symptomatic anemia	2 to 4	3 to 12	20 to 80	0.4 to 1.0	0.4 to 1.0	Normal or slightly increased	0	Normal	Normal; occasionally decreased in severe forms; increase in stage of regeneration	Normal or occasionally increased	Few in severe forms
Chlorosis	2 to 5	2 to 12	13 to 80	0.4 to 0.8	0.4 to 1.0	Normal	0	Relative increase	Increased	Normal	Few in severe type
Pernicious anemia	0.4 to 4.0	1.5 to 14	10 to 95	1.15 to 2.00	1.15 to 2.00	Leukopenia	A few	Relative increase	Decreased	Decreased	Many; espec. megalocytes.
Aplastic anemia	0.8 to 4.0	2.0 to 12	13 to 80	0.7 to 1.2	0.7 to 1.2	Leukopenia	0	Relative increase marked	Greatly decreased	Increased	0
Sickle-cell anemia	1.5 to 4.0	4.5 to 12	30 to 80	0.8 to 1.2	0.8 to 1.2	Normal to 20,000	0	0	Normal	Decreased	Large number
Agranulocytosis	4 to 5.5	12 to 16.5	80 to 110	0.8 to 1.2	0.8 to 1.2	Leukopenia	0	Greatly increased	Normal	?	None or few.
Pseudoleukemia, von Jaksch	2 to 3	6 to 9	40 to 60	?	?	Normal to 50,000	Moderate number 5–10	Relative increase	Often increased	Normal (?)	Moderate number
Acute lymphocytic leukemia	1 to 4	2.5 to 12	17 to 80	0.8 to 1.4	0.8 to 1.4	50,000 to 350,000 leukopenia not uncommon	Occasional	80–99 mostly large type	Greatly decreased	Normal (?)	Few; occasionally moderate number
Acute myelocytic leukemia	1 to 9	2.5 to 12	17 to 80	0.8 to 1.4	0.8 to 1.4	50,000 to 100,000 leukopenia uncommon	10–50	Relative decrease	Decreased	Normal (?)	Occasional
Chronic myelocytic leukemia	1 to 4	2.0 to 12	13 to 80	0.8 to 1.4	0.8 to 1.4	100,000 to 200,000	30–50	Relative increase of large type	Greatly increased or normal or occasionally decreased	Normal (?)	Moderate number

anemia developing with the use of goat's milk has been mentioned elsewhere (p. 82). A diet greatly deficient in vitamins may result in poor assimilation of iron.

Another class of cases is that in which anemia seems to depend upon long-continued albuminous discharge, as seen in nephritis, chronic suppurative processes, and chronic diarrhea; part of the explanation in some of these conditions being faulty intake and assimilation of minerals, and also the lack of function of blood-forming organs. Anemia develops in chronic heart-disease, and in the debility incident to rapid growth and overwork.

3. *Toxic and Infectious Causes.*—Here may be included the action of metallic poisons such as lead; toxins produced in various diseases, especially diphtheria, malaria, tuberculosis, syphilis, pyelitis and other suppurative processes; intestinal parasites some of which also add the factor of hemorrhage; and various hemolytic agents such as obtain in certain forms of icterus. Some of these causes act by destruction of red blood-cells; others by depression of blood-formation.

Symptoms.—Except after hemorrhage the symptoms of anemia usually come on gradually. Premature infants, for example, do not show anemia at birth, but the diminution in hemoglobin and red cells reaches its height at about the third or fourth month. An unexplained form of marked anemia in the new-born has already been mentioned (p. 226). With anemia there gradually develops pallor of skin and mucous membranes. The amount of fatty tissue is not necessarily diminished; but the musculature becomes flabby, and there is a tendency to fatigue and often dyspnea, anorexia, and gastro-intestinal disturbances. Anemic murmurs may be heard over the heart and in the vessels of the neck. There may be cardiac hypertrophy; splenic enlargement; coldness of the hands and feet; nervous symptoms as fretfulness, irritability, headache, insomnia, and neuralgic pains; and syncopal attacks. Infants with severe anemia may become edematous.

The Blood.—Hemoglobin may be greatly reduced and the red blood-cells likewise. The stained red cells appear paler than normal and in severe cases show anisocytosis, poikilocytosis, and some may even be nucleated. The leukocytes may be moderately increased in number, but are generally unaffected unless by the primary disease. Severe secondary anemia may lead to the appearance of myelocytes in small numbers in the blood.

Course and Prognosis.—The prognosis of secondary anemia depends in general upon its cause, the removal of which is necessary for cure. Few patients die directly from anemia, but oftener from complicating disease, resistance being lowered by the condition of the blood.

Diagnosis.—The differential diagnosis from other forms of anemia will be discussed when considering these. The causes of secondary anemia fall, as indicated above, into three groups; hemorrhage, destruction of blood, poor formation of blood. Some assistance can be gained by a study of the icterus index (p. 659), which if high—in the absence of injury to the liver or of biliary obstruction—indicates blood-destruction, especially when reticulocytes are not increased in number.

Treatment.—Search and removal of the cause is the first object sought. Diet is an important consideration. An excess of milk must be avoided in the diet of older children, and mineral-containing foods added as early as permissible to the diet of infants. The food should conform to the digestive ability of the individual patient, and it is often better to administer iron and other drugs which stimulate blood-formation than to run the risk of establishing by a forced diet any gastro-intestinal disturbance, or of increasing one which is already present. There is some evidence, too, that a diet reasonably high in vitamins assists in the assimilation of iron (Simmonds, Becker and McCollum;[17] Maurer et al.[18]). Among foods which are helpful in anemia because they contain iron or copper are the following: Liver, kidney, egg-yolk, brains, sweetbreads, oysters, lamb, and chicken. Most studies, including our own[19] have not shown that liver has any great value in secondary anemia. It should be stated that liver-extract contains little iron (Elvehjem[20]). Fruits generally are rich in iron, copper and manganese, and especially valuable are apricots and peaches, which are as efficient dried as fresh. Prunes are also quite effective promoters of hemoglobin-regeneration, and somewhat less so are raisins, currants, and fresh grapes (Robscheit-Robbins and Whipple[21]). Certain foods as wheat, peas, navy-beans, and blueberries are rich in manganese and may be of value in anemia (see Hodges and Peterson,[22] Editorial[23]). Table 72 compiled from a number of sources shows the iron content of certain foods:

TABLE 72.—IRON CONTENT OF VARIOUS FOODS

Food.	Amount.	Gm. of iron in amount shown.	Food.	Amount.	Gm. of iron in amount shown.
Applesauce	1 tbsp.	.00003	Apricots, canned	One	.0003
Apricots, dried	One	.00009	Asparagus, fresh	5 stalks 8″	.001
Bacon	1 sm. slice	.0001	Banana	1 medium	.0008
Beans, string	1 ounce	.00023	Beets	One, 2″ diam.	.0003
Bread, wh. wheat	4″ × 4″ × 5/8″	.00036	Carrots	1 ounce	.0001
Celery	1 ounce	.00008	Chicken, creamed	1 tbsp.	.00117
Chocolate cake	3″ × 4 3/4″ × 1″	.0019	Corn flakes	1 cup	.0C015
Eggs, white	One	.00003	Eggs, yolk	One	.00129
Farina	1 ounce	.00003	Ham, boiled	4″ × 5″ × 5/8″	.001
Kidney, beef	One	.0012	Lamb chop	1 medium	.0015
Lamb, shoulder	3″ × 3″ × 1 1/2″	.0022	Liver, beef	4″ × 2 1/2″ × 1/2″	.0079
Macaroni	1 ounce	.00004	Mackerel, fresh	1 ounce	.00016
Milk, whole	1 ounce	.00005	Orange	1/2 large	.00014
Orange juice	1 ounce	.00005	Oyster	One	.00113
Peaches	1 medium	.0004	Peas, green	1 ounce	.0003
Potatoes, baked	One, 2 1/2″ diam.	.0013	Prunes	One	.0005
Raisins	1 ounce	.00035	Shredded wheat	1 biscuit	.0013
Spinach	1 ounce	.0009	Steak, club	2″ × 3″ × 2″	.0016
Tomatoes, canned	1 ounce	.0001	Tomatoes, fresh	One, 2 1/2″ diam.	.0004
Turkey roast	4″ × 3″ × 1/2″	.006			

Guerithault[24] found the following amounts of copper per kilogram of fresh material: Apples 1.4 mg., asparagus 7.0, bananas 2.4, barley 6.5, beans (kidney) 10.0, beef 2.1, beets 3.2, cabbage 1.8, carrots 2.2, celery 2.0, cherries 1.4, egg-yolk 1.8, egg-white 0.0, flour (wheat) 2.0, grapes 1.4, lettuce 2.0, milk (cow's) 0.6, oats 17.1, oranges 3.1, peas 7.2, potatoes 1.9, rice 6.4, spinach 1.8, tomatoes 2.0, wheat 7.2, wheat-germ 48.0.

Iron is a useful drug. H. S. Mitchell and Vaughn[25] found most productive of hemoglobin-formation ferric acetate, ferric albuminate, and ferric citrate. A number of other preparations of iron are of value, as the chloride, lactate, saccharated carbonate, and the mass. ferricarb. (Vallet's mass.) or pil. ferri carb. (Blaud's pill). A number of studies (Hart et al.;[26] Elvehjem;[20] Waddell et al.;[27] Keil and Nelson[28]) have shown that copper added to iron enhances its hematopoietic action. Copper must be given in small amounts. A useful preparation employed at the Children's Hospital, Cincinnati, is as follows: A solution is made containing 12 per cent of ferric ammonium citrate and 0.8 per cent copper sulphate ($CuSO_4.5H_2O$). The usual dose of this is 0.5 cc. per kilogram of body-weight per day (3.7 minims per pound) which would be equivalent to about 10 mg. of iron and 1 mg. of copper per kilogram per day. The action of copper is rapid and it should be discontinued when no longer needed, since it is possible that a toxic effect might eventually be brought about. In many cases arsenic is of avail, usually administered with iron. During active infection and fever iron and the other minerals may be little absorbed (Mackay[29]) nor can these be expected to do much good in metabolic diseases and chronic infections in which there is no real deficiency of them.

In obstinate cases of anemia, the following preparation is useful hypodermically: Ferri citras viridas, grain 1 (0.065); sodii cacodylas, grain $\frac{1}{2}$ (0.03); aqua minims 15 (0.9). This should be sterilized and kept in ampoules; the doses mentioned being administered every second or third day. Infants may receive $\frac{1}{2}$ to 1 grain (0.03 to 0.065) of the iron and $\frac{1}{2}$ to $\frac{1}{8}$ grain (0.005 to 0.008) of the cacodylate. Laurens and Mayerson,[30] Foster,[31] and others have shown experimentally that some erythropoietic and hemoglobin-stimulating action follows ultraviolet irradiation. Extracts of bone-marrow, hemoglobin, and many other substances are sometimes employed but possess no advantage over the simpler preparations mentioned above. In severe cases transfusions are of great service and stimulate blood-regeneration more rapidly than do any other means. Iron may be given intraperitoneally (Grulee and Sanford[32]), although this is seldom necessary.

Leishman's Anemia.—*Kala-azar.*—This is a form of infectious secondary anemia seen in tropical countries and in the Mediterranean basin, especially liable to attack children in the first three years of life. Talbot and Lyon,[33] and Faber and Schussler[34] have reported cases occurring in the United States. The cause is a flagellated micro-organism of the Leishmania group. The **symptoms** are irregular fever of sudden onset, emaciation, cachexia, great enlargement of the spleen and later of the liver, pigmented and perhaps icteric skin, and swelling of the joints. There is anemia of the secondary type and the leukocytes may be diminished in number, although the lymphocytes are relatively increased. Eosinophilia is usually absent. Antimony has been used in the **treatment** and in some cases splenectomy performed.

CHLOROSIS

(Chlorotic Anemia; Infantile Chlorosis; Oligochromemia)

This has often been regarded as a special type of anemia, occurring almost exclusively in females and not before the age of puberty. In this form it is becoming increasingly uncommon. The symptoms of chlorosis in general do not differ materially from those of other forms of severe anemia and the blood-picture, which consists of great diminution of hemoglobin with comparatively little decrease in the number of red cells, may occur at any time of life. Then it differs little from secondary anemia as already described, and the treatment of it is similar, with special emphasis on the curative value of iron.

SICKLE-CELL ANEMIA

(Drepanocytic Anemia)

This seems to be a distinct clinical entity, characterized by the occurrence of sickle-shaped red cells. It was first described by Herrick.[35] A large number of cases have been reported, and reviews are given by Steinberg,[36] and Fradkin and Schwartz.[37]

Etiology.—The great majority of cases occur in the negro race. Cooley and Lee[38] report an instance in a Greek child, and Stewart[39] in one of Cuban descent. The occurrence of sickle-cells in the blood is not necessarily accompanied by anemia, Cooley and Lee[40] and Levy[41] finding this phenomenon in 7.5 per cent and 5.6 per cent respectively of negro children, most of whom were normal. This condition might be called sicklemia or preferably "sacklemia" (Cooley and Lee[40]).

Sickle-cell anemia affects all ages and the peculiar changes in the blood have been found at birth. Sex exerts no influence. There is a strong familial and hereditary tendency, and it is usually possible to find sickle-cells, although not necessarily with anemia, in other members of the patient's family. The cause of the condition is unknown, although it appears to be a hereditary defect. Cooley[42] believes that it is a form of hemolytic anemia.

Pathologic Anatomy.—There have been found hyperplasia of the lymphoid tissue; enlargement of the liver with round-celled infiltration and phagocytosis of the red cells by the Kupffer cells; usually diminution in the size of the spleen with increase in reticulum and perhaps atrophy of the Malpighian bodies, and, according to Rich,[43] a characteristic lesion with malformation of the sinuses around them; a hyperplasia of the bone-marrow. Iron pigment is found in the spleen, liver, and kidneys, and calcium deposits in the spleen and kidneys.

Symptoms.—In the latent phase there may be few or no symptoms, and, as stated, sickling of cells may be discovered without the patient ever having had the characteristic anemia. There may be found general adenopathy and slight enlargement of the liver and sometimes of the spleen. During the active stage all the general signs of anemia are present, and, in addition, there may be pains in the muscles and joints, and nausea and

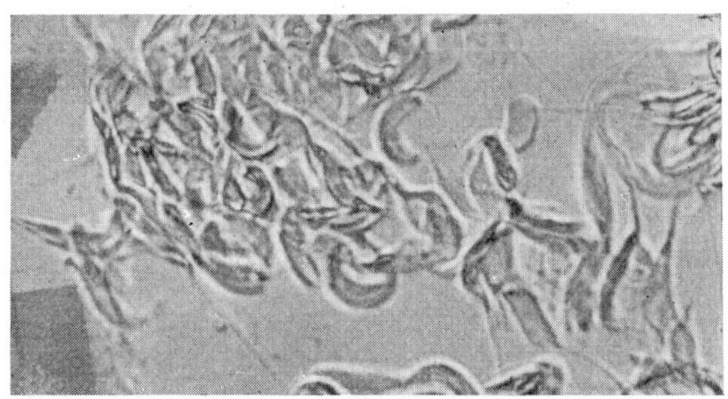

Fig. 250.—Showing sickling of cells in a sealed wet preparation; three days after preparation was made. Negro boy of eighteen months, in Cincinnati General Hospital.

vomiting, the last accompanied by abdominal pain usually in the region of the spleen ("*abdominal crisis*"). Slight fever may occur. The urine both during the active and latent phases may contain urobilin, but no bile. The roentgenograms may show thickening of the cranial bones and decrease in the width of the medullary cavities of the long bones (Moore[44]). The **blood** in the latent phase may show no anemia, but the characteristic sickle-shaped and elongated or oat-shaped red cells are always present, together with phagocytosis of these by the mononuclear and polymorphonuclear leukocytes. In wet preparations of blood sickling often appears only when these have been sealed and allowed to stand for several hours. Some sickling may be observed also in the stained specimen of blood. A large percentage of the cells may assume the characteristic shape (Fig. 250). There may be polychromatophilia, poikilocytosis, and reticulocytosis. Many nucleated red cells may be present and often in enormous numbers, and myelocytes may be found. The leukocytes may increase up to about 20,000 per cubic millimeter, the differential count showing nothing characteristic. An indirect van den Bergh reaction may be present, and an increased amount of bilirubin in the blood, and there is usually found decreased fragility of the red cells. Lawrence,[45] Hunter and Adams,[46] and others found elliptical and oval red cells in the peripheral blood of white subjects, some of whom showed no anemia. This should be differentiated from sickle-cell anemia.

Prognosis.—Death may occur during the acute phase. Patients who have frequent attacks of anemia with sickle-cells in the circulating blood, *i. e.*, as shown on the stained smear, are liable to die before reaching adult life. Some of the cases apparently remain entirely latent, although minor causes, such as acute infections and the like, are prone to precipitate active phases. In one patient from our clinic (Cook[47]) death resulted from a subarachnoid hemorrhage.

Treatment.—This consists in the ordinary measures indicated for anemia. In severe cases transfusion may be advisable. Splenectomy has sometimes resulted in improvement of the anemia and the general condition, but does not cause disappearance of the sickle-cell taint. The operation has been performed by Hahn and Gillespie,[48] Bell et al.,[49] Stewart,[39] Hahn,[50] and Landon and Lyman.[51]

PERNICIOUS ANEMIA

(Addison-Biermer Anemia)

The first recorded case of this was by Combe[52] in 1822, and the first clear description of the disease was given by Addison[53] in 1855. The condition is rarely seen in early life, although possible cases have been reported by Monti and Berggrün,[54] Cabot,[55] Fanconi,[56] Christiansen,[57] Faber,[58] Frank,[59] Orrico[60] and others. Some of the reported cases in childhood have been atypical and were probably secondary anemias. At least one case in an infant and another in an older child have come under our observation in which the diagnosis was reasonably certain. It seems most likely that this type of anemia is dependent upon failure of the primitive cells in the bone-marrow to progress toward mature erythrocytes (Minot, Murphy and Stetson[61]); due, perhaps, to lack of stroma-building material (Whipple[62]). The achylia gastrica present in pernicious anemia is in some way related, but whether it is primary or secondary is not known. A pernicious type of anemia occurs sometimes in such conditions as infestation with the dibothriocephalus latus and other intestinal parasites; atrophy of the gastric mucous membrane; sprue; and sometimes in syphilis and severe rickets. An excellent review of pernicious anemia is given by Cornell.[63] **Pathologically** there are found extreme pallor of all the internal organs, with capillary hemorrhages, fatty degeneration of the cardiac muscle and often of the liver and kidneys, an unusual deposit of iron in the liver and other organs, atrophy of the tongue and the gastric mucous membrane, degenerative changes in the central nervous system especially in the posterior and lateral columns of the cord, and hyperplasia of the bone-marrow. The **symptoms** develop slowly or sometimes rapidly, and are those characteristic of any severe anemia. The skin and mucous membranes are pale, the former exhibiting a slightly yellow tint. Hemorrhages from the skin and mucous membranes are quite common. There is almost always inflammation of the tongue, with later an atrophic glossitis. Achylia is almost a constant symptom often antedating the blood changes, and it may persist even during remissions. The urine may contain urobilin. When there are changes in the posterior column of the spinal cord, loss of sense of position occurs in the lower extremities; when in the lateral column, spastic paraplegia. In the **blood** the characteristic features are great reduction of hemoglobin and in the number of erythrocytes. There is a high color-index. The size of the red cells is variable, but they average larger than normal. There is a decided preponderance of megalocytes, this constituting one of the chief characteristics of the disease; but microcytes are common, and there may be normoblasts and megaloblasts. The leukocytes are normal in number or perhaps diminished, especially those of the polymorphonuclear type; and a few myelocytes may be found. The platelets may be diminished; there is an increased amount of bilirubin in the blood; and the fragility of the red cells is decreased. Without treatment the **course** is usually progressive, although exacerbations and temporary remissions occur. With the administration of liver the **prognosis** has been greatly improved, and apparently symptomatic cure can be brought about. The **diagnosis** rests upon the symptoms and examination as detailed above. It should be remembered that megaloblasts in small numbers may occur in other severe anemias, especially in young children. The occurrence of a very marked response to liver-therapy in any severe anemia, with a great increase of reticulocytes, suggests that it may be of the pernicious type. In **treatment** careful search should be made for any factor which might cause a severe anemia simulating the pernicious type. Medicinally arsenic is the drug of choice, but iron and copper should also be administered. Minot and Murphy,[64] and Minot et al.[65] have shown that feeding with liver causes an increase in the reticulocytes and a remission of the acute symptoms, and that it appears to be a specific for the disease. Kidney and beef are less effective than liver. Cohn, Minot, Murphy et al.,[66] and West[67] have isolated potent fractions of liver which are also effective. Continued administration of liver between remissions is necessary. Dessicated swine-stomach (*ventriculin*) has been found by Sturgis and Isaacs[68] to be effective, as has also fresh raw swine-stomach (Conner[69]). Liver has been prepared for intravenous use (Castle and Taylor[70]). A specific hematopoietic substance has been discovered in normal gastric juice when given intramuscularly (Morris et al.[71]). A preparation on the market known as *extralin* contains the extracts from both liver and stomach. Splenectomy should not be performed.

APLASTIC ANEMIA

This uncommon form of anemia was first described by Ehrlich.[72] Cases in children have been reported and collected by Hirschfeld,[73] Kleinschmidt,[74] Heubner,[75] Smith,[76] Herrman,[77] and Gibson.[78] There is a so-called idiopathic form, but aplasia or failure of function of the blood-forming tissues may follow a variety of causes, as poisoning by benzol or arsenic, sepsis, and excessive exposure to the roentgen-ray; and milder degrees of it occur in chronic disease or starvation. (See also Agranulocytosis, below.) In the terminal stage of pernicious anemia and of the leukemias aplasia of the bone-marrow may take place. The characteristic **lesion** consists in disappearance of the erythroblastic tissue of the bone-marrow. The **symptoms** are those of severe and rapidly developing anemia, with a tendency to hemorrhage into the skin and mucous membranes. Urobilin is not found in the urine. The **blood** shows great diminution of red cells, but there are few if any nucleated red cells and no poikilocytosis, anisocytosis, or polychromatophilia. The color-index is usually low. There is marked leukopenia, due largely to the diminution of polymorphonuclear cells. Platelets are diminished and coagulation-time and bleeding-time are prolonged. The **course** is rapid and death usually occurs in a few weeks or months, although recovery has been reported by Beneke,[79] Parkinson,[80] Herrman,[77] Gibson,[78] and Birk.[81] **Treatment** is supportive with frequent transfusions of blood. Gibson[78] advises the use of epinephrine, and Upham and Nelson[82] that of raw fetal liver.

AGRANULOCYTOSIS

This condition, sometimes termed *malignant neutropenia,* does not appear to be a distinct entity. Its cause is unknown, although in some cases it is claimed that infection is operative, especially with the organisms of Vincent's angina (p. 537). In many symptoms it is allied to aplastic anemia, and some cases which have been classified as this would now be designated agranulocytosis. In one form, termed *agranulocytic angina* and first described by Schultz,[83] there is ulceration of the tonsils and nasopharyngeal lymphoid tissue, and a leukopenia with a marked relative lymphocytosis. Irregular fever may be a symptom. Agranulocytosis may, however, occur without the angina. The **blood-picture** differs from that of aplastic anemia (p. 1029) in that there is little if any diminution in red cells, hemoglobin and platelets. **Prognosis** is extremely serious, although some cases recover. **Treatment** is similar to that for aplastic anemia. Jackson[84] obtained good results by intravenous and intramuscular injections of nucleotides. Cases in children have been reported and collected under the term agranulocytosis by Dwyer and Helwig,[85] Dodd and Wilkinson,[86] Tokue and Yasumoto,[87] Christof,[88] Railliet and Ginsbourgh,[89] Bigler and Brennemann,[90] Dameshek and Ingall,[91] Baldridge and Needles,[92] Empey and Proescher,[93] and others.

ACUTE HEMOLYTIC ANEMIA

A peculiar form of anemia is described by Lederer[94] in which there is a marked and rapidly progressing anemia with its accompanying symptoms, fever, enlargement of the liver and spleen, and leukocytosis. The cause is unknown. Transfusion of unmodified blood gives remarkedly good results.

PSEUDOLEUKEMIC ANEMIA

(Splenic Anemia; Anemia Splenica Infantum; Anemia Infantum Pseudoleukaemica; von Jaksch's Anemia; Erythroblastic Anemia)

The relationships of this not infrequent disorder are subject to much discussion, and it has been variously regarded as a primary blood-disease; as related to leukemia or pernicious anemia; as allied to diseases of the spleen; as the result of some infectious or toxic cause; as the accompaniment of such diseases as syphilis and rickets; or as a hemolytic type of anemia. It can safely be stated that its **cause** is unknown. Probably it is in reality a symptom-complex which includes a group of as yet unclassified disorders, rather than an independent disease. Von Jaksch,[95] after whom the condition is sometimes named, did not describe all the features later associated with it. It is probable that as knowledge increases distinct forms of anemia will be separated from the classification of pseudoleukemic anemia; such, for example, as the erythroblastic anemia of Cooley which is discussed later. At present there remain certain cases which must be considered here. These are seen usually in the first two or three years of life, but seldom before six months. There may be a familial tendency. While they occur with syphilis and rickets, this is by no means constant, and there is no relation to the severity of these diseases. Digestive disturbances sometimes precede. **Pathologically** the striking feature is the enlarged, hard spleen, which shows no characteristic changes. The liver is enlarged, and there may be moderate hypertrophy of lymphoid tissue. The condition of the bone-marrow varies, but it may be hyperplastic. The **symptoms** are slow in onset, but finally severe anemia and all its accompanying symptoms develop. Sometimes the patient remains well-nourished. The abdomen is decidedly enlarged, principally due to the increased size of the spleen, the lower edge of which may extend to the crest of the ileum. The liver may be enlarged and the superficial lymph-nodes palpable. The **blood** shows marked reduction of hemoglobin and red cells, with a low color-index. There are usually found megalocytes, microcytes, poikilocytes, and polychromatophilia. Nucleated red cells may be present in large numbers. The leukocytes vary from 15,000 to 50,000 per cubic millimeter but their number has no constant relation to the severity of the condition. Lymphocytes may be relatively increased. Myelocytes are nearly always present in considerable numbers, and often early forms of these are seen. In 1 case we[96] found the myelocytic cells as high as 45 per cent. The blood-changes have no relation to the size of the spleen. The **course** is slow, lasting over months or a year or more. The **prognosis** is uncertain. It is generally stated that 25 per cent or more of the patients die, usually from bronchopneumonia, diarrhea, or some other complication. The **diagnosis** from myelocytic luekemia is made by the greater proportion of leukocytes and myelocytes in that disease, and its more rapid course and universally fatal ending; from lymphocytic leukemia by the two last features and the great relative and absolute increase of lymphocytes which that disease exhibits. Splenic enlargement may accompany syphilis, rickets, and secondary anemias, but without the blood-changes of pseudoleukemic anemia. Hygienic, dietetic, and medicinal **treatment** of the condition is similar to that for secondary anemia. Splenectomy has been performed, but it is not curative and is not to be recommended.

Erythroblastic Anemia (*Cooley's anemia*).—Better described here than elsewhere is that form of anemia particularly studied by Cooley and his co-workers,[97] which they considered to be an erythroblastic anemia and later regarded as a hemolytic anemia having points of resemblance to congenital hemolytic anemia and sickle-cell anemia. It occurs particularly in members of the Mediterranean races, as Italians and Greeks. There is a definite familial tendency. It begins in the first year of life. The *blood* contains an increase of reticulocytes, and there are nucleated red cells which increase remarkably after splenectomy. There is no increase in fragility. Leukocytosis is present. Urobilin may be found in the urine. The van den Bergh reaction is indirect and the icterus index increased. The skin shows a muddy discoloration; there are thick cranial bones and prominent malar eminences giving a mongoloid appearance. The bone-marrow is hyperplastic, and there is rarefaction of the long and flat bones which is demonstrable roentgenologically. The prognosis is poor, the patient seldom living to adult life. Splenectomy has been performed but the effect of this on the condition is still uncertain.

LEUKEMIA

This affection was described independently by Craigie[98] and by Bennett[99] and also by Virchow[100] in 1845. The name indicates the light color of the blood. The two principal varieties, myelocytic and lymphocytic, were separated by the studies of Ehrlich and his pupils.[101]

Etiology and Pathology.—Leukemia is uncommon in early life, but it may occur even in infancy, and a leukemic condition of the blood in the new-born has been reported (Siefart,[102] Pollmann,[103] Adler,[104] Stransky[105]), in some of these cases the mother having the disease. The myelocytic form is much less common in childhood than the lymphocytic. Cases of the latter in early life have been reported and collected by Benjamin and Sluka,[106] Babonneix and Tixier,[107] Veeder,[108] Smith,[109] Gautier and Thevenod,[110] Wollstein and Bartlett,[111] Thorpe,[112] Hyland,[113] Pearce,[114] and White and Burns.[115] Most of these reported cases were in the first two or three years of life, after which time lymphocytic leukemia becomes much more common. The case of White and Burns was in an infant who died at the age of three weeks. Instances of myelocytic leukemia in early life are reported and collected by Benjamin and Sluka,[106] Adler,[104] Pisek,[116] Knox,[117] Ross,[118] Horwitt,[119] Opitz,[120] Wollstein and Bartlett,[111] Stransky,[105] Karelitz,[121] Ramsay,[122] Salomonsen,[123] Lengsfeld,[124] Pourtales[125] and others. We have seen 1 case in a child two years of age. The reports quoted are those chiefly of the acute form of myelocytic leukemia. The chronic variety is still more rare in childhood although instances are reported

(Thursfield,[126] Dupérié and Cadenaule,[127] and Esp[128]) and we have observed 3 cases. Heredity has seemed to exert an influence in some instances of leukemia, although any such factor is denied by many authors. Males are oftener attacked than females, in the proportion of 2:1. Although many hypotheses have been offered, the direct cause and nature of leukemia are unknown. Microscopic studies of the spleen show fibrosis and inflammation, with infiltration by lymphocytes and myelocytes, and the same is true of the lymph-nodes of the body. The bone-marrow is always involved. Many other tissues of the body may exhibit a lymphoid infiltration.

Classification.—There is reason to believe that the different types of leukemias are closely allied, and that in all there is a general disorder of the hematopoietic system, although in some cases and types there is a greater affection of the bone-marrow and in others of the lymphoid tissues. From a clinical point of view there is permissible a classification into: (*A*) Myelocytic leukemia (myelemia, splenomedullary, splenomyelogenous, or myeloid leukemia); (*B*) Lymphocytic leukemia (lymphemia, lymphatic or lymphoid leukemia).

Symptoms. 1. Acute Lymphocytic Leukemia.—This form may develop insidiously, but more often acutely, and sometimes with abruptness. Not infrequently the first suggestive symptom is hemorrhage into the skin or mucous membrane. There may early be ulceration of lymphoid tissue in the nasopharynx. Moderate painless enlargement of the lymph-nodes may be found, especially in the cervical region. There are irregular fever, debility, and increasing anemia. Pain in the joints may occur, and diarrhea develop. The spleen and liver become moderately enlarged in nearly all cases. As the disease advances hemorrhages from the gums, nose, mouth, or kidneys, and into the skin persist and may be severe; anemia and debility increase; fever continues; the lymph-nodes usually grow slowly in size; and edema may develop. While the lymph-nodes seldom increase greatly, we have seen as an early symptom marked enlargement of the tracheobronchial nodes demonstrated by physical examination and roentgenograms. In some cases leukemic infiltration of the skin is present; and papular, bullous or other eruptions are not uncommon. There may be infiltration of lymphoid tissue in other regions, as the eyelids, orbit, and retina; the last showing on ophthalmoscopic examination hemorrhagic areas with a white center. In rapid cases the suddenness of onset and the course resemble the result of an infection. The **blood** shows great reduction in hemoglobin and red cells. Normoblasts and megaloblasts may be present, sometimes in considerable numbers. The white cells may be increased from 50,000 up to 400,000 or more per cubic millimeter. The increase is in the lymphocytes, these constituting from 70 to 90 per cent or more of the total white cells. The lymphocytes are usually of the larger variety. There is no increase in eosinophiles or basophiles, and myelocytes are absent or found only in small numbers. Great variation in the number of lymphocytes occurs from time to time; a diminution being especially prone to happen if acute infection develops, or toward the end of the disease. Not infrequently a leukopenia exists almost throughout the course, although usually there is a terminal leukocytosis. The bleeding-time is prolonged and the platelets generally markedly diminished.

2. Acute Myelocytic Leukemia.—The onset is variable, sometimes with increasing debility and similar symptoms; sometimes with hemorrhage. Ulceration of the mouth and throat has been reported. Fever is present, and the spleen may be moderately enlarged. Leukocytosis is moderate and there may even be leukopenia; but always there is a characteristic excess in the percentage of the myelocytes, equaling from 10 to 50 per cent of the

white cells; and the number of lymphocytes is diminished. Eosinophiles and mast-cells may be absent. The platelets are decreased in number.

3. Chronic Myelocytic Leukemia (Fig. 251).—Here often the first symptom to attract attention is enlargement of the abdomen due to the splenomegaly, which may become very great. There is sometimes pain in the splenic region or in the bones. The lymph-nodes are moderately enlarged, and the liver slightly or greatly so. Fever is absent or occurs irregularly. Anemia becomes decided. Hemorrhage is usually a late rather than an early symptom. Priapism may occur, due to myelogenous infiltration

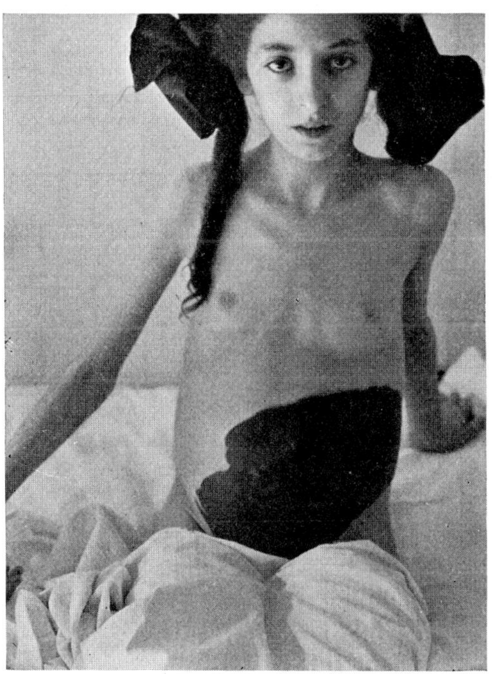

Fig. 251.—Chronic myelocytic leukemia. Girl of thirteen years, first seen June 1, in the Children's Medical Ward of the Hospital of the University of Pennsylvania. Had suffered from loss of health and weight for five months. Spleen filled the entire left side of the abdomen, leukocytes 190,400, with 56 per cent polymorphonuclears and 21 per cent said to be myelocytes. Daily radiologic treatment instituted. Feb., leukocytes 14,000, and spleen could not be palpated with certainty, general health excellent. Later relapsed in spite of renewed radiologic treatment, failed in health, and died in the autumn two and a quarter years after first seen. Black area shows position and size of spleen soon after treatment was commenced.

of the penis. The **blood** shows considerable reduction in hemoglobin and red cells; normoblasts are present in large numbers; megaloblasts may be found; polychromatophilia and granular degeneration are observed; but poikilocytosis, microcytosis and megalocytosis are less common. Leukocytosis usually reaches 200,000 or more per cubic millimeter. The increase is in all varieties but with a large proportion of myelocytes, which constitute from 30 to 50 per cent or more of the white cells. Increase of the lymphocytes is usually in the larger forms. A characteristic is the occurrence of mast-cells in fairly large quantity. The percentage of eosinophiles may be above normal. The number of platelets varies considerably. It is stated that the number of leukocytes found in the saliva varies in this and in other forms of leukemia inversely to that in the blood (Isaacs and Danielian[129]). Blood-phosphorus may be greatly increased (Buckman et al.[130]).

4. Chronic Lymphocytic Leukemia.—This variety is rarely encountered in early life, in the sense of a long-continued disorder, and the disease seldom lasts longer than three months.

5. Atypical Leukemia.—Some of the variations in types have already been noted, such, for example, as the so-called *aleukemic leukemia* or *aleukemic stages* in which there is a leukopenia rather than a leukocytosis. In our experience such cases have been relatively common. So-called "*mixed forms*" have been described, in which both myelocytic and lymphocytic cells have been present; but, as stated, the leukemias apparently constitute a general group with involvement of all of the hematopoietic system. The mixed cases usually terminate as myelocytic types and, as shown by newer staining methods, were probably so from the beginning. In the category of atypical cases some writers place *chloroma* (p. 1017). *Pseudoleukemic anemia* has by some writers been incorrectly considered merely an infantile form of leukemia. The term *leukanemia* has been applied to the state in which there appears to be a combination of the blood-pictures and symptoms of leukemia and of pernicious anemia; most of these cases probably being atypical instances of leukemia. Another confusing condition, which is intermediate between leukemia and lymphosarcoma and termed by Sternberg[131] *leukosarcoma,* is characterized by an invasive type of lymphoid tumor and a blood-picture resembling leukemia. *Monocytic leukemia* has been reported by Dameshek,[132] and Clough.[133] An uncommon form, of which a few cases have been described in childhood (Bass[134]), is termed *eosinophilic leukemia,* there being great increase of the eosinophilic polymorphonuclear cells.

Course and Prognosis.—The duration of acute lymphocytic leukemia is rarely longer than two or three months. Death is due to exhaustion; anemia from repeated hemorrhage; or some complication, as diarrhea, nephritis, tuberculosis, intracranial hemorrhage, or especially bronchopneumonia. Acute myelocytic leukemia likewise runs a rapid course to a fatal ending. Chronic myelocytic leukemia in childhood causes death in six to eight months or occasionally not for a year or two; there sometimes being remissions. Diminution in the number of white cells may indicate improvement, or may be a poor prognostic sign; and leukopenia sometimes accompanies a complication of a severe sort. Recoveries from leukemia have been reported, but are probably instances of unusually long remissions or of mistaken diagnosis.

Diagnosis.—The mere presence of a high polymorphonuclear leukocytosis is no proof of the existence of leukemia, nor is leukopenia proof of its absence. The relative rather than the absolute number of lymphocytes is important diagnostically. A great increase of lymphocytes is characteristic of lymphocytic leukemia. The presence of mast-cells and of a high percentage of myelocytes marks the myelocytic type. The blood in secondary anemia with leukocytosis often presents in children a relative increase of lymphocytes, but never to the degree seen in leukemia; while in pseudoleukemic anemia, although the number of leukocytes is augmented and myelocytes are present, the total quantity of white cells is much less than is usual in leukemia, and the myelocytes and mast-cells are few as compared with myelocytic leukemia. In both these forms of anemia the percentages of red cells and hemoglobin are usually lower than in leukemia. Rarely sarcomatous tumors of the thymus gland or of lymphoid tissue produce a condition of the blood like that of leukemia. Pertussis, while showing an actual and relative increase of lymphocytes, can seldom cause diagnostic difficulty. Glandular fever with its increased percentage of mononuclear cells and its enlarged spleen and superficial lymph-nodes may cause confusion, but this disease does not produce hemorrhages and other symptoms of leukemia, and the outcome is favorable. We have seen the diagnosis of purpura disproven by the examination of the blood. Difficulty might arise in distinguishing the aleukemic stage of leukemia from aplastic anemia (p. 1029) or agranulocytosis (p. 1029). Continued study may be necessary to diagnose some of the atypical forms of leukemia described. A diagnosis of the disease cannot be made from a single blood-examination because of the variation in the total and, to a less extent, in the differential white cell count. The oxydase granule-staining method is helpful in distinguishing the different forms of cells. It may be stated that in leukemia there is often a high metabolic rate, probably attributable to the rapid formation of the enormous number of young cells.

Treatment.—This is unsatisfactory and has no effect on the ultimate outcome. Both arsenic and benzol in full doses may cause diminution in the number of leukocytes, but have no demonstrable good effect on the general condition, except perhaps in the chronic myelocytic form which is so uncommon in childhood. Radiologic treatment over the spleen and the long bones helps to prolong life in the chronic forms, but probably hastens the end in the acute forms. (For review of this phase of the subject see Farley.[135]) Extirpation of the spleen is not to be recommended. Lucherini[136] and Anding[137] apparently influenced the course of leukemia by inoculating the patient with malaria. Pearce[138] reported apparent recovery in acute lymphocytic leukemia from the intramuscular injection of spleen-extract. We have tried this in 2 instances without result; such being also the experience of Gonce et al.[139]

Diseases of the Hemorrhagic Diathesis

Here are grouped a number of conditions, some of which are not clearly affiliated, while others shade into each other to a certain extent, and may also bear a close relationship to other affections. Hemorrhagic disorders of the new-born have been considered elsewhere (p. 219), and the hemorrhagic tendency in scurvy has been described (p. 458). There is often an intimate connection between forms of erythema and of purpura; while in nearly all of the infectious diseases a hemorrhagic tendency may at times develop; and the same is true of sepsis, leukemia, pernicious anemia, aplastic anemia, some forms of icterus, and greatly debilitated states produced in any way.

HEMOPHILIA

This is an inherited constitutional tendency to repeated, severe, and even uncontrollable hemorrhage produced by slight trauma or occurring spontaneously, the patient being known as a "bleeder."

Etiology and Pathologic Anatomy.—The disease is passed from generation to generation entirely through the female ("conductor"), although the males of the family are those affected, and the females seldom if ever. Its transmission appears to be according to Mendelian laws, and is a sex-linked recessive characteristic; careful studies of families of bleeders, such as the one reported by Klug,[140] in which the history of the family for one hundred years was known, supporting this view. Usually half the daughters of a conductor will be conductors, and half of her sons will have the disease. In rare instances it seems possible that males could transmit the condition (Mills[141]). It would be theoretically possible for a female to have the disease if she were the offspring of a hemophilic male and a female conductor. Clough,[142] however, states that no authentic case of hemophilia in a female is on record. Isolated instances of hemophilia are reported, but are probably either mistakes in diagnosis, or a more complete history would have shown the influence of inheritance.

Among causes suggested are abnormal fragility of the walls of the small blood-vessels; high blood-pressure with abnormally small vessels; diminished coagulability; destruction of blood by some toxic or infectious agent; chemical alteration in the walls of the blood-vessels. None of these, however, has been conclusively proven. According to Howell,[143] Addis,[144] Hurwitz and Lucas,[145] and others the delayed coagulation in the blood has been supposed to depend upon a defect in prothrombin, the antithrombin being present in normal amount. Howell and Cekada,[146] however, later reported cases with normal prothrombin. Minot and Lee,[147] Howell and Cekada,[146] and others believe that the platelets are at fault; these being abnormally resistant and slow in disintegration. Mills[148] found the thrombin not converted into prothrombin by the antithrombin. It would appear that there is no deficiency of fibrinogen. **Pathologically** there is no characteristic change found.

Symptoms.—As a rule the disease does not manifest itself before about the age of two years, although it has been seen in infancy and reported even in the new-born. Some of these early cases were undoubtedly instances of hemorrhagic disease of the new-born, which has no relationship to hemophilia. In fact new-born infants of a hemophilic inheritance rarely exhibit the symptoms of the disease at this period of life. The first appearance of hemophilia seldom if ever comes on after childhood is passed. The symptoms consist solely in hemorrhage, the patient being healthy in other respects, except for the anemia produced if the bleeding is frequent and extensive. Hemorrhage may take place spontaneously or, more frequently, as the result of trauma. The trauma may be very slight, such as an insignificant blow, the extraction of a tooth, the use of a toothbrush, or bruising. The spontaneous hemorrhages may occur in any region of the body. They may be preceded by malaise, irritability, headache, or other vague symptoms; or may come on without warning. They are most frequent from the nose and mouth, but may occur from any other mucous membrane; or may be subcutaneous, producing hematoma or ecchymosis; or, in unusual instances, take place from the cutaneous surface or into muscles or serous cavities. A characteristic seat is into one of the joints, most frequently the knee or elbow. The **blood** may exhibit the features of secondary anemia, and there is always greatly delayed coagulation-time. The blood for examination should be obtained preferably from a vein, in order to avoid the influence on coagulation of the tissue-juice. There may be a slight diminution of the polymorphonuclear cells. The number of blood-platelets, the amount of blood-calcium, the bleeding-time (p. 149), and the capillary-resistance test are normal.

Course and Prognosis.—The condition is essentially chronic, with a decided inclination to periodicity; the isolated occurrence of severe or persistent hemorrhage not being sufficient to justify the diagnosis of hemophilia. The duration of a single hemorrhage is uncertain and variable. The danger to life is not often immediate from the size and rapidity of the bleeding, but from its persistence and the consequent amount of blood lost. The first hemorrhage is seldom fatal. In less severe attacks there is often a remarkably rapid restoration to normal health. The prognosis on the whole is unfavorable, studies showing that 85 per cent of the patients die as the result of the disease, many of them in childhood. The earlier in life the affection begins the more unfavorable the prognosis. The longer life continues the greater the possibility of the hemorrhagic disposition disappearing; this sometimes ceasing entirely after puberty, although as a rule such is not the case. Repeated hemorrhages into a joint may cause chronic arthritis.

Diagnosis.—Without a family history of the disorder the diagnosis is uncertain, since other causes produce repeated hemorrhages. The possibility, but very great improbability, of hemophilia occurring in the female has been mentioned. It is difficult to classify some of the reported instances of familial tendency to bleeding affecting females as well as males, such as those reported by Little and Ayres;[149] and equally so to place the long familial history with normal coagulation time recorded by von Willebrand.[150] As stated, hemorrhagic disease in the new-born is not related to hemophilia; the subjects of the former not exhibiting this disease later, and hemophilia rarely, if ever, appearing in the new-born. From purpura, hemophilia is distinguished by the presence in the blood of a normal number of platelets, and by the delayed coagulation-time. It is an interesting observation that in hemophilia hemorrhage from a needle-prick for the purpose of obtaining blood can usually be arrested without difficulty.

Treatment.—In the way of **prophylaxis** marriage of the females should be discouraged in families known to be bleeders. Even in the case of a child with hemophilic antecedents, who has as yet shown no symptoms, operations should be avoided as far as possible, and accidents which might produce hemorrhage guarded against. Vaccination, however, has not been found to be dangerous. Little benefit can be expected from the administration of calcium, since the blood is not deficient in this mineral. Ovarian extract has been given on the basis that females do not manifest the disease, and ovarian implantation has also been performed (Nieham,[151] Birch,[152] Foord and Dysart[153]). Good results have been claimed from both these measures. We have had some success with the procedure proposed by Vines[154] and used by Mills,[155] and Eley and Clifford,[156] in which the patient is sensitized to a foreign protein, such as sheep serum. A subcutaneous injection of 4 cc. is given, followed in seven to ten days by an intradermal injection of a similar serum. The injection may be repeated every week or so or perhaps at much longer intervals, in order to keep the patient sensitive. This treatment, is, however, only partly effective,—controlling or preventing chiefly the hemorrhage which might otherwise follow minor injuries.

In the treatment of **actual hemorrhage,** the bleeding part should be kept elevated, and compresses, tampons or the cautery used, according to the situation and the demands. Trial may also be made locally of epinephrine, thromboplastin, cephalin, calcium chloride, gelatin, fresh thymus extract, or chloride of iron. The subcutaneous injection of epinephrine, pituitrin, peptone, platelet-extract, fibrogen and gelatin respectively have their adherents. The subcutaneous or intravenous injection of serum from another human, or from the rabbit or the horse, increases the coagulability of the blood, and is one of the best procedures. When the loss of blood has been great, transfusion should certainly be done. After recovery from an attack tonic remedies are indicated as in any form of anemia.

PURPURA

By this title is designated the occurrence of more or less scattered effusions of blood beneath or into the skin, from the mucous membranes, or into the internal organs. The various affections which manifest this symptom are intimately associated with each other. In some the purpura is secondary or symptomatic, while in others it is primary or idiopathic in the sense that it is not associated with any other discoverable morbid state. A convenient classification is into (1) Symptomatic Purpura and (2) Idiopathic Purpura.

1. Symptomatic Purpura.—Here hemorrhages are usually situated only in the skin, but to this there are exceptions. The purpura is merely a secondary symptomatic manifestation. It does not differ in appearance

from that of the idiopathic form. Necrotic areas may develop in some cases with greatly lowered vitality. Causes may be divided into (*a*) infectious; (*b*) toxic; (*c*) cachetic; (*d*) neurotic; and (*e*) mechanical;—although the distinctions are by no means sharp.

(*a*) **Infectious Purpura.**—This is a not infrequent form observed in septicemia; pyemia; acute miliary tuberculosis; malignant endocarditis; and many of the eruptive and other infectious fevers, especially variola, cerebrospinal fever, and typhus fever. We have twice seen purpura in cases without symptoms of meningitis, in which meningococci were found in the blood; and they have been recovered also from the hemorrhagic spots (Netter, Salanier and Wolfrom[157]). Typical cases of rheumatism rarely exhibit any purpuric eruption, and the so-called "rheumatic purpura" is probably not rheumatic in nature (p. 1040). In infectious purpura the spots may vary in size from those of a petechial character to widespread subcutaneous and submucous hemorrhages.

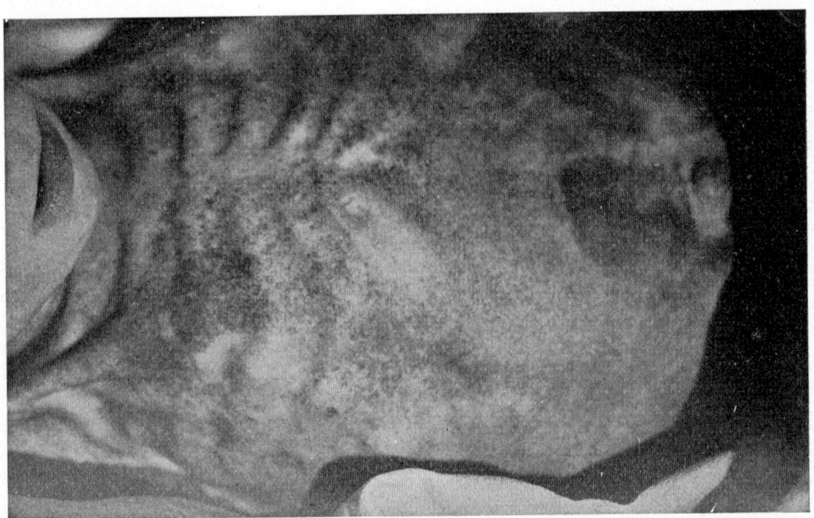

Fig. 252.—Cachectic purpura on chest. From a marantic infant of ten months in the Children's Hospital of Philadelphia. Died a week after admission.

(*b*) **Toxic Purpura.**—In this class may be included endogenous toxins as in cases of icterus; or exogenous poisons as in snake-bite, and in the administration of certain drugs and other substances as antipyrine, the iodides, copaiba, quinine, phosphorus, benzol, arsenic, potassium chlorate, belladonna, and foreign sera (*anaphylactoid purpura*).

(*c*) **Cachetic Purpura.**—Here should be noted purpura occurring in greatly debilitated states (Fig. 252), as produced by chronic diarrhea or other digestive disturbances and avitaminosis; or resulting from empyema, tuberculosis, prolonged bronchopneumonia, and malignant growths. Here, too, is best placed purpura seen in leukemia, pernicious anemia, aplastic anemia, pseudoleukemic anemia, scurvy, Hodgkin's disease, Gaucher's disease, and Banti's disease. In cachetic purpura the spots are usually small and occur chiefly on the abdomen and chest.

(*d*) **Neurotic Purpura.**—This form is very uncommon in early life. It may appear in hysteria, myelitis, locomotor ataxia, and some other nervous disorders.

(*e*) **Mechanical Purpura.**—This may occur in pertussis from the violence of the cough; in epilepsy; when a limb is released from bandages; on the first use of the legs after a long illness; or whenever there has been venous stasis from any cause.

The condition of the *blood* in symptomatic purpura varies to some extent with the cause. There is usually no alteration in the number of platelets in cases of hemorrhagic conditions dependent upon scurvy, Hodgkin's disease, pseudoleukemia, jaundice, and hemophilia. The platelets are generally diminished in number in purpura connected with severe infections, cachetic states, pernicious anemia, aplastic anemia, leukemia, and the introduction of poisons or foreign sera.

2. IDIOPATHIC PURPURA (*Morbus maculosus Werlhofii*).—Once considered as distinct, the different forms of this are now believed to be but variations in degree and localization of a single process. For convenience the division may be made into (*a*) purpura simplex; (*b*) purpura rheumatica; (*c*) purpura hemorrhagica; (*d*) Henoch's purpura; and (*e*) purpura fulminans.

Etiology and Pathologic Anatomy.—Primary purpura is oftenest seen in children after the age of three and up to that of ten years. It may occur even in the new-born, and then be associated with thrombopenia (Waltner,[158] Greenwald and Sherman[159]). Glanzman,[160] Rothman and Nixon,[161] and others report instances in which there was a strong hereditary tendency. There is little difference in the frequency in the sexes. Among predisposing causes are debility, unhygienic conditions, digestive disorders, and anemia; but frequently purpura develops in children apparently in the best of health. The nature of any direct exciting cause is unknown. That the blood-vessels are affected in some manner appears certain, but it is not clear whether this is an acute degenerative process, a bacterial embolism, a result of a toxin, or a vasomotor disturbance. It is possible that the cause differs with the case. The etiologic relationship of changes in the blood to the eruption is uncertain. Pathologically there is nothing characteristic found except hemorrhage in various localities. The *blood* changes are chiefly those of secondary anemia. There may be a moderate leukocytosis at times. The condition of the blood-platelets and the bleeding-time will be referred to in considering the different varieties. The coagulation-time is not altered, although in some cases the clot retracts poorly.

The special symptoms, course, and prognosis may be studied more satisfactorily under the different clinical types.

(*a*) **Purpura Simplex.**—This is the mildest and most frequent form of idiopathic purpura. There may be slight indisposition for a few days, shown by loss of appetite, headache, diarrhea, vomiting, and moderate fever; but often the attack begins suddenly with the appearance of numerous, scattered, discrete, small, pin-head and split-pea sized or larger, rounded, purple spots on some region of the body. The favorite sites are the extensor surfaces of the upper and especially the lower extremities; but the trunk may also be involved when the eruption is widespread. The face and hands generally escape. The spots often come out in crops, closely following each other, or sometimes in the form of recrudescences of the disease after intermissions. In some cases there is edema in the affected region; or the individual purpuric spots may be edematous (*purpura urticans*), and larger than in the ordinary form (Fig. 253). Sometimes urticaria and exudative erythema also develop, but this is less frequent than in rheumatic purpura.

Attending the eruption there may be slight fever, but oftener none, or slight pain in the muscles and joints. The number of blood-platelets and the bleeding-time are usually not altered. The *duration* is from one to three weeks, or often longer, depending upon whether one or several crops of spots develop. Recurrences are liable to take place some weeks or months after the attack is over. The *prognosis* is entirely favorable, except for the occasional passing of purpura simplex into a severer type.

(*b*) **Purpura Rheumatica** (*Peliosis rheumatica; Schönlein's*[162] *disease; Arthritic purpura; Anaphylactic purpura*).—The characteristic of this type of purpura is the combination of the cutaneous eruption with pain and swelling of the joints, and often with urticaria and exudative erythema. The title "rheumatic" is misleading, as predicating an association with rheumatism, against the existence of which connection there is abundant evidence. The disease is less common in children than in young adults, and somewhat oftener seen in males than in females. There are frequently decided *prodromal symptoms;* an exaggeration of those described under purpura simplex. In addition sore throat is a common early symptom, and there may be vague, not well localized pains in the limbs. Then appears the purpuric eruption, similar to or often of smaller size than that in

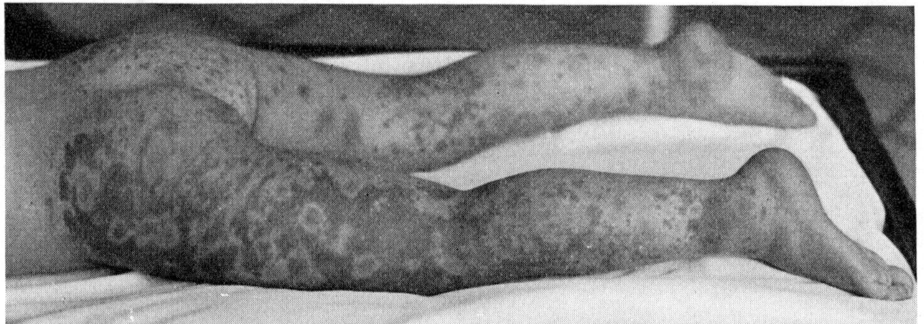

Fig. 253.—Male, four years of age, in Children's Hospital, Cincinnati. Bleeding-time, coagulation-time and retractility of clot all normal. No bleeding from mucous membranes. There was some edema of the skin and the rash was of the purpura urticans type.

purpura simplex, and sometimes with vesiculation. It is much oftener seen in the lower extremities, especially about the affected joints, but may appear on any part of the body. It is, as stated, frequently combined with urticaria (*purpura urticans*), and in other cases with erythema multiforme, or, less often, erythema nodosum. At times the amount of the edema is decided, and this may involve the face and eyelids. Developing at about the same time with the eruption are pain and swelling in the joints, oftenest the knees or ankles, and usually multiple. The swelling is periarticular as well as from serous effusion into the joint itself. The *general symptoms* are febrile in nature, but are usually not severe. The bleeding-time and the number of platelets are generally normal. Complications are not common, although exceptionally endocarditis and pericarditis have been noted. The *duration* of the disease is variable, lasting two weeks or longer, depending on whether crops of eruption continue to appear. A tendency to repeated attacks is observed. The *prognosis* is favorable.

(*c*) **Purpura Haemorrhagica** (*Thrombopenia*).—To this variety some writers apply especially the sub-title *morbus maculosus Werlhofii* (Werlhof[163]), others using this latter term as a synonym for idiopathic purpura of any sort. In purpura haemorrhagica there is sometimes a hereditary influence. It is rather sharply distinguished from other types of idiopathic purpura by the decided diminution in the number of platelets, which frequently are fewer than 100,000 per cubic millimeter, in place of the approximate normal of 450,000. The diminution of platelets is probably due to their excessive destruction by the reticulo-endothelial system (de Sanctis and Allen[164]). The bleeding-time, too, is prolonged several minutes to many hours, and a hemorrhagic area is liable to form in the skin around the puncture. The leukocytes may be normal in number, or there may be either leukopenia or leukocytosis. There are not only the subcutaneous hemorrhages of purpura simplex, but from the beginning hemorrhage into and from the mucous membranes and into the internal organs. Vague prodromal symptoms of indisposition may last for some days, but oftenest the attack begins abruptly. The eruption is in part similar to that of purpura simplex; in part consists of ecchymoses of a size as large as, or larger than, the hand. It may be situated in any part of the body, including the face. In the most severe cases a large area of cutaneous surface, as perhaps an entire extremity, is edematous and purple-red from confluence of the hemorrhagic spots, and may occasionally exhibit vesiculation. The occurrence of erythema and urticaria is rare. The joints may be involved, but less often than in purpura rheumatica.

Contemporaneously with the cutaneous eruption bleeding, which may be slight or severe, takes place from the mucous membranes. Hemorrhage from the nose is the most frequent; hematuria is common; bleeding may occur also from the intestine; or there may be hematemesis, or, less often, hemorrhage from the genitals, the ears, or the lungs. Sometimes hemorrhage from mucous membranes may be the only symptom of the disease. Ecchymoses may appear upon the visible mucous membranes. The tendency to bleeding is so great that slight pressure upon, or scratching of, the skin may produce subcutaneous effusion or the free escape of blood from the surface; and a needle-prick may be followed by bleeding which is controlled with great difficulty. The *general symptoms*, as fever and the like, vary with the severity of the attack. The amount of blood lost in various ways may be so great that severe anemia and even collapse result. Some cases may pass into a typhoid state; or cerebrospinal symptoms may be present, dependent upon intracranial or intraspinal hemorrhage or upon anemia. The spleen is palpable in about a third of the cases. Albuminuria may occur, and edema, especially of the face and feet, may be present. Nephritis may develop. Vomiting is common. The *duration* of the disease in favorable instances is two weeks or longer. There is always great danger of recurrence, and this may take place again and again, prolonging the course for weeks or even months. The *prognosis* of purpura haemorrhagica in general is good, and the majority of cases recover. Death may take place from exhaustion following loss of blood, or from intracranial hemorrhage, or in the typhoid state.

(*d*) **Purpura Abdominalis** (*Henoch's Purpura*[165]).—This type is observed chiefly in children and adolescents. It begins with the *symptoms* usual to rheumatic purpura, including the involvement of the joints, the urticaria and erythema, and the purpuric eruption, except that the last may early be slightly developed. Then, with an increase of these, severe abdominal manifestations suddenly appear, among them being very obstinate vomiting, paroxysmal attacks of intense abdominal pain, complete loss of appetite, constipation followed by diarrhea, tenesmus with bloody stools, not infrequently nephritis, enlargement of the spleen, and hemorrhage from the mucous membranes. The abdomen is hard and tender, particularly in the region of the transverse colon; the condition suggesting intestinal obstruction, especially intussusception. There is generally fever, and the patient rapidly becomes much debilitated. The single attack lasts only a few days, but is then followed in the course of a few days more, or perhaps a week or month, by another attack, and so on; the course being sometimes protracted. Generally there are less than half a dozen attacks, the intensity growing gradually less, but there may be a great many. The predisposition to recurrence is marked. In certain cases resembling Henoch's purpura there seems to be an association with allergy; at least the attacks can be brought on in subjects otherwise known to be allergic by the ingestion of certain foods, as eggs (Alexander and Eyermann[166]). Not all the characteristic features are seen in each case, or even in each attack in the same individual. The cause of the abdominal pain is not understood. It may be a thrombosis of the intestinal vessels, or effusion of blood into the mucous membrane of the stomach and intestine, or localized edema in these regions. The prognosis must be guarded, but the majority of the cases in children recover.

(*e*) **Purpura Fulminans** (Fig. 254).—This very unusual condition, to which the title was given by Henoch,[167] is seen oftenest in children, and is like purpura simplex in the limitation of the hemorrhage to the skin; but unlike it in the rapid development, and in the extent and amount of the hemorrhage. The onset is very sudden, with chilliness, high fever, great prostration, and vomiting. Ecchymoses of large size, often symmetrically placed, appear with remarkable rapidity, in the course of a few hours completely covering large areas chiefly on the extremities. The skin is hard,

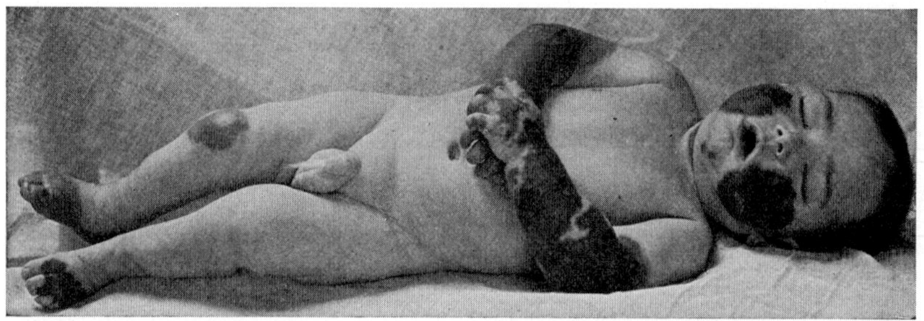

Fig. 254.—Purpura fulminans. Infant in the Children's Hospital of Philadelphia. Time and method of onset not clearly discoverable. Patient exhibited edema and large dark-purple effusions of blood. Mucous membranes apparently uninvolved. Necropsy negative.

edematous, and may exhibit bullae containing a bloody, serous fluid. Gangrene may develop (Beinhauer[168]). The spleen is generally enlarged, and there is often albuminuria. Death takes place in from twelve to twenty-four hours, or sometimes after three or four days, with cerebral symptoms ending in coma.

Diagnosis of Purpura.—This is difficult only when there is hemorrhage from mucous membranes but not into the skin. Symptomatic purpura is recognized by its development after or in connection with some of the conditions mentioned as causative factors, while idiopathic purpura is distinguished by the absence of any such cause. Confusion might be possible between a purpura fulminans and some of the malignant, rapidly fatal, hemorrhagic secondary cases associated with the infectious fevers. These latter are characterized by the higher temperature, the prodromes, and the probable presence of some distinguishing symptoms of the causative disease. The hemorrhagic condition seen in lymphocytic leukemia and aplastic anemia is recognized by an examination of the blood. Scorbutus might suggest a primary purpura with articular involvement; but the onset in scurvy is slower, the history distinctive, the gums are spongy, and the painful regions are the shafts of the bones, not the articulations. Henoch's purpura may be mistaken for intussusception, acute colitis, or gastric or duodenal ulcer; and this has, in fact, happened and operations been performed. On the other hand, a number of cases of intussusception occurring as a complication of Henoch's purpura have been reported (Morse and Stone[169]). A recurring purpura hemorrhagica can be positively distinguished from hemophilia by the fact that in the latter the coagulation-time of the blood is greatly delayed, the bleeding-time is not prolonged, the blood-platelets are not diminished, and that simple puncture of the skin with a needle does not cause obstinate hemorrhage unless a vein has been actually wounded. The reverse in all these particulars is true of purpura haemorrhagica. It should be borne in mind, however, that there appear to be exceptional borderline cases between thrombopenia and hemophilia. Thus Opitz and Frei[170] report an instance in a female infant in which, with a diminution of platelets and a greatly prolonged bleeding-time, there was no coagulation even after two hours. They entitle the condition "pseudo-hemophilia." Somewhat similar cases have been recorded by others (Rabe and Salomon;[171] Weil and Ischl-Wall[172]). We have seen an instance of haemorrhagic purpura in which the coagulation-time was prolonged. It is further to be borne in mind that in the hemorrhagic disease of the new-born both coagulation-time and bleeding-time may be prolonged.

The various types of primary purpura appear to shade into each other or to constitute forms of one disease. Purpura simplex is characterized by subcutaneous hemorrhages only; purpura rheumatica by the combination of these with urticaria and allied conditions, and with involvement of the joints; purpura haemorrhagica by the existence of hemorrhage from the mucous membranes as well as in the skin; Henoch's purpura by the combination of the symptoms of rheumatic purpura with abdominal crises and hemorrhage from the mucous membranes; purpura fulminans by its rapid, fatal course, with the extensive hemorrhage occurring only in the skin.

There is sometimes made a division of purpura into the thrombopenic (thrombocytopenic) and the nonthrombopenic forms; the former consisting of purpura haemorrhagica and the latter all other varieties. This is hardly acceptable, since diminution of platelets may occur in secondary forms of purpura, especially those associated with severe infectious and toxic states, marked anemias, and leukemia. Rosenthal[173] would classify purpura into three groups, those with (1) diminution in platelets, (2) alteration in functions of platelets without diminution, and (3) changes in the capillaries. In view of the uncertainty regarding pathogenesis it seems better to follow an etiologic and symptomatic classification as used in this chapter.

Treatment.—The treatment of secondary purpura is that of the primary disease. Measures to improve any resultant anemia or the general health are indicated. Rest is the most important treatment for idiopathic cases, and this should be sufficiently prolonged; too early activity often resulting in a return of the purpura. Various remedies have been advised, among them sulphuric acid, ergotine, epinephrine, hydrastine, gallic acid, turpentine, and arsenic. The last is perhaps one of the best. There is no reason why calcium should be of benefit, since in purpura there is no lack of this mineral. The treatment must, in the main, be symptomatic. Hemorrhage from the nose may demand local measures, as the application of a solution of epinephrine, or perhaps the plugging of the posterior nares. Severe bleeding from any region may be treated by the application of such organic derivatives as thromboplastin and cephalin, or by the hypodermic administration of epinephrine, fibrinogen, gelatin thoroughly sterilized, pituitrin, or of normal human blood-serum or that of other animals. Transfusion of uncitrated whole blood is preferable, since this offers a method of increasing the number of blood-platelets. Some investigators have warned against a foreign serum in purpura hemorrhagica, since violent reactions may occur. Such patients may also be extremely sensitive to tuberculin. Removal of the spleen in the thrombopenic cases was first recommended by Kaznelson,[174] on the theory that the spleen exerted a thrombolytic action. Among others who have studied this procedure are Brill and Rosenthal,[175] Giffin and Halloway,[176] Williamson,[177] Spence,[178] Quénu,[179] and Washburn.[180]

The consensus of opinion is that about 75 to 80 per cent of the patients are greatly benefited or cured. It should be noted that the operation does not always restore, except temporarily, the number of platelets to normal; although in spite of this symptomatic cure may result. Some of the failures of splenectomy have been attributed to the presence of accessory spleens (Morrison, Lederer and Fradkin[181]). In one of our[182] cases platelets were brought to normal number in the circulating blood by repeated radiologic treatment over the spleen. Exposure of the body to ultraviolet irradiation has been claimed to accomplish this restoration to normal (Sooy and Moise[183]), but has seemed to have relatively little effect in our experience. For the pain and vomiting of Henoch's purpura the application of an ice-bag to the abdomen may be tried, and if necessary, a hypodermic injection of morphine and atrophine given.

References

1. Quart. J. Med., 1931, **24,** 285. 2. Fletcher and Mitchell, Am J. Dis. Child., 1927, **34,** 807. 3. Mitchell, Am. J. Dis. Child., 1915, **9,** 358. 4. Deutsch. med. Wchnschr., 1904, **30,** 54; 92. 5. Ztschr. f. klin. med., 1920, **89,** 1. 6. The Blood Picture, 1929. 7. Am. J. Dis. Child., 1930, **40,** 70. 8. Arch. Pediat., 1932, **49,** 207. 9. Compt. rend. soc. de biol., 1892, **44,** 384. 10. Am. J. Med. Sc., 1923, **166,** 469. 11. Ztschr. f. Kinderh., 1925, **40,** 225. 12. Quart. J. Med., 1908, **2,** 85; Polycythaemia, Erythrocytosis, and Erythraemia, 1921. 13. Medicine, 1928, **7,** 291. 14. Therap. Monatshr., 1918, **32,** 322. 15. J.A.M.A., 1929, **93,** 1205. 16. Ann. Int. Med., 1932, **5,** 1367. 17. J.A.M.A., 1927, **88,** 1047. 18. Am. J. Syph., 1928, **12,** 328. 19. Griffith and Scott, M. J. and Rec., 1928, **128,** 121. 20. J.A.M.A., 1932, **98,** 1047. 21. Am. J. Physiol., 1927, **80,** 400. 22. J. Am. Dietet. A., 1931, **7,** 6. 23. J.A.M.A., 1931, **97,** 180. 24. Ref. McCollum and Simmonds, Newer Knowledge of Nutrition, 1929, p. 140. 25. J. Biol. Chem., 1927, **75,** 123. 26. J. Biol. Chem., 1928, **77,** 797. 27. J. Biol. Chem., 1929, **83,** 243; 251. 28. J. Biol. Chem., 1931, **93,** 49. 29. Nutritional Anemias in Infancy. Med. Res. Counc., London, 1931, 157. 30. J. Nutrition, 1931, **3,** 465. 31. J. Nutrition, 1931, **4,** 517. 32. Am. J. Dis. Child., 1931, **41,** 53. 33. Am. J. Dis. Child., 1918, **16,** 154. 34. J.A.M.A., 1923, **80,** 93. 35. Arch. Int. Med., 1910, **6,** 517. 36. Arch. Path., 1930, **9,** 876. 37. J. Lab. and Clin. Med., 1930, **15,** 519. 38. Am. J. Dis. Child., 1929, **38,** 103. 39. Am. J. Dis. Child., 1927, **34,** 72. 40. Am. J. Dis. Child., 1926, **32,** 334. 41. Arch. Path., 1929, **1,** 820. 42. Am. J. Dis. Child., 1928, **36,** 1257. 43. Bull. Johns Hopkins Hosp., 1928, **43,** 399. 44. J. Missouri M. A., 1929, **26,** 561. 45. J. Clin. Investig., 1927, **5,** 31; Am. J. M. Sc., 1931, **181,** 240. 46. Ann. Int. Med., 1929, **2,** 1162. 47. J. Med. Cincinnati, 1930, **11,** 541. 48. Arch. Int. Med., 1927, **39,** 233. 49. Am. J. Dis. Child., 1927, **34,** 923. 50. Am. J. M. Sc., 1928, **175,** 206. 51. Am. J. M. Sc., 1929, **178,** 223. 52. Trans. Med.-Chir. Soc., Edinb., 1824, 1, 194. 53. Constitutional and Local Effects of Diseases of the Suprarenal Capsules. 54. Die chronische Anämie im Kindersalter, 1892. 55. Osler and McCrae, Modern Medicine, 1915, **4,** 620. 56. Jahrb. f. Kinderh., 1927, **117,** 257. 57. Hospitalstidende, 1927, **70,** 875. 58. Am. J. Dis. Child., 1928, **36,** 1121. 59. Arch. f. Kinderh., 1928, **86,** 13. 60. Arch. latino-am. de pediat., 1929, **22,** 125. 61. Am. J. M. Sc., 1928, **175,** 581. 62. Arch. Int. Med., 1922, **29,** 711; Am. J. M. Sc., 1928, **175,** 721. 63. Medicine, 1927, **6,** 375. 64. J.A.M.A., 1926, **87,** 470. 65. Am. J. M. Sc., 1928, **175,** 581; 599. 66. J. Biol. Chem., 1927, **74,** 69. 67. Proc. Soc. Exper. Biol. and Med., 1927, **24,** 665. 68. J.A.M.A., 1929, **93,** 747. 69. J.A.M.A., 1930, **94,** 388. 70. J.A.M.A., 1931, **96,** 1198. 71. J.A.M.A., 1932, **98,** 1080. 72. Charité Ann., 1887, **13,** 300. 73. Folia haematolog., 1911; Arch. **12,** 349. 74. Jahrb. f. Kinderh., 1915, **81,** 1. 75. Folia haematolog., 1915, Arch., **19,** 347. 76. Am. J. Dis. Child., 1919, **17,** 174. 77. Am. J. Dis. Child., 1922, **23,** 484. 78. Lancet, 1926, **2,** 948. 79. Therap. d. Gegenw., 1917, **19,** 14. 80. Brit. J. Child. Dis., 1919, **16,** 1. 81. München. med. Wchnschr., 1930, **77,** 575. 82. J. Missouri M. A., 1930, **27,** 1. 83. Deutsch. med. Wchnschr., 1922, **48,** 1495. 84. J.A.M.A., 1931, **97,** 1436. 85. Am. J. Dis. Child., 1928, **35,** 1041. 86. J.A.M.A., 1928, **90,** 663. 87. Am. J. Dis. Child., 1929, **38,** 1037. 88. Wien. klin. Wchnschr., 1929, **42,** 335. 89. Bull. et mém. soc. méd. d. hôp. de Paris, 1930, **54,** 1318. 90. Am. J. Dis. Child., 1930, **40,** 515. 91. Am. J. M. Sc., 1931, **181,** 502. 92. Am. J. M. Sc., 1931, **181,** 533. 93. Am. J. Dis. Child., 1932, **43,** 947. 94. Am. J. M. Sc., 1925, **170,** 500; Am. J. M. Sc., 1930, **179,** 228. 95. Wien. klin. Wchnschr., 1889, **2,** 435; 456. 96. Griffith, Arch. Pediat., 1924, **41,** 511. 97. Am. J. Dis. Child., 1927, **33,** 786; **34,** 347; 1928, **36,** 1257. 98. Edinburgh M. and S. J., 1845, **64,** 400. 99. Edinburgh M. and S. J., 1845, **64,** 413. 100. Froriep's Notizen, 1845, **36,** 151. 101. Farbenanalytische Untersuchungen zur Histologie und Klinik des Blutes, Gesammelte Mittheilungen, 1891, 1. 102. Monatschr. f. Geburtsh. u. Gynäk., 1898, **8,** 215. 103. München, med. Wchnschr.,

1898, **45,** 44. 104. Jahrb. f. Kinderh., 1914, **80,** 290. 105. Rev. franç. de pédiat., 1926, **2,** 26. 106. Jahrb. f. Kinderh., 1907, **65**; Ergänzungsheft, 253. 107. Arch. de méd. d. enf., 1909, **12,** 662. 108. Arch. Pediat., 1911, **28,** 43. 109. Am. J. Dis. Child., 1921, **21,** 163. 110. Nourrisson, 1924, **12,** 1. 111. Am. J. M. Sc., 1925, **169,** 819. 112. Arch. Pediat., 1927, **44,** 126. 113. Am. J. Dis. Child., 1930, **39,** 59. 114. Brit. M. J., 1930, **2,** 282. 115. Am. J. Dis. Child., 1931, **41,** 866. 116. Arch. Pediat., 1916, **33,** 638. 117. Am. J. Dis. Child., 1916, **11,** 462. 118. Lancet., 1916, **2,** 940. 119. Arch. Pediat., 1922, **39,** 819. 120. Med. Klin. 1924, **20,** 891; Monatschr. f. Kinderh., 1930, **48,** 193. 121. Am. J. Dis. Child., 1927, **33,** 394. 122. Arch. Dis. Childhood, 1927, **2,** 119. 123. Acta paediat., 1930, **9,** 497. 124. Jahrb. f. Kinderh., 1930, **126,** 289. 125. Arch. Pediat., 1931, **48,** 463. 126. Garrod, Batten and Thursfield.-Dis. of Childr., 1913, 519. 127. Gaz. hébd. d. sc. méd. de Bordeaux, 1926, **47,** 754; Bull. et. mém. soc. de méd. et chir. de Bordeaux, 1927, p. 312. 128. Acta paediat., 1929, **9,** 89. 129. Am. J. M. Sc., 1927, **174,** 70. 130. Arch. Int. Med., 1925, **35,** 389. 131. Beitr. z. path. Anat. u. z. allg. Path., 1905, **37,** 437; 1915, **61,** 75. 132. Arch. Int. Med., 1930, **46,** 718. 133. J.A.M.A., 1931, **96,** 2150; Tr. A. Am. Phys., 1931, **46,** 258. 134. Am. J. Dis. Child., 1931, **41,** 1394. 135. Medicine, 1928, **7,** 65. 136. Policlinico, 1925, **32,** 1745. 137. Odesskii meditz. J., 1927, p. 7; Ref. J.A.M.A. 1928, **90,** 816. 138. Brit. M. J., 1930, **2,** 282. 139. Am. J. M. Sc., 1932, **183,** 850. 140. Deutsche Ztschr. f. Chir., 1926, **199,** 145. 141. J.A.M.A., 1930, **94,** 1571. 142. Dis. of the Blood, 1929. 143. Arch. Int. Med., 1914, **13,** 76. 144. J. Path. and Bact., 1911, **15,** 427. 145. Arch. Int. Med., 1916, **17,** 543. 146. Am. J. Physiol., 1926, **78,** 500. 147. Arch. Int. Med., 1916, **18,** 474. 148. Am. J. M. Sc., 1926, **172,** 71. 149. J.A.M.A., 1928, **91,** 1251. 150. Finska Läkaresallsk. Handl., 1926, **68,** 87; Ref. Am. J. Dis. Child., 1926, **32,** 763. 151. Schweiz. med. Wchnschr., 1930, **60,** 18. 152. Proc. Soc. Exper. Biol. and Med. 1931, **28,** 752; J.A.M.A., 1931, **97,** 244. 153. J.A.M.A., 1932, **98,** 1444. 154. Quart. J. Med., 1920, **13,** 257. 155. Am. J. Physiol., 1926, **76,** 632. 156. Am. J. Dis. Child., 1931, **42,** 1331. 157. Brit. J. Child. Dis. 1917, **14,** 104. 158. Jahrb. f. Kinderh., 1924, **106,** 307. 159. Am. J. Dis. Child., 1929, **38,** 1245. 160. Jahrb. f. Kinderh. 1918, **88,** 1; 113. 161. J.A.M.A., 1929, **93,** 15. 162. Allg. u. spec. Path. u. Therap. 3d. ed., part 2, 48. 163. Opera omnia, collegit et auxit, Hanover, J. E. Wichmann, 1775. 164. Am. J. Dis. Child., 1931, **41,** 552. 165. Berl. klin. Wchnschr. 1874. **11,** 641. 166. J.A.M.A., 1929, **92,** 2092. 167. Berl. klin. Wchnschr. 1887, **24,** 8. 168. Am. J. Dis. Child., 1929, **38,** 1013. 169. Arch. Pediat., 1909, **26,** 287. 170. Jahrb. f. Kinderh., 1921, **94,** 374. 171. Deutsch. Arch. f. klin. Med., 1920, **132,** 240. 172. Presse. méd., 1923, **31,** 243. 173. J. Lab. and Clin. Med., 1928, **13,** 303. 174. Wien. klin. Wchnschr., 1916, **29,** 1451. 175. Arch. Int. Med., 1923, **32,** 939. 176. Am. J. M. Sc., 1925, **170,** 186. 177. Arch. Dis. Childhood, 1926, **1,** 39. 178. Brit. J. Surg., 1928, **15,** 466. 179. Rev. de chir. Paris, 1929, **67,** 24. 180. J.A.M.A., 1930, **94,** 313. 181. Am. J. M. Sc., 1928, **176,** 672. 182. Griffith, Arch. Pediat., 1924, **41,** 527. 183. J.A.M.A., 1926, **87,** 94.

CHAPTER II

DISEASES OF THE SPLEEN AND RETICULO-ENDOTHELIAL SYSTEM

ACUTE ENLARGEMENT OF THE SPLEEN

ENLARGEMENT of the spleen is common in many acute and chronic diseases, particularly in early life. Temporary enlargement of moderate degree is a frequent attendant upon most of the acute infectious diseases, especially typhoid fever, malaria, acute tuberculosis, measles, and sepsis. At necropsy the spleen is found congested, deep-red, and soft, and the Malpighian bodies may be increased in size. In sepsis and occasionally in typhoid fever infarcts and sometimes abscesses may be present.

In palpating for the spleen the child should be on its back or its right side, the physician's warmed finger-tips resting closely but lightly beneath the left costal border in the mid-axillary line. During inspiration the spleen can then be palpated if enlarged. The abdominal walls should be relaxed, and the flexing of the child's thighs and the diverting of its attention may aid in accomplishing this. If the enlargement is not at first discovered, the

TABLE 73.—DIFFERENTIATION OF CERTAIN CONDITIONS ATTENDED BY SPLENOMEGALY

	Age.	Onset.	Enlargement of spleen.	Enlargement of liver.	Enlargement of superfic. lymph-nodes.	Icterus.	Ascites.	Hemorrhage.
Pseudoleukemia, von Jaksch....	Six months to three years.	Insidious and slow	++	+	+	Rare	0	0
Acute lymphocytic leukemia....	Common in infancy and childhood	Rapid	+	Slight	+	0	0	0
Acute myelocytic leukemia......	Rare in infancy and childhood	Rapid	Slight	Slight or 0	Slight	0	0	++
Chronic myelocytic leukemia....	Rare in infancy and childhood	Insidious	+++	+ to ++	+	0	Rare; late	+
Banti's disease..................	Usually adult or late childhood	Insidious and slow	++	++; later shrinks	0	+; late	++; late	+; especially from stomach; late
Gaucher's disease..............	Begins in infancy	Insidious and very slow	+++	++; late	0; or slight	Rare; but skin is often brownish	0	Rare
Hemolytic icterus..............	New-born or any age	In exacerbations	++	Slight	0	+ to ++	0	Occasionally
Hodgkin's disease...	Childhood	Insidious and slow	++; late	++ slight	++; particular group involved	0; except by pressure of glands	0	Rare; late
Niemann-Pick's disease.........	Early infancy	Slow	+++	+++	++	Discoloration of skin	0	0
Schüller-Christian's disease	Early childhood	Slow	Slight; occasionally great	Slight	0	Perhaps	0	0

	White blood cells, number.	Myelocytes per cent.	Lymphocytes per cent.	Platelets number.	Fragility, red blood cells.	Course.	Prognosis.	Remarks.
Pseudoleukemia, von Jaksch	Normal to 50,000	5 to 10	Relative increase	Often increase	Normal	One to two years	25 per cent mortality	
Acute lymphocytic leukemia	50,000 to 350,000; or leukopenia	Occasionally	80 to 99; mostly large type	Greatly decreased	Normal	Six weeks	100 per cent mortality	
Acute myelocytic leukemia	50,000 to 100,000; or occasionally leukopenia	10 to 50	Relative decrease	Decreased	Normal	Six months to two years	100 per cent mortality	
Chronic myelocytic leukemia	100,000 to 200,000	30 to 50	Relative increase	Increased, normal, or decreased	Normal		100 per cent mortality	
Banti's disease	Leukopenia	0	Relative decrease	Decreased or normal	Normal; may be decreased	Five to ten years	Fairly favorable with operation	
Gaucher's disease	Leukopenia	0	Normal	Usually decreased	Normal	Many years	Die from intercurrent infection	Familial but not hereditary. Perhaps involvement of bones.
Hemolytic icterus	Normal	A few occasionally	Normal	Normal	Increased	Throughout life	Favorable	Reticulocytes 15–20 per cent or more.
Hodgkin's disease	Leukopenia or moderate increase	0; occasionally a few	Relative decrease	Increased	Normal	Two to three years or longer	100 per cent mortality	
Niemann-Pick's disease	15,000 to 20,000	0	Normal	Normal	Normal	Two years	100 per cent mortality ?	Jewish race; familial; Mongoloid appearance; more frequent in girls.
Schüller-Christian's disease	Normal to 20,000	0	Normal	Normal	Normal	Several years ?	May be spontaneous remission	Involvement of cranium; exophthalmos; diabetes insipidus; no racial or familial tendency.

hand should be kept in position and the pressure gradually increased, the finger-tips pushing upward under the costal border, while the other hand supports the posterior left lower chest. Inasmuch as even the normal spleen may sometimes be detected in this way, to constitute a moderate enlargement the organ should protrude an inch below the border of the ribs. Percussion of the spleen is unsatisfactory in infancy, and positive conclusions cannot be drawn from it alone.

Rupture of the Spleen.—This is a rare sequel of acute enlargement in typhoid fever or malaria. It may also result from trauma. Immediate operation is necessary.

CHRONIC ENLARGEMENT OF THE SPLEEN

This is dependent upon a variety of causes. Diverse pathologic conditions result, some of which are discussed each under its individual title. The enlargement may be of moderate size or very great. Among the causes may be mentioned severe anemias, leukemia, pseudoleukemic anemia, Leishman's anemia, Hodgkin's disease, rickets, hereditary syphilis, miliary tuberculosis, malaria, hemolytic icterus, passive congestion in cardiac disease, amyloid degeneration, Bilharzia, morbid growths, Banti's disease, and the various disturbances of lipoid metabolism to be described in this chapter. A synopsis of certain features of some of the splenomegalies is found in Table 74.

1. Banti's Disease

The title "splenic anemia" sometimes used for this condition is too indefinite. Furthermore it is confusing, since it has also been applied to pseudoleukemic anemia (p. 1030), and to other conditions which are now recognized as entities. The condition was first differentiated from other splenomegalies by Banti.[1] The **cause** is unknown, and there is no evidence of inheritance. The increased amount of pigment in the spleen, and the recoveries which have followed splenectomy indicate that the principal elements producing the symptoms reside in this organ. Banti's disease develops usually in young adult males, and seldom before later childhood. A few cases at an earlier age have been reported and collected by Smith,[2] Canelli,[3] and di Meuron.[4] **Pathologically** there is increased fibrous tissue in the spleen; the Malpighian bodies are small and few in number; infarcts are sometimes found; and an increased amount of pigment is usually present. Later there is added hepatic cirrhosis. The splenic vein, portal veins, and neighboring vessels are dilated and exhibit degenerative changes. There is no enlargement of the lymphatic nodes. Characteristic **symptoms** are splenic enlargement, anemia, and hepatic cirrhosis. The slow course is divided into three stages. In the *first*, or pre-ascitic stage, lasting several years there are increasing weakness and pallor; digestive disturbances and abdominal pain; a hard, smooth, progressively enlarging spleen; a tendency to hemorrhage, especially from the stomach; and moderate anemia of the chlorotic type. Very often, however, the anemia and hemorrhagic tendency do not develop until later. In some cases there is delay in sexual development. There is an excess of urobilin in the urine. The number of white cells is always finally below normal, and there may be a marked leukopenia. The neutrophiles are relatively increased, the eosinophiles disappear, and the platelets are diminished. The red cells may show decreased fragility. Rosenthal[5] believes that there are two divisions of Banti's disease. In the first, or thrombocytopenic, group the platelets are diminished before splenectomy but normal after it; in the second, or thrombocythemic, group they are normal before operation but much increased after it. The *second* stage of Banti's disease is of a few months' duration, and is characterized by scanty urine with an increase of urobilin, digestive disturbances and diarrhea, and slight augmentation of the size of the liver. The *third* stage is that of developing hepatic cirrhosis; with ascites, occasionally slight jaundice, bile in the urine, emaciation, anemia, and finally shrinking of the liver. Although the **course** is slow, lasting perhaps ten years or more, the ultimate **prognosis** is unfavorable, unless splenectomy is performed. The patient may die before the stage of cirrhosis. Recovery is, however, possible with operation, even after hepatic cirrhosis has commenced. The **diagnosis** is made by exclusion of other causes of splenomegaly. Secondary anemia accompanied by splenic enlargement might sometimes cause confusion for a while, although there is seldom leukopenia as in Banti's disease. Pseudoleukemic anemia, leukemia, and pernicious anemia all exhibit their characteristic blood-changes. Hemolytic icterus early has discoloration of the skin, often appears at an earlier period of life, and has increased fragility of the red cells. Gaucher's disease begins in infancy and childhood; its course is extremely slow; it exhibits often a familial occurrence; jaundice and ascites are absent; a brownish discoloration of the skin may occur; and the spleen is generally larger than in Banti's disease and the anemia less. In portal hepatic cirrhosis the enlargement of the spleen is a secondary affection, the course is shorter, and the anemia is less marked. In Hanot's cirrhosis the liver is greatly enlarged and there is a chronic icterus. Enlargement of the liver and spleen due to syphilis is associated with other signs of this disease. The only **treatment** is splenectomy, which should be performed early and before the liver has become involved. It is especially likely to be of benefit in cases with thrombocytopenia (Rosenthal[5]). The difficulty in distinguishing Banti's disease from syphilitic enlargement of the spleen demands that syphilitic treatment should be given a trial in all cases with serologic evidence of this disease. Radiologic treatment of the spleen may be tried if splenectomy is not performed. In the ascitic stage salts of mercury may be administered (p. 826).

2. Chronic Thrombosis of the Splenic Vein

This is a rare condition causing splenomegaly in infancy and childhood. It may be associated with, and apparently in some cases is due to, cavernous malformation about the portal vein. Among other causes considered have been congenital narrowing or other malformation of the vessels, and sclerosis of the vessels; and, in cases when the portal vein appears to be primarily at fault, the factor of an umbilical infection has been invoked. Vomiting of blood is a marked feature. Leukopenia and anemia may be present. The liver enlarges little if any, and ascites rarely develops. The course is chronic with remissions. The condition has been mistaken for Banti's disease; which, however, rarely occurs in childhood, has a large liver, and eventually is associated with ascites. Splenectomy has been performed. Spontaneous cure may come about through canalization of the thrombus. Cases belonging in this category have been reported by Wallgren,[6] Smith and Howard,[7] Wilson and Lederer,[8] Holzmann,[9] Vertan,[10] and others.

3. Hemolytic Icterus

The forms of this have been discussed under Diseases of the Liver (pp. 661–664). Certain of them may be mentioned here because of their association with splenomegaly. In the 1st, the *acquired* or *Hayem*[11] type, there is no familial history, the disease may develop at any age, and the course is chronic. There are decided anemia, chronic acholuric icterus, a large hard spleen, slight enlargement of the liver, and increased fragility of the red cells. The 2d, the *familial, congenital,* or *Minkowski,*[12] type, has a decided familial tendency; is observed oftenest congenitally or in the new-born, although it may not appear for several years; the jaundice is chronic, moderate, and acholuric; the urine contains urobilin, but no biliary coloring matter; and the fragility of the red cells is increased. The characteristic feature is the large number of reticulated red cells, which may form 15 or more per cent of the total count. The spleen is enlarged, the liver not involved, the anemia moderate. The general condition of the patient is little if any affected. There may be delay in sexual development. In both types mentioned there may be exacerbations with temporary decrease in the number of red cells. They may be **diagnosed** from Banti's disease by the increased fragility of the red cells, and in the Minkowski type by the familial character and usually early development. The **prognosis** is favorable as to continuance of life, especially in the familial type; but unfavorable for recovery from symptoms. Splenectomy has been performed with favorable results. It is not, however, to be advised unless the general health is suffering. Radiologic treatment of the spleen is said to be helpful.

4. Morbid Growths of the Spleen and Miscellaneous Splenomegalies

Morbid growths of the spleen are of exceptional occurrence. Sarcoma is that oftenest seen, being usually secondary. Fibroma has been reported; and cysts (dermoid, lymphangiomatous, echinococcic, or simple) may occur. A type of splenomegaly in children is described by Hitzrot[13] which he does not think fits into any particular group. Sato and Takahashi[14] report a case with congenital splenomegaly having associated porphyrinuria (see also p. 811).

DISTURBANCES OF THE RETICULO-ENDOTHELIAL SYSTEM

(Xanthomatosis: Lipoidosis)

Here may be considered a group of affections which recent studies have apparently shown to be related. Concerned in pathogenesis is the reticulo-endothelial system. This consists in the reticulum cells of the spleen, lymphoid tissue, and bone-marrow; the endothelial cells of the capillaries of these organs as well as of the liver, the suprarenals, and other tissues; phagocytic cells in the connective tissue; and certain monocytic cells derived from some of these sources and present, at times, in the blood-stream (p. 1020). In xanthomatosis the reticulo-endothelial system is infiltrated by lipoids and other metabolic products, where the so-called "macrophages" of this system appear in some instances to store them and to form nodular growths. The cause of the disturbance of lipoid metabolism is unknown. An important paper on this subject is by Rowland,[15] who groups together certain syndromes to be considered in this section; namely Gaucher's disease, Niemann-Pick's disease, Schüller-Christian's disease; and, in addition, amaurotic family idiocy (Tay-Sach's disease) (p. 908), and certain other disorders, often designated xanthoma, in which there is the deposit of lipoid material in the skin, muscle, and other tissues. Different forms of lipoids or combinations of them appear to be operative in these several allied disorders. The relation of multiple myeloma (p. 1017) to xanthomatosis is undetermined. A number of other students of this subject are in agreement with Rowland, and there are constantly being emphasized links between the syndromes mentioned.

1. Gaucher's Disease

This affection was first described by Gaucher[16] under the title of "primary epithelioma of the spleen." Hoffman and Makler[17] tabulate 89 cases with bibliographies; and Reiss and Kato[18] have included 24 further reports, and add 3 cases personally observed. The 2 cases reported by Knox, Wahl and Schmeisser[19] are probably better classed as instances of Niemann-Pick's disease. The **pathogenesis** has been discussed above. The condition is often distinctly familial but not hereditary, and is more frequent in females. The principal **lesions** consist in the deposit in the spleen of masses of large, multinuclear cells of endothelial character (*Gaucher cells*); these occurring also in the liver, bones, bone-marrow, lymphatic tissues, and suprarenals. The disease begins insidiously in infancy or early childhood, although it is probably congenital. About a third of the cases show symptoms before puberty. The chief **symptom** is a progressive enlargement of the spleen, which is hard, smooth, and finally reaches an enormous size. The liver after a time enlarges also, but there is usually no ascites. The general health is in no way affected at first, but later a mild anemia of the chlorotic type develops. Leukopenia is a characteristic symptom; the differential count is normal; the platelets may be diminished. There is in about half the cases a brownish discoloration of the skin, especially of the face and extremities; and, less frequently, a yellowish wedge-shaped thickening of the conjunctiva on each side of the cornea. The superficial lymphatic nodes may be slightly enlarged. There may be submucous or subcutaneous hemorrhages; but the gastric hemorrhage so characteristic of Banti's disease is absent. There may be pain in the bones and pathologic fractures, particularly in the femur, and the roentgenograms may show rarefaction of the bones. Abdominal pain may occur, due to perihepatitis. In infants all of these symptoms may be absent, especially the anemia, the hemorrhages, and the pigmentation of the skin. Mental deficiency may be associated, and there are sometimes nervous symptoms, as rigidity, strabismus, and opisthotonos. The disease may last for years, the average **duration** of life being twenty years or more. Death occurs from some intercurrent infection. The **diagnosis** from Banti's disease is discussed elsewhere (p. 1048). In Gaucher's disease the liver is not enlarged as much as the spleen, while in Niemann-Pick's disease the enlargement of the liver is especially marked. In the differential diagnosis from Niemann-Pick's disease splenic puncture, puncture of the bone-marrow, or biopsy of a lymph-node may show in Gaucher's disease the typical Gaucher cell, and in Niemann-Pick's disease the so-called "foam cell." In Niemann-Pick's disease there is also said to be a higher cholesterol and total fatty acid content of the blood. It is claimed by Bloom and Kern,[20] MacFate,[21] Epstein and Lorenz,[22] and others that chemical analysis of the tissues demonstrates that in Gaucher's disease and Niemann-Pick's disease different lipoids are at fault. In **treatment** splenectomy has been many times performed and apparently brings about improvement. Too much cannot be hoped for, since the seat of the disease is not in the spleen alone.

2. Niemann-Pick's Disease

(Lipoid Histiocytosis; Splenohepatomegaly)

This condition was first described by Niemann,[23] and Pick[24] distinguished it from Gaucher's disease. The literature on the subject is reviewed and cases reported by Corcan, Oberling and Dienst;[25] Abt and Bloom;[26] Baty;[27] Smetana;[28] Goldstein and Wexler;[29] Wascowitz;[30] Poncher;[31] Knox and Ramsey;[32] and others. Pathologic studies have been made by Bloom[33] and by Sobotka et al.[34] The disease is more frequent in girls than in boys in the ratio of about 4 to 6:1, and its incidence is almost entirely confined to the Jewish race. More than one child in a family may be attacked. It is probably congenital, or at least symptoms begin in the first few weeks of life. **Pathologically** the condition is characterized by large numbers of so-called "foam cells" which are found throughout the body, especially in the spleen, lymphatic tissue, bone-marrow, suprarenals, and thymus; and also in the kidney, heart-muscle, and other tissues. **Symptoms** consist in enormous enlargement of the liver and spleen, and there is a general adenopathy. Mental as well as physical retardation is found, and in several reported cases there has been a cherry-red spot in the macula lutea, as in amaurotic family idiocy (p. 908). A brownish discoloration of the skin develops, and there may be a mongoloid appearance. Irregular and intermittent fever is present, and a mild leukocytosis (15,000 to 20,000). The urine shows nothing abnormal. There is an increase in the cholesterol and total fatty acids of the blood. Death usually occurs before two years of age. In differential **diagnosis** Niemann-Pick's disease is distinguished from congenital hemolytic jaundice by the fact that in the latter there is fragility of the red cells, the urine contains urobilin, and jaundice is present; from Gaucher's disease by the fact that in this the increase in the size of the liver occurs late and there is a leukopenia (see also p. 1051); from pseudoleukemic anemia by the characteristic blood-picture of that disease.

3. Schüller-Christian's Disease

(Hand's Disease; Rowland's Disease)

The association of diabetes insipidus with exophthalmos and areas of softening in the cranium was first described by Hand[35] in 1893 and believed by him to be due to tuberculous infection. He[36] later described two other such instances, one of them previously published by Kay.[37] Schüller[38] reported similar cases, as did Christian.[39] We[40] reported an instance of the syndrome under the title "xanthoma tuberosum." In the meantime similar cases had been noted by Pusey and Johnstone[41] and by Dietrich.[42] Rowland's[15] report cites 14 and Sosman's[43] 45 collected cases. This condition, while similar to Gaucher's disease and Niemann-Pick's disease in **pathogenesis,** differs in that there is no racial or familial tendency. It attacks chiefly young children. **Symptomatically** there is involvement of the bones of the skull with rarefaction and thinning of areas of it, and occasionally involvement of other bones; frequently exophthalmos; often diabetes insipidus due to lipoid infiltration of the pituitary region (see also p. 503); perhaps jaundice, stomatitis, looseness of teeth, dwarfism, and infantilism. The spleen is usually slightly, if at all, enlarged, the liver moderately so. Occasionally there is considerable splenomegaly and also enlargement of the liver. The symptoms vary according to the location of the tumor-like xanthomatous deposits. Local trauma or infection may initiate the deposit of the lipoid material. Spontaneous remission may occur. The blood may show a hypercholesteremia. The leukocytes may be normal in number, or a mild leukocytosis may exist. The **diagnosis** of the condition from other forms of xanthomatosis is chiefly by the diabetes insipidus and the involvement of the cranial bones. Chloroma (p. 1017) can be differentiated by the leukemia-like blood-picture in this disorder. In **treatment** a low-fat diet may be tried, thyroid extract administered, and radiologic treatment of the involved areas given. If polyuria and polydipsia are extreme, pituitary extract may be given subcutaneously. (See treatment of diabetes insipidus, p. 503.)

References

1. Lo Sperimentale, 1894; Sez. Biol., **48,** 407. 2. Brit. J. Child. Dis., 1920, **17,** 34. 3. Pediatria, 1921, **29,** 833. 4. Arch. de méd. d. enf., 1923, **26,** 416. 5. J.A.M.A., 1925, **84,** 1887. 6. Acta paediat., suppl., 1927, **6,** 1. 7. Am. J. Dis. Child., 1927, **34,** 585. 8. Am. J. Dis. Child., 1929, **38,** 1231. 9. Monatschr. f. Kinderh., 1929, **45,** 294. 10. Zentralbl. f. Chir., 1930, **57,** 1342. 11. Presse méd., 1888, **5,** 121. 12. Verhandl. d. Cong. f. inn. Med., 1900, **18,** 316. 13. Ann. Surg., 1928, **88,** 361. 14. Am. J. Dis.

Child., 1926, **32**, 325. 15. Arch. Int. Med., 1928, **42**, 611. 16. Thèse de Paris, 1882, Ref., Krumbhaar, Am. J. M. Sc., 1915, **150**, 227. 17. Am. J. Dis. Child., 1929, **38**, 775. 18. Am. J. Dis. Child., 1932, **43**, 365. 19. Bull. Johns Hopkins Hosp., 1916, **27**, 1. 20. Arch. Int. Med., 1927, **39**, 456. 21. Arch. Path., 1928, **6**, 1054. 22. Ztschr. f. physiol. Chem., 1930, **192**, 145. 23. Jahrb. f. Kinderh., 1914, **79**, 1. 24. Ergebn. d. inn. Med. u. Kinderh., 1926, **29**, 519; Med. Klin., 1927, **23**, 1483. 25. Rev. franç. de pédiat., 1927, **3**, 789. 26. J.A.M.A., 1928, **90**, 2076. 27. Am. J. Dis. Child., 1930, **39**, 573. 28. Virchow's Arch. f. path. Anat., 1930, **274**, 697. 29. Arch. Ophth., 1931, **5**, 704. 30. Am. J. Dis. Child., 1931, **42**, 356. 31. Am. J. Dis. Child., 1931, **42**, 77. 32. Ann. Int. Med., 1932, **6**, 218. 33. Arch. Path., 1928, **6**, 827. 34. Arch. Path., 1930, **10**, 677. 35. Arch. Pediat., 1893, **10**, 673. 36. Am. J. M. Sc., 1921, **162**, 509. 37. Pennsylvania M. J., 1905–6, **9**, 520. 38. Fortschr. a. d. Geb. d. Roentgenstrahlen, 1915–16, **23**, 12; Brit. J. Radiol., 1926, **31**, 156; Wien. med. Wchnschr., 1921, **71**, 510. 39. Contrib. to Med. and Biol. Research, Sir W. Osler Volume, N. Y., 1919, **1**, 391. 40. Griffith, Arch. Pediat., 1922, **39**, 297. 41. J. Cutan. Dis. incl. Syph., 1908, **26**, 552. 42. Virchow's Arch. f. path. Anat., 1913, **212**, 119. 43. J.A.M.A., 1932, **98**, 110.

CHAPTER III

DISEASES OF THE LYMPH-NODES AND LYMPH-VESSELS

THERE exists in early life a predisposition to enlargement of the lymph-nodes. This may be secondary to some disease elsewhere, the glands affected being usually those into which the lymphatics from the diseased regions drain; but not infrequently it is dependent upon chronic ill-health, and the tendency is often seen also in children who appear in other respects to be entirely well. Certain children, especially some of those formerly classed as "scrofulous," but more properly as "lymphatic," exhibit a special proneness to lymphatic involvement, which may be both familial and inherited. The disorder denominated the Lymphatic Diathesis has been described elsewhere (p. 482), as have been briefly the normal relationships of the superficial glands (p. 43).

HODGKIN'S DISEASE

(Pseudoleukemia; Adenie; Lymphadenoma; Anaemia Lymphatica; Lymphoblastoma; Malignant Lymphoma)

Hodgkin's disease appears to be the least objectionable of the titles applied to this malady, first described by Hodgkin[1] in 1832.

Etiology and Pathology.—The affection is not common. It begins oftenest after childhood, although its occurrence up to ten years of age was reported by Longcope[2] in 15 per cent of 150 collected cases. Burnam[3] states that only 2.45 per cent of 173 cases observed in Baltimore were under ten years. Corbeille[4] found that in 33 cases under fifteen years of age one half had developed the first symptoms in the first five years. Priesel and Winkelbauer[5] reported a proved case in an infant dying at four and one-half months of age, whose mother had the disease. The cause and nature are unknown. Inflammation of the mouth or throat, trauma, or some infectious malady may precede the glandular swelling. Tuberculosis was brought into prominence as a possible cause especially by Sternberg,[6] but most authorities do not accept this view. Among other assigned causes, the proof of which is lacking, are infections of some sort, parasitic infestation, the possible influence of avian tubercle-bacilli (L'Esperance[7]), and that the disease is of the nature of a malignant growth. It would seem best to exclude from the category of Hodgkin's disease all cases in which the lymph-glands show evidence of syphilis or tuberculosis.

Pathologic Anatomy.—There is hyperplasia of the lymphoid tissues everywhere, more marked in some regions than in others; and in fact practically every part of the body may be involved, including the liver, spleen, lungs, the bones, and the nervous system. (See Symptoms.) The glands may reach in some places the size of an egg. Generally they remain discrete and do not invade surrounding tissue. The spleen is enlarged in about 75 per cent of the cases. Histologically the lymph-nodes show proliferation of reticulo-endothelial cells; eosinophilic cells; lymphoid cells; and the peculiar type of giant cells often designated the "Dorothy Reed[8] cell." Later there is connective tissue overgrowth.

Symptoms.—The onset is usually slow, the first symptom being enlargement of some group of nodes, much oftenest those on one or both sides of the neck. In Burnam's[3] cases primary involvement was in the nodes in the neck in 86.1 per cent, mediastinal nodes in 7.5, and abdominal in 6.1. The swelling is at first soft, later hard; not adherent to the skin or the tissues beneath, and not tender or painful (Fig. 255). The aggregation of numerous nodes in close juxtaposition may produce a mass the size of a fist or larger. The lymphoid tissue of the tongue and throat may also show hyperplasia. Generally months or years pass before any further extension occurs, and then a progressive enlargement of the nodes in other regions of the body will be noticed; the axillary ones usually being involved before the inguinal. The spleen and liver exhibit enlargement on palpation. Very rarely lymphomatous growths appear in the skin.

The general condition of health is at first little if at all affected; but later secondary symptoms appear. One of these is anemia, which is usually not severe. There is no constant change in the leukocytes. Oftenest there is a polymorphonuclear leukocytosis, especially later in the disease; sometimes a leukopenia; occasionally an eosinophilia. It has been claimed by Bunting[9] that the platelets are constantly increased in number, but others have not found this. Fever of an irregular type is present in most cases; sometimes continuous, sometimes with periods of intermission. Pressure-symptoms of the most varied kind are liable to develop, their nature depending upon the region of the body where overgrowth of tissue occurs. As stated, any part of the body may be involved and sometimes one region predominantly. It is possible for the primary involvement to be anywhere. There may be edema and pain in the arms from pressure upon the vessels and nerves in the axilla, or the lower limbs may be affected in a corresponding way by the enlarged inguinal glands; cough, dyspnea or dysphagia may be caused by hypertrophy of the mediastinal glands; jaundice by interference with the discharge of bile; disturbance of urination by pressure on the ureter; nervous symptoms from involvement of the brain or spinal cord. Among other symptoms sometimes present are albuminuria, pleural or pericardial effusion, rapid action of the heart, pigmentation of the skin, pruritus, boils, tenderness along the course of the bones, rarefaction of bone, nodules on the skin and mucous membranes. Herpes along the course of a nerve has been described (Pancoast and Pendergrass[10]). As the disease advances the masses of glands may reach an enormous size; the spleen may become greatly enlarged; there are progressive cachexia and emaciation; and death occurs from exhaustion, amyloid degeneration, pneumonia, or as a result of the pressure somewhere in the body.

Course and Prognosis.—The average duration of life, according to studies such as those of Burnam[3] and Corbeille,[4] is less than two years. In some instances the course is very rapid, and in others it may last several years, being greatly influenced by the treatment. It is doubtful whether any cases have really recovered. Intermissions are not uncommon, during which swelling of the lymph-nodes diminishes, fever ceases, and other symptoms improve.

Diagnosis.—From *tuberculosis* Hodgkin's disease is to be distinguished by the absence in the latter of matting together of the glands or of suppuration; and by the final wide diffusion of the process, tuberculous adenitis being more localized. Early in the course distinction from tuberculous cervical adenitis may be difficult. Diagnostically a tuberculin-reaction is helpful only if it is negative. Biopsy may be necessary to establish the differential diagnosis. *Lymphocytic leukemia* can be differentiated by the characteristic blood-changes. Skworzoff[11] reported cases of Hodgkin's disease combined with acute myeloid leukemia. *Lymphosarcoma* is distinguished by the penetration of the process into tissues outside the gland, this rarely occurring in Hodgkin's disease; and by the absence of splenomegaly. Both lymphosarcoma and Hodgkin's disease may exist in the same patient (Levin[12]). The lymph-node enlargement in the *lymphatic diathesis*

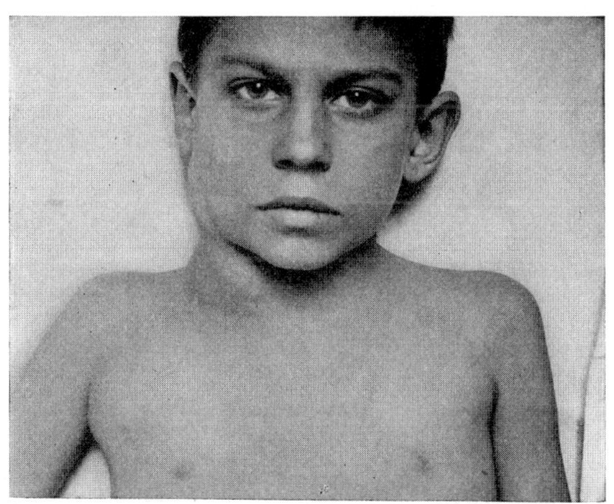

Fig. 255.—Hodgkin's disease. Shows glandular enlargement right side of neck and axilla. Anthony P. Aged nine and one-half years. Children's Medical Ward of the Hospital of the University of Pennsylvania. Swelling of right side of neck began two years previously, and two months ago rapid increase occurred. *Examination in Hospital.*—Hard mass of glands on the right side of the neck and at the anterior portion of the right axilla. Scattered glands in left side of neck, left axilla, above clavicles and in groins. Spleen greatly enlarged. Red blood-cells 3,200,000. Leukocytes 4700. Hemoglobin 40 per cent. Roentgenogram showed a tumor-mass in the mediastinum. Diagnosis confirmed by biopsy. Great improvement under roentgenological treatment.

or in the course of some other disorders is of moderate degree and not progressive in its extension.

Treatment.—In addition to the general tonic and hygienic treatment and the measures indicated for anemia, the therapy consists in the use of the roentgen-ray or of radium. This should be started early, before extensive fibrosis of the involved tissues develops. Great improvement can be secured, which, however, is only temporary. Removal of affected glands is liable to be followed by a return of the disease in greater force. Benefit has been claimed from the injection of a vaccine prepared from the micro-organisms obtained from the affected glands (Billings and Rosenow,[13] Hatcher and Lemmon[14]). Coley[15] advises, in addition to radiologic treatment, injections of the toxins of the bacillus of erysipelas and bacillus prodigiosus. Lortat-Jacob and Schmite[16] claimed that there was benefit following the injection with serum from another patient with Hodgkin's disease who had received radiotherapy.

ACUTE SIMPLE ADENITIS

All children have a marked susceptibility to lymph-node enlargement, and a special tendency to this sometimes appears to be hereditary and familial. (See also Lymphatic Diathesis p. 482.) Acute adenitis is encountered most often in the first two years of life, although common throughout childhood. In later childhood many cases are observed due to the acute infectious diseases. Debilitated health is a powerful predisposing cause. Local irritation or infection leads to inflammation of the nodes into which the lymphatics of the region drain. For example, affection of the mouth or throat produces enlargement of the nodes below the jaw; that of the scalp and ear involvement of the occipital, posterior auricular, or superficial cervical nodes; that of the lower extremities or genitalia enlargement of the femoral nodes or those in the groin. Disorders of the intestine are followed by an involvement of the mesenteric group, and respiratory infections may produce enlargement of the tracheobronchial nodes. Any of the pyogenic bacteria may be the active agent, oftenest the staphylococcus or the streptococcus. The **prognosis** for final recovery is favorable, but uncertain as regards the development of suppuration. Adenitis seen in the infectious diseases seldom goes on to suppuration except in scarlet fever. Of the cases due to other causes the majority occurring in infancy suppurate. Often a swollen gland will remain in a quiescent state for a week or more and then rapidly proceed to suppuration. It seems probable that nonsuppurative tracheobronchial adenitis may produce fever of low grade lasting for some weeks. The **duration** of adenitis in cases which do not suppurate is from a few weeks to two or three months before complete recovery. Suppurative cases generally show signs of this in the second or third week. The recovery after the abscess has been incised is generally rapid.

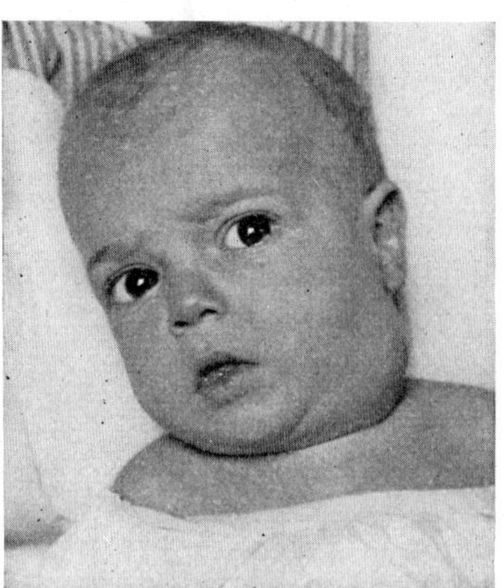

Fig. 256.—Simple cervical adenitis. Infant of five months in the Children's Hospital of Philadelphia, with suppurative adenitis. Incision later.

One of the most common errors in **diagnosis** is that of mistaking cervical adenitis for mumps. In this disease, however, the center of swelling is over the parotid gland, whereas in adenitis it is below or at the angle of the jaw. It has repeatedly happened that mesenteric adenitis produces symptoms suggesting appendicitis. The distinction between simple and tuberculous adenitis is discussed elsewhere (p. 1063). In **treatment** either hot or cold applications may aid in aborting an attack, the result varying with the case. Poultices may be employed, and although they may in some cases increase the liability to suppuration, in others they rapidly favor dissipation of the swelling. Ointments of iodine and of guaiacol may possess some value, as may gentle massage with a stimulating liniment. Suppuration demands incision as soon as an area of softening has developed. Radiologic treatment especially of the cervical adenitis, has been quite widely used. It usually causes rapid resolution, or it may result in acceleration of suppuration. It has been advocated that tonsils, if present, be removed during the attack of acute adenitis. This seems to us to be a dangerous procedure and we have, in fact, seen septicemia follow it.

ACUTE EPIDEMIC INFECTIOUS ADENITIS

(Glandular Fever; Acute Infectious Mononucleosis; Acute Benign Lymphoblastosis)

"Glandular fever" was first described under that title by E. Pfeiffer.[17] There appears to be a form of acute epidemic adenitis which is not necessarily a specific disorder, but a symptom especially of such diseases as grippe or other maladies which in themselves are epidemic, and which have as part of their course inflammation of the nasopharynx. The lymph-nodes most often and predominantly attacked are the cervical ones, but sometimes there is an accompanying involvement of the nodes in various parts of the body.

The condition termed "acute infectious mononucleosis," in which there is a characteristic blood-change first described by Türk,[18] might with reason be regarded as an entity. This may be encountered both in infancy and childhood. Sporadic cases occur, but epidemic influence is often present. We have seen an epidemic in an infant's home where of 25 inmates 15 were affected. The incubation period ranges from about five to fourteen days (Baldridge et al.,[19] Davis[20]).

The **symptoms** of acute epidemic adenitis consist in sudden onset, with fever, pain in the neck and perhaps in the abdomen, pain in the bones, and sometimes vomiting. Mild inflammation of the nose and throat may be present. Within a few hours or a day or two after the onset the cervical nodes enlarge, often with involvement of the axillary and inguinal group, sometimes with the mesenteric, and occasionally with enlargement of the liver and spleen. The nodes are tender, but seldom reach any great size, and only rarely suppurate. Substernal pain may occur, presumably due to involvement of the bronchial nodes. A leukocytosis of about 15,000 to 20,000 is present, but usually not until after the first week. There is a relative lymphocytosis which may commence before the leukocytosis, and which may persist for several months after the acute symptoms subside. This blood-picture led to the employment of the term "mononucleosis" by Sprunt and Evans.[21] That these cells belong to the lymphocytic series rather than the myelocytic is indicated by studies with the peroxidase stain. The lymph-node swelling lasts two or three weeks or longer, although the constitutional symptoms may disappear earlier. Frequently there may be return of fever and general symptoms on one or two occasions before final convalescence is established. Exceptionally a nephritis of the acute hemorrhagic type occurs as a complication. Mononucleosis could be confounded with an acute lymphocytic leukemia, although the severe hemorrhagic manifestations of this disorder and marked anemia are not present. Furthermore, complete recovery invariably takes place. Treatment is symptomatic.

CHRONIC SIMPLE ADENITIS

This common disorder may remain after one or more attacks of acute adenitis; or may be chronic from the beginning, attending some persistent source of irritation, as pediculi, chronic otitis media, etc., and especially the presence of adenoid or tonsillar hypertrophy. Impaired health is a frequent cause, chronic lymphadenitis being common under circumstances in which children receive poor food or insufficient air. Tracheobronchial adenitis may attend chronic bronchitis or remain after an acute respiratory infection. Chronic lymphatic enlargement is one of the symptoms of the lymphatic diathesis (p. 482). Syphilis is a not infrequent cause of localized moderate enlargement of the lymph-nodes, and exceptionally of extensive multiple adenitis in later childhood. The exciting cause of adenitis is a chronic toxic or mechanical influence, or a bacterial involvement; the latter being of low virulence and insufficient to cause suppuration. Practically the only **symptom** is the enlargement of the nodes. A single node or oftener a whole group may be involved, or sometimes nodes in various parts of the body. The adenitis is oftenest situated in the neck. The condition may last several months and then disappear, or may be very persistent. Chronic tracheobronchial adenitis, not tuberculous, is probably of frequent occurrence. Its local symptoms and physical signs do not differ from those produced by tuberculosis, except that pressure-symptoms are less frequent. The roentgenological distinction lies in the fact that the presence of calcification signifies that the process is tuberculous. (See also p. 1063.) In **diagnosis** distinction can be made from lymphocytic leukemia by examination of the blood. Hodgkin's disease results in greater enlargement of the nodes, especially in certain local groups. In **treatment** the first object is removal of the source of irritation. In addition measures must be employed to improve the general health. Cod liver oil may be of service, and sometimes arsenic or iodide of iron. A change of climate may be most beneficial. Local measures may perhaps be of aid, as in acute adenitis (p. 1056).

TUBERCULOUS ADENITIS

Etiology.—This common disorder attacks children oftener than adults. In infancy the internal lymph-nodes, such as the tracheobronchial and the mesenteric, are those usually affected, while in childhood and later the external glands, especially the cervical groups, are those oftenest involved. Children born of tuberculous parents have a tendency to develop tuberculous adenitis, and the same is true of subjects of the exudative diathesis or of lymphatism. Tuberculous adenitis is also liable to occur as a sequel to attacks of the infectious disorders, especially pertussis and measles. Diseases of the bronchial mucous membrane or of the intestine are readily followed by tuberculosis of the tracheobronchial or the mesenteric glands respectively. A gland attacked by a simple inflammation may become tuberculous later.

Pathologic Anatomy.—The tuberculous gland on section reveals scattered, minute, grayish spots, the foci of tuberculous infiltration; and still later by fusion of these foci the whole section becomes grayish, and finally the gland caseates. Meantime the surrounding tissue grows inflamed and adherent, and a number of nodes of the group are matted together. Aided by the softening process an abscess may be produced; or the gland may remain caseous and be encapsulated by fibrous tissue; or may be replaced chiefly by connective tissue. Tubercle bacilli are found in the early stages, but in a thoroughly caseous node they may be difficult to discover. The so-called pus of a suppurating gland is sterile in uncomplicated cases. The breaking down of tubercles and of the tissue of the nodes is, however, often associated with pyogenic infection. Suppurating nodes may rupture externally; or into a lymph-vessel or blood-vessel and produce tuberculous meningitis, tuberculous bronchopneumonia, or general miliary infection. In other cases fibrous overgrowth is more prominent from the beginning, and there is less matting of the nodes, and little adherence to contiguous structures.

Symptoms. **1. Generalized Tuberculous Adenitis.**—Tuberculosis developing in nearly all the lymph-nodes of the body is of uncommon occurrence. It may appear without warning in children previously in good health, or oftener may be seen in those already debilitated; or it may come on suddenly as a sequel to some localized tuberculous process. The onset is sudden, with malaise, loss of appetite, fever and emaciation. The glands rapidly hypertrophy, either simultaneously or oftener successively, and may reach a large size, filling the sides of the neck, the axillae and the groins. At necropsy widespread involvement of the internal lymphatic glands also is discovered, and sometimes the enlargement is found to be chiefly here.

2. Localized Tuberculosis of the External Lymph-nodes.—This occurs most frequently in the cervical nodes, those of them attacked being determined by the lymphatics through which the bacilli chance to enter. The infection is generally derived from the nasopharynx. That it can be an ascending infection from tuberculous tracheobronchial glands is doubtful. Involvement of the cervical nodes is one of the forms of tuberculosis frequently dependent upon the bovine type of bacillus. (See p. 409.) Oftenest affected are the deep cervical and the submaxillary groups and those below the parotid glands. The first *symptom* noted is the presence of small, hard nodules (kernels) in the neck, appearing at the angle of the jaw, or along the anterior or posterior border of the sternocleidomastoid muscle. The swelling has come on gradually and without any constitutional disturbance. Usually the enlargement is present on both sides, although more on one than the other (Fig. 257). The glands are not tender and appear at first to be distinct from one another. Increase in size goes on slowly, and the nodes finally are no longer distinctly separated from each other, and some tenderness may develop. The skin is freely movable over them. The degree of enlargement varies from time to time, any condition which lessens the general health being liable to increase the swelling. If the process advances to softening and discharge, the skin over the swelling becomes adherent, the surrounding tissue is swollen and indurated, and the abscess finally discharges on the surface of the neck and leaves a sinus, which heals only after all the glandular tissue has broken down and been evacuated, and results in much disfigurement. In this way one gland after another may break down and discharge, either through the old opening or oftener through new ones, and the process may be long continued. During the period of active inflammation the patient has fever and the general health suffers.

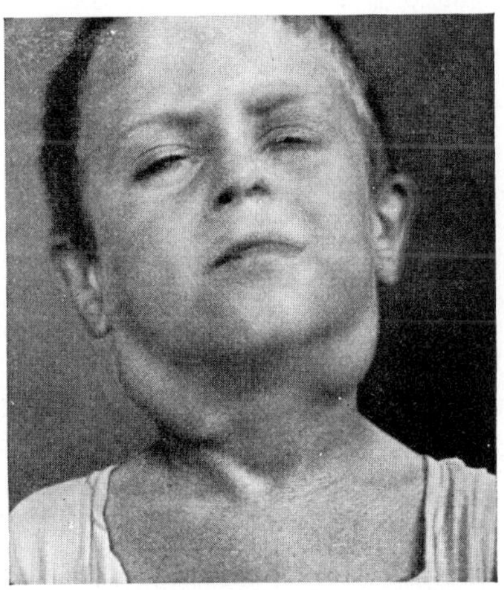

Fig. 257.—Tuberculous adenitis. (*Courtesy of Dr. H. R. Wharton.*)

Not all tuberculous glands undergo this course, and resolution can take place; or the glands may remain indurated and adherent to each other without suppurating. Tuberculous infiltration may extend from the cervical glands to those just above the clavicle, the posterior part of the neck, or the axilla; or this last-mentioned region or the groin may exceptionally be the first or the only part affected.

In addition to the presence of the enlarged glands, and not caused by this, there may be a group of symptoms to which the title *scrofula* has often been applied. These children are anemic, flabby, and stupid in appearance. There is a tendency to blepharitis, and to ulcerative or phlyctenular keratitis. Constant thick discharge from the nose is frequent, producing swelling and redness and often eczema of the upper lip; and chronic purulent otitis media is often present (Fig. 258). The teeth are frequently carious, and obstinate cutaneous lesions may occur. Whether all the lesions referred to depend upon the actual presence in them of tubercle bacilli, or whether the mere existence of such bacilli elsewhere in the body, oftenest in the tracheobronchial glands, brings about in some way, presumably through a toxin, an unhealthy state of the tissues in general; or whether again some of these symptoms belong rather to the exudative-lymphatic diathesis in combination with a complicating tuberculosis, has been a matter much discussed. It seems better to do away with the term scrofula entirely and to regard the complex of symptoms as one of tuberculosis occurring in a subject with the exudative-lymphatic diathesis (pp. 481, 482).

3. Tuberculosis of the Tracheobronchial Nodes.—The glands which may be affected consist of the groups about the trachea or the large bronchial tubes, and the chains extending along the smaller bronchi into the lungs (Fig. 87, p. 418). Generally all the groups are involved, but not all to the same extent. Tuberculosis of these glands is one of the most common forms of the infection found at necropsy upon infants and children. It

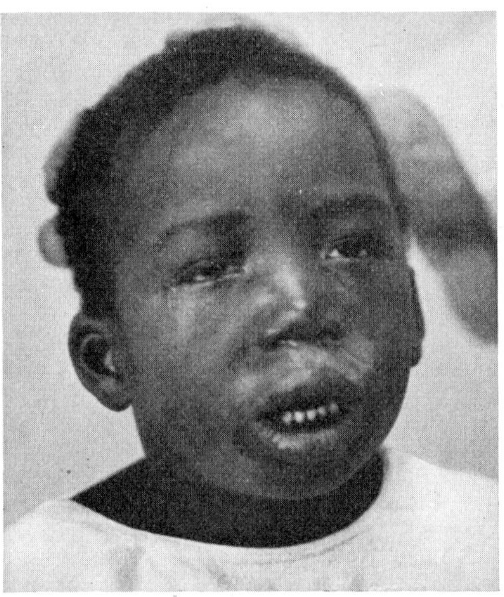

Fig. 258.—Patient in Cincinnati General Hospital, four years of age. Known to have a pulmonary tuberculous lesion since about three months of age which at the time of this picture was not active. Has phlyctenular conjunctivitis and keratitis and an irritating discharge from the nose. Tuberculin-test strongly positive, Wassermann negative.

may exist apparently alone, although probably secondary to an undiscovered pulmonary lesion, but is often associated with definite clinical pulmonary tuberculosis of some sort; or it may be followed finally by tuberculous meningitis or miliary tuberculosis. A few or, frequently, many of the glands of the chain show enlargement, often chiefly on the right side, and generally of moderate degree. Sometimes, however, a large mass is produced by the matting together of a number of glands. Suppuration does not often occur except in infancy, and encapsulation with caseation or calcification is the usual outcome, the glands lying dormant, although always a source of danger as the focus for widespread infection of the lungs or other parts of the body.

Clinically, however, tuberculosis of the bronchial lymph-nodes is not a common disease. General *symptoms* are absent or are very indefinite. They consist in the gradual development of deterioration of health, shown by loss of appetite and of flesh, pallor, and low irregular fever. Sometimes the onset is more sudden and the fever higher, particularly if suppuration is occurring. None of these symptoms can be called characteristic, since they could be produced by tuberculosis elsewhere in the body. Local evidences are uncommon, and present only if the glands attain large size and cause local interference, or if an abscess has formed. Such symptoms develop usually only in early and later childhood, infants with the disease dying of other tuberculous manifestations before the glandular ones appear.

A caseous suppurating gland may rupture into a large bronchus or into the trachea and produce asphyxia, or may break into the mediastinum and penetrate in different directions or open externally, or may perforate one of the large blood-vessels. The trachea, bronchi, esophagus, vena cava, or pneumogastric or recurrent laryngeal nerve may be compressed by enlarged glands. Interference with the nerve produces an irritating, hacking, paroxysmal cough suggesting pertussis. It may be absent for considerable periods and then return, depending upon a changing degree of glandular enlargement. It accounts, too, for the production of dyspnea. Pressure on the trachea may produce a noisy cough and prolonged dyspneic, noisy respiration. This comes on in paroxysms with cyanosis, strongly suggesting asthma or spasmodic croup. Between the paroxysms the stridor is diminished in intensity or even disappears. Pressure upon the large veins may give rise to a murmur audible over the upper part of the sternum when the head is thrown back. This, the *Eustace Smith sign*, is often absent; and may occur in other conditions. If the compression is great, there may be cyanosis and edema of the face and dilatation of the superficial veins. Among other physical signs, which have been described as occurring if the mass is of large size, is dulness on percussion posteriorly beside the spinal column over the roots of the lungs between the third and the sixth dorsal vertebrae. This sign is, however, often absent, and according to Armand-Delille and Lestocquey,[22] who checked their physical findings by necropsies, such dulness never occurs. In front there may be dulness over the upper part of the sternum, but it is difficult to distinguish this from that caused by an enlarged thymus or disease of the lung itself. If one main bronchus is compressed, the lung on this side may give a percussion-note of diminished resonance. Percussion-dulness over the apices of the lungs, or in the spinous fossae, supposed to be dependent upon pulmonary involvement, may be the result of the pressure of enlarged tuberculous bronchial glands. Auscultation is sometimes of value. If a main bronchus is compressed there may be feeble respiration in the clavicular region. Posteriorly there may be tracheal or bronchial respiration along the spine below the level of the third dorsal vertebra. *D'Espine's*[23] sign, in which spoken or whispered pectoriloquy, or rather a whispered echo after the spoken voice, is heard below the level of the seventh cervical or first dorsal vertebra is of doubtful significance and of little value in our opinion, and this is the view of practically all those who have studied the sign in its relation to roentgenograms and necropsies. It must be admitted that in spite of the numerous physical signs which may occur, in the majority of cases no certain conclusions can be reached, except by the employment of roentgenograms. Even these must be carefully correlated with other signs and symptoms, since they may not prove that the shadow about the hilus is caused by tuberculous adenitis rather than by simple enlargement of the nodes; or, indeed, that it is due to glandular enlargement of any kind.

4. Tuberculosis of the Mesenteric Nodes.—"Tabes mesenterica," as this condition is sometimes called, is discovered at necropsy in from about 15 to 40 per cent of tuberculous children according to different studies (Freeman[24]). Apparently the mesenteric adenitis is always secondary to a tuberculous lesion of the intestine at the portal of entry. (See p. 410.) It may be secondary also to active tuberculous disease of the intestine. The enlarged glands may be numerous, discrete, and rather small; or much larger, fused, and forming masses of considerable size. The retroperitoneal nodes may be involved as well. Resolution or, oftener, caseation takes place; suppuration or calcification is not frequent. Some degree of localized peritonitis is liable to be present in well-marked cases.

Clinically the disease is uncommon. The general *symptoms* are often masked by those accompanying intestinal ulceration. There is impairment of the general health, with wasting, anemia, loss of appetite and strength, irregular fever, and slight abdominal pain. Tympanitic distention of the abdomen, and the occurrence of diarrhea or constipation belong rather to symptoms of intestinal tuberculosis than to those of mesenteric involvement; or the distention may indicate tuberculous peritonitis. Fatty stools may occur as the result of interference with the absorption of fat (Talbot[25]).

The most characteristic of the local symptoms is the discovery by palpation of the enlargement of the nodes. As a rule, they cannot be felt, on account either of the moderate degree of hypertrophy or of the abdominal distention. In some cases enlarged glands can be distinctly felt in the deeper parts of the abdomen near the spinal column; or, in great hypertrophy, close to the abdominal walls. Rectal examination may aid in revealing the tumors. Calcification in the nodes may sometimes be shown by roentgenograms (Dunham and Smythe[26]). Very exceptionally other local symptoms of different sorts may result from pressure of the growths upon internal organs, such as the portal vein, the vena cava, or the thoracic duct; or there may be intestinal obstruction, or ulceration into arteries. An error in diagnosis which has repeatedly occurred is the mistaking for an appendicitis an acute tuberculous inflammation of the glands near the cecum.

Course and Prognosis of Tuberculous Adenitis.—In *generalized tuberculous adenitis* recovery takes place only exceptionally. Death is due to increasing cachexia or some complicating tuberculous condition. This occurs often after an illness of only a few weeks or months, although sometimes a somewhat more chronic form of the disease develops.

The course of *cervical adenitis* is usually much prolonged and the duration uncertain, one node after another breaking down, often with the lapse of months between these occurrences. There is also the possibility of different groups of nodes becoming involved, the infection spreading from the carotid group to those about the clavicle and even downward to the intrathoracic group. The more favorable cases terminate in resolution after several months. Suppuration will take place in over half the cases unless treatment is well carried out. The affected nodes may be quiescent for several years and then produce pus more or less rapidly. Neglected suppurating cases will retain a discharging sinus for long periods, or leave ulcers which are most resistant to treatment, and finally heal with irregular and disfiguring scars. The prognosis for life is favorable, with unusual exceptions dependent upon extension to nodes elsewhere. The prognosis of tuberculosis of the *axillary* and *supraclavicular* glands is not quite so favorable, as there is greater danger of the involvement of the pleura or lung.

In *tuberculosis of the tracheobronchial lymph-nodes*, the duration cannot be estimated, because the time of onset of the enlargement can seldom be determined. The course is subacute or chronic. It is certain that the inflammation may be long-continued, and that recovery may take place. As a matter of fact this is a frequent mode of acquiring immunity to later infection by the tubercle bacillus (p. 419). There is always, however, danger of the extension of the tuberculous process to other regions by way of the blood-vessels, and this is particularly true under the age of six years, at which time softening of the glands is liable to occur. An abscess may rupture into the pericardium or pleura, or pus may escape into the trachea and cause sudden, fatal asphyxia.

The course of *tuberculosis of the mesenteric nodes* is very similar to that of the disease situated in the bronchial group. It may continue for years without symptoms; and even with symptoms present the condition may last for months, with death finally from exhaustion. Yet occasionally symptoms disappear even with palpable tumors remaining. Calcification of tuberculous nodes seen on the roentgenogram, while demonstrating attempt at healing, does not guarantee quiescence of the lesions.

Diagnosis.—*General glandular tuberculosis* is to be distinguished from leukemia, lymphosarcoma, and Hodgkin's disease. The first is readily recognized by examination of the blood; the second by enlargement of one group of nodes only, at least at the onset; the third by the absence of inflammation and of fusion of the nodes, and the slower onset and longer course. The diagnosis of *cervical tuberculous adenitis* from simple acute adenitis is generally not difficult. The former in general runs a slower course; the nodes on both sides of the neck are enlarged; the whole group is more or less involved; there is more matting together of the nodes; softening is slower, and the pus formed is of more cheesy character. The absence of a tuberculin-reaction speaks strongly for simple adenitis. Simple chronic adenitis occasions more diagnostic difficulty; yet here, too, there is no fusion of the nodes or adherence to the overlying skin; softening does not occur; duration is shorter; a discoverable irritating cause is often present; and the tuberculin-test is negative, unless there is tuberculosis elsewhere in the body. In Hodgkin's disease the course is very slow; caseation or suppuration does not occur; groups of nodes elsewhere than in the neck are involved at the same time or in succession; and the constitutional symptoms are eventually more severe. In all the conditions so far mentioned, biopsy may be necessary to establish the differential diagnosis. If calcification of cervical nodes can be demonstrated on the roentgenogram, the diagnosis of tuberculosis may be made.

The diagnosis of *tracheobronchial tuberculous adenitis* is one made usually by exclusion. The combination of mild, irregular fever which extends over a long time, with wasting, anemia, malaise, and the like, is strongly suggestive in the absence of other discoverable cause. There may also be the symptoms of pressure previously described, and the physical signs which, as stated, are difficult to elicit. Roentgenograms of the chest should always be taken when there is suspicion of tuberculous adenitis; calcification indicating that the process is a tuberculous one. It should be mentioned here that certain pear-shaped or circular shadows often diagnosed as calcified lymph-nodes are in reality densities cast by blood vessels (McPhedran[27]). The differentiation of tracheobronchial adenitis from thymic enlargement is sometimes difficult in the roentgenogram. The former, however, occurs at a later age. The diagnosis of *tuberculosis of the mesenteric nodes* is difficult in the absence of local manifestations. Here again there may be wasting and irregular fever, and often, too, a complicating disturbance of intestinal function. When calcified the mesenteric nodes may be demonstrated on the roentgenogram. Abdominal masses due to enlarged mesenteric nodes must be differentiated from fecal masses, cysts, tuberculous peritonitis, new growths, and occasionally from a subacute intussusception. Fecal masses can be removed by proper treatment. Tuberculous peritonitis gives generally more numerous masses nearer to the abdominal wall; but involvement of the peritoneum is likely to be a complication of disease of the mesenteric nodes. Abdominal neoplasms must be differentiated by their position and their history.

Treatment.—All the measures recommended for the treatment of tuberculosis in general should be employed in lymph-node tuberculosis (p. 424), and the use of ultraviolet irradiation is especially applicable.

Infectious and other acute diseases should be avoided as far as possible, since under their influence the tuberculous process is liable to grow worse. Special symptoms as fever, cough, and the like demand symptomatic treatment. In the case of the cervical nodes it is important to remove all such sources of local irritation as carious teeth, chronic otitis, and the like, including perhaps removal of adenoids and tonsils. Operation on the nodes can usually be avoided by proper general treatment. If softening occurs and spontaneous rupture of the node is likely it is better to open and drain, removing as much of the diseased tissue as possible. It is well to operate, if possible, before the glands become adherent to the surrounding tissues. The operative scar will be less disfiguring than that resulting from a continuing sinus. The value of tuberculin in the treatment of tuberculous glands is much questioned. Radiologic treatment of tuberculous nodes is of decided value and aids in their resolution. It may be combined with aspiration of any glands which have reached the stage of liquefaction.

DISEASES OF THE LYMPHATIC VESSELS

A diffuse **lymphangiectasis** is rarely seen. It may be either congenital or acquired. An interesting case of the former with necropsy study is reported by Rich and Dembo.[28] In tropical climates lymphangiectasis may result in an **elephantiasis** depending upon the presence of filaria. In other regions elephantiasis may be produced by inflammation of the lymphatic vessels. It is occasionally seen in children. At this age, too, the congenital variety may give rise to local overgrowth and cause gigantism of the part. Some cases of hemihypertrophy are of this nature (p. 1091). Affections of the **thoracic duct** are very rare, the most frequent being the production of chylous ascites or chylous pleural effusion, depending upon some damage to the duct by tumors or in other ways. (See pp. 681, 761.)

MORBID GROWTHS OF THE LYMPHATIC GLANDS AND VESSELS

Those of any form are rare in early life. Primary **lymphosarcoma** is occasionally seen in the cervical or in the tracheobronchial nodes. It grows rapidly and soon invades the surrounding tissues, this distinguishing it from Hodgkin's disease. Unless relieved by operation the patient dies in a few weeks or months. Cavernous **lymphangioma** of the tongue has been reported as a congenital occurrence producing macroglossia. It is an angiomatous dilatation of the lymphatic vessels. A similar condition is occasionally observed in the lips, mouth, neck, axilla, or behind the knee. A **cystic lymphoma** also occurs, oftenest in the neck. (See Hygroma, p. 546.) **Adenocarcinomatosis** in a young child has been reported (Lyon, Klumpp and Ferguson[29]).

References

1. Med.-Chir. Trans., 1932, **17**, 68. 2. Osler and McCrae, Mod. Med., 1928, **5**, 227. 3. J.A.M.A., 1927, **87**, 1445. 4. Minnesota Med., 1928, **11**, 678. 5. Virchow's Arch. f. path. Anat., 1926, **262**, 749. 6. Ztschr. f. Heilk., 1898, **19**, 21. 7. J. Immunol., 1930, **18**, 127. 8. Johns Hopkins Hosp. Rep., 1902, **10**, 133. 9. Johns Hopkins Hosp. Bull., 1911, **22**, 114; 369. 10. Am. J. M. Sc., 1924, **168**, 326. 11. Frankfurt. Ztschr. f. Path., 1930, **40**, 81. 12. J.A.M.A., 1931, **96**, 421. 13. J.A.M.A., 1913, **61**, 2122. 14. J.A.M.A., 1915, **65**, 1359. 15. Ann. Surg., 1928, **88**, 641. 16. Paris méd., 1927, **65–66**, 2, 452. 17. Jahrb. f. Kinderh., 1889, **29**, 257. 18. Wien. klin. Wchnschr., 1907, **22**, 15. 19. Arch. Int. Med., 1928, **38**, 413. 20. J.A.M.A., 1929, **92**, 1417. 21. Bull. Johns Hopkins Hosp., 1920, **31**, 410. 22. Am. J. Dis. Child., 1929, **38**, 1125. 23. Bull. de l'acad. de méd., 1907, 3s, **57**, 167; Brit. M. J., 1910, **2**, 1136. 24. Med. News, 1906, **86**, 969. 25. Am. J. Dis. Child., 1912, **4**, 49. 26. Am. J. Dis. Child., 1926, **31**, 815. 27. Am. J. M. Sc., 1927, **173**, 245. 28. Am. J. Dis. Child., 1927, **33**, 249. 29. Am. J. Dis. Child., 1929, **37**, 134.

SECTION XI

DISEASES OF THE DUCTLESS GLANDS AND THE INTERNAL SECRETIONS

Knowledge of the functions of the internal glands is gained in several ways:—By observation of patients and animals who have disease of them; by the effects of implantation of these glands or the injection of extracts of them; by the results of total or partial removal of the glands; by the recovery from the glands, or from the blood or lymph draining them, of physiologically active substances. The spleen, although a ductless gland, has been more conveniently considered elsewhere. It must be admitted that present knowledge is quite incomplete, although much has been assumed. There are certain definite syndromes which can be associated with disease of some of these organs. The custom, however, of attributing to the endocrine system various symptoms for which other explanation is lacking, is greatly to be deprecated. In many cases there is an interrelationship of the different glands, and the action of one is opposed to or increased by that of another. It must also be emphasized that knowledge of the action of certain internal secretions does not necessarily lead to the ability to apply that knowledge therapeutically. The statements which follow are to be accepted as provisional and subject to modification.

CHAPTER I

DISEASES OF THE THYROID GLAND

Congestion of the thyroid gland, with temporary enlargement, may occur in girls during the establishment of menstruation, and continue for some months. It may also be seen with affections of the heart and in febrile infectious disorders; this type of congestion sometimes being associated with hypersecretion of the gland. Temporary congestion may result from over-exertion, constriction of the neck, or long crying. A tense swelling may sometimes develop on forced expiration, or with crying (Orgel[1]). School-epidemics of congestion have been observed. There are no symptoms characteristic of congestion and no particular treatment is required.

Thyroiditis is uncommon, particularly in infancy. It may be primary as a result of trauma or of some undiscoverable cause; or oftener secondary, occurring in the course of some acute febrile disease or infectious fever, sepsis, or rheumatism. Inflammation usually involves one lobe only, or one more than the other. There are local symptoms of swelling, tenderness, and pain on swallowing; and constitutional ones with fever. Generally resolution occurs after a few days, or suppuration may take place. In the latter instance, it is possible that there may be sufficient destruction of tissue to cause subsequent hypothyroidism. Treatment consists in that usual for inflammation, and incision if suppuration takes places.

GOITER

Etiology.—This disease was known to the ancients, and as early as the twelfth century was treated by giving iodine-containing substances, as seaweed and burnt sponge (McClendon[2]). It consists of a chronic enlargement of the thyroid gland, either congenital or acquired, endemic or sporadic. Congenital goiter is not uncommon. According to Skinner[3] it was first described by Fodéré in 1796, and cases have been reported and collected by Demme,[4] Porter and Vonderlehr,[5] Skinner[3] and others. Slight enlargement of the gland is, in fact, common in new-born infants in regions where goiter prevails; this often disappearing after a few months. At times, however, it may be so large that severe pressure-symptoms may develop. Goiter is endemic in certain widely scattered regions of the world, and in the United States is found with greater frequency in the Pacific Northwest and in the Great Lakes basin. Less important foci occur in other regions. There have been many studies which show that some enlargement, usually slight, may be observed, in the regions in the United States where goiter prevails, in from 30 to 80 per cent of school-children examined; and even along the sea coast, where the disease occurs only sporadically, the enlargement may be detected in 20 per cent of the children. The frequency increases as puberty approaches. Females are attacked two or three times more often than males. It is not a truly hereditary disease, for, although affected mothers not infrequently give birth to goitrous infants, this can be prevented by the administration of iodine to the mother during pregnancy. In older children the development of the disease can be avoided by systematic prophylactic treatment with iodine. Acute diseases, especially the communicable ones, may be followed by enlargement of the thyroid gland, but this is only temporary (Oleson[6]). A number of studies, as those of Marine and his coworkers,[7] and McClendon,[2,8] appear to have demonstrated that goiter is an expression of iodine-starvation which leads to a compensatory hypertrophy. Such factors as puberty, infections, intoxications, defective utilization of iodine, or low intake of iodine may, therefore, result in goiter. Analyses of the soil and water in regions where goiter is endemic usually reveal a low iodine-content. To the hypothesis that lack of iodine is the sole cause there are dissenting opinions. McCarrison,[9] for example, believes that an infectious agent may be responsible; and more recently Hellwig[10] again brings up the question and suggests that, in addition to a deficiency of iodine, there is also a positive etiologic factor of some sort which has an influence. **Pathologically** the changes found are follicular, cystic, colloid, or fibroid; the last two being uncommon in early life. Generally the involvement of the gland is only partial, and occurs oftenest on the right side or in the isthmus.

Symptoms.—With the usual slight swelling of the thyroid gland found in children in goitrous districts there are no symptoms, although cretinism or mild degrees of hypothyroidism may be associated. In 100 cases of simple goiter studied by Topper and Mulier[11] the basal metabolic rate was normal in 74 cases; increased to 10 per cent above normal in 17; and decreased to 10 per cent below normal in 9. Oleson and Fernald[12] observed no effect of goiter on intelligence, except, perhaps, some slight impairment of it in those with marked enlargement. There may be some physical retardation, Oleson and Taylor[13] finding in a study on a relatively small number of patients that children with enlarged thyroids, while of greater weight than those with normal glands, were inferior in other physical measurements. Simple goiter may sometimes become so large that there are symptoms of a mechanical nature produced, as interference with respiration and compression of the veins. Rarely there may be such complications as atelectasis, pulmonary edema, bronchopneumonia, cardiac dilatation, and softening of the tracheal cartilage. Moderate enlargement of the thyroid may be visible if there is not much subcutaneous fat.

Prognosis.—This on the whole is favorable. In most instances the goiter remains small or diminishes under treatment or spontaneously; this being true also of congenital cases. Pressure-symptoms may possibly be fatal unless relieved.

Diagnosis.—Other tumors in the neck are uncommon in children. The high position of the gland in the short neck of infants should be remembered. Goiter is to be distinguished from congestion of the thyroid by its persistence, and by the frequent limitation of it to part of the gland.

Treatment.—Surgical treatment of goiter is to be employed only when other means have failed or pressure symptoms demand it. Continued administration of iodine is the best remedy. In the prevention of goiter in districts where it is endemic the best procedure is to give once a week a tablet containing 10 mgm. (0.15 grain) of iodine. This should be administered to all children around the age of puberty, especially girls, and it would probably be well to start it in all children at the age of four or five years. The danger of iodine causing thyroid overactivity is very slight in children, if it exists at all. There are other methods of giving iodine, such as the administration of 1 oz. (29.5) of the syrup of iodide of iron or of hydriodic acid spread over a period of two or three weeks and given twice yearly (Marine and Kimball[14]). Two grams (31 grains) of sodium iodide may be employed, administered over a period of about two weeks twice daily. Iodized salt has been used, in which sodium or potassium iodide has been added in about the proportion of 0.01 per cent. In some districts iodine in the concentration of about 1 part to 100,000,000 parts has been added to the drinking water of the community for a period of two weeks each autumn and spring. As stated, the administration of the 10 mgm. of iodine in tablets is the preferable method. Prophylactic treatment is especially important in pregnant women and lactating mothers. As a source of iodine dried sea-kelp (Kelplek) is sometimes used, but possesses no particular advantage.

In cases of colloid goiter the dosage of iodine should be somewhat larger, giving perhaps the 10 mg. amount two or three times a week every other month. Marine and Kimball[14] advise giving 0.1 to 0.2 Gm. (1.5 to 3.0 grains) of desiccated thyroid daily for a period of two weeks, and if there has been no change in pulse-rate or other evidence of injury, this treatment is repeated. After an interval of one to two weeks syrup of hydriodic acid is administered in a daily dose of 2 to 4 cc. (32 to 64 minims) for a period of two weeks. This combined course of treatment may be repeated three times a year. The administration of thyroid products would, of course, be contra-indicated if there is evidence of hyperthyroidism. It should be stated that the slight enlargement of the thyroid, which is that oftenest observed, is without significance and causes no symptoms, and that the only treatment needed is the administration of the small doses of iodine recommended.

SPORADIC CRETINISM

(Infantile Myxedema, Athyriosis, Hypothyroidism, Myxidiocy, Congenital Myxedema)

Endemic cretinism is confined to certain regions in Europe. Many of its subjects also exhibit goitrous enlargement of the thyroid, or are born of parents with this. On the other hand, there are often endemic cretins who do not suffer from goiter, and the two conditions are not necessarily combined. The symptoms are so much those of sporadic cretinism that the description will be limited here to the latter.

Sporadic cretinism was shown by Borneville and d'Olier[15] to be identical with the myxedema of adults, to which attention was first called by Gull.[16] It is uncommon, and differs from the endemic form in that goiter is not often present, there is usually no hereditary or familial tendency, and but one case may occur in a family.

Etiology.—Females are somewhat more often attacked than males. The cause is a deficiency of the internal secretion of the thyroid gland. This depends oftenest upon absence or atrophy of the organ, but, as stated, may occur in hypertrophied glands, the function of which, however, is impaired. The disease is usually congenital, although there may be delay in the appearance of symptoms even as late as the latter part of the first year,—this perhaps depending in some instances upon thyroid secretion in the mother's milk, or received through the placenta and effective for some time; or in others upon the fact that the thyroid is active temporarily. Hypothyroidism when not congenital (*acquired cretinism, juvenile myxedema*) may depend upon a lesion of the gland occurring during the course of an acute infectious disease; upon injury; be associated with sporadic goiter; be the result of thyroidectomy; or be brought about by an unknown cause.

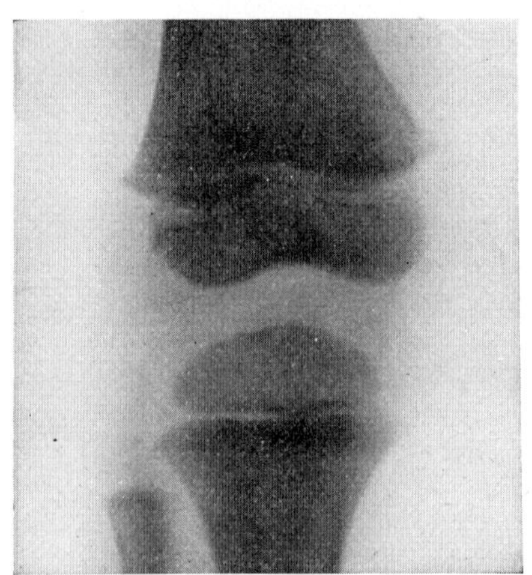

Fig. 259.—Roentgenogram of normal bones in a child of three years. Shows the good development of the epiphyseal centers in contrast with cretinism. (See Fig. 260.)

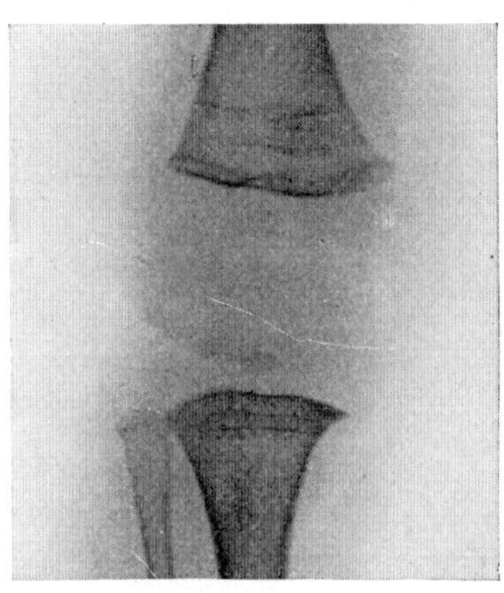

Fig. 260.—Roentgenogram of bones in cretinism. Child of three years in the Children's Hospital of Philadelphia. Shows markedly retarded development of the epiphyseal centers, with slimness of the cortex of the diaphyses.

Pathologic Anatomy.—The thyroid gland is generally atrophied or absent, but may be enlarged and of the colloid type. The liver and spleen are often enlarged. The skin and mucous membrane are thickened by myxedematous changes, which are often spoken of as fatty in nature; but which may be due to abnormal deposits of protein (Boothby et al.[17]). The entire process of osseous development is slow, both in the epiphyses and diaphyses (Figs. 259, 260), and in the flat bones also. There is sometimes hyperplasia of the pituitary, pineal, and thymus glands.

Symptoms.—These vary depending upon the age at which hypothyroidism develops and its degree. In the congenital cases they are usually not observed before six months of age, and in mild cases not until during the second or third year. The appearance of a congenital cretin is characteristic. There is general stunting of growth; the extremities are short; the head appears large; the fontanelle is late in closing; the hair of the scalp is coarse and scanty; the forehead low; the eyes far apart; the palpebral fissure narrow and the eyelids swollen; the bridge of the nose broad and flat and the alae thick; the tongue is thick and broad and often protrudes from the mouth; the lips are thick; the teeth late in appearing and frequently carious. The face appears blotched and sallow, and often exhibits deep creases in the forehead and elsewhere, and the whole expression is blank and apathetic; the neck is short and thick; there are often fleshy deposits above the clavicles and sometimes also between the scapulae and in the axillae; the abdomen is prominent, and umbilical hernia is common; the hands are broad, with short fingers, and often are cold and cyanotic, and corresponding changes occur in the feet. The skin of the body is harsh and dry, thickened, and appears to be edematous, but does not pit on pressure; there is little perspiration; subcutaneous fat is abundant. The basal metabolism is low and the body-temperature subnormal. Constipation and anemia are common (Figs. 261; 262). As age advances there is no sexual development; muscular movements are few and made slowly; standing and walking are learned late, and sometimes never. Intelligence is extremely backward, although a hoarse speech may finally be acquired. The disposition is apathetic but good-natured, and much of the time is spent in sleep.

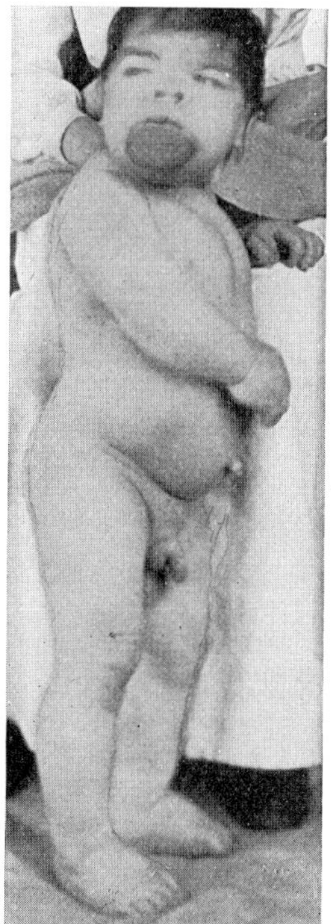

Fig. 261.—Cretinism. Patient, aged fourteen years in the Children's Ward of the Hospital of the University of Pennsylvania. Severe advanced case.

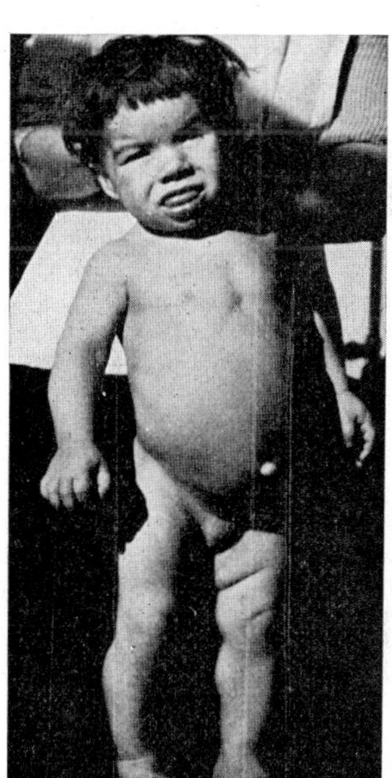

Fig. 262.—Cretinism. Patient, aged four years in Children's Hospital of Philadelphia. Takes little interest in surroundings and cannot walk or talk.

Great variation is seen in the degree of these symptoms. In mild cases (*cretinoid; hypothyroidism*) in which some function of the thyroid gland remains, the degree of lack of bodily and intellectual development is not so marked. In some cases the patient has seemed fairly normal until about four or five years, and then, following some acute disease or without discoverable reason, begins to show the symptoms of hypothyroidism. McCarrison,[18] and Kraus, Brock, and Sloane[19] have observed a so-called *nervous* form of cretinism in which, with the usual symptoms, there are associated spastic paraplegia, athetosis, ataxia, or convulsions.

Course and Prognosis.—Without treatment many cretins die in childhood, generally of some complication. Some, however, and presumably those with a certain degree of thyroid function, live for many years. The earlier treatment is started, the better the results (Figs. 263, 264). Even after a delay of several years the improvement is sometimes remarkable. In no cases can optimum normal physical and mental development be expected, and this applies even to cases in which the thyroid medication has been started in the first few months of life.

Diagnosis.—The condition causing most confusion is *mongolian idiocy*. In both this and cretinism the tongue is protruded, the palpebral fissure narrow, and the intelligence subnormal. The tongue of the mongolian idiot, however, is not really enlarged; the eyes often have the oriental slant; the child is restless rather than apathetic; the hands have not the broad, squat form of the cretin, and often exhibit incurving of the little

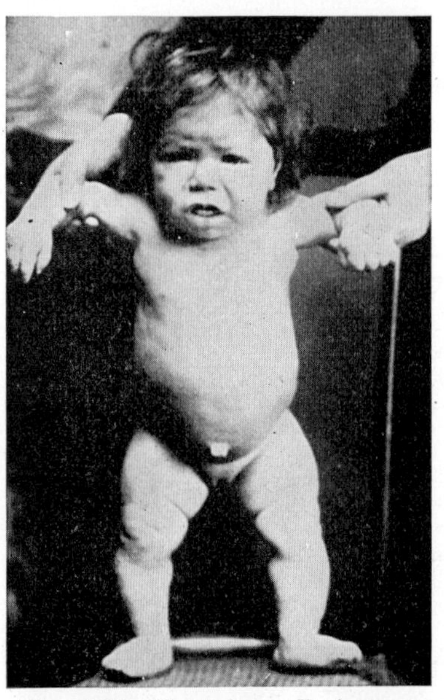

Fig. 263.—Cretinism. Patient, aged two years and one month. Before treatment. (*Courtesy of Dr. A. H. Davisson.*)

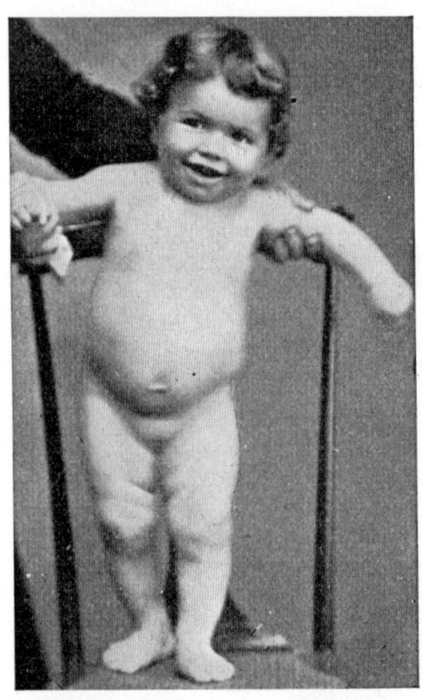

Fig. 264.—Cretinism. Same case as in Fig. 263, now aged three years and two months. Condition after thirteen months of treatment with thyroid extract.

finger; there is no uniform delay in ossification, at least not to the degree in cretinism; and the basal metabolism is usually normal or but slightly decreased. *Achondroplasia* produces shortness of the extremities combined with a large head and flattening of the bridge of the nose; but there is no other resemblance to cretinism, and the mental development, while sometimes slow, is eventually normal. *Rachitis* may show stunted growth, large open fontanelles, and delayed dentition; but in no other respects bears any resemblance to cretinism. *Infantilism* of other sorts may be mistaken for the cretinoid type because of the dwarfism present, but usually exhibits definite characteristics, and there is absence of myxedema, the cretinoid facies and other features of hypothyroidism (p. 1068).

Treatment.—This consists in the oral administration of a reliable thyroid extract. The amount required varies with the individual case, and, when possible, the basal metabolic rate should be ascertained from time to time. Symptoms of overdose of thyroid extract are rapid loss of weight, fever, rapid cardiac action, nausea, restlessness, perspiration, faintness, and sleeplessness. There is relatively little danger should overdosage occur, and perhaps the usual mistake is giving too small amounts. The initial dose should not be over $\frac{1}{4}$ grain (0.016) twice daily, or $\frac{1}{10}$ grain (.0065) in the first few months of life, and the amount may be steadily increased to a dosage of 5 grains (0.32) if no unfavorable symptoms appear. Response to the medication is shown in the course of a few weeks by disappearance of subnormal temperature, a moderate loss of weight, and diminution in the size of the tongue. The teeth make their way through the gums; increase in length of the body begins; the child commences to walk; the character of the hair changes; constipation ceases; and intellectual power is improved. Physical development generally takes place before intellectual. Treatment must be continued throughout life, although often with lessened dosage, and perhaps with occasional intermissions. Hypothyroid patients are unusually susceptible to morphine.

In the prevention of cretinism it is especially important that in districts where goiter is prevalent, iodine should be administered to pregnant women and nursing mothers.

EXOPHTHALMIC GOITER

(Graves' Disease; Basedow's Disease; Hyperthyroidism; Thyrotoxicosis)

Etiology.—Although cases had been reported earlier, Graves[20] in 1835 was the first to describe the condition fully. It is not common in childhood, but cases have been published or statistics collected by Barret,[21] Buford,[22] Cole,[23] Heiman,[24] Helmholz,[25] Ginsburg,[26] Greene and Mora,[27] and others. Most of the cases are in older children, many of them about the age of puberty; but the malady has been said to appear even congenitally (White[28]). An instance in an infant of nine months was noted by Klaus.[29] We have seen not more than a dozen cases, the youngest patient being one of four years. Inheritance appears sometimes to play a rôle, the parents having had simple or exophthalmic goiter, or having been neuropathic or alcoholic. It is maintained by some that there is a constitutional anomaly in the person predisposed to hyperthyroidism (Warthin,[30] Moschcowitz[31]). That the disease is a pure thyroid disturbance has been questioned, and Marine[32] with others believes that there is deranged function of the visceral nervous system, the hyperthyroidism being a physiologic attempt to overcome disturbed tissue-oxidation. Other endocrine glands have been implicated, such as the thymus, the suprarenals, and the sex-glands. Females are much oftener attacked. The condition may have been preceded by shock, fright, trauma, or infectious diseases; these causes being exciting rather than primary. Occasionally hyperthyroidism exists as a complication of simple goiter. In the literature there is much discussion concerning the differentiation between exophthalmic goiter and toxic adenoma. Some authors distinguish the former by the fact that there is a diffuse, soft enlargement of the thyroid with great vascularity, and that exophthalmos is present in addition to the other symptoms of nervousness, tachycardia, and increased metabolism. In toxic adenoma, which occurs rarely if at all in childhood, there is nodular and often asymmetrical thyroid enlargement, the ocular signs are absent, and the onset is slower.

The **symptoms** are much as observed in adults. Most frequently present in children are tachycardia, enlargement and pulsation of the thyroid gland, and exophthalmos, the last often slight. Tremor is less common than in adults; or there may be coarser movements. Among other symptoms are vomiting and diarrhea; anemia; emaciation; headache; elevation of temperature; and excessive perspiration, flushing, pigmentation, or other cutaneous manifestations. The heart may suffer from myocardial change, and there be extra systoles, auricular fibrillation, or murmurs. There may be retraction (Stellwag's sign) or lagging (von Graefe's sign) of the upper eyelids. The psychic state may not be disturbed as much as in adults, but there is some irritability, restlessness, and insomnia. Hyperglycemia and glycosuria may occur. The basal metabolic rate is increased in proportion to the severity of the disease; 20 to 50 per cent increase representing a mild form and over 75 a severe one. Increased excretion of calcium and probably of phosphorus occurs; this probably explaining the osteoporosis which may develop (Aub et al[33]). Rarely in childhood is there neuritis or chronic arthritis.

This description applies to more fully developed cases; but more often in children there may be milder degrees of hyperthyroidism with any one of the three chief manifestations being the first to appear, and perhaps for a time the only one. The severity of all of the symptoms mentioned may vary with the case. The **course** in early life may be chronic, but the onset is oftenest sudden with the complete picture attained in a few weeks. So, too, recovery may occur rapidly; but even when delayed takes place finally in over half the cases. In other instances great improvement comes about; but the enlarged thyroid and some of the other symptoms persist, and there is a tendency to relapse. In the more chronic cases there is a gradual development of anemia, emaciation, pigmentation, and the other symptoms mentioned. Even after all other symptoms have disappeared, exophthalmos may continue. Rarely a myxedematous condition may finally develop, due to atrophy of the gland. Death from the disease itself is exceptional in early life. The **treatment** consists in rest, fresh air, avoidance of exertion and excitement, warm baths or packs, and the control of such symptoms as cardiac failure and the like. Sedatives may be indicated. Nourishment must be maintained, and, in fact, there is an increased susceptibility to acidosis on starvation; probably because of the decreased ability to store carbohydrates. While partial thyroidectomy has been performed in children, this is usually unnecessary, due to the favorable course. Exposure of the gland to the roentgen-ray or to radium may have a beneficial effect. (For radium treatment in children, see Ginsburg.[26]) The use of iodine in hyperthyroidism has been much discussed. Its greatest value seems to be as a pre-operative measure, since it causes a lowering of the metabolic rate, although this is usually only temporary. It may be given as Lugol's solution 15 minims (0.9) twice a day for ten days or two weeks before operation. Iodine has also been used continuously or intermittently for several months without operation and good results reported (Thompson et al.[34]).

OTHER DISORDERS OF THE THYROID GLAND

Tumors are rare, although primary sarcoma has been reported, as also carcinoma. Secondary growths are somewhat more frequent. Enchondroma has been seen. Aberrant thyroid tissue in the neck may develop into tumor-masses or cysts. This has been observed in tumors of the lingual thyroid attached to the hyoid bone, or situated deep in the tongue. We have seen faulty diagnoses of congenital laryngeal stridor and enlarged thymus made when the symptoms were due to thyroglossal cysts. **Tuberculosis** may involve the thyroid gland; hereditary **syphilis** may produce a goitrous enlargement; and **cysts** other than those occurring in goiter may be found.

DISEASES OF THE PARATHYROID GLANDS

These glands, usually four in number, first described by Remak,[35] are attached to the lateral lobes of the posterior aspect of the thyroid. The parathyroid hormone is concerned with calcium-equilibrium rather than with the absorption of this mineral (Stewart and Percival[36]). The removal or injury of the parathyroids leads to hypocalcemia. There may be additional functions, such as a possible relation to the action of vitamins on the body. In certain chronic tetanies with a persistent low level of calcium in the blood, and in which it is presumed that hypoparathyroidism is present, in addition to increased mechanical and electrical excitability of the nerves and attacks of laryngospasm, there will be found carpopedal spasm and generalized convulsions, defects of the enamel of the teeth, and opacity of the crystalline lens of the eye (Barker[37]). In a case apparently of this type, although without any suggestion of cataract, we were able temporarily to increase the blood-calcium and relieve the symptoms by the administration of parathyroid extract. Overaction of the gland, stimulated, perhaps, by tumor-formation, may result in hypercalcemia. Excessive elimination of calcium salts occurs in the urine; the serum-calcium is increased; and osseous dystrophies of varied types, such as fibrosis and cystic change, occur. In distinguishing hyperparathyroidism from renal rickets (p. 822) it should be remembered that the former leads to a high blood-calcium and a low blood-phosphorus and the latter a reverse of this relationship. Collip[38] has extracted the active principle (hormone) of the parathyroid gland. Injection of this will restore a lowered blood-calcium to normal. Overdose of it produces hypercalcemia, diarrhea, drowsiness, muscular flaccidity, increased viscosity of the blood, and certain other symptoms. The extract has been used in infantile tetany (p. 874), in injury to or after removal of the parathyroids, and in osteitis fibrosa.

The relation of the parathyroids to the usual infantile tetany is not satisfactorily determined, although in this condition there is usually no lesion of these glands discovered (p. 869). They are sometimes enlarged in osteitis fibrosa.

References

1. Am. J. Dis. Child., 1925, **29,** 41. 2. Physiol. Rev., 1927, **7,** 189. 3. J.A.M.A., 1924, **82,** 1190. 4. Gerhardt's Handb. d. Kinderkr., 1878, **3,** H. 2, 369. 5. Am. J. Dis. Child., 1921, **22,** 477. 6. Pub. Health Rep., 1928, **43,** 3009. 7. Medicine, 1924, **3,** 453; 1927, **6,** 1127. 8. J.A.M.A., 1923, **80,** 600. 9. Lancet, 1913, **1,** 219; 365; Brit. M. J., 1927, **1,** 94. 10. Arch. Path., 1931, **11,** 709. 11. Am. J. Dis. Child., 1930, **40,** 974. 12. Pub. Health Rep., 1926, **41,** 971. 13. Pub. Health Rep., 1926, **41,** 1881. 14. Arch. Int. Med., 1918, **22,** 41; 1920, **25,** 661. 15. Prog. méd., 1880, **8,** 709. 16. Tr. Clin. Soc., London, 1874, **7,** 180. 17. Ergebn. d. Physiol., 1925, **24,** 773. 18. Proc. Roy. Soc. Med., Sec. Med., 1902; **2,** 1. 19. Am. J. M. Sc., 1929, **178,** 548. 20. London M. and S. J., 1835, **7,** 513. 21. Thèse de Paris, 1901. 22. J.A.M.A., 1922, **78,** 1533. 23. Arch. Pediat., 1923, **40,** 703. 24. Am. J. Dis. Child., 1923, **26,** 216. 25. J.A.M.A., 1926, **87,** 157. 26. Am. J. Dis. Child., 1929, **37,** 923. 27. Surg., Gynec., and Obst., 1931, **53,** 375. 28. Proc. Roy. Soc. Med., 1912, **5,** Obst. Sec., 247. 29. Prag. med. Wchnschr., 1914, **39,** 515. 30. Ann. Int. Med., 1928, **2,** 553. 31. Arch. Int. Med., 1930, **46,** 610. 32. Medicine, 1926, **6,** 127; Am. J. M. Sc., 1930, **180,** 767. 33. J. Clin. Investigation, 1929, **7,** 97. 34. Arch. Int. Med., 1930, **45,** 481. 35. Untersuch. über d. Entwick. d. Wirbelthieres, 1851, **35,** 194; Ref. McCullogh, Arch. Int. Med., 1928, **42,** 546. 36. Biochem. J., 1927, **21,** 301; Physiol. Rev., 1928, **8,** 283. 37. Am. J. Dis. Child., 1928, **35,** 872. 38. J. Biol. Chem., 1925, **63,** 395; 439.

CHAPTER II

DISEASES OF THE THYMUS GLAND

THE physiologic function and the diseases of the thymus gland are but little understood. Its dimension and weight appear to vary so greatly within normal limits, that the determination at necropsy that the condition is abnormal can be made only when the variations from the average are extreme. Equally disputed is the power of the thymus gland to produce symptoms, either mechanically or by a disturbance of its internal secretion. (See pp. 43, 482.) It is believed that the gland possesses such a secretion, and among the properties assigned to it are that it influences the development of the bones, as in rickets; by the production of a toxin is the cause of sudden death in the lymphatic diathesis; is a factor in the cause of exophthalmic goiter; increases the coagulability of the blood; is an important regulator of blood-pressure; produces symptoms suggesting tetany; exerts some action upon the development of the nervous system and the sexual organs; has some general influence over growth; is of importance in the production of chlorosis and the primary myopathies; and acts as a reservoir of phagocytic cells. It is at least certain that much further investigation is required before any of these functions can be accepted. Some of the conclusions drawn from animal experimentation may not be applicable to man. Studies on dogs do not appear to prove that the thymus is an essential or even an important organ (Park and McClure[1]).

ABSENCE AND ATROPHY OF THE THYMUS GLAND

There may rarely be congenital **absence** of the thymus gland. This is generally associated with other malformations of some sort, especially anencephalus, or with defective mentality. **Atrophy** of the gland is a natural occurrence as adult life is reached; but it may be seen also in the new-born (Durante[2]), and is found often in the case of infants dying in a state of malnutrition. The assumption has sometimes been made that thymic atrophy was the cause of the general wasting; but it is much more probable that it is merely a part of it. There are, in fact, no special symptoms connected with atrophy of the gland.

ENLARGEMENT OF THE THYMUS GLAND

Etiology and Pathology.—(See p. 43.) More or less **persistence** of the thymus gland during adolescence and into adult life is often observed. Some endocrinologists claim that there is associated with this a type of person who is tall, slender and loose-jointed; exhibits fine texture of the skin, scanty hair, poor resistance to infection; who has thin-walled blood vessels; and who becomes easily fatigued and shows inferiority in the development of circulatory and endocrine organs. This association is not generally accepted. A true **hyperplasia** in early life is common, and not infrequently seen even after this period. The gland may sometimes be so much enlarged that it nearly covers the heart, and projects well beyond the internal borders of the lungs, and occasionally weighs as much as 30 or 40 Gm. (1.05 or 1.4 oz.) or more. The subject of the causes and clinical manifestations of hyperplasia is a matter of much discussion. As already stated, the range of size of the gland within normal limits is so wide that it is difficult to determine the exact definition of what is and what is not hypertrophy. (See p. 43.) It is only, therefore, in cases where the size and weight of the organ are exceptionally great that we can with certainty maintain its existence (Fig. 265). This hypertrophy is generally the result of a simple hyperplasia, but it may depend upon a thymitis or exceptionally upon hemorrhage or edema. Its cause is far from being understood. That the condition is a frequent one in lymphatism has already been pointed out (p. 482); but a very large thymus gland may occur in children who have no symptoms of this disorder. Enlargement has been found in combination with a number of morbid conditions, among them exophthalmic goiter, acromegaly, epilepsy, leukemia, pylorospasm, and Hodgkin's disease, although any etiologic connection of the hypertrophy with these conditions is not clear. There may be an association of the thymus with the thyroid, spleen, pituitary body, adrenals, and other internal glands. Whether the thymic hyperplasia is a compensatory process in diseases of these organs, or whether it is due to an accompanying disturbance of the thymic function is a matter for further study.

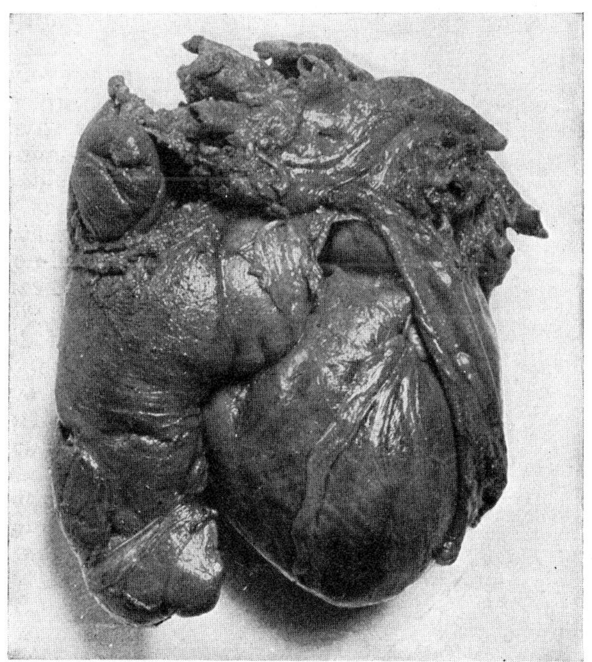

Fig. 265.—Enlarged thymus gland. Infant of three and one-half months dying after a few hours illness. Rapid respiration and cyanosis, but no symptoms of obstruction. Necropsy showed the thymus gland measuring 7 cm. (2.76 in.) in length, $3\frac{1}{2}$ cm. (1.38 in.) in breadth and 2 cm. (0.78 in.) in thickness. (*Courtesy of Dr. Eleanor Jones.*) (*See also, Arch. Pediat.*, 1903, **20,** 596.)

Symptoms.—Unless greatly enlarged the thymus cannot be accurately outlined by percussion. The supposedly normal limits of dulness up to six years of age are shown in Fig. 266. The normal thymus may occasionally be palpated at the episternal notch. The roentgenographic study of the thymus is not simple, and the shadow cast does not correspond to the gland as seen at necropsy (Benjamin and Gött[3]), although this discrepancy may in part be due to shrinkage. Furthermore, as shown by Gerstenberger;[4] Blackfan and Little,[5] and others, the roentgenographic shadow increases on deep inspiration; dorsal flexion of the head may diminish it; and other distortions may occur with changes in position. A further difficulty in interpretation of percussion-dulness or of the roentgenogram is the determining what constitutes enlargement. Some roentgenographers have endeavored to fix certain limitations which would define thymic enlargement. Certainly, however, a shadow beyond these can occur without there being any symptoms whatever. Occasionally a lateral view on the roentgenogram may show an apparent compression of the trachea. A study of the literature, together with our own experience, appears to us to justify the statement that there is little if any correlation between the size of the roentgenographic shadow and clinical symptoms which could be attributed to enlargement of this organ.

Plater[6] in 1614 noted the presence of a tumor apparently of the thymus in an infant dying suddenly; and Kopp[7] in 1830 maintained the existence of a "thymic asthma" dependent upon the pressure of such a gland upon the trachea. This view held sway until the classical studies by Friedleben,[8] which indicated that there was no connection between enlargement of the thymus gland and asthma or sudden death. A reversion of sentiment in favor of compression by the gland occurred under the influence of Grawitz;[9] but only a short time later Paltauf[10] advanced the theory of the existence of what he called the "status lymphaticus." According to this view, enlargement of the thymus gland is but a part of the general involvement of the lymphatic system occurring in the lymphatic diathesis (p. 482); and the symptoms depend upon a neurosis and not upon the thymus itself, or certainly not upon its enlargement and compression thus caused. Paltauf's opinions found much acceptance, although many now would agree with the conclusion of Boyd[11] and others that the condition described by Paltauf really represents the normal thymus and lymphoid tissue of a well-nourished child. Cases continued to be reported indicating the possibility of pressure by the thymus gland, and the production of symptoms, or even of death, brought about in this way. Many of these do not stand analysis, and careful study would reveal that the actual cause of death in most reported cases was incorrectly attributed to the thymus. It would appear too dogmatic to deny entirely that the so-called "thymus-death" as well as certain symptoms, may not occasionally be connected with thymic hyperplasia. These symptoms may be of different sorts and produced in different ways:

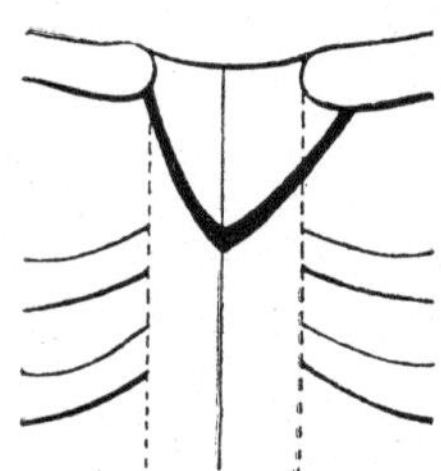

Fig. 266.—Diagram showing normal thymus dulness. (*Blumenreich, Virchow's Arch.*, 1900, **160**, 34.)

1. *Pressure upon the Trachea.*—There is no doubt that such pressure may occur, and that symptoms are produced by it, although not nearly so often as supposed by some. This is supported by the evidence that thymectomy or radiologic treatment may cause diminution or cessation of such symptoms as stridor and cyanosis, and that roentgenograms demonstrate a decrease in size coincident with the clinical improvement. It must be recognized that while the clinical evidence is that symptoms can be produced by pressure of an enlarged thymus gland upon the trachea, this is certainly an unusual occurrence. There seems to be no proportionate relationship between the size of the thymus and the likelihood of pressure-symptoms developing; and it is not even certain that the enlarged thymus, if producing the symptoms at all, is not doing it in some other way than mechanically. In all undoubted cases of pressure of the thymus upon the trachea, the symptoms are of a *chronic* nature with a more or less persistent tracheal stenosis; and such cases are certainly of infrequent occurrence. Cases of *congenital laryngeal stridor* have been claimed by Hochsinger[12] to be the result of pressure of an enlarged thymus gland. Some of these are possibly due to thymic enlargement; others certainly depend upon different causes. (See p. 701.) Attacks of holding the breath have also been attributed to a thymic disorder (p. 893).

2. *Pressure upon Other Organs.*—Theories have been advanced that symptoms may result from pressure of the thymus gland upon the large vessels within the thorax, upon the nerves, or upon the heart itself. These have not obtained general acceptance and lack sufficient anatomic confirmation.

3. *Symptoms other than those of Pressure Attributed to Thymic Hyperplasia.*—Here may be discussed the not infrequent cases of sudden death occurring sometimes entirely without warning, and in which hypertrophy of the thymus or other lymphoid structures or both may be discovered. (See Lymphatism, p. 483.) Whether the thymus gland has anything directly to do with this is doubtful. Although a disturbance of the function of the thymus and an intoxication by its secretion are conceivable, as Escherich[13] believed, this has never been proven. Svehla,[14] Basch,[15] and others have claimed decided, although varying, effects in animals from the injection of an extract of the thymus gland, and a condition of hyperthymization has been spoken of. On the other hand, injections made by Fischl[16] were entirely without serious action. The sudden death is ascribed to cardiac failure. It has also been claimed that death is due to a fall in blood-pressure, the result of failure of proper adrenalin production (Hymanson[17]). In some cases of sudden death associated with what appears to be an overgrowth of lymphoid tissue throughout the body, we have found intracranial hemorrhage. Aldrich[18] considers it possible that the suprarenal involution which occurs in the new-born may result in vagotonia and thymic hypertrophy. Hammar[19] in a study of a series of so-called thymus-deaths in children found no characteristic morphologic changes, no marked variations in size of the gland, and no ground for assuming the action of either an increased or a diminished function. Many other observations, such as those of Boyd,[11] would support Hammar's conclusions.

Rachford,[20] Pitfield,[21] Barbour,[22] Rubin,[23] and Aldrich[18] have claimed a connection between the thymus and some instances of pylorospasm; radiologic treatment of the former being beneficial to the latter. Our own experience does not support this relationship.

Prognosis and Treatment.—The prognosis of stridor dependent upon pressure of the thymus on the trachea is usually good. There is a tendency to recover as the child grows older, and even in severe cases there is usually time for successful treatment. This consists in exposure to the roentgen-ray, as first suggested by Friedlander.[24] The criterion for treatment is the presence of symptoms of stridor and cyanosis not explicable on any other basis, rather than the size of the thymus shown on the roentgenogram. The symptoms sometimes appear worse for twenty-four hours or longer after the treatment, presumably due to swelling of the gland. Structures other than the thymus, especially the thyroid region, should be protected against the ray during the exposure, since it is possible that subsequent bad effects might be brought about. It is also questionable whether over-treatment of the thymus with too rapid and too great destruction of it, might not lead to subsequent lack of general development. Any proof of these bad effects is difficult to secure, although spoken of by a number of clinicians. Thymectomy is no longer performed to any extent. Parker[25] and Klose[26] collected instances in which this operation was done. It should be stated that the indiscriminate exposure to the roentgen-ray of every new-born infant who supposedly has an abnormally large thymic shadow, yet is without clinical symptoms, is a procedure to be deprecated as not only unnecessary but possibly harmful.

Diagnosis.—The difficulty of deciding by percussion or by roentgenographic examination whether a thymus is abnormally enlarged has been discussed. Thymic hypertrophy, when it is a manifestation of lymphatism, is associated with other symptoms of this, as enlargement of the tonsils, adenoids, and superficial lymph-nodes, and a lymphocytosis. Congenital laryngeal stridor usually causes much noisier respirations than in thymic asthma, and is without cyanosis. Other conditions from which thymic stridor must be differentiated, often by laryngoscopic examination, are certain intrinsic tumors of the throat and larynx, as papilloma; diaphragm-like deformity below the glottis (Kennedy and New[27]); bilateral abductor paralysis; and thyroglossal or other cysts of the tongue. Tongue-swallowing (p. 526) should be thought of in differential diagnosis; also mediastinal tumors or enlarged tracheobronchial glands producing pressure. The relief which may attend intubation in laryngeal affections is an aid in differentiation, since this is of no benefit in cases of pressure by the thymus. The finding of an enlarged thymus gland or even general lymphoid hypertrophy at necropsy after sudden death has occurred does not in itself prove that these were responsible. All other possible factors must be looked for.

OTHER DISORDERS OF THE THYMUS GLAND

Acute thymitis is a rare affection, the result oftenest of pyemia. General **tuberculosis** of the body may exhibit miliary tubercles or caseous foci in the thymus gland; and **syphilis** may produce gummata there, or often a small-celled infiltration with consecutive fibrosis. The so-called "Dubois'[28] abscesses" are probably only cystic degeneration of the Hassall bodies dependent upon hereditary syphilis, but they may occasionally occur in nonsyphilitic infants (Benjamin[29]). **Hemorrhage** into the gland is rare. Of this 19 cases were collected by Wahl and Walthall[20] in addition to two of their own. **Tumors** of the thymus, either primary or secondary, are unusual. Leukemia may involve the gland; and lymphoma, lymphosarcoma, carcinoma, and teratoma have been recorded.

References

1. Am. J. Dis. Child., 1919, **18,** 317. 2. Compt. rend. soc. biol., 1896, **48,** 285. 3. Jahrb. f. Kinderh., 1912, **75,** 367. 4. Am. J. Dis. Child., 1921, **21,** 534. 5. Am. J. Dis. Child., 1921, **22,** 459. 6. Observat. in homin. affect. pleurisque, 1614, lib. **3,** 172. 7. Denkwürdikeiten, 1830, 1. 8. Die Physiologie der Thymusdrüse, 1858. 9. Deutsch. med. Wchnschr., 1888, **14,** 429. 10. Wien. klin. Wchnschr., 1889, **2,** 877; 1890, **3,** 172. 11. Am. J. Dis. Child., 1927, **33,** 867. 12. Wien. med. Wchnschr., 1903, **53,** 2106. 13. Berl. klin. Wchnschr., 1896, **33,** 645. 14. Wien. med. Blätter 1896, **19,** 723. 15. Wien. klin. Wchnschr., 1903, **16,** 893. 16. Jahrb. f. Kinderh., 1914, **79,** 385; 589. 17. Arch. Pediat., 1928, **45,** 592. 18. J.A.M.A., 1930, **94,** 1119. 19. Ztschr. f. Kinderh., Orig., 1916, **13,** 153; Endocrinology, 1921, **5,** 543. 20. Arch. Pediat., 1917, **34,** 803. 21. New York M. J., 1917, **105,** 988. 22. Arch. Pediat., 1927, **44,** 314. 23. J.A.M.A., 1928, **90,** 1694. 24. Am. J. Dis. Child., 1913, **6,** 38. 25. Am. J. Dis. Child., 1913, **5,** 89. 26. Therapeut. Monatsh., 1915, **29,** 6. 27. J.A.M.A., 1931, **96,** 1286. 28. Gaz. méd. de Paris, Ser. 3, 1850, **5,** 392. 29. Am. J. Dis. Child., 1930, **39,** 586. 30. Am. J. Dis. Child., 1922, **24,** 27.

CHAPTER III

DISEASES OF THE PITUITARY, PINEAL AND SUPRARENAL GLANDS

DISEASES OF THE PITUITARY GLAND

THE pituitary body consists of three parts. The secretion from the anterior lobe is necessary to life and contains two hormones; (1) sex-gland stimulating, and (2) growth-promoting. The posterior lobe possesses a hormone which raises blood-pressure and one which influences uterine contractions and smooth muscle in general; and also contains substances which exert a diuretic-antidiuretic action, and have an effect on the metabolism of carbohydrate and of fat. It is sometimes claimed that the pars intermedia secretes some of the active substances found in the posterior lobe, these passing through the latter on their way to the 3d ventricle. Apparently the hypothalamic region is connected in some way with the pituitary gland, and involved in its activity. There is evidently a close relationship between the functions of the pituitary and those of other glands of internal secretion, as the thyroid, pineal, suprarenals, and the sex-glands.

Acromegaly is to be regarded as dependent upon an excess of secretion of the anterior lobe of the pituitary, but does not appear before the age of puberty. The condition of **gigantism** is the counterpart of acromegaly, when hypersecretion of the pituitary is present before ossification is complete. There then occurs a delay in ossification and a subsequent increase in the size of the skeleton. Such patients are liable to be without great strength, and to have some degree of mental deficiency. At necropsy there is usually found involvement of the pituitary and neighboring structures by a tumor, oftenest fibroma or myxoma. In some cases radiologic treatment of the tumor is of benefit.

Hypopituitarism may produce a form of infantilism. (Fröhlich's Syndrome, see p. 1088.) Hypopituitarism may occur as a sequel to hyperpituitarism, or the symptoms may be combined, so that the title *dyspituitarism* could be employed. A condition described by Simmonds[1] is probably due to atrophy or insufficiency of the anterior lobe. Seventy cases of this are reviewed by Calder,[2] but only 9 of these occurred in childhood and only a few in adolescence. A case in a boy ten years of age is reported by Kurokawa.[3] It is seen in both sexes. The chief symptoms are emaciation; trophic changes in the skin, teeth and hair; listlessness and somnolence; general muscular weakness; subnormal temperature; lowered basal metabolic rate; and impotence;—in fact, all the symptoms of premature senility. (See also Progeria, p. 1086.)

DISEASES OF THE PINEAL GLAND

The functions of this body and its relation to glands of internal secretion and to other body-processes and structures are little understood. It is claimed by some that it does not produce an internal secretion, but that it has a neuro-regulatory influence of some sort. Certainly disturbances of it, which are almost invariably due to tumors (teratoma, sarcoma, cyst, glioma, pinealoma, and carcinoma), lead to overgrowth of the sex-glands and premature development of puberty. The condition has been studied especially by Bailey and Jelliffe,[4] Jelliffe,[5] Morse,[6] Zandrèn,[7] Laurensich,[8] Horrax and Bailey,[9] and Haldeman;[10] the last author summarizing 113 reported cases. In cases of pineal tumor occurring after puberty trophic changes may not come about, since involution of the pineal body begins to take place at about that age. The syndrome occurs most often in boys, or, according to Horrax and Bailey,[9] only in them. In addition to the general symptoms of brain-tumor which may be present, there take place abnormal development of the body; early growth of hair on the pubis, and sometimes elsewhere, as on the face; obesity; marked overgrowth of the penis and sometimes of the testicles and breasts; and perhaps alteration of the voice (*macrogenitosomia praecox*). (Fig. 267.) Mentality is usually unaffected, except as the result of intracranial pressure. Sometimes there is mental precocity. Some of the symptoms may be due to lesions of neighboring structures rather than of the pineal body itself. Radiologic treatment of the pineal region may be tried. Pineal extract has no effect.

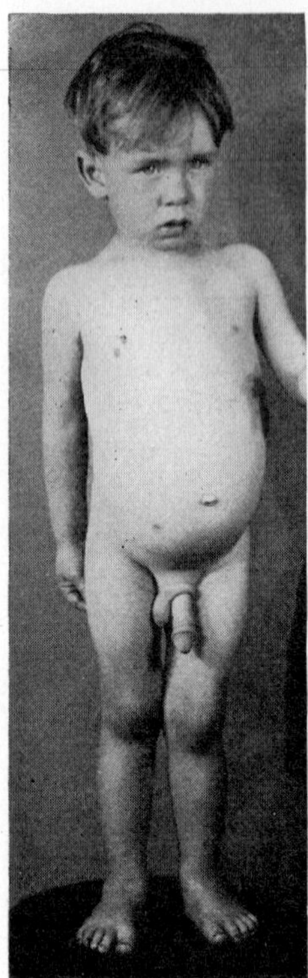

Fig. 267.—Patient seen with Dr. Stewart Matthews, Wyoming, Ohio. Age at the time two and one-half years. Weight and measurements those of a child of four years of age. Anterior fontanelle did not close until twenty-seven months of age. Began to have polyuria and polydipsia at about one year of age. Now has marked symptoms of diabetes insipidus. Penis began to enlarge at about two years of age. Has deep voice. Eyegrounds normal. Roentgenogram of skull shows a calcified mass in the region of the pineal gland. Diagnosis, brain-tumor involving pituitary and pineal region.

At nine years of age child still alive; has no marked failure of vision; is mentally backward; is overweight and height for his age; has pubic and axillary hair.

DISEASES OF THE SUPRARENAL GLANDS

The medulla of these bodies arises from the sympathetic system; the cortex from the primitive mesodermal epithelium. There is relationship between the secretion of the suprarenals and those of other internal glands, as the thyroid, thymus, pituitary, and the sex-glands. It has been found experimentally that removal of the medulla of the suprarenal is not necessarily fatal, whereas removal of the cortex is invariably so (Stewart and Rogoff;[11] Kovács[12]). The secretion of the cortex (interrenal tissue) appears to have some effect on general and sexual growth; hypersecretion producing precocious sexual development, and hyposecretion infantilism. Goldzieher,[13] Hartman, Brownell and Hartman,[14] and Swingle and Pfiffner[15] have prepared extracts of the cortex ("cortin," "interrenin"), which are active experimentally and in the control of Addison's disease.

ADDISON'S DISEASE

This affection, uncommon at any age, is still more so in childhood, but cases in early life have been collected and reported by Monti,[16] Fleming and Miller,[17] Felberbaum and Fruchthandler,[18] Croom,[19] Chemin,[20] Rolleston and Boyd,[21] Cannata,[22] and Peutz.[23] Most of these cases were in children about the age of puberty, and not all of them were confirmed by necropsy. In some instances there has appeared to be an hereditary influence. **Pathologically** the lesions in the suprarenals nearly always consist of tuberculous changes. In some cases there has been found atrophy, fatty degeneration, amyloid degeneration, gummatous degeneration, or the presence of morbid growths. For these rare nontuberculous cases the term *hyposuprarenalism* or *suprarenal cortical insufficiency* has sometimes been employed. A case of this type in a child is reported by Peterman.[24] The essential lesion in Addison's disease, as in hyposuprarenalism of any type, appears to be destruction of the cortex rather than of the medulla. In some instances there has also been found fatty degeneration or atrophy of the semilunar ganglion and solar plexus; these tissues being embryologically related to the suprarenal body. The **symptoms,** which are usually insidious in onset, although sometimes acute, consist of increasing debility; cardiac weakness; low blood-pressure; anorexia; irritability or apathy; anemia; hypoglycemia; and pigmentation of the skin of a yellow or sometimes almost black color, and most marked about the genitalia, umbilicus, axillae, nipples and flexor surface of the articulations, and involving also the mucous membranes. The pigmentation may sometimes be almost absent, and in other cases generalized rather than confined to the areas mentioned. It is usually seen first on the face and hands and may not appear until late in the disease, although commonly an early manifestation. Among other symptoms sometimes occurring are headache, vertigo, convulsions, paralytic manifestations, and vague pains especially in the abdomen. The **duration** of the disease is variable; sometimes a few months; oftener a year or more. The **prognosis** is poor, but cases of undoubted Addison's disease have recovered. The **diagnosis** rests upon the symptoms described. Pigmentation of the skin resembling Addison's disease may occur in other conditions, as malaria or after the continued administration of arsenic. In some cases calcification of the suprarenals due to tuberculosis may be seen on the roentgenogram (Rolleston and Boyd[21]). The **treatment** is symptomatic. The dehydration which sometimes comes about should be combated by injection of glucose and normal saline solutions; the former being especially indicated because of the hypoglycemia. The ordinary preparations of suprarenalin or adrenaline when given by mouth are inert, and when administered hypodermically are of little avail. Extracts of the suprarenal cortex have had definite effect in alleviating the symptoms and prolonging life (Rogoff and Stewart;[11] Rowntree, Greene, Swingle and Pfiffner[25]).

TUMORS OF THE SUPRARENAL GLANDS

Considerable confusion exists in terminology, classification, and especially in the understanding of the pathologic characteristics of suprarenal tumors. There have been reported sarcomas, neuroblastomas, adenomas, and mixed tumors. Many formerly classified as sarcomas are now termed neuroblastomas (neurocytomas). There may be a tentative division into benign and malignant tumors. The benign group includes hyperplasia, adenoma, and ganglioneuroma; these not metastasizing, although the ganglioneuromas perhaps showing local invasion. The so-called "paragangliomas" (chromaffin tumors) consist of small, usually nonmalignant, pigmented nodules. The *malignant* tumors are of two types, the neuroblastoma and allied growths arising in the medullary portion, and the hypernephroma originating in the cortex.

Benign tumors are without characteristic **symptoms.** Malignant tumors produce manifestations varying in their nature and the portion of the organ involved. The neuroblastomas show a special tendency to metastasis, whereas the cortical hypernephromas produce precocious sexual development.

(*A*) Nonepithelial Tumors of the Suprarenal Gland.—Growths of this nature are usually neuroblastomas, although rarely lymphosarcoma or fibrosarcoma is encountered. While uncommon, they are seen oftenest in children, and more in males than in females. The primary lesion arises in the medullary portion of the gland. Metastatic growths resemble the primary tumor in character.

While some of these suprarenal tumors have no special characteristics, the following rather distinct types can be recognized:

1. Neuroblastoma of the Suprarenal Glands with Cranial Metastasis.—This is often referred to as "sarcoma." The syndrome was first described by Hutchinson.[26] Cases have also been reported and collected by Tileston and Wolbach,[27] Frew,[28] Weber,[29] Benedixen and Lamb,[30] Sturtevant and Kelly,[31] Holmes and Dresser,[32] Greig,[33] and others. We have seen 5 cases of this condition, 3 confirmed by necropsy. The first *symptoms* are often misleading and not referred to the abdomen, and the tumor here may not be discovered until late in the course. Perhaps the initial manifestation may be a discoloration of the eyelids, or exophthalmos on one or both sides, the result of metatastic growths in the bones of the orbit. Tumors then develop elsewhere in the cranium, especially in the temporal region. Much less commonly there is metastasis to other bones. As the disease advances exophthalmos increases, and there may be ulceration of the cornea and blindness, and evidences of increased intracranial pressure. In *diagnosis* the possibility of scurvy with orbital hemorrhage must be ruled out. Chloroma is differentiated by the characteristic blood-picture of that affection. Cases are described, as those of Volpe and Bloise,[34] in which primary lymphosarcoma of the perirenal lymph-nodes showed metastasis to the cranium and other symptoms resembling neuroblastoma of the suprarenals. The only *treatment* except symptomatic is exposure to the roentgen-ray or radium, which temporarily causes recession of the growths.

2. Neuroblastoma of the Suprarenal Gland and Liver.—This type was studied especially by Pepper[35] and cases have been reported or collected by Frew,[28] Kwartin and Twiss,[36] van Veen,[37] and Capon.[38] The *lesions* consist in neoplastic growths in the suprarenal and the liver. The malignancy is great and the *course* rapid, death often occurring in a few weeks or months. The liver becomes extensively infiltrated, and in the suprarenal the growth is hemorrhagic. There is great abdominal distention, but no jaundice, pigmentation of the skin, or ascites; and little pain.

3. Neuroblastoma of the Suprarenal Gland with Metastasis to the Long Bones.—This condition, as described by Scudder,[39] might be regarded as a third type. It occurs chiefly, or perhaps only, in adults, and exhibits a special tendency to metastasis in the long bones, although other tissues may occasionally be involved as well.

(*B*) Cortical Hypernephroma.—Cases of this have been reported and collected by Guthrie and Emery,[40] Glynn,[41] Jump et al.,[42] Ambrožič and Baar,[43] Hoag,[44] Collett,[45] and others. Males are more frequently affected. The tumor grows more slowly than neuroblastoma and has less tendency to metastasize. The *symptoms* appear to depend in part upon disturbed internal secretion of the gland. They consist chiefly in the early appearance of pubic, axillary, and facial hair; occasionally hyperplasia of the genital organs; and as a rule the production of obesity, and sometimes of unusual physical growth. It is noteworthy that there is a development of male sexual characteristics only; females showing a tendency to male characteristics, as in unusual size of the clitoris and the usual absence of early increase in size of the breasts. Males do not show any of the feminine sex-characteristics, but rather a general early somatic precocity. There is no characteristic mental change. The cases have been divided by Guthrie and Emery[40] into two types from which, however, there are distinct departures.

1. The Precociously Obese Type.—This may affect males or females. There is not true precocity of development of the generative organs, although there is well-advanced growth of body-hair on the pubis and elsewhere. There is deposit of fat; the increase being especially prominent in the abdomen, chest, mammary glands, cheeks, and neck; the extremities remaining thin. The face is dusky and congested and often exhibits stellate venules. There may be pigmentation, but no bronzing of the skin (Fig. 268). The distribution of this fat is different from that of hypopituitarism, which is more particularly in the breasts, mons veneris and hips. The obesity of pineal disease is less marked, and that disorder usually presents the evidence of intracranial tumor.

2. The Infant Hercules Type.—This is usually seen in males. There is unusual development of the muscular and skeletal system with actual sexual precocity; and obesity is absent.

As stated, some cases, such as those of Jump et al.[42] and of Ambrožič and Baar[43] (Fig. 269), occupy intermediate positions or are variants or combinations of the types described.

The *prognosis* of cortical hypernephroma is unfavorable, the patient dying before or shortly after puberty. In *diagnosis* the chief feature is the presence of precocious hirsuites without true early sexual development (although the latter may sometimes occur), combined with the discovery of an abdominal tumor. Diseases of the pineal gland, ovaries, or testes may produce sexual precocity, but often without hirsuites; while that of the pituitary body, although causing somatic overgrowth, exhibits delay in sexual development. *Treatment* consists in early surgical removal if but one gland is involved.

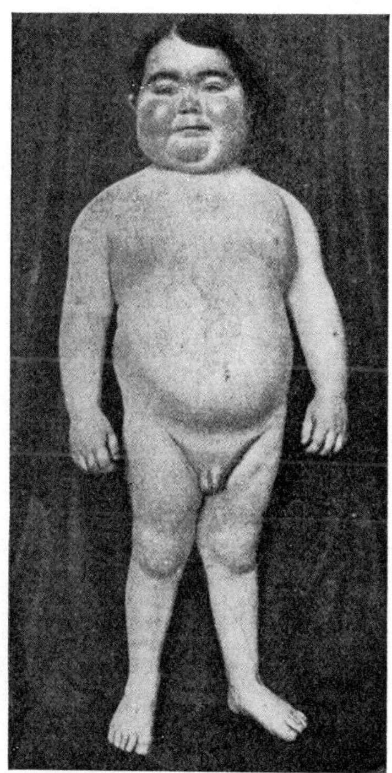

Fig. 268.—Cortical hypernephroma with precocious obesity. Boy, aged four and three-fourth years. Stoutness with growth of hair on face and pubis began two years before, cheeks large and bright red, whole upper part of the body fat, buttocks and legs not especially so, but muscular; genital organs of size for age. Died of acute tuberculosis. Necropsy showed hypernephroma. (*Guthrie and Emery, Tr. Clin. Soc., London,* 1907, **40**, 182.)

In this connection reference must be made to the fact that vestiges of suprarenal tissue may be found in other body-structures, as the kidneys, ovaries, testes, broad ligaments, spermatic veins, and elsewhere; and that a tumor of the nature of hypernephroma may develop with these remains as its base. Most frequent of these is renal hypernephroma, which, in fact, is of more common occurrence than the suprarenal growth, at least after childhood is passed. This tumor does not produce alteration in sexual characteristics.

HEMORRHAGE INTO THE SUPRARENAL GLAND

This affection, uncommon at all periods, is rarely seen after the first year of life. Systematic necropsies, however, show that it occurs more frequently than supposed, especially in the new-born. Cases have been reported and collected by Hamill,[46] Rabinowitz,[47] Corcoran and Strauss,[48] Goldzieher and Greenwald,[49] Arnold,[50] and others. Among etiologic factors mentioned are long-continued or difficult labor, septic infection through the umbilicus, eclampsia or infections of the mother; and when occurring in older infants or children the cause may be thrombosis of the suprarenal veins, syphilis, hemophilia, purpura haemorrhagica, acute infectious diseases especially diphtheria, or burns. **Pathologically** the hemorrhage may be very large, and bilateral or unilateral, in the latter event being oftenest upon the right side. It is situated especially in the medulla. In severe cases the entire gland is transformed into a sac containing blood. Blood may escape into the peritoneal cavity, and there has been noted at times thrombosis of the renal vein or of the inferior cava. The **symptoms** are obscure, but the diagnosis may sometimes be made during life by the discovery of an abdominal tumor, combined with sudden onset of abdominal pain, fever, cyanosis, anemia, perhaps purpura, and collapse. Death may

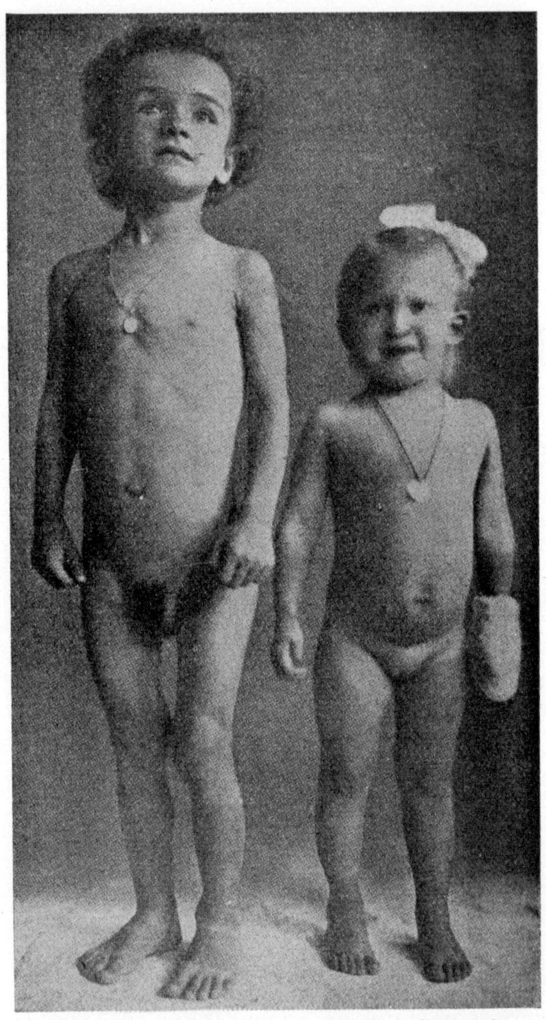

Fig. 269.—Overgrowth seen in cortical hypernephroma. Girl of three years of age resembling in size child of six years. Development of genital hair. Girl on right is normal one of equal age. (*Ambrožič and Baar, Ztschr. f. Kinderh.* 1920, **27**, 135.)

occur in a few days, sometimes with symptoms of peritonitis; oftener it seems entirely sudden. The condition has been reported as occurring almost epidemically. The **prognosis** is poor, but recovery can occur if there is not too extensive destruction of suprarenal tissue. The injection of epinephrine seems to be without much effect, but it has been recommended that the extracts of the cortex (interrenin or cortin; p. 1081) be employed.

OTHER LESIONS OF THE SUPRARENAL GLANDS

Symptoms similar to those of hypernephroma may result from a benign **hyperplasia** of the suprarenal cortex. In pseudohermaphroditism of the female type, with development of organs suggesting the male characteristics, there may be associated congenital hyperplasia of the suprarenal cortex. **Hypoplasia, atrophy** or **absence** of the glands may be found, perhaps associated with failure of development of the brain, especially anencephalus. **Syphilis** may produce interstitial changes in the glands, and **tuberculosis,** as stated, is the most frequent cause of Addison's diseases.

References

1. Deutsch. med. Wchnschr., 1914, **40,** 322. 2. Bull. Johns Hopkins Hosp., 1932, **50,** 87. 3. J. Pediat. (Tokyo), 1926, p. 1815; Ref. Am. J. Dis. Child., 1927, **33,** 834. 4. Arch. Int. Med., 1911, **8,** 851. 5. Nelson's Looseleaf Medicine **3,** 257. 6. Arch. Pediat., 1913, **30,** 179. 7. Acta med. Scandinav., 1921, **54,** 323. 8. Pediatria, 1923, **31,** 817. 9. Arch. Neurol. and Psychiat., 1925, **13,** 423; 1928, **19,** 394. 10. Arch. Neurol. and Psychiat., 1927, **18,** 724. 11. Am. J. Physiol., 1919, **48,** 397; 1926, **78,** 683; 1928, **84,** 660; J.A.M.A., 1929, **92,** 1569. 12. Beitr. d. path. Anat. u. d. allg. Path., 1928, **79,** 213. 13. Klin. Wchnschr., 1928, **7,** 1124. 14. Am. J. Physiol., 1930, **95,** 670. 15. Am. J. Physiol., 1931, **96,** 153. 16. Kinderheilkunde im Einzeldarstellungen, 1903, **3,** 567. 17. Brit. M. J., 1900, **1,** 1014. 18. New York M. J., 1907, **86,** 256. 19. Lancet, 1909, **1,** 603. 20. Thèse de Paris, 1910. 21. Brit. J. Child. Dis., 1914, **11,** 105. 22. Pediatria, 1922, **30,** 585. 23. Nederl. Tijdschr. v. Geneesk., 1927, **71,** 3295. 24. Am. J. Dis. Child., 1929, **37,** 1239. 25. J.A.M.A., 1931, **96,** 231; **97,** 1446. 26. Quart. J. Med., 1907–08, **1,** 33. 27. Am. J. M. Sc., 1908, **135,** 871. 28. Quart. J. Med., 1911, **4,** 123. 29. Brit. J. Child. Dis., 1920, **17,** 133. 30. J. Lab. and Clin. Med., 1926, **12,** 130. 31. Am. J. Dis. Child., 1927, **33,** 590. 32. J.A.M.A., 1928, **91,** 1246. 33. Edinburgh M. J., 1929, **36,** 25. 34. Arch. de méd. d. enf., 1927, **30,** 73. 35. Am. J. M. Sc., 1901, **121,** 287. 36. Am. J. Dis. Child., 1927, **34,** 61. 37. Nederl. Tijdschr. v. Geneesk., 1928, **72,** 4393. 38. J. Path. and Bact., 1928, **31,** 659. 39. Pub. Massachusetts Gen. Hosp., 1907, **1,** No. 3, 82. 40. Clin. Soc. Trans., London, 1907, **40,** 175. 41. Quart. J. Med., 1912, **5,** 157. 42. Am. J. M. Sc., 1914, **147,** 568. 43. Ztschr. f. Kinderh., 1920, **27,** 135. 44. Am. J. Dis. Child., 1923, **25,** 441. 45. Am. J. Dis. Child., 1924, **27,** 204. 46. Arch. Pediat., 1901, **18,** 81. 47. Am. J. M. Sc., 1923, **166,** 513. 48. J.A.M.A., 1924, **82,** 626. 49. Am. J. Dis. Child., 1928, **36,** 324. 50. Am. J. Dis. Child., 1930, **40,** 1053.

CHAPTER IV

DISORDERS ATTRIBUTED TO THE INTERNAL SECRETIONS AND ALLIED CONDITIONS

Certain disturbances of growth or nutrition which appear to be the result of a diseased state of one or more of the glands of internal secretion have been discussed in the previous chapter. Other conditions now to be mentioned seem, in some instances, to be also dependent upon alteration of internal secretions; although in some which will be included here for convenience the connection is quite doubtful.

INFANTILISM

While all forms of infantilism have not been shown to be dependent upon disorders of internal secretion, some of them unquestionably are, and all may be studied together. The term "infantilism" designates a continuance to some extent of the bodily and often of the psychic characteristics of infancy and childhood, and it may be employed, too, where there is a persistence of characteristics belonging to a time of life earlier than the actual age of the patient. In dwarfism (*nanism*) there may be an arrest of growth but not of development, as in cases of severe rickets, achondroplasia, chondrodystrophy, etc. There may also be infantilism without dwarfism, as in some instances of pituitary infantilism. A distinction between infantilism and dwarfism would be that in the former there is delay in or absence of sexual development, but this is not an all-inclusive differentiation, since certain of the dwarfs may be of the so-called "asexual type," and, on the other hand, the infantile characteristics may occasionally be shown in other ways than the undeveloped sexual apparatus. Infantilism may be divided into: (*A*) *The Essential group*, including ateliosis and progeria; the causes being unknown, and (*B*) *The Symptomatic group;* the cause being probably some disturbance of function to which the infantilism is secondary.

(*A*) Essential Infantilism. **1. Ateliosis.**—There is in this an inherited and familial predisposition. The arrested development, occurring generally in infancy or early childhood, results in dwarfing; the infantile characteristics existing at the time of onset persisting to a great extent. The limbs are short, the head large, the face small, and there is a general roundness of form. Gilford[1] divides the cases into two types, not always sharply differentiated. In *asexual* ateliosis there is marked delay in general bodily development, shown in some parts more than in others, the sexual organs being the most backward of all. Usually intelligence is normal. When the time for puberty arrives no change in the sexual characteristics takes place. In *sexual* ateliosis the infantile features continue until puberty, which is often delayed, and then the sexual organs and powers develop normally. In contrast to the asexual form there is then the development of epiphysial and osseous changes proper for this period and the patient becomes a miniature man or woman; although in physiognomy, proportions, and size still a child. Many professional dwarfs belong to one or the other of these classes; as, for instance, General and Mrs. Tom Thumb, and others.

2. Progeria.—The term designates premature old age. The first reports of cases of progeria appear to have been by Gilford.[2] Curtin and Kotzen[3] found 10 more or less characteristic recorded instances. There exists decided infantilism with premature senility, as shown by the early development of gray hair or of baldness, arteriosclerosis, emaciation, trophic changes in the skin and nails, etc. Also found may be a large skull with open fontanelles, a prominent nose and small facial bones, prominent abdomen with obliteration of the umbilicus, and enlarged epiphyses and joints. Death usually occurs by twenty years of age from cardiac syncope. Progeria should be distinguished from hereditary ectodermal dysplasia (p. 518). A form of premature senility may be brought about by pituitary disturbance (p. 1079).

(*B*) Symptomatic Infantilism.—The lack of development here is less marked than in ateliosis; there is absence of familial predisposition; and the cases are secondary to some morbid condition. Various types have been described, but there are two principal forms:

1. The Lorain Type.[4]—In this the subject is small, but as age increases there is nothing of the child-form except the shortness in height and the failure of development of the genitalia or sexual characteristics commensurate with the age. The head is small; the limbs slender, but long in comparison with the trunk. The intellect may be normal or retarded (Fig. 270). The proportions are those of a miniature adult. Among etiologic factors are hereditary syphilis; the lymphatic diathesis; any cause producing chronic malnutrition; congenital or acquired cardiac disease; arterial hypoplasia; chronic poisoning by tobacco, opium, lead, etc.; metabolic poisons, as produced by chronic renal insufficiency or other chronic autointoxication. The type has sometimes been considered one of the forms of hypopituitarism. In many cases no cause can be discovered.

2. The Brissaud Type.[5]—In this the body is small, the head large, the abdomen prominent, the limbs short and rounded, the trunk relatively large, and there is a tendency to obesity. The sexual organs are undeveloped and the mentality retarded (Fig. 271). The condition has sometimes been attributed to hypothyroidism (*myxedematous infantilism*) and this factor is probably present in some instances. Others have considered it

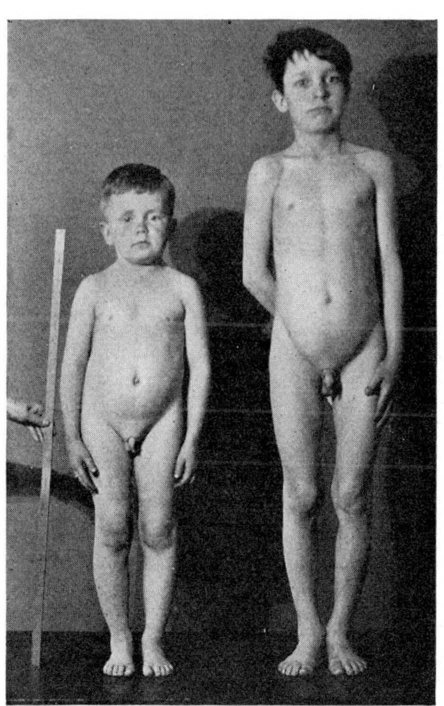

Fig. 270.

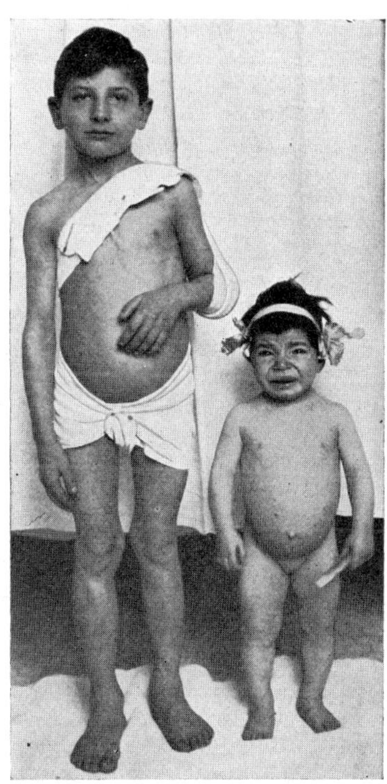

Fig. 271.

Fig. 270.—Infantilism, Lorain type. Boy, ten years. Patient in Children's Hospital, Cincinnati. Picture shows contrast with normal-sized child of same age. There are seven normal siblings. Metabolism normal for size, low for age. Mentality normal for ten years. Wassermann and tuberculin tests negative. Roentgenologic examination negative. Height 41.5 in. (105.4), weight 40.25 lb. (18.3 kg.).

Fig. 271.—Infantilism, Brissaud type. Girl, seven years. Patient University of Pennsylvania Hospital, Philadelphia. Child normal to twenty-one months when had pertussis. Since then has grown little. Said to be normal mentally. Examinations showed extremities short for size of thorax, legs bowed, skin harsh and dry, head large, hair of scalp short and moderately harsh, eyes somewhat far apart, palpebral fissures narrowed, tongue looks slightly larger than normal, but does not protrude, thyroid gland cannot be felt, and thyroid region seems less full than normal. Slight subcutaneous deposits of fat in supraspinous fossae, abdomen greatly distended. Temperature averages below normal. Height 29 in. (74 cm.), weight 20 lb. (9072 Gm.). Feces negative for bacillus bifidus, bacillus infantilis, coccal forms and fermentative forms. Roentgenogram negative. Condition practically uninfluenced by thyroid extract, thymus extract and pituitary extract. Photograph shows comparison with boy of same age and of normal development, with a height of 48 in. (122 cm.). (*Griffith, Am. J. Dis. Child.*, 1918, **16**, 103.)

dependent upon disturbed pituitary secretion. The administration of thyroid extract, while sometimes beneficial, does not give such marked results as in true cretinism, and little if any benefit is derived from the feeding of pituitary extract.

Certain other forms of symptomatic infantilism can be classified more definitely on an etiologic basis:

3. Intestinal Infantilism.—In this type (Fig. 272), studied by Herter[6] and others, there are present the symptoms of chronic intestinal indigestion (celiac disease) (p. 609); this condition being marked and leading to stunting of growth, often with delayed sexual development. As pointed out particularly by Parsons[7] there may be with it a form of rickets or osteoporosis associated with genu valgum and a low blood-phosphorus, due probably to a deficient absorption of calcium and phosphorus from the intestine, the result of impaired absorption of fat and vitamins.

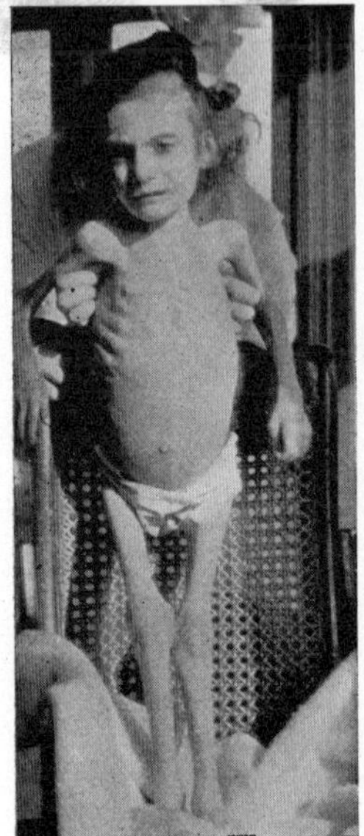

Fig. 272.—Intestinal infantilism; showing dwarfing and extreme emaciation from chronic intestinal indigestion. Girl, aged seven years four months. Patient in Children's Hospital of Philadelphia, Sept., 1923 with chronic intestinal indigestion. Weight 18 lb. Suffered from more or less constant diarrhea with large, loose, offensive, undigested stools of light color not much mucus but without excess of fat. Bacteriologic examination revealed no characteristic organisms. Dietetic treatment of various sorts entirely without influence. Death after several months.

4. Pancreatic Infantilism.—This form was so named by Bramwell.[8] It is allied to, if not identical with, intestinal infantilism. Bramwell's case appeared to improve following the administration of a pancreatic extract.

5. Pituitary Infantilism.—This is often called "Fröhlich's[9] syndrome" or "dystrophia adiposogenitalis" (Bartels[10]). It is believed to depend upon tumor or disturbed function of the anterior lobe of the pituitary gland. The symptoms, apart from those of increased intracranial pressure when tumor is present, are connected with development. Some cases are not associated with tumor, but appear to be due to a simple hypopituitarism. Much is still lacking in our knowledge of the relationship of the pituitary body to the symptoms attributed to it (p. 1079). In Fröhlich's syndrome the sexual organs remain infantile in character; or, in patients in whom the disease begins in adult life, undergo a reversion to some extent to the infantile condition. There is no axillary or pubic hair. The marked obesity present is general, although more pronounced in the trunk, mammae, mons veneris, and hips. Polyuria and polydipsia may sometimes be observed. There is often an unusual tolerance for carbohydrates, as shown by the blood-sugar curve (p. 154). Basal metabolism may be below normal. The temperature is often subnormal. There may be general sluggishness and asthenia. The condition may occur in more than one child in the same generation. Retarded skeletal development is a feature, but it is possible for the reverse of this to occur, as observed in 1 of our own cases (Fig. 273); this perhaps depending upon activation of the anterior lobe combined with insufficiency of the posterior lobe (Cushing[11]). At times there may be associated mental deficiency, retinitis pigmentosa, and polydactylism, as in the 4 cases in a family reported by Solis-Cohen and Weiss.[12] Weiss[13] later reported 2 somewhat similar cases in a family, in which, instead of retinitis, there was nerve-deafness. Other cases, often familial, have been described; 36 according to Bing,[14] and 48 according to Weiss,[13] and the condition has been supposed to be due to defective development of the forebrain rather than to pituitary deficiency alone. This has also been called "cerebral adiposity" or the *Laurence-Moon-Biedl syndrome* (Laurence and Moon;[15] Biedl[16]).

Among other forms of infantilism may be mentioned **hepatic infantilism,** in which infantilism and stunted growth are associated with cirrhosis of the liver (Lereboullet;[17] Göttche;[18] Exchaquet[19]). In some of these cases there is a familial tendency. Hypoglycemia and hypercholesterolemia have been found. Another variety is **renal infantilism,** dependent upon chronic renal insufficiency and not infrequently associated with a form of rickets (renal rickets (see p. 821)). **Cardiac infantilism** may be dependent upon congenital heart disease (Herrman[20]), or upon hypoplasia of the heart and arteries, as in some cases of the Lorain type (Weber[21]). Infantilism may be associated with **status lymphaticus. Diseases of the thyroid gland** produce stunting of growth and failure of development, as in cretinism, the Brissaud type of infantilism, and probably in other forms. It is possible that the **thymus gland** or the **suprarenals** may be operative in certain cases of infantilism. The **testes** have an influence upon the development of sexual characteristics, and some cases of infantilism may depend upon disturbance of the internal secretion of these organs; although this may be associated with gigantism rather than with dwarfism. The interdependence of various internal glands in the production of infantile characteristics needs further study. **Simple correlated infantilism** or *nanism* may be associated with achondroplasia, muscular dystrophy, hydrocephalus, microcephalus, and mongolism.

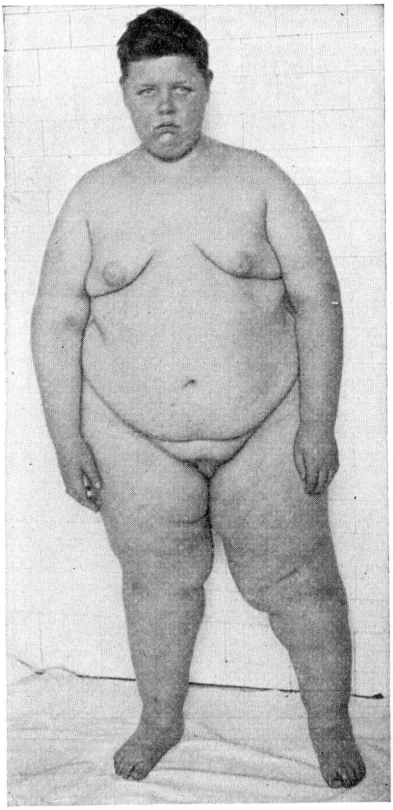

The **treatment** of infantilism is directed to the cause. For example, in cretinism thyroid extract should be given, and it may be tried also in the Brissaud type. Pituitary extract may be administered in Fröhlich's syndrome with the hope of benefit. In the Herter type the intestinal condition should be corrected if possible. For the last Miller[22] recommends the use of bile salts, although Parsons[7] and others have shown that these are not absent from the intestinal tract.

Fig. 273.—Pituitary infantilism. Boy, aged eleven years. Admitted to the University of Pennsylvania Hospital. The tendency to obesity appeared at the age of eleven months, and has increased since then. Is mentally bright. Height 5 ft., 1 in. (160 cm.), weight 251 lb. (113,851). Penis small for his age and very small in comparison with his other development, buried in fat, testicles descended and very small, almost no trace of pubic hair. Roentgenogram showed sella turcica definitely smaller than normal, indicating a small pituitary body. Sugar-tolerance increased, but this diminished markedly after continued administration of pituitary extract. Prolonged treatment practically without effect on the obesity. (*Griffith, Am. J. Dis. Child.*, 1918, **16**, 103.)

OBESITY

Not all cases of adipositas are dependent upon disordered internal secretions, but as others of them are, they may all be considered here. The boundaries between the development of abundant adipose tissue which is within physiologic limits, and pathologic obesity are not sharply defined. Striking examples of congenital obesity are collected and reported by Braoude,[23] including a case of Chambers weighing 16 lb. (7257) at birth. Belcher[24] records the case of a new-born infant weighing 25 lb. (11,349) and measuring 28 in. (71) in length. Foscue[25] reports three babies from one mother all weighing over 13 lb., one of them 14 lb. 6 oz. (6520). Some of these should be regarded as being precociously large rather than obese (p. 1091). After the period of infancy is passed, decided obesity is not common in early life. A few instances of hemiobesity have been reported, as the case of Shaw[26] and that of Hutchison.[27] Heredity is an uncommon **cause** in children, although its influence is frequently seen in adults. The commonest factor is diet, which may be active even in breast-fed infants, as shown by Heubner[28] and others. In the obesity of later childhood, seen rather oftener in females, diet plays a prominent part also, the food being excessive in fat or carbohydrate or in total caloric value. The factor of exercise is important, a child who is very active tolerating an amount of food which in a less energetic subject might produce obesity. Apart from this some persons appear to store fat to a greater extent than others, although the cause of this metabolic difficulty is unknown (Cannon[29]). According to Newburgh[30] the basal metabolism of obese persons per square meter of body surface is normal. This author also claims that all obesity is "simple obesity," in the sense that the increase in weight merely represents an inflow of energy greater than the outflow. In addition to the causes mentioned obesity is an attendant upon pituitary disturbance, hypernephroma; and sometimes upon lymphatism, cretinism (here largely dependent upon myxedema), pineal tumor, hypogonadism, etc. It sometimes follows encephalitis. The **symptoms** consist of the deposition of fat, which is distributed differently from that seen in middle age. There is not the special tendency to abdominal fat, but the face is full and round, the cheeks and eyelids full, the upper and lower part of the trunk affected alike, the mammae in both sexes large from the deposition of fat, and the extremities fat. This description does not necessarily apply to obesity dependent upon disordered internal secretions, as in Fröhlich's syndrome (p. 1088), hypernephroma (p. 1082), etc. The **treatment** apart from cases due to diseases of the internal glands consists chiefly in a modification of the diet of such a nature that the tendency to obesity may be checked, but the normal strength and development of the patient maintained. In some instances of obese breast-fed infants the excessive deposit of fat will disappear when weaning takes place. In general the amount of carbohydrate, and especially of fat, in the diet, should be reduced, and perhaps the total amount of nourishment as well. These changes should be made gradually, watching carefully the alterations in weight. Green vegetables and fruit should replace to a considerable extent the starchy foods. There must always be the ingestion of a sufficient amount of protein to assure maintenance and growth. A diminution in the quantity of liquid ingested may be of service. Increased exercise should be insisted upon. Thyroid extract should be administered only in cases where hypothyroidism is suspected, or where the basal metabolism can be carefully watched. The obesity of hypopituitarism may possibly be affected by giving pituitary extract, and sometimes thyroid extract as well.

LIPODYSTROPHIA PROGRESSIVA

This uncommon affection was described under this title by Simons,[31] although similar cases had been earlier reported by Campbell,[32] and Barraquer,[33] and 1 was studied by Osler in 1895 (Weber[34]). Reports and reviews are those by Feer,[35] Herrman,[36] Weber,[37] Boissonas,[38] Carreau,[39]

Klien,[40] Schwenke,[41] Reuben et al.,[42] Coates,[43] Pollock and Gill,[44] Kerley and Blanchard,[45] Bilderback,[46] and Parmelee.[47] The last mentioned author, who reports 6 cases, states that 75 had previously been recorded, but this figure probably does not include all the reported instances. We have seen 3 cases which have not been reported. The **cause** is obscure, but it has been surmised that the endocrine glands are at fault or that there has been an encephalitic or toxic affection of the thalamic or subthalamic regions of the midbrain. Usually, however, nothing is discovered at necropsy. The condition is more common in females and usually begins in later childhood. Rarely if ever is more than one person in a family attacked. The **symptoms** consist in progressive and finally complete wasting of the subcutaneous fat of the face, arms and trunk. The skin is entirely normal. The face is usually first to be affected, and the advance to other regions is slow. A characteristic is the overdevelopment of the fat of the buttocks, hips and thighs, and to a less extent of the calves. This generally does not begin until several years after the onset of the disease. The general health is in no way involved, nor is the duration of life curtailed. Calcareous deposits may occur in the skin. **Treatment** has been of no avail.

HEMIHYPERTROPHY AND HEMIATROPHY

In **hemihypertrophy,** which is almost invariably congenital, a part or the whole of one side of the body is larger than the other; the latter being of normal appearance. It has been considered by some as a unilateral gigantism, and it has been suggested, although not proved, that it may depend upon some disorder of the glands of internal secretion or of the sympathetic nervous system. Females are oftener affected. The right side is involved more frequently than the left. Rarely the two sides tend to become more equal in development as the child grows older. Mental defect is sometimes observed. The paired internal organs may also show a difference in size. Malformation of other sorts may be present. In some cases hemihypertrophy may develop because of congenital arteriovenous fistula, as reported by Horton,[48] and as we have seen in one typical instance. Cases of hemihypertrophy have also been reported by Houzel, Schekter and Babonneix;[49] Lance,[50] and others. Fenner[51] published an observation in which the hypertrophy of the lower left leg was apparently dependent upon a fibrosarcoma. Further reports and reviews have been made by Coston,[52] Stanton and Tuft,[53] Fenstrup,[54] Wakefield,[55] Kitaigorodskaja,[56] Stoesser,[57] and Gesell.[58] The last author reports 2 cases and reviews 53 previously recorded instances of total hemihypertrophy. In true hemihypertrophy the skeletal system is involved as well as other tissues, whereas in certain other conditions due to local influences, as mentioned above, or in elephantiasis (p. 1064) or Milroy's disease (p. 1094), the bones are not affected.

In **hemiatrophy,** which is also congenital and rarely seen, all or nearly all of one side of the body is smaller than normal. In some cases there is atrophy of the face on one side and of the body on the other. Cases have been recorded by Rachford,[59] Garzon,[60] Weber,[61] (whose case was connected in some way with congenital multiple chondromata), Tobias,[62] Pollak,[63] and others. There appears to be an etiologic connection in most cases with disease of the sympathetic nervous system. A partial review of the literature is given by Kraus and Perkins.[64] Progressive facial hemiatrophy is described elsewhere (p. 983).

PRECOCITY

Mental precocity has already been discussed (p. 902). Here is considered only precocious development of the body or its functions, in whole or in part. This is seen oftener in females, and is then represented either by precocious menstruation alone (p. 854); or by a more general precocious maturity, perhaps accompanied by general somatic overdevelopment. Excessive birth-weight has been referred to under Obesity (p. 1090). In male subjects there may be emission of semen as early as two or three years of age (Neurath;[65] Reuben and Manning[66]).

In typical cases of premature menstruation or precocious maturity there is no discoverable cause. There are, however, others in both sexes in which the premature sexual development is dependent upon disorder of such internal glands as the suprarenal, pineal, and the gonads. Gigantism can be called a form of somatic precocity, although in such cases there may be sexual underdevelopment.

References

1. Lancet, 1914, **1,** 587. 2. Practitioner, 1904, **73,** 188. 3. Am. J. Dis. Child., 1929, **38,** 993. 4. Preface de la Thèse de Faneau de la Cour., Paris, 1871; Ref. Apert in Traité d. mal. de l'enf. (Grancher, etc.), 1904, **1,** 993. 5. Leçons sur l. mal. nerv., 1895, 625. 6. Trans. Assn. Am. Phys., 1910, **25,** 528; Intestinal Infantilism, 1908. 7. Birmingham M. Rev., 1913, **74,** 33; Arch. Dis. Childhood, 1927, **2,** 198; Am. J. Dis. Child., 1932, **43,** 1293. 8. Scottish M. and S. J., 1904, **14,** 321. 9. Wien. klin. Rundsch., 1901, **15,** 883. 10. Ztschr. f. Augenheilk., 1906, **16,** 407; 530. 11. The Pituitary Body, 1912, 177. 12. Am. J. M. Sc., 1925, **169,** 489. 13. Endocrinology, 1931, **15,** 435; Am. J. M. Sc., 1932, **183,** 268. 14. Norsk. Mag. f. Laegervidensk., 1931, **92,** 956. 15. Brit. Ophthalm. Rev., 1866, **2,** 32. 16. Deutsch. med. Wchnschr., 1922, **48,** 1630. 17. Les cirrhoses biliaires, 1902, 76. 18. Monatschr. f. Kinderh., 1927, **35,** 305. 19. Arch. de méd. d. enf., 1931, **34,** 656. 20. Arch. Pediat., 1922, **39,** 45. 21. Brit. J. Child. Dis., 1913, **10,** 203. 22. Lancet, 1920, **2,** 894. 23. Thèse de Paris, 1900. 24. J.A.M.A., 1916, **67,** 950. 25. Med. Rec., 1921, **100,** 1076. 26. Proc. Roy. Soc., 1914, **8,** 1, 15. 27. Brit. J. Child. Dis., 1904, **1,** 258. 28. Kinderheilk., 1911, **2,** 52. 29. Physiol. Rev., 1929, **9,** 399. 30. J.A.M.A., 1931, **97,** 1659. 31. Ztschr. f. d. ges. Neurol. u. Psychiat., Orig., 1911, **5,** 29. 32. Trans. Clin. Soc., London, 1907, **40,** 272. 33. Neurol. Zentralbl.,1 907, **26,** 1072. 34. Ref. Weber., Proc. Roy. Soc. Med., 1913, **6,** Neurol. Sec., 130. 35. Jahrb. f. Kinderh., 1915, **82,** 1. 36. Arch. Int. Med., 1916, **17,** 516. 37. Quart. J. Med., 1917, **10,** 131; Brit. J. Child. Dis., 1917, **14,** 81; 179. 38. Rev. Neurol., 1919, **26,** 721. 39. Arch. lat.-am. de pediat., 1921, Nov.–Dec., Ref. Arch. de méd. d. enf., 1923, **26,** 511. 40. München. med. Wchnschr., 1921, **68,** 206. 41. Deutsch. med. Wchnschr., 1922, **48,** 292. 42. Arch. Pediat., 1924, **41,** 480; 1928, **45,** 127. 43. Brit. J. Child. Dis., 1925, **22,** 194. 44. Arch. Pediat., 1927, **44,** 42. 45. Arch. Pediat., 1927, **44,** 232. 46. J.A.M.A., 1929, **93,** 1052. 47. J.A.M.A., 1932, **98,** 548. 48. J.A.M.A., 1932, **98,** 373. 49. Bull. soc. de pediat. de Paris, 1928, **25,** 409. 50. Bull. soc. de pediat. de Paris, 1928, **25,** 418. 51. M. J. and Record, 1926, **123,** 501. 52. Med. Rec., 1920, **97,** 222. 53. J.A.M.A., 1923, **80,** 1432. 54. Acta paediat., 1926, **6,** 205. 55. Ann. Int. Med., 1927, **1,** 292. 56. Jahrb. f. Kinderh., 1929, **125,** 38. 57. Am. J. Dis. Child., 1928, **35,** 885. 58. Arch. Neurol. u. Psychiat., 1921, **6,** 400; Am. J. M. Sc., 1927, **173,** 542. 59. New York M. J., 1920, **112,** 677. 60. Arch. lat.-am. de pediat., 1916, Nov.–Dec.; Ref. Arch. de méd. d. enf., 1917, **20,** 654. 61. Brit. J. Child. Dis., 1920, **17,** 85. 62. Arch. Pediat., 1928, **45,** 673. 63. Arch. f. Dermat. u. Syph., 1930, **159,** 188. 64. Arch. Neurol. and Psychiat., 1927, **18,** 249. 65. Erbeg. d. inn. Med. u. Kinderh., 1909, **4,** 46. 66. Arch. Pediat., 1922, **39,** 769.

SECTION XII

DISEASES OF THE SKIN, EYE AND EAR

CHAPTER I

DISEASES OF THE SKIN

DERMATOLOGY as it applies to early life is so large a subject, and requires such special knowledge, that no attempt can be made here to consider it at any length. Only those disorders will be discussed which are entirely or largely limited to infancy and childhood, or which are of frequent occurrence at this period or exhibit special features incident to it. The involvement of the skin in various diseases, as typhoid fever, meningococcic meningitis, purpura, the eruptive fevers and the like, has been mentioned in the appropriate sections. Congenital anomalies and defects of the skin are rare and of academic interest only. Ectodermal dysplasia has been described elsewhere (p. 518).

SUBCUTANEOUS EMPHYSEMA

Developing in the eyelids this may result from fracture of the orbit, permitting air to enter from the sinuses. In the neck it may follow tracheotomy, deep ulceration in the mouth and pharynx, esophageal wounds or gastric ulcer; or oftener emphysema of the mediastinum. Appearing primarily in the thorax, it may be the result of rupture of a pulmonary lesion, usually tuberculous, combined with local obliteration of the pleural sac; but is more often caused by thoracentesis under the same condition of obliteration. The direct cause may be violent cough or severe dyspnea. Subcutaneous emphysema may also come about through infection with gas-producing organisms. It may rarely occur in the new-born; then perhaps due to trauma of labor.

EDEMA

Cutaneous edema is but a symptom produced by a large number of etiologic factors. Rarely there is *fetal edema* in which the infant is still-born or lives at most a few days. *Oedema neonatorum* and *fetal erythroblastosis* are described elsewhere (pp. 245, 246). Edema from *nephritis* (p. 817) may occur even in infancy; and the influence of *gastro-intestinal diseases* and of *syphilis* in the production of dropsy should not be forgotten. Occasionally there has been observed edema having the distribution and appearance of nephritis, yet without albumin or casts in the urine. We[1] have reviewed this subject elsewhere. *Cardiac edema* is common. *Marantic* edema is frequent in greatly debilitated infants; and also in older children who are exhausted from any cause. The edema of malnutrition, in some instances at least, depends upon a low serum-protein; the low osmotic pressure permitting excessive infiltration of fluid from capillaries into intercellular tissue. The best treatment for this is transfusion of blood. Allied to marantic edema is that due to *excessive amounts of starch* (p. 467). *Severe anemia* is another cause, as is *purpura.* There is described an *essential edema,* sometimes congenital, in which ascites is combined with hydrothorax and perhaps general anascarca without discoverable cause. Rost[2] reports a case belonging in this category.

Localized edema is seen in *erysipelas*, *eczema*, and *cutaneous infections*. It may occur in the face in *measles;* about the eyelids in severe *pertussis;* and in various parts of the body from *mechanical interference* with the circulation, as by tumors or enlarged glands. Circumscribed swelling is characteristic of *angioneurotic edema* (p. 1095). Tetany is frequently accompanied by edema of the hands and feet, and sometimes, perhaps, by generalized edema (Shannon[3]). *Elephantiasis* is another cause of localized edema. *Persistent localized edema*, either congenital or acquired, may occur. In some instances this is hereditary in character (*Milroy's*[4] *disease*). This form of congenital edema has a definite familial tendency; is very persistent; is limited to one or both lower extremities; is permanent and yields to pitting; is without constitutional symptoms; and the swollen limb is painless. A case of this was seen at the Cincinnati General Hospital and reported by Higgins.[5] Other instances have been recorded (see Stoesser[6]). We[1] encountered a case of edema of the left leg and face, not pitting on pressure, beginning at the age of three months, and still persisting when the patient was examined at the age of four years. A somewhat similar condition was reported by Marcus,[7] which he attributed to anomalous development of the lymphatic system; and a case of this localized edema was recorded by Leopold and Rogatz,[8] thought to be due to maldevelopment of the sympathetic nervous system. Apert and Bach[9] refer to an instance of edema of the face of unknown origin disappearing with thyroid treatment.

URTICARIA

Hives is a common affection which makes its appearance at any age. It may occur even in the first few weeks or months of life, and in exclusively breast-fed infants; then perhaps being due to the transmission of allergins through the mother's milk. There is some relation to other allergic, or presumably allergic, disorders, as hay fever, asthma, angioneurotic edema, eczema, and erythema multiforme; these conditions perhaps alternating with attacks of urticaria. A hereditary predisposition is seen in some instances. Attacks may attend indigestion, but, independently of this, many children exhibit idiosyncrasy to articles of the diet which act as the exciting causes. These articles vary with the individual, but among those oftenest causing urticaria are shell-fish, strawberries or other fruit, eggs, and the like. (See Allergy, p. 484.) Urticaria may be initiated by intestinal worms; various medicaments, (p. 1097); the hypodermic injection of foreign protein; exposure to pollens or animal emanations; the presence on the skin of parasites; the cutaneous irritation produced by certain caterpillars and moths, jelly-fish, nettles, and the like. Attacks may occur in hypersensitive persons on exposure to light, heat, cold, freezing, burns and scratching. The **symptoms** in typical cases consist in the production of pale-red or white, round, oval or sometimes irregular flattened elevations, varying much in size. They may appear suddenly and last but a few hours. The lesions are few or many, and may come out in crops. They are attended by itching and burning. Especially in young children, and most of all in infants, there may be a modification of the rash with a tendency to form papules, papulo-vesicles, vesicles, and sometimes pustules (*urticaria papulosa, lichen urticatus*, etc.). In *urticaria pigmentosa* the urticarial wheals persist as pigmented areas. Ray and Kiyasu[10] have collected 282 such cases reported in patients under fifteen years of age.

The **prognosis** is favorable and the duration in the ordinary form is usually only a few days; but this may extend into weeks and the disease is sometimes very persistent; while in other cases there is a great tendency to recurrence. The **diagnosis** of the ordinary form is easy, but it is necessary to exclude the bites and stings of insects. Urticaria papulosa is difficult of recognition, unless the wheals can be found, and these are often of very temporary duration.

Treatment.—Prophylaxis consists in removing the cause of the attacks, or perhaps in desensitization (p. 487). It may be necessary to remove one article of diet after another, until the offending substance is discovered. Treatment of the attack consists in giving a saline purge; the administration of full doses of an alkali as sodium bicarbonate; and the employment of sedatives if necessary. Internally there have been advised salicylates; calcium; and, in chronic cases, atropine and arsenic. Severe cases sometimes respond well to the hypodermic administration of adrenaline, and ephedrine administered orally has been recommended. During the attack many substances are recommended for use locally to allay the itching. A good preparation is a solution of bicarbonate of soda which is applied and allowed to dry. A powder of camphor dr. 1 (3.9); zinci oxidum oz. ½ (15.5); amylum oz. ½ (15.5) frequently gives relief. In older children lotions containing small amounts of carbolic acid may be employed, if the lesions are not too numerous and extensive (p. 1099).

ANGIONEUROTIC EDEMA

(Acute Circumscribed Edema; Giant Urticaria)

Angioneurotic edema, as it was entitled by Quincke,[11] is a vasomotor neurosis; in some instances, at least, apparently of an allergic nature (p. 484). A good bibliography on the subject is given by Dunlap and Lemon.[12] It is not common at any time of life and least in infancy and early childhood. It is frequently hereditary in nature. The attacks may depend upon exposure to cold, digestive disturbances, or the action of certain articles of diet. The **symptoms** consist in the sudden development of localized, nonpitting edema, situated oftenest on the face, genitalia, or the extremities. Sometimes the mucous membranes, as of the tongue, pharynx or larynx are involved. The duration is generally from a few hours to a few days, and there is decided tendency to recurrence. The **treatment** consists in removing the cause if this can be found; the employment of the same measures as recommended for urticaria (see above); and, if the study of the patient indicates, desensitization to the initiating substance. (See Allergy, p. 487.)

ERYTHEMA

Some of the various forms of this seen in early life require consideration.

Erythema Simplex consists of simple redness in localized small or larger areas, sometimes with edema, but without true inflammation. It may result from exposure to the sun's rays (*erythema solare; sun-burn*), from heat applied in other-ways, or from exposure to cold (*erythema pernio; chilblain; frost-bite*). (See p. 1099.) The **treatment** consists in local soothing ointments, as those of zinc oxide or boric acid. Frequently powders are more satisfactory, as those of bismuth, zinc oxide, or starch; or a wash may be used, as one of pulv. zinc. carb. praecip., pulv. zinc. ox., pulv. amyli, glycerin, each 4 dr. (15.6); water to make 1 pint (473).

Erythema Intertrigo.—This is a severer form of erythema, not infrequently passing into an eczema. It results from friction between two moist surfaces, or the continued contact of soiled diapers, particularly if there is an abnormal condition of the feces or urine present. The **treatment** consists in cleanliness and dryness, and the application of powders or lotions as in erythema simplex. Sometimes a stiff zinc paste containing lanoline and with starch added, is useful. It is often beneficial to expose the parts carefully to the sun's rays or to artificial heat; and the mere fact that the diapers are not used for a few days, but the buttocks exposed to warm air, will frequently result in cure of obstinate irritation.

Erythema Multiforme (*Erythema Exudativum*).—This differs from the two types just described in that a certain degree of inflammation is present. The **cause** is uncertain, but is perhaps a toxemia, and in some instances it is of an allergic nature. The disease is common, especially in autumn and spring. It may be associated with disordered digestion, and not infrequently with urticaria and purpura rheumatica (p. 1040). Psychic or reflex nervous influences may occasion it in some instances; in others it may follow the ingestion of certain drugs (p. 1097). The **symptoms** in typical cases consist in the development of bright-reddish, and later bluish or purplish, somewhat elevated patches, or of papules or vesicles, scattered or grouped, and often somewhat symmetrically arranged. The favorite seats are on the dorsum of the hands, the forearms, the tibial regions, and the face or neck, but sometimes the eruption is widespread. The rash may appear in one or in numerous crops. Occasionally mucous membranes are attacked. At the onset there may be slight fever or rheumatic or abdominal pain, but oftener no general symptoms. Locally there may be moderate itching and burning.

A number of varieties are described; all, however, only modifications of the one disease. *Erythema papulatum* exhibits flat, reddish to purplish papules; *erythema tuberculatum* has similar but larger or more prominent lesions; *erythema iris* shows areas of concentric rings of vesiclo-papules or papules, the lesions at the center of the group fading while fresh ones develop on the periphery; *erythema circinatum* is in the form of concentric patches, not vesicular, with the center fading while the periphery extends; and *erythema marginatum* exhibits a large irregular, gyrate periphery, with faded center. The **duration** of erythema multiforme may be from a few days to a few weeks, but occasionally is chronic, with frequent recurrences over a period of years. The **diagnosis** rests especially upon the acute course, the multiform character of the eruption, the absence of severe itching, and the tendency to recurrence. The **treatment** consists in the administration of a laxative, the restriction of the diet, the administration of alkalies, and rest. Salicylates are sometimes given, but do not appear to be of much value. If there is much local itching a dusting powder or a lotion may be employed, as advised for erythema simplex (p. 1095). If an allergic relationship is discovered, the offending substance should be eliminated and perhaps desensitization carried out. (See Allergy, p. 487.)

Erythema Scarlatiniforme.—This disorder has been described in the section on differential diagnosis of scarlet fever (p. 263). Here it should be stated that a scarlatiniform rash may occur in a number of conditions, as the prodromal rash of varicella, variola, typhoid fever, grippe, and diphtheria; may attend tonsillitis, rheumatism, and sepsis (due to streptococci, staphylococci and other organisms); may be produced by drugs, as belladonna and quinine; or may follow injections of foreign serum. The giving of an enema may occasionally be followed by the appearance of a scarlatiniform rash. There are well-marked cases in which no cause is discoverable. In none of the conditions mentioned is the rash accompanied by the appearance of the throat and tongue seen in typical scarlet fever; and desquamation, if it occurs at all, appears after only a few days and is slight in character. There is no contagiousness.

An exception to these statements is seen in the condition known as *recurrent desquamative scarlatiniform erythema.* This has a widespread, intense rash, with moderately severe constitutional symptoms, and an abundant, lamellar desquamation, with the skin of the hands and feet occasionally shed in the form of casts. Such an attack may last in all three or four weeks. It may sometimes be impossible to make a certain diagnosis from scarlatinia in the first attack, but recurrences are prone to occur, and the diagnostic difficulty is then removed.

Erythema Nodosum.—This not common variety of erythema is seen oftenest in young adults and children, especially in females. Raggio[13] reports it in an infant of nineteen months. We have never observed it in infancy. It sometimes occurs in the course of such conditions as malaria, scarlatina, syphilis and diphtheria; may follow or be accompanied by gastro-intestinal disturbances; or may be associated with rheumatism. Ernberg;[14] Hambro;[15] Wallgren;[16] Dickey,[17] and many others have observed a close association with tuberculosis, based upon a positive tuberculin-reaction, roentgenograms of the bronchial glands, the later development of active tuberculosis, and the obtaining of tubercle bacilli in the sputum or by lavage of the stomach. (See p. 421.) By some the disease is regarded as an allergic manifestation of tuberculosis. (See p. 422.) A confusing observation is that of Magni,[18] who found that during the course of erythema nodosum children who had previously had a negative tuberculin-reaction showed a positive one, which later again became negative. Certain authors have considered the condition a specific infectious disease (nodal fever); others as one which is not due to tuberculosis, but predisposes to it. It probably fairly represents prevailing opinions to say that many cases are associated with early tuberculous infection elsewhere in the body, but that there are others which may occur without this factor being present. The **symptoms** may begin with slight constitutional disturbances, as fever and pain in the joints; or without these there may suddenly develop large, nodular swellings, varying in number from a few up to a dozen or more, and in circumference from that of a cherry to that of a hen's egg. They are of a reddish tint, turning often to bluish or purplish as they progress, and then suggesting the color of a fading bruise. They are shining, without sharply defined borders, painful and tender, and at first hard, although later they may become softer. They are seen most frequently upon the anterior tibial region of both legs, less often on the arms and forearms. Any constitutional symptoms present disappear after a few days. The individual nodes last about a week, but there is a tendency for the lesions to appear in crops. Recurrence is uncommon. Erythema nodosum has been reported in epidemic form (Wallgren[19]). The **prognosis** is favorable, although very rarely severe and even fatal cases have been recorded. The lesions never suppurate. The differential **diagnosis** from erythema multiforme is made by the nodular character and limited distribution of the lesions. From bruises, abscesses, and gummata erythema nodosum is distinguished by the sudden onset, the symmetrical distribution of the lesions, their number, and the absence of suppuration. **Treatment** consists chiefly in rest. If pain is severe, salicylates or other analgesics may be given, or hot fomentations applied. A roentgenogram of the chest should always be taken and, in any event, the child should be closely observed after an attack for evidence of tuberculous disease.

DRUG-ERUPTIONS

Here may be grouped a number of eruptions produced by the absorption of ingested drugs. Many of these are to be classed as erythemata; others more properly as dermatitis. Only those especially liable to occur in early life will be mentioned.

Antipyrine sometimes produces a macular rash much suggesting measles. Occasionally it may give rise to an urticarial, vesicular, or hemorrhagic eruption. The administration of *arsenic* may occasionally be followed by an eruption of almost any type, in some instances extensively pigmented. *Belladonna* in full doses produces an intense scarlatiniform erythema, most marked in the upper parts of the body, and especially well-shown on the forehead. The *bromides* may occasion lesions of various sorts; vesicular, acneform, pemphigoid, large papular or echthymatous (Fig. 274). The mucous membranes are occasionally attacked. It is possible for the drug to affect the infant through the milk of the mother. *Chloral* may cause a scarlatinal eruption; sometimes one of some other nature. The *iodides* give rise oftenest to an acneform eruption; less frequently to other rashes—bullous, erythematous, purpuric, papular or vesicular. *Opium* occasionally produces erythema or urticaria. *Quinine* in certain cases is the cause of a desquamative scarlatiniform erythema. The *salicylates* sometimes cause erythematous or purpuric rashes. *Santonin* rarely is followed by urticaria. *Sulphonal* may bring about a rubeoloid or scarlatiniform erythema, and phenobarbital a similar, or an urticarial, rash. *Hexamethylenamine* may cause a maculo-papular rash. *Phenolphthalein* occasionally produces an urticarial eruption. *Ephedrine* has been reported as the cause of an erythematous and also of a purpuric eruption.

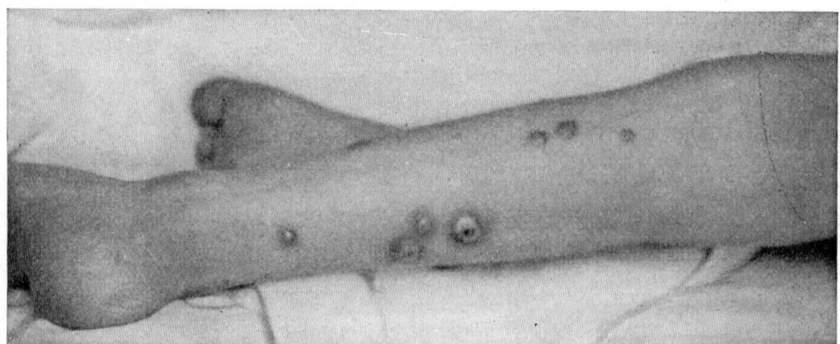

Fig. 274.—Bromide eruption. Ecthymatous eruption following the administration of potassium bromide in a case of cerebrospinal fever. From a patient in the Children's Hospital of Philadelphia.

Finally in this category are to be included the eruptions following the *injection of sera* (see Allergy, p. 485), as seen, for instance, in that of diphtheria-antitoxin. There may exceptionally be a widespread erythema soon after the injection is given. Generally, however, the cutaneous symptoms appear from the fifth to the ninth day after the injection, and consist oftenest in an extensive development of urticaria, or in other frequent cases in an eruption resembling erythema multiforme, or one of either a scarlatiniform or rubeoloid type. Usually a rise of temperature accompanies the appearance of the rash and articular pain and constitutional symptoms may be present. (See p. 485.)

DERMATITIS

Inflammation of the skin is chiefly the result of the action of external influences. The causes are heterogenous, and the intensity of the inflammation differs greatly in the various forms. The following types may be enumerated:

Dermatitis Venenata.—Here are included the eruptions produced by the local effect of some substance poisonous to the skin of the individual. In many instances there exists a distinct idiosyncrasy. Most frequently in children the poison-ivy (*Rhus toxicodendron*) or sometimes some other species of sumach is the cause. The **symptoms** consist in burning and itching, soon followed by erythema and edema, and then by the development of numerous vesicles and bullae, which rupture readily and discharge yellowish serum drying in soft crusts. The most common situations are those most exposed to direct contact with the poison, or through transmission by the hands; viz. the hands, face and external genitals. Not infrequently the swelling of the face is so great that the eyes are almost or quite closed. A slight febrile reaction may be present, and the general discomfort is often intense. At the end of about a week the acute symptoms are usually over.

Of the numerous other plants which are productive of a dermatitis in susceptible persons, the primrose (*primula*) stands next in frequency. The eruption may be like that of the poison-ivy rash or be bullous or urticarial in nature. Among other substances used locally and capable of giving rise to dermatitis venenata may be mentioned croton oil and tartar emetic, either of which produces a pustular eruption; iodoform, causing an erythematous or vesicular dermatitis; carbolic acid, occasioning an erythematous eruption followed in severe cases by actual loss of substance, as in a burn; and mercury which sometimes produces a severe inflammation.

The **diagnosis** of dermatitis venenata from eczema is not always easy. It rests chiefly upon the very acute onset and the limitation to the exposed regions. The **treatment** will be considered especially as it applies to the commonest form, poison ivy rash. Other varieties are benefited by the same applications. A large number of remedies have been suggested. At the first appearance of the rash washing the entire body with a strong alkaline soap or a solution of sodium bicarbonate may in some cases prevent further involvement of the skin. The employment of lotio nigra followed by zinc ointment has long been popular, as have diluted liquor plumbi subacetatis, tincture of the chloride of iron, or a saturated solution of boric acid. With all these it is necessary, but difficult, to keep the surface of the skin constantly moist, as by the wearing of a mask for the face; otherwise when dry the skin feels more tense and inflamed than ever. The addition of a little glycerin to the lotion may prevent this. In other cases the application of an oily substance often gives greater relief. For this purpose petrolatum alone may be used, or with the addition of 2 grains (0.13) of menthol to the ounce (31); or, in the case of older children, with a small lesion, 5 to 10 grains (0.32–0.65) of carbolic acid (p. 181) instead of menthol. For the cases in which the eruption is chiefly erythematous, powders may be of benefit, such as zinc oxide, boric acid, bismuth or talc, alone or in combination, and with camphor added. In the treatment of dermatitis venenata due to rhus or other plant-poisoning, Strickler[20] has had success by using toxin (antigen). The specific antigen of the plant is employed, and from 3 to 5 injections of a solution of this are given intramuscularly, beginning with about 0.3 cc. to 0.5 cc. (5.4 to 8 minims) and increasing up to 1 to 2 cc. (16 to 32 minims). The first 2 injections are given at twenty-four hour intervals and the later ones every second or third day. Schamberg[21] has been able to desensitize persons against ivy-poison by oral administration of the tincture. Intramuscular injections may also be employed in prevention. Both these measures, if protective, are so only for one season and should be repeated each year.

Dermatitis Actinea.—This is merely the condition of sunburn in which the parts are more swollen than in erythema, and in which vesicles and bullae appear. The same local treatment may be applied as in dermatitis venenata.

Dermatitis Congelationis (*Chilblain, Frost-bite*).—Severe degrees of this disorder are entirely in the domain of surgery. In milder degrees the condition depends upon exposure to moderate cold, often combined with a state of lowered general resistance, or on individual predisposition. The **lesions** consist in the development of circumscribed burning and itching areas of a dusky-red color, hard, and somewhat elevated. They occur oftenest upon the hands and feet, the ears, cheeks and nose. They may last for days or longer, and may then disappear entirely; or return whenever the parts are exposed to cold or to heat. In the **treatment** of the initial lesion, the frozen part should be rubbed with snow or cold water until the circulation is well-established, and the patient kept away rom the heat. Later there should be efforts made to prevent recurrence by the wearing of warm clothing and the protection of the parts against cold. Locally benefit sometimes follows painting the chilblains with a mixture of tincture of iodine fl. dr. 1 (3.7), flexible collodion fl. oz. 1 (30). Should bullae have formed, these should be opened, if not already broken, and the parts dressed with carbolized petrolatum (grains 10 (0.65); oz. 1 (31)).

Dermatitis Gangrenosa.—The rare disease going by this name develops oftenest in debilitated infants, especially those recovering from varicella. (See p. 303.) In other instances it may arise without other previous cutaneous disorder, various pyogenic germs seeming to be active factors. The **lesions** consist of multiple areas of cutaneous gangrene. Constitutional **symptoms** may be absent in the mildest cases, but oftener they are severely septic, and in the majority of instances death from sepsis occurs. **Treatment** in addition to local antisepsis is as in other septic conditions.

Dermatitis Exfoliativa Neonatorum (*Ritter's Disease*).—This affection was first described by Ritter[22] who reported upon 297 cases occurring in infants up to the age of five weeks. A similar condition has been reported as exceptionally occurring in early childhood (Baümler[23]). The disease in the experience of most physicians is decidedly uncommon. Its **cause** is not known. It has been considered closely related to pemphigus or impetigo contagiosa. It has been observed chiefly in asylums for infants, and has occurred epidemically. The **symptoms** rarely begin before the end of the first week and after the normal desquamation of the skin following birth is over. There then appears an intensely red area, oftenest about the mouth, with the formation of fissures here. The redness rapidly increases in degree and spreads until the whole body is covered. Meanwhile the skin is thickened and edematous, and the epithelium separates in large pieces, the surface beneath often being moist. Sometimes a few bullae are present. The mucous membranes of the mouth, nose and conjunctiva may exhibit erosion. Constitutional symptoms, including fever, are generally absent. The duration of the disease is one to two weeks in favorable cases; but in others may be lengthened by continued desquamation. About 50 per cent of the cases die from debility, or from the occurrence of gastro-enteritis, pneumonia, or purulent invasion of the skin or umbilicus. The fissuring is distinguished from that of hereditary syphilis by the absence of other evidence of that disease. The widespread, macular, papular, or chiefly squamous erythema sometimes seen in the new-born is distinguished from exfoliating dermatitis chiefly by the fact that there is no fissuring. The constitutional **treatment** is supportive, including transfusion of blood; and the local consists in protecting the skin and keeping it soft with petrolatum, zinc oxide, or Lassar's paste (zinc oxide oz. ½ (15.5), amylum oz. ½ (15.5), petrolatum oz. 1 (31.1).

ERYTHRODERMIA DESQUAMATIVA

(Leiner's Disease)

The first detailed description of this affection, probably not uncommon, was by Leiner.[24] It appears in early infancy at the end of the first or second month of life, and begins as a seborrhea of the scalp or as erythematous spots on the trunk. In well-developed cases the entire cutaneous surface becomes intensely red and covered with large yellow or whitish scales, which are readily removable, leaving the surface dry beneath. The nails are involved. There is usually no fever or other constitutional disturbance, except loss of weight and the uniform presence of diarrhea. There is no itching. The **cause** would appear to be an autointoxication of some sort. The **prognosis** is usually favorable and recovery takes place in a few weeks. The **diagnosis** is to be made from Ritter's disease, in which the condition begins around the mouth, there is often moist exudation under the epidermis, no seborrhea of the head, and the onset and course are more acute than in Leiner's disease. In **treatment** bran-baths may be tried and a simple ointment applied. Blood-transfusion has given good results, as have also intramuscular injections of maternal blood.

MILIARIA

(Prickly Heat)

This may be seen in the course of acute febrile diseases, especially typhoid fever, rheumatism, and scarlatina (see Scarlatina miliaris, p. 255); but may also occur in debilitated states attended by free perspiration. Other causes are exposure to heat, the wearing of too warm clothing, and hard exercise. The disease may be divided into several forms. In the first **sudamia** or **miliaria crystallina,** there are large numbers of discrete, usually closely placed, minute, transparent vesicles with clear contents, found principally upon the trunk. No inflammatory element is present. **Inflammatory miliaria** may be divided into several subvarieties: *Miliaria vesiculosa* (numerous vesicles situated upon a red base); *Miliaria rubra* (vesicles so packed that the whole affected skin has a red appearance); *Miliaria alba* (basal congestion slight, and vesicles less translucent); *Miliaria papulosa* or *lichen tropicus* (numerous crowded, minute, papules, with interspersed tiny vesicles). There is no sharp distinction between these various forms. The onset of miliaria of the inflammatory type is sudden, and the eruption usually widespread. Itching and burning may be slight, but are often intense. The rash lasts a few days, or may be continued almost indefinitely by the development of new crops. As recovery takes place fine desquamation may follow. In severe or long-continued cases, eczema or secondary pustular lesions may develop. The **diagnosis** is to be made especially from eczema. In this latter disease, however, the causes mentioned are absent, the onset less sudden, the lesions larger, and rupture of the vesicles and oozing occurs. The **treatment** consists in the removal of the cause; the prohibition of too warm clothing; the insuring of cleanliness by frequent bathing; and keeping the skin dry by the application of a nonirritating powder, as talc or powdered cornstarch. The skin of some infants is intolerant of wool even in wintertime, and undergarments of other material must be employed. If the rash is already present there may be recommended a solution of bicarbonate of soda (1:200); a calamine lotion (calamine, zinc oxide each dr. 2 (7.8), water fl. oz. 4 (118)); or lotio nigra. Among powders may be mentioned lycopodium; zinc and starch; and a camphor-zinc-and starch powder (p. 1095), which is often efficacious.

SEBORRHEA

This consists in abnormal increase in the secretion of the sebaceous glands. Attacking the scalp it is frequent in early life, and particularly in infancy. The **cause** is unknown, but the view prevails that it is dependent upon the action of bacteria. Probably debility, anemia, indigestion, and the like predispose to its development. *Seborrhea oleosa* is seen in older children approaching puberty; producing an oily state of the nose and forehead, the front of the chest, and the scalp. *Seborrhea sicca* is common particularly in infants. The deposit is a mixture of seborrheal secretion with epithelial cells and dirt; and forms a thick, oily, yellowish crust (milk-crust). It is most marked on the vertex, but may cover the greater portion of the scalp and even attack the forehead, nose and chest. Removal of the crusts shows the skin apparently normal, unless the case has existed for some time, when there may be redness and infiltration of it. The deposit is easily removed, but the final cure is often only slowly attained, since relapse readily occurs. In older children the deposit on the scalp is in the form of small, whitish scales (dandruff). The crusted and scaly condition, especially on the scalp, is to be **diagnosed** from eczema by the absence of all evidence of inflammation. Should this symptom be present, the condition is to be regarded as seborrheic eczema. In the treatment of milk-crust, the first step is that of softening the mass by the application of a bland oil or petrolatum, and then dislodging it by washing with hot soapy water. All violence, such as the use of a fine tooth-comb, is to be avoided. After cleansing, an ointment is required, as of resorcin (grains 5 (0.32), or salicylic acid (grains 10 (0.65), or yellow oxide of mercury (grains 5 (0.32) combined with petrolatum oz. 1 (31)). The washing process should be repeated as soon as fresh crusts are seen. In older children, and in the case of the oily form of seborrhea, weak lotions of carbolic acid, sulphur or resorcin may be preferable, and the use of one of the superfatted soaps, medicated with resorcin, salcylic acid, or sulphur, alone or combined, may be beneficial.

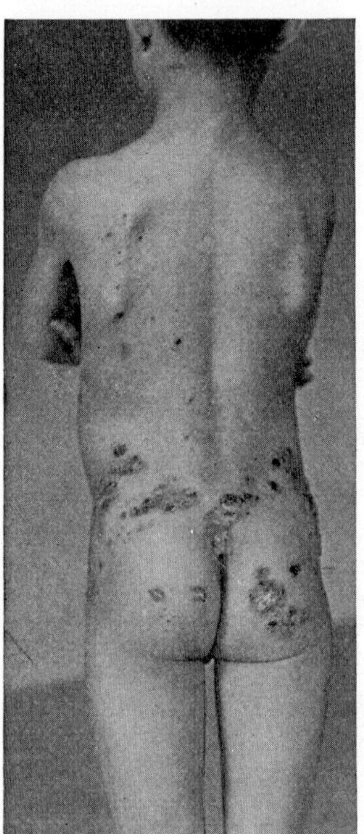

Fig. 275.—Psoriasis. From a patient in the Children's Hospital of Philadelphia.

PSORIASIS

About half the cases of this begin in childhood (Nielsen[25]). It has been seen in the first year of life and even in the first few weeks (Rille,[26] Davis[27]). A familial tendency has occasionally been observed. The disease is commonest in winter, and the patient may be free from it in the summer, to suffer a recurrence with the return of cold weather. Its **cause** is unknown. The eruption begins as more or less rounded spots, pinhead sized, which extend at the periphery until they attain an area of a rounded or irregular form and of an inch (2.5) or more in diameter. At the beginning they may be smooth and red, but soon they are covered with a crust of silvery scales. They are always sharply circumscribed. Scraping of the lesions removes the scales, and reveals a red, dry base, upon which numerous bleeding points develop if the scraping is continued. Often the centers of the larger areas show a tendency to recovery, thus leaving the outer scaling border in the form of a ring. The spots may be few or many, and they involve by preference the extensor surface of the limbs (especially about the joints), the trunk and the scalp. The nails may sometimes be brittle and opaque or pitted. The face, palms and soles are not often attacked. Itching and other subjective manifestations are insignificant. The disease is essentially chronic, new lesions developing slowly or rapidly during an indefinite period. Although yielding to treatment, or disappearing spontaneously, recurrence is almost sure to take place, perhaps after months or years.

In children, especially in the first attack, the lesions are often small, smooth, and do not show the characteristic silvery scaling until gentle scraping is employed. Eczema is **diagnosed** in that it itches severely, has a less sharply circumscribed border, and any crusting present is yellowish, or in the case of seborrheic eczema, greasy. In **treatment** the administration of arsenic is favored. Salicylates are also recommended. Alteration of the diet may be tried, Schamberg[28] reporting excellent results from a low-protein intake. Removal to a warm climate may be serviceable. External treatment is important. Among remedies which have been extensively used are preparations of salicylic acid, sulphur, ammoniated mercury, tar, chrysarobin, and pyrogallol. The last two are often irritating, especially with children. A warm bath should precede the application of the medication. Injection of foreign protein, such as horse-serum, has been claimed to be curative in some instances. Sachs[29] reported good results following intravenous injections of sodium salicylate.

ECZEMA

Etiology.—The causes of eczema, one of the most common diseases of early life, are (1) constitutional and (2) local. The majority of cases start in the first two years of life; many in the first four months. Males are somewhat oftener affected.

Of *constitutional* causes one of the most prominent, especially in infancy, is a sensitive character of the skin, often inherited. There may also be an inherited predisposition to allergy. There is active, too, the influence of the exudative diathesis (p. 481). Eczema in infancy may be replaced by asthma later, and there may be a relationship to allergic manifestations as hay-fever, urticaria and angioneurotic edema. White[30] claims that infants who develop eczema have often been especially prone to colic (enterospasm) in the first four months of life. Gastro-intestinal disturbances give rise to attacks; and without indigestion, certain articles of food produce eczema in some children because of allergy or sensitivity to them (p. 484). Many articles of food may be operative in individual cases; most frequently eggs, milk, wheat, barley, orange, tomatoes, peas, potatoes and spinach. Excessive quantities of carbohydrates and fats appear to have an effect in some cases. Urbach and Sicher[31] and others claim that the action of carbohydrate is not a general one, but is due to a local metabolic disturbance of carbohydrate in the skin. Others have observed abnormally high blood-sugar and a decreased sugar-tolerance (Ayres,[32] Holdin-Davis and Wells[33]). Finkelstein[34] thought that the salts of milk had an influence. It has been shown by many studies, as those of Schloss,[35] O'Keefe et al.,[36] and Smyth et al.,[37] that about 50 per cent of cases of eczema in infants and children react to cutaneous protein-tests of various kinds. It should be said that in eczema, cutaneous rather than intracutaneous tests are preferable, since they may more closely determine the source of the cutaneous irritation. It is to be borne in mind also that a positive cutaneous protein-test does not prove that the substance used is causative, nor, on the other hand, does a negative reaction demonstrate that allergy may not exist (p. 486); and, further, that dietetic articles other than those containing protein seem in some cases to possess a specific causative action. The attempt by means of protein-testing to discover the allergic cause of eczema is often disappointing. It would appear evident that the term "eczema" is a broad one and covers many forms of dermatitis. The influence of diet is undoubtedly great, and overfeeding of any sort, as well as specific proteins which vary with the individual case, may produce the disease. Well-nourished breast-fed or bottle-fed babies are liable to develop eczema more frequently than underfed atrophic ones. In fact, loss of weight due to illness or starvation sometimes causes improvement in the cutaneous condition. As discussed under Allergy (p. 485) human milk may possibly transmit proteins and in this way breast-fed infants acquire sensitivity, or the transmission of sensitivity may have been by the placental route. Perhaps certain drugs which would cause eczema may be transmitted by breast-milk.

Local irritation is a frequent factor. This may depend upon uncleanliness; irritating discharge from the nose or ear; prolonged contact of wet diapers; the presence of pediculi or of scabies; exposure to cold or high winds; irritating clothing, especially woolen, or garments containing aniline dyes; the local action of drugs, as formaldehyde, sulphur, iodoform, etc. Eczema may follow miliaria, intertrigo, seborrhea; or result from the use of strong alkaline soaps, or even too frequent bathing in simple water.

Symptoms.—These may be divided into (1) those seen in infants, and (2) those occurring in older children.

1. Eczema in Infancy.—Over half of all cases of eczema begin in the first six months of life. The situation is oftenest the face or head, which may be partially or completely covered by the eruption. The next most favorite regions are the genitalia, folds of the joints, breasts, abdomen and back. Much less often eczema is universal in distribution. In typical cases the disease begins as an erythema or a papular redness, with severe itching. The affected area soon becomes moist and shows a multitude of vesicles, many of them ruptured and discharging a sticky fluid. Often the whole area exhibits a swollen, weeping surface, rendered visible after the removal of the thick, yellowish crusts which form upon it. Secondary infection may cause the production of pustules, or the discharge of pus from the raw surface. This is especially common in early life. Extreme itching results in scratching, which is followed by the effusion of blood. The skin is much swollen, and the neighboring lymph-nodes enlarge and perhaps suppurate. The milder cases suffer little from constitutional symptoms, but in others sleepless days and nights and constant crying produced by the itching result in debility and impaired nutrition.

Not all cases exhibit these typical manifestations. The eczema may be less acute and the skin dry, red, swollen, scaling and cracked. There is severe itching as in the moist type. This "icthyoid" form is seen oftener on the trunk and extremities than on the face. The moist type and the dry type may appear at different times in the same locality.

2. Eczema in Older Children.—After infancy eczema approaches the adult type in proportion as the age increases. Certain varieties are of special interest. There is to be noted the eczema of the eyelids and of the nostrils and upper lip common in children with tuberculous cervical glands (*scrofulous eczema*). There is also at this time of life less tendency to involve the face; the flexures of the joint being favorite seats. The scalp, especially in the occipital region, is often affected from the irritation set up by pediculi. Independently of these there is frequently seen a pustular eczema of the scalp characterized by the development of crusts. The neighboring lymph-nodes are enlarged. In other cases eczema tends to be of a papular type, with intense itching.

Course and Prognosis.—In most cases acute eczema is easy to relieve, but there is great tendency to relapse. Some cases appear absolutely resistant to treatment. After the first or, perhaps, the second year of life, however, eczema has a tendency to disappear of itself, especially when the child is put on a diet which is not so largely of milk. On the whole the prognosis for complete recovery from the disease is unfavorable during the first year; and in eczema developing or continuing after the second year recurrences are frequent. Severe cases may exhibit fever and nervous symptoms, and develop a toxic state which may prove fatal. At such a time the rash frequently improves greatly; a condition to which the laity sometimes applies the term "striking-in." There are instances in which nephritis develops; and others in which sudden death takes place, perhaps due to status lymphaticus. After the eczema improves, other allergic manifestations may develop.

Diagnosis.—Eczema is distinguished from *erythema* by the evidence of cutaneous infiltration; from severe forms of *dermatitis* by the less violent sudden onset, the longer course, and the localization; from *seborrhea* by the presence of a red inflamed area under the crusts; from *miliaria* by the slower onset and the tendency to rupture of the vesicles. *Scabies* resembles eczema in the severity of the itching, but is most frequent on the flexor surfaces, the arm-pits, the hands, and between the fingers and toes; and careful examination will reveal burrows. *Erysipelas* presents greater swelling, less uniform fine vesiculation, and fever. *Impetigo* is distinguished by the fact that the crusts are produced by separate isolated pustules. In *syphilis* the lesions are larger, more discrete, less scaly and of a darker red or often a coppery tint, and do not itch; and other symptoms of the disease are generally present.

Treatment. **Constitutional.**—The nature of the cause and of the lesions must be taken into consideration. The digestive condition should be studied and such foods excluded as appear to be factors; overfeeding avoided; and constipation relieved. In very moist types reasonable limitation of fluid may be of assistance, but this must be done cautiously. If the digestive condition permits, concentrated feedings may be tried (p. 103). There appears to be no basis for the limitation of salt in the diet; at least there is no demonstrable disturbance of chloride metabolism in eczema (Burgess[38]). The use of acid-milk (p. 104) has been found of benefit by some pediatrists as, for instance, Scheer[39] and Sandels.[40] In breast-fed babies the milk may be too rich or in too great quantity. In cases of suspected allergy from breast-milk, cutaneous tests should be made and the proteins to which the infant reacts should be removed from the mother's diet. The same considerations apply in artificially-fed infants; namely, that the food may be in too great quantity or that some particular protein may be operative. In older children it may be necessary to reduce the total amount of food, and a trial may be made of the omission of eggs, milk, and the like; if possible basing the elimination upon the results of cutaneous tests. At any age alteration of the diet should not be such that general nutrition is impaired. It is not advisable to remove all milk from the diet, but where a positive cutaneous reaction to cow's milk has been found, goat's milk may be tried (p. 82), or the cow's milk-protein may be modified by peptonization or prolonged boiling, or dried milk may be given. For some of the cases sensitive to cow's milk a milk-free food, the protein of which is derived from soy bean, may be employed. (Hill and Stuart.[41] See p. 111.) This is sold under the trade-name of Sobee. Its percentage strength when diluted is very similar to that of milk. In addition to the elimination of the offending protein, or in conjunction with it, desensitization may be carried out (p. 487). Yet therapy conducted on the theory of protein-desensitization is often disappointing, even in the presence of positive cutaneous reactions. Some children are anemic and flabby and will be benefited by cod-liver oil and the administration of iron, copper and perhaps arsenic. Sojourn at the seashore helps in some cases, but in others appears to make the condition worse. Roentgen-ray and ultraviolet irradiation is seldom curative, but may have some beneficial effect. Huldschinsky[42] advises painting the eczematous area with a 3 per cent solution of silver before the exposure to ultraviolet irradiation.

Constipation should be corrected. In certain cases, especially of the moist type, atropine seems helpful. Thyroid extract may have an effect in cases with a coincident hypothyroidism, but otherwise should not be given. The intense itching in some cases indicates the administration of sedatives; for which symptom, too, Pilcher[43] found that epinephrine given subcutaneously was of benefit.

Local Treatment.—Local causes as irritation by the clothing, exposure to cold and wind, or excessive perspiration, must be removed. Scratching must be prevented by mechanical restraint if necessary. Pasteboard splints, or those constructed from wooden tongue-depressors and adhesive plaster, bound around the elbows are useful. In eczema of the buttocks care should be taken that the diapers are not washed with strong soda. Exposure of the buttocks to dry heat, with the diaper left off, is often beneficial.

Before local treatment of any kind is given the region should be freed of crusts. Sometimes the employment of soap and water or even of plain water for this purpose is contraindicated, and starch-water or boric acid solution is to be preferred; or some oily substance, as petrolatum or cold cream. The choice of local applications is wide. Some cases are most benefited by ointments or pastes, as one of acid boric grain 20 (1.3), ung. zinci oxidi oz. 1 (31); or bismuth subnitrate dr. 1 (3.9), ung. aquae rosea oz. 1 (31). Menthol, 1 to 2 grains (0.065 to 0.13), may be added to relieve the itching, or for older children small amounts of carbolic acid, cautiously (p. 181). Any application must be in sufficient quantity and frequently enough renewed to keep in constant contact with the part. Lassar's paste (p. 1100) is an excellent basis for medication of different sorts, or may be used alone. Any ointment or paste may be spread upon a linen mask and applied to the face. Elsewhere on the body it may be spread thickly on a soft cloth and secured with bandages. Some cases do better with lotions, as, for example, one of a saturated solution of boric acid; or calamine grains 20 (1.3), zinc oxide grain 30 (1.9), aqua rosea fl. oz. 1 (30). Aqua camphorae may be used as a diluent to relieve the itching, with 10 minims (0.62) of glycerin added to prevent too rapid drying. The affected part should be kept constantly moist. Medication may also be applied in the form of a mucilage and allowed to dry on; using, for instance, Pick's[44] formula (tragacanth 5, glycerine 2, boiling water 100) to which any drug selected may be added. The addition of 2 per cent boric acid aids in preserving it. In many cases of vesicular eczema with oozing, powders are still better, using, for example, one composed of bismuth subcarbonate grain 20 (1.3), talc oz. ½ (15.5), amylum oz. ½ (15.5). Crude coal-tar, recommended by White[45] and others, often does good. It may be employed pure or in the form of an ointment consisting of crude coal tar and powdered zinc oxide each 1 part, corn-starch and petrolatum, each 8 parts. For less acute and more prolonged cases of vesicular eczema, and for those of a papular or squamous form, more stimulating medication is needed, employing, for example, oil of cade fl. dr. ½ (1.9), flexible collodion fl. oz. 1 (30); the mixture being painted over the diseased region and allowed to dry, and fresh applications made as it peels. In other cases coal-tar may be applied as a lotion (coal-tar 1 part; tincture of soap-bark 6 parts). In pustular cases one of the best remedies is ammoniated mercury from 5 to 20 grains (0.32 to 1.3), lanolin and petrolatum each oz. ½ (15.5).

HERPES SIMPLEX

(Fever Blisters)

Herpes has been believed to be caused by a filterable virus, and it is claimed that it is transmissible to animals by inoculation. It is associated with so many conditions that this virus must be widespread. Its portal of entry is probably the mucous membrane of the nose and throat. (For relation to epidemic encephalitis, see p. 399). The disease is rare in early childhood. The apparent **causes** of the eruption are various, among them being slight febrile disturbance, respiratory infections, indigestion, exposure to cold winds or an excess of sunshine. Often no cause can be discovered. With certain diseases, as croupous pneumonia, cerebrospinal fever, influenza, certain acute forms of jaundice and malaria, there is a special tendency for herpes to develop. Herpetiform eruptions also occur at times after the ingestion of arsenicals, morphine, lead, and iodine; and during the reaction following vaccine or serum injections (Goodpasture[46]). The **symptoms** manifest themselves as vesicles of pin-head or slightly large size, situated upon a slightly reddened base and oftenest upon the skin close to the lips or the neighboring portion of the face. Sometimes the distribution is wider, and the mucous membranes of the mouth and throat, or, in fact, almost any portion of the cutaneous or mucous surface may be involved. (See Herpetic Stomatitis, p. 521.) Preceding the appearance of the vesicles a slight burning sensation may be experienced. The duration of the attack is a few days or a week, the vesicles forming crusts which leave no scarring. Many persons have a peculiar disposition to recurrence. Herpes zoster is distinguished from herpes simplex by the location of the former along the course of the nerves, and by the accompanying pain. In **treatment** the vesicles may be covered with zinc ointment, or calamine lotion or boric acid and camphor-water may be employed. (See p. 1106.)

HERPES ZOSTER

(Shingles; Zona)

This occurs not infrequently in early life. It depends upon inflammation of a root-ganglion or the sensory nerve connected with it, the eruption being merely the cutaneous manifestation. The possible relationship to varicella has been discussed elsewhere (p. 301). In contradistinction to herpes simplex, shingles has not been transmitted to lower animals, but Kundratitz[47] claims to have produced the disease experimentally in two infants by inoculation. The **symptoms** consist of neuralgic pain, accompanied or followed in a few hours or longer by the appearance of vesicles scattered along the course of one nerve, or sometimes more than one. The vesicles usually appear upon one side of the body only. They are split-pea in size, grouped, and situated on a pinkish red base of a color more intense than in herpes simplex. Burning and some itching may be experienced. In children the pain may be slight or absent. Sometimes fever, malaise and nausea precede the eruption. The vesicles soon become dried into crusts, which persist for a week or more and leave temporary staining of the skin. Only rarely does suppuration occur. The usual situation is on the trunk in the course of the intercostal or abdominal nerves; but the lesions may also appear on the buttocks, thighs, neck and forehead. In the last situation they may involve the eye. In children it is uncommon for tenderness of the skin or severe neuralgic pain to continue after the eruption has disappeared. In **treatment** the affected part should be protected from irritation, best by bandaging after applying a dusting powder of oxide of zinc and starch. The employment of menthol locally in some form is serviceable. It has also been claimed that the administration of sodium iodide orally and of pituitary extract intramuscularly is beneficial.

PEMPHIGUS NEONATORUM

True pemphigus is a rare disorder, seen after the period of early infancy, and need not receive further consideration here. The condition designated *pemphigus neonatorum* is closely allied to, if not a form of, contagious impetigo (*impetigo bullosa*, p. 1110). It is an infectious and somewhat epidemic and contagious disorder occurring in the first two weeks of life, especially in institutions for infants, and apparently dependent upon pyogenic infection, oftenest the staphylococcus aureus. The organisms may possibly be derived from the mother's milk, or, in some cases, from her vaginal secretion. The disease may attack others than the new-born, and even rarely adults (Heinmüller[48]). Occasionally it may be truly congenital in the sense that the infant is born with one or more of the characteristic vesicles. Predisposing factors seem to be excessive moisture of the skin and irritation. Negroes and other dark skinned races have a comparative

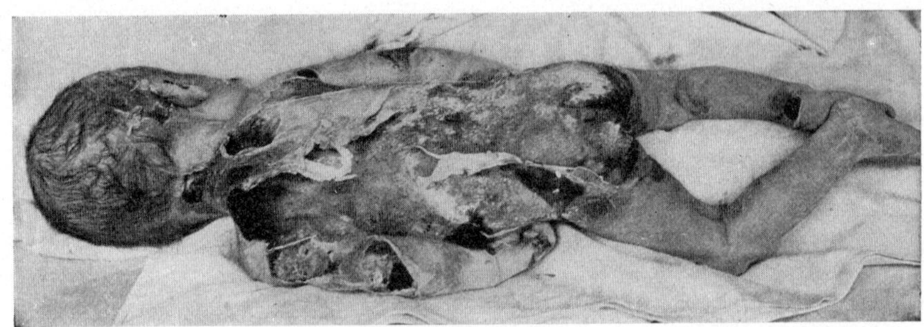

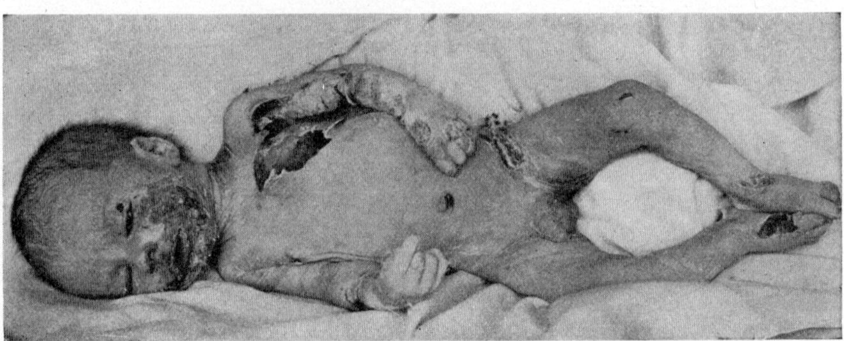

Fig. 276.—Pemphigus neonatorum. Infant born Jan. 19th in the Maternity Ward of the Hospital of the University of Pennsylvania. Normal except abrasion of right ear. *Jan. 20th.* —Slight extension of crusting from ear to scalp. *Jan.* 21.—Blebs on right hand and wrist. *Jan.* 22.—Entire right side of scalp involved, with skin coming off in places. *Jan.* 23.—Extensive desquamation over scalp and cheeks on right side. Numerous blebs size of a dollar on the abdomen, many of them confluent. *Jan.* 24.—Photograph taken on this date. Peeling of skin leaving moist surface over the entire back and to some extent on the abdomen and face. Some on the arms and legs. *Jan.* 25.—Died.

immunity. The **symptoms** of the malady are represented by the appearance of scattered bullae increasing in size to $\frac{1}{2}$ in. (1.3) or less in diameter, with a slightly reddened base, and seen oftenest at first upon the hands or face. These rupture in a few days, or dry and form crusts, but in some cases other crops appear. The general health is little affected at first. Another variety, *syphilitic pemphigus*, occurs in the new-born and involves especially the palms and soles (p. 429). The **prognosis** of pemphigus neonatorum is uncertain. In milder cases recovery takes place after a few weeks. Severe cases may run a rapid, fatal course, the bullae coalescing, the epidermis stripping from extensive inflamed raw-looking moist areas (Fig. 276), fever and septic symptoms developing with decided debility, and death occurring in a week or less. In **diagnosis** the distinction is to be made between the nonsyphilitic and the syphilitic forms by the involvement of the palms and soles in the latter, and other symptoms of this disease. *Dermatitis exfoliativa neonatorum* is closely allied etiologically to pemphigus neonatorum and the two conditions may appear in the same epidemic. It is distinguished from pemphigus by the fissuring about the mouth, the lesser tendency to moisture of the denuded surface, and the usual absence of bullae. The **treatment** consists in opening the bullae, protecting the affected parts, and the application of powders of zinc oxide and starch, or a weak ammoniated mercury ointment. Ultraviolet irradiation seems to be of some benefit. Taylor[49] advises for prophylaxis the use in nurseries of a powder containing three parts of mercurous chloride, two parts of talc, and one part of zinc oxide. In epidemics in nurseries great care must be practised in asepsis and isolation.

FURUNCULOSIS. MULTIPLE CUTANEOUS ABSCESSES

These two conditions are closely allied and depend upon the entrance into or beneath the skin of pyogenic germs, especially the staphylococcus aureus. Individual tendency to furunculosis is seen in some children, otherwise healthy. Generally, however, especially in cases with numerous small suppurating cutaneous foci, there are evidences of indigestion or improper diet; or the subjects may be debilitated by some recent disease; or there is local irritation, as from eczema or impetigo. White infants are more commonly affected than colored ones. To a certain extent the condition is auto-inoculable. In typical **furuncles,** or boils, the hair-follicles or sweat-glands are involved. They may occur at any age, are single or numerous, acuminated, and with a central slough. **Multiple subcutaneous abscesses** are peculiar to infancy, and are localized in the subcutaneous tissue. They suppurate, but are without the characteristics of the furuncle. Intermediate between these forms are the numerous cases seen especially in infancy, but sometimes later, with many widespread, small, suppurative foci, which do not have the character of the furuncle, yet do not occupy the subcutaneous tissue, but rather the substance of the skin itself. Considerable constitutional disturbance attends the production of furuncles, as well as of large subcutaneous abscesses; while the small numerous abscesses of the intermediate type generally exhibit little fever, and the constitutional symptoms are those of the primary disease. The **prognosis** of these purulent processes is generally good, although with widespread and constantly recurring suppurating foci in debilitated infants there may follow great exhaustion and even death. The **treatment** of furuncles and abscesses consists in incision and drainage. It is often well to allow these processes to become somewhat advanced before opening, since at that time the pus is more or less sterile and there is less liability of local infection in contiguous areas of the skin. It may be indicated to hasten softening of the infected foci by the use of hot compresses or antiseptic poultices. The general treatment consists in regulation of the diet and the treatment of any anemia and debility present. It is questionable whether the administration of yeast or of calcium sulphide possesses specific action in combating furunculosis. The general cutaneous surface, and especially the area in the neighborhood of suppurating foci, should be washed frequently with alcohol or a 1:5000 solution of bichloride of mercury to prevent auto-inoculation. Exposure to sunlight or artificial ultraviolet irradiation may be of some assistance. For recurring cases vaccine treatment, preferably with autogenous vaccines, should be tried.

IMPETIGO CONTAGIOSA

The disease is both contagious and auto-inoculable, and depends upon the action of pyogenic bacteria, oftenest the staphylococcus aureus, perhaps at times with a streptococcus. It is most frequent in infants and young children. Generally several children in a family are attacked, or a considerable number when the outbreak is in institutions. Those with impaired health are most liable to become affected. In the typical form the **lesions** usually start as small vesicles or vesico-papules, but soon increase in size, perhaps to ½ in. (1.3) in diameter. They are not fully distended, and their contents are a yellowish, seropurulent fluid, which in two to five days dries into yellowish crusts. These crusts seem to be "stuck on" in the center, with the edges slightly raised. The eruption develops especially on the face, scalp and hands; but may spread by auto-inoculation to other regions, particularly the legs, feet and forearms. Lesions may be quite numerous or few only, and are generally discrete, although coalescence may occur. Slight evidence of inflammation is seen in the skin surrounding the lesions. There is little itching, and no constitutional symptoms are present. Neighboring lymph-nodes may become inflamed. Variations from this typical condition may be seen, in which the deeper portion of the skin becomes involved. By confluence of several lesions there may develop a raw area healing in the center, but with a circinate border (*impetigo circinata*). In *impetigo bullosa* (p. 1108) the lesions may remain bullous on the extremities and the genitalia; and in some cases only bullae may be found anywhere, at times very large, and without tendency to the formation of crusts. Mucous membranes are occasionally attacked in this variety.

The **prognosis** in the ordinary form is favorable, and, under treatment, recovery takes place in a few weeks. The course may be prolonged by auto-inoculation. The bullous form is often tedious and may terminate fatally. In cachectic subjects the lesions of impetigo may assume an ecthymatous character. In **diagnosis** from eczema it should be remembered that the latter exhibits smaller vesicles and crusts, itching, and distinct infiltration and edema of the skin. The bullous form of impetigo may suggest varicella, but differs from it in its longer course, the greater size of the lesions, and the absence of the areola. The **treatment** consists in opening the vesicles and bullae, removing the crusts by warm water and soap, and the constant application of an antiseptic ointment, as ammoniated mercury (grains 15 to 20) (1 to 1.3): oz. 1 (31). The areas may be touched with 20 per cent solution of silver nitrate after removal of the crusts (Morrow[50]). An excellent treatment is the painting of the lesions with 20 per cent alcohol to which 5 per cent gentian violet has been added (Smith and Burky[51]). The skin surrounding the area should be frequently washed with alcohol or a 1:5000 solution of bichloride of mercury or a superfatted sulphur soap. Underclothing should be changed frequently. The greatest difficulty obtains in preventing the spread of impetigo, especially in nurseries for new-born infants. Isolation and asepsis in the care of individual infants are necessary.

NEVUS

(Angioma; Birth-mark; Mole)

Under the term "nevus" are included several varieties of congenital growths of the skin, either vascular, pigmented, or of other nature. The most important, **vascular nevus,** is present at birth, or develops soon after, and consists of small, reddish or bluish spots which are flat or slightly elevated, pinhead size or larger, and which disappear on pressure. They are composed of small dilated capillaries (*telangiectasis*). Larger areas of a similar nature constitute the "port-wine stain," **naevus flammeus.** In another form, **angioma cavernosum,** the arterioles are distinctly dilated, there is overgrowth of surrounding connective tissue, the affected area is elevated, and the color is purplish. The **pigmented nevus,** or *mole,* is oftenest situated on the face, neck or back. Not uncommonly it is covered by coarse hair. The mole is composed of overgrowth of cuboidal epithelial cells, together with deposit of pigment in the rete and corium.

The **prognosis** of nevus is variable. Some of the smaller may disappear as the child grows older. Eczema or ulceration may develop under the influence of irritation, while in other cases rapid extension in size and malignant transformation occur. This is particularly true of thickened nevi of a cavernous nature. Moles have little tendency to alter, but the hypertrophic form may take on carcinomatous changes. Port-wine stains offer little hope of spontaneous improvement. In **treatment** small vascular nevi and moles may be let alone unless in a position where they cause disfigurement. If rapid growth of a nevus or mole begins, surgical removal is to be recommended. Depending on the type and location of a nevus various methods may be employed for its removal; these including electrolysis, the application of carbon dioxide snow, and exposure to the roengen-ray or radium.

CAROTINEMIA

To this condition Hess and Meyers[52] called attention in the United States, although it had been noted in Europe for some years,[53] and has been reported in several other countries. It consists of a yellowish discoloration of the skin and urine following the ingestion of vegetables and other foods containing large amounts of carotin. It has been observed in new-born infants when the mother during pregnancy has been on a high vegetable diet (DeBuys[54]). There is a marked individual susceptibility, some children developing the discoloration readily and others not at all, in spite of the administration of large amounts of carotin-containing substances. Foods containing the pigment in large amounts are carrots, spinach, egg-yolk, oranges and squash. It is also present in pumpkins, yellow turnips, parsnips, lettuce and kale. There are no general symptoms. The discoloration varies from a canary-yellow tinge to a deep orange, and tends to appear particularly on the palms, soles, forearms and the nasolabial folds. The sclera is never discolored. The blood-serum and the urine show the yellow tint. **Diagnosis** is made from jaundice by the lack of discoloration in the sclera and of other symptoms of jaundice, as itching, slow pulse, and the like. **Treatment** is unnecessary. When the carotin-containing foods are stopped the color slowly disappears.

VERRUCAE

(Warts)

Verrucae may appear in two forms; the ordinary wart (*verruca vulgaris*), and the plane wart (*verruca plana juvenilis*). They appear to be infectious and auto-inoculable, but beyond this the cause is unknown. **Verruca vulgaris** consists of one or more hard elevations of varying size; flat, filiform, or lobulated, and occurring oftenest on the hands, scalp, or face. They grow rapidly or slowly, and last months or years, and often finally disappear without treatment. **Verruca plana juvenilis** appears in the form of pinhead sized or larger, slightly elevated, yellowish or pale-brown growths; usually very numerous, and situated chiefly on the face, hands and forearms. The **treatment** is often difficult. Internally arsenic or mercurous iodide has been in favor, especially for the plane wart. Locally verruca vulgaris may be touched with strong nitric or with trichloracetic acid, carefully avoiding the spread of this to the surrounding skin. Freezing with carbonic dioxide snow or the employment of the roentgen-ray may be of service. A 2 to 4 per cent ointment of salicylic acid may be employed for the plane wart.

LENTIGO

(Freckles)

This common condition, consisting of numerous small deposits of pigment in the skin, is of importance only from an esthetic point of view. Lentigo appears oftenest in blondes, generally not before the age of three years, and tends to disappear as the patient grows older (Fig. 280). It develops especially in summer on parts exposed to the sun's rays. In the way of **treatment** prevention may be attempted, if deemed desirable, by the wearing of a veil or a broad-brimmed hat. For the removal of the freckles a lotion may be employed consisting of compound tr. benzoin and glycerin, each fl. dr. 1 (1.8), and aq. rosae fl. oz. 3 (89); or one of sodium biborat. dr. 1 (3.9) acid acet. dil. fl. oz. ½ (14.8), aq. rosae fl. oz. ½ (14.8). A solution of bichloride of mercury grains 6 (0.39) in water fl. oz. 4 (118) may be tried, but with caution against too vigorous an action. The application of buttermilk has been a domestic remedy.

ICHTHYOSIS

There will be described here only the ichthyosis affecting the new-born infant (*Congenital ichthyosis*). In this the whole surface of the body is

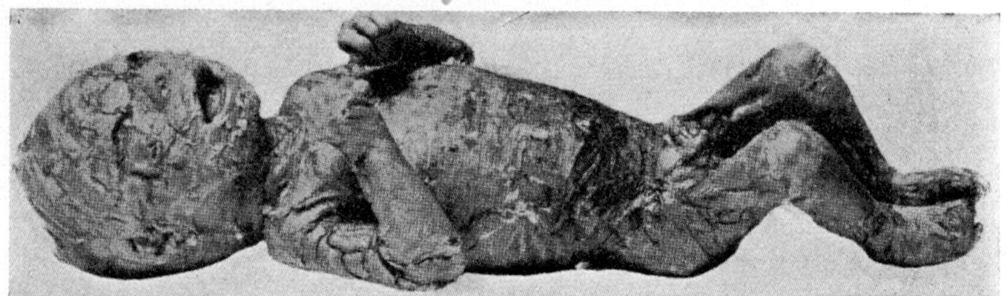

Fig. 277.—Congenital ichthyosis. Shows the thickened, hardened and fissured skin with epithelial plates. Child died on eighth day of life. (*Hess and Schultz, Am. J. Dis. Child.*, 1921, **21,** 359.)

found covered at birth with thick, plate-like masses of scales, and exhibits numerous furrows and fissures (Fig. 277). The skin is dry and thickened and the normal folds largely obliterated. The ears and nose may be nearly closed by the epithelial scales; ectropia is present; nursing is difficult or impossible; and death usually takes place from inanition in a few days or weeks. A less severe degree of congenital or fetal ichthyosis may be observed in which life continues for a long time.

KERATOSIS PALMARIS ET PLANTARIS

This rather uncommon anomaly of the skin may be congenital or appear in childhood. There is hereditary influence in some cases. Usually the palms and soles are symmetrically affected, and in some cases other parts of the body. There are areas of horny tissue, sometimes ⅛ in. (0.3 cm.) or more in thickness, with sharply marked borders and without any evidence of inflammation. The affection is sometimes combined with ichthyosis. Some relief can be obtained by the application of preparations of salicylic acid and treatment by the roentgen-ray.

MOLLUSCUM CONTAGIOSUM

This infectious disorder more often attacks children than adults, and sometimes occurs endemically in schools and institutions. The nature of the virus is not known. The lesions, which may be few or numerous, consist of small, shining, yellowish or whitish nodules of pinhead size up to that of a pea, with a minute opening at the slightly depressed center (Fig. 278). They are situated oftenest on the eyelids, forehead, neck and genitals. New lesions develop as the older ones disappear by shrinking or by discharge of the central mass. **Treatment** consists in the application of sulphur ointment, or one of ammoniated mercury (2 to 4 per cent).

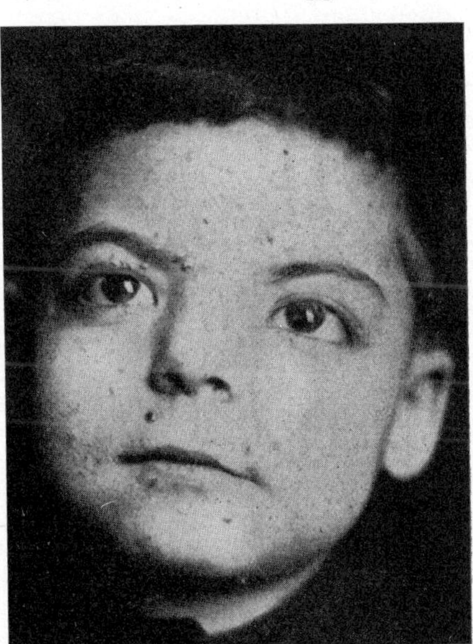

Fig. 278.—Molluscum contagiosum. From a patient in the Children's Hospital of Philadelphia. Scattered lesions are seen chiefly on the eyelids and about the mouth.

TUBERCULOSIS OF THE SKIN

The subject, although important, can receive but brief mention here. The lesions are divided into those which are produced by tubercle bacilli, and others, the *tuberculides,* which appear to be the result of the toxin of tuberculosis present elsewhere in the body. It is maintained by some that all of the lesions are in reality the product of local action of the germs.

1. Lupus Vulgaris.—This often begins in childhood; is seen most frequently among the poor; and is not often observed in this country, although common in Europe. Debilitated health predisposes to it, as does the occurrence of some one of the infectious diseases, especially those which have cutaneous manifestations. In most cases tuberculosis exists in the family, or is present elsewhere in the body of the patient. Clinically the **lesion** appears as a brownish-red, slightly elevated, flattened, indurated area. This is composed of small, confluent nodules of pinhead size, or slightly larger. The characteristic brownish-red color and nodular character are well shown if a flat piece of glass is pressed upon the patch. Later the diseased area may become ulcerated and crusted, or may exhibit the development of cicatricial tissue, or of growths of a warty nature, situated oftenest upon the extremities. The patches are commonly single, but may be numerous over the body. The disease appears most frequently on the face, particularly on the end of the nose or on the cheeks. Mucous membranes, principally of the nose and mouth, may be attacked primarily or secondarily. The **course** is slow, perhaps years being required to produce a patch of much size. There are periods, too, in which the growth is quiescent. The **prognosis** on the whole is unfavorable. The lesion spreads from its periphery, and extensive destruction of tissue may finally ensue. The outlook is better in children than in adults because of the lesser degree of involvement when coming under observation. Tuberculosis may develop elsewhere in the body, if not already present. **Treatment** is best carried out by a dermatologist. Various remedial measures have been employed, including the use of the roentgen-ray, ultraviolet irradiation, excision, and cauterization.

The choice of these depends largely upon the character and position of the lesion. Also used are gold and sodium thiosulphate, and the injection of tuberculin.

2. Scrofuloderma.—This term designates cutaneous **lesions**, actually tuberculous in nature, and dependent upon adjacent tuberculous bone or lymph-nodes. They appear as hard, pointed swellings of the skin of a purplish-red color. They may also develop as subcutaneous tuberculous infiltrations occurring independently of any underlying primary lesion. The mass soon softens and opens by one or several small ulcers. When more than one, they are connected with each other by sinuses as well as with any underlying tuberculous focus present. The area grows by the enlargement of the ulcer, or by the formation of new ones. The lesions are found oftenest in the neck and groin, or in other positions where caseous lymph-nodes or necrotic bone-tissue exists. In infants they are most frequent on the face. The **course** of the disease is chronic with little tendency to healing. The **diagnosis** is based upon the symptoms described, together with the presence of neighboring or more distant tuberculous foci. **Treatment** consists in removing any underlying osseous or lymph-node disease present. The employment of the roentgen-ray is often of benefit to the cutaneous lesion, as is also the application of iodoform or boric acid preparations; and treatment with tuberculin has been employed. Of greatest importance is the improvement of the general health.

3. Lichen Scrofulosorum.—The title designates a form of cutaneous tuberculous disease seen especially in children. It is one of those generally called a "tuberculide." Material obtained from biopsy of the lesions usually does not cause tuberculosis in injected guinea pigs. The disease sometimes follows an attack of one of the exanthemata. Frequently other forms of tuberculosis in the patient are discoverable. The **lesions** are pinhead-sized nodules of a yellowish-brown or reddish color, firm, but little elevated; and occurring isolated, or oftener in patches up to 1 or 2 in. (2.5 to 5.1) in diameter. There may be a great many or a limited number of such groups. They are situated chiefly on the trunk and produce no subjective symptoms. We have seen the number increase greatly within less than twenty-four hours following the intracutaneous injection of tuberculin. The **course** is chronic. It may continue for months or even years, the original patches gradually disappearing, usually without a trace, but new ones developing. The **diagnosis** rests upon the occurrence on the trunk, the absence of itching, the age of the patient, and often the evidence of tuberculosis elsewhere in the body. **Treatment** consists in improving the general health, and the application of an ointment containing thymol or subacetate of lead.

4. Acne Scrofulosorum (*Papulo-necrotic tuberculide, Acne necrotica*).—This affection is allied to the lichen scrofulosorum just described, and often associated with it. The **lesions**, which continue to appear in crops, are larger in size, and are firm, hard, papular, bluish-red, and crusted at the summit. Other tuberculous manifestations are nearly always present. The **course** is chronic, and as the lesions heal small scars remain. Under **treatment** the eruption disappears, but is liable to return. The treatment is that recommended for lichen scrofulosorum.

RINGWORM

(Tinea)

Etiology.—The parasitic disorder bearing the name of ringworm, or tinea, was shown by Sabouraud[55] to be causable by more than 40 species of fungi belonging to the same family. But two types need to be mentioned: the *microsporon Audouini*, a small-spored fungus, and the *trichophyton*, a large-spored fungus. The latter is further divided into endothrix and ectothrix, according as the fungus is found within the shaft of the hair or on its surface. The microsporon is usually the type attacking the scalp; while elsewhere on the body the trichophyton is nearly always the active agent. Ringworm of the scalp is largely limited to children between the ages of five and ten years, and is rarely seen after puberty; while ringworm of the body can occur at any age, although oftenest in children.

Ringworm is distinctly contagious, being spread directly or through clothing, toilet articles, and the like. Its primary source not infrequently is a domestic animal. The microsporon Audouini is a human species, but occasionally other species of this genus may be acquired from the dog, cat or horse. The trichophyton is commonly acquired from these animals.

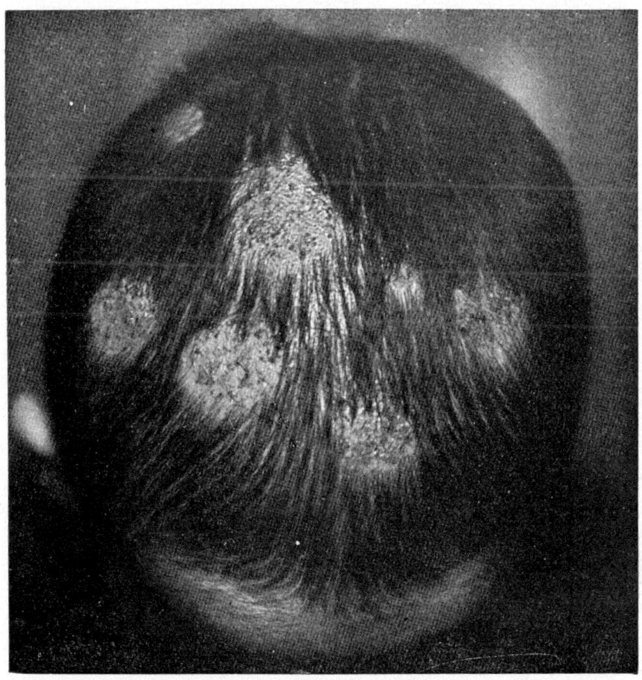

Fig. 279.—Ringworm (tinea tonsurans) of somewhat inflammatory type. (*Stelwagon, Diseases of the Skin, 8th Ed.*, 1171.)

Symptoms.—The disease is divided into (1) Tinea tonsurans, or ringworm of the scalp, and (2) Tinea circinata, or ringworm of the general body-surface.

1. Tinea Tonsurans.—In this common affection there are found one or more gray, scaly spots from a fraction of an inch up to 2 in. (5.1) or more in diameter, which are partly denuded of hair and exhibit a number of broken-off, opaque, brittle, thickened hair-stumps (Fig. 279). The hairs can readily be pulled out with forceps; and sometimes have been broken off close to the skin, producing the "black-dot" variety of ringworm. Scaling may be so abundant that the stumps of the hair are largely concealed, or so slight that it is scarcely apparent. Some of the latter cases with very few hair-stumps may suggest alopecia areata (*tinea decalvans*). Sometimes inflammation produces deep-seated, boggy, suppurating lesions (*tinea kerion*).

2. Tinea Circinata.—The lesions here are situated oftenest upon the face, neck, hands and forearms, and rarely on the palms and soles. They may occur with or without involvement of the scalp. They appear as scaly, pink, slightly elevated, and distinctly circumscribed small spots. These enlarge into ring-shaped areas by extension of the periphery, this being a trifle elevated and reddened in color, while the center is paler or whitish (Fig. 280). There are usually only one or two patches, but the number may reach ten or more. They vary in size from ½ in. (1.3) up to several inches in diameter. Generally they are discrete. Considerable itching may be present. Any degree of inflammation is uncommon. The trichophyton sometimes attacks the nails, which grow opaque and brittle.

Course and Prognosis of Ring Worm.—Several weeks or months are required before the patches of *tinea tonsurans* reach their full development. New spots may appear and confluence of the affected areas may occur. The ultimate prognosis is good, but untreated cases may last for years. The disease finally disappears, and the hair grows again as the patient reaches puberty. Recovery may take place within a few months when treatment is

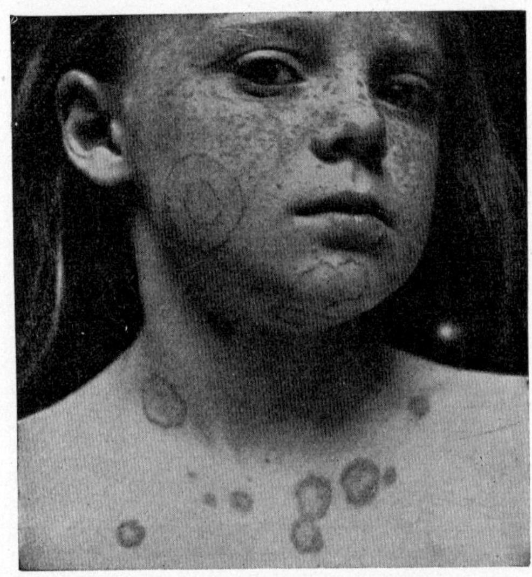

Fig. 280.—Ringworm of the body. Showing the rather uncommon occurrence of a double ring. Illustration also shows a marked example of freckles. (*Stelwagon, Diseases of the Skin, 8th Ed.*, 1163.)

energetic and only a few areas are involved. The occurrence of kerion is often curative. *Tinea circinata* likewise develops slowly, and after the patch reaches its maximum size it tends to remain stationary for a time and then to disappear. Treatment is usually efficacious after a few days or weeks. Recovery from both forms of tinea is commonly without permanent traces of injury.

Diagnosis.—The recognition of tinea circinata is based upon the circinate character with a pale healing center. The diagnosis of tinea tonsurans must sometimes be made from alopecia areata and favus. The former never exhibits any broken stumps of hair, and the skin is smooth. Favus is recognized by the sulphur-yellow, cup-shaped crusts. The scaling and loss of hair in seborrhea is diffuse and without broken hairs. While psoriasis produces rounded patches, these are widely scattered and have none of the characteristics of tinea. Microscopical examination of the hair after previous treatment with liquor potassae reveals the characteristic spores and mycelial threads. A method of diagnosis of tinea tonsurans has been followed by Ray [56] and others, having been originally employed by Margot and Devèze.[57]

This consists in passing ultraviolet rays through a deep-violet glass filter containing nickle oxide, known as Wood's glass, which causes the infected hair to fluoresce.

Treatment.—In tinea circinata any scaling should be removed with soap and water and the area treated with a parasiticide, as tincture of iodine $\frac{1}{2}$ strength, painted on the spots daily for three or four days. There may also be used an ointment of precipitated sulphur grain $\frac{1}{2}$ (1.9) in Lassar's paste oz. 1 (31) (p. 1100).

Treatment for tinea tonsurans is discouraging, although successful if persisted in. The hair should be cut close or shaved over the entire head and kept so; or certainly over and in the neighborhood of the patch. The scalp should be washed with soap and water, and all broken or loose hairs be pulled out with forceps, and after this the parasiticide well rubbed in for five or ten minutes once or twice daily. To prevent spread of the infection to others, the patient should wear a close-fitting skull-cap of some material which can be boiled, and the greatest care taken that soap, towels, hairbrushes, etc. are individual ones. Among remedies most frequently recommended may be mentioned ointment of sulphur grains 30 (1.9): oz. 1 (31); tincture of iodine; ointments of oil of cade or other tarry substance, or of ammoniated mercury, salicylic acid or chrysarobin. An efficacious treatment for tinea tonsurans is the employment of the roentgen-ray, by means of which depilation is produced, the fungus coming out with the hair, and cure being obtained in three to four months (Sabouraud and Noire[58]). Also recommended is thallium acetate, administered orally in 1 dose (8 mg. per kilo, (.056 grain per pound) of body weight), with a maximum dose of 0.3 Gm. (4.6 grains). The drug should not be given in divided doses, since when so employed it may cause severe poisoning and even death. (See p. 515.)

FAVUS

Tinea favosa is rare in this country, and seen chiefly in immigrants from Russia, Poland and other lands where the disease is common. It may appear at any age, but is uncommon on the scalp after puberty. It is caused by a fungus, the Achorion Schönleinii, and is decidedly contagious. It may be acquired from other persons, or from dogs, cats, mice, rabbits, fowls, and less often horses and cattle. The fungus consists of mycelium and spores. These can readily be seen under the microscope when a portion of the crust has been previously soaked in liquor potassae for a few minutes. In children the **lesions** are usually on the scalp. Here it first appears as one or more small yellowish spots, which soon enlarge and become sulphur-yellow cups, from the depressed center of each of which a hair projects. The spot grows in size and the cups become more or less confluent into yellowish crusts of an inch (2.5) or more in diameter. New points of infection may appear until much of the scalp is involved. A peculiar mousy or musty odor may be produced. Beneath the yellowish deposits there is slight inflammation. The hairs over the seat of the disease are dull and fall out, or break off readily. Upon the body favus is less common and generally a sequel to involvement of the scalp. Favus is practically without subjective symptoms, except a varying degree of itching. The **course** of the disease on the scalp is slow, months being required before much spread takes place. On other areas of the body the extension may be rather rapid. The **prognosis** for the body-surface is good; but for the scalp is unfavorable. In the latter situation the disease is extremely resistant to treatment, and there may be permanent loss of hair in the affected region. The local **treatment** is the same as for ringworm.

TINEA VERSICOLOR

This depends upon the presence of the microsporon furfur. It is not often seen in children. It is only slightly contagious. The fungus consists of mycelium and spores which grow in the horny layers of the epithelium. The occurrence of free perspiration is an important predisposing cause. The disease appears as faint yellowish or brownish spots, little if at all elevated, slightly scaly, fusing into larger areas, and situated chiefly upon the thorax and arms. Slight itching may be present. The discoloration is readily removed by scraping, leaving no redness of the skin beneath. The course is slow. The disorder is easily cured, although relapses readily occur. The **treatment** consists in the application of an ointment of precipitated sulphur (1:16), or of a lotion of hyposulphite of soda (1:32). The remedy is applied at least twice a day. Relapse is to be guarded against by frequent changing and thorough disinfection of the underclothing.

SCABIES

Scabies, or the itch, is the result of infection of the skin by the acarus scabiei or sarcoptes scabiei, which attacks only the human race. A somewhat similar affection may rarely be acquired from domestic animals. The disease appears at any age; and, while contagious, requires for its spread close contact with an infected person, or with body-clothing or especially bed-clothing. The characteristic **symptom** is the presence of irregular elevated lines on the skin; the burrows made by the female parasite in the corneous layer. These lesions vary in size, the largest being about $\frac{1}{2}$ in. (1.3) in length, and exhibit minute blackish or brownish spots, which are the eggs and excreta of the mite. At the end of the burrow is a small elevated whitish spot beneath the skin; the female insect, which is about $\frac{1}{70}$ (0.036) of an inch in length. The burrows are often outnumbered by secondary inflammatory lesions; namely the papules, pustules, vesicles and excoriations. The lesions of scabies predominate in or are limited to certain regions of the body, although this is not so often the case in infants. These are the lateral surfaces of the fingers, the wrists, about the elbows, the axillae, the lower part of the abdomen, the inner side of the thighs, the ankles, the feet, the penis, and in females the nipples; in short, regions where the skin is warmest and most delicate. The face always escapes, except in nursing infants infected from the mother's nipple. The lesions may be few or many, and are often obscured by dirt or the excoriation from scratching. Itching is intense, particularly at night-time when, under the influence of the heat of the bed, young acari migrate from the burrows. Eczema frequently develops as a complication. Urticaria, too, may occur. The **prognosis** is good under efficient treatment. Otherwise there is no tendency to recovery. **Diagnosis** is often difficult. It rests upon the occurrence of several cases in one family; the intense itching, especially at night; the characteristic distribution of the lesions; and particularly the discovery of the burrows. In **treatment** the patient should be thoroughly scrubbed with soap and water and given a hot bath. The parasiticide is then well rubbed in over the entire body except the head; and in cases occurring in infancy in which the face is involved, this part also must receive treatment. The anointing is repeated once or twice a day for three or four days, after which a hot bath is given and a complete change of bed-clothing and underclothing made. Should any burrows remain, a second course of treatment must be administered. The discarded clothing should be destroyed or disinfected. Search for itch in other members of the family should be made. As a parasiticide there may be used an ointment of precipitated sulphur of the strength of 1:8, or in younger children 1:24. Another serviceable remedy is balsam of Peru, which may be combined with the sulphur ointment. The treatment of scabies may produce a moderate amount of eczematous disturbance of the skin, which should not be mistaken for the disease itself, lest too much irritating treatment be given.

PEDICULOSIS

The causative parasite here is of three species; *pediculus capitis*, the most common, which attacks the scalp; *pediculus corporis* or *vestimenti*, inhabiting especially the underclothing; and *pediculis pubis*, attacking the pubic hair, but also the eyebrows, eyelashes, the stiff hairs on the body, and occasionally the scalp. The last species will receive no further consideration here. The chief **symptom** of **pediculosis capitis** is the itching, which causes the child to scratch frequently at his head. This is often most marked in the occipital region, and not infrequently accompanied there by eczema or pustular lesions. The latter may even occur on the face and neck. The lymph-nodes of the neck, especially the occipital, may become secondarily enlarged. Examination reveals large numbers of the ova or "nits" firmly attached by one end to the hair. They are small, pinhead size, oval bodies, whitish in color or straw-yellow if the shell is empty or the embryo dead. Live pediculi may be seen on the scalp. **Pediculosis corporis** is often attended by intense itching and scratching, especially at night, probably due to the dislodging of some of the lice from the clothing during undressing. The lesions are most abundant where the clothing is tightly pressed upon the skin; as for instance over the shoulders and back, and around the neck and waist. The lice, if not numerous, are found only on the underclothing, and particularly in the seams. In the **treatment** of **pediculosis capitis,** especially in girls with long hair, it is advantageous, but not often necessary, to cut this closely. If there is not too much cutaneous inflammation, the hair and scalp may be soaked with kerosene and the head then wrapped in a towel to prevent the oil extending to the face and neck, where it might cause irritation. The towel can be left in place for twelve hours and the scalp then thoroughly washed. Needless to say, the patient should be kept far removed from the kitchen or from an open flame of any kind during this time. A useful mixture to destroy both the lice and the ova is glacial acetic acid minims 20 (1.23), bichloride of mercury grain $\frac{1}{2}$ (0.032), and water fl. oz. 1 (30). The application should be preceded by washing of the scalp and hair with soap and water, and the treatment given daily for a week. Another remedy is tincture of cocculus Indicus diluted with two or three parts of alcohol and used daily. If there is much irritation of the scalp an ointment is to be preferred, as of ammoniated mercury grains 20 to 40: oz. 1 (1.3 to 2.6:31). In the treatment of **pediculosis corporis** disinfection of the body is not necessary, but an antipruritic lotion may be applied, such as menthol grain $\frac{1}{4}$ (0.016), boric acid grains 15 (0.972), powdered talc dr. 2 (7.77), and water fl. oz. 1 (29.57). The underclothing must be destroyed or disinfected. Even the outer clothing may need baking.

BITES AND STINGS OF OTHER INSECTS

A number of other insects than the pediculus may excite disturbance of the skin. The **flea** (*pulex irritans*) produces a small erythematous elevation often with an urticarial wheal, this having a minute central hemorrhagic point, which distinguishes it from urticaria. Many persons are entirely insensitive to the bite of this insect; others very susceptible. *Treatment* consists in the employment of lotions, as of thymol, which are distasteful to the insect as well as a relief to itching. The wearing of cheese-cloth bags of camphor or pyrethrum under the clothing may drive the parasites away. The **bedbug** (*cimex lectularius*) causes an inflamed lesion with a purpuric tendency. The bite of the **mosquito,** the **black fly,** and the **gnat** produce erythematous spots or wheals which cause intense itching and may persist for days, or be but transitory. The exposed parts are attacked. A central point shows that the condition is a bite, and serves to distinguish it from other lesions. **Treatment** consists in the use of antipruritic lotions suitable for urticaria or eczema. Camphor in oil, carbolic acid in alcohol (2 per cent) (not for infants), and ammonia-water are serviceable applications. Ointments to prevent the biting may be employed, containing tar, menthol, pennyroyal, citronella, and the like. **Mites** (*chiggers, grain-mites*) burrow under the skin and often lead to secondary infection from scratching. They should be treated with an ointment having a fatty base to which sodium chloride has been added. The sting of the **wasp** or **bee** causes decided swelling, redness and pain. If the stings are numerous constitutional symptoms may be severe. There may be applied the antipruritic applications noted above, or a paste of soap or of bicarbonate of soda. In the United States the usual **spider** which causes poisoning (*arachnoidism*) is the lactrodectus mactans (the black-widow or hour-glass spider). The bite of other spiders may occasionally be irritating. General constitutional as well as local symptoms may develop. Among other sources of cutaneous irritation are the **sand-flea,** various **ticks** in addition to those mentioned, and the hairs of certain **caterpillars** or **moths,** especially the brown-tail moth.

References

1. Griffith and Newcomet, Med. News, 1897, Oct. 2. 2. Am. J. Dis. Child., 1927, **34,** 773. 3. Arch. Pediat., 1929, **46,** 549. 4. Omaha Clinic 1892, **5,** 101; New York M. J., 1892, **56,** 505; J.A.M.A., 1928, **91,** 1172. 5. J. Med. Cincinnati, 1927, **8,** 199. 6. Am. J. Dis. Child., 1928, **35,** 885. 7. Arch. Pediat., 1929, **46,** 507. 8. Am. J. Dis. Child., 1930, **39,** 1045. 9. Arch. de méd. d. enf., 1928, **31,** 611. 10. Am. J. Dis. Child., 1929, **38,** 1020. 11. Monatschr. f. prakt. Dermat., 1882, **1,** 129. 12. Am. J. M. Sc., 1929, **177,** 259. 13. Arch. latino-am. de pediat., 1928, **22,** 599. 14. Jahrb. f. Kinderh., 1921, **95,** 8. 15. Acta tuberc. Scandinav., 1927, **3,** 1. 16. Am. J. Dis. Child., 1928, **36,** 702; 1928, **38,** 829; 1931, **41,** 816. 17. Am. J. M. Sc., 1930, **180,** 489. 18. Riv. di clin. pediat., 1927, **25,** 27. 19. Jahrb. f. Kinderh., 1927, **117,** 313. 20. J. Cutan. Dis., 1918, **36,** 327; J.A.M.A., 1921, **77,** 910; 1923, **80,** 1588. 21. J.A.M.A., 1919, **73,** 1213. 22. Centralb. f. Kinderh., 1878, **2,** 3; Archiv. f. Kinderh., 1880, **1,** 53. 23. Jahrb. f. Kinderh., 1929, **123,** 170. 24. Brit. J. Child. Dis., 1908, **5,** 244; Arch. f. Dermatol. u. Syph., 1908, **89,** 65. 25. Monatschr. f. prakt. Dermatol., 1892, **15,** 325. 26. Wien. med. Wchnschr., 1895, **45,** 2097. 27. Brit. J. Child. Dis., 1914, **11,** 22. 28. J.A.M.A., 1932, **98,** 1633. 29. Wien. klin. Wchnschr., 1921, **34,** 185. 30. Am. J. Dis. Child., 1929, **38,** 935. 31. Wien. klin. Wchnschr., 1928, **41,** 1481. 32. Arch. Derm. and Syph., 1925, **11,** 623. 33. Brit. J. Derm. and Syph., 1925, **37,** 364. 34. Med. Klin., 1907, **3,** 1098. 35. Tr. Am. Pediat. Soc., 1915, **27,** 62; Am. J. Dis. Child., 1920, **19,** 433. 36. Boston M. and S. J., 1921, **185,** 194; J.A.M.A., 1922, **78,** 483; J.A.M.A., 1929, **92,** 883. 37. J.A.M.A., 1931, **97,** 1291. 38. Arch. Derm. and Syph., 1929, **20,** 59. 39. München. med. Wchnschr., 1928, **75,** 852. 40. Arch. f. Kinderh., 1929, **88,** 146. 41. J.A.M.A., 1929, **93,** 985. 42. Klin. Wchnschr., 1929, **8,** 71. 43. J.A.M.A., 1927, **89,** 110. 44. Arch. f. Derm. u. Syph., 1891, **23,** 633. 45. Boston M. and S. J., 1918, **178,** 5; Arch. Derm. and Syph., 1921, **4,** 796; 1925, **12,** 896; 1926, **13,** 242. 46. Medicine, 1929, **8,** 223. 47. Ztschr. f. Kinderh., 1925, **39,** 379. 48. Monatschr. f. Kinderh., Orig., 1916, **14,** 7. 49. Am. J. Dis. Child., 1929, **38,** 437. 50. J.A.M.A., 1917, **69,** 176. 51. Bull. Johns Hopkins Hosp., 1924, **35,** 78. 52. J.A.M.A., 1919, **73,** 1743. 53. Editorial, J.A.M.A., 1920, **74,** 32. 54. Tr. Mississippi State M. A., 1923, 133; Ref. J.A.M.A., 1929, **93,** 30. 55. Les Teignes, 1910. 56. Am. J. Dis. Child., 1929, **38,** 339. 57. Bull. soc. de sc. méd. et biol. de Montpellier, 1924–25, **6,** 375. 58. Presse méd., 1904, **11,** 825.

CHAPTER II

DISEASES OF THE EYE

THIS topic is of so special a nature that only a few phases of it can be discussed, and those briefly. Ophthalmia neonatorum has been described elsewhere (p. 242), as has nystagmus (p. 857); and various affections of the eye connected secondarily with other diseases have been referred to under these separate topics.

BLEPHARITIS

This disorder depends upon general poor health, the exudative diathesis, eye-strain, and the occurrence of any acute disease which produces inflammation of the eyes. The **symptoms** consist in redness, swelling, scaling, and sometimes small crusted ulcerations of the margins of the lids, which causes these to become matted together during sleep. Conjunctivitis is liable to be present. The disease is often resistant to **treatment.** Efforts should be made to remove the cause. Application of petrolatum will prevent adherence of the eyelids. Boric acid lotions and instilling a 25 per cent solution of argyrol are of value, as is, especially, the anointing of the edges of the lids with a combination of yellow oxide of mercury grain 1 (0.065) and petrolatum dr. 1 (3.9).

HORDEOLUM

(Stye)

This is a localized inflammation of the edges of the eyelids often associated with blepharitis and perhaps involving the meibomian gland. Some children are remarkably predisposed to the disease. The lesion is a hard, tender, painful swelling, finally with a yellow point of suppuration. **Treatment** consists in hot fomentations, the application of yellow oxide of mercury as in blepharitis, and perhaps the incision of the stye when sufficiently softened.

CONJUNCTIVITIS

Among the various causes of this are exposure to wind and dust; misplaced eyelashes; foreign bodies and other traumata; eyestrain; nasal catarrh; cutaneous and other disorders affecting the eyelids; acute infectious diseases, especially grippe and measles; and impairment of health, as in tuberculous or lymphatic subjects. Bacteria of various sorts are found on the conjunctiva in health. Some of these are not pathogenic; others are the specific cause of inflammation in some instances.

Symptoms.—There are several varieties of the disease: **Catarrhal conjunctivitis** is the simplest form and is not due to any specific micro-organism. The symptoms consist in conjunctival injection of one or both eyes, photophobia, itching or other discomfort about the eyes, and increased secretion. The last may be serous or mucopurulent; free or scanty. The disease is not contagious and the inflammation usually disappears in a few days. **Acute contagious conjunctivitis,** "pink-eye," is a severer form of conjunctivitis, very contagious, occurring often epidemically at any age and oftenest in autumn and spring, and dependent upon the action of the Koch-Weeks bacillus. The symptoms, which are commonly more intense than in the simple form, begin in about thirty-six hours after exposure. Both eyes are attacked simultaneously, or one soon after the other. The duration is from four to ten days and the prognosis is good. Among forms of acute conjunctivitis dependent upon other causes are **influenzal conjunctivitis,** seen most frequently in infants and children, and **pneumococcic**

conjunctivitis, occurring at any age, but chiefly in early life. The latter is to an extent contagious. **Gonococcic conjunctivitis** is also to be mentioned, both it and the pneumococcic form tending to purulent secretion. **Angular conjunctivitis** is a more chronic form, of insidious onset and less common in children, depending upon the Morax-Axenfeld diplobacillus. There is aching and a sensation as of sand in the eyes, with redness of the edges of the lids, especially at the canthi, and congestion of the conjunctiva in the vicinity. The secretion is soapy, grayish, scanty, not purulent, and adheres to the edges of the lids, or is seen at the internal canthus. The course is tedious and the disease may last for months, even under treatment. Phlyctenules and corneal ulceration may occur as complications. **Vernal conjunctivitis** is characterized by the tendency to develop each year with the oncoming of warm weather, and may be related to and associated with hay-fever. The condition is most common in childhood and usually yields readily to treatment, but returns the succeeding year, and so on during several years. There are photophobia and lachrymation, mucous secretion with injection and thickening of the conjunctiva, and the formation of gray flattened nodules, especially on the palpebral conjunctiva. **Pseudomembranous conjunctivitis** may be either diphtheritic in nature, or depend upon a variety of other germs, and sometimes occurs in connection with measles, grippe and scarlet fever. It is commonest in early childhood. The diphtheritic form is contagious.

Treatment of Conjunctivitis.—The treatment of *catarrhal conjunctivitis* consists in removing the cause and allaying the inflammation. The latter may be accomplished by frequent bathing with hot or cold water, guarding the eye from light with an eyeshade or with dark glasses, and frequent douching with normal salt-solution or a solution of boric acid grain 10 (0.65): fl. oz. 1 (30), or of borax grain 6 (0.39): aq. rosea and aq. camphorae each fl. oz. $\frac{1}{2}$ (14.8). Instilling daily a few drops of a 5 or 10 per cent solution of argyrol is of service. In some instances benefit may come from the daily use of stronger astringent solutions, such as zinc sulphate (grain 2 (0.13): fl. oz. 1 (30)). The edges of the lids may be smeared with petrolatum. *Acute contagious conjunctivitis* demands similar treatment, a zinc sulphate solution or one of argyrol or other organic silver preparation being effective. For *angular conjunctivitis* the best treatment is the solution of sulphate of zinc mentioned. *Vernal conjunctivitis* requires the use of dark glasses, boric acid eyewash, and yellow oxide of mercury ointment. In treatment of *pseudomembranous conjunctivitis* there should be employed ice compresses, frequent flushing with boric acid solution or a solution of bichloride of mercury (1:10,000), and the instillation of argyrol (10 to 25 per cent) or silver nitrate (0.5 per cent). Diphtheria-antitoxin should be given promptly in all cases suspected of being diphtheritic. Atropine should be instilled, and the sound eye guarded by an occluding bandage.

PHLYCTENULAR CONJUNCTIVITIS AND KERATITIS

This affection is claimed by many authors to be a manifestation of the presence of the toxin of tuberculosis. Tuberculosis is frequently discoverable elsewhere in the body of the patient with the disease, and the tuberculin-reaction is almost invariably positive, and often markedly so. It would appear, however, that a small percentage of the cases should be regarded as nontuberculous. It is sometimes seen in children with the exudative diathesis, and there is often an intimate association with eczema. It is a possibility that the disease is a tuberculous process especially tending to develop in cases of lymphatism (p. 482).

Symptoms.—The phlyctenules consist of an infiltration of round-cells producing minute, gray, translucent elevations surrounded by injected vessels. In **phlyctenular conjunctivitis** one or more of these are situated on the bulb of the eye, near or on the corneal margin, or occasionally on the tarsal conjunctiva, while in **phlyctenular keratitis** they are on the cornea itself. As the disease progresses an ulcer forms, which leaves no scar in the conjunctival cases, but which on the cornea may on healing leave a small opacity. There is lachrymation and pain, and photophobia is a prominent symptom, especially in keratitis. The **prognosis** of the conjunctival cases is always good, and recovery occurs in from one to two weeks. In severe cases of keratitis, however, scarring may be decided and interfere with vision; and in some instances perforation of the cornea may occur. Cases of keratitis when associated with the so-called "scrofulous" symptoms (p. 1059) are often long-continued and resistant to treatment. In milder cases the **treatment** consists in frequent employment of soothing eye-lotions, as in any form of conjunctival inflammation, and in guarding the eye from light. Ointment of yellow oxide of mercury (grain 1 (0.065):dr. 1 (3.9)) should be introduced into the eye once a day after acute symptoms have moderated, or calomel may be dusted over the lesions. When the cornea is involved an ophthalmologist should be consulted. Instillation of a solution of cocaine or a similar drug may relieve the pain and the resulting blepharospasm, and permit of inspection and treatment. Atropine should be instilled in sufficient strength and frequency to keep the pupil dilated. The possible association of tuberculosis should lead to a careful study of the patient, and hygienic and dietetic treatment carried out as indicated. Change of climate may be advisable. Treatment with injections of tuberculin often seems of great benefit (Casparis[1]).

STRABISMUS

Squint or cross-eye need receive no technical discussion here, and the treatment should be carried out by those specially trained. The pediatrist must urge early treatment, since the loss of vision increases with the duration of the condition. The measures employed are correction of the refractive error, occlusion of the sound eye, and training of the fusion faculty. Operation may be necessary in some cases. In the first five or six months of life, when there is normally some inco-ordination of the ocular muscles, it may be difficult in some cases to determine that permanent squint is present. As soon, however, as the diagnosis is made, and certainly in the first year of life, treatment should be commenced. It should be remembered that syphilis may be the cause of some cases of paralysis of the cranial nerves.

Reference

1. Am. J. Dis. Child., 1927, **34**, 779.

CHAPTER III

DISEASES OF THE EAR

OTITIS

Inflammation of the ear in some of its forms is extremely frequent in early life, and associated with many conditions. Reference has repeatedly been made to it in discussing several topics. It may be divided into inflammation of (1) the external ear, (2) the middle ear, and (3) the internal ear.

1. Otitis Externa.—The disease is of three forms (*a*) *Diffuse inflammation* depending upon pyogenic infection sometimes arising spontaneously, sometimes following trauma; (*b*) *Pseudomembranous otitis*, generally caused by the diphtheria bacillus; and (*c*) *Acute circumscribed inflammation* or *furuncle*. The **symptoms** in the *diffuse form* are pain, itching, swelling, and narrowing of the external canal; and often a discharge, which is usually thin and viscid. The *pseudomembranous form* is rare. There are swelling of the auricle and narrowing of the canal by the pseudomembranous exudate, and there appears a thin, or later a purulent, discharge from the meatus, which causes excoriation of the neighboring skin, followed by a pseudomembranous deposit there. The constitutional symptoms are severe. The *furuncle* is not common in children. It produces swelling, great tenderness in the canal, and sometimes temporary impairment of hearing. Pus forms after several days and is discharged, unless earlier relieved by treatment. In **treatment** of otitis externa the cause should be removed if possible. In diffuse inflammation moist heat is employed by douching with a hot boric acid solution. In the pseudomembranous form diphtheria antitoxin should be given and locally warm antiseptic applications employed, such as weak solutions of bichloride of mercury, carbolic acid, or hydrogen peroxide. For furunculosis an ointment of yellow oxide of mercury may be tried, and this should be continued for several days after the disease appears to be over. Generally incision of the furuncle is needed.

2. Otitis Media.—The large majority of cases of otitis media occur in infancy and childhood. Cold weather predisposes to it. The inflammation is nearly always secondary to disease elsewhere. It is a frequent finding at necropsy. The middle ear is usually involved by extension through the Eustachian tube, secondary to a catarrhal inflammation of the nasopharynx. This occurrence is rendered particularly easy in early life by the short length and relatively greater diameter of the tube. It is especially common if adenoid hypertrophy is present. It may be produced by the nasal douche or syringe forcing secretion through the eustachian tube into the middle ear. Among diseases which are often accompanied by otitis are pneumonia, especially bronchopneumonia; and acute infectious diseases, particularly scarlet fever, measles and grippe. It occurs frequently, too, in marantic infants with tuberculosis, syphilis or gastro-intestinal disturbances. A causative relation of otitis media to gastro-enteritis is maintained by some pediatrists. (See Gastro-enteritis p. 583.)

The direct **cause** in the purulent cases is the action of the staphylococcus, pneumococcus, streptococcus, influenza bacillus, and other germs; alone or in combination. In chronic cases the tubercle bacillus is sometimes found, and not uncommonly the diphtheria bacillus is present in chronic discharge from the ear.

In the way of **symptoms** the disease may be divided into catarrhal and purulent forms, either of which may be acute or chronic. One or both ears may be involved, although not necessarily to the same degree or simultaneously. Unless frequent examination of the drums is made, otitis may not be diagnosed until perforation occurs; the symptoms being masked by those of the primary disease or being supposed to depend upon other causes. In cases in which this masking does not occur, one of the most characteristic symptoms is fever, which may reach 103 or 104 F. (39.4 or 40 C.), usually with decided fluctuations in its course. With the fever there is pain in the ear, as indicated by children who can speak, and sometimes equally well by infants through the putting of the hand to the side of the head; and the tenderness shown when the ear is pressed upon. The pain is continuous or intermittent and is often worse at night. The last is probably the result of the alternate chilling and heating produced by the child turning upon the pillow. On examination of the ear there is found decided redness of the tympanic membrane, and later a yellow discoloration with distinct bulging. Impairment of hearing is common, and liable to persist for some days after the acute symptoms are over. Leukocytosis is present.

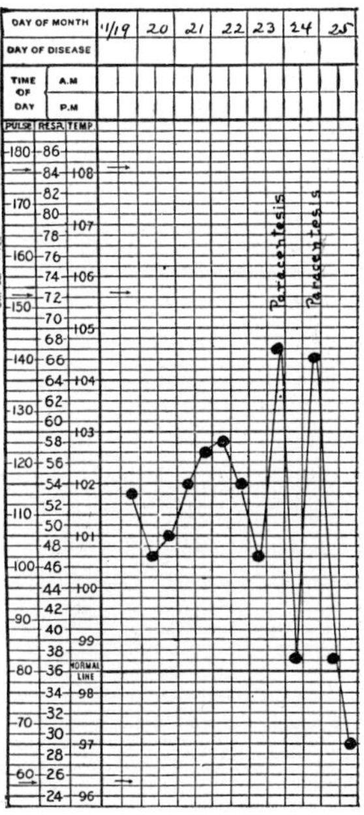

Fig. 281.—Otitis media. Mike P., aged fifteen months. A poorly nourished infant, ill one week with cough, fever and diarrhea. Admitted to the Children's Hospital of Philadelphia, Nov. 19. Congestion of the drum-membrane discovered, leukocytes 27,400; Nov. 23, bulging of drum-membrane, paracentesis done, with prompt fall of temperature; Nov. 24, rise of temperature, paracentesis again performed, followed by disappearance of fever.

There are many variations from the typical symptoms. In atrophic infants suffering from gastro-intestinal disturbances there may be no symptoms connected with the ear, and diagnosis is not made until spontaneous rupture occurs. In other cases there is decided fever, but no evidence of pain or tenderness about the ear. In fact, the only suspicious symptom may be the continued fever without discoverable cause, and the correct diagnosis can be made only by otoscopic examination. In some cases the symptoms strongly suggest meningeal irritation.

In the majority of recognized cases the disease does not go on to suppuration and perforation, but resolution and absorption of the fluid take place. This often occurs after one or two days. In other cases the course is prolonged; exacerbations alternate with periods of improvement; and after all the acute symptoms have disappeared, rupture of the drum occurs.

In severe acute purulent cases perforation and discharge of pus may occur within a few hours from the onset. The fever in suppurative cases is often high and shows a decided tendency to irregularity, and all the local symptoms are exaggerated. Usually after the free discharge of pus the temperature falls, unless there is involvement of the mastoid region (Fig. 281).

In some perforating cases the diseases passes into a *chronic purulent otitis media.* This is especially common in patients with tuberculosis, and also after measles, diphtheria, and scarlet fever. In tuberculous subjects the purulent discharge may continue indefinitely, perhaps with intermissions; there is no pain or fever, but complications readily develop. The discharge from the ear may be very offensive, especially when there is necrosis of bone. Double or multiple perforation of the drum-head is pathognomonic of tuberculosis. *Chronic catarrhal otitis media* is generally bilateral. It may follow repeated attacks of acute otitis, or arise insidiously as a sequel to chronic infection in the nasopharynx. As stated, some cases of this chronic form may be due to diphtheritic infection. There are deafness and ringing in the ears, but generally no pain. The eustachian tube may be partly closed. Deafness generally increases progressively.

Complications and Sequels of Otitis Media.—*Mastoiditis* occurs with especial readiness in early life. The mastoid process contains one large cell connected with the tympanic cavity, instead of numerous small, closed cells as in adult life, and consequently the pus enters the mastoid antrum with ease. Mastoiditis is seen most often in the second year, but may occur in very young infants. A mild mastoiditis is probably almost a constant attendant upon purulent otitis at any age, but usually does not produce marked symptoms, inasmuch as the pus is discharged through the auditory canal. The symptoms in well-marked cases consist of pain and tenderness in the mastoid region; and perhaps later edema and swelling of the skin here, with a pushing of the auricle away from the ear. The disease should be suspected when the temperature continues elevated after the drum has been opened, or when the flow of pus from the auditory canal ceases but other symptoms of otitis persist. It may develop while otitis is still active, or oftener two or three weeks after the discharge from the ear commenced. *Thrombosis of the lateral sinus* may be a sequel to mastoid disease, and occur after operation on the mastoid process or independently of this. The symptoms have been described elsewhere (p. 933). *Meningitis* of a serous nature may develop due to the neighboring presence of pus; or pus actually make its way through the wall of the mastoid process, or from the roof of the tympanic cavity, to the meninges, and produce a localized or a general septic meningitis. In other instances meningitis results from the rupture of an otitic cerebral abscess, or follows septic thrombosis of the lateral sinus. It is not a frequent complication, especially in infancy. The symptoms have been described elsewhere (p. 922). An interesting symptom (*Gradenigo's syndrome*) sometimes develops in otitis media due to extension of inflammation into the petrous tip of the mastoid. The localized meningitis produced here exerts pressure on the 6th nerve and results in a paralysis or paresis of the external rectus of the eye, accompanied by severe temporo-parietal pain. Occasionally the 3d and 4th nerves are also involved. *Abscess of the brain* is an uncommon complication produced in the same way as septic meningitis. It may be combined with sinus-thrombosis. It is found oftenest in the temporo-sphenoidal lobe or in the cerebellum (see Abscess of the Brain, p. 938); in the former region when the disease began in the middle ear in the latter when there is chronic suppuration in the labyrinth. *Facial paralysis* may develop in the course of purulent otitis media, being produced by involvement of the facial nerve in its canal. (See Facial Neuritis, p. 980.)

The **prognosis** of otitis media varies with the variety. In acute catarrhal otitis it is nearly always good, and in the acute purulent form is likewise generally excellent if no complications arise, and if the disease does not pass into the chronic form. The outcome of chronic catarrhal otitis is uncertain and often unfavorable as regards hearing. Chronic purulent otitis runs a long and uncertain course.

Treatment.—This varies with the type of otitis. *Prevention* is of great importance. When there is a tendency to recurrence any diseased condition of the nose and throat should receive treatment; this perhaps including the removal of the tonsils and adenoids. During infectious fevers the mouth and nasal passages should be kept as clean as possible, but there should be borne in mind the danger of driving infectious material into the eustachian tube and middle ear from too vigorous spraying or douching.

In *acute otitis* pain may be relieved by the external application of a hot-water bag, or by douching the ear with water or boric acid solution at a temperature of 110 F. (43.33 C.). A few drops of a mixture of cocaine and adrenaline is often useful, instilled in the auditory canal, using 3 to 5 minims (0.18 to 0.3) of a 4 per cent solution of cocaine in a 1:1000 solution of adrenaline chloride; or a 5 per cent solution of phenol in glycerine may be satisfactorily employed in the same way. The nose should receive treatment recommended for acute rhinitis. (See p. 687.) Internal measures, such as the administration of analgesics, may be indicated; and any disease to which the otitis is secondary appropriately treated. Salicylates have been claimed to increase the congestion of the middle ear. In the meantime the ear should be frequently examined, and if marked bulging is present paracentesis performed. It is always better to open an ear drum rather than to allow it to perforate spontaneously, since healing comes about more rapidly with the former. There is much discussion among otologists as to whether frequent douching should be carried out after an acute otitis has discharged. Probably the best procedure is to keep the canal as clean as possible, but to accomplish this without using much force in douching it. Any other treatment than that mentioned should be decided upon by those specially qualified. This applies particularly to *chronic purulent otitis.* In this form autogenous vaccines may possibly be of service, but sometimes cure may only result after an operation upon the mastoid cells. Search should always be made to determine whether the condition is tuberculous, and cultures taken to eliminate the possibility of diphtheritic infection. Decision regarding the treatment of *mastoiditis,* and whether it is to be surgical in nature, should certainly be referred to an aural surgeon.

3. OTITIS INTERNA (*Inflammation of the Labyrinth*) is uncommon. It may occasionally result from extension of inflammation from the middle ear. In other cases it follows an acute infectious disease, as cerebrospinal fever, scarlet fever and mumps. The acute symptoms are usually masked by those of the primary disorder. Later there may be discovered vertigo and partial deafness, and frequently nystagmus. Occurring early in life and in both ears labyrinthitis is one of the causes of deaf-mutism (see p. 889).

FOREIGN BODIES IN THE EAR

These may find entrance either accidentally, or may have been pushed into the ear by the patient. Among foreign bodies found in the auditory canal are insects or their eggs, peas, pieces of wood, buttons, and the like. Moulds of different sorts may grow in the canal. If the object has not penetrated far there are no symptoms, or only a moderate sense of tickling or discomfort, combined with impairment of hearing if the passage is entirely occluded. If deeper in the canal severe pain may be present, or inflammation may be produced and a liquid discharge take place. If the object has been pushed far in, the drum may be injured and otitis media follow. In **treatment,** a living insect may usually be driven out by the instillation of oil. For other objects injections of warm water will generally be successful if the body is still in the membranous portion of the canal. The stream of water should be directed forward and downward. A long, fine nozzle should be used. An anesthetic may be given if necessary. Some foreign bodies, as seeds or other substances which absorb water, may be made smaller by the dehydration produced through the instillation of alcohol or glycerin. Often removal must be accomplished by forceps, a loop of fine wire, or other instrument.

INDEX

NOTE.—When more than one reference is given for a subject, **bold-face** type indicates where the subject is discussed *in extenso*.